Handbuch der experimentellen Pharmakologie
Handbook of Experimental Pharmacology

Heffter-Heubner New Series

XXXII/2

Add: Vol 32. Pt. 2. Insulin. 1975.

Insulin

Part 2

Contributors

N. Altszuler, J. Brange, S. E. Brolin, F. v. Bruchhausen, W. Burgermeister, T. Clausen, P. Cuatrecasas, P. M. Dean, H. Ditschuneit, J. Ellerman, F. Enzmann, J. D. Faulhaber, K. Federlin, A. W. Forst, G. M. Grodsky, J. Hanoune, S. Hansen, A. Hasselblatt, L. G. Heding, C. Hellerström, B. Hellman, H. R. Henrichs, J. L. Izzo, K. H. Jørgensen, R. L. Jungas, H. Kasemir, W. Kemmler, L. Kerp, F. Krug, W. J. Malaisse, F. M. Matschinsky, E. K. Matthews, C. Pace, U. Panten, M. Pingel, F. Raybaud, S. Sailer, Y. Sakamoto, J. Schlichtkrull, H.-H. Schöne, C. D. Seufert, H. D. Söling, S. Stillings, I.-B. Täljedal, G. P. E. Tell, P. Volfin, I. G. Wool, W. Zawalich

Editors

Arnold Hasselblatt and Franz v. Bruchhausen

With 181 Figures

Springer-Verlag Berlin · Heidelberg · New York 1975

Professor Dr. med. ARNOLD HASSELBLATT
Institut für Pharmakologie und Toxikologie
D-3400 Göttingen, Geiststrasse 9

Professor Dr. med. FRANZ VON BRUCHHAUSEN
Pharmakolog. Institut der FU
D-1000 Berlin 33, Thielallee 69/73

ISBN 3-540-07006-0 Springer-Verlag Berlin · Heidelberg · New York

ISBN 0-387-07006-0 Springer-Verlag New York · Heidelberg · Berlin

Library of Congress Cataloging in Publication Data
Main entry under title:
Insulin II (Handbuch der experimentellen Pharmakologie.
New series; v. 32 pt. 2)
1. Insulin. I. Altszuler, Norman. II. Bruchhausen, F. von,
1929 – ed. III. Hasselblatt, A., 1929 – ed. IV. Series. [DNLM:
1. Insulin. QV34 H236 Bd. 32 T. 1] QP 905. H 3. vol. 32, pt. 2
[QP 572.15] 615'.1'08s [615'.365] 75-4788
ISBN 0-387-07006-0

Type-setting and printing: Joh. Roth sel. Ww., Graphische Kunstanstalt, München
Binding: Konrad Triltsch, Graphischer Betrieb, Würzburg

Preface

The present subvolume was assigned to other editors than those of the first part, which may also serve to explain the delay in publication.

The compilation of a volume on insulin for the *Handbook of Experimental Pharmacology* appeared to us an enticing task, for two reasons in particular. Insulin has now been in use for 50 years and can be classified among the old-established and almost sacrosanct drugs; for this very reason the knowledge of this hormone, its mode of action, and quality of effect demands special attention. No limitation on its use can yet be foreseen. Recent work on the formation, secretion and probable activity in the organism of a hormone like insulin, which is produced within the body, opens up prospects of penetrating the mysteries of both the work and the regulatory possibilities of this small "drug factory" within the organism, the pancreatic islet. It may be more than just coincidence that this peptide hormone was called after its place of fabrication. Furthermore, the work done on insulin has stimulated other studies for the assessment and elucidation of other hormonal systems.

It was not the intention of the editors to compile all known effects of insulin in the present volume, as it was felt that such an attempt would result merely in a list of facts that would be of questionable value and certainly incomplete. Whenever data are derived from animal experiments, the experimental procedure itself influences the results. To quote one example, insulin may evoke severe hypoglycemia, which in turn sets off a series of secondary effects like the release of catecholamines, growth hormone, glucagon, and corticosteroids, to mention only a few. All of these hormones will affect metabolism and may interfere with the activities of insulin that are the subject of the study. Results quoted without reference to the experimental procedure employed may therefore yield contradictory information, so adding to the impression that the literature on insulin is not only vast but also "complex".

We were quite aware of the fact that it was necessary to organize our material very carefully and to obtain the help of experts in editing a handbook volume covering such a variety of problems.

As anticipated, the various authors adopted an individual approach. The secretion of insulin and the wide range of its effects does indeed offer great scope for fruitful research. The contributors to this volume were free to present their work as they wished and to report in considerable detail the kind of information they considered most relevant. The editors were confident that a stimulating and reliable picture of the secretion of insulin and its effects would finally emerge from this approach to the problem.

It was felt that in presenting the data together with the ideas and notions underlying the experimental approach, we could benefit further research. Progress in research certainly depends on new concepts, but perhaps even more on the measures taken to put them to the test. The history of the discovery of insulin provides a lesson in how new perspectives are opened up by pursuing the way indicated by the experimental results. The work of BANTING and BEST is an oft-quoted example of such a breakthrough.

What is mentioned less frequently is that 32 years elapsed between the preparation of the first pancreatic extract that was active in both animals and man and the discovery of MERING and MINKOWSKY in 1889 that the removal of the pancreas gland induces diabetes. MINKOWSKI (1893) went further and found that diabetes could be prevented by implanting tissue from the pancreas gland under the skin of the abdomen. In 1900 SCHULZE ligated the pancreatic duct and, as the islets survived, he classified them as blood vessel glands of the same type as the pituitary. SSOBOLEW suggested in 1902 that glands from newborn animals be used for the organotherapy of diabetes and expressed the hope that this approach would help those suffering from diabetes. There is at least some probability that, had the physiological and biochemical research based on this morphologist's ideas continued, it might have led to the discovery of insulin at an earlier date than 1921. A joint effort, like the material of the present volume, may perhaps encourage a coordinated approach to the unsolved problems we face today.

A rather large amount of space had to be devoted to the description of insulin secretion. Now the time has come to draw up a balance sheet, which also includes many question marks concerning future work on this interesting field of research. A similar stage has been reached as regards the problem of proinsulin. However, we thought it better to deal with these questions at the relevant points in the different chapters rather than to give proinsulin a special position within the volume.

The editors wish to express their gratitude for all the encouragement and support they received from the colleagues and friends who have contributed to this volume. Most authors tried to incorporate very recent results; this may explain why some of the manuscripts were completed at a later date than others. Anybody who has ever taken part in a contest will know that, although every contestant is doing his best, the competitors do not all finish together. Now that the volume is completed, we sincerely thank all those who participated in this joint enterprise.

Göttingen and Berlin
March 1975

ARNOLD HASSELBLATT
FRANZ V. BRUCHHAUSEN

Contents

Secretion of Insulin

II. Hexoses and Insulin Secretion. F.M. MATSCHINSKY, J. ELLERMAN, S. STILLINGS, F. RAYBAUD, C. PACE and W. ZAWALICH. With 18 Figures

III. Amino Acids and Insulin Secretion. U. PANTEN. With 4 Figures

IV. Participation of the Adenylate Cyclase System. W. J. MALAISSE

Pharmacokinetics of Insulin

Effects of Insulin and Proinsulin

Immunopathology of Insulin

Determination and Preparations of Insulin

List of Contributors

ALTSZULER, N., New York University, School of Medicine, 550 First Avenue, New York, N.Y. 10016

BRUCHHAUSEN, F. VON, Pharmakologisches Institut der Freien Universität, Thielallee 69—73, D – 1000 Berlin 33

CLAUSEN, T., Aarhus University, Institute of Physiology, DK – 8000 Aarhus C

CUATRECASAS, P., The Johns Hopkins Univ., School of Medicine, 725 North Wolfe Street, Baltimore, Md. 21205

DITSCHUNEIT, H., Zentrum für Innere Medizin und Kinderheilkunde der Univ., Steinhövelstraße 9, D – 7900 Ulm/Donau

FAULHABER, J.D., Zentrum für Innere Medizin der Universität, Steinhövelstraße 9, D – 7900 Ulm/Donau

FEDERLIN, K., Zentrum für Innere Medizin und Kinderheilkunde der Universität, Steinhövelstraße 9, D – 7900 Ulm/Donau

FORST, A.W., Pharmakologisches Institut der Universität, Nußbaumstraße 26, D – 8000 München 15

GRODSKY, G.M., Metabolic Research Unit, 1143 – HSW, University of California, San Francisco, Cal. 94143

HASSELBLATT, A., Institut für Pharmakologie und Toxikologie der Universität, Geiststraße 9, D – 3400 Göttingen

HELLERSTRÖM, C., Histological Department Biomedicum, Box 571, S – 75123 Uppsala

HELLMAN, B., University of Umea Department of Histology, S – 90187 Umea 6

HENRICHS, H.R., Medizinische Univ.-Klinik, Hugstetter Straße 55, D – 7800 Freiburg/Brsg.

IZZO, J.L., University of Rochester, School of Medicine and Dentistry, 260 Crittenden Boulevard, Rochester, N.Y. 14620

JUNGAS, R.L., Department of Physiology, U. Conn. Health Center, Farmington, Conn. 06032

KEMMLER, W., Institut für Diabetesforschung, Kölner Platz 1, D – 8000 München 40

MALAISSE, W.J., Laboratory of exp. Medicine, 115 Boulevard de Waterloo, B – 1000 Bruxelles

MATSCHINSKY, F.M., Washington Univ. Medical School, Department of Pharmacology, 660 S. Euclid Avenue, St. Louis, Miss. 63110

MATTHEWS, E.K., University of Cambridge, Department of Pharmacology, Hills Road, Cambridge, CB 2 2QD

PANTEN, U., Institut für Pharmakologie und Toxikologie der Universität, Geiststraße 9, D – 3400 Göttingen

SAILER, S., Medizinische Klinik, Anichstraße 35, A – 6020 Innsbruck

SCHLICHTKRULL, J., Novo Research Institute, Novo Alle, DK – 2880 Bagsvaerd

SCHÖNE, H.-H., Farbwerke Hoechst AG, D – 6230 Frankfurt/Main-Hoechst

SÖLING, H.D., Medizinische Univ.-Klinik, Humboldtallee 1, D – 3400 Göttingen

VOLFIN, P., Institut de Biochimie Centre Universitaire, F – 91405 Orsay

WOOL, I.G., University of Chicago, Department of Physiology, 920 East 58th Street, Chicago, Ill. 60637

Secretion of Insulin

A. The Kinetics of Insulin Release*

GEROLD M. GRODSKY

With 8 Figures

I. Introduction

Insulin release is the result of a series of phenomena including: (1) synthesis of proinsulin in the endoplasmic reticulum, (2) transport of proinsulin to the Golgi apparatus, (3) formation and maturation of granules, (4) conversion of proinsulin to insulin during steps 2 and 3, (5) transfer or conversion of granules to a labile form, and (6) release of insulin from the cell. Glucose, the primary physiologic modulator of insulin release, is known to affect several of these processes. It increases proinsulin synthesis both at transcriptional (HOWELL *et al.*, 1965; SANDO *et al.*, 1972; LIN *et al.*, 1972; LERNMARK and HELLMAN, 1970; JARRETT *et al.*, 1968; MORRIS and KORNER, 1970; TANESE *et al.*, 1970; BURR *et al.*, 1969; KIPNIS and PERMUTT, 1972) and translational levels (KIPNIS and PERMUTT, 1972). As a result of these effects on hormonogenesis, or by independent mechanisms, it also increases packaging in the Golgi (LEE *et al.*, 1970). Glucose also stimulates release of stored insulin, independent of its action on insulinogenesis (GRODSKY and BENNETT, 1963; GRODSKY *et al.*, (2) 1967), by at least two mechanisms: it causes instantaneous release and, in addition, stimulates provision to or potentiation of the release system, thereby making more insulin available for secretion. Since all of these phenomena may vary in their time course and magnitude of their contribution to insulin release, variable patterns of hormone secretion during glucose stimulation can be expected.

Initial studies employing *in vitro* perfused preparations showed that the pancreas, when subjected to a rapid constant stimulation with glucose, releases insulin in a multiphasic pattern (Fig. 1) characterized by a rapid transient release and a second sustained secretion (GRODSKY *et al.*, 1968; CURRY *et al.*, 1968; LAUBE *et al.*, 1971). Similar patterns have been produced in other *in vitro* pancreatic systems (LACY *et al.*, 1972), from the *in situ* perfused pancreas of the dog (COLWELL *et al.*, 1970; KANAZAWA *et al.*, 1966), and in man (CERASI and LUFT, 1967; MALHERBE *et al.*, 1970; BLACKARD and NELSON, 1970; TURNER *et al.*, 1971). In man, these

* Originally submitted, April 1973.

patterns are modified somewhat by glucose administration over many hours (Porte and Bagdade, 1970; Goodner *et al.*, 1969; Perley and Kipnis, 1966; Basabe *et al.*, 1970). Furthermore, changes in the basal set of kinetic patterns can occur with prolonged dietary modification or in endocrinologic states associated with insulin resistance (Porte and Bagdade, 1970). The current presentation, however, will be restricted to the kinetic patterns seen during acute stimulation.

Table 1. *Characteristics of multiphasic response*

	1st Phase	2nd Phase
Pancreatic insulin	1—2%	20% (1 h)
Puromycin	no effect	Partial inhibition
Actinomycin	no effect	Partial inhibition
Pyruvate	no effect	Stimulation
Diazoxide	Partial inhibition	Complete inhibition
Dilantin	Partial inhibition	Complete inhibition
Tolbutamide	Stimulation	Minor effect
Visual (EM)	Granule secretion only	New granules in Golgi

II. Dissociation of Different Phases of Insulin Secretion

Table 1 summarizes observations indicating that the two phases of insulin release reflect different, though possibly related, phenomena. In contrast to the first phase, the second is partially inhibited by puromycin (Grodsky *et al.*, (2) 1967; Curry *et al.*, 1968) or cycloheximide (Basabe *et al.*, 1970), suggesting that it involves protein synthesis, though not necessarily insulinogenesis. In static incubations, insulin secretion can be inhibited by oligomycin or antimycin A indicating an energy dependence of the system (Lambert *et al.*, 1969; Georg *et al.*, 1971). In dynamic systems, ATP or phosphocreatinine levels are unchanged during the first phase of insulin release (Krzanowski *et al.*, 1971) and exogenous energy substrates (citrate or pyruvate) were shown to preferentially enhance the second phase (Burr *et al.*, 1970). Thus, the second phase is more dependent on a continuous source of energy and the first either requires little energy or is well compensated.

Both phases differ in their sensitivity to various agents. Differential inhibition of the second phase can be achieved by dilantin or diazoxide (Levin *et al.*, (1) 1972; Basabe *et al.*, 1971) and preferential stimulation of the first occurs with tolbutamide (Grodsky *et al.*, (2) 1967; Curry *et al.*, 1968; Loubatieres *et al.*, (1) 1970), secretin (Lerner and Porte, 1970), or glyceraldehyde (Grodsky, unpublished observations).

Structural differences in the islets can be determined electronmicroscopically during the different phases of insulin release (Lee *et al.*, 1970). At peak release in the first phase, the Golgi apparatus appears normal and there is evidence of undissolved insulin granular material secreted into the extracellular fluid; at 60 min, there is increased Golgi activity with appearance of new granules in this organelle.

Although the two phases may reflect different targets for glucose action, the primary action of glucose on both may be the same. Dose responses obtained *in vitro* in the perfused pancreas (Grodsky, 1972) and in man (Cerasi *et al.*, (1) 1972; Karam *et al.*, 1971) show that insulin release from either phase is the same sigmoidal function of glucose concentration; though more insulin is released in

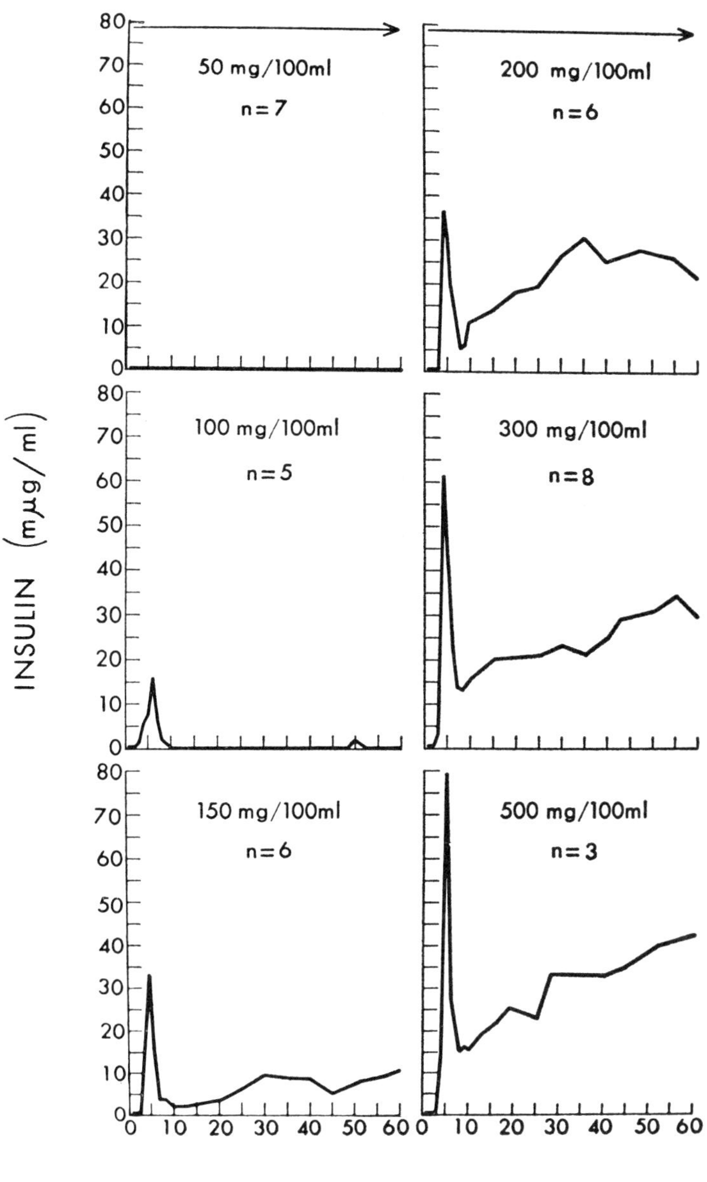

Fig. 1. Effect of constant infusion of glucose on insulin release from the *in vitro* perfused pancreas of the rat. (Taken from GRODSKY, 1972)

the second phase at each glucose concentration, the minimum sensitivity, half-maximum, and maximum effect of glucose on both are identical (Fig. 2). A primary action of glucose in the β cell may involve calcium since glucose increases calcium uptake (MALAISSE-LAGAE and MALAISSE, 1971) and calcium is required for both phases of insulin release (GRODSKY and BENNETT, 1966; CURRY *et al.*, 1968).

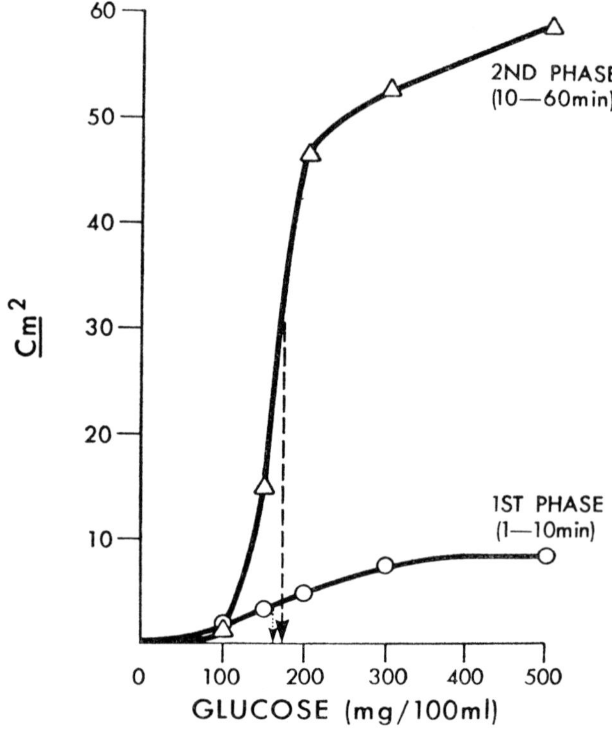

Fig. 2. Total insulin secreted during first and second phases of insulin release at various glucose concentrations. (Data taken from Fig. 1)

III. Influence of Non-glucose Stimulators

A variety of agents not only have their own characteristic effects on dynamic insulin release but in addition enhance the effectiveness of glucose, thereby stimulating the characteristic biphasic response to glucose. The response to these stimulating agents, therefore, can be highly dependent on the level of effective glucose. Sulfonylureas, in the absence of glucose, produce or stimulate first spike response as noted above. *In vitro*, combinations of sulfonylurea and glucose enhance insulin release (Loubatieres *et al.*, (1) 1970; Malaisse *et al.*, 1972) but not beyond a maximum glucose response. In the presence of marginal stimulating concentrations of glucose, typical biphasic responses of higher glucose concentrations are produced by sulfonylureas, indicating these agents enhance glucose action rather than the reverse (Grodsky *et al.*, (1) 1971). Similar results have been obtained *in vivo* (Siegal *et al.*, 1971; Cerasi *et al.*, 1969), the sulfonylureas being comparatively ineffective when hypoglycemia is previously induced. *In vitro*, arginine causes a small nonphasic insulin release (Levin *et al.*, (2) 1972; Hertelendy *et al.*, 1968) when added alone, but it also amplifies the biphasic response to glucose (Levin *et al.*, (2) 1972; Iversen, 1971). In man, a biphasic response to arginine is observed (French *et al.*, 1971; Floyd *et al.*, 1970; Fajans *et al.*, 1972), but not when glucose availability is reduced with mannoheptulose (Fajans *et al.*,

1972) or by previously induced hypoglycemia (EFENDIC *et al.*, 1971). Also, agents increasing cAMP, such as theophylline or glucagon, are either inactive or cause a small nonphasic secretion in the absence of glucose (CHARLES *et al.*, 1973; BURR *et al.*, 1970; GRODSKY *et al.*, (1) 1967; COLL-GARCIA and GILL, 1969; BASABE *et al.*, 1971; TURTLE *et al.*, 1967; SUSSMAN and VAUGHAN, 1967; LANDGRAF *et al.*, 1971), but amplify the characteristic phases of glucose-stimulated insulin release, even beyond the maximum glucose effect (LANDGRAF *et al.*, 1971; CHARLES *et al.*, 1973). *In vivo*, biphasic response to cyclic-AMP elevation has been noted in the presence of glucose but not during hypoglycemia (GOLDFINE *et al.*, 1972). Gastrointestinal factors, such as secretin, also have interrelating effects with glucose (KIKUCHI *et al.*, 1971; MOODY *et al.*, 1970), though LERNER and PORTE (1971) (1) have suggested that the action of secretin on the first phase of insulin release may be uniquely different from that of glucose. Potentiating effects of xylitol on glucose responses in man have also been noted (TURNER *et al.*, 1971).

Beta-adrenergic blockers and epinephrine, known to decrease cyclic-AMP and calcium uptake (MALAISSE *et al.*, 1970), inhibit both phases of glucose-mediated insulin release *in vitro* and in man (CERASI *et al.*, (2) 1972; LOUBATIERES *et al.*, (2) 1970; BURR *et al.*, (2) 1971; LERNMARK and HELLMAN, 1970).

IV. Role of Insulinogenesis

The nature of the mechanisms that are responsible for both phases of glucose-stimulated insulin release is unclear. Observations that puromycin (CURRY *et al.*, 1968) or cycloheximide (BASABE *et al.*, 1970) cause partial inhibition in the second phase suggested that glucose stimulation of insulinogenesis was involved. This possibility was supported by the fact that glucose can stimulate insulinogenesis (HOWELL *et al.*, 1965), and the dose relationship of glucose to insulin synthesis is a sigmoidal curve almost identical as that for insulin release (LIN *et al.*, 1972). We have emphasized, however, that insulinogenesis may not be responsible for the second phase since inhibition by puromycin or cycloheximide is only partial (about 20%) (GRODSKY *et al.*, 1971 (2)). Also, in early experiments using the perfused pancreas with recirculating perfusate, concentrations of dinitrophenol sufficient to block protein synthesis had no detectable effect on glucose-stimulated insulin release (GRODSKY and BENNETT, 1963). Although increased synthesis at the translation level can be detected within 15 min (KIPNIS and PERMUTT, 1972), most investigators using static preparations (SANDO *et al.*, 1972; MORRIS and KORNER, 1970; TANESE *et al.*, 1970; SORENSEN *et al.*, 1970) have shown that little *de novo* synthesized insulin is released from the pancreas before 2 h of glucose stimulation. SANDO and GRODSKY (1973) compared the isotopic characteristics of stored and secreted insulin and proinsulin at identical periods in time using a dynamic perifused islet system. At 60 min of glucose stimulation, when the second phase was approaching steady state, the contribution of newly synthesized insulin was calculated to be less than 0.5%. Based on the turnover rate of endogenous proinsulin, the maximum rate of insulin synthesis was estimated at 15 pm/h/100 islets or approximately one-fifth the secretion rate. Thus, it was concluded that *de novo* insulin synthesis was not responsible for the second phase although it could play a progressively greater role with prolonged glucose stimulation. Observations that colchicine, an inhibitor of microtubular elements or the sorbitol pathway but not of protein synthesis, blocks both phases, support this conclusion (GABBAY and TZE, 1972). Since parachloromercuribenzoate causes biphasic release, both phases may reflect membrane changes (BLOOM *et al.*, 1972).

V. Kinetic Characteristics of Insulin Response to Glucose

Many characteristics of the dynamic response to glucose are illustrated in Fig. 1 and/or have recently been described (Grodsky, 1972). Even at high glucose concentration, the total amount of insulin released in the first phase (or spike) is less than 1—2% of pancreatic insulin content, indicating response is not the result of depletion of total stored insulin. The amount of insulin released during the initial spikes is greater with increasing glucose concentration; at all concentrations, however, the qualitative character of spikes is similar; secretion rates rise and fall within 3—4 min and the ratio of maximum secretion height to total insulin release is constant. When glucose was administered as a series of continuous increasing steps (staircase), each step elicited an additional spike of insulin release. Such studies also emphasize that insulin release is not determined by the absolute increment of the stimulus in a linear fashion, since the amount of secreted insulin differed for each step though the glucose increments were the same.

Under conditions where glucose concentration is suddenly reduced to a less effective concentration, a short refractory period or negative spike of insulin release can be produced (Grodsky *et al.*, (2) 1967) (Fig. 3). Negative spikes were also observed when arginine was suddenly removed from a combined glucose-arginine stimulus (Levin *et al.*, (2) 1972).

Both *in vitro* and *in vivo* experiments show that prolonged glucose stimulation of 1 h or more, even when followed by a brief rest, results in a pancreas hypersensitive to further stimulation (Grodsky *et al.*, 1969; Grodsky, 1972; Perley and Kipnis, 1966; Porte and Pupo, 1969) (Fig. 4). Thus, prolonged glucose potentiates the release mechanism, making additional insulin available for a given glucose stimulation.

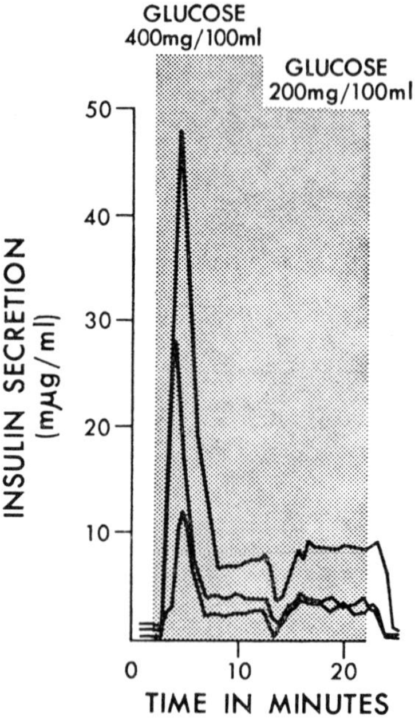

Fig. 3. Response of the *in vitro* perfused rat pancreas to decreased glucose concentration. (Data taken from Grodsky *et al.*, 1967)

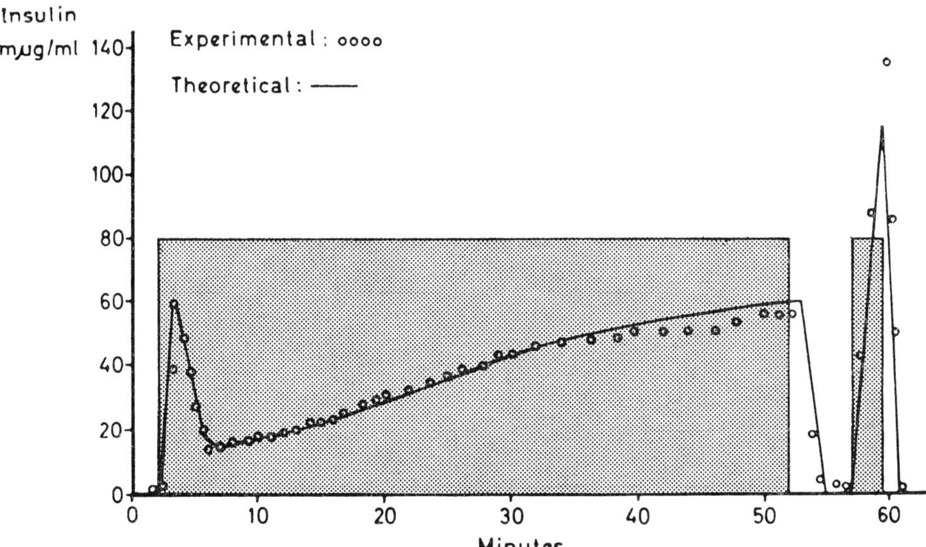

Fig. 4. Effect of prolonged glucose infusion and restimulation on insulin secretion from the *in vitro* perfused pancreas of the rat. Shaded area represents period of glucose stimulation at 300 mg/100 ml. (Taken from GRODSKY *et al.*, 1969)

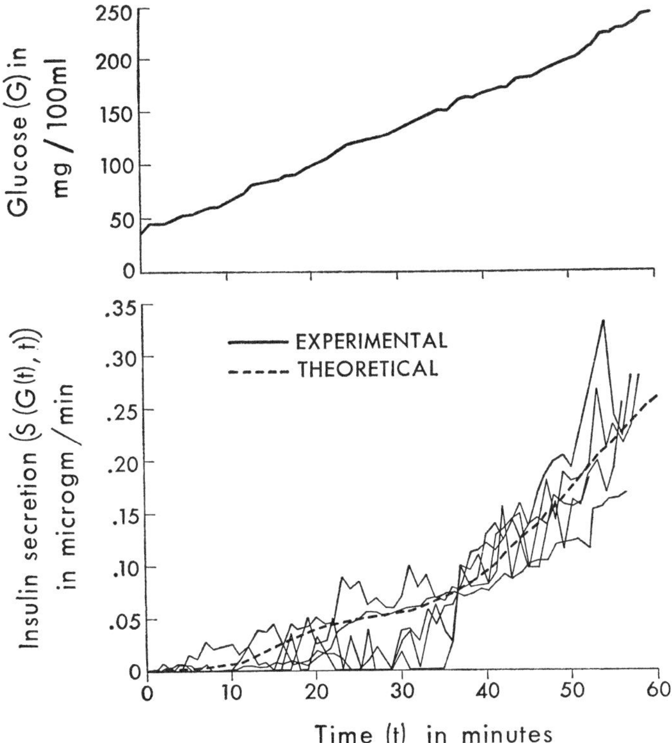

Fig. 5. Effect of gradually increasing glucose concentration on insulin secretion from the *in vitro* perfused pancreas of the rat. (Taken from GRODSKY, 1972)

Though prolonged glucose can potentiate the pancreas, causing hyperresponsiveness to a subsequent stimulus, brief stimulation by glucose sufficient to elicit the first spike of insulin release often causes a temporary refractory period (GRODSKY *et al.*, (2) 1967; GRODSKY, 1972).

As shown in Fig. 5, the multiphasic character of insulin release depends on the rate of glucose presentation. The slower the rate, the less discernible the first phase appears (GRODSKY *et al.*, (2) 1971; GRODSKY, 1972; CURRY, (1) 1971). These experiments illustrate that the comparatively slow rise in glucose which occurs in man postprandially or after an oral glucose tolerance test may not produce detectable phases of insulin secretion. The two phases, however, may still contribute to the overall secretion pattern even though overlap of the two does not permit their easy distinction. Within experimental error, it is probable that the minimal detectable threshold to glucose is not rate-sensitive, but is the same (70—90 mg/ml) whether glucose is presented rapidly as a single step or in slowly increasing concentrations (GRODSKY, 1972).

The time required to reach the first peak of insulin release is finite and can vary with the stimulating agent employed; thus glucose at all concentrations requires more time than the sulfonylureas (CURRY, (2) 1971). The prior infusion of a subthreshold concentration of glucose, however, causes the glucose-induced insulin peak to occur faster (LANDGRAF *et al.*, 1971).

Finally, certain combinations of non-glucose stimulators, which produce atypical secretion patterns, often produce a rapid spike of insulin release or "off response" after the stimulus is terminated (LANDGRAF *et al.*, 1971).

VI. Theoretical Models for Insulin Secretion

On the basis of characteristic secretion patterns *in vitro* and in man, it has been proposed that insulin may be stored in more than one compartment or pool which differ in labilities to stimulating agents (GRODSKY *et al.*, 1969; PORTE and PUPO, 1969). Glucose is proposed to have a dual effect, both on release of insulin from the labile compartment and on the provision of additional insulin to the secretory system (GRODSKY *et al.*, 1969). However, this model, assuming a single homogeneous labile compartment, when subjected to mathematical analysis, did not replicate the consistent rapid spikes of early insulin release seen during the first phase at all glucose concentrations[1] (Fig. 1). A similar model described recently by BERGMAN (BERGMAN and URGUHART, 1971) was similarly incapable of producing these responses. Recently the computerized two-compartmental model was expanded to include a threshold or sensitivity distribution hypothesis (GRODSKY, 1972). This hypothesis (Fig. 6) proposes that labile insulin (or a metabolic signal controlling insulin release) is not stored in homogeneous form but exists as a bell-shaped distribution of packets with different thresholds to glucose. These packets respond quickly when their threshold levels to glucose are reached or exceeded. The mathematical derivative of the sigmoid dose-response curves generates this bell-shaped distribution function (Fig. 7). Thus, low concentrations of glucose cause immediate release of the few packets capable of responding to that concentration. Most respond through the glucose range 110—250 mg/100 ml and

1 If increased glucose (or one of its metabolic signals) acts by simple mass action to increase the number of collisions on a single homogeneous compartment, a continuous submaximal glucose stimulation (e.g. 100 mg/100 ml) would have been expected to cause a moderate release of insulin; declining only when total insulin in the labile compartment became slowly exhausted. Total insulin released during the first phase at all glucose concentrations would eventually be identical and the pattern of release would become increasingly sharp with increasing glucose concentration.

only a comparatively few remain with thresholds above 300 mg/100 ml. The model also provides for the dual effect of glucose: (1) stimulation of the immediate release of stored labile insulin characterized by initial spike responses at any glucose concentration (Fig. 1), and (2) the provisionary or potentiating effect in which additional insulin or signal is provided to the secretory system causing the gradual increase in hypersensitivity to glucose with prolonged glucose infusion. Many observations support the proposal that insulin may exist in more than one storage form. The large stable compartment in the model would reflect the typical storage granules. The small labile compartment could include: beta-cell granules aligned along microtubules (LACY *et al.*, 1968; ORCI *et al.*, 1973); pale granules which are increased in conditions associated with increased insulin secretion (LAZARUS and VOLK, 1970); or the small microvesicles located in or around the Golgi apparatus. Also, the labile storage form could simply represent a geographical localization of granules at a site readily available to stimulating agents. Within any of these proposed storage systems a Gaussian normal distribution of packets differing in maturation, localization, or glucose sensitivity is not unlikely. Concurrent with our development of the threshold distribution hypothesis for insulin storage, MATTHEWS and DEAN (DEAN and MATTHEWS, 1972) observed that an increased *number* of beta cells initiate action-potential discharges with increasing glucose concentration, suggesting the threshold sensitivity characteristic could be among beta cells rather than within single cells. The possibility that stimulating agents differ from glucose regarding the threshold distributions on which they can act may explain the apparent additional pools of releasable insulin postulated for growth hormone (MERIMEE and FINEBERG, 1973) or secretin (LERNER and

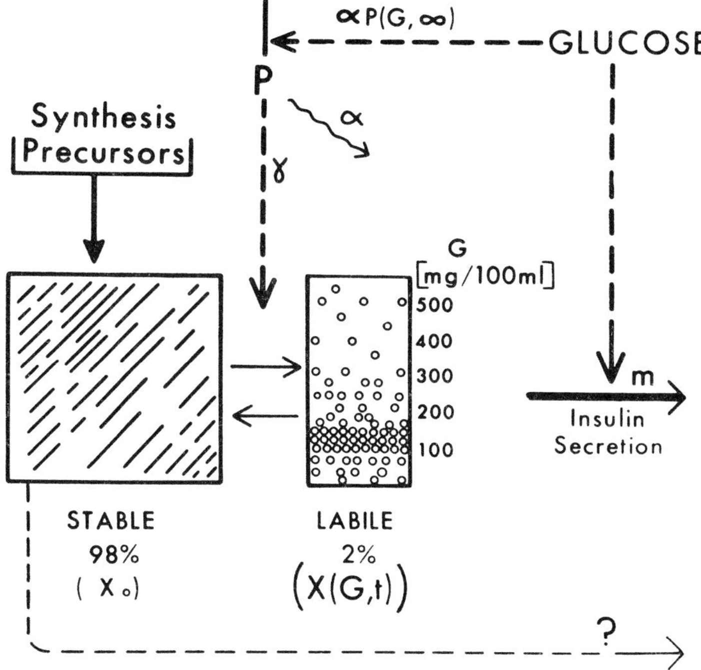

Fig. 6. Compartmental model for insulin release incorporating a threshold sensitivity hypothesis. (Taken from GRODSKY, 1972)

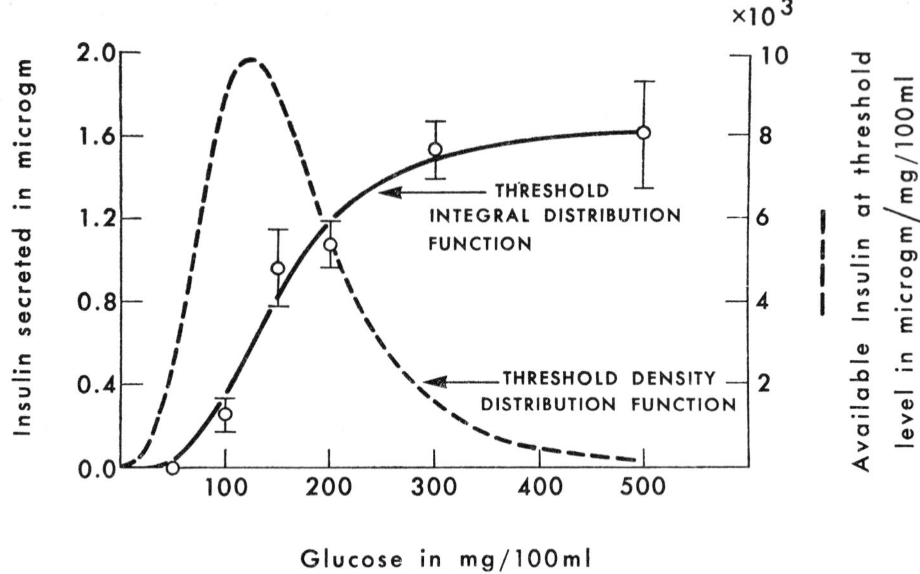

Fig. 7. Total insulin secreted from the *in vitro* perfused pancreas during the first phase (open circles — data from Fig. 1). Solid line is a lognormal approximation to the experimental values. Broken line is its mathematical derivative. (Taken from GRODSKY, 1972)

PORTE, (1) 1971). A two-compartmental model is also useful to explain the inhibition, escape, and rebound patterns seen with inhibitors of insulin release such as epinephrine (ROBERTSON *et al.*, 1971; BURR *et al.*, (3) 1971), and diazoxide or dilantin (ANDERSON *et al.*, 1971; LEVIN *et al.*, (1) 1972). Though the model describes compartmentation and threshold distribution of packets at the level of stored insulin, the data could be explained by a similar distribution of a metabolic signal whose mobilization directly controls insulin release.

The existence of unit packets has been proposed to play a role in the release of acetylcholine (KATZ, 1969), suggesting that the threshold distribution hypothesis for packet storage of hormones may have general applicability to many neurologic and endocrine systems.

It is emphasized that alternate explanations for the multiphasic release of insulin by glucose are equally possible. Not all patterns fit the compartmental model (at least without additional modification). For example, the model does not explain the negative spikes observed when stimulation is suddenly, though not completely, reduced (Fig. 3) (GRODSKY *et al.*, (2) 1967; LEVIN *et al.*, (2) 1972). This type of experiment strongly supports an earlier suggestion (GRODSKY *et al.*, (2) 1967) that the first phase of insulin release results from a stimulator-induced feedback inhibition. This could take the form of a complex series of metabolic interrelationships resulting in a transient rise and fall of the metabolic signal which causes parallel changes in insulin secretion. Another variant of stimulator-induced feedback inhibition is that in which the signal for insulin release is the *difference* in concentration of an agent across a biological barrier. Such a signal would be rapidly terminated either by equilibration of the stimulator across the barrier or by neutralization of its action by movement of other substances. For example, a rapid differential of glucose concentration could activate the beta-cell plasma membrane (possibly by depolarization). A change of membrane permeability could permit cation flux which would neutralize the glucose effect and terminates the initial spike discharge of insulin. Such a "delta" hypothesis is attractive in view of the observations that, (1) glucose, initiates electrical activity in the beta cell (DEAN and MATTHEWS, 1972; PACE and PRICE, 1972), (2) activators of ATPase inhibit insulin release (LEVIN *et al.*, (1) 1972) while inhibitors such as ouabain increase it (BURR *et al.*, (1) 1971; HALES and MILNER, 1968), (3) release is highly dependent on potassium, sodium, and calcium (HALES and MILNER, 1968; GRODSKY and BENNETT, 1966), and (4) glucose promptly increases the intracellular level of calcium ion (MALAISSE-LAGAE and MALAISSE, 1971). A simple "delta" model, employing a nonlinear glucose-insulin dose-response and a comparatively independent but interrelated provisionary or potentiating action of glucose, has been developed and computerized in association with M. O'CONNOR and H. LANDAHL and is shown in Fig. 8. Current experiments indicate this model can duplicate many of the characteristic secretion patterns obtained with glucose presented as single steps, staircases, or ramp functions. However, its limitations may be detected when it has been subjected to as rigorous testing as the compartmental computer model.

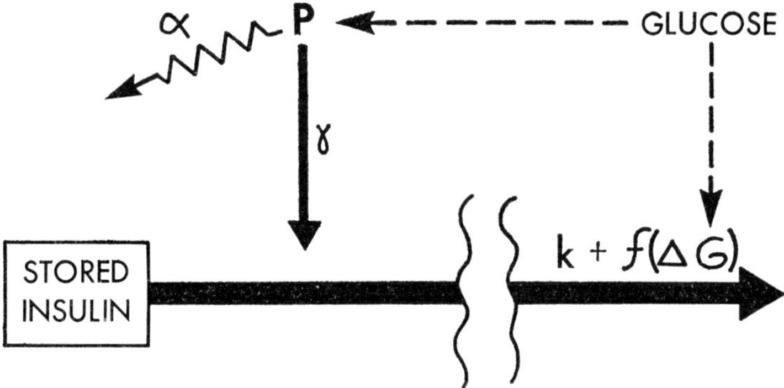

Fig. 8. Schematic representation of a "delta" model for insulin release

It has been suggested that the phasic response of glucose-stimulated insulin release may simply result from a feedback inhibition by insulin itself (IVERSEN and MILES, 1971), a suggestion consistent with observations that added insulin can inhibit further insulin release (RAPPAPORT *et al.*, 1972; SODOYEZ *et al.*, 1970; IVERSEN and MILES, 1971). Studies in the dynamic perfused pancreas do not exclude the possibility that perfused insulin can have a mild inhibitory effect on insulin release but do suggest that phasic responses to glucose are not caused primarily by this phenomenon (GRODSKY *et al.*, 1973).

VII. Application in Man

Although the underlying mechanisms remain unclear, two important characteristics of glucose action should be considered for analysis of glucose-stimulated insulin secretion curves of man. First, glucose not only stimulates immediate release, but with time it increases potentiation or provision of additional insulin to the release system (GRODSKY *et al.*, 1969; PORTE and PUPO, 1969). Thus, during glucose stimulation the sensitivity of the pancreas is continually changing, release being potentiated the longer the time of exposure to the stimulus. A mild defect in insulin release, but with comparatively normal potentiation or provisionary action of glucose, can be introduced into compartmental models to mathematically reproduce the classic initial impairment followed by hyperinsulinism seen in some mild diabetics during oral glucose tolerance tests. Such a defect in the first phase of insulin release has been demonstrated during intravenous glucose tolerance tests (SIMPSON *et al.*, 1966; VARSANO-AHARON *et al.*, 1970; BLACKARD and NELSON, 1971; LERNER and PORTE, JR., (2) 1971; SELTZER *et al.*, 1967). Recent studies in the mild diabetic, in which constant elevated glucose is maintained, show that both the immediate release and provisionary phases may be impaired. This suggests impairment may be due to a general insensitivity to glucose rather than a differential defect at one of the target phenomena of the glucose action (CERASI *et al.*, (1) 1972). Identical results were obtained in the *in vitro* perfused pancreas of the diabetic Chinese hamster (FRANKEL *et al.*, 1973).

Second, the response of the pancreas to glucose is not linear but is sigmoidal (Fig. 2). At fasting basal glucose levels (80—100 mg/100 ml), glucose is a poor modulator of insulin release, which may explain why basal insulin secretion appears regulated by other factors (PORTE and BAGDADE, 1970; GOODNER *et al.*, 1969). Small increments of glucose above normal fasting sugar levels, however, can cause manyfold changes in secretion rate. Often studies of the effect of *in vivo* agents on insulin release may be misinterpreted because only "minor" changes of blood glucose are noted and not considered significant.

Finally, new evidence indicates that multiphasic insulin secretion may not only reflect different pancreatic phenomena governing insulin release but may also be advantageous for effective and prompt regulation of circulating glucose (ALBISSER *et al.*, 1974; CHERRINGTON *et al.*, 1974).

References

ALBISSER, A.M., LEIBEL, B.S., EWART, T.G., DAVIDOVAC, Z., BOTZ, C.K., ZINGG, W.: An artificial endocrine pancreas. Diabetes **23**, 389 (1974)

ANDERSON, J.H., BYRD, G.W., BLACKARD, W.G.: Hyperresponsiveness to tolbutamide of dogs pretreated with diazoxide. Metabolism **20**, 1023 (1971)

BASABE, J., LOPEZ, N., VICTORA, J., WOLFF, F.: Studies of insulin secretion in the perfused rat pancreas. Effect of diazoxide and A025. Diabetes **19**, 271 (1970)

BASABE, J., LOPEZ, N., VICTORA, J., WOLFF, F.: Insulin secretion studied in the perfused rat pancreas. II. Effect of glucose, glucagon, 3′5′-adenosine monophosphate, theophylline, imidazole and phenoxybenzamine; their interaction with diazoxide. Diabetes **20**, 457 (1971)

BERGMAN, R.N., URGUHART, J.: The pilot gland approach to the study of insulin secretory dynamics. Recent Progr. Hormone Res. **27**, 583 (1971)

BLACKARD, W.G., NELSON, C.: Portal and peripheral vein immunoreactive insulin concentrations before and after glucose infusion. Diabetes **19**, 302 (1970)

BLACKARD, W.G., NELSON, C.: Portal vein insulin concentrations in diabetic subjects. Diabetes **20**, 286 (1971)

BLOOM, G.D., HELLMAN, B., IDAHL, L.-A., LERNMARK, A., SEHLIN, J., TÄLJEDAL, I.-B.: Effects of organic mercurials on mammalian pancreatic β-cells. Insulin release, glucose transport, glucose oxidation, membrane permeability and ultrastructure. Biochem. J. **129**, 241 (1972)

BURR, I.M., BALANT, L., STAUFFACHER, W., RENOLD, A.E.: Perifusion of rat pancreatic tissue in vitro: substrate modification of theophylline-induced biphasic insulin release. J. clin. Invest. **49**, 2097 (1970)

BURR, I.M., STAUFFACHER, W., BALANT, L., RENOLD, A.E., GRODSKY, G.M.: Acta Diabetologica Latina: Pharmacokinetics and Mode of Action of Oral Hypoglycemic Agents (Third Capri Conference, May 2—3, 1969), Vol. 6 (Supple. 1): 580, September 1969

BURR, I.M., MARLISS, E.B., STAUFFACHER, W., RENOLD, A.E.: (1) Differential effect of ouabain on glucose-induced biphasic insulin release in vitro. Amer. J. Physiol. **221**, 943 (1971)

BURR, I.M., BALANT, L., STAUFFACHER, W., RENOLD, A.E.: (2) Adrenergic modification of glucose-induced biphasic insulin release from perifused rat pancreas. Europ J. clin. Invest. **1**, 216 (1971)

BURR, I.M., MARLISS, E.B., STAUFFACHER, W., RENOLD, A.E.: (3) Diazoxide effects on biphasic insulin release: "Adrenergic" suppression and enhancement in the perifused rat pancreas. J. clin. Invest. **50**, 1444 (1971)

CERASI, E., CHOWERS, I., LUFT, R., WIDSTROM, A.: The significance of the blood glucose level for plasma insulin response to intravenously administered tolbutamide in healthy subjects. Diabetologia **5**, 343 (1969)

CERASI, E., LUFT, R.: "What is inherited — what is added" hypothesis for the pathogenesis of diabetes mellitus. Diabetes **16**, 615 (1967)

CERASI, E., LUFT, R., EFENDIC, S.: (1) Decreased sensitivity of the pancreatic beta cells to glucose in prediabetic and diabetic subjects: A glucose dose-response study. Diabetes **21**, 224 (1972)

CERASI, E., LUFT, R., EFENDIC, S.: (2) Effect of adrenergic blocking agents on insulin response to glucose infusion in man. Acta endocr. (Kbh.) **69**, 335 (1972)

CHARLES, M.A., FANSKA, R., SCHMID, F., FORSHAM, P.H., GRODSKY, G.M.: Adenosine 3′5′-monophosphate in pancreatic islets: Glucose-induced insulin release. Science **179**, 569 (1973)

CHERRINGTON, A.D., KAWAMORI, R., PEK, S., VRANIC, M.: Arginine infusion in dogs; Model for the roles of insulin and glucagon in regulating glucose turnover and free fatty acid levels. Diabetes **23**, 805 (1974)

COLL-GARCIA, E., GILL, J.R.: Insulin release by isolated pancreatic islets of the mouse incubated in vitro. Diabetologia **5**, 61 (1969)

COLWELL, A.R., ZUCKERMAN, L., BERGER, S.: Pancreatic insulin secretion following intrapancreatic infusion of amino acids. Diabetes **19**, 217 (1970)

CURRY, D.L.: (1) Insulin secretory dynamics in response to slow-rise and square-wave stimuli. Amer. J. Physiol. **221**, 324 (1971)

CURRY, D.L.: (2) Is there a common beta cell insulin compartment stimulated by glucose and tolbutamide? Amer. J. Physiol. **220**, 319 (1971)

CURRY, D.L., BENNETT, L.L., GRODSKY, G.M.: Dynamics of insulin secretion by the perfused rat pancreas. Endocrinology **83**, 572 (1968)

DEAN, P.M., MATTHEWS, E.K.: The biological properties of pancreatic islet cells; Effect of diabetogenic agents. Diabetologia **8**, 173 (1972)

EFENDIC, S., CERASI, E., LUFT, R.: Role of glucose in arginine-induced insulin release in man. Metabolism **20**, 568 (1971)

FAJANS, S.S., FLOYD, J.C., KNOPF, R.F., PEK, S., WEISSMAN, P., CONN, J.W.: Amino acids and insulin release in vivo. Israel J. med. Sci. **8**, 233 (1972)

FLOYD, J.C., FAJANS, S.S., PEK, S., THIFFAULT, C.A., KNOPF, R.F., CONN, J.W.: Synergistic effect of certain amino acid pairs upon insulin secretion in man. Diabetes **19**, 102 (1970)

FRANKEL, B.J., GERICH, J.E., HAGURA, R., FANSKA, R.E., GRODSKY, G.M.: Abnormal release of insulin and glucagon from the in vitro perfused pancreases of nonobese, genetically diabetic, Chinese hamsters. Clin. Res. **21**, 273 (1973)

FRENCH, J.W., BAUM, D., PORTE, D.: Multiphasic insulin response to arginine. Proc. Soc. exp. Biol. (N.Y.) **137**, 858 (1971)

GABBAY, K.H., TZE, W.J.: Inhibition of glucose-induced release of insulin by aldose reductase. Proc. nat. Acad. Sci. (Wash.) **69**, 1435 (1972)

GEORG, R.H., SUSSMAN, K.E., LEITNER, J.W., KIRSCH, W.M.: Inhibition of glucose and tolbutamide-induced insulin release by iodoacetate and antimycin A. Endocrinology **89**, 169 (1971)

GOLDFINE, I.D., CERASI, E., LUFT, R.: Glucagon stimulation of insulin release in man: Inhibition during hypoglycemia. J. clin. Endocr. **35**, 312 (1972)

GOODNER, C.J., CONWAY, M.J., WERBACH, J.H.: Control of insulin secretion during fasting hyperglycemia in adult diabetics and in non-diabetic subjects during infusion of glucose. J. clin. Invest. **48**, 1878 (1969)

GRODSKY, G.M.: Unpublished observations

GRODSKY, G.M.: A threshold distribution hypothesis for packet storage of insulin and its mathematical modeling. J. clin. Invest. **51**, 2047 (1972)

GRODSKY, G.M., BENNETT, L.L.: Insulin secretion from the isolated pancreas in absence of insulinogenesis: Effect of glucose. Proc. Soc. exp. Biol. (N.Y.) **114**, 769 (1963)

GRODSKY, G.M., BENNETT, L.L.: Cation requirements for insulin secretion in the isolated perfused pancreas. Diabetes **15**, 910 (1966)

GRODSKY, G.M., BENNETT, L.L., SMITH, D.F., SCHMID, F.G.: (1) Effect of pulse administration of glucose or glucagon on insulin secretion in vitro. Metabolism **16**, 222 (1967)

GRODSKY, G.M., BENNETT, L.L., SMITH, D., NEMECHEK, K.: (2) The effect of tolbutamide and glucose on the timed release of insulin from the isolated perfused pancreas. In: Tolbutamide After Ten Years, p. 11. W. J. H. BUTTERFIELD and W. WESTERING, editors. Amsterdam: Excerpta Medica 1967

GRODSKY, G.M., CURRY, D.L., BENNETT, L.L., RODRIGO, V.V.: Factors influencing different rates of insulin release in vitro. In: Mechanism and Regulation of Insulin Secretion, p. 140. R. LEVINE and E.F. PFEIFFER, editors. Milano: Casa Editrice 1968

GRODSKY, G.M., CURRY, D., LANDAHL, H., BENNETT, L.L.: Further studies on the dynamic aspects of insulin release in vitro with evidence for a two-compartmental storage system. Acta diabet. lat. **6**, (Supple. 1), 554 (1969)

GRODSKY, G.M., FANSKA, R., SCHMID, F.G.: Evaluation of the role of exogenous insulin on phasic insulin secretion. Diabetes **22**, 256 (1973)

GRODSKY, G.M., LEE, J.C., FANSKA, R., SMITH, D.: (1) Insulin secretion from the in vitro perfused pancreas of the rat: Effect of Ro-6-4563 and other sulfonylureas. International Symposium on Recent Hypoglycemic Sulfonylureas: Mechanisms of Action and Clinical Indications, p. 83. U.C. DUBACH and A. RICKERT, editors. Bern: Huber 1971

GRODSKY, G.M., LICKO, V., LANDAHL, H.: (2) Variable sensitivity of the perfused rat pancreas to glucose. In: Recent Advances in Endocrinology, p. 421. VII. Pan American Congress of Endocrinology, Sao Paulo. Amsterdam: Excerpta Medica 1971

HALES, C.N., MILNER, R.D.G.: The role of sodium and potassium in insulin secretion from rabbit pancreas. J. Physiol. (Lond.) **194**, 725 (1968)

HERTELENDY, F., MACHLIN, L.J., TAKAHASHI, Y., KIPNIS, D.M.: Insulin release from sheep pancreas in vitro. J. Endocr. **41**, 605 (1968)

HOWELL, S.L., PERRY, D.G., TAYLOR, K.W.: Secretion of newly synthesized insulin in vitro. Nature (Lond.) **208**, 487 (1965)

IVERSEN, J.: Secretion of glucagon from the isolated, perfused canine pancreas. J. clin. Invest. **50**, 2123 (1971)

IVERSEN, J., MILES, D.W.: Evidence for a feedback inhibition of insulin on insulin secretion in the isolated, perfused canine pancreas. Diabetes **20**, 1 (1971)

JARRETT, R.J., KEEN, H., TRACK, N.S.: Insulin biosynthesis and RNA metabolism studied in isolated islets of Langerhans. Diabetologia **4**, 394 (1968)

KANAZAWA, Y., KUZUYA, T., IDE, T., KOSAKA, K.: Plasma insulin responses to glucose in femoral, hepatic, and pancreatic veins in dogs. Amer. J. Physiol. **211**, 442 (1966)

KARAM, J.H., CHING, K.N., BURRILL, K., SCHMID, F.G., GRODSKY, G.M.: Stepwise stimulation of insulin secretion: Evidence for multicompartmentalization and multiphasic insulin release in man. Diabetes **20** (Supple. 1), 323 (1971)

KATZ, B.: The release of neural transmitter substances. Liverpool: Liverpool University Press 1969

KIKUCHI, M., KUZUYA, T., IDE, T.: Plasma insulin response to intravenous administration of tetragastrin (C-terminal tetrapeptide amide of gastrin) in man. Metabolism **20**, 433 (1971)

KIPNIS, D.M., PERMUTT, M.A.: Inductive effects of glucose on the insulin secretory and synthetic apparatus of the pancreatic β-cell. Israel J. med. Sci. **8**, 224 (1972)

KRZANOWSKI, J.J., FERTEL, R., MATSCHINSKY, F.M.: Energy metabolism in pancreatic islets of rats. Studies with tolbutamide and hypoxia. Diabetes **20**, 598 (1971)

LACY, P.E., HOWELL, S.L., YOUNG, D.A., FINK, C.V.: New hypothesis of insulin secretion. Nature (Lond.) **219**, 1177 (1968)

LACY, P.L., WALKER, M.M., FINK, C.J.: Perifusion of isolated rat islets in vitro. Participation of the microtubular system in the biphasic release of insulin. Diabetes **21**, 987 (1972)

LAMBERT, A.E., ORCI, L., KANAZAWA, Y., RENOLD, A.E.: Biosynthesis and release of insulin in organ cultures of fetal rat pancreas. Acta diabet. lat. **6** (Supple. 1), 505 (1969)

LANDGRAF, R., BRANTBURG, J., MATSCHINSKY, F.: Kinetics of insulin release from the perfused rat pancreas caused by glucose, glucosamine and galactose. Proc. nat. Acad. Sci. (Wash.) **68**, 536 (1971)

LAUBE, H., FUSSGÄNGER, R., GOBERNA, R., SCHRÖDER, K., STRAUB, K., SUSSMAN, K., PFEIFFER, E.F.: Effects of tolbutamide on insulin and glucagon secretion of the isolated perfused rat pancreas. Horm. Metabol. Res. **3**, 238 (1971)

LAZARUS, S.S., VOLK, B.W.: Ultrastructural aspects of the function of rabbit β-cells. In: The Structure and Metabolism of the Pancreatic Islets, p. 159. S. FALKMER, B. HELLMAN, and I.-B. TALJEDAL, editors. New York: Pergamon Press 1970

LEE, J.C., GRODSKY, G.M., BENNETT, L.L., SMITH-KYLE, D.F., CRAW, L.: Ultrastructure of β-cells during the dynamic response to glucose and tolbutamide in vitro. Diabetologia **6**, 542 (1970)

LERNER, R.L., PORTE, D.: Uniphasic insulin responses to secretin stimulation in man. J. clin. Invest. **49**, 2276 (1970)

LERNER, R.L., PORTE, D.: (1) Secretin and glucose: Stimulation of rapid insulin response from separate functional pools. Clin. Res. **19**, 478 (1971)

LERNER, R.L., PORTE, D.: (2) Relationships between intravenous glucose loads, insulin responses and glucose disappearance rate. J. clin. Endocr. **33**, 409 (1971)

LERNMARK, A., HELLMAN, B.: Effect of epinephrine and mannoheptulose on early and late phases of glucose-stimulated insulin release. Metabolism **19**, 614 (1970)

LEVIN, S.R., CHARLES, M.A., SMITH, D., GRODSKY, G.M.: (1) Contrasting effects of diphenylhydantoin (DPH) and diazoxide (Dz) upon the first and second phases of insulin secretion in the isolated, perfused rat pancreas. Diabetes **21**, 327 (1972)

LEVIN, S.R., GRODSKY, G.M., SMITH, D., HAGURA, R., FORSHAM, P.: (2) Relationships between glucose and arginine in the induction of insulin secretion in the isolated perfused rat pancreas. Endocrinology **90**, 624 (1972)

LIN, B.J., NAGY, B.R., HAIST, R.E.: Effect of various concentrations of glucose on insulin biosynthesis. Endocrinology **91**, 309 (1972)

LOUBATIERES, A., MARIANI, M.M., CHAPAL, J.: (1) Combined effects of tolbutamide and of glucose on the secretion of insulin by isolated and perfused rat pancreas. Diabetologia **6**, 54 (1970)

LOUBATIERES, A., MARIANI, M.M., CHAPAL, J.: (2) Insulino-sécrétion etudiée sur le pancréas isolé et perfusé du rat. II. Action des catécholamines et des substances bloquant les récepteurs adrénergiques. Diabetologia **6**, 533 (1970)

MALAISSE, W.J., BRISSON, G., MALAISSE-LAGAE, F.: The stimulus-secretion coupling of glucose-induced insulin release. I. Interaction of epinephrine and alkaline earth cations. J. Lab. clin. Med. **76**, 895 (1970)

MALAISSE, W.J., MAHY, M., BRISSON, G.R., MALAISSE-LAGAE, F.: The stimulus-secretion coupling of glucose-induced insulin release. VIII. Combined effects of glucose and sulfonylureas. Europ. J. clin. Invest. **2**, 85 (1972)

MALAISSE-LAGAE, F., MALAISSE, W.J.: Stimulus-secretion coupling of glucose-induced insulin release. III. Uptake of ^{45}calcium by isolated islets of Langerhans. Endocrinology **88**, 72 (1971)

MALHERBE, C., HELLER, F., DE GASPARO, M., DE HERTOGH, R., HOET, J.J.: Insulin response during prolonged glucose infusion. J. clin. Endocr. **30**, 535 (1970)

MORRIS, G.E., KORNER, A.: The effect of glucose on insulin biosynthesis by isolated islets of Langerhans of the rat. Biochim. biophys. Acta (Amst.) **208**, 404 (1970)

MERIMEE, T.J., FINEBERG, S.E.: Pancreatic compartmentalization of insulin — Evidence for pituitary control. Diabetes **22**, 25 (1973)

MOODY, A.J., MARKUSSEN, J., FRIES, A.S., STEENSTRUP, C., SUNDBY, F.: The insulin releasing activities of extracts of pork intestine. Diabetologia **6**, 135 (1970)

ORCI, L., AMHERDT, M., MALAISSE-LAGAE, F., ROUILLER, C., RENOLD, A.E.: Insulin release by emiocytosis: Demonstration with freeze-etching technique. Science **179**, 82 (1973)

PACE, C.S., PRICE, S.: Electrical responses of pancreatic islet cells to secretory stimuli. Biochem. biophys. Res. Commun. **46**, 1557 (1972)

PERLEY, M., KIPNIS, D.M.: Effect of glucocorticoids on plasma insulin. New Engl. J. Med. **274**, 1237 (1966)

PORTE, D., BAGDADE, J.D.: Human insulin secretion: An integrated approach. Ann. Rev. Med. **21**, 219 (1970)

PORTE, D., PUPO, A.A.: Insulin responses to glucose: Evidence for a two pool system in man. J. clin. Invest. **48**, 2309 (1969)

RAPPAPORT, A.M., OHIRA, S., CODDLING, J.A., EMPEY, G., KALNINS, A., LIN, B.J., HAIST, R.E.: Effects on insulin output and on pancreatic blood flow of exogenous insulin infusion into an 'in situ' isolated portion of the pancreas. Endocrinology **91**, 168 (1972)

ROBERTSON, R.P., LERNER, R.L., PORTE, D.: Control of insulin secretion in the basal state. Clin. Res. **19**, 142 (1971)

SANDO, H., BORG, J., STEINER, D.F.: Studies on the secretion of newly synthesized proinsulin and insulin from isolated rat islets of Langerhans. J. clin. Invest. **51**, 1476 (1972)

SANDO, H., GRODSKY, G.M.: Dynamic synthesis and release of insulin and proinsulin from perifused islets. Diabetes **22**, 354 (1973)

SELTZER, H.S., ALLEN, E.W., HERRON, A.L., BRENNAN, M.F.: Insulin secretion in response to glycemic stimulus: Relation of delayed initial release to carbohydrate intolerance in mild diabetes mellitus. J. clin. Invest. **46**, 323 (1967)

SHERWOOD, L.M., MAYER, G.P., RAMBERG, C.F., KRONFOLD, D.S., AURBACH, G.D., POTTS, J. T.: Regulation of parathyroid hormone secretion: Proportional control by calcium, lack of effect of phosphate. Endocrinology **83**, 1043 (1968)

SIEGAL, A.M., KREISBERG, R.A., OWEN, W.C.: Potentiation of "Acute Phase" insulin release in healthy subjects. Clin. Res. **19**, 52 (1971)

Simpson, R.G., Benedetti, A., Grodsky, G.M., Karam, J.H., Forsham, P.H.: Stimulation of insulin release by glucagon in non-insulin-dependent diabetics. Metabolism **15**, 1046 (1966)

Sodoyez, J.C., Sodoyez-Goffaux, F., Foa, P.P.: Feedback regulation of insulin secretion by insulin: Role of 3′,5′-cyclic AMP. In: The Structure and Metabolism of the Pancreatic Islets, p. 445. S. Falkmer, B. Hellman, I.B. Taljedal, editors. Oxford: Pergamon Press 1970

Sorensen, R.L., Steffes, M.W., Lindall, A.W.: Subcellular localization of proinsulin to insulin conversion in isolated rat islets. Endocrinology **86**, 88 (1970)

Sussman, K.E., Vaughan, G.D.: Insulin release after ACTH, glucagon and adenosine 3′,5′-phosphate (cyclic AMP) in the perfused isolated rat pancreas. Diabetes **16**, 449 (1967)

Tanese, T., Lazarus, N.R., Devrim, S., Recant, L.: Synthesis and release of proinsulin and insulin by isolated rat islets of Langerhans. J. clin. Invest. **49**, 1394 (1970)

Turner, R.C., Schneeloch, B., Nabarro, J.N.: Biphasic insulin secretory response to intravenous xylitol and glucose in normal, diabetic and obese subjects. J. clin. Endocr. **33**, 301 (1971)

Turtle, J.R., Littleton, G.K., Kipnis, D.M.: Stimulation of insulin secretion by theophylline. Nature (Lond.) **213**, 727 (1967)

Varsano-Aharon, N., Echemendia, E., Yalow, R.S., Berson, S.A.: Early insulin responses to glucose and to tolbutamide in maturity-onset diabetes. Metabolism **19**, 409 (1970)

B. Insulin Synthesis in β-Cells

I. Role of Proinsulin in Insulin Biosynthesis*

WOLFGANG KEMMLER

With 8 Figures

1. Introduction

The biosynthesis of insulin and the historical development of its investigation was discussed in general by HUMBEL in this handbook (Insulin Part I). With the demonstration of the single chain polypeptide as the biosynthetic precursor of insulin by STEINER and OYER (1967) first in a human islet cell adenoma and, later, in normal rat islets (STEINER *et al.*, 1967), the unique problem of the biosynthesis of the two chain polypeptide insulin seemed to be solved. The special difficulty in the understanding of the biosynthesis of insulin has been the mechanism of correct formation of this two-chain structure and particularly of the three pairs of disulfide bonds. The role of proinsulin as biosynthetic precursor of insulin is now well established in different species, such as the rat (STEINER *et al.*, 1967; ORCI *et al.*, 1971; TANESE *et al.*, 1970), codfish (GRANT and REID, 1968), anglerfish (YAMAJI 1972; TRACATELLIS and SCHWARTZ, 1970), beef (TUNG and YIP, 1968), pork (CHANCE *et al.*, 1968) and rabbit (BODER *et al.*, 1969). However, this discovery raised many new questions regarding the detailed mechanism of proinsulin synthesis, intracellular transport, conversion to intermediate forms, insulin and C-peptide by an intracellular proteolytic process and, finally, secretion of the conversion products and their significance within the circulation. Defects in these mechanisms may play a role in the pathogenesis of diabetes mellitus and their elucidation may therefore be of great importance.

The purpose here is to summarize the knowledge accumulated since 1967 on the intracellular events in the biosynthesis of insulin which lead to the secretion of insulin and other conversion products of proinsulin. In the next chapter the secretion of these products, their biological activity and peripheral metabolism will be discussed.

Many excellent review articles appeared on this prohormone, the reader is referred to the more recent and most complete of them (CHANCE 1971; STEINER *et al.*, 1969; STEINER *et al.*, 1972; RUBENSTEIN *et al.*, 1972c; KITABCHI *et al.*, 1972b).

2. Chemical Structure and Properties of Proinsulin and Related Compounds

In the following, a short description of the chemical properties of proinsulin and related compounds will be given which are necessary for the understanding of the physiological mechanisms discussed below. For detailed information on this matter see the review articles by CHANCE (1971) and KITABCHI *et al.* (1972b).

* This work is based on the literature available in May 1973

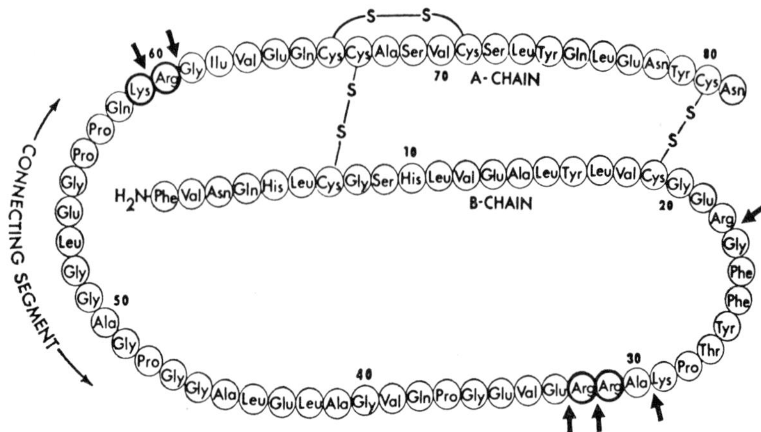

Fig. 1. Structure of bovine proinsulin showing sites of cleavage by trypsin. (From KEMMLER *et al.*, 1971a)

Figure 1 shows the primary structure of bovine proinsulin. Proinsulin is a polypeptide containing the A- and B-chain of insulin and in addition the connecting peptide or C-peptide which links the carboxyl-terminal end of the B-chain with the amino terminal end of the A-chain. Two pairs of basic residues (Arg-Arg between C-peptide and B-chain, Lys-Arg between C-peptide and A-chain) link the C-peptide with the insulin portion of the molecule. This principal structure of mammalian proinsulins was also indirectly confirmed for human proinsulin (OYER *et al.*, 1971) despite the impossibility of preparing sufficient amounts of proinsulin from human pancreas for direct sequence studies.

The primary structure of proinsulin from other than mammalian species is not known. YAMAJI *et al.* (1972) studying the biosynthesis of insulin in anglerfish isolated an intermediate product which let suggest that fish proinsulin might differ from mammalian proinsulin in its general structure. The authors found only one basic residue linking the C-peptide with the A-chain of the insulin portion.

Proinsulin has a molecular weight of approximately 9000, thus it is about $1^1/_2$ times the size of insulin. The isoelectric point is almost identical for both molecules (STEINER *et al.*, 1972). Physicochemical studies by FRANK and VEROS (1968, 1970) indicate that the insulin portion of proinsulin probably has the same conformation as native insulin. Immunological studies which will be discussed in the next chapter, support this idea. Investigation of the three dimensional structure of the proinsulin crystals will help to clarify this question. Preliminary X-ray studies were reported by FULLERTON *et al.* (1970). Proinsulin cocrystallizes and coprecipitates together with insulin during the usual preparation procedures of insulin. Regular crystalline insulin, therefore, is a source of proinsulin as well as several other related proteins (CHANCE, 1971; STEINER *et al.*, 1968; SCHMIDT and ARENS, 1968).

The intermediates or partly cleaved forms are of interest since they may reflect different states of the degradation of proinsulin *in vivo*. Whether all of those are natural products of the conversion is still a matter of discussion. Their relevance for the converting mechanism will be described later. In bovine crystalline insulin two principal intermediates can be detected, each one missing one of the two pairs of basic residues (Fig. 2). Table 1 shows the characteristics of the proinsulin and insulin-like components found in porcine crystalline insulin prepara-

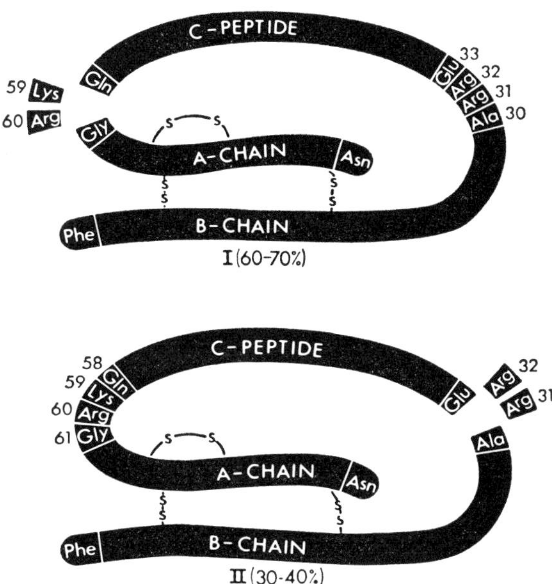

Fig. 2. Structure of the two principal intermediate forms isolated along with proinsulin from crystalline bovine insulin. (From STEINER *et al.*, 1970)

tions (CHANCE, 1969). Only one of the two major intermediate forms shown in Fig. 2 could be found in crystalline porcine insulin, and in addition other proinsulin-like components have been characterized: Split proinsulin, probably a product of chymotryptic activity with a split between Leu_{54}—Ala_{55} in the C-peptide and desnonapeptide proinsulin. The latter component may be derived from proinsulin either by chymotryptic hydrolysis of desdipeptide proinsulin or by tryptic hydrolysis of split proinsulin (CHANCE, 1971). The insulin-like components monoarginine-insulin and diarginine-insulin refer to insulin with one or two arginine residues attached to the B-chain. The description of the preparation and chemical characterization of bovine and porcine intermediate fractions is published elsewhere. For detailed information the reader is referred to these original articles (CHANCE, 1971; NOLAN *et al.*, 1971; STEINER *et al.*, 1968).

The amino acid sequence of the connecting peptide has been elucidated for beef (NOLAN *et al.*, 1971; STEINER *et al.*, 1971; SALOKANGAS *et al.*, 1971), horse (TAGER and STEINER, 1972), rat (TAGER and STEINER, 1972, SUNDBY and MARKUSSEN, 1972; MARKUSSEN and SUNDBY, 1972), sheep, dog and monkey (CHANCE *et al.*, 1968; PETERSON and STEINER, (1972) and man (OYER *et al.*, 1971; KO *et al.*, 1971). In Steiner's laboratory two different proinsulin molecules in rat pancreas could be demonstrated (CLARK and STEINER, 1969), each one corresponding to one of the two insulin molecules of that species (SMITH, 1966). The two C-peptides found in the rat are also different in structure. Figure 3 shows the amino acid sequence of nine mammalian connecting peptides.

It is remarkable that in contrast to the amino acid sequence of the different insulin molecules (SMITH, 1966), the sequences of the C-peptides vary to a great extent between different species, differing over all up to about 50% of their residues. There is also a variation in length from 26—31 residues. Despite these considerable structural differences the peptides exhibit some homology which

	1	2	3	4	5	6	7	8	9	10	11	12	13	14	15	
NH_3^+ -	Glu -	Ala -	Glu -	Asp -	Leu -	Gln -	Val -	Gly -	Gln -	Val -	Glu -	Leu -	Gly -	Gly -	Gly -	MAN
NH_3^+ -	Glu -	Ala -	Glu -	Asp -	Pro -	Gln -	Val -	Gly -	Gln -	Val -	Glu -	Leu -	Gly -	Gly -	Gly -	MONKEY
NH_3^+ -	Glu -	Ala -	Glu -	Asp -	Pro -	Gln -	Val -	Gly -	Glu -	Val -	Glu -	Leu -	Gly -	Gly -	Gly -	HORSE
NH_3^+ -	Glu -	Val -	Glu -	Asp -	Pro -	Gln -	Val -	Pro -	Gln -	Leu -	Glu -	Leu -	Gly -	Gly -	Gly -	RAT I
NH_3^+ -	Glu -	Val -	Glu -	Asp -	Pro -	Gln -	Val -	Ala -	Gln -	Leu -	Glu -	Leu -	Gly -	Gly -	Gly -	RAT II
NH_3^+ -	Glu -	Ala -	Glu -	Asn -	Pro -	Gln -	Ala -	Gly -	Ala -	Val -	Glu -	Leu -	Gly -	Gly -	Gly -	PIG
NH_3^+ -	Glu -	Val -	Glu -	Gly -	Pro -	Gln -	Val -	Gly -	Ala -	Leu -	Glu -	Leu -	Ala -	Gly -	Gly -	COW, LAMB
NH_3^+ -	Asp -	Val -	Glu -									- Leu -	Ala -	Gly -	Ala -	DOG

16	17	18	19	20	21	22	23	24	25	26	27	28	29	30	31		
- Pro -	Gly -	Ala -	Gly -	Ser -	Leu -	Gln -	Pro -	Leu -	Ala -	Leu -	Glu -	Gly -	Ser -	Leu -	Gln -	CO_2^-	MAN
- Pro -	Gly -	Ala -	Gly -	Ser -	Leu -	Gln -	Pro -	Leu -	Ala -	Leu -	Glu -	Gly -	Ser -	Leu -	Gln -	CO_2^-	MONKEY
- Pro -	Gly -	Leu -	Gly -	Gly -	Leu -	Gln -	Pro -	Leu -	Ala -	Leu -	Ala -	Gly -	Pro -	Gln -	Gln -	CO_2^-	HORSE
- Pro -	Glu -	Ala -	Gly -	Asp -	Leu -	Gln -	Thr -	Leu -	Ala -	Leu -	Glu -	Val -	Ala -	Arg -	Gln -	CO_2^-	RAT I
- Pro -	Gly -	Ala -	Gly -	Asp -	Leu -	Gln -	Thr -	Leu -	Ala -	Leu -	Glu -	Val -	Ala -	Arg -	Gln -	CO_2^-	RAT II
- Leu -	Gly -			- Gly -	Leu -	Gln -	Ala -	Leu -	Ala -	Leu -	Glu -	Gly -	Pro -	Pro -	Gln -	CO_2^-	PIG
- Pro -	Gly -	Ala -	Gly -	Gly -	Leu -						- Glu -	Gly -	Pro -	Pro -	Gln -	CO_2^-	COW, LAMB
- Pro -	Gly -	Glu -	Gly -	Gly -	Leu -	Gln -	Pro -	Leu -	Ala -	Leu -	Glu -	Gly -	Ala -	Leu -	Gln -	CO_2^-	DOG

Fig. 3. Amino acid sequences of nine mammalian C-peptides. Certain residues in those C-peptides showing amino acid deletions were positioned to obtain optimal homolgy with the 31-residue peptides. Those residues appearing to be invariant in this scheme are underlined. (From TAGER and STEINER, 1972)

might be important for their function to facilitate the formation of the native structure of insulin by influencing the correct folding of the proinsulin polypeptide chain. In all C-peptides studied so far there are no aromatic, histidine or cysteine residues. At either end of the connecting peptide are regions with a high proportion of polar residues and in the center of the molecules high concentrations of glycine residues surrounded by residues which are largely nonpolar (OYER *et al.*, 1971).

3. Secretory Cycle of the ß-Cell

The current view on intracellular events resulting in the secretion of insulin from the β-cell is that both proinsulin and insulin, like all other proteins produced for the secretion into the extracellular medium, are transported through a series of compartments in the cell in a precise time sequence from the site of synthesis to the plasma membrane.

The principal concept of synthesis, transport and secretion of secretory proteins is based on the now classical studies performed by PALADE and co-workers

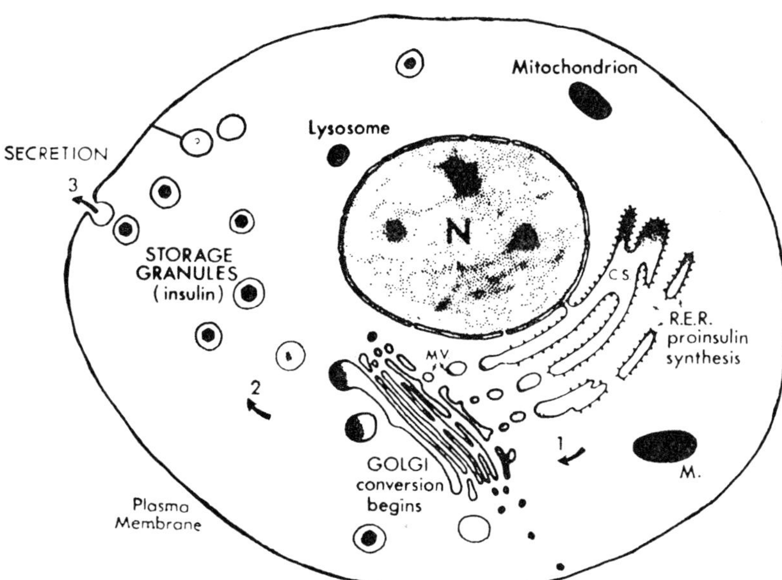

Fig. 4. Proposed secretory cycle in the β-cell. Proinsulin is synthesized in the ribosomes of the rough endoplasmic reticulum (R.E.R.). Proinsulin is then transferred to the cisternae of the R.E.R. and transported to the Golgi complex via smooth microsomes. Secretion granules are formed from the condensing vacuoles of the Golgi apparatus where the newly synthesized proteins are stored and transported to the plasma membrane. From our knowledge up to now it can be concluded that the conversion of proinsulin starts in the Golgi region and continues in newly formed secretion granules (see text). Finally the conversion products are secreted from the cell by emiocytosis. (From STEINER *et al.*, 1972)

with pancreatic zymogen proteins (JAMIESON and PALADE, 1967a, 1967b, 1968a, 1968b, 1971). Zymogen proteins synthesized in the membrane bound ribosomes are first transferred by "vectorial discharge" into the cisternae of the rough endoplasmic reticulum (R.E.R.). The contents are then transported by an energy dependent process via the smooth microsomes to the periphery of the Golgi complex. The transport to the Golgi apparatus takes about 10 min. Between 10 and 20 min after synthesis the proteins are found in the Golgi region. The condensing vacuoles of the Golgi complex are then transformed to zymogen granules, where the new proteins begin to accumulate after 40 min. The granules are finally discharged after about 60 min by exocytosis. That endocrine cells follow a similar pattern of the secretory cycle for their secretion products was demonstrated first with pituitary cells (SMITH and FARQUHAR, 1966; McShan and HARTLEY, 1965). It is of importance to note that the secretory proteins are always compartmentalized during their transport through the cell.

Several lines of evidence indicate that a similar sequence of events occurs in the pancreatic β-cell. Earlier, ultrastructural (WILLIAMSON *et al.*, 1961) and fractionation experiments (BAUER *et al.*, 1966) suggest that insulin or its precursor is synthesized in the ribosomes. In a recent study PERMUTT and KIPNIS (1972) found that at least 85% of proinsulin synthesis occurs on membrane bound polysomes. After synthesis, a rapid translocation of proinsulin from the R.E.R. into membrane-limited vesicles or granules was observed in fractionation studies (GRANT *et al.*, 1970a; SORENSEN *et al.*, 1970). As we will see later, the fractionation techniques available do not allow the separation of clean subcellular fractions in β-cells in contrast to exocrine cells, therefore a detailed localisation of the proteins during their transport through the β-cell is not possible. However, the time course of the progression of labelled proteins in β-cells has been studied recently by autoradiographic technique by Howell *et al.* (1969) and was shown to be similar to that seen in pancreatic acinar cells. Figure 4 shows the proposed secretory cycle in the β-cell.

4. Localization of the Converting Process

The conversion of proinsulin to insulin and C-peptide must occur during their transport through the β-cell. Early studies with isolated rat islets indicate that the site of conversion of proinsulin to insulin and C-peptide is within the β-cell and not in the surrounding medium (Steiner, 1967; Steiner *et al.*, 1969). During incubation of isolated rat islets with ^{3}H-labelled leucine, incorporation of the labelled amino acid into proinsulin can be observed after 1—2 min already, whereas small amounts of labelled insulin begin to accumulate after a delay of 10—15 min, a time lag consistent with the requirement for transfer of proinsulin to the Golgi region (Fig. 5). The half-time of proinsulin was calculated to be about 1 h (Steiner, 1967).

On comparing these kinetics with the time-course of intracellular transport we already can conclude that the transformation of proinsulin starts in the Golgi region and continues in the newly formed secretory granules. Another indirect evidence for this localization of the conversion process was found by Clark

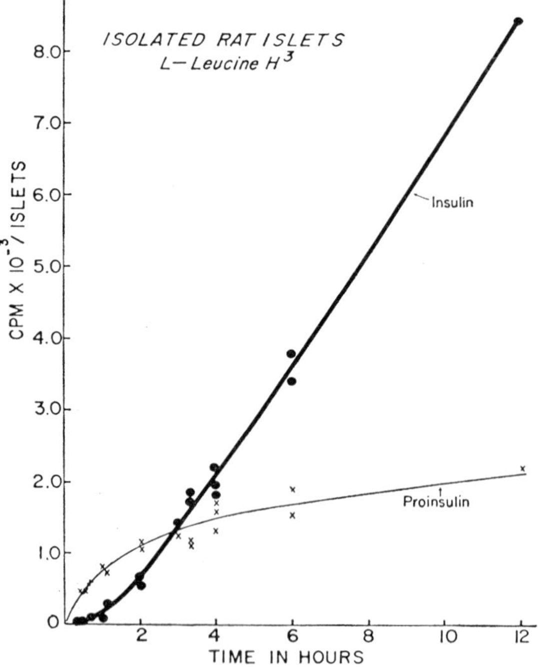

Fig. 5. Time course of incorporation of ^{3}H-labelled leucine into proinsulin and insulin in isolated rat islets. Groups of islets were incubated with ^{3}H-leucine for different time periods and the proportion of labelled proinsulin/insulin was determined after extraction of the islets together with medium and separation of the components by gel-chromatography. (From Steiner *et al.*, 1967)

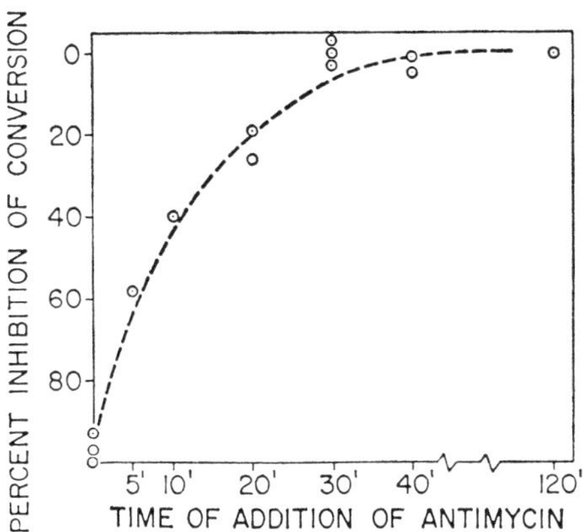

Fig. 6. Inhibition of proinsulin conversion by antimycin A. Isolated islets were incubated with ^{3}H-phenylanine for 5—10 min (pulse) as described by CLARK and STEINER (1969). Groups of islets were then transferred to fresh medium with or without antimycin A (chase), which was added at the times shown. The islets were extracted after 2 h chase period and the amount of proinsulin and insulin determined. On the ordinate, zero per cent inhibition of conversion means that the conversion measured was the same as in control groups of islets without antimycin A incubated for 2 h. 100% inhibition means that no further conversion was observed in the islet group extracted after the pulse period. (From CLARK, 1969)

(1969). The transport of newly synthesized protein from the smooth microsomes to the Golgi region is the only energy dependent step of the intracellular transport (JAMIESON and PALADE, 1968a). Antimycin A, a potent inhibitor of energy metabolism, used in pulse-chase experiments with isolated rat islets is able to inhibit the conversion of proinsulin if added to the islets within the first 30 min after synthesis of proinsulin. When added later, no inhibition was observed (Fig. 6). These data support the idea that newly formed proinsulin must reach the Golgi region before it can be converted. However, the transformation itself is not energy dependent (CLARK, 1969; KEMMLER *et al.*, 1971b).

In a recent study by HOWELL (1972) these results were confirmed. The author investigated the role of ATP in the translocation of proinsulin in rat islets using dinitrophenol as inhibitor of energy metabolism. He found that addition of dinitrophenol to the islets strongly reduced the conversion process to about 15—20% of the control. In addition it was observed by autoradiographic technique that dinitrophenol stopped the granule formation from the Golgi apparatus. The reduced but still significant conversion after addition of the inhibitor let the author suggest that secretory granule formation is not necessary for the initiation of the transformation. This however does not exclude the possibility that conversion occurs also in the secretory granules after it has been started in the Golgi apparatus. On the other hand, the initiation of proinsulin transformation in secretory granules cannot definitely be ruled out by these data. Dinitrophenol sharply reduced the conversion to 15—20%. This small remaining conversion rate could be accomplished in a few secretory granules formed after addition of the inhibitor but not detectable by autoradiographic technique, which is limited in its sensitivity.

In order to localize the conversion process more directly, fractionation studies of isolated islets were used (KEMMLER and STEINER, 1970; KEMMLER *et al.*, 1973).

Isolated islets were first incubated with tritium-labelled leucine for 30 min (pulse) and, after washing further, incubated with an excess of unlabelled leucine (chase) for 15 min. The islets were homogenized and the still intact cells, cell debris, and nuclei were separated by a short centrifugation. A crude granule fraction was obtained by centrifugation of the remaining homogenate on a discontinuous sucrose gradient. The granule fraction was collected on a cushion of dense sucrose and suspended in an appropriate incubation medium at pH 6.3. This fraction when examined by electron microscopy, contained granules as well as mitochondria and microsomal membrane material. Upon 1 h of incubation of this fraction at 37° C, proinsulin was converted to insulin at a rate comparable to that obtained during incubation of intact islets. The conversion is demonstrated in Fig. 7. The fractions were extracted by a modification of the procedure of DAVOREN (1962). Proinsulin and insulin were separated by gel chromatography on Bio Gel P-30. Externally added ^{131}I-labelled bovine proinsulin or ^{3}H-labelled rat proinsulin were not converted at all, indicating that the conversion is going on within the subcellular particles. Addition of soybean trypsin inhibitor (STI) to

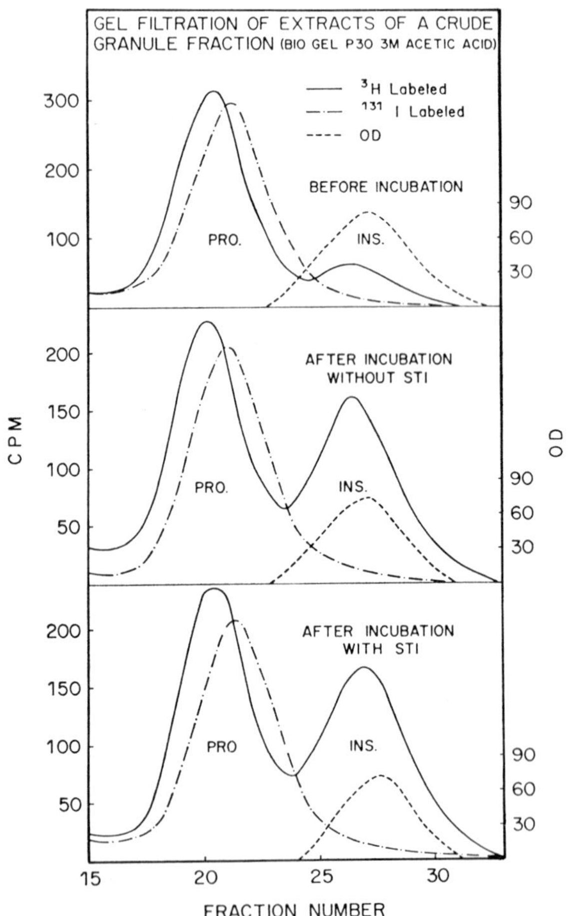

Fig. 7. Conversion of proinsulin to insulin in a crude granule fraction from rat islets *in vitro*. For details see text. (From KEMMLER and STEINER, 1970)

the incubation medium had no effect on the conversion rate, indicating that contamination of the islets with trypsin containing acinar tissue is not responsible for the observed transformation. From these experiments it can be concluded that the transformation of proinsulin occurs within subcellular particles of the β-cell and that it is not dependent on the integrity of the cell. From the length of pulse and chase period and the known timecourse of intracellular transport it can be concluded that most of the labelled precursor protein has reached the Golgi region or newly formed secretory granules before the observed conversion starts. Other experiments with the same system but varying pulse chase times supported the idea that the conversion starts in the Golgi region and continues in newly formed secretion granules (KEMMLER *et al.*, 1973). The distribution of labelled proinsulin and insulin in subcellular fractions from rat islets, studied by SORENSON *et al.* (1970), are also consistent with this interpretation. Recently the same group of investigators observed a conversion of proinsulin to insulin in a granula-rich subfraction of rat islets essentially confirming our results in a similar system (SORENSON *et al.*, 1972). GRANT *et al.*, (1970a) have reported the conversion of a fish proinsulin in isolated subcellular fractions from codfish islets.

Although insulin-containing fractions of secretion granules have been separated from islet tissue from both fish (SORENSON *et al.*, 1969; GRANT *et al.*, 1971) and mammals (HOWELL *et al.*, 1969; COORE *et al.*, 1969), it has been impossible so far to obtain highly purified preparations. Our own efforts to further fractionate the crude granule preparation with various techniques to produce a pure granule or Golgi fraction were also only partly successful (KEMMLER *et al.*, 1973). This technical limitation has hampered efforts to precisely localize the conversion process and to define the orderly sequence of movement of proinsulin and of the conversion products in the β-cell during its secretory cycle.

5. The Nature of the Proinsulin Converting Enzymes

Proinsulin with its four basic residues linking the C-peptide with the insulin portion of the molecule is a good substrate for pancreatic trypsin, the point of attack of trypsin being the carboxyl side of basic residues (STEINER and OYER, 1967; CHANCE *et al.*, 1968). Figure 1 shows the cleaving sites by trypsin in bovine proinsulin. Very rapid cleavage occurs at the Arg_{60}—Gly_{61}—bond in the carboxylterminal region and the Arg_{32}—Glu_{33}—bond in the aminoterminal region of proinsulin connecting peptide. The first products of trypsin cleavage are therefore insulin bearing two carboxylterminal Arg-residues and C-peptide with carboxylterminal Lys-Arg residues. Slower cleavage then proceeds between the terminal basic residues and at the Lys_{29}—Ala_{30}—bond within the insulin molecule to yield de-alanated insulin (NOLAN *et al.*, 1971; CHANCE, 1969). Native insulin cannot be formed by trypsin cleavage alone.

In the case of many fish proinsulins, trypsin alone or a similar enzyme could apparently accomplish the conversion into native insulin, as these insulins are similar in structure to mammalian de-alanyl insulin (SMITH, 1966; GRANT *et al.*, 1970). Recently YAMAJI *et al.* (1972) could demonstrate that trypsin alone is indeed able to convert anglerfish proinsulin *in vitro*. For the conversion of mammalian proinsulins it was postulated by different authors that it could be accomplished by a combined action of trypsin and carboxypeptidase-B, the latter removing preferentially basic carboxylterminal residues from proteins. In this hypothetical conversion process carboxypetidase-B would split the remaining Arg residues from the mono-or diarginine insulin formed by trypsin, thereby liberating native insulin with the Ala residues at the carboxyl end of the B-chain (NOLAN *et al.*, 1971; STEINER *et al.*, 1971; STEINER *et al.*, 1968; KEMMLER *et al.*, 1971b).

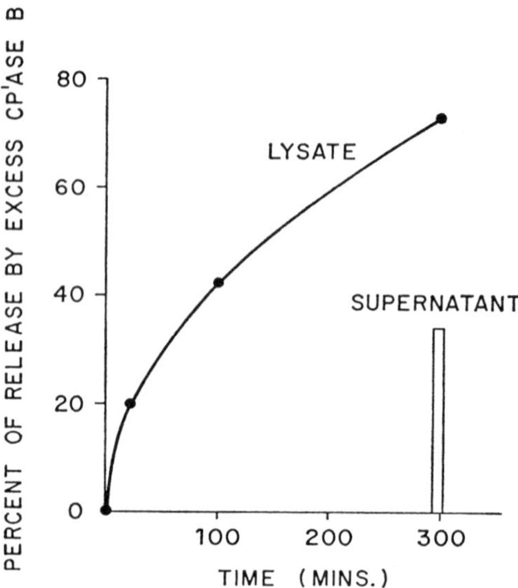

Fig. 8. Release of free ^{3}H-arginine during incubation of the ^{3}H-arginine labelled substrates prepared by mild trypsin treatment of ^{3}H-arginine labelled rat proinsulin with an islet granule lysate. The amount of arginine liberated was determined by gel chromatography after different time intervals and was expressed as the percentage of the radioactive arginine that was released by excess carboxypetidase-B. (From KEMMLER *et al.*, 1973)

In *in vitro* experiments it could be demonstrated that indeed the combined action of TPCK (L-1-tosylamido-2-phenylethyl chloromethyl ketone) — treated trypsin with an excess of DFP (diisopropylfluorophosphate) — treated carboxypeptidase-B results in a rapid and quantitative transformation of the proinsulin to native insulin and C-peptide with the liberation of 3 residues of free Arg and 1 residue of free Lys. Further cleavage at the Lys_{29}-Ala_{30} in the B-chain or at other sites was not observed under the conditions employed (KEMMLER *et al.*, 1971c).

Several observations indicate the existence of a similar enzyme system *in vivo*. Products of such proposed stepwise transformation were isolated and characterized by several groups of investigators as we have seen. Intermediates I and II (Fig. 2) were found in great abundance in a crude proinsulin fraction from bovine pancreas (NOLAN *et al.*, 1971). Desdipeptide proinsulin was also found in crystalline porcine insulin preparations together with small amounts of mono- and diarginine insulin (see Table 1, CHANCE, 1971). TRACK and KANAZAWA (1972) characterized mono- and diarginine insulin in fetal calf pancreas. The occurence of intermediate fractions in the biosynthesis of insulin was observed in rat islets (CLARK, 1969) and also in a crude granule fraction isolated from rat islets and incubated *in vitro* (KEMMLER *et al.*, 1973). GUTMAN *et al.* (1972) found arginine insulin and desdipeptide insulin in the circulation of human subjects after stimulation of insulin secretion with glucose or tolbutamide under certain conditions. The demonstration of these intermediate fractions is consistent with the idea of a stepwise conversion of proinsulin in which more than one enzyme might be involved. It seems likely that all fractions are natural products of the transformation process.

In rat proinsulin (TAGER *et al.*, 1973) and perhaps also in other species (CHANCE, 1971) chymotryptic cleavage may also occur within the C-peptide but this does not appear to be essential for the conversion process.

Table 1. *Proteins isolated from a porcine insulin preparation*

Proteins	Biological Activity by Mouse Convulsion Assay: Units/mg*	Relative activity (equimolar)	Immunological Activity**: Relative cross-reactivity to insulin antisera (equimolar)	Relative cross-reactivity to purified porcine proinsulin antisera (equimolar)
Proinsulin-like				
Proinsulin	3.0 ± 0.8 (150 mice)	18%	45%	100%
Split proinsulin (Leu_{54}-Ala_{55} bond split)	3.4 ± 0.5 (150 mice)	20%	45%	107%
Desdipeptide proinsulin (Lys_{62}-Arg_{63} absent)	10.3 ± 0.5 (150 mice)	58%	61%	84%
Desnonapeptide proinsulin [nonapeptide (B_{55}-$_{63}$) absent]	12.0 ± 2.4 (150 mice)	62%	61%	107%
Insulin-like				
Diarginine insulin (Arg_{31}-Arg_{32} attached to Ala_{30})	16.2 ± 3.2 (600 mice)	62%	80%	0%
"Monoarginine" insulin (Arg_{31} attached to Ala_{30})	17.6 ± 2.4 (150 mice)	66%	67%	0%
"Single-component" insulin (single band by electrophoresis)	27.0 ± 4.6 (900 mice)	100%	100%	0%
Monodesamido insulin (Asp instead of Asn at A_{21})	26.5 ± 6.1 (300 mice)	98%	80%***	No data

Data from CHANCE (1971). * Sample concentrations were estimated by optical density using OD_{276} mμ for porcine insulin = 1.052 and for porcine proinsulin = 0.667 (1 mg/ml concentration). Assays were provided through the courtesy of Mr. R. M. Ellis of the Lilly Research Laboratories. ** Relative crossreactivities based on molar concentrations at points where 40% of the respective labelled antigens were still bound to the antiserum. ***Data for monodesamido insulin were obtained in separate experiments.

To prove our hypothesis regarding the nature of the converting enzymes it would be necessary to demonstrate trypsin-like and carboxypeptidase-B-like activity in homogenates of islets or β-granules. Unfortunately a direct demonstration of a trypsin-like enzyme activity was thus far not possible. Disruption of rat islets or human islet cell tumor tissue by homogenization, sonication or freeze-thawing destroys the converting activity (CLARK, 1969). Similarly, isolated crude granule preparations almost completely lose the ability to convert endogenously labelled proinsulin after lysis by freeze thawing, detergent treatment, sonication or homogenization (KEMMLER and STEINER, 1970). Complete abolishment of the conversion of codfish proinsulin was also observed in granule fractions from codfish islets after treatment with deoxycholate (GRANT and COOMBS, 1970). Our failure to detect proinsulin converting activity in lysed granules may be due to trivial causes such as enzyme instability, substrate dilution or others. On the other hand it could mean that the converting enzyme(s) is part of the membrane of the Golgi apparatus, or granules, or membrane bound. Recent studies by SMITH (1972) using electron microscopic histochemical localisation techniques, have demonstrated the deposition of an electron-dense tryptic reaction product within secretory granules, especially those surrounding the Golgi apparatus in rat β-cells.

While we were not able to demonstrate trypsin-like converting activity in lysed granule preparations, we clearly could detect carboxypeptidase-B-like activity. The problem was to find a system sensitive enough to detect very small amounts of enzyme activity. As substrate we prepared products of mild trypsin treatment of ^{3}H-arginine-labelled rat proinsulin. By carboxypeptidase-B-treatment in excess, 62% of the ^{3}H-arginine could be liberated from the material produced indicating that the major part of the insulin prepared consisted either of Di-Arg- or Mono-Arg-insulin and that the formed C-peptide had one or two basic residues still attached. During incubation of these substrates with a lysed granule preparation described above, liberation of free mono-^{3}H-arginine could be observed indicating the presence of carboxypeptidase-B-like acitivity (Fig. 8; KEMMLER *et al.*, 1973).

In another series of experiments with ^{3}H-arginine-labelled proinsulin, we examined specifically the fate of the 4 basic residues linking the C-peptide and insulin during the transformation process. It was found that mono-arginine is the conversion product, and no dipeptide, neither Arg-Arg nor Arg-Lys, could be detected. These results rule out the existence of a novel dipeptidase that could excise the basic regions as simple units from proinsulin (KEMMLER *et al.*, 1973).

It was hoped that the effect of several known protease inhibitors would help to further characterize the converting enzyme system. In experiments with intact rat islets performed by CLARK (1969) none of the following serine protease inhibitors showed any effect on the transformation of proinsulin to insulin: PTI (basic pancreatic trypsin inhibitor), DFP (diisopropylfluorophosphate), NPGB (p-nitrophenyl-p-guanidino benzoate), TLCK (1-chloro-3-tosylamido-7-amino-2-heptanone), NEP (O-ethyl-O-p-nitrophenylphenyl-propylphosphonate). Similarly, preincubation of the above described crude granule fraction for 1 h at room temperature with N-ethylmaleimide, sodium iodoacetate, DFP, Benzamidine, NPGB and TLCK in relatively high concentration also failed to inhibit significantly the observed *in vitro* conversion. However, p-chloromercuribenzoate (PCMB) in relatively high concentration (1 mM), completely inhibited the conversion (KEMMLER *et al.*, 1973). These results may indicate that the converting enzyme system does not belong to the trypsin-related serine proteases nor to the group of proteases with a thiol group in the active center. On the other hand it is not known whether these substances are able to cross the membrane of the granules or intact islets. In contrast to these results GRANT and REID (1968) reported an inhibition of the conversion of cod proinsulin in cod fish islets with NEP and DFP. DFP also caused an inhibition of the transformation in a subcellular fraction of cod fish islets (GRANT, 1971, GRANT *et al.*, 1971).

The most extensive studies on intracellular digestion of proteins were performed by DE DUVE and co-workers (DE DUVE, 1969). The acid proteases, the cathepsins, contained in the lysosomes of most cell types, are relatively nonspecific in their action (COFFEY and DE DUVE, 1968). Their participation in the conversion process seems rather unlikely. The only role that has thus far been determined for lysosomes in the β-cell is the disposal of secretory granules produced in excess of demand (CREUTZFELDT *et al.*, 1969). Partly purified cathepsin-B from calf liver cleaved proinsulin and insulin more extensively than did trypsin. There was no indication of insulin formation from proinsulin (KEMMLER, unpublished results). Cathepsin-B, a thiol enzyme, is the only lysosomal protease known with trypsin-like activity (SNELLMAN, 1969).

YIP (1971) reported the isolation of an anionic trypsin-like enzyme from bovine pancreas that converts proinsulin to insulin. This enzyme apparently cleaves at the carboxyl side of the alanine residue at the end of the B-chain and splits between Gly-Arg at the end of the A-chain to liberate insulin. Whereas free arginine could be detected, no free lysine was found. From the data presented the endproduct of this proteolytic action is C-peptide with lysine or lysine and arginine still bound to the carboxyl terminus. Since free C-peptide without basic residues is the product of the conversion *in vivo* (Steiner *et al.*, 1971), possibly other enzymes in addition, or different enzymes, participate in the conversion *in vivo*. On the other hand, anionic trypsins are known to occur in the pancreatic juice (Voytek and Gyessing, 1971), which suggests a possible exocrine origin of this material. The role of this enzyme found by Yip (1971) *in vivo* has yet to be established.

While our results all support the hypothesis that trypsin-like and carboxypeptidase-B-like activities normally participate in the conversion, we were thus far not able to resolve the question about the exact nature of these proteolytic enzymes.

6. The Products of Conversion and Their Intracellular Fate

The most important product of conversion, insulin, is stored in the β-granules as shown in immunohistochemical studies (Misugi *et al.*, 1970) and by correlating the degree of β-granulation with the insulin content of the pancreas (Hartcroft and Wrenshall, 1955). Proinsulin is not the storage form. The content of proinsulin in the β-cell is less than 10% of total immunoreactive insulin in all species studied (Sando *et al.*, 1972; Lockwood and Misbin, 1972; Chance, 1971; Steiner *et al.*, 1968; Rastogi *et al.*, 1970).

Another major conversion product is the C-peptide. C-peptide is retained in the β-cell after the transformation and was found in bovine and human pancreas on an equimolar basis with insulin as expected from the stoichiometry of the cleavage process (Clark *et al.*, 1969; Steiner *et al.*, 1971). In recent studies with isolated crude granule fractions we could demonstrate that the C-peptide is retained in equimolar amounts with insulin also in subcellular particles after the conversion (Kemmler *et al.*, 1973). The explanation for these observations may be that the major conversion products, insulin and C-peptide, are stored together in the secretory granules. Thus at times of granule discharge by emiocytosis, equivalent amounts of C-peptide and insulin would be liberated. In the next chapter we will see that this is indeed what could be observed by measuring proinsulin, insulin and C-peptide in the circulation.

It is of interest that after a very long incubation (16 h) of the already described crude granule fraction, when about 70% of the labelled material is converted to insulin and C-peptide, the remaining 30% consist of intermediate forms and almost no proinsulin can be detected anymore (Kemmler *et al.*, 1973). Therefore it seems possible that mature granules, ready for emiocytosis, contain intermediate fractions instead of proinsulin which might be released into the circulation.

The fate of arginine and lysine is less clearly understood. Diffusion of these basic amino acids from the granule and their replacement by hydrogen ions may result in a slow decrease in pH within the granules which may influence the formation of zinc insulin crystals.

7. Significance of Proinsulin for the Biosynthesis of Insulin

Proinsulin fulfills a clear biosynthetic need for the correct formation of the disulfide bonds within in the insulin molecule. This pairing of the cysteine residues is evidently accomplished by the folding of the single chain polypeptide. As mentioned earlier specific structures, which can be demonstrated in all the C-peptides of different species, might be important for this folding process (Oyer *et al.*, 1971). Anfinsen and co-workers proposed the concept that the formation of the tertiary structure of proteins is solely dependent on its primary structure leading to the energetically favored conformation (EPSTEIN *et al.*, 1963). Thus spontaneous folding of unfolded proinsulin should ensure the correct formation of its native structure. This hypothesis was tested in *in vitro* experiments by STEINER and CLARK (1968). Fully reduced and therefore unfolded proinsulin was allowed to reoxidize in the presence of free thiol. 80% of the proinsulin regained its native structure spontanously, as measured by immunoassay. Intermediate fractions cleaved at either side of the A- or B-chain showed no greater refolding ability than reduced insulin chains (NOLAN *et al.*, 1971). The recombination rate of separated insulin chains under optimal conditions is mostly less than 10% (HUMBEL *et al.*, 1972).

But this function of proinsulin can not fully explain its existence. The discovery of proinsulin was followed by a search for other precursors of peptide hormones in many laboratories. As a result the number of prohormones characterized is steadily increasing. SACHS *et al.*, (1969) found evidence for a precursor form of vasopressin in hypothalamic tissue, but this protein has not yet been isolated.

The existence of a precusor of parathyroid hormone is well documented (COHN *et al.*, 1972; KEMPER *et al.*, 1972; HAMILTON *et al.*, 1971). The evidence suggests that the precursor consists of parathyroid hormone with additional peptide material attached through a basic residue that serves as cleavage site (HABENER *et al.*, 1973).

Studies by YALOW and BERSON (1970) and GREGORY and TRACY (1972) indicate the existence of a precursor of gastrin. Cleavage by trypsin results in the formation of the native hormone. Recently "big ACTH" was demonstrated by YALOW and BERSON (1973) in human plasma and pituitary extracts, which is also susceptible to tryptic cleavage. The characterization let suggest that "big ACTH" contains ACTH covalently linked to the carboxyl group of a basic amino acid of a larger more acidic peptide. Several laboratories have provided evidence that glucagon also is derived from a higher molecular weight precursor form (NOE and BAUER, 1971; TUNG and ZEREGA, 1971; NOE and BAUER, 1973). TAGER and STEINER (1973) were able to isolate a minor component form of crystalline glucagon that consists of glucagon with 8 additional amino acids. A basic residue links again the additional peptide to the hormone. This component was considered to be a intermediate form of proglucagon. Another possible prohormone is the pituitary peptide β-lipotropin which contains the amino acid sequence of β-MSH linked to the remainder of the polypeptide chain at either end through a pair of basic amino acids (CHRETIEN and LI, 1967).

All of these data let suggest that most of the small peptide hormones are derived in the biosynthesis from larger precursor molecules and that similar modes of intracellular cleavage may also be involved. However, precursor forms are not restricted to hormones. It was shown that proteolytic cleavage of larger polypeptides occurs in the formation of the capsule proteins of several animal viruses and bacteriophage heads (JACOBSEN and BALTIMORE, 1968; KIEHN and HOLLAND, 1970; LAEMMLI, 1970). Recently a precursor protein was also found for collagen (BELLAMY and BORNSTEIN, 1971; CHURCH *et al.*, 1971). Procollagen is cleaved by an extracellular protease which seems not to be trypsin like (LAPIERRE *et al.*, 1972).

From these data it can be concluded that precursors might play a more general role in the biosynthesis of proteins. Precursors were demonstrated for single chain polypeptides which do not contain disulfide bonds. A requirement for single chain precursors for the correct folding of these proteins seems therefore unneccessary. What accounts so well for the existence of proinsulin does not hold for other precursors as well. Thus far a teleological explanation for the presence of precursor molecules in protein biosynthesis remains to be found.

II. Secretion of Proinsulin and C-Peptide and their Significance*

WOLFGANG KEMMLER

With 6 Figures

1. Secretion of Proinsulin and C-Peptide In Vitro

Recent studies on insulin secretion response in different systems have demonstrated a biphasic pattern consisting of a small initial peak of insulin release followed by a slower more sustained rise after glucose stimulation (CERASI and LUFT, 1967; GRODSKY *et al.*, 1970; PORTE and PUPO, 1969; see also the chapter by GRODSKY in this volume). This observation suggests a two-compartmental model for insulin secretion, the first peak representing the release of stored material, while the second is composed mainly of newly synthesized insulin, as it can be partly suppressed by inhibitors of protein synthesis such als cycloheximide and puromycin. Experiments designed to study the kinetics of proinsulin and insulin secretion from isolated islets, or other systems *in vitro*, could answer the question whether there exists such a preferential release of newly synthesized material. If so, we would expect a marked release of proinsulin after stimulation. Such experiments which have been undertaken by several groups of investigators do not allow a definite conclusion since the results are conflicting.

Proinsulin and intermediate fractions were demonstrated to be secretion products of isolated rat islets (TANESE *et al.*, 1970; CLARK and STEINER, 1969). Proinsulin and insulin release was stimulated by glucose concentrations above 5.3 mmoles/liter, theophylline, tolbutamide and dibutyryl cyclic AMP. The latter substances showed a stimulating effect only in the presence of glucose. Glucose stimulation alone led to a preferential release of insulin, when the ratios of islets to medium for insulin and proinsulin plus intermediates were calculated. Each of the other substances, together with glucose, showed still a preferential release of insulin to a slight degree; however, the relative proportion of proinsulin to insulin increased considerably. The medium contained roughly equal amounts of insulin and proinsulin (TANESE *et al.*, 1970). These results may indicate that the stronger the stimulation of secretion the more newly synthesized material is secreted. Preferential release of proinsulin was observed even after glucose stimulation alone with rat islets by CLARK and STEINER (1969) and by LAZARUS *et al.* (1970a) with human insulinoma tissue and several insulin secretagogues. BURR *et al.* (1969) measured the proinsulin and insulin release from a perifused rat pancreas

* This work is based on the literature available in May 1973

preparation before and after stimulation with glucose. After 60 min of stimulation the portion of proinsulin secreted increased ten fold above prestimulation levels, representing up to 17% of the total immunoreactive insulin. All these results are consistent with the idea of preferential secretion of newly synthesized material after stimulation.

SANDO *et al.* (1972) on the other hand, could not demonstrate a significant secretion of newly synthesized material after stimulation. These authors calculated the total amounts and specific activities of proinsulin and insulin in rat islets and in medium samples, after pulse labelling the islets with ^{3}H-Leucine for 1 h and subsequent chase periods for several hours, with low and high glucose concentrations in the medium. Additional experiments were performed with dibutyryl cyclic AMP and cycloheximide in the incubation fluid. The experiments were designed in such a way that mainly the second phase of insulin secretion was studied. It was interesting to find that with isolated islets, cycloheximide did not lower the release of insulin, in contrast to the effect shown by the drug in perfused pancreas preparations (GRODSKY *et al.*, 1970). SANDO *et al.*, (1972) found no increase in the proportion of proinsulin to insulin in the medium during a 2 h incubation period with high glucose concentrations, and also after addition of dibutyryl cyclic AMP. In terms of both concentration and radioactivity, proinsulin was always found to be 6—7% that of the insulin on a molar basis, in both the medium and the islets. The ratio of labelled proinsulin to insulin was slightly lower in the medium than in the islets. The specific activity of proinsulin was about the same in both medium and islets and was much higher than that of insulin. Neither high glucose nor cycloheximide did alter the specific activity of proinsulin. These results indicate that stimulation of secretion does not change the mode of release; they demonstrate however, that during all states of release the proinsulin and insulin must derive from granules containing a high proportion of proinsulin and newly synthesized material. There is no preferential secretion of the "oldest" secretion granules before the release of newer ones. The ratio of the specific activities of insulin in the medium to that in the islets rose slightly after incubation with high glucose. Maximal release of newly synthesized material after glucose stimulation occured between the 3rd and 4th hour of incubation, confirming the results of HOWELL and TAYLOR (1967). Addition of dibutyryl cyclic AMP with high glucose increased the rate of insulin secretion but did not change the patterns of release.

These results suggest that newly synthesized material may be preferentially released to a slight degree; however, the authors calculated that 90% of the insulin is derived from preexisting granule stores. The secretion of small amounts of newly synthesized proinsulin and insulin suggests that newly formed secretory granules mix with "older" granule populations and undergo release randomly rather than preferentially. These observations taken together argue against the two-compartmental model of insulin secretion.

The results of the experiments of SANDO *et al.* (1972) support the hypothesis that there is no alternate or "non granule" route of insulin secretion. Again the authors found no discharge of newly synthesized material during the first hour of labelling the islets, confirming the results of STEINER *et al.*, (1970), HOWELL and TAYLOR (1967) and TANESE *et al.* (1970). This long delay argues against a direct fast transport from the rough endoplasmic reticulum to the plasma membrane. On the other hand, if a non-granule secretion were to occur, the secreted material should consist mainly of proinsulin rather than insulin. In the experiments however, as mentioned above, the ratio of proinsulin to insulin in the medium was always lower than that in the islets.

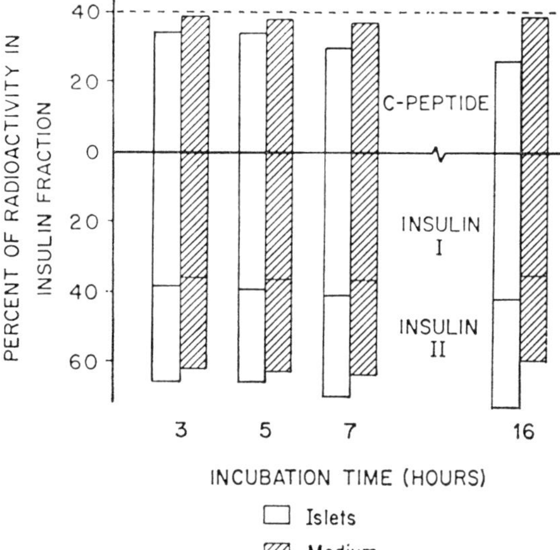

Fig. 1. After incubation of the islets with medium containing ^{3}H-leucine for the times indicated, medium and islets were extracted seperately. After filtration on Bio-Gel P-30 columns the two rat insulins and C-peptides were separated by polyacrylamide gel electrophoresis. Each bar segment indicates the percent of radioactivity found in the two insulins and the combined C-peptides; each bar spans 100%. The dotted line indicates the theoretical value for an equimolar amount of C-peptide. (From STEINER *et al.*, 1970)

The C-peptide was also shown to be a secretory product of rat islets *in vitro* (CLARK and STEINER, 1969). Labelled material corresponding to free C-peptide can be detected in the medium after incubation of islets when an appropriate precursor, such as leucine or proline, is used. C-peptide appears in the medium in equimolar amounts with insulin (Fig. 1). From these results it can be concluded that the C-peptide is retained in the secretory granules after transformation of proinsulin and is subsequently liberated with insulin into the medium. The findings are consistent with the observations made in experiments with isolated crude granule fractions as mentioned in the previous chapter, and have been confirmed by measurements of the secretion products *in vivo* described on the following pages.

2. Immunological Methods for the Determination of Circulating Proinsulin and Related Peptides

Proinsulin, C-peptide, and probably different intermediate forms are secreted by the β-cell into the circulation (see the next chapter). With the exception of only one antiserum described in the litterature antisera prepared against one of these compounds crossreact with at least one of the substances. This fact makes the immunological measurement of proinsulin and C-peptide a complex and interesting field of study (see also the chapter by DITSCHUNEIT in this volume and the review articles by CHANCE (1971) and KITABCHI *et al.* (1972b).

All *insulin antisera* known crossreact with proinsulin. Studies comparing the physical properties of proinsulin and insulin reported in the previous chapter, showed that the insulin part of the proinsulin molecule has nearly the same conformation as native insulin (FRANK and VEROS, 1968, 1970). Therefore it seems likely that these two proteins crossreact immunologically if the binding sites for insulin antibodies are not masked in the proinsulin molecule. The degree of cross-

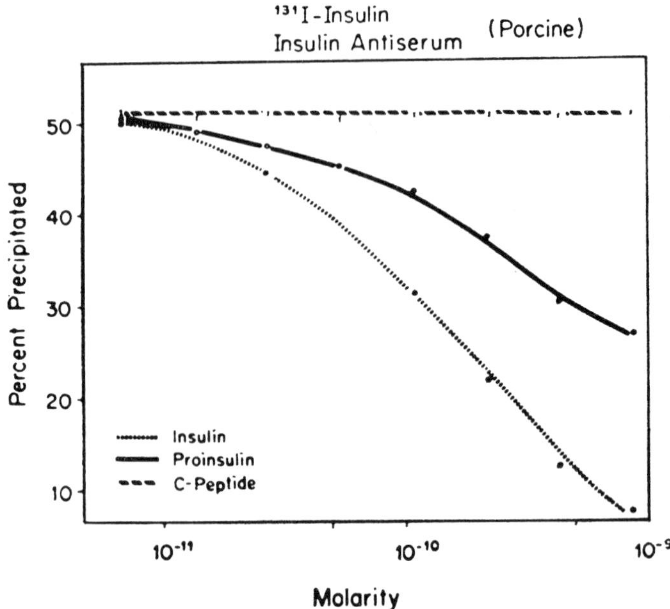

Fig. 2. Reaction of homologous insulin, proinsulin and C-peptide standards with porcine insulin antisera. Radio-immunoassay was performed by a modification of the method of MORGAN and LAZAROW (1963). The ordinate indicates the percentage counts in the precipitate (antibody bound) after addition of the rabbit antiguinea pig globulin serum. (From RUBENSTEIN *et al.*, 1970a)

reactivity varies to a great extent with the antiserum and technique (WRIGHT and MAKULU, 1969). Most investigators find that proinsulin binds $^1/_2$—$^1/_4$ as well to an insulin antiserum as insulin (CHANCE, 1971; KITABCHI, 1970; RUBENSTEIN *et al.*, 1969a; 1970a; STOLL *et al.*,1970a; MELANI *et al.*, 1970c; GUTMAN *et al.*,1971). But there are special antisera described which react with insulin and proinsulin to the same degree (GORDEN and ROTH, 1969; STOLL *et al.*, 1969; GOLDSMITH *et al.*, 1969). Insulin antisera also crossreact with intermediate fractions (KITABCHI *et al.*, 1972c) but not with C-peptide (RUBENSTEIN *et al.*, 1970a) (Fig. 2).

Proinsulin antisera are not specific either. They crossreact with C-peptide, insulin and intermediate forms to a variable degree as shown by RUBENSTEIN *et al.* (1970a). The crossreaction of proinsulin antisera with insulin can be suppressed by several techniques. Preincubation of these antisera with large amounts of insulin results in a "coated antibody" which binds proinsulin and C-peptide selectively (RUBENSTEIN *et al.*, 1969c). YIP and LOGOTHETOPOULOS (1969) removed the insulin binding portion by passing the antisera over a column of Sephadex-insulin. It may be assumed that these treated antibodies react with the C-peptide moiety of proinsulin only. Indeed, STOLL *et al.* (1970a) using such a modified antiserum, found that the C-peptide was bound three times as well as proinsulin on a weight basis, indicating equal reactivity on a molar basis.

Antibodies directed against proinsulin are much more species specific than the corresponding insulin antibodies. Antiserum to highly purified bovine proinsulin shows strong reaction only with bovine proinsulin and weak crossreaction with human or porcine proinsulin. Similarly, porcine proinsulin antiserum reacted poorly with human and bovine proinsulin (RUBENSTEIN and STEINER, 1970). Furthermore, if the insulin binding part of the proinsulin antibody is suppressed

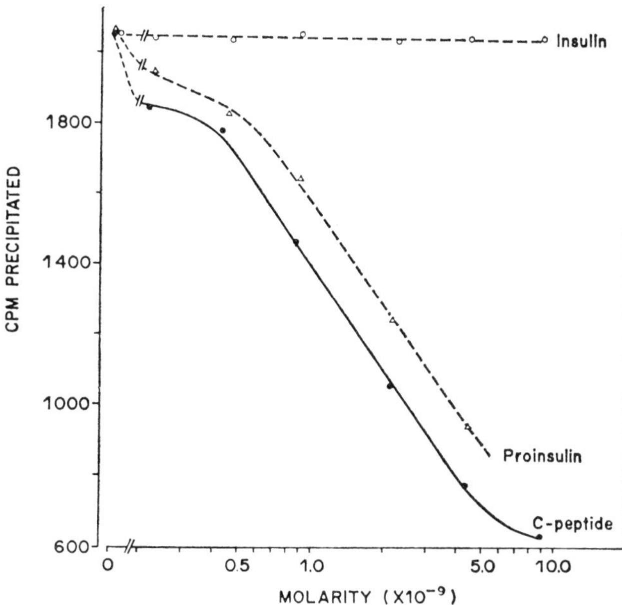

Fig. 3. Immunoassay of human C-peptide, proinsulin, and insulin using human C-peptide antiserum and (^{131}I) tyrosylated human C-peptide. (From MELANI *et al.*, 1970a)

or separated by the techniques described above, there remains very little crossreactivity between proinsulin antisera against the proinsulin of one species and the proinsulin molecules of an other species, as demonstrated by RUBENSTEIN *et al.* (1970a). These findings are not surprising in view of the marked differences in the structure of C-peptides of different species. Therefore, C-peptide molecules of different species are immunologically highly specific towards proinsulin antisera. Human C-peptide for instance does not react with porcine or bovine pro insulin antisera (RUBENSTEIN *et al.*, 1970a). From these data it can be concluded that for optimal assay conditions of the different proinsulins, the specific proinsulin antibody will be needed as mentioned by RUBENSTEIN *et al.* (1970a).

C-peptide antisera to human C-peptide, as developed by MELANI *et al.* (1970d) crossreact with human proinsulin to about 50%. In contrast, porcine and bovine insulin, proinsulin and C-peptide, and human insulin did not react with these antibodies.

Because of the crossreactions described the direct measurement of proinsulin, insulin, or C-peptide in blood with one of the usual antisera directed against one of these compounds is not possible. There is one exception: a proinsulin antiserum was obtained by STOLL *et al.* (1970b) which crossreacts neither with insulin nor C-peptide. This unique antibody must be directed against the regions of basic amino acids connecting C-peptide and insulin in the proinsulin molecule. By the use of this antiserum it was possible to measure proinsulin directly in serum.

But usually the different components have to be separated before measurement. Gel filtration is commonly used to separate proinsulin, insulin and C-peptide after extraction from serum or plasma. There are several other methods described for the separation of these compounds, such as thin layer chromatography (RYAN and ROBBINS, 1969) or polyacrylamide gel electrophoresis (HINZ *et al.*, 1970). All these methods have the disadvantage of being time-consuming. A simple and promising technique of separating proinsulin from insulin was developed by KITAB-

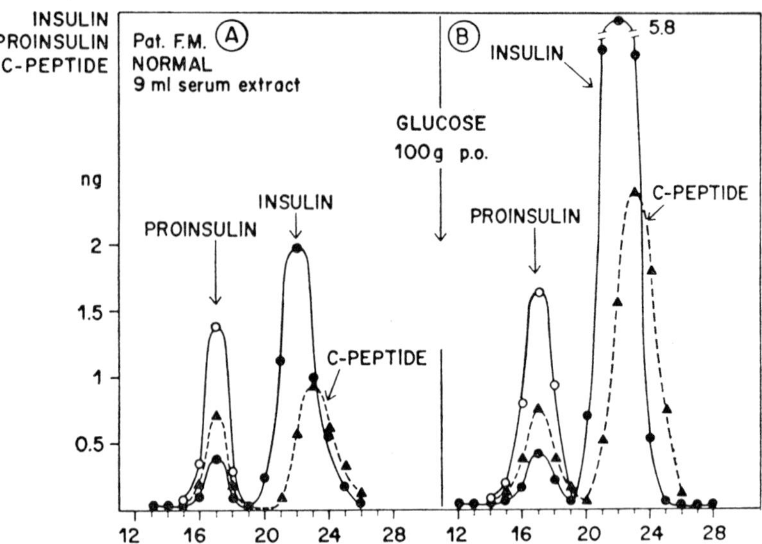

Fig. 4. Elution profile of serum taken from a healthy fasted subject, before and after glucose administration. After acid-ethanol extraction and gel filtration on a Bio-Gel P-30 column, the fractions were assayed by two different immunoassay systems: 1. Insulin assay: insulin standard ●—●; proinsulin standard ○—○. 2. C-peptide assay (described under Methods for the determination of circulating proinsulin and related peptides): C-peptide standard ▲---▲ (From MELANI *et al.*, 1970a)

CHI and co-workers. Insulin is degraded in this system by a proteolytic enzyme, "insulin specific protease", which degrades insulin but not proinsulin (BRUSH, 1971). The details of this method are described by KITABCHI *et al.* (1971).

With the separation of the components, not all the difficulties in measuring circulating proinsulin and C-peptide are solved. Human proinsulin is not available in sufficient quantities neither for immunization nor for the use as standard in an immunoassay for all investigators. The amount of proinsulin in human blood is usually determined with an immunoassay system using anti-bovine or -porcine insulin sera and the corresponding insulin as standard. The crossreactivity of insulin antisera with proinsulin varies to a great extent as we have seen, proinsulin reacting mostly less well than insulin. Therefore, in such a system proinsulin and intermediate fractions are underestimated and their levels as measured in different laboratories with different antisera, are not comparable.

Thus the levels of proinsulin in human blood described in the literature show great variations as will be seen later. Only the use of human proinsulin as standard can help to determine absolute proinsulin levels (MELANI *et al.*, 1970c). In order to make the results of different laboratories comparable, it would be necessary to test each insulin antibody used once against human proinsulin to elucidate its crossreactivity, as long as sufficient amounts of human proinsulin for standards are not available. Porcine or bovine proinsulin cannot be used as standards since their immunoreactivity differs from that of human proinsulin as we have seen.

Intermediates occuring in the blood give false results of absolute proinsulin levels even if human proinsulin is used as standard, since they react immunologically differently from proinsulin (KITABCHI *et al.*, 1972c; CHANCE, 1971). Several intermediates are not seperated from proinsulin by gel chromatography (STEINER *et al.*, 1969).

The only technique for the separation of intermediates from proinsulin known for human blood was developed by LAZARUS *et al.* (1971) using polyacrylamide gel electrophoresis after gel chromatography. Intermediate fractions do occur under certain circumstances in human blood (GUTMAN *et al.*, 1972; LAZARUS *et al.*, 1972). Therefore the measurement of absolute levels of proinsulin in human blood needs very timeconsuming and laborious separation techniques which are not practical as a routine assay.

C-peptide in human blood can be measured by a specific immunoassay developed by MELANI *et al.* (1970a). Guinea pigs injected with human C-peptide coupled to rabbit albumin developed antibodies which reacted specifically with human proinsulin and C-peptide. (^{131}I)-tyrosylated human C-peptide was used as tracer (Fig. 3). With this system and human proinsulin as standard, absolute levels of proinsulin in human blood can also be determined (MELANI *et al.*, 1970c). However, prior separation of proinsulin from C-peptide by gel chromatography is necessary. C-peptide was measured earlier by RUBENSTEIN *et al.* (1969b) using a bovine proinsulin antiserum in which the insulin binding part was suppressed before use.

The detection of proinsulin, intermediate fractions and C-peptide in the circulation shed new light on the immunoassay for the determination of insulin in blood. The direct measurement of immunoreactive insulin (IRI) in blood without prior fractionation does not distinguish between proinsulin, intermediates and insulin. Thus the assay is not as specific as it was thought to be before the discovery of the prohormone. Furthermore, the immunoassay of insulin in plasma containing the prohormone and intermediate fractions leads to quantitative errors. As we have seen earlier the degree of cross-reactivity of different insulin antibodies with proinsulin

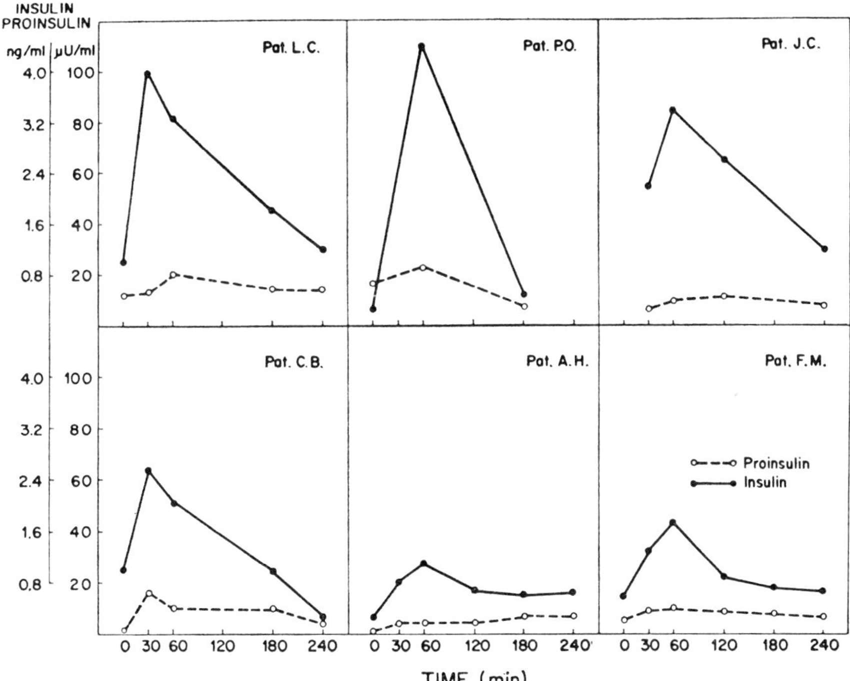

Fig. 5. Absolute concentrations of serum proinsulin and insulin in six normal subjects after oral administration of 100 g glucose. Porcine insulin -^{131}I and porcine insulin antiserum were used for immunoassay. The insulin values were read from a standard of human insulin and the proinsulin values from a standard of human proinsulin. (From MELANI *et al.*, 1970c)

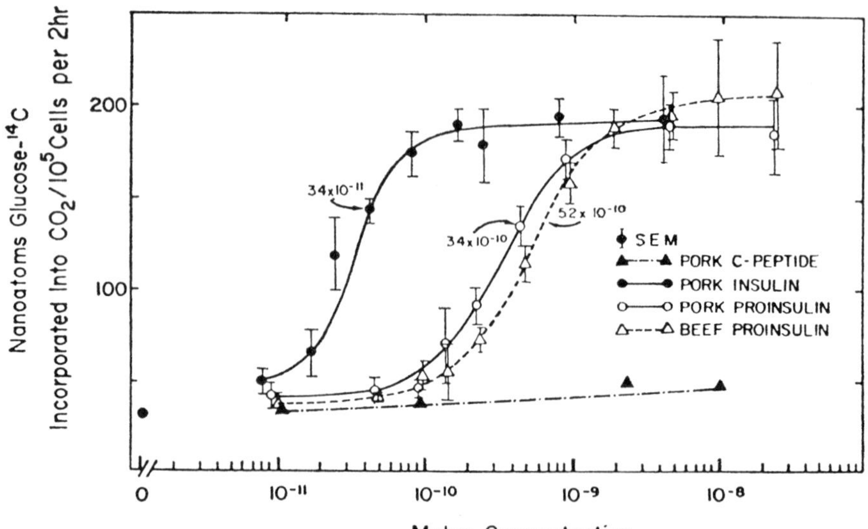

Fig. 6. Dose response curve for pork insulin, pork proinsulin, beef proinsulin, and pork C-peptide. Isolated rat fat cells were incubated with glucose -U-^{14}C with 0,55 mM glucose for 2 h in Krebs-Ringer-biocarbonate buffer pH 7.4 with 4% bovine serum albumin, under 5% CO_2 95% Oz. Arrows point to the concentration of each compound at half-maximum stimulation. (From KITABCHI, 1970)

shows a wide variation. Therefore the amount of total IRI in blood containing proinsulin like components (PLC) measured in different laboratories with different antibodies can not be absolutely comparable. In addition WRIGHT and MAKULU (1970) demonstrated that the degree of crossreactivity of insulin antibodies with proinsulin depends on the method used for immunoassay. GORDON and ROTH (1969) showed by indirect methods that the quantitative error involved in the direct measurement of insulin depends also on the relative amount of proinsulin and insulin in the blood. As the authors had no human proinsulin and insulin to test their respective influence on the immunoassay directly, they studied an analogous system by using a mixture of bovine and porcine insulin. The different reactivity of these insulins in the immunoassay system was thought to be roughly analogous to the reactivity of proinsulin and insulin. The mixture of the two insulins therefore approximates the situation encountered in plasma containing insulin and proinsulin. The authors found that at relatively low concentrations of insulin in the mixture the error encountered in measurements of total insulin levels was neglegible, regardless of the ratio beef to pork. As the total concentration of insulin (beef plus pork) is increased, the proportion of the apparent to actual insulin concentration falls progressively. For plasma containing insulin and proinsulin the following can be concluded from these experiments: the error will be increased by antibodies which discriminate well between insulin and proinsulin, by high proportions of proinsulin in the sample, and by a low position of the sample on the standard curve of the immunoassay.

3. Secretion of Proinsulin and C-Peptide In Vivo

a) Proinsulin

Shortly after the discovery of proinsulin two groups of investigators described independently the occurrence of a substance in human serum which was crossreacting immunologically with insulin but which exhibited a higher molecular weight (RUBENSTEIN *et al.*, 1968). This material, coeluting with proinsulin on gel chromatography, was presumed to be proinsulin by RUBENSTEIN *et al.* (1968). ROTH *et al.* (1968) referred to it as "big insulin", differentiating it from "little insulin" or native insulin. A similar material was also found in human urine (RUBENSTEIN *et al.*, 1968; CONSTAN *et al.*, 1970). Figure 3 shows the elution profile of extracted human serum from a healthy fasted subject before and after glucose administration.

α) Normal subjects and animals

Now is it generally recognized that "big insulin" is identical with proinsulin or proinsulin-like material (LAZARUS *et al.*, 1970a; SHERMAN *et al.*, 1971; SHERMAN *et al.*, 1972; MELANI *et al.*, 1970c). The chemical isolation and direct identification of this circulating material remains still to be accomplished, but there is enough indirect evidence to characterize it as proinsulin-like material: identical elution pattern on gel filtration (MELANI *et al.*, 1970c; SHERMAN *et al.*, 1971) and identical migration pattern on polyacrylamide gel electrophoresis (GUTMAN *et al.*, 1972) immunological identity in serial dilutions with human proinsulin (MELANI *et al.*, (1970c), crossreaction with antiserum directed against human C-peptide and bovine insulin (MELANI *et al.*, 1970c), conversion to insulin-like material upon exposure to trypsin (MELANI *et al.*, 1970c), and low insulin-like biological activity (SHERMAN *et al.*, 1971). Yet the possibility cannot be ruled out that the material may consist to a smaller or larger extent of different intermediate forms (see below); therefore it seems advisable to refer to it as proinsulin-like components (PLC). Proinsulin-like components were also found in serum of porc (STOLL *et al.*, 1970a), dog (ROTH *et al.*, 1968), and calf (YIP and LOGOTHETOPOULOS, 1969).

The concentration of PLC in serum of fasted healthy human subjects ranges between 0.05 and 0.4 ng/ml, corresponding to 5—48% of the insulin concentration (MELANI *et al.*, 1970c). These values may represent true proinsulin and not PLC levels in serum. First they are measured with a human proinsulin standard in two different assay systems, the insulin and C-peptide system (Fig. 3). Secondly it was shown by GUTMAN *et al.* (1972) that in normal healthy subjects no intermediate fractions can be found in serum. The oral glucose tolerance test (Fig. 4) gives the following results: the absolute level of PLC and insulin increased, but there was a delay in the increase of PLC as compared to that of insulin, and the PLC increase was of lesser magnitude than that of insulin. When the proinsulin values are expressed as a percentage of insulin the percent PLC tends to decrease in the first 2 h after oral glucose. Towards the end of the test it returned to fasting levels. These changes are mainly due to changes of the insulin concentration. Striking changes in PLC concentrations were not observed (MELANI *et al.*, 1970c).

Other investigators reported varying fasting levels of PLC in normal human subjects. SHERMAN *et al.* (1972) found 20% or less of total IRI, GORDEN *et al.* (1971a) approximately 20%; in another report 10—40% (GORDEN *et al.*, 1970). GUTMAN *et al.* (1971) observed 0—17%. KITABCHI *et al.* (1971), measuring the PLC directly in the plasma by the use of the insulin degrading enzyme, found much higher levels of 26—76%. Whether this discrepancy with other investigators is caused by the difference of the methods used remains unclear since direct comparison of the same sera in three laboratories, using the method developed by KITABCHI and co-workers and the usual column fractionation procedure, showed close agreement (KITABCHI *et al.*, 1971). In all these determinations, the true values of PLC are underestimated since insulin standards were used in the immunoassays. However, from all data in the litterature it can be concluded that PLC may represent an appreciable amount of IRI in normal subjects. The physiological significance of these high levels is still unclear.

After oral glucose, Gorden *et al.* (1970), Gorden and Roth (1969) and Kitabchi *et al.* (1971) observed a pattern of PLC response in normal healthy subjects which was similar to that shown by Melani *et al.* (1970c) as cited earlier. Stimulation of insulin secretion with other stimuli such as tolbutamide or arginine yielded a response similar to that of glucose stimulation (Gorden and Roth, 1969). In contrast, Stoll *et al.* (1970a) found in swine a rapid and sharp rise in PLC after glucose or glucagon administration with a biphasic pattern but it must be emphasized that in the system used by these authors, C-peptide was measured as part of the PLC. C-peptide is secreted together with insulin in equimolar amounts as will be seen later and therefore the PLC measured by these authors evidently mimic the insulin secretion pattern.

β) Pathological states

The levels of PLC in the circulation and their clinical significance were studied in a wide variety of pathological states; diabetes mellitus of course was the most interesting. There is no indication so far that any state of human diabetes mellitus is associated with high levels of PLC in the circulation (Rubenstein and Steiner, 1970; Goldsmith *et al.*, 1969; Gorden and Roth, 1969). The concept was tempting that a possibly hereditary enzyme defect in the conversion of proinsulin to insulin which may lead to a biologically less potent hormone, might play a role in the etiology of diabetes mellitus. However, this could not be supported by experimental data. Similarly, Poffenbarger *et al.* (1971) studied hereditary diabetes in hyperinsulinemic mice and found neither abnormal levels of PLC nor any abnormality in the biosynthesis of insulin in the islets of these animals.

In obese patients with hyperinsulinemia, Melani *et al.* (1970c) found higher fasting levels of PLC than in normal subjects and a greater increase of these components after oral glucose administration in absolute levels. However, the relative proportions of PLC and insulin were in the same range as observed in the normal control group. Gutman *et al.* (1971) observed a similar pattern in obese subjects after stimulation with tolbutamide. In contrast, Gorden and Roth (1969) found an elevation in percent "big insulin" at early times after oral glucose administration which was roughly proportional to the increase in percent of the ideal body weight in eight out of ten obese subjects, whereas at a later point the percent PLC in obese fell within the same wide range as in thin subjects.

Goldsmith *et al.* (1969) studied patients with various conditions reported to be associated with insulin insensitivity such as myotonic dystrophy, hypertriglyceridemia, thyroid deficiency and uremia, and found normal PLC levels in plasma after administration of oral or intravenous glucose, not exceeding 20% of the total IRI. Gordon and Roth (1969) on the other hand, observed in acromegalic patients high proportions of PLC in the early phase of oral glucose tolerance test, and they found the same pattern in obese patients. Patients with functional hypoglycemia were studied by Gutman *et al.* 1971) which showed normal levels of PLC, whereas Duckworth and Kitabchi (1972) recently observed two patients which developed hypoglycemia during oral glucose tolerance tests and PLC levels comprising more than 50% of total IRI. Patients with hypokalemia resulting from different chronic diseases associated with insulinopenia and glucose intolerance showed significant proportions of PLC (10—65% of total IRI) after glucose administration (Gorden *et al.*, 1972). The increased percentage of biologically less active PLC may contribute in these cases to the abnormality in glucose tolerance. Thus there are several pathological states reported with relatively high proportions of PLC in the circulation. But so far there exist only few reports and some of them are contradictory.

On the other hand elevated PLC levels in the circulation are of definite clinical interest in patients with islet cell tumors. Increased levels of PLC in patients with insulinomas were reported by a number of investigators (MELANI *et al.*, 1970b; GOLDSMITH *et al.*, 1969; GUTMAN *et al.*, 1971; GORDEN *et al.*, 1971a; BLACKARD *et al.*, 1970; PEARSON *et al.*, 1972; KITABCHI *et al.*, 1971; SHERMAN *et al.*, 1972; LAZARUS *et al.*, 1970a, 1972).

The values of PLC in patients bearing insulinomas range from 8—89% of total IRI in the literature; a value of more than 25% (measured against an insulin standard) in a patient with hypoglycemia can be used as additional aid in the diagnosis of the tumors. In the most extensive study reported recently on 19 patients with benign islet cell adenomas, SHERMAN *et al.* (1972) found that the fasting PLC levels were clearly elevated (greater than 25% of total IRI) in two thirds of the patients. In most cases with high PLC levels high IRI levels were also found: among the seven patients with normal IRI levels (20 μU/ml or less) only in two did the PLC exceed 25%. In those cases with slight hypoglycemia and normal IRI, the estimation of PLC would be diagnostic of the presence of an insulin producing tumor (SHERMAN *et al.*, 1972). This diagnostic aid might be of clinical importance in many cases since high IRI levels are not an invariable finding in patients with islet cell tumors. BERSON and YALOW (1962) reported that only 7 out of 15 patients exhibited fasting values above 100 μU/ml. Similar results were obtained by SAMOLS and MARKS (1963) who found elevated IRI levels in only 50% of the patients investigated. The patients with malignant islet cell tumors showed all abnormally elevated PLC levels (SHERMAN *et al.*, 1972; GUTMAN *et al.*, 1971; BLACKARD *et al.*, 1970; GORDEN *et al.*, 1971; PEARSON *et al.*, 1972).

Most of the patients with islet cell tumors demonstrate the same quantitative dynamics with regard to the PLC/IRI ratio after stimulation of secretion as normal healthy subjects. Acute administration of different secretagogues such as glucose, leucine or sulfonylureas causes mostly release of insulin resulting first in a decrease of the percent PLC with a subsequent increase due to an absolute increment of PLC and a fall of insulin at later times after stimulation (MELANI *et al.*, 1970b; GORDEN *et al.*, 1971a; SHERMAN *et al.*, 1972).

The effect of stimuli of insulin secretion in patients with insulinomas is quantitatively different from that in normal patients. In these patients tolbutamide is more effective than glucose or leucine in stimulating insulin secretion, whereas in normals glucose is the most effective stimulus (BERSON and YALOW, 1962; SAMOLS and MARKS, 1963). Thus tumor bearing patients exhibit glucose tolerance tests of a diabetic type and hyperreactivity to tolbutamide (FAJANS *et al.*, 1961). Two recent reports demonstrate also a qualitatively different response to the different stimuli. GUTMAN *et al.* (1971) observed in a patient with benign insulinoma that tolbutamide apparently released PLC with 75% of total IRI, whereas the proportion of PLC after glucose stimulation was only 5%. In contrast, PEARSON *et al.* (1972) reported a case of islet cell carcinoma where glucose, but not tolbutamide caused a release of PLC. These results indicate that islet cell tumors and even islet cell adenomas are heterogeneous and variable in their function which perhaps reflects variable degrees of cytodifferentiation of their cells seen in islet cell tumors as well as in other neoplastic tissues (MUNGER, 1972).

Malignant islet cell tumors show variable reactions to the administration of streptozotocin. In some cases the drug is without any effect on IRI or PLC levels (SHERMAN *et al.*, 1972; PEARSON *et al.*, 1972), in others both components are lowered (SHERMAN *et al.*, 1972). In one interesting case reported by BLACKARD *et al.* (1970), therapy with streptozotozin was followed by a decrease of PLC only, the total IRI remained unchanged. This theraphy however caused a dramatic clinical response with cessation of hypoglycemic attacks. The administration of diazoxide in cases of malignant islet cell tumors leads to a fall in both PLC and IRI levels (Sherman *et al.*, 1972).

What causes the high proportion of PLC in most of the patients with islet cell tumors is yet an unanswered question. Melani *et al.* (1970b) found that PLC represented 52% of the IRI in the adenoma tissue removed from a patient with preoperative plasma levels of 77% PLC. After removal of the tumor the PLC fell to about 10% of total IRI. Sherman *et al.* (1972) observed that islet cell tumors from hamsters contained 32% PLC and the animals bearing these adenomas had also very high PLC proportions of total plasma IRI. These relatively high PLC levels in the tumor tissue and plasma compared to that in normals might be caused by a relative deficiency of the converting enzyme system or a defective release and storage mechanism. There is no indication for an absolute deficiency of the converting enzymes in any tumor or nontumor case reported in the literature. Lazarus *et al.* (1970) observed normal conversion rates of proinsulin to insulin in pieces of human insulinoma tissue, in spite of high plasma PLC levels of the patient before the tumor was removed, indicating that the failure is probably in the release and storage mechanism and not in the conversion. It is even unclear whether the PLC measured in tumor patients consists of normal proinsulin and known intermediates. Gorden *et al.* (1971b) found evidence for a unique form of circulating insulin in an islet cell carcinoma which has a higher molecular weight, an enhanced biological activity and which reacts with insulin antibodies but is different from proinsulin and intermediate forms.

Thus detailed studies of more cases are necessary in order to understand the significance of the elevated PLC levels found in most of the patients with insulin producing tumors.

b) Intermediate Forms

Lazarus *et al.* (1972) and Gutman *et al.* (1972) reported the occurence of intermediate forms in the circulation. In three normal healthy subjects the PLC peak eluted from gel chromatography and further fractionated by polyacrylamide gel electrophoresis consisted entirely of proinsulin, and no intermediates could be detected in the basal state or after tolbutamide or glucose stimulation. In all three obese patients tested and in one case of islet cell carcinoma the PLC was heterogeneous, a significant proportion consisting of intermediates after stimulation of insulin secretion. It remains to be studied whether these intermediates might play a role in the pathophysiology of obesity.

c) C-Peptide

Rubenstein *et al.* (1969b) were the first to identify C-peptide in the circulation by examining serum of the cow. Melani *et al.* (1970a) developed the immunoassay for human C-peptide described earlier (Fig. 3). The authors found C-peptide and insulin in equimolar amounts under several conditions in the circulation: in the fasting state, after stimulation with secretagogues, and in patients with islet cell adenomas. These results suggested that C-peptide and insulin are excreted in equivalent amounts during emiocytosis of the beta granules. This interpretation would agree with the studies on isolated secretion granule fractions and on the *in vitro* secretion studies mentioned earlier. However, the hypothesis is based on the assumption that the half life of these proteins in the circulation is similar, which is still unknown.

With the recently developed immunoassay for human C-peptide it is possible to study the beta-cell function in insulin treated diabetics (Block *et al.*, 1972). In juvenile diabetics the authors were unable to detect any C-peptide immunoreactivity thus indicating complete absence of secretory capacity. In maturity onset diabetics, however, even under insulin therapy, the measurements suggest that in the majority of cases the secretion of proinsulin, insulin, and C-peptide continues for years.

4. Peripheral Degradation of Proinsulin

The relatively high concentration of PLC in the circulation in normal healthy subjects could be explained by two different mechanisms which also might be combined in their effect. The PLC content of the pancreas was measured by different laboratories and was found to be about 1% of the total pancreatic IRI in rat and bovine pancreas (Steiner *et al.*, 1968), 0.26—1.6% in human fetal pancreas (Rastogi *et al.*, 1970), about 7% in adult and fetal porcine pancreas (Lockwood and Misbin, 1972) and about 10% in porcine pancreas (Chance, 1971). To reach the relatively high plasma concentrations mentioned earlier (from 15—45% of total IRI in normal fasting human subjects, Melani *et al.*, 1970c) PLC must either be preferentially released from the β-cell, or its disappearance rate from the circulation must be different from that of insulin. It is obvious that the existence of significant differences in peripheral metabolism and distribution of proinsulin and insulin may influence their relative blood levels. From the *in vitro* studies by Sando *et al.* (1972) which have been described earlier in this text, it can be assumed that there is no preferential release of PLC from the beta cell. However, these data are at variance with observations by others (Tanese *et al.*, 1970; Clark and Steiner, 1969; Lazarus *et al.*, 1970a; Burr *et al.*, 1969). The peripheral degradation of PLC might therefore explain the high proinsulin levels, but it is also of interest in relation to its biological activity. As we will see later, it is still a matter of controversy if proinsulin has a intrinsic biological activity, or has to be degraded to insulin before it is active on the target tissue.

Tompkins *et al.* (1971) calculated that proinsulin and insulin are distributed in approximately the same space. The immunological half disappearance time, t 1/2, of human insulin and porcine proinsulin in man was calculated by the authors to be 25 min for proinsulin and 4 min for insulin. Stoll *et al.* (1970c) found similar half lifes for porcine proinsulin in baboons (18 min) and swine (22 min). In these species, the t 1/2 for insulin was calculated to be about one half of that of proinsulin. The values determined by Rubenstein *et al.* (1970b) in dogs are comparable.

The localization and the product of peripheral degradation of PLC are as yet not well understood, and the available data are widely divergent. Liver is the major organ that removes insulin from the circulation (Izzo *et al.*, 1967). Stoll *et al.* (1970c) and Rubenstein *et al.* (1972b) therefore studied the hepatic extraction of proinsulin by the isolated perfused rat liver. Rubenstein *et al.* (1972b) found that the hepatic removal of proinsulin was considerably slower, averaging 10—15 times less than that of insulin; the t 1/2 of insulin being 14—17 min in that system. Similarly Stoll *et al.* (1970c), could not demonstrate any significant clearance of proinsulin or C-peptide in the liver perfusion system in contrast to that of insulin. It is noteworthy that both groups of investigators found no indication for any conversion of proinsulin to insulin in their system, whereas the transformation to intermediate fractions could not be ruled out by the techniques used.

This slow hepatic clearance rate could eventually explain the prolonged half time of proinsulin in the circulation. Rubenstein *et al.* (1970b) concluded from their experiments on the renal extraction of proinsulin in dogs that this organ might play an important role in peripheral proinsulin metabolism. The authors determined a renal arterio-venous concentration difference of 23—50% of the prevailing arterial proinsulin level.

Several groups of investigators studied the degradation of proinsulin and insulin by organ homogenates. In the most extensive experiments KITABCHI and STENTZ (1972) investigated the degradation activities of homogenates of different rat tissues. They found that with the exception of pancreas and kidney, none of the ten different organs studied was able to degrade proinsulin more than 5—10% of the rate at which insulin was degraded. The degrading activity was mainly in the soluble fraction of these organs. Pancreas and kidney exhibited a ratio of insulin to proinsulin degradation of about 20%. The partly purified insulin specific protease of the kidney had similar characteristics to that of muscle (BRUSH, 1971) and liver (BURGHEN *et al.*, 1972). It is of interest to notice that, as judged from the kinetics of degradation which was measured immunologically, in none of the organs there was evidence for a specific conversion of proinsulin to insulin.

MASHITER and KING (1969) however, in contrast to the data presented by KITABCHI and STENTZ (1972) and RUBENSTEIN *et al.* (1972b), found evidence for a specific conversion of proinsulin to insulin by organ homogenates. Homogenates of rat liver, spleen, muscle and kidney were incubated with proinsulin and the insulin immunoreactivity measured after varying times. The immunoreactivity rose markedly in the first min, then after about 7 min a rapid decline took place. The interpretation of these results by the authors was that proinsulin was first converted to insulin with higher immunoreactivity, and then further degraded to less reactive material. However, neither this final material nor the insulin formed were directly characterized, therefore the interpretation remains doubtful.

CHALLONER (1971) studied the degradation of proinsulin and insulin to TCA soluble material in intact adipose tissue and fat homogenates. Surprisingly, the degradation rate by intact fat cells and their homogenates was the same for both proteins, whereas homogenates of fat pieces showed about half of the degradative activity for proinsulin as compared to insulin. Kunitz pancreatic trypsin inhibitor (KPTI) was able to inhibit the degradation of proinsulin in homogenates of fat pieces and not that of insulin. These differences await further clarification. Since the products of degradation were not fully characterized, it remains open whether a specific conversion of proinsulin to insulin took place, or whether an unspecific degradation was in fact observed.

The question whether proinsulin can be converted to insulin or intermediates in the blood, was investigated by injecting radioactively labelled proinsulin intravenously or intramuscularly into rats (RUBENSTEIN *et al.*, 1969a; LAZARUS *et al.*, 1970b). In none of the experiments the degradation to insulin could be observed. Even at time intervals after injection, when profound hypoglycemia could be measured in the animals, no conversion to insulin or intermediates could be detected with the aid of gel chromatography and polyacrylamide gel electrophoresis. The mechanism by which proinsulin produces hypoglycemia appears therefore to be a direct one.

The only careful direct characterization of the degradation products of proinsulin in intact target tissue was reported by LAZARUS *et al.* (1970b). Labelled proinsulin was incubated *in vitro* with rat hemidiaphragm. Only 7% of the proinsulin was degraded within 60 min. Polyacrylamide gel electrophoresis and gel chromatography were performed and neither the formation of insulin nor that of intermediates could be detected. The presence of Kunitz pancreatic trypsin inhibitor (KPTI) had neither a qualitative nor quantitative effect on degradation.

In conclusion, the longer half life of proinsulin than that of insulin could explain the relatively high levels of PLC in the blood as compared to its content in pancreas. No organ could be detected which is specifically able to degrade proinsulin.

The occurrance of insulin or intermediate fractions as a product of peripheral degradation in blood, intact target tissue or organ homogenates seems highly unlikely from the present studies. All except one group of investigators cited earlier agree in that they found no evidence for a specific degradation to insulin or intermediates in the periphery. In contrast, the study by MASHITER and KING (1969) which suggests such a conversion, is based on indirect evidence.

In the next section experiments with protease inhibitors will be discussed which have also been interpreted as evidence for or against peripheral conversion of proinsulin to insulin.

5. Biological Activity

a) In-Vivo Studies

The biological significance of proinsulin in the circulation has interested a large number of investigators.

Proinsulin has an insulin-like biological effect *in vivo*. CHANCE *et al.* (1968) were the first reporting an insulin-like effect of proinsulin in the mouse convulsion assay, proinsulin beeing about 20% as potent as insulin in equimolar amounts. The same authors found that proinsulin with an activity of 3 units/mg as calculated from the mouse convulsion assay gave a moderatly prolonged hypoglycemic effect in rabbits similar to NPH-insulin (CHANCE, 1971); a similar prolonged hypoglycemic activity was observed by PULS and KRONEBERG (1969) in rats and mice. Surprisingly, the effect of proinsulin was stronger in fasted than in fed rats. The activity on the blood sugar was more protracted and the onset more delayed than that of insulin when given in equimolar amounts. Nephrectomcy, pancreatectomy or 2/3 hepatectomy did not change the activity. STOLL *et al.* (1971) observed the same pattern of proinsulin action in baboons and swine when proinsulin was given in equipotent doses as calculated from the respective activities in the mouse convulsion assay. GALLOWAY *et al.* (1969) studied the effect of the prohormone in healthy male volontears and found a weak hypoglycemic activity which was also slightly delayed in onset and of longer duration than that of insulin. The prolonged action of proinsulin observed by all investigators could be explained by the already described longer half-life of proinsulin; the delay of onset was interpreted by some authors as indicating the necessary conversion to insulin or intermediates. However, such an explanation seems unlikely from the data presented in the last section. WILLMS *et al.* (1969) reported that proinsulin is without any hypoglycemic activity in eviscerated, hepatectomized rats. This lack was interpreted as beeing due to the failure of the operated animals to convert proinsulin to insulin. These results were contradicted by PENHOS *et al.* (1970) who reinvestigated the effect of proinsulin on hepatectomized eviszcerated rats in view of the finding of the same group that proinsulin is not converted to insulin in the periphery (LAZARUS *et al.*, 1970b). The authors found that proinsulin had the expected effect on hypoglycemia also in operated animals when given in equipotent doses as insulin as calculated from their respective activities in the mouse convulsion assay. Thus PENHOS and coworkers concluded that proinsulin conversion by the removed organs does not appear to be a prerequisite for proinsulin action. If indeed proinsulin has an intrinsic *in vivo* effect in causing hypoglycemia then in any case the prohormone is much less potent than insulin.

REES and MADISON (1969), however, reported a qualitatively and quantitatively equal *in vivo* effect of proinsulin and insulin on hepatic glucose output, and on arterial glucose and fatty acid concentrations by measuring the *in vivo* effects of the two hormones in a dog liver perfusion system. In most other studies reported in the literature on the biological activity of the prohormone *in vivo* and *in vitro*, its effect was qualitatively equal but quantitatively less than that of insulin; therefore this interesting experiments need to be reinvestigated in other species expecially in man. Qualitatively similar effects of proinsulin and insulin were observed by RUDORFF *et al.* (1970a, 1970b) on the inhibition of glucose formation from alanine and incorporation of alanine into protein in isolated perfused liver of normal and alloxan diabetic rats. There was no initial lag period observed in the action of the prohormone, which was interpreted as indicating that conversion to insulin is not necessary for this action.

Other *in vivo* studies were carried out by FINEBERG and MERIMEE (1970) with the human forearm-perfusion system. Proinsulin administered in equimolar amounts was less potent than insulin in stimulating glucose and potassium uptake by muscle and, in general, also on the suppression of fatty acid release from muscle and fat tissue. However, the biological potency of proinsulin on fatty acid release was greater in fat than in muscle tissue compared to that of insulin and in one of the two individuals tested even greater.

b) In-Vitro Studies

In vitro studies on the biological effect of proinsulin were carried out by a number of investigators. The incorporation of glucose ^{14}C into lipids and its oxidation to carbon dioxide under the influence of proinsulin was studied in rat fat cells and fat pads by SHAW and CHANCE (1968), KITABCHI (1970, see Fig. 5), GLIEMANN and SORENSON (1970), TOOMEY *et al.* (1970), LAVIS *et al.* (1970), CHALLONER and YU (1970). The antilipolytic effect in rat fat tissue was investigated by CHALLONER and YU (1970), STEELE *et al.* (1970), and TOOMEY *et al.* (1970). FAULHABER *et al.* (1972) examined the biological activity of proinsulin on human adipose tissue slices. Proinsulin exerts the same qualitative biological effects on fat tissue as insulin but its potency is reduced; the ratio of effectiveness insulin to proinsulin varies to a great extend in the reports, ranging when used in equimolar amounts with insulin from 10—84. In all studies proinsulin was found to be less than 10% as potent as insulin. Figure 6 shows the dose response curves for pork insulin and proinsulin, beef proinsulin, and pork C-peptide in the rat fat cell assay.

Interestingly, the differences in potency of proinsulin and insulin are the same on lipid and glucose metabolism (CHALLONER and YU, 1970; LAVIS *et al.*, 1970). The dose response curves of the two hormones are parallel and the maximum effect is the same (CHALLONER and YU, 1970; GLIEMANN and SORENSON, 1970). Furthermore, the biological response of the prohormone and insulin administered in equipotent doses showes the same time curves (GLIEMANN and SORENSON, 1970; KITABCHI, 1970). Proinsulin and insulin are neither suppressing nor potentiating their respective effects on the target tissue (KITABCHI, 1970; LAVIS *et al.*, 1970). Proinsulin intermediate fractions are biologically more active than proinsulin itself on fat tissue (KITABCHI *et al.*, 1972b).

SHAW and CHANCE (1968), LAVIS *et al.* (1970) and LAZARUS *et al.* (1970b) studied the biological effect of proinsulin on rat hemidiaphragm *in vitro*. On muscle tissue, when the glucose uptake and carbon dioxide production from glucose is measured, proinsulin is also less potent than insulin, being 8—25% as active as insulin. In one report on *in vitro* studies KONSENK *et al.* (1971) found proinsulin and insulin equipotent when administered in equimolar amounts. The authors measured the sodium transport stimulated by proinsulin and insulin across isolated toad skin segments.

The question is still open whether the biological activity of proinsulin is an intrinsic one or whether the prohormone has to be converted to insulin before it can act on the target tissue. From the studies on the peripheral degradation mentioned earlier a prior conversion seems unlikely. However, the divergent and conflicting results of the experiments with protease inhibitors on the biological activity leave this question still open to discussion. In some reports, the biological activity of proinsulin could be suppressed by the addition of KPTI (Kunitz pancreatic trypsin inhibitor). Such an effect indicating a protein splitting system necessary for the activation of proinsulin was observed by SHAW and CHANCE (1968), LAZARUS *et al.* (1970b) and CHALLONER and YU (1970). The authors measured the activity on rat fat pads or rat hemidiaphragm. In contrast, GLIEMANN and SORENSON (1970) using rat fat pads could not find any inhibitory activity of KPTI. The discrepancy in these studies cannot be explained. LAZARUS *et al.* (1970b) were not able to explain the effect of KPTI in their study on hemidiaphragm since they found no evidence for a conversion in careful analysis of the degradation products, and could not observe any correlation of the effect to the antitryptic activity of the inhibitor. KPTI has no influence on the biological activity of proinsulin on isolated fat cells (GLIEMANN and SORENSON, 1970; KITABCHI 1970; STEELE *et al.*, 1970; CHALLONER and YU, 1970; TOOMEY *et al.*, 1970). Interestingly no other protease inhibitor such as trasylol or soybean trypsin inhibitor (STI) used in all systems studied caused an effect on the biological activity of proinsulin.

Thus the divergent and yet unexplained results of the experiments with the inhibitor KPTI and the studies of MASHITER and KING (1969) on peripheral degradation of proinsulin, discussed earlier, give the only indication for a peripheral conversion of proinsulin to insulin. The results taken together are not conclusive enough to make an intrinsic low biological activity of proinsulin doubtful. Further experiments on the eventual conversion of proinsulin to intermediate fractions are however needed.

Recent studies on insulin binding are consistent with the hypothesis that proinsulin binds to the same receptors than insulin but the binding is relatively weak. Furthermore the lower affinity of proinsulin to the receptor sites, compared to that of insulin, corresponds very well with its lower biological activity observed *in vitro* either when studied with fat cell membranes, liver cell membranes, or isolated "receptors" from fat cells and liver cells (CUATRECASAS, 1971, 1972; FREYCHET *et al.*, 1971). Proinsulin even displaced labelled insulin from the receptor sites 10% as well as cold insulin in human lymphocytes, a tissue where both hormones show no biological effect (GAVIN *et al.*, 1972).

Porcine or bovine C-peptide have no insulin-like activity in rat fat cells or fat pads (GLIEMANN and SORENSON, 1970; KITABCHI, 1970; see Fig. 6). The known differences of the primary structures of the C-peptides of different species could explain the failure of heterologous C-peptide to react; on the other hand, the binding of C-peptide to insulin receptor sites seems highly unlikely in view of its structure. C-peptide has no inhibitory effect either on proinsulin or insulin action (GLIEMANN and SORENSON, 1970; KITABCHI, 1970). Whether the C-peptide has any peripheral function remains to be tested in systems different from those where insulin is active.

6. Prospects and Conclusions

Since the discovery of proinsulin in 1967 important new knowledge has been accumulated on the principles of insulin biosynthesis from its precursor form. The physiological importance of the prohormone was demonstrated in all species studied.

Proinsulin and the conversion products other than insulin, such as C-peptide and intermediate forms, are chemically well characterized in the meantime. We do not know very much about the intracellular events leading to the conversion. In view of isolated products of the conversion a hypothesis can be developed on the enzymatic process which might be involved in the transformation. *In vitro* and *in vivo* studies on the conversion process support the view that a combined action of two enzymes, a trypsin-like and a carboxypeptidase-B-like protease might be responsible for the conversion *in vivo*. However, the direct characterization of the converting enzymes thus far has not been possible. From the data on other prohormones we can conclude that the proteolytic mechanism liberating the hormone from the precursor might be the same for all prohormones. Possibly the characterization of this common converting enzyme will be easier in other endocrine tissue than in islets of Langerhans.

The half time of proinsulin was calculated to be 1 h. This time course of the conversion seems not to be variable. Thus far we do not know any condition where the kinetics of this process are altered. However, only very few studies were performed concerning this problem. The conversion rate seems not to be influenced by the secretion of insulin. Insulin secretagogues like cyclic AMP (TANESE *et al.* 1970), tolbutamide (TANESE *et al.*, 1970; SCHATZ *et al.*, 1972), glibenclamide (SCHATZ *et al.*, 1972) and glucose (SCHATZ *et al.*, 1972; STEINER *et al.*, 1972), do not change the conversion rate of proinsulin.

The exact localization of the conversion process within the β-cell is not known. All indirect data accumulated support the idea that the conversion starts in the Golgi complex and continues in the secretory granules. Methodological difficulties did not allow the direct localization in isolated pure subcellular fractions of islets of Langerhans.

The observations on the secretion of proinsulin, C-peptide and insulin *in vivo* and *in vitro* are consistent with the idea that small amounts of proinsulin which escaped conversion, intermediate fractions and the final conversion products insulin and C-peptide are packaged together in the secretory granules and released from the β-cell by emiocytosis. However, much more detailed studies are necessary to understand the qualitative and quantitative aspects of secretion of these compounds. Very little is known about the intracellular fate of the secretory granules from the time of their formation from the Golgi complex to the emiocytosis. It is not known if the granules need to reach a certain state of maturaty before they can secrete their content. Thus it is still not clear whether there exists a preferential release of newly synthesized material deriving from "younger" granules under certain conditions of stimulation of insulin secretion. The data in the literature on this question are controversial. Even a non-granule route of insulin secretion can not be totally ruled out thus far.

The immunological determination of PLC in blood in the presence of insulin remains an interesting field of study. The detailed characterization of PLC especially of the intermediate forms in the circulation under pathological and physiological conditions needs much further work.

The physiological significance of the relatively high fasting levels of proinsulin in the circulation is unknown. Proinsulin is biologically less active than insulin in most test systems. On the basis of the available information the prohormone has intrinsic activity and does not require conversion to insulin. However, its biological function *in vivo* needs to be evaluated further especially in the liver and fat tissue. Proinsulin might be responsible for basal insulin-like anabolism in the post absorptive state.

It was hoped that the detailed knowledge of the mechanism involved in insulin biosynthesis might help to find defects in the insulin production as pathogenetic factor of diabetes mellitus. A tempting idea for the pathogenesis of diabetes mellitus would be a genetic defect of the converting enzyme of proinsulin leading to abnormal, biologically less potent conversion products. If there exists such an abnormal product is not known. Some studies indicate the occurence of a biologically less active insulin in diabetics (ELLIOT *et al.*, 1965; O'BRIEN *et al.*, 1967; ROY *et al.*, 1968). In a more recent study the data supported the idea that the observed abnormal insulin might be identical with proinsulin (ELLIOT, 1969). The same group of investigators, however, demonstrated an abnormal insulin in human pancreas which has other characteristics than proinsulin (ROY *et al.*, (1971). On the other hand KIMMEL and POLLAK (1967) found no evidence for abnormal insulin components in diabetic patients.

It was also not possible to demonstrate an defect in the conversion rate in diabetic patients resulting in the preferential release of the normal biologically less active proinsulin. The PLC levels of diabetic patients are not elevated. Thus a defect in the biosynthesis of insulin seems not to be responsible for the diabetic state. Abnormal PLC levels are well documented in many cases of islet cell adenomas and carcinomas and can be helpfull for the diagnosis of these tumors. Elevated PLC levels are reported also in several other disorders such as different states of hypokalemia. Intermediate fractions were found in obese people and not in normals, but only few cases are studied. Complete elucidation of the role of PLC in various diseases must await investigations of larger numbers of patients. New and easier techniques for the determination of PLC in blood need to be developed for this purpose.

Nothing is known about the role of the C-peptide in the circulation. This peptide has no biological activity in all test systems studied. But thus far the peptide was tested only for insulin-like activity. As the C-peptide is secreted with insulin in equimolar amounts one function might be the feedback regulation of insulin secretion.

Our information on the peripheral degradation of both proinsulin and C-peptide is very limited. At least in the rat no single organ exhibits any special ability to degrade the prohormone.

Finally the teleological question why the precursor exists is only partly answered. As we have seen the correct folding of the disulfide bonds in the insulin molecule can not fully explain the existence of proinsulin since other prohormones were found in the meantime, which do not contain disulfide bonds. Much more work needs to be done to understand this new important principle of precursor formation in the biosynthesis of protein hormones.

References

(Concluded May 1973)

BAUER, G.E., LINDALL, A.W., DIXIT, P.K., LESTER, G., LAZAROW, A.: Studies on insulin biosynthesis — subcellular distribution of leucine-H^3 radioactivity during incubation of goosefish islet tissue. J. Cell Biol. **28**, 413—429 (1966)

BELLAMY, G., BORNSTEIN, P.: Evidence for procollagen, a biosynthetic precursor of collagen. Proc. nat. Acad. Sci. (Wash.) **68**, 1136—1142 (1971)

BERSON, S.A., YALOW, R.S.: Immunoassay of plasma insulin. Ciba Foundation Colloquia on Endocrinology, vol. 14, pp. 182—211, immunoassay of hormones. Ed. by G.E.W. WOLSTENHOLME. M.P. CAMERON, Boston: Little, Brown & Comp. 1962

BLACKARD, W.G., GARCIA, A.R., BROWN, C.L.: Effect of streptocotozin on qualitative aspects of plasma insulin in a patient with a malignant islet cell tumor. J. clin. Endocr. **31**, 215—219 (1970)

BLOCK, M., MAKO, M.E., STEINER, D.F., RUBENSTEIN, A.H.: Circulating C-peptide immunoreactivity. Studies in normals and diabetic patients. Diabetes **21**, 1013—1026 (1972)

BODER, G.B., ROOT, M.A., CHANCE, R.E., JOHSON, J.S.: Extended production of insulin by isolated rabbit pancreatic islets: Evidence for biosynthesis of insulin. Proc. Soc. exp. Biol. (N.Y.) **131**, 507—513 (1969)

BRUSH, J.T.: Purification and characterization of a protease with specificity for insulin from rat muscle. Diabetes **20**, 140—145 (1971)

BURGHEN, G.A., KITABCHI, A.E., BRUSH, J.S.: Purification and properties of a rat liver protease with specificity for insulin. Endocrinology **91**, 633—642 (1972)

BURR, J.M., STAUFFACHER, W., BALANT, L., RENOLD, A.E., GRODSKY, G.: Dynamic aspects of proinsulin release from perfused rat pancreas. Lancet **1969 II**, 882—883

CERASI, E., LUFT, R.: The plasma insulin response to glucose infusion in healthy subjects and in diabetes mellitus. Acta endocr. (Kbh.) **55**, 278—345 (1967)

CHALLONER, D.R.: Degradation of porcine insulin and proinsulin by rat adipose tissue. Diabetes **20**, 276—281 (1971)

CHALLONER, D.R., YU, P.: Differential effect of porcine proinsulin on rat epidydimal fat cells and fat pieces. Diabetes **19**, 289—295 (1970)

CHANCE, R.E.: Characterization of porcine proinsulin. In: Recent progress in hormone research. Ed. by E.B. ASTWOOD, vol. 25, pp. 272—278. New York: Academic Press 1969

CHANCE, R.E.: Chemical, physical, biological and immunological studies on porcine proinsulin and related polypeptides. In: Proceedings of the Seventh Congress of the International Diabetes Federation, Buenos Aires. Excerpta Med. **119**, 292—305 (1971)

CHANCE, R.E., ELLIS, R.M., BROMER, W.W.: Porcine proinsulin: characterization and amino acid sequence. Science **161**, 165—167 (1968)

CHRÉTIEN, M., LI, C.H.: Isolation, purification and characterization of γ-lipotropic hormone from sheep pituitary glands. Canad. J. Biochem. **45**, 1163—1174 (1967)

CHURCH, R.L., PFEIFFER, S.E., TANGER, M.L.: Collagen biosynthesis: synthesis and secretion of a high molecular weight collagen precursor (procollagen). Proc. nat. Acad. Sci. (Wash.) **68**, 2638—2642 (1971)

CLARK, J.L.: Studies on rat proinsulin and insulin. (Ph. D. Dissertation). Chicago, Ill.: Univ. of Chicago 1969

CLARK, J.L., CHO, S., RUBENSTEIN, A.H., STEINER, D.F.: Isolation of a proinsulin connecting peptide fragment (C-peptide) from bovine and human pancreas. Biochem. biophys. Res. Commun. **35**, 456—461 (1969)

CLARK, J.L., STEINER, D.F.: Insulin biosynthesis in the rat: demonstration of two proinsulins. Proc. nat. Acad. Sci. (Wash.) **62**, 278—285 (1969)

COFFEY, J.W., DE DUVE, C.: Digestive activity of lysosomes. I. The digestion of proteins by extracts of rat liver lysosomes. J. biol. Chem. **243**, 3255—3263 (1968)

COHN, D.V., MACGREGOR, R.R., CHU, L.L., KIMMEL, J.R., HAMILTON, J.W.: Calcemic fraction-A: Biosynthetic peptide precursor of parathyroid hormone. Proc. nat. Acad. Sci. (Wash.) **69**, 1521—1525 (1972)

CONSTAN, L.L., MAKO, M., RUBENSTEIN, A.H., STEINER, D.F.: Urinary Proinsulin. Diabetes **19**, 359—360 (1970)

COORE, H.G., HELLMAN, B., PIHL, E., TÄLJEDAL, I.-B.: Physicochemical characteristics of insulin secretion granules. Biochem. J. **111**, 107—116 (1969)

CREUTZFELDT, W., CREUTZFELDT, H., FRERICHS, H., PERINGS, E., SICKINGER, K.: The morphological substrate of the inhibition of insulin secretion by diazoxide. Horm. Metab. Res. **1**, 53—64 (1969)

CUATRECASAS, P.: Properties of the insulin receptor of isolated fat cell membranes. J. biol. Chem. **246**, 7265—7274 (1917)

CUATRECASAS, P.: Isolation of the insulin receptor of liver and fat cell membranes. Proc. nat. Acad. Sci. (Wash.) **69**, 318—322 (1972)

DAVOREN, P.R.: The isolation of insulin from a single rat pancreas. Biochem. biophys. Acta (Amst.) **63**, 150—153 (1962)

DE DUVE, C.: The lysosome in retrospect. In: Lysosomes in biology and pathology, vol. 1, pp. 3—40. Ed. by J.T. DINGLE, H.B. FELL. London: North Holland 1969

DUCKWORTH, W.C., KITABCHI, A.E.: Hyperproinsulinemia in hypoglycemic subjects. Horm. Metab. Res. **4**, 133—135 (1972)

ELLIOT, R.B.: "Abnormal" insulin, "proinsulin" and "big insulin" in diabetes. Lancet **1969 II**, 1076—1077

ELLIOT, R.B., O'BRIEN, D., ROY, C.: An abnormal insulin in juvenile diabetes mellitus. Diabetes **14**, 780—787 (1965)

EPSTEIN, C.J., GOLDBERGER, R.F., ANFINSEN, C.B.: The genetic control of tertiary protein structure. Studies with model systems. Cold Spr. Harb. Symp. quant. Biol. **28**, 439—446 (1963)

FAJANS, S.S., SCHNEIDER, J.M., SCHTEINGART, D.E., CONN, J.D.: The diagnostic value of sodium talbutamide in hypoglycemic states. J. clin. Endocr. **21**, 371—386 (1961)

FAULHABER, J.D., MÜLLER, E., DITSCHUNEIT, H.: Effect of proinsulin on human adipose tissue slices. Israel J. med. Sci. **8**, 754—755 (1972)

FINEBERG, S.E., MERIMEE, T.J.: Proinsulin: metabolic effects in the human forearm. Science **167**, 998—999 (1970)

FRANK, B.H., VEROS, A.J.: Physical studies on proinsulin-association behavior and conformation in solution. Biochem. biophys. Res. Commun. **32**, 155—160 (1968)

FRANK, B.H., VEROS, A.J.: Interaction of zinc with proinsulin. Biochem. biophys. Res. Commun. **38**, 284—289 (1970)

FREYCHET, P., ROTH, J., NEVILLE, D.M.: Insulin receptors in the liver: specific binding of [125 J] insulin to the plasma membrane and its relation to insulin bioactivity. Proc. nat. Acad. Sci. (Wash.) **68**, 1833—1837 (1971)

FULLTERTON, W.W., POTTER, R., LOW, B.W.: Proinsulin: crystallization and preliminary X-ray diffraction studies. Proc. nat. Acad. Sci. (Wash.) **66**, 1213—1219 (1970)

GALLOWAY, J.A., ROOT, M.A., CHANCE, R.E., RATHMACHER, R.P., CHALLONER, D.R., SHAW, W.N.: In vivo studies of hypoglycemic activity of porcine proinsulin. Diabetes **18**, S. 1, 341 (1969)

GAVIN, J.R., ROTH, J., JEN, P., FREYCHET, P.: Insulin receptors in human circulating cells and fibroblasts. Proc. nat. Acad. Sci. (Wash.) **69**, 747—751 (1972)

GLIEMANN, J., SORENSEN, H.H.: Assay of insulin-like activity by the isolated fat cell method. IV. The biological activity of proinsulin. Diabetologia **6**, 499—504 (1970)

GOLDSMITH, S.J., YALOW, R.S., BERSON, S.A.: Significance of human plasma insulin sephadex fractions. Diabetes **18**, 834—839 (1969)

GORDEN, P., ROTH, J.: Circulating insulins: "big" and "little". Arch. intern. Med. **123**, 237—247 (1969)

GORDEN, P., ROTH, J.: Plasma insulin: fluctuations in the "big" insulin component in man after glucose and other stimuli. J. clin. Invest. **48**, 2225—2234 (1969)

GORDEN, P., SHERMAN, B., ROTH, J.: "Big" insulin (circulating proinsulin-like components): a high proportion of the basal insulin. Diabetes **19**, S. 1, 360 (1970)

GORDEN, P., SHERMAN, M., ROTH, J.: Proinsulin-like component of circulating insulin in the basal state and in patients and hamsters with islet cell tumors. J. clin. Invest. **50**, 2113—2122 (1971 a)

GORDEN, P., FREYCHET, P., NANKIN, H.: A unique form of circulating insulin in human islet cell carcinoma. J. clin. Endocr. **33**, 983—987 (1971 b)

GORDEN, P., SHERMAN, B.M., SIMOPOULOS, A.P.: Glucose intolerance with hypokalemia: an increased proportion of circulating proinsulin-like component. J. clin. Endocr. **34**, 235—240 (1972)

GRANT, P.T.: The conversion of proinsulin into insulin in the β-cells of mammals and fishes. Biochem. J. **125**, 49—50 (1971)

GRANT, P.T., REID, K.B.M.: Biosynthesis of an insulin precursor by islet tissue of cod (Gadus callarias). Biochem. J. **110**, 281—288 (1968)

GRANT, P.T., REID, K.B.M., COOMBS, T.L., YOUNGSON, A., THOMAS, N.W.: Distribution and radioactivity of acid-ethanol soluble protein, proinsulin and insulin in subcellular fractions from islet tissue of the cod (Gadus callarias). In: Structure and metabolism of the pancreatic islets, pp. 349—361. Ed. by S. FALKMER, B. HELLMAN, J.B. TÄLJEDAL. Oxford: Pergamon Press 1970

GRANT, P.T., COOMBS, T.L.: Proinsulin, a biosynthetic precursor of insulin. In: Essays in biochemistry, vol. 6, pp. 69—92. Ed. by P.N. CAMPBELL, F. DICKENS. London-New York: Academic Press 1970

GRANT, P.T., COOMBS, T.L., THOMAS, N.W., SARGENT, J.R.: The conversion of [14C] proinsulin to insulin in isolated sub-cellular fractions of fish islet preparations. In: Subcellular organization and function in endocrine tissues, vol. 19, pp. 481—495. Ed. by H. HELLER, K. LEDERIS, Memoirs Soc., Endocrinol., Cambridge: Univ. Press 1971

GREGORY, R.A., TRACY, H.J.: Isolation of two "big gastrins" from Zollinger-Ellison tumor tissue. Lancet **1972 II**, 797—799

GRODSKY, G.M., LONDAHL, H., CURRY, D., BENNETT, L.: In vitro studies suggesting a two-compartmental model for insulin secretion. In: Structure and metabolism of the pancreatic islets, pp. 409—420. Ed. by S. FALKMER, B. HELLMAN, J.B. TÄLJEDAL. Oxford: Pergamon Press 1970

GUTMAN, R.A., LAZARUS, N.R., PENHOS, J.C., RECANT, L., FAJANS, S.S.: Proinsulin (PI) and proinsulin-like material (PI-L-M) in serum of patients with islet cell tumors. Diabetes **19**, S. 1, 360 (1970)

GUTMAN, R.A., LAZARUS, N.R., PENHOS, J.C., FAJANS, S.S., RECANT, L.: Circulating proinsulin-like material in patients with functioning insulinomas. New. Engl. J. Med. **284**, 1003—1008 (1971)

GUTMAN, R.A., LAZARUS, N.R., RECANT, L.: Electrophoretic characterization of circulating human proinsulin and insulin. Diabetologia **8**, 136—140 (1972)

HABENER, J.F., KEMPER, B., POTTS, J.T., Jr., RICH, A.: Bovine proparathyroid hormone: structural analysis of radioactive peptides formed by limited cleavage. Endocrinology **92**, 219—226 (1973)

HAMILTON, J.W., MAC GREGOR, R.R., CHU, L.L., COHN, D.V.: The isolation and partial purification of a non-parathyroid hormone calcemic fraction from bovine parathyroid glands. Endocrinology **89**, 1440—1447 (1971)

HARTCROFT, W.S., WRENSHALL, G.A.: Correlation of beta cell granulation with extractable insulin on the pancreas. Diabetes **4**, 1—7 (1955)

HINZ, M., KATSILAMBROS, N., PFEIFFER, E.F.: Determination of insulin and proinsulin after separation by continuous flow elution from polyacrylamide electrophoresis. Horm. Metab. Res. **2**, 123—124 (1970)

HOWELL, S.L., TAYLOR, K.W.: The secretion of newly synthesized insulin in vitro. Biochem. J. **102**, 922—927 (1967)

HOWELL, S.L., KOSTIANOVSKY, M., LACY, P.E.: Beta granule formation in isolated islets of Langerhans: a study by electron microscopic radioautography. J. Cell Biol. **42**, 695—705 (1969)

HOWELL, S.L., FINK, C.J., LACY, P.E.: Isolation and properties of secretory granules from rat islets of Langerhans. I. Isolation of a secretory granule fraction. J. Cell Biol. **41**, 154—161 (1969)

HOWELL, S.L.: Role of ATP in the intracellular translocation of proinsulin and insulin in the rat pancreatic B-cell. Nature (Lond.) **235**, 85—86 (1972)

HUMBEL, R.E., BOSSARD, H.R., ZAHN, H.: Chemistry of insulin. In: Handbook of physiology, the endocrine pancreas, pp. 111—132. Ed. by D.F. STEINER, N. FREINKEL. Baltimore: Williams and Wilkins 1972

IZZO, J.L., BARTLETT, J.W., RONCONE, A., IZZO, M.J., BALE, W.F.: Physiological processes and dynamics in the disposition of small and large doses of biologically active and inactive ^{131}J-insulin in the rat. J. biol. Chem. **242**, 2342—2355 (1967)

JACOBSON, M.F., BALTIMORE, D.: Morphogenesis of poliovirus. I. Association of the viral RNA with coat protein. J. molec. Biol. **33**, 369—378 (1968)

JAMIESON, J.D., PALADE, G.E.: Intracellular transport of secretory proteins in the pancreatic exocrine cell. I. Role of the peripheral elements of the Golgi complex. J. Cell Biol. **34**, 577—596 (1967a)

JAMIESON, J.D., PALADE, G.E.: Intracellular transport of secretory proteins in the pancreatic exocrine cell. Transport to condensing vacuoles and zymogen granules. J. Cell Biol. **34**, 597—615 (1967b)

JAMIESON, J.D., PALADE, G.E.: Intracellular transport of secretory proteins in the pancreatic exocrine cell. 3. Dissociation of intracellular transport from protein synthesis. J. Cell Biol. **39**, 580—588 (1968a)

JAMIESON, J.D., PALADE, G.E.: Intracellular transport of secretory proteins in the pancreatic exocrine cell. 4. Metabolic requirements. J. Cell Biol. **39**, 589—603 (1968b)

JAMIESON, J.D., PALADE, G.E.: Condensing vacuole conversion and zymogen granule discharge in pancreatic exocrine cells. metabolic studies. J. Cell Biol. **48**, 503—522 (1971)

KEMMLER, W., STEINER, D.F.: Conversion of proinsulin to insulin in a subcellular fraction of rat islets. Biochem. biophys. Res. Commun. **41**, 1223—1229 (1970)

KEMMLER, W., PETERSON, J.D., RUBENSTEIN, A.H., STEINER, D.F.: On the biosynthesis, intracellular transport and mechanism of conversion of proinsulin to insulin and C-peptide. Diabetes **21**, S. 2, 572—581 (1971a)

KEMMLER, W., CLARK, J.L., BORG, J., STEINER, D.F.: On the nature and subcellular localization of the proinsulin converting enzymes (Abstract). Fed. Proc. **30**, 1210, part II (1971b)

KEMMLER, W., PETERSON, J.D., STEINER, D.F.: Studies on the conversion of proinsulin to insulin. I. Conversion in vitro with trypsin and carboxypeptidase-B. J. biol. Chem. **246**, 6786—6791 (1971c)

KEMMLER, W., STEINER, D.F., BORG, J.: Studies on the conversion of proinsulin to insulin. III. Studies in vitro with a crude secretion granule fraction isolated from rat islets of Langerhans. J. biol. Chem. **248**, 4544—4551 (1973)

KEMPER, B., HABENER, J.F., POTTS, J.T., RICH, A.: Proparathyroid hormone: identification of a biosynthetic precursor to parathyroid hormone. Proc. nat. Acad. Sci. (Wash.) **69**, 643—647 (1972)

KIEHN, E.D., HOLLAND, J.J.: Synthesis and cleavage of enterovirus polypeptides in mammalian cells. J. Virol. **5**, 358—367 (1970)

KIMMEL, J.R., POLLACK, H.G.: Studies of human insulin from non-diabetic and diabetic pancreas. Diabetes **16**, 687—694 (1967)

KITABCHI, A.E.: The biological and immunological properties of pork and beef insulin, proinsulin and connecting peptides. J. clin. Invest. **49**, 979—987 (1970)

KITABCHI, A.E., DUCKWORTH, W.C., BRUSH, J.S.: Direct measurement of proinsulin in human plasma by the use of an insulin-degrading enzyme. J. clin. Invest. **50**, 1792—1799 (1971)

KITABCHI, A.E., DUCKWORTH, W.C., Benson, B.: In vivo effects of insulin and proinsulin on diaphragm and epidydimal fat pads in rats. Diabetes **21**, 935—938 (1972a)

KITABCHI, A.E., DUCKWORTH, W.C., STENTZ, F.B., YU, S.: Properties of proinsulin and related polypeptides. CRC Critical Reviews in Biochemistry, pp. 59—94 (1972b)

KITABCHI, A.E., STENTZ, F.B.: Degradation of insulin and proinsulin by various organ homogenates of rat. Diabetes **21**, 1091—1101 (1972)

KO, A.S.C., SMYTH, D.G., MARKUSSEN, J., SUNDBY, F.: The amino acid sequence of the C-peptide of human proinsulin. Europ. J. Biochem. **20**, 190—199 (1971)

KONSEK, J.P., RUBENSTEIN, A.H., EHRLICH, E.N.: Biological action of proinsulin on ventral toad skin in vitro. Endocrinology **89**, 847—851 (1971)

LAEMMLI, U.K.: Cleavage of structural proteins during the assembly of the head of bacteriophage T4. Nature (Lond.) **227**, 680—685 (1970)

LAPIÈRE, C.M., LENAERS, A., KOHN, L.D.: Procollagen peptidase: An enzyme excising the coordination peptides of procollagen. Proc. nat. Acad. Sci. (Wash.) **68**, 3054—3058 (1971)

LAVIS, V.R., ENSINCK, J.W., WILLIAMS, R.H.: Effect of insulin and proinsulin on isolated fat cells and hemidiaphragms from rats. Endocrinology **87**, 135—142 (1970)

LAZARUS, N.R., TANESE, T., GUTMAN, R.A., RECANT, L.: Synthesis and release of proinsulin and insulin by human insulinoma tissue. J. clin. Endocr. **30**, 372—381 (1970a)

LAZARUS, N.R., PENHOS, J.C., TANESE, T., MICHAELS, L., GUTMAN, R.A., RECANT, L.: Studies on the biological activity of porcine proinsulin. J. clin. Invest. **49**, 487—496 (1970b)

LAZARUS, N.R., GUTMAN, R.A., RECANT, L.: A method for electrophoretic characterization on polyacrylamide gels of circulating insulin immunoreactive substances. Analyt. Biochem. **40**, 241—246 (1971)

LAZARUS, N.R., GUTMAN, R.A., PENHOS, J.C., RECANT, L.: Biologically active circulating proinsulin-like materials from islet cell carcinoma patient. Diabetologia **8**, 131—135 (1972)

LOCKWOOD, D.H., MISBIN, R.J.: Proinsulin content of adult and fetal pancreatic tissue extracted after rapid freezing in situ. Horm. Metab. Res. **4**, 232—234 (1972)

MARKUSSEN, J., SUNDBY, F.: Rat-proinsulin C-peptides. Europ. J. Biochem. **25**, 153—162 (1972)

MASHITER, K., KING, T.M.: Changes of immunoreactivity of proinsulin induced by rat tissue extracts. Nature (Lond.) **224**, 696—697 (1969)

MCSHAN, W.H., HARTLEY, M.W.: Production, storage and release of anterior pituitary hormones. Ergebn. Physiol. **56**, 246—296 (1965)

MELANI, F., RUBENSTEIN, A.H., OYER, P.E., STEINER, D.F.: Identification of proinsulin and C-peptide in human serum by a specific immunoassay. Proc. nat. Acad. Sci. (Wash.) **67**, 148—155 (1970a)

MELANI, F., RYAN, W.D., RUBENSTEIN, A.M., STEINER, D.F.: Proinsulin secretion by a pancreatic beta-cell adenoma. Proinsulin and C-peptide secretion. New Engl. J. Med. **282**, 713—719 (1970b)

MELANI, F., RUBENSTEIN, A.H., STEINER, D.F.: Human serum proinsulin. J. clin. Invest. **49**, 497—507 (1970c)

MELANI, F., RUBENSTEIN, A.H., OYER, P.E., STEINER, D.F.: Identification of proinsulin and C-peptide in human serum by a specific immunoassay. Proc. nat. Acad. Sci. (Wash.) **67**, 148—155 (1970d)

MISUGI, K., HOWELL, S.L., GREIDER, M.H., LACY, P.E., SORENSON, G.D.: The pancreatic beta cell. Demonstration with peroxidase-labelled antibody technique. Arch. Path. **89**, 97—102 (1970)

MORGAN, C.R., LAZAROW, A.: Immunoassay of insulin: Two antibody system. Plasma insulin levels of normal, subdiabetic and diabetic rats. Diabetes **12**, 115—126 (1963)

MUNGER, B.L.: The biology of secretory tumors of the pancreatic islets. In: Handbook of Physiology, Section 7, Endocrinology, vol. 1, Endocrine pancreas, pp. 305—314. Ed. by D.F. STEINER, N. FREINKEL. Baltimore: Williams and Wilkins 1972

NOE, B.D., BAUER, G.E.: Evidence for glucagon biosynthesis involving a protein intermediate in islets of the anglerfish (Lophius americanus). Endocrinology **89**, 642—651 (1971)

NOE, B.D., BAUER, G.E.: Further characterization of a glucagon precursor from anglerfish islet tissue. Proc. Soc. exp. Biol. (N.Y.) **142**, 210—213 (1973)

NOLAN, C., MARGOLIASH, E., PETERSON, J.D., STEINER, D.F.: The structure of bovine proinsulin. J. biol. Chem. **246**, 2780—2796 (1971)

O'Brien, D., Shapcott, D.J., Roy, C.C.: Further studies on an abnormal insulin of diabetes mellitus. Diabetes **16**, 572—575 (1967)

Orci, L., Lambert, A.E., Kanazawa, Y., Amherdt, M., Roullier, C.H., Renold, A.E.: Morphological and biochemical studies of β-cells of fetal rat endocrine pancreas in organ culture. J. Cell. Biol. **50**, 565—582 (1971)

Oyer, P.E., Cho, S., Peterson, J.D., Steiner, D.F.: Studies on human proinsulin. Isolation and amino acid sequence of the human pancreatic C-peptide. J. biol. Chem. **246**, 1375—1386 (1971)

Pearson, M.J., Larkins, R.G., Martin, F.J.R.: "Big" insulin and the treatment of an islet cell carcinoma with streptozotocin. Metabolism **21**, 551—558 (1972)

Penhos, J.C., Voyles, N., Lazarus, N.R., Tanese, T., Gutman, R.A.: Hypoglycemic action of porcine proinsulin in eviscerated functionally hepatectomized rats. Horm. Metab. Res. **2**, 43—44 (1970)

Permutt, M.A., Kipnis, D.M.: Insulin biosynthesis: studies of islet polyribosomes. Proc. nat. Acad. Sci. (Wash.) **69**, 505—509 (1972)

Peterson, J.D., Steiner, D.F.: Determination of the amino acid sequences of the monkey, sheep, and dog proinsulin C-peptide by a semi-micro. Edman degradation procedure. J. biol. Chem. **247**, 4866—4871 (1972)

Poffenbarger, P.L., Chick, W.L., Lavine, R.L., Soeldner, J.S., Flewelling, J.H.: Insulin biosynthesis in experimental herediatary diabetes. Diabetes **20**, 677—685 (1971)

Porte, D., Jr., Pupo, A.A.: Insulin response to glucose; evidence for a two pool system in man. J. clin. Invest. **48**, 2309—2319 (1969)

Puls, W., Kroneberg, G.: Experimentelle Untersuchungen über die blutzuckersenkende Wirkung von Rinderproinsulin. Diabetologia **5**, 325—330 (1969)

Rastogi, G.K., Letarte, J., Fraser, T.R.: Proinsulin content of pancreas in human fetuses of healthy mothers. Lancet **1970 I**, 7—9

Rees, K.O., Madison, L.L.: The effect of proinsulin on hepatic glucose output, arterial glucose and free fatty acid concentrations in dogs. Diabetes **18**, S. 1, 341 (1969)

Roth, J., Gorden, P., Pastan: "Big insulin": a new component of plasma insulin detected by immunoassay. Proc. nat. Acad. Sci. (Wash.) **61**, 138—145 (1968)

Roy, C.C., Shapcott, D.J., O'Brien, D.: The case for an abnormal insulin in diabetes mellitus. Diabetologia **4**, 111—117 (1968)

Roy, C.C., Gotlin, R., Shapcott, D., Montgomery, A., O'Brien, D.: Effects of insulin from normal and diabetic human pancreas on RNA labelling in fibroblast cultures. Diabetes **20**, 10—14 (1971)

Rubenstein, A.H., Cho, S., Steiner, D.F.: Evidence for proinsulin and insulin in urine and serum. Lancet **1968 I**, 1353—1355

Rubenstein, A.H., Melani, F., Pilkis, S., Steiner, D.F.: Proinsulin: secretion, metabolism, immunological and biological properties. Postgrad. Med. **45**, Suppl., 476—481 (1969a)

Rubenstein, A.H., Clark, J.L., Melani, F., Steiner, D.F.: Secretion of proinsulin C-peptide by pancreatic β-cells and its circulation in blood. Nature (Lond.) **224**, 697—699 (1969b)

Rubenstein, A.H., Steiner, D.F., Cho, S., Lawrence, A.M., Kirsteins, L.: Immunological properties of bovine proinsulin and related fractions. Diabetes **18**, 598—605 (1969c)

Rubenstein, A.H., Mako, M., Welbourne, W.P., Melani, F., Steiner, D.F.: Comparative immunology of bovine, porcine, and human proinsulin and C-peptides. Diabetes **19**, 546—553 (1970a)

Rubenstein, A.M., Mako, M., Steiner, D.F., Brown, D., Pullman, T.N.: The venal extraction and excretion of proinsulin (Abstract). J. Lab. clin. Med. **76**, 868—869 (1970b)

Rubenstein, A.H., Steiner, D.F.: Human proinsulin: some considerations in the development of a specific immunoassay. In: Early Diabetes, pp. 159—169. Ed. by R. Camerini-Davalos, R. Levine. New York: Academic Press 1970

Rubenstein, A.H., Block, M.B. Starr, J., Melani, F., Steiner, D.F.: Proinsulin and C-peptide in blood. Diabetes **21**, S. 2, 661—672 (1972a)

Rubenstein, A.H., Pottenger, L.A., Mako, M., Getz, G.S., Steiner, D.F.: The metabolism of proinsulin and insulin by the liver. J. clin. Invest. **51**, 912—921 (1972b)

Rubenstein, A.H., Melani, F., Steiner, D.F.: Circulating proinsulin: immunology, measurement, and biological activity in Handbook of Physiology, Section 7, Endocrinology, vol. 1, pp. 515—528. Ed. by D.F. Steiner, N. Freinkel. Baltimore: Williams and Wilkins 1972c

Rudorff, K.H., Albrecht, G., Staib, W.: Effect of insulin and proinsulin on the metabolism of alanine in the rat liver. Horm. Metab. Res. **2**, 49—50 (1970a)

RUDORFF, K.H., ALBRECHT, G., STAIB, W.: Über den Einfluß von Insulin und Proinsulin auf die Gluconeogenese aus Alanin in der isoliert perfundierten Leber normaler und alloxandiabetischer Ratten. Hoppe-Seylers Z. physiol. Chem. **351**, 975—982 (1970b)

RYAN, W.G., ROBBINS, P.: Thin layer sephadex chromatography of insulin and proinsulin (Abstract). Clin. Res. **17**, 394 (1969)

SACHS, M., FAWCETT, P., TAKABATAKE, Y., PORTANOVA, R.: Biosynthesis and release of vasopressin and neurophysin. Recent Progr. Hormone Res. **25**, 447—484 (1969)

SALOKANGAS, H., SMYTH, D.G., MARKUSSEN, J., SUNDBY, F.: Bovine proinsulin: amino acid sequence of the C-peptide isolated from pancreas. Europ. J. Biochem. **20**, 183—189 (1971)

SAMOLS, E., MARKS, V.: Insulin assay in insulinomas. Brit. med. J. **1963 I**, 507—510

SANDO, H., BORG, J., STEINER, D.F.: Studies on the secretion of newly synthezised proinsulin and insulin from isolated rat islets of Lagerhans. J. clin. Invest. **51**, 1476—1485 (1972)

SCHATZ, M., MAIER, V., HINZ, M., NIERLE, C., PFEIFFER, E.F.: The effect of tolbutamide and glibenclamide on the incorporation of [^{3}H] leucine and on the conversion of proinsulin to insulin in isolated pancreatic islets. FEBS Letters **26**, 237—240 (1972)

SCHMIDT, D.D., ARENS, A.: Proinsulin vom Rind. Isolierung, Eigenschaften und seine Aktivierung durch Trypsin. Hoppe-Seylers Z. physiol. Chem. **349**, 1157—1168 (1968)

SHAW, W.N., CHANCE, R.E.: Effect of porcine proinsulin in vitro on adipose tissue and diaphragm of the normal rat. Diabetes **17**, 735—745 (1968)

SHERMAN, B.M., GORDON, P., ROTH, J., FREYCHET, P.: Circulating insulin: the proinsulin-like properties of "big" insulin in patients without islet cell tumors. J. clin. Invest. **50**, 849—858 (1971)

SHERMAN, B.M., PEK, S., FAJANS, S.S., FLOYD, J.C., CONN, J.W.: Plasma proinsulin in patients with functioning pancreatic islet cell tumors. J. clin. Endocr. **35**, 271—280 (1972)

SMITH, L.F.: Species variation in the amino acid sequence of insulin. Amer. J. Med. **40**, 662—666 (1966)

SMITH, R.E.: Summary of discussion. Diabetes **21**, S. 2, 581—583 (1972)

SMITH, R.E., FARQUHAR, M.G.: Lysosome function in the regulation of the secretory process in cells of the anterior pituitary gland. J. Cell Biol. **31**, 319—347 (1966)

SNELLMAN, D.: Cathepsin B., the lysosomal thiol proteinase of calf liver. Biochem. J. **114**, 673—678 (1969)

SORENSEN, R.L., LINDALL, A.W., LAZAROW, A.: Studies on the isolated goosefish insulin secretion granules. Diabetes **18**, 129—137 (1969)

SORENSEN, R.L., STEFFES, M.W., LINDALL, A.W.: Subcellular localisation of proinsulin and insulin conversion in isolated rat islets. Endocrinology **86**, 88—96 (1970)

SORENSEN, R.L., SHANK, R.D., LINDALL, A.W.: Effect of pH on conversion of proinsulin to insulin by a subcellular fraction of rat islets. P.S.E.B.M. **139**, 652—655 (1972)

STEELE, A.A., BROWN, J.D., STONE, D.B.: Antilypolytic effect of porcine proinsulin. Diabetes **19**, 91—97 (1970)

STEINER, D.F.: Evidence for a precursor in the biosynthesis of insulin. Trans. N.Y. Acad. Sci. Ser. II, **30**, 60—68 (1967)

STEINER, D.F.: Proinsulin and the biosynthesis of insulin. New Engl. J. Med. **280**, 1106—1113 (1969)

STEINER, D.F., CHO, S., OYER, P.E., TERRIS, S., PETERSON, J.D., RUBENSTEIN, A.H.: Isolation and characterization of proinsulin C-peptide from bovine pancreas. J. biol. Chem. **246**, 1365—1374 (1971)

STEINER, D.F., CLARK, J.L.: The spontaneous reoxidation of reduced beef and rat proinsulins. Proc. nat. Acad. Sci. (Wash.) **60**, 622—629 (1968)

STEINER, D.F., CLARK, J.L., NOLAN, C., RUBENSTEIN, A.H., MARGOLIASH, E., ATEN, B., OYER, P.E.: Proinsulin and the biosynthesis of insulin. In: Recent progress in hormone research, vol. 25, pp. 207—282. New York: Academic Press 1969

STEINER, D.F., CLARK, J.L., NOLAN, C., RUBENSTEIN, A.H., MARGOLIASH, E., MELANI, F., OYER, P.E.: The biosynthesis of insulin and some speculations regarding the pathogenesis of human diabetes. In: The pathogenesis of diabetes mellitus. Proceedings of the Thirteens Nobel Symposium, pp. 123—132. Ed. by E. CERASI, R. LUFT. Stockholm: Almqvist & Wiksell 1970

STEINER, D.F., CUNNINGHAM, D., SPIGELMAN, L., Aten, B.: Insulin biosynthesis: evidence for a precursor. Science **157**, 697—700 (1967)

STEINER, D.F., HALLUND, O., RUBENSTEIN, A.H., CHO, S., BAYLISS, C.: Isolation and properties of proinsulin, intermediate forms, and other minor components from crystalline bovine insulin. Diabetes **17**, 725—736 (1968)

STEINER, D.F., KEMMLER, W., CLARK, J.L., OYER, P.E., RUBENSTEIN, A.H.: The biosynthesis of insulin: Handbook of Physiology, Section 7, Endocrinology, vol. 1, pp. 175—198. Endocrine pancreas. Ed. by D.F. STEINER, N. FREINKEL. Baltimore: Williams and Wilkins 1972

Steiner, D.F., Oyer, P.E.: The biosynthesis of insulin and a probable precursor of insulin by a human islet cell adenoma. Proc. nat. Acad. Sci. (Wash.) **57**, 473—480 (1967)

Stoll, R.W., Ensinck, J.W., Williams, R.H.: Immunological and biological activities of the heterogenous components of insulin. Diabetes **18**, 392—396 (1969)

Stoll, R.W., Touber, J.L., Ensinck, J.W., Williams, R.H.: Substances immunologically related to proinsulin or connecting peptide in swine plasma. Horm. Metab. Res. **2**, 153—156 1970a

Stoll, R.W., Touber, J.L., Ensinck, J.W., Williams, R.M.: Proinsulin and connecting peptide in swine plasma. Clin. Res. **18**, 172 (1970b)

Stoll, R.W., Touber, J.L., Menahan, L.H., Williams, R.H.: Clearance of porcine proinsulin and insulin and connecting peptide by isolated rat liver. Proc. Soc. exp. Biol. (N.Y.) **133**, 894—896 (1970c)

Stoll, R.W., Touber, J.L., Winterscheid, L.C., Ensinck, J.W., Williams, R.M.: Hypoglycemic activity and immunological half life of porcine insulin and proinsulin in baboons and swine. Endocrinology **88**, 714—717 (1971)

Sundby, F., Markussen, J.: Rat proinsulins and C-peptides. isolation and amino-acid compositions. Europ. J. Biochem. **25**, 147—152 (1972)

Tager, H.S., Steiner, D.F.: Primary structure of the proinsulin connecting peptides of the rat and the horse. J. biol. Chem. **247**, 7936—7940 (1972)

Tager, H.S., Emdin, O.S., Clark, J.L., Steiner, D.F.: Studies on the conversion of proinsulin to insulin. II. Evidence for a chymotrypsin-like cleavage in the connecting peptide region of insulin precursors in the rat. J. biol. Chem. **248**, 3476—3482 (1973)

Tager, H.S., Steiner, D.F.: Isolation of a glucagon-containing peptide. Primary structure of a possible fragment of proglucagon. Proc. nat. Acad. Sci. (Wash.) **70**, 2321—2325 (1973)

Tanese, T., Lazarus, N.R., Devrim, S., Recant, L.: Synthesis and release of proinsulin and insulin by isolated rat islets of Langerhans. J. clin. Invest. **49**, 1394—1404 (1970)

Tompkins, C.V., Srivastava, M.C., Sönksen, P.H., Nabarro, J.D.N.: A comparative study of the distribution and metabolism of monocomponent human insulin and porcine proinsulin in man. Biochem. J. **125**, 64 (1971)

Toomey, R.E., Shaw, W.N., Reid, L.R., Young, W.K.: Comparative study of the effects of porcine proinsulin and insulin on lipolysis and glucose oxidation in rat adipocytes. Diabetes **19**, 209—216 (1970)

Track, N.S., Kanazawa, Y.: Fetal calf pancreas; its suitability for studies of (pro)insulin biosynthesis. Horm. Metab. Res. **4**, 421—426 (1972)

Trakatellis, A.C., Schwartz, G.P.: Biosynthesis of insulin in anglerfish islets. Nature (Lond.) **225**, 548—549 (1970)

Tung, A.K., Yip, C.C.: The biosynthesis of insulin and proinsulin in fetal bovine pancreas. Diabetologia **4**, 68—70 (1968)

Tung, A.K., Zerega, F.: Biosynthesis of glucagon in isolated pigeon islets. Biochem. biophys. Res. Commun. **45**, 387—395 (1971)

Voytek, P., Gjessing, E.C.: Studies of an anionic trypsinogen and its active enzyme from porcine pancreas. J. biol. Chem. **246**, 508—516 (1971)

Williamson, J.R., Lacy, P.E., Grisham, J.W.: Ultrastructural changes in islets of the rat produced by tolbutamide. Diabetes **10**, 460—469 (1961)

Willms, B., Appels, A., Söling, H., Creutzfeldt, W.: Lack of hypoglycemic effect of bovine proinsulin in eviscerated hepatectomized rats. Horm. Metab. Res. **1**, 199—200 (1969)

Wright, P.H., Makulu, D.R.: Some immunological properties of insulin and proinsulin. Diabetes **18**, S. 1, 339 (1969)

Wright, P.H., Makulu, D.R.: Reactions of proinsulin and its derivatives with antibodies to insulin. Proc. Soc. exp. Biol. (N.Y.) **134**, 1165—1169 (1970)

Yalow, R.S., Berson, S.A.: Size and change distinctions between endogenous human plasma gastrin in peripheral blood and heptadecapeptide gastrin. Gastroenterology **58**, 609—615 (1970)

Yalow, R.S., Berson, S.A.: Characteristics of "big ACTH" in human plasma and pituitary extracts. J. clin. Endocr. **36**, 415—423 (1973)

Yamaji, K., Tada, K., Trakatellis, A.C.: On the biosynthesis of insulin in anglerfish islets. J. biol. Chem. **247**, 4080—4088 (1972)

Yip, C.C., Logothetopoulos, J. A specific anti-proinsulin calf serum. Proc. nat. Acad. Sci. (Wash.) **62**, 415—419 (1969)

Yip, C.C.: A bovine pancreatic enzyme catalyzing the conversion of proinsulin to insulin. Proc. nat. Acad. Sci. (Wash.) **68**, 1312—1315 (1971)

C. Biochemistry and Biophysics of Insulin Secretion

I. Energy Metabolism of the B-Cell

Claes Hellerström and Sven E. Brolin *

With 5 Figures

1. Introduction

It has been well documented that both the biosynthesis and secretion of proteins represent energy-dependent manifestations of cellular activity. Thus, when amino acids are assembled into protein molecules metabolic energy is used for the formation of peptide bonds, and this energy demand may be considerable in cells with high turnover rates of proteins. The secretion process is a complex sequence of intracellular events which commences with the unidirectional transport of the newly formed proteins from the site of synthesis on the polysomes to the Golgi region, where the protein is condensed and packed into secretory granules. The granules are subsequently stored in the cytoplasm, moved towards the plasma membrane and finally discharged across the membrane into the extracellular space. Each of these steps may be regarded as potentially energy-dependent; this has been particularly well demonstrated for the transport step between the endoplasmic reticulum and the Golgi region (Jamieson and Palade, 1968; Howell, 1972). The energy needed for these processes is supplied by hydrolysis of high-energy phosphate bonds such as occur in adenosine triphosphate or phosphocreatine.

Detailed knowledge concerning energy requirements for the various steps in the synthesis and secretion of insulin by the B-cell is still lacking. Nevertheless, a great deal of information is available about both the metabolism and the secretory responses of the B-cell. It is the purpose of this chapter to review current knowledge on the metabolic properties of these cells in mammals and to discuss briefly possible links between energy metabolism and insulin secretion. Since the expansion of this field of research has been so critically dependent on the devel-

* The work of the authors included in this review was supported by the Swedish Medical Research Council, the Swedish Board for Technical Development, the Swedish Diabetes Association, Nordisk Insulinfond, and the US Public Health Service.

The survey of the literature for this review was concluded in December 1972.

opment of new tools and technics, often on a microscale, some attention will be devoted also to methodology.

2. Methodological Problems in the Study of Islet Metabolism

a) Preparation of Islet Samples

The dispersion of the endocrine pancreas into numerous small portions, comprising in all only 1—2% of the pancreatic parenchyma, has seriously hampered metabolic studies of the mammalian B-cell. Attempts were made early to solve the problem by the use of fish islets, since in some species of bony fish these consist of a few macroscopically visible cell aggregates, the Brockmann bodies, located in the mesentery close to the spleen and intestinal wall (LAZAROW *et al.*, 1957; FALKMER, 1961; LAZAROW, 1963; HUMBEL and RENOLD, 1963). This pioneering work provided important information on the metabolic behaviour of islet cells *in vitro* and greatly stimulated interest in further biochemical exploration of islet metabolism. However, the results of the investigations may not have been entirely representative of the mammalian B-cell, since fish islets contain a substantial admixture of non-B-cells (FALKMER, 1961; LAZAROW, 1963) and also because the evolutionary distance between fish and mammals is considerable.

As early as 1911 BENSLEY reported the successful isolation of a few islets from the pancreas of the guinea pig, but it was not until 1962 that it became possible to utilize isolated mammalian islet cells for metabolic research. At this time LACY (1962) and LACY and WILLIAMSON (1962) applied the microtechnics developed by LOWRY (1953) to isolate B-cells from rabbit pancreas for subsequent determination of enzyme activities and insulin content. The samples were dissected from unstained, lyophilized sections of pancreas and had a dry weight in the range 0.02—0.2 μg. The analytical procedures applied to these tissue specimens were sensitive enough to provide accurate information on both the hormone content and the activities of a number of oxidative enzymes. Further refinements of ultramicrotechnics make it now possible to measure also nucleotides and metabolites in islet cells prepared by this technic.

While freeze-dried samples of islets are suitable preparations for studies of enzyme activities or metabolite levels, direct determinations of metabolic rates must be performed with fresh, surviving islet cells. There are now several technics available for isolation of surviving islets, and all are based on either a microdissection procedure or enzymatic digestion. In 1964 HELLERSTRÖM reported a technic for microdissection of fresh islets from the pancreas of rat, mouse, and guinea pig. The fresh pancreas is removed and placed in a chilled physiologic medium and islets are isolated from the surrounding acinar cells with the aid of simple tools such as watchmaker's forceps and hypodermic needles. The entire isolation procedure is performed under rigorous control of medium composition and temperature, and after isolation the islets are handled with the aid of braking pipettes (HOLTER and LINDERSTRÖM-LANG, 1943). It has been shown conclusively that islets isolated with this technic are functionally and metabolically active for hours after isolation (HELLERSTRÖM, 1966, 1967; LERNMARK, 1971). In an alternative technic described by KEEN *et al.* (1965) the exocrine pancreas of rats is rendered atrophic by ligation of the pancreatic duct before islets are removed by microdissection.

Although microdissection is a simple and rapid technic for obtaining viable islets it is rather tedious if a large number is required. In this situation is seems preferable to apply the enzymatic technic first described by MOSKALEWSKI (1965) and subsequently modified in different ways (LACY and KOSTIANOVSKY, 1967;

Howell and Taylor, 1968; Lindall *et al.*, 1969; Ballinger and Lacy, 1972). In all these refinements attention is focused on large-scale isolation of islets and, in the experience of the present authors, more than a thousand islets may be obtained within a reasonable period of time. The technic involves three essential steps: (I) distension of the pancreas by injection of a physiologic medium either via the main pancreatic duct or directly under the pancreatic capsule, (II) digestion of the finely diced gland in a solution of collagenase, and (III) separation of the isolated islets from the remaining pancreatic fragments either individually with pipettes or glass rods or in bulk by density-gradient centrifugation. It is generally agreed that this method provides islets that are well suited for a variety of metabolic studies.

Mammalian pancreatic islets are mainly composed of B-cells, but also A_1- and A_2-cells, endothelium, and fibrocytes are present, and these latter cells may comprise as much as 30—40% of the entire cell population (Hellerström *et al.*, 1964; Lacy and Greider, 1972). The ideal tool for metabolic studies *in vitro* of the B-cell would obviously be a pure suspension of surviving B-cells. Although, at present, technics for large-scale preparation of such cells are not available, there are methods for the isolation of individual B-cells which may be of potential value in this context. Petersson (1966) showed that single islet cells could be prepared by gently squashing of isolated islets. Such cells were subsequently used for estimations of the dry weights of both A_2- and B-cells. This technic has now been developed further so that suspensions of dissociated cells can be prepared after mild enzymatic digestion of islets with trypsin (Petersson *et al.*, unpublished data).

Dispersion of islet cells can also be accomplished by trypsination of whole pancreas. Several investigators have used this approach in order to obtain a mixed islet-acinar cell suspension for subsequent monolayer cell culture (Hilwig *et al.*, 1968; Macchi and Blaustein, 1969; Lambert *et al.*, 1972). In the modification of Lambert *et al.* (1972), separation of fibroblasts from the islet and acinar cells is accomplished by first allowing the fibroblasts to attach themselves to the bottom of the culture dish and subsequently decanting off the still freely suspended epithelial cells into a new culture vial. Further enrichment of endocrine cells occurs during the period of culture because the acinar cells degenerate and disappear. The cultured cells maintain the capacity for replication and survive for up to 8—10 days before overgrowth of fibroblastoid cells seemingly inevitably occurs. Studies of endocrine cell function in such cultures have shown that both glucagon and insulin are released into the medium and that the release mechanisms respond normally to physiologic stimuli (Lambert *et al.*, 1972). This technic would seem to be of great potential value for establishing a pure line of B-cells for long-term culture *in vitro*.

In most studies of cell metabolism the actual metabolic measurements are expressed in relation to the amount of biological material used for the analyses. It may be difficult, however, to obtain reliable values in some cases from studies of isolated pancreatic islets, because these are available generally only in submilligram quantities. Very sensitive microtechnics must therefore be employed, which place great demands on analytical accuracy. Nevertheless, even in face of these difficulties there is now much quantitative information available expressed in different terms, e.g. with reference to islet size, islet-DNA content, or islet dry weight. Some of these reference quantities have been summarized in Table 1. It should be emphasized that reference to well defined quantities, such as for example dry weight or DNA content, is much to be preferred to the often used number of islets.

Table 1. *A summary of published data on volume, weight, and cell number of isolated pancreatic islets in laboratory animals and in man*

Reference quantity	Dimension	Species	Authors
Volume	2 nl/islet	Mouse	ASHCROFT *et al.* (1970)
Dry weight	0.5 μg/islet	Mouse	ASHCROFT *et al.* (1970)
Dry weight	0.67 ± 0.02 μg/islet	Mouse	HEDESKOV *et al.* (1972)
Dry weight	0.2—4 μg/islet	Mouse	HELLERSTRÖM (1964)
Dry weight	3—80 μg/islet	Mouse[a]	HELLERSTRÖM (1964)
Dry weight	0.3—102 μg/islet	Guinea pig	HELLERSTRÖM (1964)
Water content	75%	Mouse[a]	MATSCHINSKY and ELLERMAN (1968)
DNA content	50 ± 0.05 ng/islet	Rat	GREEN and TAYLOR (1972)
DNA content	16.4 ± 1.7 ng/islet	Mouse	HEDESKOV *et al.* (1972)
Protein content	780 ± 70 ng/islet	Rat	GREEN and TAYLOR (1972)
Protein content	540 ± 50 ng/islet	Man	ASHCROFT *et al.* (1971)
Insulin content	56 ± 1.5 ng/islet	Rat	GREEN and TAYLOR (1972)
Insulin content	3764 ± 384 μU/μg[b]	Rat	LACY and WILLIAMSON (1962)
Insulin content	204.3 ± 80.3 ng/μg[c]	Mouse	ANDERSSON and HELLERSTRÖM (1972)
Number of cells	2200/μg[b]	Rat	LACY and WILLIAMSON (1962)
Number of cells	5700/islet	Rat	GREEN and TAYLOR (1972)
Number of cells	5500/μg[b]	Mouse[a]	PETERSSON (1968)
Number of cells	2200/islet	Mouse	HEDESKOV *et al.* (1972)

[a] Obese-hyperglycemic mouse (*obob*)
[b] Value calculated per μg dry islet weight
[c] Value calculated per μg islet protein

b) Microchemical Assay

Since each molecule of an enzyme is able to convert numerous substrate molecules, determinations of enzyme activities in tissue samples require only limited amounts of cells. In biochemical analyses of the minute islet specimens the conversion of pyridine nucleotides can be utilized for assay according to LOWRY and PASSONNEAU (1972) of both dehydrogenase reactions and a number of reactions coupled to these. This means that not only enzymes but also metabolite levels can be determined. Measurements of dehydrogenase activities require addition to the reaction mixture of the relevant nucleotide and substrate, whereas assays of metabolites require addition of enzyme and nucleotide. In each kind of assay the amount of converted nucleotide can be determined by its fluorescence after treatment with strong alkali. This, naturally, must be preceded by destruction of the unconverted part of the added nucleotide.

In assays of metabolite levels in the islet samples the conversion of pyridine nucleotide is limited by the amount of metabolite available. For this reason the converted form may be too small for direct fluorimetric determination. There are at present two means to overcome this complication. One is to apply a chemical amplification by means of enzymatic cycling as described by LOWRY *et al.* (1961) and exemplified in Fig. 1. The other analytical procedure does not require amplification and utilizes bioluminescence developed in reactions between the nucleotides and extracts of fireflies or light-producing bacteria (STREHLER and TOTTER, 1952, 1954; MCELROY and SELIGER, 1963; HASTINGS, 1966). These reactions have recently been employed for microchemical assay in tissue samples, e.g. islets of Langerhans (WETTERMARK *et al.*, 1970; BROLIN *et al.*, 1971). The actual measurements are performed by evaluation of light emission with highly sensitive instruments. The time courses of the light emission in different analyses of islet samples are shown in Fig. 2. The sensitivity is such that metabolites at or below the picomole level can be detected. Hitherto bioluminescence has been employed in islet research for a number of nucleotides, enzymes, and metabolites (ASHCROFT

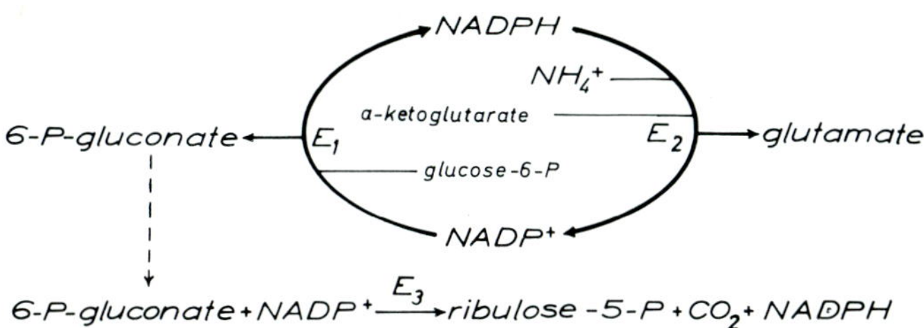

E_1 - glucose-6-P dehydrogenase
E_2 - glutamate dehydrogenase
E_3 - 6-P-gluconate dehydrogenase

Fig. 1. Example of assay by means of enzymatic cycling. The cycling mixture is composed of two dehydrogenases, their substrates in excess together with appropriate additives and the nucleotide to be measured, which in this case may be either NADPH or $NADP^+$. A chemical amplification is obtained by the conversions resulting in accumulation of reaction products as indicated by arrows (left and right). After destruction of the cycling enzymes and NADPH, one of the accumulated products is estimated in a separate dehydrogenase reaction, driven with $NADP^+$ added in excess. NADPH formed in this reaction serves as measurable product

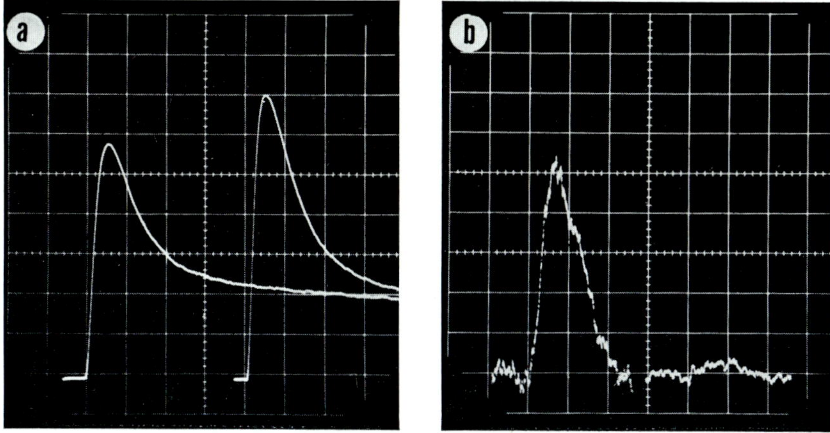

Fig. 2. Oscillograms showing photokinetic analyses of nucleotides in samples of pancreatic islets. The light flash is initiated by fast injection of the sample extract into a reaction mixture in front of a photomultiplier. After passing through a cathode follower the signal from the phototube is displayed on an oscilloscope and photographed. *a*. Assay of ATP in an islet sample of 110 ng, using the firefly luciferin-luciferase system. The left curve represents the sample and the right an ATP standard of 1.8 picomoles. Time scale 2 s per main division. Vertical scale 100 mV per main div. *b*. Assay of NADH after selective enzymatic oxidation of NADPH, using the light emission of luciferase from *Achromobacter fischerii*. The signal is obtained with 0.11 picomoles NADH extracted from an islet sample of 660 ng. Time scale same as in *a*. Vertical scale 50 mV per main div

et al., 1972a; Kilbert *et al.*, 1972; Berne *et al.*, 1973; Borglund, 1973a, b). For example, the light produced from firefly luciferase by ATP has been utilized in analyses not only of ATP itself, but also of ADP and AMP after preceding phosphorylation.

3. Enzymatic Equipment and Nucleotide Levels of the B-Cells

In quantitative enzymatic studies of the islet B-cells the regulation of insulin release by glucose has attracted much attention. Up to now the activity pattern has been recorded for enzymes active in glycolysis and also for a number of enzymes active in other metabolic pathways of the B-cells. A summary of the present knowledge in this field is given below.

a) Phosphorylation of Glucose

The islets possess a higher capacity for phosphorylation of glucose than either the exocrine pancreas or liver (BROLIN *et al.*, 1966). In detailed studies of sugar phosphorylation in mouse islets ASHCROFT and RANDLE (1970) demonstrated two components of hexokinase which differed with regard to their K_m values. The high K_m variety required a glucose concentration above the physiological level to achieve the maximum rate and could therefore, like liver glucokinase, exert a

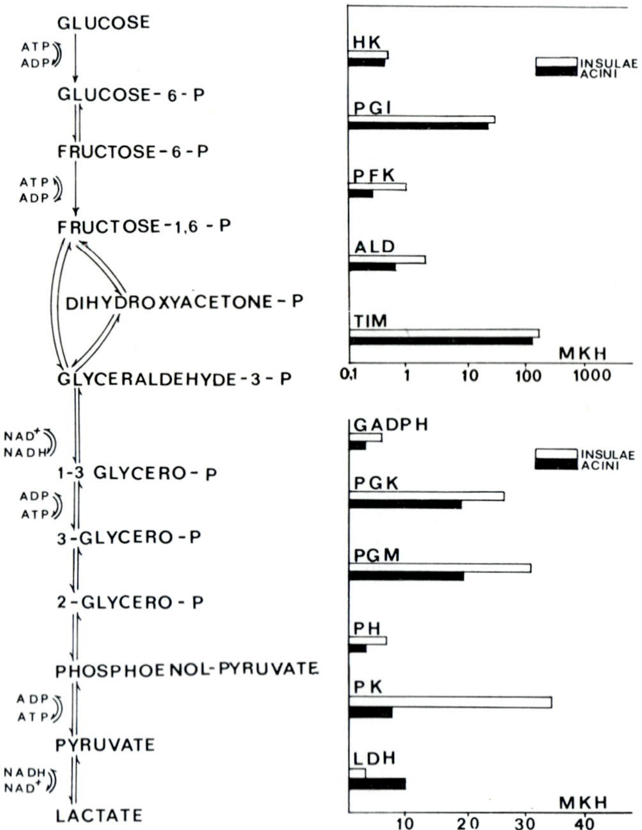

Fig. 3. Enzymatic activities in the glycolytic degradation of glucose. The activity pattern of islets and acini from NZO mice is given as MKH values (moles per kilogram dry weight per hour). Note the logarithmic scale for the initial steps. Abbrevations: HK, hexokinase; PGI, phosphoglucoisomerase; PFK, phosphofructokinase; ALD, aldolase; TIM, triosephosphate isomerase; GAPDH, glyceraldehydephosphate dehydrogenase; PGK, phosphoglycerate kinase; PGM, phosphoglyceromutase; PH, phosphopyruvate hydratase; PK, pyruvate kinase; LDH, lactate dehydrogenase. Data from BROLIN *et al.* (1966), BROLIN and BERNE (1967) and BROLIN *et al.* (1967a)

Table 2. *A summary of some data on metabolic rates of pancreatic islets isolated from the pancreas of mice*

Metabolic parameter	Glucose concentration (mM)	Metabolic rate (μmoles/g dry islet per h)	Reference
Glucose utilization	3.3	37.8[a]	Ashcroft *et al.* (1972c)
Glucose utilization	16.7	162.2[a]	Ashcroft *et al.* (1972c)
Glucose phosphorylation	0.5	57[b, c]	Matschinsky and Ellerman (1968)
Glucose phosphorylation	100	111[b, c]	Matschinsky and Ellerman (1968)
Glucose oxidation	4.5	8	Ashcroft *et al.* (1970)
Glucose oxidation	16.7	44	Ashcroft *et al.* (1970)
Glucose oxidation	3	8.8[b]	Hellman *et al.* (1971d)
Glucose oxidation	20	63.4[b]	Hellman *et al.* (1971d)
Glucose oxidation	3.3	7.8[b, d]	Hellerström and Gunnarsson (1970)
Glucose oxidation	16.7	30.0[b, d]	Hellerström and Gunnarsson (1970)
Lactate production, aerobic	3.3	10[e]	Ashcroft *et al.* (1970)
Lactate production, aerobic	16.7	29[e]	Ashcroft *et al.* (1970)
Lactate production, anaerobic	0	25[e, f]	Hellerström and Gunnarsson (1970)
Lactate production, anaerobic	16.7	60[e, f]	Hellerström and Gunnarsson (1970)
Glucose metabolism via the pentose phosphate shunt	2.8—16.7	3.9	Ashcroft *et al.* (1972)
Islet oxygen uptake	0	254[b, d]	Gunnarsson and Hellerström (1973)
Islet oxygen uptake	16.7	384[b, d]	Gunnarsson and Hellerström (1973)
Islet oxygen uptake	2.5	132[d]	Hedeskov *et al.* (1972)
Islet oxygen uptake	16.7	239[d]	Hedeskov *et al.* (1972)

[a] Recalculated, assuming a dry islet weight of 0.5 μg (Ashcroft *et al.*, 1970)
[b] Obese-hyperglycemic mouse (*obob*)
[c] Freeze-dried islet sections assayed at +22—26° C
[d] Incubation of islets performed in phosphate-buffered medium
[e] Lactate expressed as glucose equivalents
[f] Recalculated as the fraction of $Q_{CO_2}^{N_2}$ which could be inhibited by 1.0 mM iodoacetate

regulatory influence. Matschinsky *et al.* (1971) found, however, only a low K_m islet hexokinase in the rat although in the mouse there were components with different K_m values. The hexokinase reaction is virtually irreversible but significant hydrolysis of glucose-6-phosphate is still possible, since glucose-6-phosphatase has been demonstrated in the islets of several species (Täljedal, 1967, 1969, 1970; Petkov, 1970). The capacity for glucose phosphorylation in mouse islets is given in Table 2 and Fig. 3. It is evident that the phosphorylating capacity as indicated by the hexokinase activity exceeds considerably the value found for total glucose utilization (see below).

b) Glycolysis

Enzymes of the glycolytic pathway have been studied extensively in the islets of the obese and hyperglycemic New Zealand mouse (NZO). As seen in Fig. 3, the islets display higher activities than the pancreatic acini except for lactate dehydrogenase, as has been demonstrated also in the rabbit, rat, and man (Lacy, 1962; Dixit and Lazarow, 1964, 1969; Kissane *et al.*, 1964). As compared to the pancreatic acini the mouse islets are enzymatically well equipped for the glycolytic formation of ATP. In man also, pyruvate kinase shows a much higher activity in the islets (Gepts and Gregoire, 1971). The activity pattern of glycolytic enzymes as given in Fig. 3 indicates that the pancreatic islets are well equipped for glucose degradation. Phosphofructokinase may be of particular importance for the metabolic flow, since it has a relatively low activity and is furthermore subjected to regulatory effects from adenine nucleotides and citrate (Passonneau and Lowry, 1964; Matschinsky *et al.*, 1968a). It is worthy of note that this enzyme operates essentially only in the forward direction; the reverse reaction being catalyzed by hexosediphosphatase. The latter is lacking in the B-cells of the mouse at least, which are therefore not capable of gluconeogenesis, since this requires backward operation in the glycolytic pathway (Brolin *et al.*, 1968).

c) Pentose Phosphate Shunt

The islets seem to be enzymatically well equipped for the oxidation of glucose-6-phosphate and 6-phosphogluconate with $NADP^+$ (Fig. 3). In contrast to NADH, however, NADPH is presumably provided for synthetic processes rather than for ATP production in the respiratory chain (Horecker, 1967). The activities of the shunt have been studied by Matschinsky *et al.* (1968b) in the obese hyperglycemic mouse (Fig. 4). They compared the islets with the exocrine pancreas, but found no significant differences. The supply of triosephosphates from the shunt to the glycolytic pathway may be limited, since transketolase and transaldolase activities are low (Fig. 4). In NZO mice the transaldolase activity of the islets is lower than that of the acini (Brolin *et al.*, 1967b).

d) Citric Acid Cycle and Respiratory Chain

The enzyme pattern of the citric acid cycle has not been completely elucidated so far, but available data suggest a high capacity for energy transfer (Fig. 4), probably higher than that of the exocrine pancreas. With regard to the formation of energy-rich phosphate bonds in the B-cells, information about the respiratory chain would be of interest. The flavoprotein succinate dehydrogenase is closely associated with the respiratory chain and, as evidenced by the marked rise in oxygen consumption of the islets after addition of succinate, this enzyme should have a high activity (Hellerström *et al.*, 1970). A further approach to evaluate the properties of the respiratory chain has been made by differential fluorometric assay of FMN and FAD levels (see below, section).

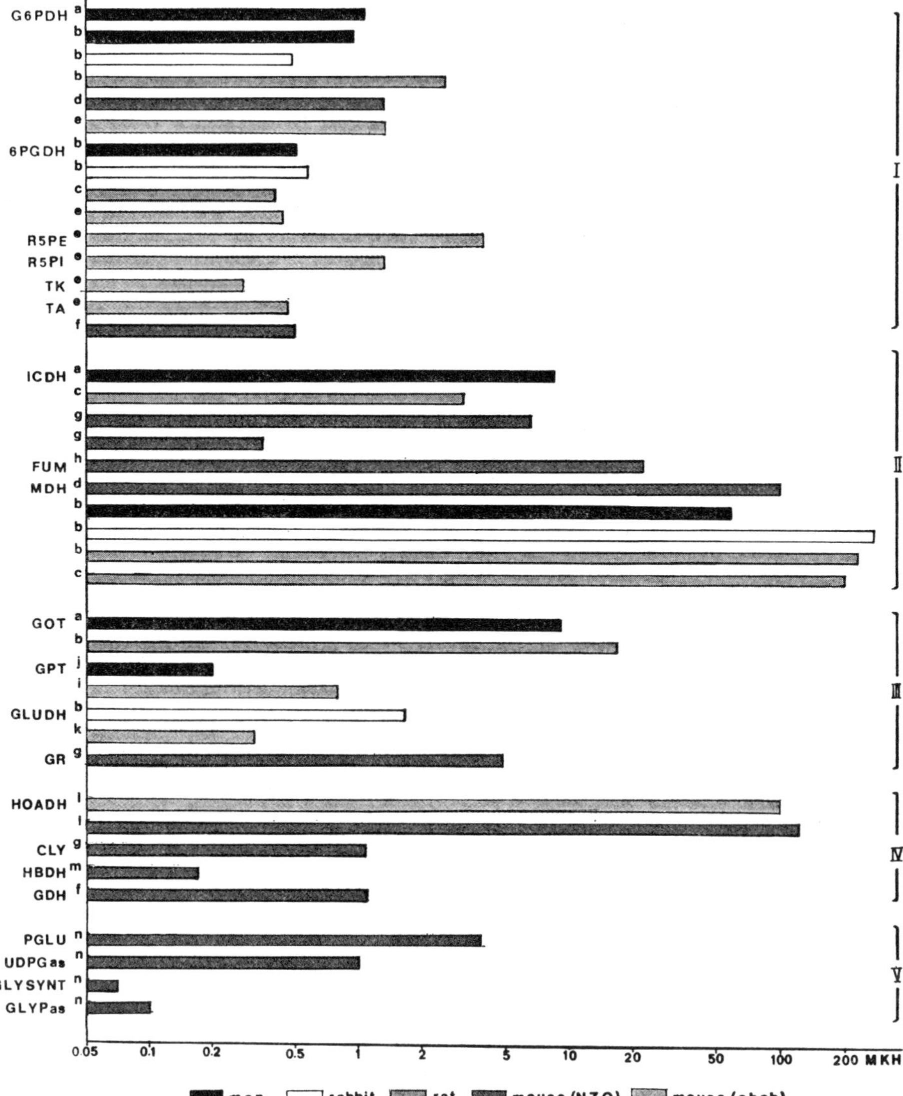

Fig. 4. Patterns of islet enzymes representing (I) the pentose phosphate shunt, (II) part of the citric acid cycle, (III) some reactions in the amino-acid metabolism, (IV) the lipid metabolism, and (V) the formation and degradation of glycogen. The activities are given in a logarithmic scale as MKH values (moles converted substrate per kilogram per hour). For the obese-hyperglycemic mouse (*obob*) the enzyme activities of the shunt were determined at 25°C instead of 38°C (G6PDH and 6PGDH excepted) and are shown doubled in the diagram to facilitate comparisons. Abbrevations: G-6-PDH, glucose-6-phosphate dehydrogenase; 6-PGDH, 6-phosphogluconic dehydrogenase; R-5PI, D-ribose-5-phosphate isomerase; R5PE, ribose-5-phosphate epimerase; TK, transketolase; TA, transaldolase; ICDH, isocitrate dehydrogenase (NAD^+ used as cofactor for the lowest value); FUM, fumarase; MDH, malate dehydrogenase; GOT, glutamic-oxalacetic transaminase; GPT, glutamic-pyruvic transaminase; GLUDH, glutamate dehydrogenase; GR, glutathione reductase; HOADH, 3-hydroxyacyl-CoA dehydrogenase; CLY, citrate lyase; HBDH, 3-hydroxybutyrate dehydrogenase; GDH, glycerol-1-phosphate dehydrogenase; PGLU, phosphoglucomutase; UDPGas, UDPG pyrophosphorylase; GLYSYNT, glycogen synthetase; GLYPas, glycogenphosphorylase. Data from [a]GEPTS *et al.* (1970); [b]KISSANE *et al.* (1964); [c]DIXIT and LAZAROW (1969); [d]BROLIN *et al.* (1964); [e]MATSCHINSKY *et al.* (1968b); [f]BROLIN *et al.* (1967b); [g]BERNE (1971); [h]unpublished material; [i]HELLMAN (1965); [j]GEPTS and GRÉGOIRE (1971); [k]HELLMAN (1967); [l]HAMMAR and BERNE (1970); [m]BERNE (1972); [n]BROLIN and BERNE (1970)

e) Amino Acids

Among the enzymes operating in the utilization of amino acids glutamic-oxalacetic transaminase shows a high activity in the islets, whereas glutamic-pyruvic transaminase displays a considerably lower activity (Fig. 4). There is a comparatively high activity of glutathione reductase, which may be of significance for the $NADP^+$-NADPH turnover.

f) Lipids and Fatty Acids

The islets seem to have a high enzymatic capacity for beta oxidation of fatty acids (Fig. 4). Comparisons have been made between samples of islets, exocrine pancreas, liver, heart, and skeletal muscle from NZO mice; the highest activities of beta-hydroxyacyl-CoA dehydrogenase being found in the islets (HAMMAR and BERNE, 1970). As demonstrated by measurements of the formation of carbon dioxide from labeled acetoacetate and beta-hydroxybutyrate (see below), ketone bodies can also be utilized as fuel by the islets. In agreement with this, the islet cells show some activity of beta-hydroxybutyrate dehydrogenase (Fig. 4). A significantly higher activity of this enzyme is, however, found in renal cortex and heart muscle, both of which are known to possess a great capacity for utilization of these ketone bodies. In cells lacking glycerokinase, formation of triglycerides requires alpha-glycerophosphate dehydrogenase, which has a lower activity in the islets than in the acini (BROLIN and BERNE, 1967). This would indicate that the B-cells use fatty acids for energy production rather than for synthesis of fat.

g) Glycogen Metabolism

Glycogen is normally present in the B-cell and may be abundant in certain diabetic states (PICTET *et al.*, 1967; MATSCHINSKY and ELLERMAN, 1968; HELLMAN and IDAHL, 1970). As evidenced by studies in NZO mice, the islets are enzymatically better equipped for the metabolism of glycogen than the acini, but the activities are low as compared to those of the liver. The activity pattern appears similar to that of other organs with glycogen synthetase and glycogen phosphorylase as rate-limiting enzymes. The values given in Fig. 4 represent measurements at maximum rates, using glucose-6-phosphate as stimulator for the synthetase and AMP for the phosphorylase. The results suggest that a substantial accumulation of glycogen in the B-cells would require stimulation of the synthesis for a

Table 3. *Nucleotide content of the islets in vivo, given as moles per kilogram dry weight*

Nucleotide	Principle of the assay Fluorescence	Photoreaction
NAD^+	0.32[a]*	1.3[b]
NADH	0.18[a]	0.17[c]
$NADP^+$	0.04[a]	
NADPH	0.05[a]	0.08[c]
ATP	11.3[a]; 6.9[d]; 20.9[e] (rat)	11.1[f]; 12.2[f] (NZO); 12.3[g]
ADP		3.4[f]; 4.7[f] (NZO); 2.0[g]
AMP		7.7[g]
FMN	0.02[h]	
FAD	0.14[h]	

Data from [a]MATSCHINSKY and ELLERMAN (1968); [b]BROLIN *et al.* (1971); [c]BERNE *et al.* (1973); [d]HELLMAN *et al.* (1969); [e]KRZANOWSKI *et al.* (1971); [f]WETTERMARK *et al.* (1970); [g]BORGLUND (1973a, b); [h]BROLIN and ÅGREN (unpublished data).

* When not otherwise stated the values refer to the obese-hyperglycemic mouse (*obob*).

considerable length of time. The maximal capacity of glycogen phosphorylase is compatible with available data on the rate of glycogen degradation.

h) The Level of Nucleotides in the B-Cells

In experiments designed to evaluate the energy flux in the B-cell it is important to have some idea of the metabolic control of energy transfer. Although enzyme activity patterns represent condensed information about the prerequisites for metabolic rates, the actual flux is controlled by a number of other factors. Among these the interconversion between nucleotides holds a central position and current information on the *in vivo* levels of various nucleotides in the B-cell is summarized in Table 3. The *in vitro* nucleotide levels have not been included in the Table since they exhibit variations depending on the experimental design. It is of interest that anoxia causes accumulation of NADH but not of NADPH (BERNE *et al.*, 1973). This finding may signify that the latter nucleotide, as in other cells, is utilized for synthetic purposes rather than for oxidative phosphorylation. From energetic aspects there may thus be fundamental differences between the glycolysis with NAD^+ as hydrogen acceptor and the shunt with $NADP^+$ as acceptor. PANTEN *et al.* (1970, 1971, 1972) reported an elegant technic for studies of changes of reduced pyridine nucleotides by continuous recording of fluorescence in microdissected, perifused mouse islets. Stimulation of insulin release by raising the glucose level was accompanied by a markedly increased fluorescence. This reduction of pyridine nucleotides was abolished by D-mannoheptulose, but enhanced by pentobarbital, another inhibitor of insulin release. Neither pyruvate nor glibenclamide altered the fluorescence. The results were interpreted to indicate that a change in the NAD^+/NADH-system of the B-cell is probably not the trigger of insulin release.

The levels of FMN and FAD are high in heart muscle and liver, and significantly lower in the pancreas, where the endocrine part shows slightly higher values than the exocrine. It is, however, conceivable that the amount of flavin groups is not rate-limiting for respiration in either component of the pancreas (BROLIN and ÅGREN, unpublished data).

4. Substrate Utilization and Metabolism in the B-Cell

a) Metabolism of Glucose

In view of the important regulative effects of glucose on insulin release, the glucose metabolism of the B-cell deserves special attention. Extensive reviews on the subject have been published recently (GRODSKY, 1970; RANDLE and HALES, 1972; MATSCHINSKY, 1972; ASHCROFT *et al.*, 1972b), and the following section therefore deals mainly with those aspects of glucose metabolism in the B-cell which are relevant to the energy requirements of this cell.

Cellular control of substrate utilization may be exerted either through transport mechanisms located in the plasma membrane or through intracellular events involving various enzymes. The uptake of D-glucose and other sugars by the B-cell has attracted much interest during recent years, and it is now generally agreed that a glucose transport system with high capacity is present in the B-cell membrane (IDAHL and HELLMAN, 1968; MATSCHINSKY and ELLERMAN, 1968; HELLMAN *et al.*, 1971a; MATSCHINSKY *et al.*, 1971). In fact, this carrier system is so efficient that transmembrane movement of glucose is probably not a rate-limiting step in the glucose utilization of the B-cell. This means that intracellular glucose levels may closely reflect fluctuations in the extracellular glucose concentration and in blood glucose levels. In agreement with this IDAHL and HELLMAN (1968), MATSCHINSKY and ELLERMAN (1968) and MATSCHINSKY *et al.* (1971)

demonstrated a significant correlation between serum glucose levels and intracellular glucose in the islets of both obese-hyperglycemic mice and rats. It is conceivable that close monitoring of blood-glucose fluctuations by the B-cell would serve the purpose of modulating the insulin release. It seems also possible that a pathologic state in the islet capillaries, such as might occur in diabetes mellitus, could easily disturb this process.

The mechanism for sugar uptake in mammalian B-cells has further been elucidated by the careful studies of HELLMAN *et al.* (1971a) using the B-cell-rich, microdissected islets of obese-hyperglycemic mice. It was demonstrated that the *in vitro* uptake of D-glucose was saturable with a maximal rate of about 400 μmoles/h per g dry weight and with a K_m around 50 mM. L-Glucose was virtually excluded from the B-cell indicating stereospecificity of a postulated carrier. Phlorizin at 10 mM blocked the uptake of D-glucose, whereas neither mannoheptulose (20 mM) nor L-glucose (4—40 mM) had any effect. Mannoheptulose itself was also found to be taken up by the B-cells, which was interpreted as further support for the view that inhibition of insulin release by this sugar is exerted by intracellular interference with B-cell metabolism (HELLMAN *et al.*, 1972).

Although early studies with isolated islets indicated that glucose and several other sugars serve as substrates in the metabolism of the B-cells, it was not until recently that total glucose utilization of these cells was evaluated in quantitative terms (SNYDER *et al.*, 1970; ASHCROFT *et al.*, 1972c). At an extracellular glucose concentration of 16.7 mM the maximal rate of utilization in mouse islets was calculated as 89 pmoles/h per islet and in rat islets as 134 pmoles/h per islet. In the mouse the half-maximal rate was achieved at about 7mM glucose. Glucose utilization showed a marked dependence on extracellular glucose concentration, and the rate increased fivefold as the glucose concentration in the medium was raised from 3.3—16.7 mM (ASHCROFT *et al.*, 1972c). It was also noted that the curve relating the glucose-utilization rate to the extracellular glucose concentration was sigmoid and similar in shape to curves describing a number of other glucose-sensitive parameters of the islets, e.g. glucose-oxidation rate and islet-glucose-6-phosphate concentration (ASHCROFT and RANDLE, 1968; LÖFFLER *et al.*, 1969; ASHCROFT *et al.*, 1970), islet 6-phosphogluconate concentration (MONTAGUE and TAYLOR, 1970), insulin release (MALAISSE, 1969; ASHCROFT *et al.*, 1972b), and the frequency of B-cells from which action potentials can be recorded (DEAN and MATTHEWS, 1970a). Altogether these important observations strongly suggest a relationship between insulin release, and the utilization and metabolism of glucose, although the nature of the underlying mechanism remains to be clarified. It is of further interest that glucose utilization in human islets has been measured recently (ASHCROFT *et al.*, 1971). Glucose utilization was increased sixfold by raising extracellular glucose from 3.3—16.7 mM and the absolute values were of the same order of magnitude as those found in mouse islets.

Phosphorylation of glucose in the pancreatic islets has been dealt with in the preceding section on the enzymatic equipment of the B-cell. With respect to further degradation of glucose in the B-cell it seems to be generally agreed that only limited amounts of glucose are metabolized via the pentose phosphate shunt and that this fraction decreases as glucose concentration increases (SNYDER *et al.*, 1970; ASHCROFT *et al.*, 1972c; LANDAU, 1972). Since, moreover, glycogen stores are small (HELLMAN and IDAHL, 1969, 1970; MATSCHINSKY *et al.*, 1971) and the turnover rate of glycogen may be low (JARRETT and KEEN, 1968; MATSCHINSKY *et al.*, 1971; KRZANOWSKI *et al.*, 1971), this suggests that the glycolytic pathway predominates in the glucose utilization of the B-cell. In agreement with this, a high rate of anaerobic glycolysis has been demonstrated in isolated islets of both mice and rats. Thus, in mice HELLERSTRÖM and GUNNARSSON (1970) using the Cartesian diver microgasometer, found a maximal $Q_{CO_2}^{N_2}$ [1] equivalent to an anaerobic glycolysis of 60 μmoles glucose/h per g dry islet weight. In isolated islets of newborn rats the corresponding value was as high as 325 μmoles/h per g with an extracellular glucose concentration of 16.7 mM (ASPLUND and HELLERSTRÖM, 1972). The anaerobic glycolytic rate in 6-day-old rats had decreased to 240 μmoles/h per g. Aerobic lactate formation is considerably lower, suggesting a marked Pasteur effect in the B-cells (ASHCROFT *et al.*, 1970). Nevertheless, at a high glucose level it may account for as much as 30—40% of total glucose utilized by the B-cell.

Oxidation of glucose by the Krebs cycle has been studied in isolated islets of rats and mice, and values for normal and obese-hyperglycemic mice are given in Table 2. Corresponding values for rat islets have been given as 42.5 pmoles/h per islet (LÖFFLER *et al.*, 1969) which would correspond to about 35 μmoles/h per g dry islet weight assuming a dry weight of 1.14 μg/rat islet (recalculated from GREEN and TAYLOR, 1972). The glucose oxidation tends to increase in a sigmoid fashion with increasing glucose concentration with a threshold in mouse islets of approximately 5 mM glucose and a K_m of about 7 mM (ASHCROFT *et al.*, 1970). Recent studies showed that mouse islets maintained in tissue culture at a high glucose level (ANDERSSON and HELLERSTRÖM, 1972) had a considerably decreased K_m-value for both glucose oxidation and insulin release (ANDERSSON, 1972; Fig. 5). Similarly, the insulin response to glucose in isolated islets of pregnant rats is considerably enhanced (GREEN and TAYLOR, 1972). It appears from these data that the glucose metabolism of the B-cell may show adaptive changes in situations with increased functional demands on this cell.

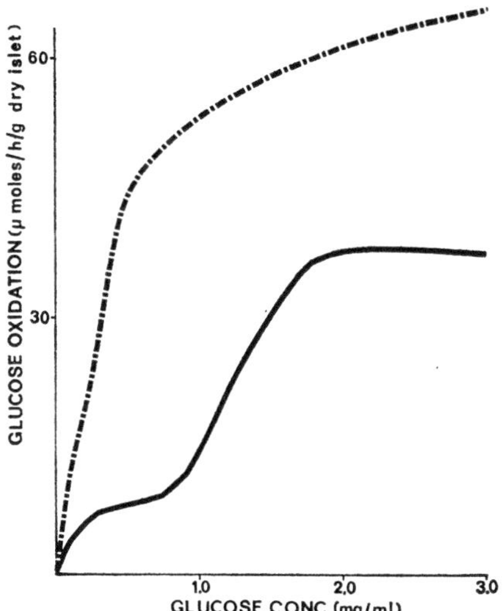

Fig. 5. Effect of glucose concentration on the rate of glucose oxidation in mouse pancreatic islets either isolated directly by collagenase (—) or after subsequent tissue culture for 6 days at a glucose concentration of 5 mg/ml (—.—.—.)

1 $Q_{CO_2}^{N_2}$ denotes liberation of CO_2 from a bicarbonate buffer due to lactic acid production from tissue samples incubated in a gas phase of 95% N_2+5% CO_2.

b) Metabolism of Non-Carbohydrate Substrates

Information on the metabolism of amino acids and fatty acids in the B-cell is so far limited. Considerable interest has, however, been devoted to the uptake and transport of amino acids into the islet cells, since it has been shown that a number of amino acids, including some which are not metabolized, are able to stimulate insulin release (Floyd *et al.*, 1968; Malaisse and Malaisse-Lagae, 1968; Milner, 1969; Edgar *et al.*, 1969; Milner, 1970; Lambert, 1970; Christensen *et al.*, 1971; Lernmark, 1972a, b). In a series of studies Hellman *et al.* (1971b, c) and Sehlin (1972a, b) demonstrated the following amino acid transport systems in the islets: an alanine-preferring system for neutral amino acids (A-system), a leucine-preferring system for neutral amino acids (L-system), a system for cationic amino acids, and a system for dicarboxylic amino acids. It was also found that amino acids transported by the L-system or by the system for cationic amino acids stimulate insulin release, whereas those transported by the A system or the system for dicarboxylic amino acids did not. The nonmetabolizable and synthetic amino acid BCH(2-amino-bicyclo [2,2,1]heptane-2-carboxylic acid) stimulated insulin release and was taken up in a similar way as L-leucine. Briel *et al.* (1972) measured the content of free amino acids in the B-cells of mice and found that most amino acids occurred in greater amounts in the islets than in the exocrine pancreas. Aspartic acid, valine, and leucine were present in tenfold amounts. Like nervous tissue, the islets contained gamma-aminobutyric acid and high levels of taurine.

Oxidation of amino acids in the B-cell was initially studied by Hellerström *et al.* (1969) and Stork *et al.* (1970) who found that leucine stimulates islet respiration and that this amino acid is readily oxidized by the B-cells. Decarboxylation of leucine seemed to be strongly depressed by various sulfonylurea drugs. Hellman *et al.* (1971d) and Sehlin (1972a, b) found that also alanine and glutamic acid may be oxidized by the islets, whereas arginine and glycine appeared to be of minor importance as fuels for the B-cell.

Fatty acids and ketone bodies may stimulate insulin secretion although this property depends to a great extent on the species (Madison *et al.*, 1964; Sanbar and Martin, 1967; Manns *et al.*, 1967; Horino *et al.*, 1968; Montague and Taylor, 1968; Malaisse and Malaisse-Lagae, 1968; Crespin *et al.*, 1969; Jenkins *et al.*, 1970; Balasse *et al.*, 1970). The oxidation of fatty acids by the islets has been measured by Edwards *et al.* (1972) in guinea pigs and by Berne (1972) in mice. The results showed that octanoate is oxidized at a high rate in both these species which is in accord with the high activity of beta-hydroxyacyl-CoA dehydrogenase found previously (Hammar and Berne, 1970). The long-chain fatty acid palmitate seemed to be oxidized at a slower but still significant rate in the B-cells of the mouse and not at all in those of the guinea pig. Also oleate was oxidized by the B-cells of the mouse. Berne (1972) also measured the conversion of beta-hydroxybutyrate and acetoacetate to CO_2 by the B-cell of the mouse. He found that both these compounds are oxidized, although not as fast as glucose at concentrations yielding maximum rates.

5. Energy Metabolism of the B-Cell in Relation to Insulin Biosynthesis and Secretion

In evaluating the energy requirements for the synthesis and secretion of insulin, knowledge of the ATP levels and the ATP turnover of the B-cell is of great importance. Direct measurements of the ATP concentrations in the B-cell have been performed and related to the functional state of the cell. Studies *in vivo* in the rat by KRZANOWSKI *et al.* (1971) suggested that levels of ATP are of the order of 16—20 μmoles/g dry islet weight and remain rather unchanged during stimulation of insulin release with glucose or sulfonylurea. These authors also demonstrated the presence of substantial amounts of phosphocreatine in the islets (about 5 μmoles/g) and, like ATP, this intermediate seemed to be maintained at a fairly constant level irrespective of the functional state of the B-cell (MATSCHINSKY *et al.*, 1971; MATSCHINSKY, 1972; MATSCHINSKY *et al.*, 1972). In the islets of mice, the ATP concentration is about half that in the rat (MATSCHINSKY and ELLERMAN, 1968; HELLMAN *et al.*, 1969; WETTERMARK *et al.*, 1970). In the mouse, ADP levels were also determined (WETTERMARK *et al.*, 1970; BORGLUND, 1973a). They were found to be of the order of 4 μmoles/g dry weight; the ATP/ADP ratio being in the range 3—4. BORGLUND (1973a, b) also measured AMP, which was found to be about 8 μmoles/g in the islets and about 4 μmoles/g in the acini of obese-hyperglycemic mice. The additional finding of marked adenylate kinase activity in the islets may explain why ATP levels are so well maintained in the B-cells *in vivo*.

In vitro studies of ATP levels in isolated islets do not entirely conform to the *in vivo* studies referred to above. Thus, HELLMAN *et al.* (1969) found that the ATP content of microdissected islets of obese-hyperglycemic mice was markedly dependent on the extracellular glucose concentration in so far as absence of glucose in the incubation medium reduced the ATP to about half the level recorded in the presence of at least 1 mg/ml of glucose. Furthermore, it was found that sulfonylureas (carbutamide or glibenclamide) significantly reduced the ATP concentration during incubation periods of 15—45 min. Similar results were recently reported by ASHCROFT *et al.* (1972d), who made the additional observation that islet ATP concentrations were maintained at a normal level *in vitro* by both glucose, mannose, leucine, and glyceraldehyde, whereas galactose, acetate, and octanoate were unable to do so. Altogether these observations suggest that ATP levels in the B-cell are not so precisely maintained *in vitro* as *in vivo*. Other factors such as, for example, differences between species and between the concentrations of glucose and sulfonylurea should, however, also be considered when the *in vivo* and *in vitro* experiments are compared.

Measurements of ATP levels in the B-cell do not by themselves provide information about the total ATP production in these cells. Such data can be calculated approximately from the respiration rates of the B-cells or from the disappearance rate of the energy pool in islets exposed to anoxia. Rates of oxygen uptake of islets isolated by microdissection from obese-hyperglycemic mice have been reported by HELLERSTRÖM (1967) and by HELLERSTRÖM *et al.* (1970) and of islets isolated by collagenase from normal mice by HEDESKOV *et al.* (1972). In obese-hyperglycemic mice there was an endogenous islet oxygen uptake of 5.7 μl/h per mg dry islet weight, corresponding to 4.3 μmoles O_2/min per g. When glucose was added to the incubation medium a maximal respiratory stimulation of about 50% was obtained at a glucose concentration of 16.7 mM, corresponding to an oxygen consumption rate of 6.4 μmoles/min per g. Measurements of both oxygen consumption and glucose oxidation in the same islets (HELLERSTRÖM and GUNNARSSON, 1970) showed that the increased respiration in the presence of glucose was sufficient to account for the observed rate of glucose oxidation and, in fact, corresponded precisely to the calculated oxygen requirement for this oxidative process. The additional oxygen uptake in the presence of glucose thus seems to be used solely for oxidation of this substrate, indicating that the islet ATP production (assuming a maximal P:O ratio for glucose of 6.34 μmoles ATP formed per μmole oxygen utilized) would increase by about 13 μmoles/min per g at a high glucose level.

Since the nature of the endogenous fuels in the B-cell is not known, only an approximate figure can be calculated for the total ATP generated in the B-cell. Assuming a mixed substrate pool consisting mainly of carbohydrates and fatty acids (HELLERSTRÖM and GUNNARSSON, 1970) with a mean P:O ratio of 6, there would be a total ATP production of about 30 μmoles/min per g in the B-cell of the obese-hyperglycemic mouse. This is, in fact, the approximate value found for the consumption of energy-rich phosphate equivalents by the B-cells in the rat during the initial 30 s of total pancreatic ischemia (KRZANOWSKI *et al.*, 1971). During this period of anoxia the ATP dropped by about 23%, phosphocreatine 65%, and glucose 17%, while glycogen remained relatively unchanged. With an ATP production of about 38 μmoles/min per g the turnover rate of ATP in the B-cells would be about 4 times/min in the mouse and half that rate in the rat.

The energy requirements of the various steps in insulin biosynthesis and secretion are as yet incompletely known. Some insight has, however, been gained by studies of the functional state of the B-cell in the presence of various metabolic inhibitors. Thus, inhibition of oxidative phosphorylation by anoxia or 2,4-dinitrophenol blocks stimulation of insulin release by a number of agents, indicating that ATP is needed for the release (COORE and RANDLE, 1964; MILNER and HALES, 1969; ALEYASSINE, 1970). Similarly, it has been shown that antimycin A, in concentrations that inhibit islet respiration completely, prevents the conversion of proinsulin to insulin (STEINER *et al.*, 1970). As suggested by HOWELL (1972), this might reflect a block in intracellular translocation of proinsulin from the rough-surfaced endoplasmic reticulum to the Golgi complex, where conversion to insulin is thought to occur. This would conform to the previous observation of a similar energy-requiring step in the intracellular transport of proteins in the exocrine pancreatic cell (JAMIESON and PALADE, 1968).

Inhibition of protein synthesis in the B-cell by cycloheximide does not significantly alter the rate of glucose utilization or glucose oxidation, or of oxygen consumption (ASHCROFT *et al.*, 1970, 1972c; HELLERSTRÖM, unpublished data). Biosynthesis of proinsulin may therefore not be a major controlling factor in the oxidative metabolism of the B-cells and would account for only a minor fraction of the ATP expenditure of these cells (cf. LIN and HAIST, 1971). Nevertheless, a more long-term decrease of the functional state of the B-cell, such as induced by total starvation, leads to a significant diminution of the oxidative metabolism of these cells (HELLERSTRÖM and GUNNARSSON, 1970).

The precise energy expenditure of the various steps in insulin secretion is difficult to assess as long as the mechanism for stimulus-secretion coupling remains unknown. Current knowledge of such mechanisms will be discussed in detail in the following chapters of this volume. In analogy with other cells, a significant fraction of ATP generated in the B-cell would be expected to be used for the maintenance of correct ionic gradients across the plasma membrane. Direct evidence for participation of ions in the release process has been obtained in a number of careful studies including those of (a) MILNER and HALES (1967a, b, 1968) and HALES and MILNER (1968a, b) on the effects on insulin secretion on changes in extracellular ionic composition, (b) GRODSKY and BENNETT (1966) and MALAISSE *et al.* (MALAISSE *et al.*, 1971a, b; MALAISSE-LAGAE and MALAISSE, 1971; MALAISSE, 1972; BRISSON *et al.*, 1972) on the significance of calcium for insulin secretion, and (c) MATTHEWS (1970) and DEAN and MATTHEWS (1970b) on the relationship between extracellular ionic composition and electrical activity of the B-cell. Ionic fluxes across the plasma membrane may therefore represent one site at which energy metabolism is linked to the release process of the B-cell. It is also conceivable that ATP is of significance at several other sites involved in insulin secretion. Thus cyclic AMP, which plays a key role in the release process, is generated from ATP. Furthermore, ATP is presumably required for phosphorylation of proteins by protein phosphokinases, which have recently been demonstrated in the islets of Langerhans (MONTAGUE and HOWELL, 1972). It seems now probable that both Ca^{++}, cyclic AMP and protein phosphokinases are of importance for activation of a microtubular system involved in the final discharge of insulin across the B-cell membrane. Although ATP is probably utilized in this system there is up to now little evidence that it is of direct regulatory significance.

References

ALEYASSINE, H.: Energy requirements for insulin release from rat pancreas in vitro. Endocrinology **84**, 84—89 (1970)

ANDERSSON, A.: Structure and metabolism of isolated pancreatic islets in tissue culture. Abstract, European Association for the Study of Diabetes, 8th Annual Meeting, Madrid 1972

ANDERSSON, A., HELLERSTRÖM, C.: Metabolic characteristics of isolated pancreatic islets in tissue culture. Diabetes **21**, Suppl. 2, 546—554 (1972)

ASHCROFT, S.J.H., BASSETT, J.M., RANDLE, P.J.: Isolation of human pancreatic islets capable of releasing insulin and metabolising glucose in vitro. Lancet **1971 I**, 888—889

ASHCROFT, S.J.H., HEDESKOV, C.J., RANDLE, P.J.: Glucose metabolism in mouse pancreatic islets. Biochem. J. **118**, 143—154 (1970)

ASHCROFT, S.J.H., RANDLE, P.J.: Glucose metabolism and insulin release by pancreatic islets. Lancet **1968 I**, 278—279

ASHCROFT, S.J.H., RANDLE, P.J.: Enzymes of glucose metabolism in normal mouse pancreatic islets. Biochem. J. **119**, 5—15 (1970)

ASHCROFT, S.J.H., RANDLE, P.J., TÄLJEDAL, I.-B.: Cyclic nucleotide phosphodiesterase activity in normal mouse pancreatic islets. FEBS Letters **20**, 263—266 (1972a)

ASHCROFT, S.J.H., BASSETT, J.M., RANDLE, P.J.: Insulin secretion mechanisms and glucose metabolism in isolated islets. Diabetes **21**, Suppl. 2, 538—545 (1972b)

ASHCROFT, S.J.H., WEERASINGHE, L.C.C., BASSETT, J.M., RANDLE, P.J.: The pentose cycle and insulin release in mouse pancreatic islets. Biochem. J. **126**, 525—532 (1972c)

ASHCROFT, S.J.H., WEERASINGHE, L.C.C., RANDLE, P.J.: Islet metabolism, ATP concentration and insulin release. Abstract, European Association for the Study of Diabetes, 8th Annual Meeting, Madrid 1972d

ASPLUND, K., HELLERSTRÖM, C.: Glucose metabolism of pancreatic islets isolated from neonatal rats. Horm. Metab. Res. **4**, 159—163 (1972)

BALASSE, E.O., OOMS, H.A., LAMBILLIOTTE, J.P.: Evidence for a stimulatory effect of ketone bodies on insulin secretion in man. Horm. Metab. Res. **2**, 371 (1970)

BALLINGER, W.F., LACY, P.E.: Transplantation of intact pancreatic islets in rats. Surgery **72**, 175—186 (1972)

BENSLEY, R.R.: Studies of the pancreas of the guinea pig. Amer. J. Anat. **12**, 297—388 (1911)

BERNE, C.: Quantitative measurements of enzymes involved in the turnover of fatty acids in the islets of New Zealand obese mice. Diabetologia **7**, 400—401 (1971)

BERNE, C.: Oxidation of fatty acids and ketone bodies in isolated pancreatic islets. Diabetologia **8**, 364 (1972)

BERNE, C., BROLIN, S.E., ÅGREN, A.: Influence of ischemia on the levels of reduced pyridine nucleotides in the pancreatic islets. Horm. Metab. Res. **5**, 141—142 (1973).

BORGLUND, E.: To be published (1973a)

BORGLUND, E.: To be published (1973b)

BRIEL, G., GYLFE, E., HELLMAN, B., NEUHOFF, W.: Microdetermination of free amino acids in pancreatic islets isolated from obese-hyperglycemic mice. Acta physiol. scand. **84**, 247—253 (1972)

BRISSON, G.R., MALAISSE-LAGAE, F., MALAISSE, W.J.: The stimulus-secretion coupling of glucose-induced insulin release. VII. A proposed site of action for adenosine-3′,5′-cyclic monophosphate. J. clin. Invest. **51**, 232—241 (1972)

BROLIN, S.E., BERNE, C.: The enzymatic activities of the initial glycolytic steps in pancreatic islets and acini. Metabolism **16**, 1024—1028 (1967)

BROLIN, S.E., BERNE, C.: The activity pattern of enzymes associated with glycogen metabolism in the islets of Langerhans. In: FALKMER, S., HELLMAN, B., TÄLJEDAL, I.-B. (eds.): The Structure and Metabolism of the Pancreatic Islets, pp. 245—252. Oxford: Pergamon Press 1970

BROLIN, S.E., BERNE, C., LINDE, B.: Measurements of enzymatic activities required for ATP formation by glycolysis in the pancreatic islets of hyperglycemic mice. Diabetes **16**, 21—25 (1967a)
BROLIN, S.E., BERNE, C., BORGLUND, E.: Enzymatic aspects of the stimulation of the B-cells by glucose. In: ÖSTMAN, J. (ed.): Proceedings of the VIth Congress of the International Diabetes Federation, pp. 140—146. Amsterdam: Excerpta Med. 1967b
BROLIN, S.E., BERNE, C., PETERSSON, B., LARSSON, A.: Histochemical staining and microchemical studies of fructose-1,6-diphosphate splitting enzymes in the pancreatic islets and liver of NZO mice. J. Histochem. Cytochem. **16**, 654—658 (1968)
BROLIN, S.E., BORGLUND, E., OHLSSON, A.: On the enzymatic activity of the pancreatic islets and acini in New Zealand obese mice. In: BROLIN, S.E., HELLMAN, B., KNUTSSON, H. (eds.): The Structure and Metabolism of the Pancreatic Islets, pp. 289—294. Oxford: Pergamon Press 1964
BROLIN, S.E., BORGLUND, E., OHLSSON, A.: The phosphorylation of glucose in pancreatic islets and acini as studied by measurements of the enzymatic activity. Acta Soc. Med. upsalien. **71**, 334—340 (1966)
BROLIN, S.E., BORGLUND, E., TEGNÉR, L., WETTERMARK, G.: Photokinetic microassay based on dehydrogenase reactions and bacterial luciferase. Analyt. Biochem. **42**, 124—135 (1971)
CHRISTENSEN, H.N., HELLMAN, B., LERNMARK, Å., SEHLIN, J., TAGER, H.S., TÄLJEDAL, I.-B.: In vitro stimulation of insulin release by non-metabolizable, transport-specific amino acids. Biochem. biophys. Acta (Amst.) **241**, 341—348 (1971)
COORE, H.G., RANDLE, P.J.: Insulin secretion from rabbit pancreas in vitro. In: BROLIN, S.E., HELLMAN, B., KNUTSSON, H. (eds.): The Structure and Metabolism of the Pancreatic Islets, pp. 295—297. Oxford: Pergamon Press 1964
CRESPIN, S.R., GREENOUGH, W.B., STEINBERG, D.: Stimulation of insulin secretion by infusion of free fatty acids. J. clin. Invest. **48**, 1934—1943 (1969)
DEAN, P.M., MATTHEWS, E.K.: Glucose-induced electrical activity in pancreatic islet cells. J. Physiol. (Lond.) **210**, 255—264 (1970a)
DEAN, P.M., MATTHEWS, E.K.: Electrical activity in pancreatic islet cells: effect of ions. J. Physiol. (Lond.) **210**, 265—275 (1970b)
DIXIT, P.K., LAZAROW, A.: Effect of alloxan on the lactic dehydrogenase (LDH) activity of the microdissected mammalian pancreatic islets. Metabolism **13**, 285—290 (1964)
DIXIT, P.K., LAZAROW, A.: Effect of alloxan on the enzymatic activity of microdissected mammalian pancreatic islets. Diabetes **18**, 589—597 (1969)
EDGAR, P., RABINOWITZ, D., MERIMEE, T.J.: Effects of amino acids on insulin release from excised rabbit pancreas. Endocrinology **84**, 835—843 (1969)
EDWARDS, J.C., HELLERSTRÖM, C., PETERSSON, B., TAYLOR, K.W.: Oxidation of glucose and fatty acids in normal and in A_2-cell rich pancreatic islets isolated from guinea-pigs. Diabetologia **8**, 93—98 (1972)
FALKMER, S.: Experimental diabetes research in fish. Acta endocr. (Kbh.) **37** (Suppl. 59), 1—122 (1961)
FLOYD, J.C., JR., FAJANS, S.S., CONN, J.W., THIFFAULT, C., KNOPF, R.F., GUNTSCHE, E.: Secretion of insulin induced by amino acids and glucose in diabetes mellitus. J. clin. Endocr. **28**, 266—276 (1968)
GEPTS, W., GRÉGOIRE, F.: Quantitative histochemistry of the endocrine pancreas. In: DUBACH, V.C. and SCHMIDT, V. (eds.): Recent Advances in Quantitative Histo- and Cytochemistry, pp. 284—311. Bern: Huber 1971
GEPTS, W., GRÉGOIRE, F., VAN ASCHE, A., DE GASPARO, M.: Quantitative enzyme pattern and insulin content of human islets of Langerhans. In: FALKMER, S., HELLMAN, B., TÄLJEDAL, I.-B. (eds.): The Structure and Metabolism of the Pancreatic Islets, pp. 283—303. Oxford: Pergamon Press 1970
GREEN, I.C., TAYLOR, K.W.: Effects of pregnancy in the rat on the size and insulin secretory response of the islet of Langerhans. J. Endocr. **54**, 317—325 (1972)
GRODSKY, G.M.: Insulin and the pancreas. Vitam. and Horm. **28**, 37—101 (1970)
GRODSKY, G.M., BENNETT, L.L.: Cation requirements for insulin secretion in the isolated perfused pancreas. Diabetes **15**, 910—913 (1966)
GUNNARSSON, R., HELLERSTRÖM, C.: Acute effects of alloxan on the glucose metabolism and insulin secretion of the pancreatic B-cell. Horm. Metab. Res. **5**, 404—409 (1973)
HALES, C.N., MILNER, R.D.G.: The role of sodium and potassium in insulin secretion from rabbit pancreas. J. Physiol. (Lond.) **194**, 725—743 (1968a)
HALES, C.N., MILNER, R.D.G.: Cations and the secretion of insulin from rabbit pancreas in vitro. J. Physiol. (Lond.) **199**, 177—187 (1968b)
HAMMAR, H., BERNE, C.: The activity of β-hydroxyacyl-CoA dehydrogenase in the pancreatic islets of hyperglycemic mice. Diabetologia **6**, 526—528 (1970)

HASTINGS, J.W.: The chemistry of bioluminescence. In: SANADI, D.R. (ed.): Current Topics in Bioenergetics, pp. 113—139. London: Academic Press 1966

HEDESKOV, C.J., HERTZ, L., NISSEN, C.: The effect of mannoheptulose on glucose- and pyruvate-stimulated oxygen uptake in normal mouse pancreatic islets. Biochim. biophys. Acta (Amst.) **261**, 388—397 (1972)

HELLERSTRÖM, C.: A method for microdissection of intact pancreatic islets of mammals. Acta endocr. (Kbh.) **45**, 122—132 (1964)

HELLERSTRÖM, C.: Oxygen consumption of isolated pancreatic islets of mice studied with the Cartesian-diver micro-gasometer. Biochem. J. **98**, 7C—9C (1966)

HELLERSTRÖM, C.: Effects of carbohydrates on the oxygen consumption of isolated pancreatic islets of mice. Endocrinology **81**, 105—112 (1967)

HELLERSTRÖM, C., GUNNARSSON, R.: Oxygen utilization and oxidative metabolism in the B-cells. In: LUFT, R., RANDLE, P.J. (eds.): On the Pathogenesis of Diabetes Mellitus, pp. 127—151. Milano: Casa Editrice "Il Ponte" 1970

HELLERSTRÖM, C., HELLMAN, B., PETERSSON, B., ALM, G.: The two types of pancreatic A-cells and their relation to the glucagon secretion. In: BROLIN, S.E., HELLMAN, B., KNUTSSON, H. (eds.): The Structure and Metabolism of the Pancreatic Islets, pp. 117—129. Oxford: Pergamon Press 1964

HELLERSTRÖM, C., WESTMAN, S., MARSDEN, N., TURNER, D.S.: Oxygen consumption of the B-cells in relation to insulin release. In: FALKMER, S., HELLMAN, B., TÄLJEDAL, I.-B. (eds.): The Structure and Metabolism of the Pancreatic Islets, pp. 315—328. Oxford: Pergamon Press 1970

HELLERSTRÖM, C., WESTMAN, S., STORK, H., SCHMIDT, F.H.: Zur Wirkung der blutzuckersenkenden Sulfonylharnstoffe auf den in-vitro-Stoffwechsel von Glukose und Aminosäuren in den B-Zellen des Pankreas von Mäusen. Arzneimittel-Forsch. **19**, 1464—1467 (1969)

HELLMAN, B.: Fluorometric assays of glutamic pyruvic transaminase activity in microdissected pancreatic islets from obese hyperglycemic mice. Acta physiol. scand. **65**, 357—363 (1965)

HELLMAN, B.: Islet morphology and glucose metabolism in relation to the specific function of pancreatic B-cells. In: ÖSTMAN, J. (ed.): Proceedings of the VIth Congress of the International Diabetes Federation, pp. 92—109. Amsterdam: Excerpta Medica Foundation 1967

HELLMAN, B., IDAHL, L.Å.: Presence and mobilization of glycogen in mammalian pancreatic B-cells. Endocrinology **84**, 1—8 (1969)

HELLMAN, B., IDAHL, L.Å.: On the functional significance of the pancreatic B-cell glycogen. In: FALKMER, S., HELLMAN, B., TÄLJEDAL, I.-B. (eds.): The Structure and Metabolism of the Pancreatic Islets, pp. 253—262. Oxford: Pergamon Press 1970

HELLMAN, B., IDAHL, L.Å., DANIELSSON, Å.: Adenosine triphosphate levels of mammalian pancreatic B-cells after stimulation with glucose and hypoglycemic sulfonylureas. Diabetes **18**, 509—516 (1969)

HELLMAN, B., IDAHL, L.Å., LERNMARK, Å., SEHLIN, J., SIMON, E., TÄLJEDAL, I.B.: The pancreatic B-cell recognition of insulin secretagogues. I. Transport of mannoheptulose and the dynamics of insulin release. Molec. Pharmacol. **8**, 1—7 (1972)

HELLMAN, B., SEHLIN, J., TÄLJEDAL, I.-B.: Evidence for mediated transport of glucose in mammalian pancreatic B-cells. Biochim. biophys. Acta (Amst.) **241**, 147—154 (1971a)

HELLMAN, B., SEHLIN, J., TÄLJEDAL, I.-B.: Uptake of alanine, arginine and leucine by mammalian pancreatic B-cells. Endocrinology **89**, 1432—1439 (1971b)

HELLMAN, B., SEHLIN, J., TÄLJEDAL, I.-B.: Transport of alpha-aminoisobutyric acid in mammalian pancreatic B-cells. Diabetologia **7**, 256—265 (1971c)

HELLMAN, B., SEHLIN, J., TÄLJEDAL, I.-B.: Effects of glucose and other modifiers of insulin release on the oxidative metabolism of amino acids in micro-dissected pancreatic islets. Biochem. J. **123**, 513—521 (1971d)

HILWIG, I., HEPTNER, W., VON WASIELEWSKI, E.: Über das Wachstum der Pankreaszellen von Säugetieren als monolayer cultures. Z. Zellforsch. **90**, 333—346 (1968)

HOLTER, H., LINDERSTRÖM-LANG, K.: On the Cartesian diver. C. R. Lab. Carlsberg, Ser. Chim. **24**, 333—478 (1943)

HORECKER, B.L.: Glucose-6-phosphate dehydrogenase, the pentose phosphate cycle and its place in carbohydrate metabolism. Amer. J. clin. Path. **47**, 271—281 (1967)

HORINO, M., MACHLIN, L.J., HERTELENDY, F., KIPNIS, D.M.: Effect of short-chain fatty acids on plasma insulin in ruminant and nonruminant species. Endocrinology **83**, 118—128 (1968)

HOWELL, S.L.: Role of ATP in the intracellular translocation of proinsulin and insulin in the rat pancreatic B-cell. Nature (New Biology) **235**, 85—86 (1972)

HOWELL, S.L., TAYLOR, K.W.: Potassium ions and the secretion of insulin by islets of Langerhans incubated in vitro. Biochem. J. **108**, 17—24 (1968)

HUMBEL, R. E., RENOLD, A. E.: Studies on isolated islets of Langerhans (Brockman Bodies) of Teleost fishes. I. Metabolic activity in vitro. Biochim. biophys. Acta (Amst.) **74**, 84—94 (1963)

IDAHL, L. Å., HELLMAN, B.: Microchemical assays of glucose and glucose-6-phosphate in mammalian pancreatic B-cells. Acta endocr. (Kbh.) **59**, 479—486 (1968)

JAMIESON, J. D., PALADE, G. E.: Intracellular transport of secretory proteins in the pancreatic exocrine cell. IV. Metabolic requirements. J. Cell Biol. **39**, 589—603 (1968)

JARRETT, R. J., KEEN, H.: Glucose metabolism of isolated mammalian islets of Langerhans; effects of glucagon, 2-deoxy-D-glucose and D-mannoheptose. Diabetologia **4**, 249—252 (1968)

JENKINS, D. J. A., HUNTER, W. M., GOFF, D. V.: Ketone bodies and evidence for increased insulin secretion. Nature (Lond.) **227**, 384—385 (1970)

KEEN, H., SELLS, R., JARRETT, R. J.: A method for the study of the metabolism of isolated mammalian islets of Langerhans and some preliminary results. Diabetologia **1**, 28—32 (1965)

KILBERT, L. H., JR., SCHIFF, M. S., FOA, P. P.: The measurement of ATP in pancreatic islets by means of luciferin — luciferase reaction. Horm. Metab. Res. **4**, 242—244 (1972)

KISSANE, J. M., LACY, P. E., BROLIN, S. E., SMITH, C. H.: Quantitative histochemistry of the islets of Langerhans. In: BROLIN, S. E., HELLMAN, B., KNUTSON, H. (eds.): The Structure and Metabolism of the Pancreatic Islets, pp. 281—287. Oxford: Pergamon Press 1964

KRZANOWSKI, J. J., JR., FERTEL, B. A., MATSCHINSKY, F. M.: Energy metabolism in pancreatic islets of rats. Studies with tolbutamide and hypoxia. Diabetes **20**, 598—606 (1971)

LACY, P. E.: Quantitative histochemistry of islets of Langerhans. I. Lactic, malic, glucose-6-phosphate and 6-phosphogluconic dehydrogenase activity of beta cells and acini. Diabetes **11**, 96—100 (1962)

LACY, P. E., GREIDER, M. H.: Ultrastructural organization of mammalian pancreatic islets. In: STEINER, D. F., FREINKEL, N. (eds.): Endocrine pancreas. Handbook of Physiology, Section 7, Vol. 1, pp. 77—89. Baltimore: Williams and Wilkins 1972

LACY, P. E., KOSTIANOVSKY, M.: Method for the isolation of intact islets of Langerhans from the rat pancreas. Diabetes **16**, 35—39 (1967)

LACY, P. E., WILLIAMSON, J. R.: Quantitative histochemistry of the islets of Langerhans. II. Insulin content of dissected B-cells. Diabetes **11**, 101—104 (1962)

LAMBERT, A. E.: Biochemical and morphological studies of cultured fetal rat pancreas. Thesis: University of Louvain 1970

LAMBERT, A. E., BLONDEL, B., KANAZAWA, Y., ORCI, L., RENOLD, A. E.: Monolayer cell culture of neonatal rat pancreas: Light microscopy and evidence for immunoreactive insulin synthesis and release. Endocrinology **90**, 239—248 (1972)

LANDAU, B. R.: Quantitation of pathways of carbohydrate metabolism. In: STEINER, D. F., FREINKEL, N. (eds.): Endocrine pancreas. Handbook of Physiology, Section 7, Vol. 1, pp. 215—218. Baltimore: Williams and Wilkins 1972

LAZAROW, A.: Functional characterization and metabolic pathways of the pancreatic islet tissue. Recent Progr. Hormone Res. **19**, 489—546 (1963)

LAZAROW, A., COOPERSTEIN, S. J., BLOOMFIELD, D. K., FRIZ, G. T.: Studies on the isolated islet tissue of fish. II. The effect of electrolytes and other factors on the oxygen uptake of pancreatic islet slices, using the Cartesian diver microrespirometer. Biol. Bull. **113**, 414—425 (1957)

LERNMARK, Å.: Isolated mouse islets as a model for studying insulin release. Acta diabet. lat. **8**, 649—679 (1971)

LERNMARK, Å.: Effects of neutral and dibasic amino acids on the in vitro release of insulin. Hormones **3**, 22—30 (1972a)

LERNMARK, Å.: Specificity of leucine stimulation of insulin release. Hormones **3**, 14—21 (1972b)

LIN, B. J., HAIST, R. E.: Respiration and insulin synthesis in the islets of Langerhans. Canad. J. Physiol. Pharmacol. **49**, 559—567 (1971)

LINDALL, A., STEFFES, M., SORENSON, R.: Immunoassayable insulin content of subcellular fractions of rat islets. Endocrinology **85**, 218—223 (1969)

LOWRY, O. H.: The quantitative histochemistry of the brain. Histological sampling. J. Histochem. Cytochem. **1**, 420—428 (1953)

LOWRY, O. H., PASSONNEAU, J. V.: A flexible system of enzymatic analysis. London: Academic Press 1972

LOWRY, O. H., PASSONNEAU, J. V., SCHULZ, D. W., ROCK, M. K.: The measurement of pyridine nucleotides by enzymatic cycling. J. biol. Chem. **236**, 2746—2755 (1961)

LÖFFLER, G., TRAUTSCHOLD, I., SCHWEITZER, T., LOHMANN, E.: Effects of glibenclamide and tolbutamide on isolated pancreatic islets of the rat. Horm. Metab. Res. **1**, Suppl., 41—44 (1969)

MACCHI, J. A., BLAUSTEIN, E. H.: Cytostructure and endocrine function of monolayer cultures of neonatal hamster pancreas. Endocrinology **84**, 208—216 (1969)

MADISON, L. L., MEBANE, D., UNGER, R. H., LOCHNER, A.: The hypoglycemic action of ketones. II. Evidence for a stimulatory feed back of ketones on the pancreatic beta cells. J. clin. Invest. **43**, 408—415 (1964)

MALAISSE, W. J.: Étude de la sécrétion insulinique in vitro. Bruxelles: Editions Arscia 1969

MALAISSE, W. J.: Role of calcium in insulin secretion. Israel J. med. Sci. **8**, 244—251 (1972)

MALAISSE, W. J., MALAISSE-LAGAE, F.: Stimulation of insulin secretion by non-carbohydrate metabolites. J. Lab. clin. Med. **72**, 438—448 (1968)

MALAISSE, W. J., MALAISSE-LAGAE, F., BRISSON, G. R.: The stimulus-secretion coupling of glucose-induced insulin release. II. Interaction of alkali and alkaline earth cations. Horm. Metab. Res. **3**, 65—70 (1971a)

MALAISSE, W. J., MAHY, M., MALAISSE-LAGAE, F.: Effect of sulfonylureas on calcium uptake and insulin secretion by islets of Langerhans. Arch. Int. Pharmac. Ther. **192**, 205—207 (1971b)

MALAISSE-LAGAE, F., MALAISSE, W. J.: Stimulus-secretion coupling of glucose-induced insulin release. III. Uptake of 45-calcium by isolated islets of Langerhans. Endocrinology **88**, 72—80 (1971)

MANNS, J. G., BODA, J. M., WILLES, R. F.: Probable role of propionate and butyrate in control of insulin secretion in sheep. Amer. J. Physiol. **212**, 756—764 (1967)

MATSCHINSKY, F. M.: Enzymes, metabolites and cofactors involved in intermediary metabolism of islets of Langerhans. In: STEINER, D. F., FREINKEL, N. (eds.): Endocrine pancreas. Handbook of Physiology, Section 7, Vol. 1, pp. 199—214. Baltimore: Williams and Wilkins 1972

MATSCHINSKY, F. M., ELLERMAN, J. E.: Metabolism of glucose in the islets of Langerhans. J. biol. Chem. **243**, 2730—2736 (1968)

MATSCHINSKY, F. M., ELLERMAN, J. E., LANDGRAF, R., KRZANOWSKI, J., KOTLER-BRAJTBURG, J., FERTEL, R.: Quantitative histochemistry of glucose metabolism in the islets of Langerhans. In: DUBACH, U. C., SCHMIDT, U. (eds.): Recent Advances in Quantitative Histo- and Cytochemistry, pp. 143—182. Bern: Huber 1971

MATSCHINSKY, F. M., LANDGRAF, R., ELLERMAN, J., KOTLER-BRAJTBURG, J.: Glucoreceptor mechanisms in islets of Langerhans. Diabetes **21**, Suppl. 2, 555—569 (1972)

MATSCHINSKY, F. M., RUTHERFORD, C. R., ELLERMAN, J. E.: Accumulation of citrate in pancreatic islets of obese hyperglycemic mice. Biochem. biophys. Res. Commun. **33**, 855—862 (1968a)

MATSCHINSKY, F. M., KAUFFMAN, F. C., ELLERMAN, J. E.: Effect of hyperglycemia on the hexose mono-phosphate shunt in islets of Langerhans. Diabetes **17**, 457—480 (1968b)

MATTHEWS, E. K.: Electrical activity in islet cells and insulin secretion. In: LUFT, R., RANDLE, P. J. (eds.): On the Pathogenesis of Diabetes Mellitus, pp. 83—89. Milano: Casa Editrice "Il Ponte" 1970

MCELROY, W. D., SELIGER, H. H.: The chemistry of light emission. In: NORD, F. F. (ed.): Advances in Enzymology. Vol. 25, pp. 119—166. New York: Interscience Publ. 1963

MILNER, R. D. G.: The mechanism by which leucine and arginine stimulates insulin release in vitro. Biochim. biophys. Acta (Amst.) **192**, 154—156 (1969)

MILNER, R. D. G.: The stimulation of insulin release by essential amino acids from rabbit pancreas in vitro. J. Endocr. **47**, 347—356 (1970)

MILNER, R. D. G., HALES, C. N.: The stimulation by potassium of insulin secretion from rabbit pancreas incubated in vitro. Biochem. J. **105**, 28 P (1967a)

MILNER, R. D. G., HALES, C. N.: The role of Ca^{++} and Mg^{++} in insulin secretion from rabbit pancreas studied in vitro. Diabetologia **3**, 47—49 (1967b)

MILNER, R. D. G., HALES, C. N.: Cations and secretion of insulin. Biochim. biophys. Acta (Amst.) **150**, 162—164 (1968)

MILNER, R. D. G., HALES, C. N.: The interaction of various inhibitors and stimuli of insulin release studied with rabbit pancreas in vitro. Biochem. J. **113**, 473—479 (1969)

MONTAGUE, W., HOWELL, S. L.: The mode of action of adenosine 3′:5′-cyclic monophosphate in mammalian islets of Langerhans. Biochem. J. **129**, 551—560 (1972)

MONTAGUE, W., TAYLOR, K. W.: Regulation of insulin secretion by short chain fatty acids. Nature (Lond.) **217**, 853 (1968)

MONTAGUE, W., TAYLOR, K. W.: The role of the pentose phosphate pathway in insulin secretion. In: FALKMER, S., HELLMAN, B., TÄLJEDAL, I.-B. (eds.): The Structure and Metabolism of the Pancreatic Islets, pp. 263—273. Oxford: Pergamon Press 1970

MOSKALEWSKI, S.: Isolation and culture of the islets of Langerhans of the guinea-pig. Gen. comp. Endocr. **5**, 342—353 (1965)

Panten, U., von Kriegstein, E., Poser, W., Schönborn, J., Hasselblatt, A.: Effects of L-leucine and alpha-ketoisocaproic acid upon insulin secretion and metabolism of isolated pancreatic islets. FEBS Letters **20**, 225—228 (1972)

Panten, U., Poser, W., Hasselblatt, A.: Fluorescence of reduced pyridine nucleotides of superfused pancreatic islets. Diabetologia **6**, 643 (1970)

Panten, U., dal Ri, H., Poser, W., Hasselblatt, A.: Eine Methode der Gewebsumströmung für Fluorescenzmessungen. Pflügers Arch. **323**, 86—90 (1971)

Passonneau, J. V., Lowry, O. H.: The role of phosphofructokinase in metabolic regulation. In: Weber, G. (ed.): Advances in enzyme regulation, Vol. 2, pp. 265—274. Oxford: Pergamon Press 1964

Petersson, B.: Isolation and characterization of different types of pancreatic islet cells in guinea-pigs. Acta endocr. (Kbh.) **53**, 480—488 (1966)

Petersson, B.: The dry mass of the pancreatic B-cells in relation to their content of secretion granules. Histochem. J. **1**, 55—58 (1968)

Petkov, P. E.: Comparative histochemical studies of mammalian pancreatic islets. In: Falkmer, S., Hellman, B., Täljedal, I.-B. (eds.): The Structure and Metabolism of the Pancreatic Islets, pp. 213—222. Oxford: Pergamon Press 1970

Pictet, R., Orci, L., Gonet, A. E., Rouiller, C., Renold, A. E.: Ultrastructural studies of the hyperplastic islets of Langerhans of spiny mice (Acomys cahirinus) before and during the development of hyperglycemia. Diabetologia **3**, 188—211 (1967)

Randle, P. J., Hales, C. N.: Insulin release mechanisms. In: Steiner, D. F., Freinkel, N. (eds.): Endocrine Pancreas. Handbook of Physiology, Section 7, Vol. 1, pp. 219—235. Baltimore: Williams and Wilkins 1972

Sanbar, S. S., Martin, J. M.: Stimulation by octanoate of insulin release from isolated rat pancreas. Metabolism **16**, 482—484 (1967)

Sehlin, J.: Transport and oxidation of glycine in mammalian pancreatic islets with reference to the mechanism of amino acid — induced insulin release. Hormones **3**, 144—155 (1972 a)

Sehlin, J.: Uptake and oxidation of glutamic acid in mammalian pancreatic islets. Hormones **3**, 156—166 (1972 b)

Snyder, P. J., Kashket, S., O'Sullivan, J. B.: Pentose cycle in isolated islets during glucose-stimulated insulin release. Amer. J. Physiol. **219**, 876—880 (1970)

Steiner, D. F., Clark, J. L., Nolan, C., Rubenstein, A. H., Margoliash, E., Melani, F., Oyer, P. E.: The biosynthesis of insulin and some speculations regarding the pathogenesis of human diabetes. In: Cerasi, E., Luft, R. (eds.): Pathogenesis of Diabetes Mellitus, pp. 57—78. Stockholm: Almqvist & Wiksell 1970

Stork, H., Schmidt, F. H., Hellerström, C., Westman, S.: Respiration of the B-cells in the presence of sulfonylureas. In: Falkmer, S., Hellman, B., Täljedal, I.-B. (eds.): The Structure and Metabolism of the Pancreatic Islets, pp. 331—336. Oxford: Pergamon Press 1970

Strehler, B. L., Totter, J.: Firefly luminescence in the study of energy transfer mechanisms. I. Substrate and enzyme determination. Arch. Biochem. **40**, 28—41 (1952)

Strehler, B. L., Totter, J. R.: Determination of ATP and related compounds; firefly luminescence and other methods. In: Glick, D. (ed.): Methods of Biochemical Analyses, pp. 341—356. New York: Interscience 1954

Täljedal, I.-B.: Some aspects of the apparent glucose-6-phosphatase activity in the pancreatic islets of mammals. Biochim. biophys. Acta (Amst.) **146**, 292—295 (1967)

Täljedal, I.-B.: Presence, induction and possible role of glucose-6-phosphatase in mammalian pancreatic islets. Biochem. J. **114**, 287—394 (1969)

Täljedal, I.-B.: Glucose-6-phosphatase in pancreatic B-cell metabolism. In: Falkmer, S., Hellman, B., Täljedal, I.-B. (eds.): The Structure and Metabolism of the Pancreatic Islets, pp. 233—244. Oxford: Pergamon Press 1970

Wettermark, G., Tegnér, L., Brolin, S. E., Borglund, E.: Photokinetic measurements of the ATP and ADP levels in isolated islets of Langerhans. In: Falkmer, S., Hellman, B., and Täljedal, I.-B. (eds.): The Structure and Metabolism of the Pancreatic Islets, pp. 275—282. Oxford: Pergamon Press 1970

II. Hexoses and Insulin Secretion

F.M. MATSCHINSKY, J. ELLERMAN, S. STILLINGS, F. RAYBAUD, C. PACE and W. ZAWALICH

With 18 Figures

1. Introduction

D-glucose seems to be the preeminent factor controlling islet-cell function as illustrated by the well-known metabolic effects of the oral and the intravenous glucose tolerance tests routinely used in the diabetic clinic. But considering the large number of other factors known to affect the secretory function of the β-cells, one is tempted to conclude, at first glance at least, that the role of glucose constitutes a relatively narrow aspect of the metabolism and function of these cells (Fig. 1). In addition to D-glucose, insulin secretion can be provoked by other hexoses and related substances (e.g. mannose, sorbitol, and glucosamine); besides carbohydrates many of the natural calorigenic molecules of low molecular weight are potent stimulators of insulin release (amino acids, fatty acids, and certain metabolites of intermediary metabolism); and finally insulin release can be modulated by an impressively large number of hormones and by neural stimuli. However, a more attentive analysis of all available information shows, that most members of the different classes of substances listed above need the presence of nonstimulatory or threshold levels of glucose for expressing their insulin-releasing action (EFENDIC *et al.*, 1969; GOLDFINE *et al.*, 1972; MATSCHINSKY *et al.*, 1972a). This implies that the glucose molecule occupies the crucial positions in islet-cell physiology attributed to it by researchers who have pioneered this field (GRAFE and MEYTHALER, 1927). The multiple functions of D-glucose and of chemically related substances in the islets of Langerhans are therefore chosen as the central theme of this chapter. There is by necessity some overlap with other chapters in

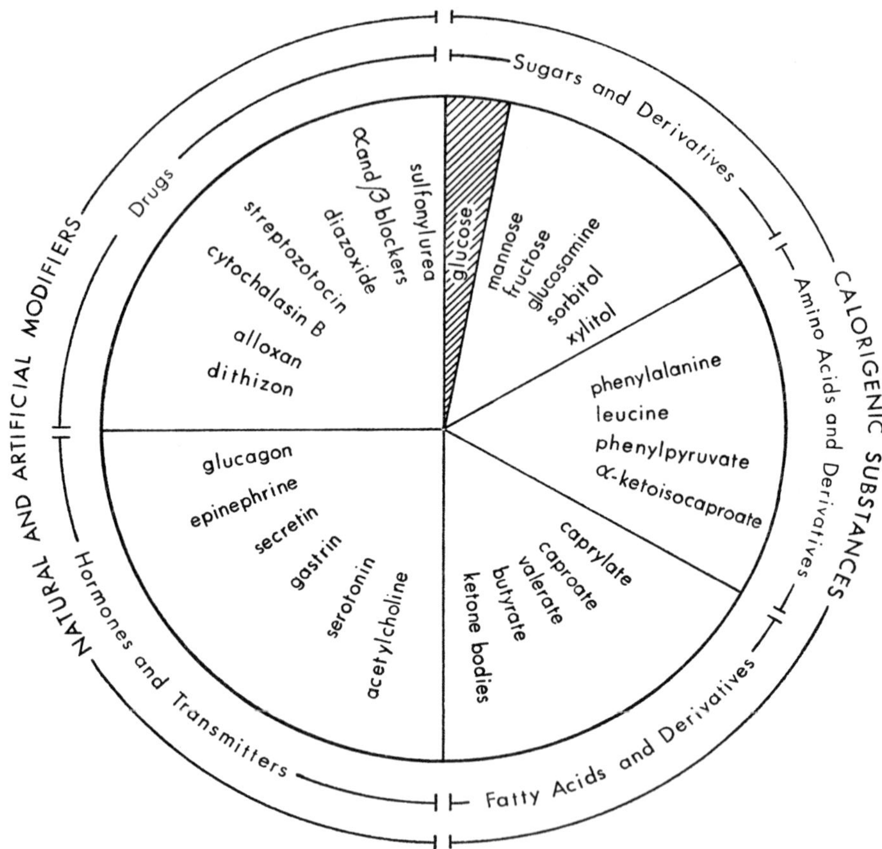

Fig. 1. The chemosensitivity of β-cells

this and the preceding volume of this handbook, but it was felt that this may actually benefit the reader. Also, since numerous comprehensive reviews concerning the metabolism and function of the islets of Langerhans have been written during the very recent past (GRODSKY and FORSHAM, 1966; WILLIAMS and ENSINCK, 1966; FAJANS *et al.*, 1967; LACY, 1967; FRASER, 1968; RANDLE *et al.*, 1968; CANDELA and COORE, 1969; FROHMAN, 1969; KIZER and BRESSLER, 1969; MAYHEW *et al.*, 1969; GRODSKY, 1970; PORTE and BAGDADE, 1970; RENOLD, 1970; RANDLE, 1970; PFEIFFER, 1971; MATSCHINSKY, 1972; RANDLE and HALES, 1972; MALAISSE, 1972), we decided to be highly selective in our choice of references and to limit our discussion to the newer developments in this field, thus, hopefully avoiding tiresome repetition.

2. Insulin Secretion Due to Hexoses and Pentoses as Well as their Derivatives and Analogues

a) Effects of Hexoses, Hexose Derivatives, and of Mannoheptulose

α) Stimulation of release

Countless reports have appeared during the last decades confirming and extending the original observations of Grafe and Meythaler who demonstrated that D-glucose acted on the islets of Langerhans and who imaginatively coined

Table 1. *Effect of various hexoses and hexose derivatives on insulin secretion*

Agent	Experimental Conditions	Species	Effect on insulin secretion	Classification of Mechanism	References (note: only the first author is listed)
Glucose	*in vivo*				
	adult — i.v. or p.o.	man, dog, sheep	agonist	not defined	Boda (1964), Grafe (1927), Kalkhoff (1964), Kilo (1967), Metz (1960), Seltzer (1964)
	fetus — i.v.	man, monkey, sheep	no effect	—	Mintz (1969), Thoreel (1970), Willes (1969)
	in vitro				
	isol. perf. pancr. — adult	dog, rat	agonist	independent releaser	Anderson (1947), Iversen (1971), Grodsky (1963), Landgraf (1971), Sussman (1966)
	pancr. pieces — adult	rat, rabbit, hamster	agonist	independent releaser	Creutzfeldt (1964), Coore (1964), Malaisse (1967a, b)
	pancr. pieces — fetal	man, rabbit, rat	no effect	—	Asplund (1970), Milner (1969), Milner (1971)
	isolated islets — adult	man, rat, mouse	agonist	independent releaser	Ashcroft (1971), Lacy (1968), Lernmark (1969)
	isolated islets — fetal	man	no effect	—	Espanosa (1970)
	organ culture — fetal	rat	agonist	dependent releaser	Lambert (1969)
	monolayer cell culture — neonatal	rat	agonist	dependent releaser	Lambert (1971)
Mannose	*in vivo*				
	adult — i.v.	man, dog	agonist	not defined	Karam (1966), Kilo (1967)
	in vitro				
	isol. perf. pancr. — adult	rat	agonist	independent releaser	Grodsky (1963), Sussman (1966)
	pancr. pieces — adult	rabbit, rat	agonist	independent releaser	Coore (1964), Malaisse (1967b)
	isol. islets — adult	rat, mouse	agonist	independent releaser	Ashcroft (1972a, b), Lacy (1968)
	organ culture — fetal	rat	agonist	dependent releaser	Lambert (1969a, b)

Table 1 (continued)

Agent	Experimental Conditions	Species	Effect on insulin secretion	Classification of Mechanism	References (note: only the first author is listed)
Fructose	*in vivo*				
	adult — i.v. or p.o.	man, dog	agonist or no effect	not defined	CORNBLATH (1963), KILO (1967), SAMOLS (1963)
	in vitro				
	isol. perf. pancr. — adult	rat	agonist or no effect	dependent releaser	GRODSKY (1963), MATSCHINSKY (1972), SUSSMAN (1966)
	pancr. pieces — adult	rabbit, rat	no effect	—	COORE (1964), LACY (1968)
	isolated islets — adult	rat, mouse	agonist	dependent releaser	ASHCROFT (1972a, b)
	organ culture — fetal	rat	agonist	dependent releaser	LAMBERT (1969a, b)
Galactose	*in vivo*				
	adult — i.v. or p.o.	man, dog	no effect	—	ISSELBACHER (1956), KARAM (1966), POZZA (1958), ROMMEL (1969), SAMOLS (1963)
	in vitro				
	isol. perf. pancr. — adult	rat	agonist or no effect	dependent releaser	GRODSKY (1963), LANDGRAF (1971), SUSSMAN (1966)
	pancr. pieces — adult	rat	no effect	—	COORE (1964), MALAISSE (1967a, b)
	isol. islets — adult	rat, mouse	agonist or no effect	dependent releaser	ASHCROFT (1972a, b)
	organ culture — fetal	rat	agonist	dependent releaser	LAMBERT (1969a, b)
Glucosamine	*in vitro*				
	isol. perf. pancr. — adult	rat	partial agonist	dependent releaser	LANDGRAF (1971), MATSCHINSKY (1972)
	pancr. pieces — adult	rat	partial agonist	independent releaser	COORE (1964)
	isol. islets — adult	rat, mouse	partial agonist	independent releaser	ASHCROFT (1972a, b)
	organ culture — fetal	rat	agonist	dependent releaser	LAMBERT (1969a, b)

Table 1 (continued)

Agent	Experimental Conditions	Species	Effect on insulin secretion	Classification of Mechanism	References (note: only the first author is listed)
N-acetyl-glucosamine	*in vitro*				
	isol. perf. pancr. — adult	rat	agonist	dependent releaser	MATSCHINSKY (1973)
	isol. islets — adult	rat, mouse	agonist	dependent releaser	ASHCROFT (1972a, b)
	organ culture — fetal	rat	agonist	dependent releaser	LAMBERT (1969a, b)
3-O-methyl-glucose	*in vitro*				
	isol. perf. pancr. — adult	rat	no effect	—	MATSCHINSKY (unpublished)
	pancr. pieces — adult	rabbit	no effect	—	COORE (1964)
	isolated islets — adult	rat, mouse	no effect	—	ASHCROFT (1972a, b)
	organ culture — fetal	rat	agonist	dependent releaser	LAMBERT (1969a, b)

the term "glucose as the hormone for insulin release" (GRAFE and MEYTHALER, 1927; GRAFE and MEYTHALER, 1928a; GRAFE and MEYTHALER, 1928b).

A wide variety of approaches was used for investigating the actions of glucose on pancreatic endocrine cells: insulin release was studied in the intact organism (e.g. FAJANS *et al.*, 1967) or *in vitro* with the isolated perfused pancreas (ANDERSON and LONG, 1947; GRODSKY *et al.*, 1963; SUSSMAN *et al.*, 1967; LANDGRAF *et al.*, 1971), with pancreas pieces (COORE and RANDLE, 1964; CREUTZFELDT *et al.*, 1964; MALAISSE *et al.*, 1967b; BURR *et al.*, 1970) and with isolated islets which were obtained by digesting the pancreas with collagenase (LACY and KOSTIANOVSKY, 1967; HOWELL and TAYLOR, 1968; LACY *et al.*, 1972) or by freehand dissection (HELLERSTRÖM, 1964). A great wealth of information about insulin release, particularly due to hexoses and their derivatives, was gathered using embryonic pancreas explants (LAMBERT *et al.*, 1969a; LAMBERT *et al.*, 1969b; KANAZAWA *et al.*, 1971).

It is mandatory to point out again and again that the population of β-cells has never been pure, whatever the experimental conditions, and that therefore uncertainties remain whether or not other elements present in the islet tissue (e.g. D cells, a_1- and a_2-cells, endothelial cells, nerve ganglion cells) might be involved in the secretory responses of the β-cells.

Disregarding the difficulty of cellular diversity of the islets of Langerhans it has been shown that hexoses and their close derivatives may cause insulin release from the β-cells by one of two possible ways (Table 1): a) independently or b) requiring the presence of one or several other effector molecules. This classification of action of sugars and sugar derivatives shows inconsistencies probably because of differences in the experimental systems and of the species employed, but constitutes a useful framework for the discussion. Almost all investigators agree that D-glucose and D-mannose belong to group *a* (MAYHEW *et al.*, 1969; GRODSKY, 1970; RANDLE and HALES, 1972). The secretory effects of various sugars and sugar derivatives comprising group *b* of the classification vary greatly depending on the test system employed. LAMBERT and his colleagues (LAMBERT *et al.*, 1969b) using embryonic rat pancreas explants found that addition of methylxanthines was required for eliciting insulin release by all hexoses and their derivatives (including D-glucose). The most remarkable feature of this system is its responsiveness to 3-O-methyl glucose and galactose. Release due to these two sugars is small but significant (3 and 15%, respectively, of the effect of equimolar levels of glucose). D-glucosamine (LAMBERT *et al.*, 1969b) and D-galactosamine (MATSCHINSKY *et al.*, unpublished experiments) apparently also belong in this group, judging from results obtained with the isolated perfused rat pancreas (LANDGRAF *et al.*, 1971; MATSCHINSKY *et al.*, 1972a, b; MATSCHINSKY *et al.*, unpublished experiments) or with isolated islets from mouse or rat (ASHCROFT *et al.*, 1972a). Galactose, fructose and N-acetylglucosamine are listed here in group b of the above classification, as indicated by findings gathered with islet preparations from adult mouse and rat or both (ASHCROFT *et al.*, 1972a) and with the isolated perfused rat pancreas (MATSCHINSKY *et al.*, 1972a, b). With the above three sugars low levels of glucose (2.75—5.5 mM) in addition to caffeine or theophylline were required for causing a secretory response. Some of the effects with galactose and 3-O-methyl glucose cited here remain controversial. In the case of galactose it was claimed in one report that release was most pronounced following rather than during exposure of the isolated perfused pancreas to the sugar alone (LANDGRAF *et al.*, 1971), in another report galactose required the presence of caffeine for exerting its action (LAMBERT *et al.*, 1969b), and in a third paper (ASHCROFT *et al.*, 1972a) caffeine plus low glucose levels were needed for rendering galactose effective. The majority of investigators concluded, however, that galactose is unable to release insulin (RANDLE *et al.*, 1968; MAYHEW *et al.*, 1969; GRODSKY *et al.*, 1963). In the case of 3-O-methyl glucose, insulin release was seen by only one group and a requirement for caffeine was noted (LAMBERT *et al.*, 1969 b). All others have failed to observe release or inhibition of release due to 3-O-methyl glucose under a wide variety of experimental conditions (RANDLE *et al.*, 1968; MAYHEW *et al.*, 1969; GRODSKY *et al.*, 1963). The following hexoses seemed consistently unable to release insulin: L-glucose, 2-deoxyglucose, gold thioglucose, and 1,5-anhydroglucitol (ASHCROFT *et al.*, 1972 a).

β) Inhibition of release by hexoses and mannoheptulose

Release due to glucose can be inhibited competitively by mannoheptulose (COORE and RANDLE, 1964), glucosamine (COORE and RANDLE, 1964), and usually but not consistently by 2-deoxyglucose (KILO *et al.*, 1963; MALAISSE, 1968; COORE and RANDLE, 1964). It is important to note that N-acetylglucosamine was unable to block glucose-provoked release (COORE and RANDLE, 1964; ASHCROFT *et al.*, 1970). The action of mannose shows the same susceptibilities to the inhibitory sugars described above for glucose action, as far as tested at least (MALAISSE, 1968). Possible interactions between other sugars, for example between glucosamine and mannoheptulose, have barely been studied. A short sentence in one paper states that the release due to glucosamine can be partially blocked by mannoheptulose (ASHCROFT *et al.*, 1972 a), and it was found in the authors' laboratory with the isolated perfused pancreas that 20—30 mM mannoheptulose partially inhibited release due to 10 mM glucosamine plus 5 mM theophylline (MATSCHINSKY *et al.*, unpublished experiments). Whether this inhibition of release indicates direct interactions of the two sugar molecules or whether it is due to a decrease of the energy potential, that might result from impaired glycolysis, is not clear.

γ) Modulation of release by 2-deoxyglucose and mannoheptulose

LAMBERT and his collaborators have demonstrated with embryonic pancreas explants that 22 mM mannoheptulose or 2-deoxyglucose potentiate the releasing action of 11 mM pyruvate or of 200 μg/ml of tolbutamide (KANAZAWA *et al.*, 1971). On the other hand, it was found by the same authors that the action of 5.5 mM glucose was inhibited by 43% in the presence of 22 mM mannoheptulose and by 55% due to 22 mM 2-deoxyglucose. These latter results are extremely puzzling since it is well established that excess mannoheptulose as used here completely blocks glucose phosphorylation in isolated islets (ASHCROFT *et al.*, 1970). One cannot help postulating that the unexpectedly high residual insulin secretion seen in these experiments might be a manifestation of agonist activity of mannoheptulose and possibly of 2-deoxyglucose. In this context it seems appropriate to refer to *in vivo* experiments, which uncovered a similar paradoxical potentiator effect of mannoheptulose: FAJANS and his collaborators found in dogs that pretreatment with mannoheptulose potentiated the insulin-releasing action of leucine and of the nonmetabolizable amino acid 2-amino bicyclo (2,2,1)-heptane-2-carboxylic acid (BCH) (FAJANS *et al.*, 1971). It seems worthwhile to pursue these leads derived from *in vivo* studies using appropriate *in vitro* systems.

δ) Insulin release due to phlorizin

As soon as the possibility of a glucoreceptor at the β-cell membrane was considered as the primary target of the glucose molecule, a search started for nonmetabolizable glucose analogues and derivatives that might stimulate insulin release. HELLMAN and his colleagues in Umea found that phlorizin caused insulin secretion at levels of 10 mM or more (HELLMAN *et al.*, 1970; HELLMAN *et al.*, 1972).

Since they also observed partial inhibition of this stimulation by mannoheptulose, they concluded that a glucoreceptor might be involved in phlorizin-stimulated release. The specificity of action was however questioned because the aglycone phloretin was similarly agonistic and, in addition, was partially blocked by mannoheptulose. Phlorizin also potentiated leucine-induced insulin release but was unable to substitute for glucose as permissive agent with arginine and theophylline as releasers. In summary then: phlorizin, a β-glucopyranoside, probably nonmetabolizable, mimics some but not all secretory properties of glucose in β-cells. It may become a useful tool in studying glucoreceptor sites in β-cells.

ε) Effects of fasting and feeding on glucose-induced insulin release

It is well documented that starvation decreases the responsiveness of β-cells to glucose (Malaisse, 1972). Kipnis (Kipnis, 1972) has demonstrated in rats that this effect of starvation can be prevented by multiple injections of glucose amounting to only a small fraction of the normal daily caloric intake. Furthermore, the reappearance of responsiveness to glucose due to realimentation was prevented by treatment with actinomycin D. These results led to the suggestion that insulin secretion due to glucose is controlled by an inducible enzyme system.

ζ) The kinetics of release and of inhibition of release due to hexoses and mannoheptulose

Release due to an extended (>10 min) square-wave stimulus of glucose is monophasic at low levels and biphasic at high levels (Cerasi and Luft, 1967; Curry et al., 1968; Landgraf et al., 1971; Grodsky, 1972). In addition, stimulation with glucose induces poststimulatory superresponsiveness due to basal glucose levels (Fig. 2). The dose-response curve for total release of insulin is extremely steep and is sigmoidal with an inflection at about 7.5 mM glucose (Fig. 3). The sigmoidal shape of the dose-response curve of insulin release due to glucose as the sole agonist has been observed with the various systems employed by different investigators (Cerasi et al., 1972; Grodsky, 1972; Malaisse, 1972; Matschinsky et al., unpublished experiments).

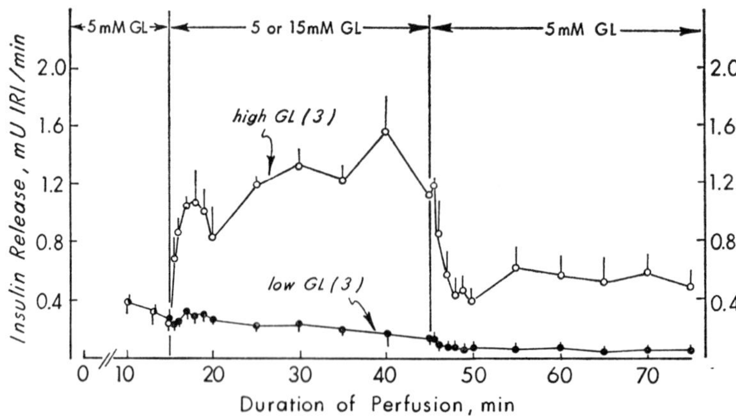

Fig. 2. Insulin release by the isolated perfused rat pancreas induced by a square-wave stimulus of glucose. In the controls 5 mM glucose was present throughout and in the experimentals the low level was present in the prestimulatory and poststimulatory periods while the stimulus was 15 mM glucose. Quantitation of immunoreactive insulin (IRI) is based on pig insulin standards. (From Matschinsky et al., unpublished experiments)

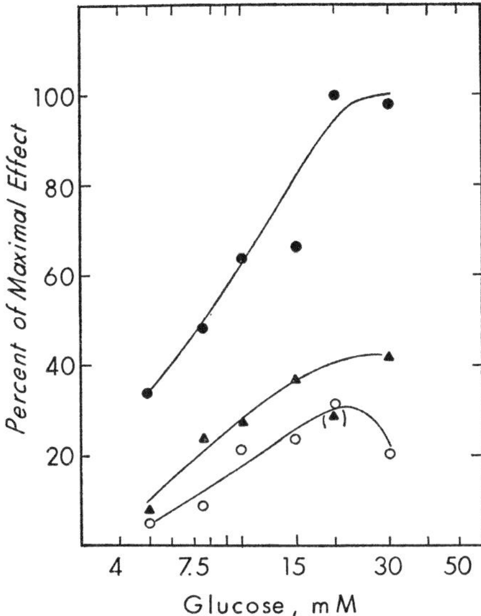

Fig. 3. Concentration dependency of glucose-induced insulin release by the isolated perfused rat pancreas. The relative potencies of glucose under three different experimental conditions are recorded: ●——● following preperfusion with 5 mM glucose, but stimulating in the presence of 5 mM theophylline. ▲——▲ following preperfusion with 5 mM glucose; ○——○ following preperfusion in the absence of glucose. The maximal rate (100%) was 28 mU of IRI released per 30 min and 100 g body weight. Quantitation of IRI is based on pig insulin standards. Each point represents the mean of 3 perfusions and was obtained by measuring the areas under the releasing profiles resulting during the period of exposure to the stimulus. (From MATSCHINSKY *et al.*, unpublished experiments)

Theophylline seems to have little effect on the affinity of the β-cells to glucose but increases the maximal response. As a result the dose-response curve seems to approach the configuration of a hyperbola, a change not readily apparent in the semilogarithmic plot used here. Stimulation of the pancreas by mannose similarly leads to a sigmoidal dose-response curve but the threshold was higher than seen with glucose (ca. 10 mM versus ca. 5 mM, respectively) and the half-maximal response was obtained at approximately 12.5 mM (MALAISSE, 1968). The kinetics of release due to mannose as the sole stimulus have to our knowledge not been investigated. It seems of considerable importance to study in detail the releasing profile and the concentration dependency of the response due to mannose.

Release due to stimulation with glucosamine plus theophylline has the following features (LANDGRAF *et al.*, 1971; MATSCHINSKY *et al.*, 1972b; MATSCHINSKY *et al.*, unpublished experiments). The onset of secretion is delayed and the islets respond with a pronounced off-effect when the two stimuli are removed (Fig. 4). The dose-response curve of release due to glucosamine plus theophylline is sigmoidal and as steep as the dose-response curve due to glucose except that higher levels of glucosamine are actually inhibitory (Fig. 5). The inflection of the curve is between 7.5 and 10 mM of the amino sugar. The development of the off-response is time-dependent, since 6—10 min of exposure to the stimuli elapse before the off-response manifests itself (Fig. 6). The off-response is similarly marked, when theophylline is discontinued without changing the glucosamine levels of the perfusate, but it is only small or not seen at all when glucosamine instead of

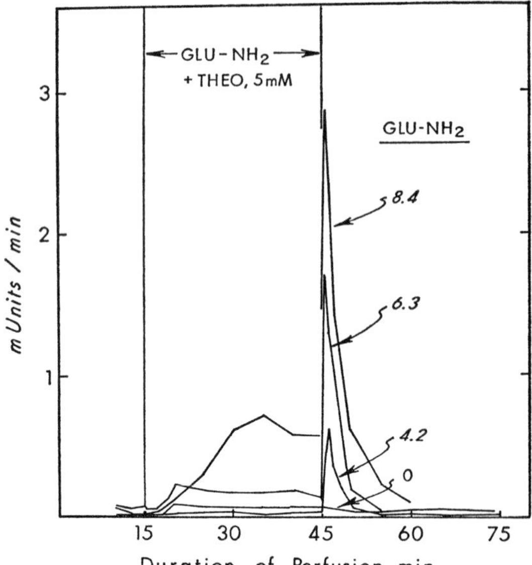

Fig. 4. Releasing profiles due to the addition of glucosamine and theophylline combined. The pancreas was perfused for 15 min with the basic perfusion medium without added fuel and the stimulants were then included for 30 min. Theophylline levels were the same in all experiments (5 mM) but glucosamine was altered as indicated. The means of 3 experiments are given. The data are based on pig insulin as standard. (From MATSCHINSKY *et al.*, unpublished experiments)

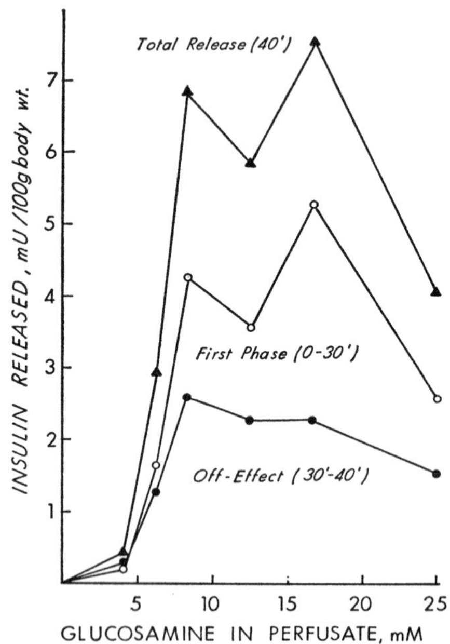

Fig. 5. Concentration dependency of glucosamine-induced insulin release. The data were obtained by measuring the areas under the releasing profiles resulting during and after exposure to the amino sugar (see Fig 4, but note: t_0 in Fig. 5 is equivalent to t_{15} in Fig. 4). Each point represents the mean of three experiments. The quantitation is based on pig insulin standards. (From MATSCHINSKY *et al.*, unpublished experiments)

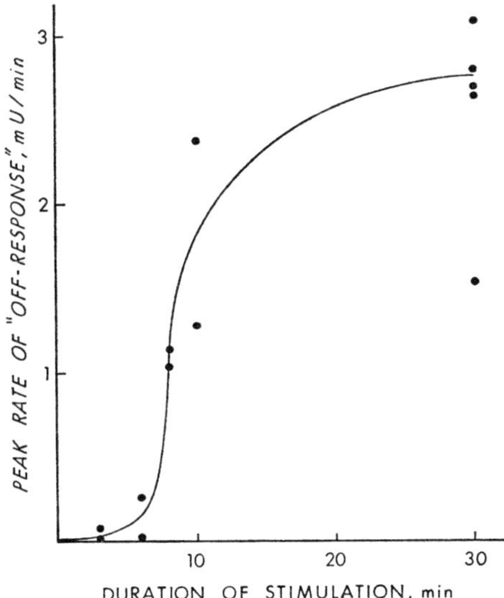

Fig. 6. Temporal development of "off-response" due to glucosamine plus theophylline. The pancreas was exposed to 5 mM theophylline plus 8.4 mM glucosamine for various lengths of time and the peak rate observed after removal of the stimulants is recorded. Each point represents one individual experiment. (From MATSCHINSKY *et al.*, unpublished experiments)

theophylline is discontinued. This indicates that theophylline functions as a partial agonist, an interpretation which is supported by results obtained when the effect of theophylline on glucose-induced insulin secretion was studied. When a square-wave pulse of 5 mM theophylline was applied while the pancreas was continuously perfused with 5 mM glucose, the previously described biphasic response, composed of a slowly rising phase and a marked off-effect, was also observed (MATSCHINSKY *et al.*, 1972b). Higher levels of glucose overcame the apparent inhibitory action of theophylline, the consequence being a pronounced potentiation of the glucose effect. Information about the kinetics of release due to hexoses (fructose and N-acetylglucosamine) which need the presence of low levels of glucose and of theophylline in order to cause release (ASHCROFT *et al.*, 1972a) is very limited. When the pancreas was exposed to a square-wave stimulus consisting of 5 mM glucose, 5 mM theophylline, and 20 mM of fructose (Fig. 7) or N-acetylglucosamine, a monophasic release of insulin occurred (MATSCHINSKY *et al.*, 1972a).

The kinetics of inhibiting glucose-provoked release by glucosamine or mannoheptulose have also received very little attention, although one might expect valuable information from such studies. It was observed for example that 20 mM glucosamine added prior to a glucose stimulus of 20 mM completely prevented release (MATSCHINSKY, unpublished experiments). However, glucosamine inhibited much less potently when release had already been initiated by 20 mM glucose (Fig. 8). In this case addition of the amino sugar caused a rapid but transient blockade of release, followed by a rebound of activity, and finally a steady release which amounted to about 50% of the rate observed in the absence of the inhibitor; when finally the inhibitor was removed a dramatic off-response occurred. The total release due to 20 mM glucose during the period of 1 h allowing for some variation between experiments was the same in the presence and absence of the

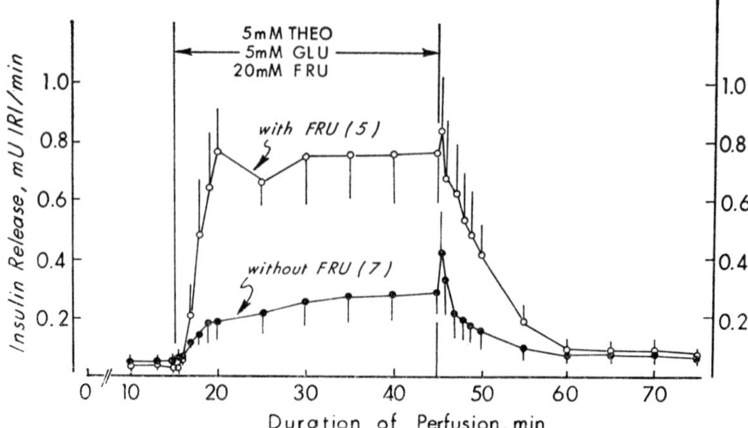

Fig. 7. The permissive effect of glucose plus theophylline on insulin release due to fructose. The means and the standard errors of the means of an indicated number of perfusions are given. In control experiments not shown here high fructose (20 mM) together with low glucose (5 mM) *or* together with theophylline (5 mM) was ineffective. (From Matschinsky *et al.*, 1972a; Matschinsky *et al.*, unpublished experiments)

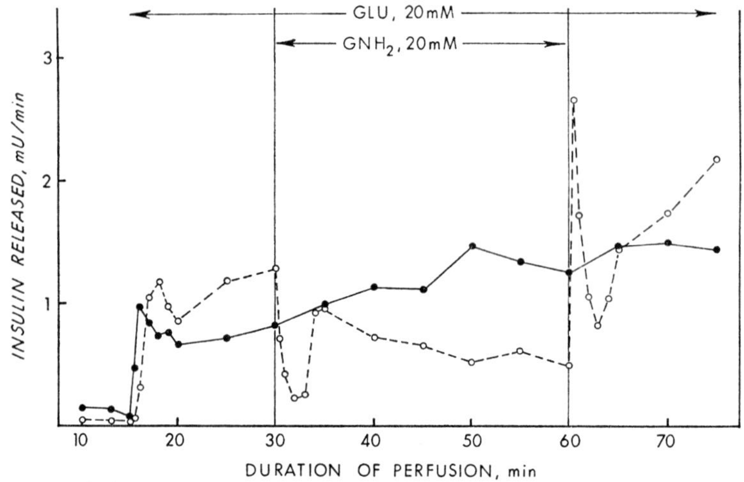

Fig. 8. Kinetics of the blockade of glucose-provoked release by glucosamine. The means of 3 perfusions are shown for each condition. ●——● controls; ○ - - - - ○ experimentals. (From Matschinsky *et al.*, unpublished experiments)

inhibitor. The phenomenon is not easily understood but the results illustrate that the chemosensitivity of the islets can be changed drastically by brief stimulation with glucose. This change of susceptibility to glucosamine is almost certainly not caused by alterations of the hexokinase system which seems to govern the metabolism of hexoses like glucose and glucosamine. Detailed biochemical studies are needed to elucidate the underlying mechanisms. Experiments like the ones described here concerning the interactions between glucose and glucosamine but using mannoheptulose, 2-deoxyglucose, and other glucose analogues might be rewarding.

b) Effects of Polyols and Pentoses

Two other classes of compounds closely related to the hexoses worth noting in this context are pentoses and polyols. Montague and Taylor have presented data indicating insulin release from rat islets due to ribose and ribitol (MONTAGUE and TAYLOR, 1968; MONTAGUE and TAYLOR, 1969; MONTAGUE and TAYLOR, 1970), and there is unanimous agreement that sorbitol and xylitol are also potent releasers, particularly in dog (KUZUYA *et al.*, 1971) and man (KUZUYA *et al.*, 1971) and monkey (WILSON and MARTIN, 1970). The detailed studies of Kuzuya and his collaborators (KUZUYA *et al.*, 1966; KUZUYA and KANAZAWA, 1969; KUZUYA *et al.*, 1969; KUZUYA *et al.*, 1971) leave little doubt about the high efficacy of the polyols. We were able to confirm the results of the Japanese investigators using the dog (MATSCHINSKY *et al.*, unpublished experiments) but were unable to observe release due to xylitol or of combinations of xylitol and theophylline using the isolated perfused rat pancreas (MATSCHINSKY *et al.*, unpublished experiments). Release due to polyols seems to be biphasic as evident from *in vivo* studies (KUZUYA and KANAZAWA, 1969). Detailed physiological and biochemical studies with sorbitol are needed since the sugar alcohol seems to penetrate only comparatively slowly into the β-cells as demonstrated with mouse islets *in vivo* (MATSCHINSKY and ELLERMAN, 1968; LANDGRAF and MATSCHINSKY, 1970). Since a procedure is available for studying insulin release from the isolated perfused dog pancreas (IVERSEN, 1970; IVERSEN and MILES, 1971) respective *in vitro* experiments with polyols seem feasible. Unfortunately it has proven impractical to prepare isolated dog islets for *in vitro* studies using the technically less demanding collagenase methods (LACY, personal communication).

3. The Permissive Action of Glucose Allowing Insulin Release Due to Calorigenic Molecules of Low Molecular Weight

a) Glucose Dependency of Release Due to Various Stimuli

Thorough investigations of possible interrelationship between glucose and other calorigenic molecules in causing insulin release have just been started. These studies are involved and time-consuming since such interactions can be elucidated only by obtaining detailed dose-response relationships using various combinations of glucose and of the compounds in question. Also, intricate interactions on the β-cells must be anticipated, since most of these naturally occurring substances are present in the serum in complex mixtures. The discussion presented here is therefore only a preliminary attempt to analyze this crucial aspect of islet physiology. In this discourse we will emphasize pertinent *in vitro* data, since the most essential variable (i.e. glucose) cannot be altered *in vivo* without provoking a vast spectrum of counter-regulatory measures in the body. We will deal here with the glucose dependency of insulin release due to amino acids, α-ketomonocarboxylic acids, α-hydroxymonocarboxylic acid, free fatty acids, and ketone bodies (FERTEL, 1972; FERTEL *et al.*, 1972; MATSCHINSKY *et al.*, 1972a). The presence of threshold levels of glucose (5 mM) permits many substances to elicit insulin release and seems to potentiate the action of others. In a comprehensive study carried out in the authors' laboratory 34 calorigenic molecules of low molecular weight were examined with the isolated perfused rat pancreas, both in the presence and absence of 5 mM glucose (Table 2). Under the conditions of the experiment only 5 of these compounds (marked in Table 2) caused significant insulin release when glucose was absent from the medium. These glucose-independent stimulators belong without exception in the class of α-ketomonocarboxylic acids. When 5 mM glucose was included in the perfusate 28 of the 34 substances tested exhibited releasing action

Table 2. *The permissive action of glucose*

Agent	Effect in the absence of glucose	Effect in the presence of glucose	Releasing profile in the presence of glucose
Amino acids			
alanine	∅	+	A
α-aminobutyrate	∅	+	A
norvaline	∅	+	A
valine	∅	∅	—
norleucine	∅	+	A
leucine*	∅	+	I
isoleucine	∅	+	B
BCH*	∅	+	I
phenylalanine	∅	+	I
arginine	∅	+	B or D
Fatty acids			
propionate	∅	∅	—
butyrate	∅	+	H
valerate	∅	+	H
isovalerate	∅	+	J
caproate	∅	+	H
isocaproate	∅	+	H
caprylate	(+)	+	H
β,β-dimethylacrylate	∅	+	H
phenylacetate	∅	+	H
Ketone bodies			
acetoacetate	∅	+	C
β-hydroxybutyrate	∅	+	C
α-Ketomonocarboxylic acids			
pyruvate	∅	(+)	—
α-O-butyrate	∅	+	A—B
α-O-valerate	∅	+	C
α-O-isovalerate	∅	+	C
α-O-caproate	+	+	C
α-O-isocaproate	+	+	C
α-O-β-methylvalerate**	∅	+	C
α-O-octanoate**	+	+	G
α-O-nonanoate**	+	+	H
phenylpyruvate	+	+	C
α-hydroxymonocarboxylic acids			
α-OH-isovalerate	∅	+	A
α-OH-caproate	∅	(+)	—
α-OH-isocaproate	∅	(+)	—
α-OH-β-methylvalerate	∅	∅	—
phenyllactate	∅	(+)	—

The results summarized in this table are taken from recent publications of the authors' laboratory (FERTEL, 1972; FERTEL *et al.*, 1972; MATSCHINSKY *et al.*, 1972a). The concentration of the stimulant was usually 5 mM and glucose was 5 mM. The explanations for the capital letters representing different releasing profiles are presented in the legend to Fig. 11. Details about the experimental procedures for obtaining these results are partially given in the legend to Fig. 11 and can be found in the above references.

* It must be noted that leucine and BCH are capable of glucose-independent action, provided the pancreas is preperfused for prolonged periods (see section C. II.).

** In these experiments the level of the stimulant was only 3 mM instead of 5 mM.

(e.g. Fig. 9). But the potency to release varied greatly. The most active substances were α-ketoisocaproate and α-ketocaproate whereas the weakest action was found with valine and with α-hydroxymonocarboxylic acids. In the series of the α-keto-monocarboxylic acids the potency increased with the length of the aliphatic

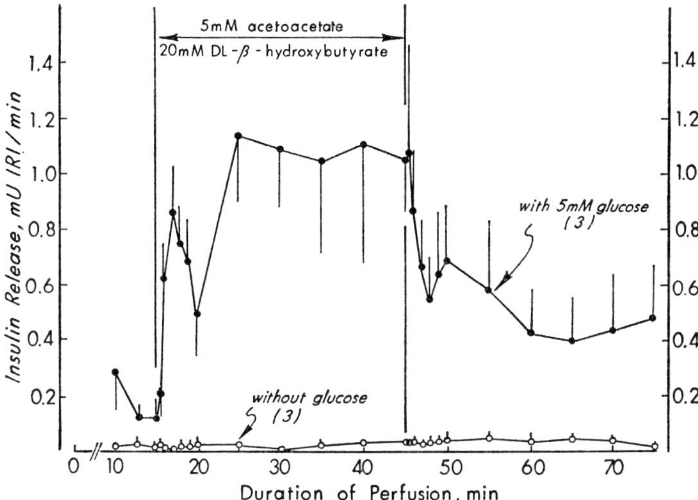

Fig. 9. The permissive effect of glucose on the insulin-releasing action of ketone bodies. The means of 3 experiments and the standard errors are given. Release was induced by a mixture of 5 mM acetoacetate and 20 mM DL-β-hydroxybutyrate, both in the absence and presence of 5 mM glucose, which was included throughout the entire period of perfusion. (From MATSCHINSKY *et al.*, unpublished experiments)

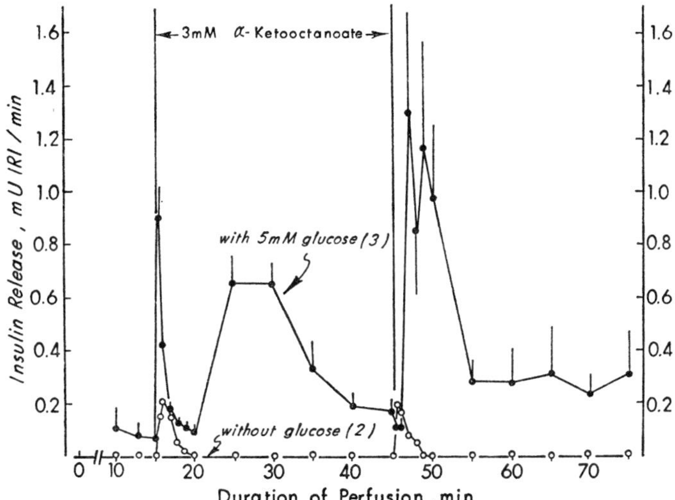

Fig. 10. Multiphasic insulin release due to α-ketooctanoate and the potentiating effect of glucose. The level of the stimulant was 3 mM. The experiment was performed both in the presence and absence of 5 mM glucose, which was present during the entire duration of the perfusion. Means and standard errors of indicated numbers of experiments are shown. (From MATSCHINSKY *et al.*, unpublished experiments)

chain, with pyruvate as the least active member of the group. The straight chain α-ketomonocarboxylic acids with 8 and 9 carbon atoms exhibited stimulatory as well as inhibitory activity (Fig. 10). One congener of the series having an aromatic radical (phenylpyruvate) was a potent glucose-independent agonist. Chain length of the aliphatic portion of the molecule had a similar influence in the series of free fatty acids, propionic acid showing the lowest and caprylic acid the highest activity. At the concentration tested here (5 mM), all fatty acids needed auxiliary amounts of glucose to show a significant releasing action and all of the active fatty acids exhibited stimulatory as well as inhibitory effects.

It is not the purpose of this review to delve deeply into the various features of and possible mechanisms explaining the differing insulin-releasing profiles elicited by the compounds discussed here. This matter is discussed in detail by Grodsky in chapter A of this volume. However, a few comments are in order because of the practical implications that arise when pertinent data from the literature are compared (also see MATSCHINSKY *et al.*, 1972a). Any substance which elicits transient on- or off-responses or both in the perfused pancreas might conceivably be considered as inactive if tested only in long-term incubations with batches of islets or pancreas pieces since the overriding effect would probably be inhibition of release. It is therefore important, if not obligatory, to gather information about the kinetics of release using the isolated perfused pancreas or one of the various systems employed for superfusion of isolated islets or of pancreas

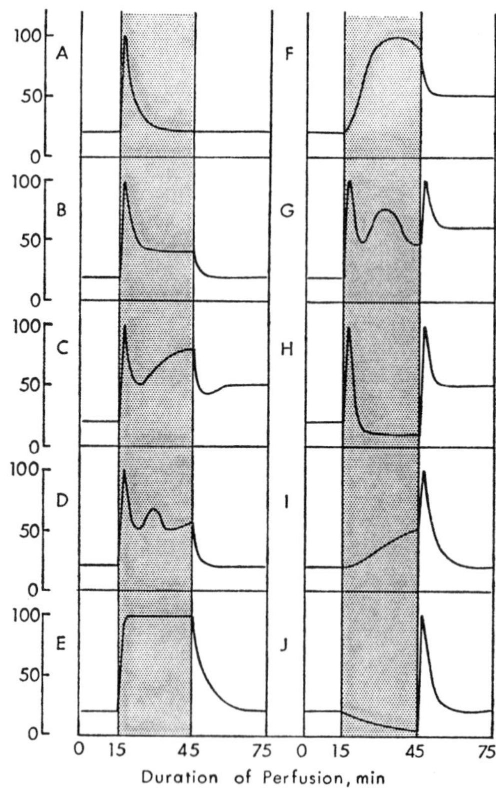

Fig. 11. Patterns of multiphasic insulin release from the isolated perfused rat pancreas. Typical secretion profiles observed with the isolated perfused pancreas are presented. The patterns are schematic drawings and small differences that exist between phenomenologically very similar responses are neglected in the idealized drawings. Relative rates of release are plotted, and for information about the conditions employed and the absolute potency of various substances the original paper should be consulted (MATSCHINSKY *et al.*, 1972a). The figure represents the keys to the last column of Table 2

fragments when the β-cytotropic properties of natural or artificial substances are to be evaluated.

We have observed at least 10 different types of releasing profiles (Fig. 11) (Matschinsky *et al.*, 1972a). These profiles should not be viewed as indicators typical for individual stimuli since the nature of the profiles is clearly concentration-dependent (Fertel, 1972; Matschinsky *et al.*, 1972a). Accordingly, only a complete family of profiles, as one obtains in classical dose-response studies, might be symptomatic for a given substance. Such comprehensive studies are scarce at this point.

The profiles discussed in the following were all obtained in the presence of 5 mM glucose and usually of 5 mM of the stimulant. Significant release was obtained only when the glucose was included in the perfusate except as noted. A peaklike monophasic on-response (Pattern A) was seen with norleucine. The well-known biphasic response (Pattern B) as usually observed with high glucose occurred with all glucose-independent stimulators (i.e. the α-ketoderivatives of caproate, isocaproate, and phenylpropionate) when tested in the absence of glucose. A biphasic pattern followed by poststimulatory superresponsiveness to basal glucose (Pattern C) was seen with many α-ketomonocarboxylic acids, with ketone bodies, and with isoleucine. Multiple peaks (Pattern D) possibly representing damped oscillatory responses were observed with high levels (10 mM) of α-ketoisocaproate. Similar kinetics with two peaks followed by depression resulted with arginine. Here the depression during the later phase of stimulation is probably due to direct inhibition by arginine (Levin *et al.*, 1972). Large monophasic patterns (E), occurred when the pancreas was stimulated with very high levels (40 mM) of α-ketoisocaproate (even in the absence of glucose), with high glucose combined with theophylline, or with high fructose combined with low glucose and theophylline. Leucine or BCH (at 20 mM) caused large monophasic release with slow onset, followed by poststimulatory superresponsiveness to basal glucose (Pattern F). A variety of profiles (Pattern G—J) indicated that certain substances exerted dual actions on the islets, i.e. were partial agonists. On removal of the agent the inhibitory function revealed itself by a dramatic off-response followed in some cases by poststimulatory superresponsiveness (Patterns G, H, and J). Isovalerate caused net inhibition of basal release and exerted stimulation only on removal (Pattern J). Most of these diverse profiles are the expression of the cooperative action of glucose and a single other calorigenic substance of low molecular weight. It was examined whether glucose exerts its permissive effect in an "all or none" or a graded fashion. The glucose-dependent stimulant β-hydroxybutyrate was chosen for that purpose (Fig. 12). Very low levels of glucose (1.25 mM) did not allow release to occur. But the responsiveness to the stimulant rose nearly linearily between glucose levels from 1.25—6.25 mM. Therefore glucose seems to function as a safety device, curbing release in case of hypoglycemia, no matter how high the serum levels of other potential insulin releasers became. Related observations have been made *in vivo* in man (Cerasi and Luft, 1969; Cerasi *et al.*, 1969; Goldfine *et al.*, 1972) and have been interpreted similarly: the releasing actions of arginine (Cerasi and Luft, 1969), tobutamide (Cerasi *et al.*, 1969), and glucagon Goldfine *et al.*, 1972) were shown to be inhibited by hypoglycemia. It seems to be important to investigate the interaction of glucose with mixtures of glucose-dependent releasers since, a priori, such mixtures might stimulate release independently of glucose. The effector action of glucose seems to be highly specific since high fructose (20 mM) and substimulatory levels of mannose (5 mM) could not substitute for glucose (Matschinsky *et al.*, 1972a). But the specificity of the permissive action of glucose has not been tested comprehensively.

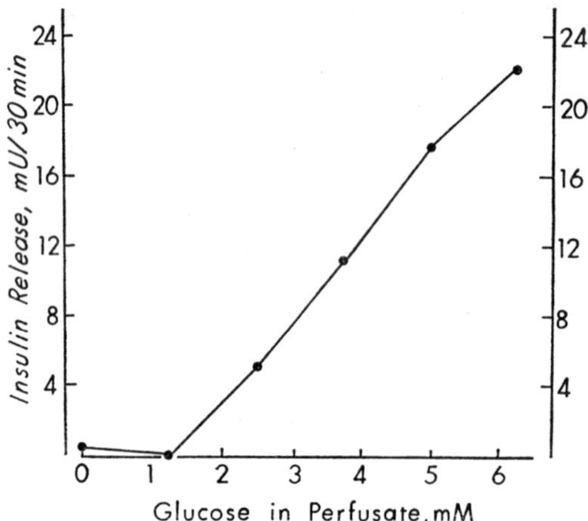

Fig. 12. The concentration dependency of the permissive action of glucose for insulin release due to DL-β-hydroxybutyrate. The isolated pancreas was continuously perfused with glucose at the indicated concentrations and insulin release was measured during 30 min of exposure to 20 mM DL-β-hydroxybutyrate. For illustration of the kinetics see the results obtained with 5 mM glucose given in Fig. 9. The increment of insulin above basal release due to the stimulant is recorded. At each glucose concentration 3 experiments were performed and the average deltas are plotted. (From MATSCHINSKY *et al.*, unpublished experiments)

b) Experimental Alterations of Chemosensitivity of Islets

It was stated earlier that unless basal levels of glucose were in the perfusate, the β-cells did not respond to leucine nor to BCH, which is considered a functional nonmetabolizable analogue of leucine. It is, however, a widely held view that islets can be readily stimulated by leucine and BCH in the absence of glucose (FAJANS *et al.*, 1971). These contradictory results prompted further investigations (MATSCHINSKY *et al.*, 1972a). It was found that the isolated perfused rat pancreas could indeed be stimulated directly by leucine and BCH, provided the organ was preperfused for prolonged periods (ca. 90 min) with saline devoid of glucose and other fuels. The responsiveness to stimulation by glucose was either maintained or actually decreased following the extended rinsing of the tissue. Currently it is not possible to decide whether the results obtained during the early or the late stage of perfusion are representative for the situation *in vivo*. High leucine sensitivity has been observed *in vivo* following treatment of man and animals with sulfonylurea derivatives (FAJANS *et al.*, 1967). Leucine hypersensitivity arises also for unknown reasons in a certain group of children and finally in patients afflicted by islet cell tumors of the pancreas (DI GEORGE and AUERBACH, 1960). It seems important to find out whether pretreatment of rats with chlorpropamide will render the leucine response of the isolated perfused pancreas entirely glucose-independent. It is presently also not clear whether arginine is a glucose-dependent or -independent stimulus. Studies with the isolated perfused pancreas performed in the authors' laboratory showed that the pancreas was not responsive to 20 mM arginine when glucose was absent, even on repeated exposure, whereas Grodsky's group demonstrated glucose-independent stimulation by arginine (LEVIN *et al.*, 1972). It is conceivable that the sensitivity of the β-cells to arginine is similarly a function of the pretreatment of the pancreas as described here for the case of leucine. Furthermore, it is not clear at this point whether the actions of other substances which are apparently glucose-dependent might similarly be affected by prolonged perfusion of the pancreas with glucose-free solutions.

The changes of chemosensitivity seen during extended perfusion of the pancreas seem important in evaluating results with leucine and possibly other substances reported in the literature. Since in most instances isolated pancreatic islets were employed the isolation of which requires lengthy procedures, or since the effect of a stimulant on pancreas pieces was usually tested after prolonged preincubation, one should not be surprised to find leucine hypersensitivity in view of the above results with the perfused pancreas (MATSCHINSKY *et al.*, 1972a). The mechanisms underlying changing chemosensitivity as defined here are presently not understood but a better knowledge of the factors involved in the process might prove rewarding in view of the fact that diabetes can be considered a special manifestation of altered chemosensitivity of the islets of Langerhans.

4. Metabolic Function of Hexoses in the Islets of Langerhans

a) Stimulation of Glycolysis and Respiration in Islets by Various Hexoses

The more general aspects of energy metabolism of the islets are discussed by C. HELLERSTRÖM in another chapter of this volume. But certain specific metabolic functions of hexoses in islet cells must be considered here in sufficient detail to allow a discussion of possible mechanisms explaining the releasing actions of hexoses.

It is now well established that exposure of islets to graded levels of glucose leads to a corresponding graded increase of glucose metabolism as manifested by increased O_2-consumption (HELLERSTRÖM, 1967; HELLERSTRÖM *et al.*, 1970; ANDERSON and HELLERSTRÖM, 1972), glucose usage (ASHCROFT *et al.*, 1972b; REESE *et al.*, 1973), lactate formation (ASHCROFT *et al.*, 1970; ASHCROFT *et al.*, 1972a; MATSCHINSKY and ELLERMAN, 1973; REESE *et al.*, 1973), and CO_2 production (ASHCROFT *et al.*, 1970; ASHCROFT *et al.*, 1972a; ASHCROFT *et al.*, 1972b). Stimulation of glycolysis is 5—7 fold on exposure to high levels of glucose as indicated by the formation of ^3H_2O from glucose labeled in the 5 position (ASHCROFT *et al.*, 1972b; PACE and MATSCHINSKY, unpublished) and by the production of lactate (ASHCROFT *et al.*, 1972a; MATSCHINSKY and ELLERMAN, 1973). Glucose at high levels becomes the preferred substrate for respiration as demonstrated by the formation of CO_2 from glucose which is greatly enhanced compared to the only moderate augmentation of oxygen consumption (HELLERSTRÖM, 1967; HELLERSTRÖM *et al.*, 1970; ANDERSON and HELLERSTRÖM, 1972). Other sugars were also tested as fuels of respiration. It was found that galactose was unable to serve as substrate (JARRETT and KEEN, 1968) but that fructose and mannose were converted to CO_2 at rates amounting to approximately 15 and 40%, respectively, of the rate observed with glucose (ASHCROFT *et al.*, 1970; JARRETT and KEEN, 1968). Since a large and variable fraction of the sugars might be converted to lactate under the conditions used for measuring the rate of CO_2 formation, the rate of lactate formation by islets was measured on exposure to 27.5 mM each of glucose, fructose, and mannose and it was found that the rates were nearly the same in all three cases, i.e. 96 ± 6.2 (3), 79.5 ± 12.8 (3), and 87.4 ± 24 (3) picomoles of lactate formed per rat islet per hour (ELLERMAN and MATSCHINSKY, unpublished). These results demonstrate that the rate of CO_2 formation is not always a valid measure of the metabolic consequences of a given substance. It is obvious that measurements of net lactate formation do not allow a conclusion as to whether the lactate is derived directly from the exogenous fuel or from endogenous sources, as for instance from glycogen stores in the islets, or whether exogenous as well as endogenous sources contribute to the lactate. But whatever the origin of the lactate, it is apparent that exposure of islets to equimolar levels of glucose, fructose, or mannose leads in all three cases to a marked stimulation of glycolysis. The molecular mechanisms which underly the stimulation of glycolysis due to exposure of high levels of sugars are not entirely clear. In earlier studies evidence was found that the islets of Langerhans were endowed with a hexokinase exhibiting a high K_m for glucose, which seemed to explain the stimulation of metabolism due to glucose (MATSCHINSKY and ELLERMAN, 1968; ASHCROFT and RANDLE, 1970). But the experimental basis of this proposal is open to criticism (MATSCHINSKY, 1972).

It seems more likely on the basis of more recent results that stimulation of glycolysis is indirect and is a consequence of Na^+-dependent transmembraneous transport systems (ASHCROFT *et al.*, 1972a; MATSCHINSKY and ELLERMAN, 1973): sugars enter the cells jointly with Na^+; the increased intracellular Na^+ level in turn drives the Na^+ pump which needs energy for its operation; the enhanced

Table 3. *Effects of phlorizin, cytochalasin B, ouabain and Na^+ deficiency on the stimulation of glycolysis by glucose and 3-O-methyl glucose*

Incubation Conditions	Glucose, 27.5 mM (16.5 mM in CB studies)	3-OMG, 27.5 mM Glucose, 5.5 mM
	lactate formation, picomoles/islet × hour	
Phlorizin		
none	78.0 ± 7.0 (3)	67.2 ± 5.3 (6)
0.5 mM	—	47.1 (2)
1.5 mM	44.5 ± 6.5 (3)	30.8 ± 2.2 (3)
4.5 mM	10.7 ± 0.7 (3)	2.2 (2)
Cytochalasin B		
none, 0.007% solvent	56.2 ± 1.4 (10)	50.8 ± 2.3 (3)
10.5 μM	38.4 ± 1.7 (3)	33.9 ± 4.9 (3)
21.0 μM	20.4 ± 3.8 (3)	18.6 ± 1.7 (3)
63.0 μM	17.7 ± 4.3 (3)	6.2 ± 1.7 (3)
Ouabain		
none	78.0 ± 7.0 (3)	67.2 ± 5.3 (6)
0.2 mM	—	44.5 ± 5.1 (3)
1.0 mM	38.2 ± 2.4 (3)	29.6 ± 6.1 (3)
5.0 mM	10.4 ± 1.5 (3)	6.6 ± 0.7 (3)
Sodium replacement		
Control *a*	65.0 ± 4.4 (5)	46.7 ± 3.4 (5)
LiCl	30.3 ± 3.5 (3)	16.4 ± 0.1 (3)
Control *b* for Li^+	61.0 ± 7.7 (3)	49 (2)
Choline chloride	28.1 ± 4.6 (3)	21.3 ± 0.7 (3)
Control *b* for choline	55.2 ± 7.0 (3)	43.8 (2)
KCl	30.0 ± 4.7 (3)	26.5 ± 6.7 (3)
Control *b* for K^+	63.0 ± 12.2 (3)	48.1 (2)

For experiments with phlorizin, cytochalasin B (CB), and ouabain, the rate of lactate formation is the average of two incubation periods. The solvent for CB (Imperial Chemical Industries, Macclesfield, England) was dimethyl formamide which at the concentrations used (0.0012 to 0.007%) inhibited lactate formation only slightly (15% or less). When studying Na^+ replacement, $KHCO_3$ was substituted for $NaHCO_3$ in all solutions and NaCl was replaced by either LiCl, choline chloride, or KCl. For efficient removal of Na^+, islets were incubated for two 30 min periods in the respective glucose-free Na^+-deficient media; lactate formation was finally determined in a third 45 min period in which 27.5 mM glucose or 3-OMG were added, the latter together with 5.5 mM glucose. Two types of controls were performed in the Na^+-deficiency studies: Type *a* controls were treated like the experimental samples, except for the presence of Na^+, i.e. no sugar was present for the first two 30 min periods. Type *b* controls were run after the periods of Na^+-deficiency to determine if the islets were still viable. For this purpose, the Na^+-deficient medium was removed, the islets were washed with 300 μl of medium containing normal NaCl and then incubated with hexoses in 100 μl of medium with normal NaCl. The means of an indicated number of experiments are recorded ± SEM for the number of samples in parentheses. (From MATSCHINSKY and ELLERMAN, 1973).

energy demand is the signal for glycolysis and respiration to increase. This concept is also consistent with the results of recent studies demonstrating that non-metabolizable sugars, for instance 3-O-methyl-glucose and D-galactose, greatly enhance lactate formation from basal glucose levels (MATSCHINSKY and ELLERMAN, 1973) and is compatible with the fact that this stimulation can be interfered with by compounds that seem to inhibit sugar transport: by phlorizin (HELLMAN *et al.*, 1970) and cytochalasin B (ESTENSEN and PLAGEMANN, 1972; KLETZIEN *et al.*, 1972), by ouabain, the classical inhibitor of Na^+-K^+-ATPase (SCHATZMAN, 1953), and by various means of Na^+ deficiency (Table 3). That the transport of Na^+ plays such a profound role in regulating energy metabolism is further established by the metabolic consequences of amino-acid transport. It was shown in our laboratory that lactate formation from basal glucose was stimulated on exposure to 10 mM of L-isoleucine, BCH, or valine. The rates of glycolysis observed in these experiments were comparable to the rates resulting from incubation of islets in high glucose (ELLERMAN and MATSCHINSKY, unpublished). Respective experiments with other amino acids or with mixtures of amino acids and employing Na^+ deficiency and ouabain as experimental tools have not been performed as yet.

b) Dissociations of Metabolic and Insulin-Releasing Actions of Hexoses

The fuel function of hexoses seems to parallel their releasing function as pointed out by many investigators in the field (GRODSKY *et al.*, 1963; JARRETT and KEEN, 1968; MALAISSE, 1968; RANDLE *et al.*, 1968; ASHCROFT *et al.*, 1970; LAMBERT, 1970; ASHCROFT *et al.*, 1972a). This apparent association of the two functions of sugars forms the foundation of the metabolism hypothesis of insulin

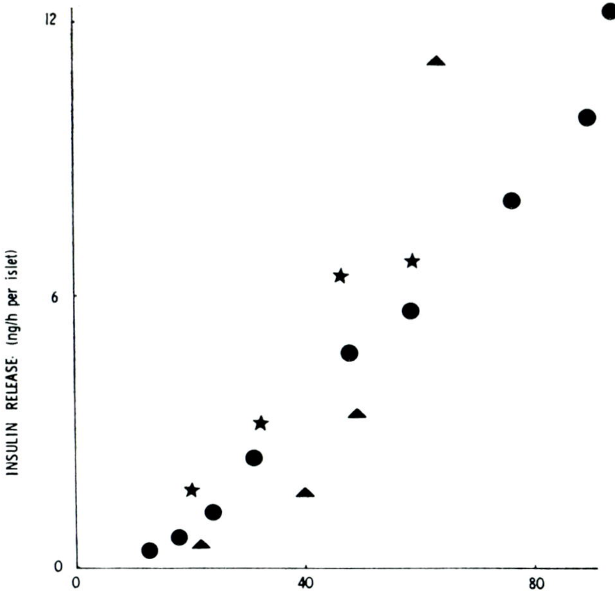

Fig. 13. Correlation between glucose utilization and insulin secretion in mouse islets. (y = 5.74× + 18.8; v = 0.94; p ≤ 0.001) ● glucose only, ▲ glucose + mannoheptulose (see text), ★ glucose + glucosamine (see text). (With permission from ASHCROFT *et al.*, 1972a)

release due to sugars (RANDLE *et al.*, 1968). This hypothesis states that glucose (or any other sugar or sugar derivative capable of stimulating release) must be metabolized and that changes of one critical metabolite or cofactor or changes of the metabolite or cofactor constellation trigger secretion in an as yet unexplained fashion. The correlation between rates of hexose oxidation and insulin secretion is indeed remarkable. This is illustrated here by one striking example (Fig. 13) (ASHCROFT *et al.*, 1972a). It was shown that a linear correlation exists between rates of glucose utilization and insulin secretion at a number of glucose concentrations between 1.8—17 mM and with varying mannoheptulose concentrations (0.5—15 mM) or glucosamine concentrations (5—20 mM) both at 18.4 mM glucose.

On thorough evaluation of all available data it cannot be overlooked, however, that the coupling between the insulin releasing and metabolic functions of hexoses is not absolute. There are several experimental conditions known in which glucose accomplishes release in spite of the fact that glucose metabolism is inhibited by various means. And, equally important, glycolysis can be stimulated without leading to release as one would expect if the theory were true. These conditions are:

1) Inhibition of glucose transport into islets
   a) By phlorizin (HELLMAN *et al.*, 1970)
2) Prevention of Na^+ entry or of the metabolic consequences of an increased Na^+ load
   a) Na^+ replacement by choline chloride (MALAISSE, 1972)
   b) Ouabain (SCHATZMAN, 1953; BURR *et al.*, 1971)
3) Inhibition of glycolysis by
   a) Iodoacetate (ALEYASSINE, 1970; MATSCHINSKY and ELLERMAN, 1973)
   b) Fluoride (ALEYASSINE, 1970)
   c) Cytochalasin B (MATSCHINSKY and ELLERMAN, 1973)
4) Stimulation of glycolysis by sugars or amino acids that do not cause release
   a) Galactose and 3-O-methyl glucose (MATSCHINSKY and ELLERMAN, 1973)
   b) Valine, D-isoleucine and b (+)-BCH (ELLERMAN and MATSCHINSKY, unpublished)

Three such examples are discussed here: cytochalasin B (20—30 μg/ml incubation fluid) substantially inhibits lactate formation from 16.5 mM glucose (75% or more, see Table 3). These concentrations potentiate insulin release due to glucose with isolated islets (MALAISSE *et al.*, 1972). Low levels of iodoacetate (0.2 mM) completely block lactate formation from glucose but do not interfere with insulin release due to glucose (MATSCHINSKY *et al.*, 1972a; MATSCHINSKY and ELLERMAN, 1973) (Fig. 14). The nonmetabolizable sugar 3-O-methyl glucose does not cause release from isolated islets or in the isolated perfused pancreas but is nevertheless a potent activator of glycolysis provided basal levels of glucose are in the medium serving as fuel for glycolysis (see Table 3). These examples serve to show that glycolysis can be inhibited without blocking glucose-provoked release and that glycolysis can be stimulated without causing release of insulin.

Studies of glucosamine metabolism by islets revealed that compared to glucose the amino sugar is a poor substrate for glycolysis, both in the presence and absence of theophylline (Fig. 15) (ELLERMAN and MATSCHINSKY, unpublished). This is further emphasized by the finding that the appearance of lactate in the incubation medium following exposure to low and high glucosamine alone or in combination with theophylline was delayed by as much as 45 min (ELLERMAN and MATSCHINSKY, unpublished). The cause of this delay is presently not known. It is not yet possible to conduct a quantitative comparison of the relative potencies of glucose and glucosamine as insulin releasers with their relative efficiency as substrates for

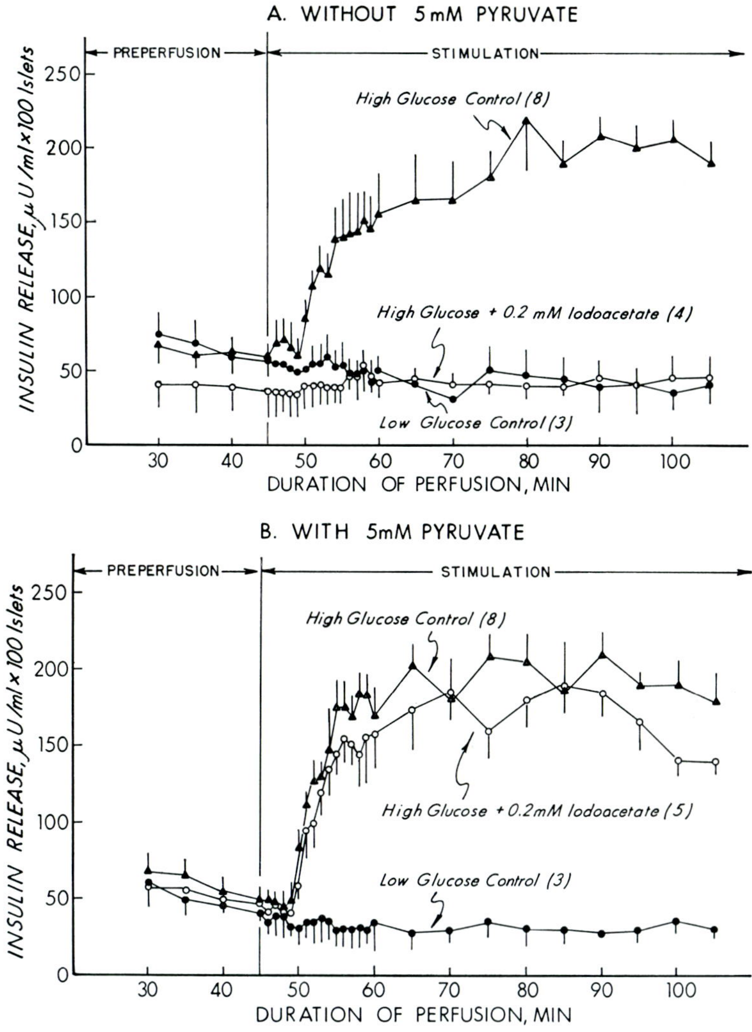

Fig. 14. Effect of iodoacetate on glucose-provoked insulin release in the presence or absence of pyruvate. Batches of 100 islets each were perfused with buffered saline containing 0.5% bovine serum albumin. The flow rate was 1 ml/min. Pyruvate was absent in A and present in B at 5 mM concentration throughout. Low glucose controls had 5.5 mM throughout. High glucose samples had 5.5 mM in the preperfusion period and 27.5 mM glucose during stimulation with or without iodoacetate present throughout as indicated. The means of indicated numbers of experiments are given. Standard errors are recorded except where this would interfere with clarity. (From MATSCHINSKY *et al.*, 1972a; MATSCHINSKY and ELLERMAN, 1973)

glycolysis, because of experimental inconsistencies between metabolic and releasing studies. But the data collected to date seem to point out that the releasing and fuel functions of glucosamine might be independent of each other (MATSCHINSKY *et al.*, 1972a). Some caution in interpreting these data is however indicated since the rate of lactate formation may not always be a valid measure of glycolytic flux. Concomitant studies using the measurement of glucose and glucosamine usage or of CO_2 production from glucose and glucosamine are needed before the evidence presented can be accepted as conclusive.

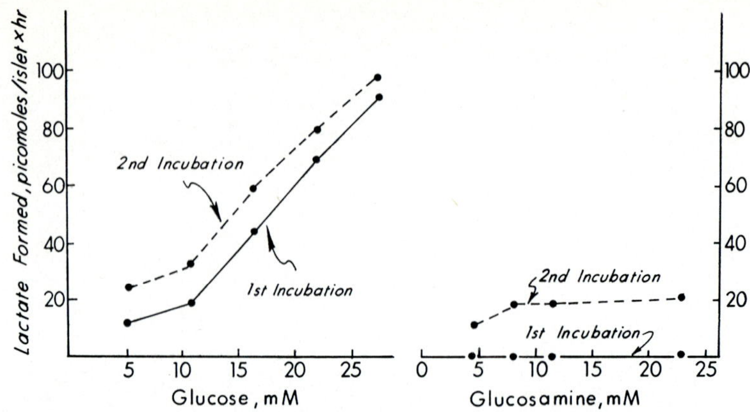

Fig. 15. Lactate formation of isolated islets stimulated by glucose and glucosamine in the presence of theophylline. Batches of 50—100 islets were incubated in the presence of indicated levels of sugar plus 5 mM theophylline. The lactate production during two consecutive incubation periods lasting 45 min each was measured by a fluorometric micromethod (MATSCHINSKY and ELLERMAN, 1973). As little as 10^{-10} moles of lactate formed by 100 islets during 45 min were accurately determined, i.e. a few picomoles/islet × hour. (From ELLERMAN and MATSCHINSKY, unpublished)

c) Dissociation of Metabolic and Permissive Functions of Glucose

It was discussed earlier that glucose plays an essential permissive role for a wide variety of stimulators of insulin release. This permissive action of glucose is usually ascribed to its fuel function. But a number of arguments can be brought forth which speak strongly against this possibility.

1) Even substances which are themselves suitable fuels for the islets (HELLMAN *et al.*, 1971) may, under certain conditions, need glucose for eliciting their action (e.g. leucine) MATSCHINSKY *et al.*, 1972a).

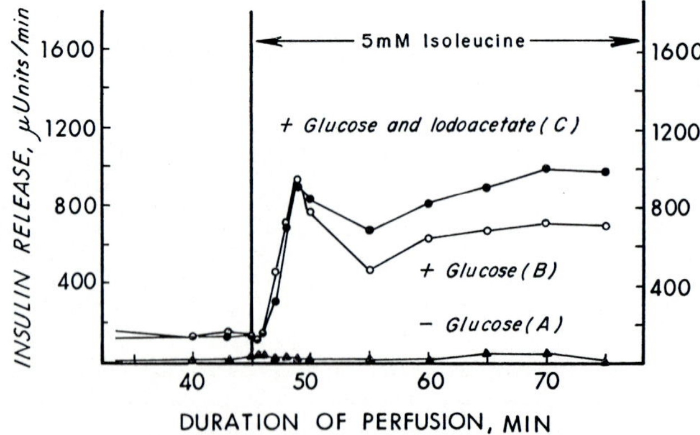

Fig. 16. Differential effect of iodoacetate on glycolytic breakdown of glucose and its regulator function. The pancreases were perfused with dextran-saline containing 0.5 mM pyruvate and 2.5 mM lactate in all three conditions (A—C), 5 mM glucose in experiment B and C and 0.2 mM iodoacetate in experiment C. At the end of the preperfusion period of 45 min L-isoleucine (5 mM) was added in all three experiments The means of 3 perfusions each are recorded. (From MATSCHINSKY *et al.*, 1972a)

2) Fructose, which is readily metabolized by islets, cannot substitute for glucose, even when increased to 20 mM. Mannose, at 5 mM, is also an ineffective substitute (MATSCHINSKY *et al.*, 1972a).

3) Iodoacetate, at a concentration which at low levels (0.2 mM) specifically blocks glycolysis, does not interfere with the permissive role of glucose (MATSCHINSKY *et al.*, 1972a).

One example is chosen here to illustrate the point: the permissive action of glucose on isoleucine-provoked insulin release (MATSCHINSKY *et al.*, 1972a) is not prevented by iodoacetate (Fig. 16).

d) The Significance of Metabolite and Cofactor Levels in Islets Exposed to Glucose and Other Substrates

The metabolism theory of glucose stimulation of insulin release implies that alterations of some metabolite of glucose or a complex change of the metabolite pattern due to glucose, rather than the glucose molecule itself, trigger insulin release from the β-cells (MATSCHINSKY and ELLERMAN, 1968; RANDLE *et al.*, 1968). To be an effective trigger, sufficient level changes of such metabolites should occur prior to the endocrine response. Also, since the endocrine response is graded one might expect the level changes of the metabolites involved to be similarly graded in nature. An extensive search for such (a) hypothetical trigger molecule(s) was undertaken and metabolites as well as cofactors of metabolism were measured in islets by a number of investigators. Such measurements were performed in batches of isolated islets exposed to glucose *in vitro* or they were performed in freeze-dried fragments of islets obtained from mouse or rat pancreas following exposure to glucose *in vivo* as well as in the isolated perfused pancreas. The initial results obtained with mouse islets about the behavior of glucose-6-P levels during hyperglycemia (MATSCHINSKY and ELLERMAN, 1968; IDAHL, 1970) seemed to support the hypothesis. It was found in these studies that this first strategic metabolite rose rapidly and significantly on exposure to glucose *in vivo*. Prolonged incubation of isolated mouse islets in high glucose similarly caused an elevation of glucose-6-P (ASHCROFT *et al.*, 1970). But when this line of study was further pursued, using the rat it was observed that changes of glucose-6-P and of other glucose metabolites occurred usually much slower than the endocrine response; and in cases when they did occur sufficiently fast, they were not always associated with release (MONTAGUE and TAYLOR, 1968; MATSCHINSKY *et al.*, 1970; MATSCHINSKY *et al.*, 1971a; MATSCHINSKY *et al.*, 1971b).

The metabolism hypothesis has received some boost from a recent report by Gabbay (GABBAY and TZE, 1972), who implicated sorbitol as a crucial metabolite of glucose in the release mechanism. He formulated this proposal, since certain inhibitors of aldose reductase (glutaric acid derivatives and colchicine) interfered with glucose-provoked insulin release. The difficulty with this hypothesis is that the aldose reductase inhibitors also interfere with release due to tolbutamide and that it neglects essential aspects of hexose-induced insulin release: mannose and glucosamine are potent stimulators of release but do not seem to serve as substrates for aldose reductase (HAYMAN and KINOSHITA, 1965); mannoheptulose, glucosamine, and 2-deoxyglucose block glucose-provoked release but seem to lack affinity to aldose reductase. The new proposal is also incompatible with the observation that a large percentage of the so-called aldose reductase inhibitors (α-ketooctanoate and caprylate, to mention just two) are in fact stimulators of insulin release (FERTEL, 1972; FERTEL *et al.*, 1972; MATSCHINSKY *et al.*, 1972a).

Possible involvement of metabolism in the release mechanism was also studied by indirect methods. PANTEN and his collaborators have used surface fluorescence measurements of the pyridine nucleotide system for this purpose (PANTEN *et al.*, 1972). They have found that isolated mouse islets exhibit rapid enhancement of fluorescence when stimulated with glucose, leucine, or α-ketoisocaproate and have taken this as evidence for direct involvement of metabolism in the release mechanism. The discussions in the preceding pages have shown that it seems possible to dissociate the metabolic and fuel function of hexoses. Analogous experiments should be performed using surface fluorescence instead of lactate formation or glucose usage as a parameter for studying the involvement of metabolism in the release mechanism. It promises to be very revealing in this connection to use nonmetabolizable releasers, as for instance α-aminoisobutyric acid (LAMBERT *et al.*, 1971), BCH (CHRISTENSEN and CULLEN, 1969; TAGER and CHRISTENSEN, 1971), and dimethylacrylic acid (RAYBAUD and MATSCHINSKY, unpublished), as agents when studying surface fluorescence. Such experiments will provide test cases for deciding whether increased surface fluorescence might be a secondary event merely manifesting enhanced usage of endogenous fuel.

5. Interactions of Hexoses and Alloxan in Islets

Alloxan, injected intravenously, leads to a rapid and highly selective destruction of the pancreatic beta-cells (DUNN *et al.*, 1943) with ensuing diabetes (DUNN and MCLETCHIE, 1943). For review of the nature of alloxan diabetes see RERUP (1970). At least three sugars, i.e. glucose, 3-O-methyl glucose and mannose are able to block the action of alloxan directly at the level of the β-cells. Alloxan might therefore be considered a useful tool for studying the chemical nature of glucose binding sites in the β-cells. A brief discussion of respective results seemed therefore an essential part of this review.

BHATTACHARYA (1953, 1954) first noted that glucose and mannose were effective antagonists of alloxan action. He suggested that alloxan induces diabetes by hexokinase inhibition. CARTER and YOUNATHAN (1962) reported that 3-O-methyl glucose, a nonmetabolizable sugar, inhibited alloxan diabetes. This observation cast considerable doubt on the hexokinase theory of alloxan action, since this sugar is not a substrate for hexokinase (SOLS and CRANE, 1954; SOLS, 1956).

SCHEYNIUS and TALJEDAL (1971) demonstrated that mannoheptulose, an inhibitor of glucose-stimulated insulin release, blocked the protective effects of glucose against alloxan diabetes, whereas mannoheptulose itself had no protective effect. These authors interpreted these data as suggesting that glucose and alloxan do not compete for a common site on the β-cell membrane and proposed that protection against alloxan diabetes by glucose might result from an indirect conformational change in the β-cell membrane induced by glucose. Protection possibly involves a specific receptor site, a transport site, or glucose metabolism. ZAWALICH and BEIDLER (1973) extended these observations and showed that mannoheptulose could also block the protective action of mannose and of 3-O-methyl glucose against alloxan diabetes. They thought that alloxan and glucose might indeed compete for a similar membrane site, either a receptor or transport site, and that this site might be involved in stimulating insulin release. If this interpretation were correct, 3-O-methyl glucose would be expected to interfere with glucose-provoked insulin release, which is apparently not the case. Applying microelectrode recording technics to the β-cells, DEAN and MATTHEWS (1970) showed that these cells were reversibly depolarized by glucose and mannose. They also reported that alloxan caused an irreversible depolarization of the β-cell membrane. This effect could be prevented by prior incubation with glucose (DEAN and MATTHEWS, 1968). In a later paper these authors (DEAN and MATTHEWS, 1972) showed that only glucose could prevent the irreversible alloxan depolarization. Mannoheptulose, glucosamine, and surprisingly, 3-O-methyl glucose were ineffective in preventing alloxan action. They argued for alloxan binding to a glucoreceptor site.

It seems of significance in this context that we observed alloxan-induced insulin secretion from the isolated perfused rat pancreas which could not be prevented by 30 mM of 3-O-methyl glucose. Apparently 3-O-methyl glucose interacts with alloxan at killing sites, leading to cell necrosis, but not at the insulin-releasing sites of alloxan responsible for depolarization of the β-cells (MATSCHINSKY *et al.*, unpublished).

While it is abundantly clear that alloxan and the hexoses glucose, mannose, and 3-O-methyl glucose interact at the level of the beta cells, the nature of the interaction remains unknown. If alloxan indeed binds to or chemically alters a glucoreceptor system involved with insulin discharge, as indicated by the discussion, it may prove to be an invaluable tool in the isolation and characterization of the receptor.

6. Electrophysiological Effects of Hexoses on Islet Cells

An important aspect in characterizing the biophysical responses of the β-cells to hexoses is the extent to which the electrical responses parallel the secretory responses. (For a more detailed discussion of the electrical phenomena of the β-cell membrane see Chapter C, VI in this volume). DEAN and MATTHEWS (1970) showed that increasing the level of glucose elicits electrical activity in a greater percentage of the population of cells impaled. Alteration of their technic to allow continuous recording of the spike activity in a single cell revealed that there was a graded increase in the frequency (spikes/second) of the electrical discharges as the level of glucose in the superfusate was raised (PACE and PRICE, 1972). This experimental approach also permitted an investigation of the immediate electrical responses of the islet cells as they were elicited by pulses of varying concentrations of stimulant compounds. Consequently, it was found that when the level of either glucose, mannose, or fructose was increased, the level of response attained its maximum intensity rapidly and a new level of activity was maintained within the time period recorded (usually five minutes.) Furthermore, when the concentration of sugar was decreased, the frequency of firing declined rapidly, reaching a new level. The transitions in the spike activity were usually completed within 2 min. Additionally, the electrical responses to a sugar were observed to be reversible whether immediately preceded by a higher or lower concentration.

Examples of the spontaneous activity of islet cells and the spike activity induced by glucose, mannose, and fructose are shown (Fig. 17, PACE, 1974). By examining the spontaneous activity of the three cells shown in the absence of sugar, it is clear that the variations in the qualitative pattern of firing are a property of the cell rather than a unique pattern induced by a given sugar.

Quantitative analysis of the electrophysiological data yielded a dissociation constant, Kd, of 8.9 mM and 11.3 mM for glucose and mannose, respectively (PACE and PRICE, 1972). These values compare favorably with the sugar levels leading to half-maximal secretory responses of rat pancreatic pieces, i.e. 9.7 and 13.9 mM for glucose and mannose, respectively (MALAISSE, 1968). Fructose is a relatively weak stimulus for insulin secretion (GRODSKY *et al.*, 1963; SUSSMAN *et al.*, 1966) and was found to be a weak stimulus for the electrical activity as well (Kd = 21.8 mM) (PACE *et al.*, 1974).

Attempts to find cells that exhibited electrical activity in response to galactose had only very limited success: only 2 out of 12 cells that responded initially to glucose (16.6 mM) also responded to galactose (16.6 mM) (PACE *et al.*, 1974). This

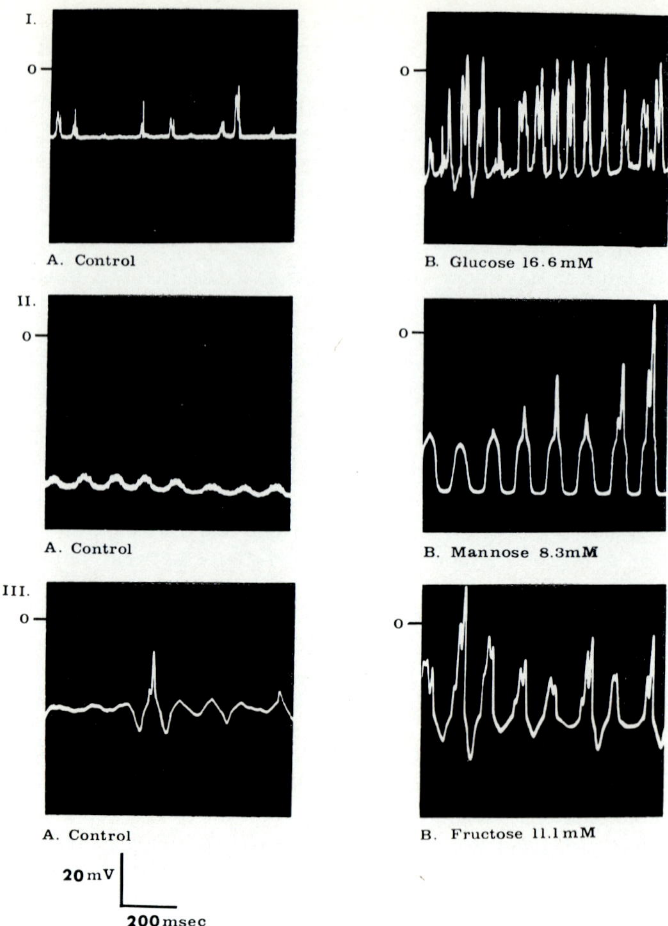

Fig. 17. Records of spontaneous activity of islet cells and of the electrical activity induced by glucose, mannose, and fructose. Each roman numeral indicates the electrical activity recorded in a single cell in the absence (A) and in the presence (B) of sugar (From PACE and PRICE, 1974)

result is intriguing in view of the fact that galactose is usually reported to be non-stimulatory (see Table 1 for references). The possibility exists that the failure of galactose to induce spike activity in a large proportion of islet cells may account for its inability to serve as a strong secretory stimulant at any concentration.

In view of the quantitative similarity of the effects of hexoses on the electrical and secretory responses, it is reasonable to consider that both phenomena are related in some manner.

7. A Possible Model Explaining the Multiple Actions of Glucose on the ß-Cells

The studies concerning the mechanism of glucose action on the β-cells have progressed to a point where it seems fruitful to formulate a working hypothesis explaining most actions of the glucose molecule. (It must be noted, however, that the hypothesis to be presented does not consider the mechanisms involved in the well-known glucose stimulation of *de novo* synthesis of insulin.)

It is obvious that a number of simplifying assumptions and definitions must be made to render such a model manageable and testable. These are: functional differences that might exist between β-cells are neglected; the influence of intercellular communication possibly connecting numerous β-cells to functional units is disregarded; the terms "glucoreceptor", "releasing site", or "permissive site" indicate molecular entities common to all β-cells rather than denoting specialized cell types within the islets.

The data collected in this review led us to believe that the β-cells are stimulated by the glucose molecule itself rather than by the energy derived from its catabolism or by possible alterations of metabolite and cofactor profiles connected with increased flux through glycolysis and citric acid cycle. Both the releasing action and the permissive action of glucose seem to be largely independent of catabolism. Reasons for adopting this version of the glucoreceptor theory are once more summarized here in concise form (Matschinsky *et al.*, 1972b).

1) A number of sugars and sugar derivatives, which are probably metabolized very slowly or not at all or which seem to penetrate the β-cells very poorly are potent stimulators or modulators of insulin release.

2) The metabolic function of glucose can be largely dissociated from its direct as well as its indirect (i.e. permissive or potentiator) releasing function.

3) Levels of metabolites and cofactors involved in glucose metabolism in pancreatic islets are precisely maintained even when the metabolic flux is increased several fold, indicating that alteration of metabolic profiles is an unlikely mechanism for triggering release due to glucose.

According to the present information there might be as many as three hexose sites in the β-cells (Fig. 18): two of these are postulated since it was found with isolated islets and with the isolated perfused pancreas that fructose, N-acetylglucosamine and, less consistently, galactose require the presence of low glucose levels *and* of methylxanthines for release to occur. The presence of a third site would most readily explain the permissive role of glucose allowing other calorigenic molecules to act. But the results would also be compatible with a model which proposes only two hexose sites, one highly specific for glucose (the permissive site) and one less specific (the releasing site).

It must also be considered that the characteristics of the sugar sites might vary greatly from one experimental system to the next. This is strikingly illustrated by the peculiarities of β-cells in tissue culture. Dr. Renold's group at Geneva found with embryonic pancreas explants that all releasing sugars merely required the presence of 10 mM caffeine for activity (Lambert *et al.*, 1969a; Lambert *et al.*, 1969b; Lambert, 1970). Stimulation of release from embryonic pancreas explants under this condition was found with the following sugars listed in their order of potency: glucose, mannose, glucosamine, fructose, N-acetylglucosamine, galactose, and 3-O-methyl glucose. (It should be noted that the potency of 3-O-methyl glucose reached only 2—3% of the potency of glucose.) It seems important to determine the relative efficacy of mannoheptulose in blocking release due to the 7 stimulatory sugars listed above. The embryonic pancreas explants would also be particularly suitable to study possible interactions among the different releasing sugars, since they are all agonists under the same conditions. Such investigations would possibly lead to information about the number of sites that might be involved in hexose-stimulated insulin release. The permissive action of glucose, which plays such a cardinal role in the adult pancreas (see this review and (Matschinsky *et al.*, 1972a)) was less apparent when the embryonic pancreas explants were employed and was observed only in the cases of tolbutamide, α-aminobutyric

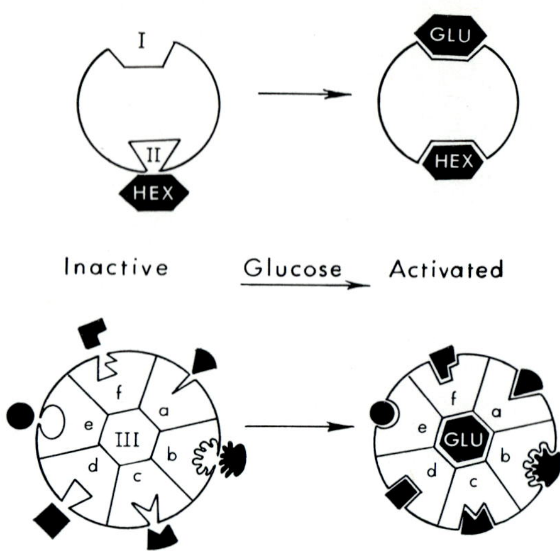

Fig. 18. Glucoreceptor sites in islets of Langerhans. The scheme shows on the top a β-cell glucoreceptor with two sites, one regulator site very specific for glucose (I) and one less specific accepting other sugars as well (II) (see also ASHCROFT *et al.*, 1972a) A general fuel receptor is depicted at the bottom with the permissive site specific for glucose (III) and a number of discriminator sites fitting a variety of low molecular stimulants (arbitrarily labeled a—f). As it stands now the results would also be compatible with a model which incorporates the general fuel receptor into a glucoreceptor (i.e. I and III are identical) or in which the general fuel receptor sites have been drawn individually each with its own permissive site for glucose (IIIa—IIIf). Addition of D-glucose converts the receptors from an inactive to an activated state allowing attachment of the stimulants (From MATSCHINSKY *et al.*, 1972a)

acid, and of lysine (LAMBERT, 1970). With several other amino acids tested (alanine, leucine, and histidine) glucose was not capable of permitting release in contrast to the highly effective caffeine. Tolbutamide, lysine, and α-aminobutyric acid represent therefore special test cases which might be used to study the permissive action of glucose in organ cultures. It is also conceivable that the paradoxical potentiation of release due to pyruvate or tolbutamide by mannoheptulose or 2-deoxyglucose (RENOLD, 1970; KANAZAWA *et al.*, 1971) involves this permissive hexose site. But the possibility has to our knowledge not been examined.

Very little is presently known about the location in the cell or about the chemical nature of the postulated hexose sites. The glucoreceptor might be located on the cell membrane and its activation might cause increased Ca^{++} uptake which leads to insulin release (MALAISSE, 1972). At low substimulatory or threshold concentration, glucose would make receptor sites accessible to other agonist molecules and the activation of such sites would again increase Ca^{++} influx with the consequence of insulin release. The mediation of stimulus-secretion coupling by Ca^{++} is the topic of a review by W. MALAISSE in this handbook (Chapter C, V).

Cerasi and Luft have speculated that glucose might act through stimulation of the β-adrenergic receptor of the β-cells, since they observed that propranolol diminished glucose-provoked release in man (CERASI and LUFT, 1969; CERASI and

Luft, 1970). This inhibition was overcome by theophylline. But this concept is not easily reconcilable with the findings made with isoproterenol. Blockade of the β-adrenergic receptors interferes with release due to isoproterenol but has little effect on glucose-provoked release (Burr *et al.*, 1970; Robertson and Porte, 1973). Respective results obtained with diabetic subjects also speak against the idea (Deckert *et al.*, 1972). The β-cells of the diabetic respond to isoproterenol even though the response to glucose is absent (Deckert *et al.*, 1972). It is, very possible that the glucoreceptors are connected with the adenyl cyclase system in a fashion not involving the β-adrenergic receptors. Recent evidence seems to support this attractive possibility since the levels of cyclic AMP rose severalfold but transiently in isolated perifused islets exposed to high glucose, as one would expect if the hypothesis were true (Zawalich *et al.*, in preparation).

The chemical characteristics of the postulated hexose sites might become more apparent if detailed dose-response studies with emphasis on the dose dependency of the kinetics of release are undertaken. Further attempts to find experimental conditions which allow a dissociation of releasing and fuel function of hexoses and thorough investigations of the biochemical correlates existing in islets under such conditions will be equally helpful for defining the glucoreceptor mechanisms of the islets more precisely.

And finally, the evidence for the presence of specific glucoreceptor molecules seems convincing enough that the application of refined methods of biochemistry (e.g. affinity chromatography (Cuatrecasas, 1972)) seems warranted in order to try the isolation of glucoreceptor molecules from islet tissue. It is encouraging that some progress has been made in the isolation and characterization of analogous glucoreceptor molecules involved in the taste of sweetness (Dastoli and Price, 1966; Price, 1969) and in chemotaxis of bacteria (Adler, 1969). Progress in β-cell research would be greatly enhanced if a high affinity ligand for the glucoreceptor could be found.

References

Adler, J.: Chemoreceptors in Bacteria. Science **166**, 1588—1597 (1969)

Aleyassine, H.: Energy requirements for insulin release from rat pancreas *in vitro*. Endocrinology **87**, 84—89 (1970)

Anderson, A.A., Hellerström, C.A.: Metabolic characteristics of isolated pancreatic islets in tissue culture. Diabetes **21**, 546—554 (1972)

Anderson, E., Long, J.A.: Effect of hyperglycemia on insulin secretion as determined with the isolated rat pancreas in a perfusion apparatus. Endocrinology **40**, 92—97 (1947)

Ashcroft, S.J.H., Bassett, J.M., Randle, P.J.: Isolation of human pancreatic islets capable of releasing insulin and metabolizing glucose *in vitro*. Lancet **1971I**, (7705) 888—889

Ashcroft, S.J.H., Bassett, J., Randle, P.J.: Insulin secretion mechanisms and glucose metabolism in isolated islets. Diabetes **21**, 538—545 (1972a)

Ashcroft, S.J.H., Hedeskov, C.J., Randle, P.J.: Glucose metabolism in mouse pancreatic islets. Biochem. J. **118**, 143—154 (1970)

Ashcroft, S.J.H., Randle, P.J.: Enzymes of glucose metabolism in normal mouse islets. Biochem. J. **119**, 5—15 (1970)

Ashcroft, S.J.H., Weerasinghe, L.C.C., Bassett, J.M., Randle, P.J.: The pentose cycle and insulin release in mouse pancreatic islets. Biochem. J. **126**, 525—523 (1972b)

Asplund, K.: The effect of glucose on the insulin secretion in fetal and newborn rats. In: The Structure and Metabolism of the Pancreatic Islets, p. 477—484 (Falkmer, S., Hellman, B., Taljedal, I.B., Eds.) Oxford: Pergamon Press 1970

Bhattacharya, G.: Protection against alloxan diabetes by mannose and fructose. Science **177**, 230—231 (1953)

Bhattacharya, G.: On the protection against alloxan diabetes by hexoses. Science **120**, 841—843 (1954)

Boda, J.M.: Effect of fast and hexose injection on serum insulin concentrations of sheep. Amer. J. Physiol. **206**, 419—424 (1964)

Burr, I.M., Balant, L., Stauffacher, W., Renold, A.E.: Perfusion of rat pancreatic tissue *in vitro*; substrate modification of theophylline induced biphasic insulin release. J. clin. Invest. **49**, 2097—2105 (1970)

Burr, J.M., Marliss, E.B., Stauffacher, W., Renold, A.E.: Differential effect of ouabain on glucose induced biphasic insulin release *in vitro*. Amer. J. Physiol. **221**, 943—947 (1971)

Candela, J.R., Coore, H.G.: Islet cell hormones: insulin secretion *in vitro*. In: Handbuch des Diabetes Mellitus, Vol. I, p. 203—220. München: J.F. Lehmann 1969

Carter, W.J., Younathan, E.S.: Studies on protection against the diabetogenic effect of alloxan by glucose. Proc. Soc. exp. Biol. (N.Y.) **109**, 611—612 (1962)

Cerasi, E., Chowers, I., Luft, R., Widström, A.: The significance of the blood glucose level for plasma insulin response to intravenously administered tolbutamide in healthy subjects. Diabetologia **5**, 343—348 (1969)

Cerasi, E., Luft, R.: The plasma insulin response to glucose infusion in healthy subjects and in diabetes mellitus. Acta endocr. (Kbh.) **55**, 278—304 (1967)

Cerasi, E., Luft, R.: Role of adrenergic receptors in glucose induced insulin secretion in man. Lancet **1969II**, 301—302

Cerasi, E., Luft, R.: Diabetes mellitus — a disorder of cellular information transmission? Horm. Metab. Res. **2**, 246—249 (1970)

Cerasi, E., Luft, R., Effendic, S.: Decreased sensitivity of the pancreatic beta cells to glucose in prediabetic and diabetic subjects. A glucose dose response study. Diabetes **21**, 224—234 (1972)

Christensen, H.N., Cullen, A.M.: Behavior in the rat of transport specific bicyclic amino acids. Hypoglycemic action. J. biol. Chem. **244**, 1521—1526 (1969)

Coore, H.G., Randle, P.J.: Regulation of insulin secretion studied with pieces of rabbit pancreas incubated *in vitro*. Biochem. J. **93**, 66—68 (1964)

Cornblath, M., Rosenthal, I.M., Reisner, S.H., Wybregt, S.H., Crane, R.K.: Hereditary fructose intolerance. New Engl. J. Med. **269**, 1271—1278 (1963)

Creutzfeldt, W., Frerichs, H., Reich, U.: *In vitro* studies on rat islets. In: The Structure and Metabolism of the Pancreatic Islets, p. 323—331 (Brolin, S.E., Hellman, B., Knutson, H., Eds.). New York: Academic Press 1964

Cuatrecasas, P.: Affinity chromatography of macromolecules. Advanc. Enzymol. **36**, 29—89 (1972)

Curry, D.L., Bennett, L.L., Grodsky, G.M.: The dynamics of insulin release by the perfused rat pancreas. Endocrinology **83**, 572—584 (1968)

Dastoli, F.R., Price, S.: Sweet-sensitive protein from bovine taste buds: Isolation and assay. Science **154**, 905—907 (1966)

Dean, P.M., Matthews, E.K.: Alloxan on islet cell membrane potentials. Brit. J. Pharmacol. **34**, 677P—678P (1968)

Dean, P.M., Matthews, E.K.: Glucose-induced electrical activity in pancreatic islet cells. J. Physiol. (Lond.) **210**, 255—264 (1970)

Dean, P.M., Matthews, E.K.: The bioelectric properties of islet cells: Effects of diabetogenic agents. Diabetologia **8**, 173—178 (1972)

Deckert, R., Lauridsen, U.B., Madsen, S.N., Deckert, M.: Serum insulin following isoprenaline in normal and diabetic persons. Horm. Metab. Res. **4**, 229—232 (1972)

Di George, A.M., Auerbach, V.H.: Leucine induced hypoglycemia, A review and speculations. Amer. J. med. Sci. **240**, 792—801 (1960)

Dunn, J.S., McLetchie, N.G.B.: Experimental alloxan diabetes in the rat. Lancet **1943II**, 384—387

Dunn, J.S., Sheehan, H.L., McLetchie, N.G.B.: Necroses of islets of Langerhans produced experimentally. Lancet **1943I**, 484—487

Efendic, S., Cerasi, E., Luft, R.: Role of glucose in arginine induced insulin release in man. Metabolism **20**, 568—579 (1971)

Ellerman, J., Matschinsky, F.M.: (unpublished)

Espinosa, M.M.A., Driscoll, S.G., Steinke, J.: Insulin release from isolated human fetal pancreatic islets. Science **168**, 1111—1112 (1970)

Estensen, R.D., Plagemann, P.G.W.: Cytochalasin B: Inhibition of glucose and glucosamine transport. Proc. nat. Acad. Sci. (Wash.) **69**, 1430—1434 (1972)

Fajans, S.S., Floyd, J.C., Jr., Knopf, R.F., Conns, J.W.: Effect of amino acids and proteins on insulin secretion in man. Recent Progr. Hormone Res. **23**, 617—662 (1967)

Fajans, S.S., Quibrera, R., Pek, S., Floyd, J.C., Christensen, H.N., Conns, J.: Stimulation of insulin release in the dog by a nonmetabolizable amino acid; comparison with leucine and arginine. J. clin. Endocr. **33**, 35—41 (1971)

Fertel, R.H.: Thesis, Part I, The effect of a-carbon substituted short-chain monocarboxylic acids on insulin release. Part II, the penetration of hexoses into the islets of Langerhans. Washington University (1972)

FERTEL, R., KOTLER-BRAJTBURG, J., HOLOWACH-THURSTON, J., MATSCHINSKY, F.M.: Insulin secretion due to alpha-keto monocarboxylic acids (alpha-KMCAs). Diabetes **21**, Suppl. 1, 359 (1972)

FRASER, R.: Insulin in blood and urine. In: Scientific Basis of Medicine Annual Reviews, pp. 206—223. London: Athlone Press 1968

FROHMAN, L.A.: The endocrine function of the pancreas. Ann. Rev. Physiol. **31**, 353—382 (1969)

GABBAY, K.H., TZE, W.J.: Inhibition of glucose-induced release of insulin by aldose reductase inhibitors. Proc. nat. Acad. Sci. (Wash.) **69**, 1435—1439 (1972)

GOLDFINE, I.D., CERASI, E., LUFT, R.: Glucagon stimulation of insulin release in man: inhibition during hypoglycemia. J. clin. Endocr. **35**, 312—315 (1972)

GRAFE, E., MEYTHALER, F.: Beiträge zur Kenntnis der Regulation der Insulinproduktion. I. Mitteilung: Der Traubenzucker als Hormon für die Insulinabgabe. Naunyn Schmiedebergs Arch. Pharmak. exp. Path. **125**, 181—192 (1927)

GRAFE, E., MEYTHALER, F.: Beiträge zur Kenntnis der Regulation der Insulinproduktion. II. Mitteilung: Die Wirkung von Kohlenhydraten (außer Traubenzucker) auf die Insulinabgabe. Naunyn Schmiedebergs Arch. Pharmak. exp. Path. **131**, 80—91 (1928a)

GRAFE, E., MEYTHALER, F.: Beiträge zur Kenntnis der Regulation der Insulinproduktion. III. Mitteilung: Die Wirkung von Anhydrokohlenhydraten, Zuckerderivaten und Zuckerspaltungsprodukten. Naunyn Schmiedebergs Arch. Pharmak. exp. Path. **136**, 360—369 (1928b)

GRODSKY, G.M.: Insulin and the pancreas. Vitam. and Horm. **28**, 37—101 (1970)

GRODSKY, G.M.: Threshold distribution hypothesis for packed storage of insulin and its mathematical modeling. J. clin. Invest. **51**, 2047—2059 (1972)

GRODSKY, G.M., BATTS, A., BENNETT, L.L., VCELLA, C., WILLIAMS, N.B., SMITH, D.F.: Effects of carbohydrates on secretion of insulin from isolated rat pancreas. Amer. J. Physiol. **205**, 638—644 (1963)

GRODSKY, G.M., FORSHAM, P.H.: Insulin and the pancreas. Ann. Rev. Physiol. **28**, 347—380 (1966)

HAYMAN, S., KINOSHITA, J.H.: Isolation and properties of les aldose reductase. J. biol. Chem. **240**, 877—882 (1965)

HELLERSTRÖM, C.A.: A method for the microdissection of intact pancreatic islets of mammals. Acta endocr. (Kbh.) **45**, 122—132 (1964)

HELLERSTRÖM, C.A.: Effects of carbohydrates on the oxygen consumption of isolated pancreatic islets of mice. Endocrinology **81**, 105—112 (1967)

HELLERSTRÖM, C.A., WESTMAN, S., MARSDEN, N., TURNER, D.: Oxygen consumption of the β-cells in relation to insulin release. In: The Structure and Metabolism of the Pancreatic Islets, p. 315—328 (FALKMER, S., HELLMAN, B., TALJEDAL, I.B., Eds.). Oxford: Pergamon Press 1970

HELLMAN, B., LERNMARK, A., SEHLIN, J., TALJEDAL, I.B.: Effects of phlorizin on metabolism and function of pancreatic β-cells. Metabolism **21**, 60—66 (1970)

HELLMAN, B., LERNMARK, A., SEHLIN, J., TALJEDAL, I.B.: The pancreatic β-cells recognition of insulin secretagogues. V. Binding and stimulatory action of phlorizin. Molec. Pharmacol. **8**, 759—769 (1972)

HELLMAN, B., SEHLIN, J., TALJEDAL, I.B.: Effects of glucose and other modifiers of insulin release on the oxidative metabolism of amino acids in microdissected pancreatic islets. Biochem. J. **123**, 513—521 (1971)

HOWELL, S.L., TAYLOR, K.W.: Potassium ions and the secretion of insulin by islets of Langerhans incubated *in vitro*. Biochem. J. **108**, 17—24 (1968)

IDAHL, L.A.: Dynamics of insulin secretion and glycolysis in isolated pancreatic islets. Diabetologia **6**, 657 (1970)

ISSELBACHER, K.J., ANDERSON, E.P., KURAKASHI, K., KALCKAR, H.M.: Congenital galactosemia: a single enzymatic block in galactose metabolism. Science **123**, 635—636 (1956)

IVERSEN, J.: Secretion of glucagon from the isolated perfused canine pancreas. J. clin. Invest. **50**, 2123—2136 (1970)

IVERSEN, J., MILES, D.W.: Evidence for a feedback inhibition of insulin on insulin secretion in the isolated perfused canine pancreas. Diabetes **20**, 1—9 (1971)

JARRETT, R.J., KEEN, H.: Oxidation of sugars, other than glucose by isolated mammalian islets of Langerhans. Metabolism **17**, 155—157 (1968)

KALKHOFF, R., SCHALCH, D.S., WALKER, L., BECK, P., KIPNIS, D.M., DAUGHADAY, W.H.: Diabetogenic factors associated with pregnancy. Trans. Ass. Amer. Phycns **77**, 270—280 (1964)

KANAZAWA, Y., KUZUYA, T., IDE, T., KOSAKA, K.: Plasma-insulin responses to glucose in femoral hepatic and pancreatic veins in dogs. Amer. J. Physiol. **211**, 442—448 (1966)

Kanazawa, Y., Orci, L., Lambert, A.E.: Organ culture of fetal rat pancreas. IV. Effects of metabolic inhibitors on insulin release. Endocrinology **89**, 576—583 (1971)

Karam, J.H., Grasso, S.G., Wegienka, J.C., Grodsky, G.M., Forsham, P.H.: Effect of selected hexoses, of epinephrine and of glucagon on insulin secretion in man. Diabetes **15**, 571—578 (1966)

Kilo, C., Devrim, S., Bailey, R., Recant, L.: Studies *in vivo* and *in vitro* of glucose-stimulated insulin release. The effects of metabolizable sugars, tolbutamide and 2-deoxy-glucose. Diabetes **16**, 377—385 (1967)

Kilo, C., Long, C.L., Jr., Bailey, R.M., Koch, M.B., Recant, L.: Studies to determine whether glucose must be metabolized to induce insulin release. J. clin. Invest. **41**, 1372—1373 (1963)

Kipnis, D.M.: Nutrient regulation of insulin secretion in human subjects. Diabetes **21**, Suppl. 2, 606—616 (1972)

Kizer, J.S., Bressler, R.: Drugs and the mechanism of insulin secretion. In: Advance in Pharmacology and Chemotherapeutics, Vol. 7, p. 91—115 (Garattini, S. *et al.*). New York: Academic Press 1969

Kletzien, R.F., Perdue, J.F., Springer, A.: Cytochalasin A and B, Inhibition of sugar uptake in cultured cells. J. biol. Chem. **247**, 2964—2966 (1972)

Kuzuya, T., Kanazawa, Y.: Studies on the mechanism of xylitol induced insulin secretion in dogs. Diabetologica **5**, 248—257 (1969)

Kuzuya, T., Kanazawa, Y., Hayashi, M., Kikuchi, M., Ide, T.: Species differences in plasma insulin responses to intravenous xylitol in man and several mammala. Endocr. jap. **18**, 309—320 (1971)

Kuzuya, T., Kanazawa, Y., Kosaka, K.: Plasma insulin response to intravenously administered xylitol in dogs. Metabolism **15**, 1149—1152 (1966)

Kuzuya, T., Kanazawa, Y., Kosaka, K.: Stimulation of insulin secretion by xylitol in dogs. Endocrinology **84**, 200—207 (1969)

Lacy, P.E.: (Personal communication)

Lacy, P.E.: The pancreatic beta cell: structure and function. New Engl. J. Med. **276**, 187—195 (1967)

Lacy, P.E., Kostianovsky, M.: Method for the isolation of intact islets of Langerhans from the rat pancreas. Diabetes **16**, 35—39 (1967)

Lacy, P.E., Walker, M.M., Fink, J.F.: Perifusion of isolated rat islets *in vitro*, participation of the microtubular system in the biphasic release of insulin. Diabetes **21**, 987—998 (1972)

Lacy, P.E., Young, D.A., Fink, C.J.: Studies on insulin secretion *in vitro* from isolated islets of the rat pancreas. Endocrinology **83**, 1155—1161 (1968)

Lambert, A.E.: Biochemical and morphological studies of cultured fetal rat pancreas. Thesis, University of Louvain, Belgium 1970

Lambert, A.E., Blondel, B., Kanazawa, Y., Orci, L., Renold, A.E.: Monolayer cell culture of neonatal rat pancreas: Light microscopy and evidence for immunoreactive insulin synthesis and release. Endocrinology **90**, 239—248 (1972)

Lambert, A.E., Jeanrenaud, B., Junod, A., Renold, A.E.: II. Insulin release induced by amino acids and organic acids, by hormonal peptides, by cationic alterations of the medium and by other agents. Biochim. biophys. Acta (Amst.) **184**, 540—553 (1969a)

Lambert, A.E., Junod, A., Stauffacher, W., Jeanrenaud, B., Renold, A.E.: Organ culture of fetal rat pancreas. I. Insulin release induced by caffeine and by sugars and some derivatives. Biochim. biophys. Acta (Amst.) **184**, 529—539 (1969b)

Lambert, A.E., Kanazawa, Y., Orci, L., Burr, I., Christensen, H.N., Renold, A.E.: Stimulation of insulin release *in vitro* by nonmetabolized amino acid analogues. Proc. Soc. exp. Biol. (N.Y.) **137**, 377—381 (1971)

Landgraf, R., Kotler-Brajtburg, J., Matschinsky, F.M.: Kinetics of insulin release from the perfused rat pancreas caused by glucose, glucosamine and galactose. Proc. nat. Acad. Sci. (Wash.) **68**, 536—540 (1971)

Landgraf, R., Matschinsky, F.M.: Penetration of xylitol into islets of Langerhans. Fed. Proc. **29**, 314 (1970)

Lernmark, A., Hellman, B.: The β-cell capacity for insulin secretion in microdissected pancreatic islets from obese-hyperglycemic mice. Life Sci. (Part II) **8**, 53—59 (1969)

Levin, S.R., Grodsky, G.M., Hagura, R., Smith, D.F., Forsham, P.: Relationship between arginine and glucose in the induction of insulin secretion from isolated, perfused rat pancreas. Endocrinology **90**, 624—631 (1972)

Malaisse, W.J.: Etude de la Secretion insulinique *in vitro*, p. 1—225. Bruxelles: Arscia 1968

Malaisse, W.J.: Hormonal and environmental modification of islet activity. Handbook of Physiology, Endocrinology I, p. 237—260, American Physiological Society, Washington 1972

MALAISSE, W.J., HAGER, D.L., ORCI, L.: The stimulus secretion coupling of glucose induced insulin release, F. The participation of the β-cell web. Diabetes **21**, Suppl. 2, 594—604 (1972)
MALAISSE, W., MALAISSE-LAGAE, F., GERRITSEN, G., DULIN, W.C., WRIGHT, P.H.: Insulin secretion *in vitro* by the pancreas of the Chinese Hamster. Diabetologia **3**, 109—114 (1967a)
MALAISSE, W.J., MALAISSE-LAGAE, F., WRIGHT, P.H.: A new method for the measurement of *in vitro* pancreatic insulin secretion. Endocrinology **80**, 99—108 (1967b)
MARTIN, J.M., BAMBERS, G.: Insulin secretion in glucosamine induced hyperglycemia in rats. Fed. Proc. **23**, 409 (1964)
MATSCHINSKY, F.M.: Enzymes, metabolites, and cofactors involved in intermediary metabolism of islets of Langerhans. Handbook of Physiology, Endocrinology I, p. 199—214, American Physiological Society, Washington 1972
MATSCHINSKY, F.M., ELLERMAN, J.: Metabolism of glucose in islets of Langerhans. J. biol. Chem. **243**, 2730—2736 (1968)
MATSCHINSKY, F.M., ELLERMAN, J.: Dissociation of the insulin releasing and the metabolic functions of hexoses in islets of Langerhans. Biochem. biophys. Res. Commun. **50**, 193—199 (1973)
MATSCHINSKY, F.M., ELLERMAN, J., KRZANOWSKI, J., KOTLER-BRAJTBURG, J., LANDGRAF, R., FERTEL, R.: Metabolic events in pancreatic islets during insulin release stimulated by glucose. Diabetes **19**, Suppl. 1, 365 (1970)
MATSCHINSKY, F.M., ELLERMAN, J., KRZANOWSKI, J., KOTLER-BRAJTBURG, J., LANDGRAF, R., FERTEL, R.: The dual function of glucose in islets of Langerhans. J. biol. Chem. **246**, 1007—1011 (1971a)
MATSCHINSKY, F.M., ELLERMAN, J., LANDGRAF, R., KRZANOWSKI, J., KOTLER-BRAJTBURG, J., FERTEL, R.: Quantitative histochemistry of glucose metabolism in the islets of Langerhans. In: Recent Advances in Quantitative Histochemistry and Cytochemistry. Methods and Applications, p. 143—182 (DUBACH, U.C., SCHMIDT, U., Eds.). Bern: Hans Huber 1971b
MATSCHINSKY, F.M., FERTEL, R., KOTLER-BRAJTBURG, J., STILLINGS, S., ELLERMAN, J., RAYBAUD, F., HOLOWACH-THURSTON, J.: Factors governing the action of small calorigenic molecules on the islets of Langerhans, 8th Midwest Conference on Endocrinology and Metabolism, Columbia, Missouri, October 1972a, 63—87
MATSCHINSKY, F.M., KOTLER-BRAJTBURG, J., ELLERMAN, J., RODGERS, M.: The mechanisms of glucosamine induced insulin release. Diabetes **21**, Suppl. 1, 328 (1972b)
MATSCHINSKY, F.M., RAYBAUD, F., ROGERS, M., STILLINGS, S.: Unpublished experiments
MAYHEW, D.A., WRIGHT, P.H., ASHMORE, J.: Regulation of insulin secretion. Pharmacol. Rev. **21**, 183—212 (1969)
METZ, R.: The effect of blood glucose concentration on insulin output. Diabetes **4**, 89—93 (1960)
MILNER, R.D.G.: The secretion of insulin from foetal and postnatal rabbit pancreas *in vitro* in response to various substances. J. Endocr. **44**, 267—272 (1969)
MILNER, R.D.G., ASHWORTH, M.A., BARSON, A.J.: Insulin release from human fetal pancreas *in vitro*. Horm. Metab. Res. **3**, 353—354 (1971)
MINTZ, D.H., CHEZ, R.A., HORGER, E.O.: III. Fetal insulin and growth hormone metabolism in the subhuman primate. J. clin. Invest. **48**, 176—186 (1969)
MONTAGUE, W., TAYLOR, K.: Pentitols and insulin release by isolated rat islets of Langerhans. Biochem. J. **109**, 333—339 (1968)
MONTAGUE, W., TAYLOR, K.: Islet cell metabolism during insulin release. Biochem. J. **115**, 257—262 (1969)
MONTAGUE, W., TAYLOR, K.W.: The role of the pentose phosphate pathway in insulin secretion. In: The Structure and Metabolism of the Pancreatic Islets, p. 263—273 (FALKMER, S., HELLMANN, B., TALJEDAL, I.B., Eds.). Oxford: Pergamon Press 1970
PACE, C., MATSCHINSKY, F.M.: (unpublished)
PACE, C.S., PRICE, S.: Bioelectrical effects of hexoses on pancreatic islet cells. Endocrinology **94**, 142—147 (1974)
PACE, C.S., PRICE, S.: Electrical responses of pancreatic islet cells to secretory stimuli. Biochem. biophys. Res. Commun. **46**, 1557—1563 (1972)
PANTEN, U., KRIEGSTEIN, E.v., POSER, W., SCHONBORN, J., HASSELBLATT, A.: Effects of L-leucine and α-ketoisocaproic acid upon insulin secretion and metabolism of isolated pancreatic islets. FEBS Letters **20**, 225—228 (1972)
PFEIFFER, E.F.: Statik und Dynamik der Insulinsekretion bei Diabetes, Proto-Diabetes und Adipositas. In: Handbuch des Diabetes Mellitus, Vol. II, p. 123—158 (PFEIFFER, E.F., Ed.). München: J. F. Lehmann 1971
PORTE, D., JR., BAGDADE, J.D.: Human insulin secretion: an integrated approach. Ann. Rev. Med. **31**, 219—240 (1970)

Pozza, G.G., Galansino, H., Hoffield, H., Foa, P.P.: Stimulation of insulin output by monosaccharides and monosaccharide derivatives. Amer. J. Physiol. **192**, 497—500 (1958)

Price, S.: Chemoreceptor proteins from taste buds. Agr. Food Chem. **17**, 709—711 (1969)

Randle, P.J.: Islet metabolism and insulin secretion. Proceedings of the 7th Congress of the International Diabetes Federation, p. 232. Buenos Aires, August (1970). (Rodriguez, P.R., Vallance-Owen, J., Eds.). Amsterdam: Excerpta Medica Foundation 1971

Randle, P.J., Ashcroft, S.J.H., Gill, J.R.: Carbohydrate metabolism and release of hormones. In: Carbohydrate Metabolism and Its Disorders, p. 427—447 (Dickens, F., Randle, P.J., Whelan, W.J., Eds.). New York: Academic Press 1968

Randle, P.J., Hales, C.N.: Insulin release mechanisms. In: Handbook of Physiology, Endocrinology I, p. 219—235, American Physiological Society, Washington 1972

Raybaud, F., Matschinsky, F.M.: (unpublished)

Reese, A.C., Landau, B.R., Craig, J.W., Gin, G., Rodman, H.M.: Glucose metabolism by rat pancreatic islets *in vitro*. Metabolism **22**, 467—472 (1973)

Renold, A.E.: Insulin biosynthesis and secretion — a still unsettled topic. New Engl. J. Med. **282**, 173—182 (1970)

Rerup, C.S.: Drugs producting diabetes through damage of the insulin secreting cells. Pharmacol. Rev. **22** (4), 485—518 (1970)

Robertson, R.P., Porte, D.: The glucose receptor: a defective mechanism in diabetes mellitus distinct from the beta adrenergic receptor. J. clin. Invest. **52**, 871—876 (1973)

Rommel, K., Melani, F., Burkhardt, H., Grimmel, K.: Einfluß der Galactose auf die Insulinsecretion beim Menschen. Diabetologia **5**, 309—311 (1969)

Samols, E., Dormandy, T.L.: Insulin response to fructose and galatose. Lancet **1963I**, 478—479

Schatzman, H.J.: Herzglykoside als Hemmstoffe für den aktiven Kalium- und Natriumtransport durch die Erythrocytenmembran. Helv. physiol. pharmacol. Acta **11**, 346—354 (1953)

Scheynius, A., Täljedal, I.B.: On the mechanism of glucose protection against alloxan toxicity. Diabetologia **7**, 252—255 (1971)

Seltzer, H.S., Harris, V.L.: Exhaustion of insulinogenic reserve in maturity onset diabetic patients during prolonged and continuous hyperglycemic stress. Diabetes **13**, 6—13 (1964)

Sols, A.: The hexokinase activity of the intestinal mucosa. Biochim. biophys. Acta (Amst.) **19**, 144—152 (1956)

Sols, A., Crane, R.K.: Substrate specificity of brain hexokinase. J. biol. Chem. **210**, 581—595 (1954)

Sussman, K.E., Vaughan, G.D., Stjernholm, M.R.: Factors controlling insulin secretion in the perfused isolated rat pancreas, p. 123. Proc. of the 6th Congress of the Int. Diabetes Federation, Stockholm. Amsterdam: Excerpta Medica 1967

Sussman, K.E., Vaughan, G.D., Timmer, R.F.: An *in vitro* method for studying insulin secretion in the perfused isolated rat pancreas. Metabolism **15**, 466—476 (1966)

Tager, H.S., Christensen, H.N.: Hypoglycemic action of 2-amino norbonane-2-carboxylic acid in the rat. Biochem. biophys. Res. Commun. **44**, 185—191 (1971)

Thoreel, J.I.: Plasma insulin levels in normal human foetuses. Acta endocr. (Kbh.) **63**, 134—140 (1970)

Willes, R.F., Boda, J.M., Manns, J.G.: Insulin secretion by the ovine fetus *in utero*. Endocrinology **84**, 520—521 (1969)

Williams, R.H., Ensinck, J.W.: Secretion, fates and actions of insulin and related products. Diabetes **15**, 623—654 (1966)

Wilson, R.B., Martin, J.M.: Plasma insulin concentrations in dogs and monkeys after xylitol, glucose or tolbutamide infusion. Diabetes **19**, 17—22 (1970)

Zawalich, W.S., Beidler, L.M.: Glucose and alloxan interactions on the pancreatic islets. Amer. J. Physiol. **224**, 963—966 (1973)

Zawalich, W., Ferrendelli, J., Matschinsky, F.M.: Involvement of cyclic AMP in glucose provoked insulin release from isolated perfused islets (in preparation)

III. Amino Acids and Insulin Secretion

Uwe Panten

With 4 Figures

1. Introduction

In man protein meals (Floyd *et al.*, 1966a; Rabinowitz *et al.*, 1966) or intravenous infusion of amino acid mixtures (Floyd *et al.*, 1966b) enhance plasma insulin levels. Evidence has been presented that the increase of blood glucose is not the major cause of insulin secretion during amino acid infusion (Fajans and Floyd, 1972). Intraduodenal administration of mixed amino acids caused higher insulin levels than intravenous administration (Raptis *et al.*, 1973), suggesting modification of amino acid-induced insulin release by gastrointestinal hormones (Marks and Samols, 1970; Fajans and Floyd, 1972; Pfeiffer *et al.*, 1973). *In vitro* experiments, however, demonstrated that several amino acids directly stimulate insulin release.

Mainly these direct effects will be reviewed in this chapter because *in vivo* effects of amino acids on insulin secretion have been discussed recently (Fajans and Floyd, 1972; Fajans *et al.*, 1972). The first section of this chapter deals with the transport and metabolism of amino acids in islet cells in order to facilitate the discussion of the possible mechanisms of amino acid-induced insulin release, which is the purpose of following sections.

The earlier literature of this area has been reviewed in several excellent articles (Kizer and Bressler, 1969; Mayhew *et al.*, 1969; Grodsky, 1970; Fajans *et al.*, 1971; Hellman and Täljedal, 1972; Malaisse, 1972).

2. Transport and Metabolism of Amino Acids by Islet Cells

a) Transport of Amino Acids

Oxender and Christensen (1963) described for Ehrlich ascites cells transport systems for neutral amino acids, the so-called alanine preferring A-system and the leucine preferring L-system. In contrast to the L-system, the A-system is sodium-dependent. Similar transport mechanisms apparently mediate amino acid uptake in pancreatic islets. Alanine (Hellman *et al.*, 1971a), glycine (Sehlin, 1972a), and α-aminoisobutyric acid (Hellman *et al.*, 1971b) are rapidly taken up by mouse islets. Their concentrative and sodium-dependent accumulation suggests the existence of the A-system in islet cells.

L- and D-leucine (Hellman *et al.*, 1971a; Hellman *et al.*, 1972) and their nonmetabolized analogues b (—)- and b (+)- 2-amino-bicyclo [2,2,1] heptane-2-carboxylic acid (BCH) (Christensen *et al.*, 1971) were concentrated only slightly by islets from obese-hyperglycemic mice. Uptake of L-leucine was sodium-independent (HELLMAN *et al.*, 1971a). Thus mouse islets show characteristics of the L-system.

Glutamate uptake by islet cells was slow and nonconcentrative (SEHLIN, 1972b).

L-arginine (HELLMAN *et al.*, 1971a) and its nonmetabolized analogue 4-amino-1-guanylpiperidine-4-carboxylic acid (GPA) (CHRISTENSEN *et al.*, 1971) were rapidly concentrated by mouse islets.

b) Synthesis and Degradation of Amino Acids

Fish islets have been shown to synthesize amino acids from glucose (HELLMAN and LARSSON, 1961; HUMBEL and RENOLD, 1963). The capacity of islet cells for transformation of α-ketoacids into amino acids seems to be high. Transaminase activity has been demonstrated in islets of different species (HELLMAN, 1965; KISSANE *et al.*, 1964; GEPTS *et al.*, 1970). When mouse islets were incubated in media containing high concentrations of α-ketoisocaproic acid (KIC), the transamination product of leucine, leucine production was enhanced severalfold (PANTEN *et al.*, 1972). Reductive amination of α-ketoglutarate in islet homogenates was increased severalfold by L-leucine (HELLMAN, 1969), probably by activation of intramitochondrial glutamate dehydrogenase (MCGIVAN *et al.*, 1973).

Decarboxylation rates of leucine in mouse islets were rather high (STORK *et al.*, 1970; ASHCROFT *et al.*, 1973), demonstrating high activities of leucine transaminase and KIC-dehydrogenase. When islets of obese-hyperglycemic mice were incubated in the presence of leucine or KIC, production of their metabolite acetoacetate was enhanced significantly (PANTEN *et al.*, 1972). Oxidation of U-^{14}C-leucine was inhibited by glucose or succinate, probably by metabolic interference (HELLMAN *et al.*, 1971c).

In the absence of glucose, mouse islets oxidized uniformly ^{14}C-labeled alanine, arginine, glycine, or glutamate only slowly (HELLMAN *et al.*, 1971c; SEHLIN, 1972a and 1972b) and addition of glucose to the incubation medium enhanced oxidation rates of only alanine and glutamate.

c) Protein Degradation

In mouse islets high peptidase activities (HELLERSTRÖM and HELLMAN, 1963; IDAHL and TÄLJEDAL, 1968) suggest that protein degradation partly regulates amino acid levels (HELLMAN and TÄLJEDAL, 1972). This is confirmed by the production of leucine and arginine by islets incubated without substrate (PANTEN *et al.*, 1972). Since the oxidation rate of arginine is very low in islet cells, arginine production may be used to measure endogenous proteolysis.

d) Amino Acid Levels

Besides protein synthesis the above-mentioned processes control amino acid levels of islet cells. Amino acid contents of incubated (BRIEL *et al.*, 1972) or perifused (PANTEN *et al.*, 1972) islets of obese-hyperglycemic mice (obob mice) have been measured using different analytical technics. Like nervous tissue (CURTIS and WATKINS, 1965; JACOBSEN and SMITH, 1968), the islets contained high amounts of γ-aminobutyric acid (GABA) and taurine. It is, however, unlikely that the sparse innervation of the islets accounts for the high concentrations of these amino acids (BRIEL *et al.*, 1972). Whether GABA or taurine play a role in the insulin release process must wait for further studies. Leucine content of perifused islets was 7 times lower than the surprisingly large amount (4.8 mmoles leucine per kg islet dry weight) of incubated islets. This difference probably results from the more rapid equilibration of the extracellular space of islets with the medium by perifusion as compared to incubation.

3. Amino Acid-Induced Insulin Secretion

a) L-Arginine and Related Substances

Of the single amino acids known to stimulate insulin secretion in humans, arginine is the most potent (FAJANS *et al.*, 1967). *In vitro*, arginine caused insulin release from pancreas pieces of rats (MALAISSE and MALAISSE-LAGAE, 1968), rabbits (EDGAR *et al.*, 1969; MILNER, 1970), or sheep (HERTELENDY *et al.*, 1968), from mouse (LERNMARK, 1972a, b; PANTEN and CHRISTIANS, 1973) or rat islets (MALAISSE-LAGAE *et al.*, 1971), or from the perfused pancreas of rats (SUSSMAN *et al.*, 1967; BASABE *et al.*, 1971; LEVIN *et al.*, 1972) or dogs (IVERSEN, 1971). Arginine has also insulinotropic effects on incubated fetal pancreatic tissue (LAMBERT *et al.*, 1969; HEINZE and STEINKE, 1972; MILNER *et al.*, 1972).

The insulinotropic effect of arginine depends on the glucose concentration the islet cells are exposed to. Intravenous infusion of arginine plus glucose induced an overadditive rise of serum insulin (FLOYD *et al.*, 1970; LEVIN *et al.*, 1971), whereas hypoglycemia inhibited the insulin response to arginine infusion (EFENDIC *et al.*, 1971). A preceding glucose infusion enhanced the respose to arginine infusion (LEVIN *et al.*, 1971). These results were confirmed by studies with the perfused rat pancreas (LEVIN *et al.*, 1972). In addition the latter authors found that low glucose concentrations (2.8—5.5 mM) changed the arginine-induced release pattern. An early discharge, a fall, and a late rise of insulin secretion took place, whereas total insulin release was not enhanced as compared to the nonphasic response to arginine in the absence of glucose. Both phases were markedly enhanced at 8.3 mM glucose.

Arginine had few additional insulinotropic effects when superimposed on near-maximal glucose concentrations (16.7—27.8 mM). The finding that arginine decreased the insulin response to high subsequent levels of glucose suggested some negative effects of arginine upon glucose-stimulated insulin secretion, which is in agreement with *in vivo* results (LEVIN *et al.*, 1971). That arginine triggers insulin release in the absence of glucose has been stated by HERTELENDY *et al.* (1968) and LEVIN *et al.* (1972). In contrast to this, several other authors (EDGAR *et al.*, 1969; MILNER, 1970; LERNMARK, 1972a; BASABE *et al.*, 1971) found that arginine required glucose to be active. These discrepancies may reflect methodological factors influencing sensitivity to arginine *in vitro*. Perhaps local effects of endogenous glucagon on the β-cells differ in the above-mentioned experiments. Glucose inhibits glucagon release from α_2-cells (FOA, 1972). On the other hand, the insulinotropic effect of glucose is enhanced by glucagon (MALAISSE, 1972).

MILNER (1970) proposed that arginine stimulates insulin secretion indirectly by eliciting glucagon from the α_2-cells. Arginine has been shown to stimulate glucagon release *in vivo* (OHNEDA *et al.*, 1968; KANETO and OSAKA, 1971) and *in vitro* (EDWARDS and TAYLOR, 1970; CHESNEY and SCHOFIELD, 1969). Glucagon enhanced cyclic AMP levels of incubated pancreatic islets (TURTLE and KIPNIS, 1967). If Milner's hypothesis is correct one would expect arginine to have effects on the adenylate cyclase-phosphodiesterase system of islet cells, causing increase of cyclic AMP. Cyclic AMP-dependent protein kinase of islets, however, was not enhanced when incubation media contained arginine, but incubation with glucagon enhanced protein kinase activity (MONTAGUE and HOWELL, 1973). In contrast to glucagon, arginine did not augment adenylate cyclase activity of islet tissue homogenates (LEVEY *et al.*, 1972; KUO *et al.*, 1973). The phosphodiesterase activity of subcellular fractions from pancreatic islets was enhanced by arginine (SAMS and MONTAGUE, 1972). Thus enzymatic studies do not support MILNER's concept.

Metabolization by the β-cells and providing energy for the release process obviously is not the mechanism of arginine-induced insulin release, because the oxidation rate of arginine by β-cell-rich islets from obese-hyperglycemic mice is very low (HELLMAN *et al.*, 1971c). This result, however, does not rule out the possibility that an early metabolite of arginine is the true trigger of insulin release, as suggested by ALSEVER *et al.* (1970). These authors found that guanidinoacetic acid, the transamidination product of arginine, was more potent than arginine in stimulating insulin secretion from the isolated perfused rat pancreas. Guanidinoacetic acid, however, was ineffective on insulin release from isolated rat islets (ALBERTI and WHALLEY, 1973).

On the other hand, arginine as such may trigger insulin secretion. This possibility is supported by the stimulation of insulin release by GPA, which was transported by the β-cells (CHRISTENSEN *et al.*, 1971; FAJANS *et al.*, 1972) and by 1-guanyl-4-piperidine-glycine (GPG) (CHRISTENSEN, 1972). Similar to arginine, GPA and GPG stimulate glucagon release (CHRISTENSEN, 1972). Both substances are nonmetabolizable arginine analogues, used as model substrates for the transport system for cationic amino acids. Therefore the receptors for arginine-induced insulin secretion may be transport sites (CHRISTENSEN *et al.*, 1971).

Decarboxylated arginine (agmatine) stimulated insulin release from isolated rat islets (ALBERTI and WHALLEY, 1973), supporting the view that receptor sites other than transport sites mediate arginine-induced insulin release. Homoarginine (CHRISTENSEN, 1972), and α-amino-γ-guanidinobutyric and α-amino-β-guanidinopropionic acid (ALBERTI and WHALLEY, 1973) stimulated insulin secretion, suggesting that the stimulatory effect of arginine is not abolished by slight changes of length of its carbon chain. On the other hand, both the α-amino and the guanidine group appear to be necessary to maintain the insulin-releasing potency of the arginine molecule, because neither N-methyl-L-arginine nor L-norvaline stimulated insulin secretion *in vitro* (LERNMARK, 1972a, b; SCHÖNBORN *et al.*, 1973a, b; ALBERTI and WHALLEY, 1973).

b) L-Leucine and Related Substances

In healthy subjects the slight hyperinsulinemia caused by L-leucine is exaggerated by pretreatment with blood sugar-lowering sulfonylureas (FAJANS *et al.*, 1963; FAJANS *et al.*, 1967). Plasma insulin of some patients suffering from idiopathic hypoglycemia (YALOW and BERSON, 1960; FAJANS *et al.*, 1967) or from functioning islet cell tumors (YALOW and BERSON, 1960; FAJANS *et al.*, 1967) was markedly elevated after administration of L-leucine. In those subjects arginine-induced insulin release was not enhanced.

The insulinotropic effect of leucine *in vitro* was demonstrated by many authors (Table 1). These experiments furthermore support the view that leucine can trigger insulin release in the absence of glucose, with a maximum effect at about 20 mM (LERNMARK, 1972b). The only reports that leucine requires glucose to be active are from EDGAR *et al.* (1969), and MALAISSE and MALAISSE-LAGAE (1968). These discrepancies may reflect different methods. It is likely that the sensitivity of pancreatic islets to leucine depends on factors like feeding of the animals, composition of media, length of preincubation, or length and mode of tissue preparation. In contrast to experiments using incubation technics (MALAISSE and MALAISSE-LAGAE, 1968; HALES and MILNER, 1968; LERNMARK, 1972b; ASHCROFT *et al.*, 1973), PANTEN *et al.* (1973) and SCHÖNBORN *et al.* (1973, 1974) found that the insulinotropic effects of leucine on perifused isolated islets or on the perfused isolated pancreas were smaller in the presence than in the absence of glucose. The latter results may reflect increased leucine sensitivity due to effective washing of the tissue. Comparing incubation with perfusion, e.g. calcium distributions, which depend on endogenous substrates and glucose, may differ. At 16.7 mM glucose

Table 1. *In vitro effect of l-leucine on insulin secretion*

Species		Basal glucose conc. mM	L-leucine conc. mM	Result*	References
Human fetus	IP	0—3.3**	5	+	MILNER *et al.* (1972)
Rabbit fetus	IP	3.3**	5	+	MILNER (1969)
Rabbit	IP	0 **	5	+	HALES and MILNER (1968)
Rabbit	IP	3.3**	5	+	HALES and MILNER (1968)
Rabbit	IP	8.3**	5	+	MILNER (1970)
Rabbit	IP	0 **	7.6	+	PFEIFFER and TELIB (1968)
Rabbit	IP	0	7.2—8.3	0	EDGAR *et al.* (1969)
Rabbit	IP	8.3	7.2—8.3	+	EDGAR *et al.* (1969)
Rat	PP	5.6	***	+	SUSSMAN *et al.* (1967)
Rat	PP	2.8	16	+	BASABE *et al.* (1971)
Rat	PP	0	10	+	LANDGRAF *et al.* (1972)
Rat	PP	0	10	+	SCHÖNBORN *et al.* (1974)
Rat	PP	5	10	0	SCHÖNBORN *et al.* (1974)
Rat	PP	5	40	+	SCHÖNBORN *et al.* (1974)
Rat	IP	0	10	0	MALAISSE and MALAISSE-LAGAE (1968)
Rat	IP	5.6	10	+	MALAISSE and MALAISSE-LAGAE (1968)
Rat	IP	0	25	+	MALAISSE and MALAISSE-LAGAE (1968)
Rat	II	0	10	+	MALAISSE-LAGAE *et al.* (1971)
Rat	II	2	5	+	GREEN and TAYLOR (1972)
Rat	CP	0****	11	+	LAMBERT *et al.* (1969)
Mouse	II	0****	2.5	+	ASHCROFT *et al.* (1973)
Mouse	II	5****	2.5	+	ASHCROFT *et al.* (1973)
Obob mouse	II	0	5	+	LERNMARK (1972b)
Obob mouse	II	10	5	+	LERNMARK (1972b)
Obob mouse	PI	0	10	+	PANTEN *et al.* (1973)
Obob mouse	PI	5	10	(+)	PANTEN *et al.* (1973)
Obob mouse	PI	5	30	+	PANTEN *et al.* (1973)

* Stimulation +; weak stimulation (+); no stimulation 0
** Media contained fumarate, pyruvate, and glutamate.
*** Leucine was applied as a pulse.
**** Media contained caffeine.
IP = incubated pancreas pieces
CP = cultured, fetal pancreatic explant
PP = perfused pancreas
II = incubated isolated islets
PI = perifused isolated islets

BASABE *et al.* (1971) demonstrated an insulinotropic effect of leucine, a finding which was not seen in a previous report (MALAISSE and MALAISSE-LAGAE, 1968). Therefore it remains unsettled whether the maximal stimulant action of glucose can be enhanced by leucine.

LUCKE *et al.* (1972) reported that mannoheptulose, an inhibitor of glucose utilization (COORE *et al.*, 1963), suppressed leucine-induced insulin release in rabbits *in vivo*. This action of mannoheptulose was not seen by FAJANS *et al.* (1971) in dogs. The latter results fit to experiments performed with pieces of rat or rabbit pancreas, or with isolated mouse or rat islets. In the absence or presence of glucose, mannoheptulose did not inhibit leucine-induced insulin release but prevented the potentiating effect of N-acetylglucosamine on insulin secretion elicited by leucine (MALAISSE and MALAISSE-LAGAE, 1968; MILNER and HALES, 1969; MALAISSE-LAGAE *et al.*, 1971; ASHCROFT *et al.*, 1973).

It has been suggested that a common extracellular space of a_2- and β-cells enabled a_2-cells to trigger a glucagon-induced insulin release (SAMOLS *et al.*, 1972). In man (FAJANS *et al.*, 1971) or dog (ROCHA *et al.*, 1972) intravenous infusion of leucine did not increase plasma glucagon. Intrapancreatically infused leucine induced a prompt but small glucagon release (KANETO and KOSAKA, 1972). *In vitro* experiments failed to demonstrate a leucine-triggered glucagon secretion in the absence of glucose, though insulin secretion was enhanced severalfold (FUSSGÄNGER *et al.*, 1972). In the presence of glucose no (CHESNEY and SCHOFIELD, 1969) or only little (FUSSGÄNGER *et al.*, 1972) glucagon was released by leucine. These results suggest that leucine does not stimulate insulin secretion via glucagon but acts directly on β-cells.

The significance of the adenylate cyclase-phosphodiesterase system of islet cells for the mechanism of leucine-induced insulin release has been considered by several authors. Glucagon, which is generally believed to enhance insulin release by elevation of cyclic AMP levels in the β-cells (MALAISSE, 1972), augmented insulin secretion in response to leucine (MALAISSE and MALAISSE-LAGAE, 1970; FAJANS *et al.*, 1971). Cyclic AMP-dependent protein kinase of incubated islets was not activated by leucine (5 mM) (MONTAGUE and HOWELL, 1973). Phosphodiesterase (SAMS and MONTAGUE, 1972) or adenylate cyclase (HOWELL and MONTAGUE, 1973; KUO *et al.*, 1973) were not activated by L-leucine (5 mM). These results argue against the view that the insulinotropic action of leucine is mainly mediated by cyclic AMP, though preliminary results from SELAWRY *et al.* (1973) demonstrate that there may be experimental conditions where leucine causes an increase of cyclic AMP levels of islet cells.

KNOPF *et al.* (1963) studied in man whether metabolization of leucine by islet cells was a prerequisite for its insulin-releasing capacity. Equimolar amounts of leucine or its catabolite a-ketoisocaproic acid (KIC) were infused intravenously to subjects pretreated with chlorpropamide. After administration of leucine, plasma levels of leucine as well as of insulin were two to three times higher than after infusion of equimolar amounts of KIC. From these results it was suggested that the insulinotropic effect of KIC resulted from its transamination to leucine *in vivo*. *In vitro* experiments, however, demonstrated that KIC rapidly released insulin by a direct effect upon islet cells (PANTEN *et al.*, 1972; FERTEL *et al.*, 1972; SCHÖNBORN *et al.*, 1973, 1974) and that the potency of KIC was higher than that of leucine. In the presence of KIC (10 mM) islets from obese-hyperglycemic mice produced 27 mmoles leucine/h/kg dry weight. This amount of leucine was released nearly completely into the medium (v. KRIEGSTEIN and PANTEN, unpublished observations), which explains the findings that, in the presence of KIC, the leucine content only increased from 0.7 to 1.7 mmoles/kg dry weight (PANTEN *et al.*, 1972). Thus elevation of leucine levels in islets is not likely to be the mechanism of KIC-induced insulin release. This is supported by the finding that even in the presence of 30 mM L-leucine 10 mM KIC induced a significant increase of insulin secretion from the perifused isolated obob-mouse islet (Fig. 1) (PANTEN *et al.*, 1973). There are some hints that mitochondrial degradation of KIC is not the cause for leucine-induced insulin release: isovaleryl-CoA is the decarboxylation product of KIC. But isovalerate did not stimulate insulin release *in vivo* (KNOPF *et al.*, 1963) or *in vitro* (PANTEN *et al.*, 1973). However, the transformation of isovalerate to isovaleryl-CoA by pancreatic islets may be rather slow, as indicated by the low rate of acetoacetate production from islets incubated in the presence of isovalerate (PANTEN *et al.*, 1972). As compared to leucine or KIC, acetoacetate or mevalonate, two final metabolites of both substances, released only insignificant amounts of insulin (FAJANS *et al.*, 1963; PANTEN *et al.*, 1972). The most important

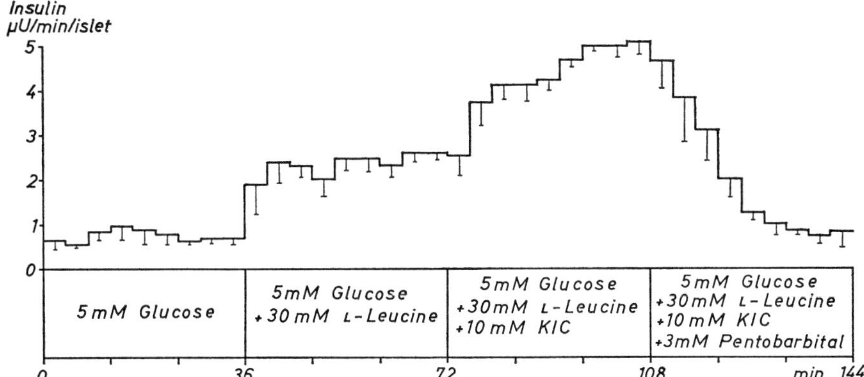

Fig. 1. Effect of KIC upon insulin release of single islets perifused with 30 mM L-leucine. The islets were microdissected from obese-hyperglycemic mice. The columns represent the mean ± s.e.m. of 3 experiments. The inhibitory effect of pentobarbital demonstrates that insulin release is an energy-consuming process. (From PANTEN *et al.*, 1973)

argument against an insulinotropic effect of leucine via its metabolization is provided by the insulin release elicited by 2-aminobicyclo [2,2,1] heptane-2-carboxylic acid (BCH). This nonmetabolized leucine analogue stimulated insulin secretion *in vivo* (CHRISTENSEN and CULLEN, 1969; FAJANS *et al.*, 1971) and *in vitro* (LAMBERT *et al.*, 1970; CHRISTENSEN *et al.*, 1971; PANTEN and CHRISTIANS, 1973; SCHÖNBORN *et al.*, 1973, 1974). Among the stereoisomers of BCH only the (—) b-form was an effective trigger of insulin release (CHRISTENSEN *et al.*, 1971). Evidence has

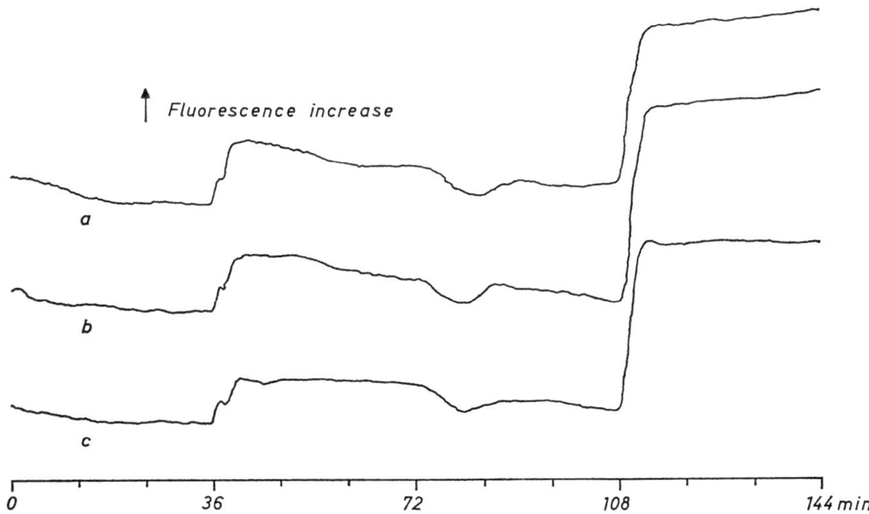

Fig. 2. a—c Fluorescence of NAD(P)H from single perifused islets. The islets (longest diameter 0.30 mm) were microdissected from obese-hyperglycemic mice. a Medium contained 10 mM L-leucine from min 36—72. b Medium contained 20 mM(±)b-BCH from min 36—72. c Medium contained a mixture (20 mM) of 5-methyl-BCH and 6-methyl-BCH from min 36—72. a—c Media contained 20 mM glucose from min 108—144. No other substrates were added to the media. (PANTEN and ISHIDA, unpublished observations)

been presented that the insulinotropic effect of (—) b-BCH is no indirect effect due to elevated leucine levels in the β-cells (PANTEN and CHRISTIANS, 1973). This view was supported by the finding that BCH did not stimulate insulin release by changes of the levels of the naturally occurring amino acids in isolated islets from obese-hyperglycemic mice (GYLFE and HELLMAN, 1972).

In isolated pancreatic islets perifused without substrate b-BCH released insulin with an initial overshoot comparable to the secretion kinetic as caused by leucine (PANTEN *et al.*, 1972; PANTEN and CHRISTIANS, 1973). The secretion profiles were accompanied by a typical twophase increase of fluorescence of reduced pyridine nucleotides (NAD(P)H) (Fig. 2). These rapid changes of islet cell metabolism probably were the consequence of the secretion process (PANTEN and CHRISTIANS, 1973). The striking similarity of leucine- or BCH-induced fluorescence traces suggest that they may be used as metabolic fingerprints to identify substances triggering insulin release by the same mechanism. This view is supported by a similar NAD(P)H-fluorescence profile when islets were perifused with methyl-BCH (Fig. 2), which stimulated insulin release from the perfused rat pancreas (JOOST and HASSELBLATT, 1974). Moreover the fluorescence trace characteristic for KIC was also seen with α-ketocaproic acid (KC), both α-ketoacids showing similar insulinotropic capacity (Fig. 3), (FERTEL *et al.*, 1972), whereas in the absence of glucose, α-ketoisovalerate did not stimulate insulin release and induced only a small increase of the NAD(P)H-fluorescence (PANTEN *et al.*, 1972). To what extent KIC- or KC-induced reduction of pyridine nucleotides is caused by mitochondrial α-ketoacid decarboxylation or by changes of islet cell metabolism due to the secretory process remains to be shown (PANTEN *et al.*, 1973).

Reduction of pyridine nucleotides of pancreatic islets, however, is no obligatory reaction accompanying amino acid-induced insulin secretion, as demonstrated by the lack of fluorescence changes when insulin release was elicited by L-arginine (PANTEN and CHRISTIANS, 1973). The latter results support the view that arginine acts upon insulin secretion by a mechanism different from the mechanism whereby leucine or BCH stimulates insulin secretion (FAJANS *et al.*, 1971). The latter authors reported evidence from *in vivo* experiments for that view: 1. Pretreatment with chlorpropamide accentuated leucine- or BCH-induced insulin secretion, but not arginine-induced insulin secretion. 2. Mannoheptulose suppressed the insulinotropic effect of arginine, but not of leucine or BCH. 3. In contrast to leucine or BCH, arginine enhanced plasma glucagon levels.

It has been proposed that leucine and BCH trigger insulin release by binding to their specific transport molecules in the β-cell plasma membrane (CHRISTENSEN and CULLEN, 1969; CHRISTENSEN *et al.*, 1971). This hypothesis was not supported by measurements of leucine or BCH uptake by pancreatic islets: only (—) b-BCH triggered insulin release, whereas (—) b-BCH as well as (+) b-BCH were rapidly taken up by islet cells (CHRISTENSEN *et al.*, 1971). HELLMAN *et al.* (1972) presented strong evidence that both L- and D-leucine were largely transported by the same system in pancreatic β-cells. But D-leucine neither stimulated insulin release nor inhibited L-leucine-induced insulin secretion (LERNMARK, 1972b; HELLMAN *et al.*, 1972), although either leucine isomer decreased the uptake of the other. Therefore the L-system probably is not the recognition site signalling insulin release in response to L-leucine or (—)b-BCH (HELLMAN *et al.*, 1972). The receptor site for insulin release obviously responds to the (—)b-BCH molecule as if it were L-leucine. The (—)b-BCH-molecule is subject to rather little distortion (CHRISTENSEN *et al.*, 1969) and can be used as a template for the positions the flexible carbon chain of L-leucine can take in space (Fig. 4) (TAGER and CHRISTENSEN, 1971a). Since a mixture of 5- and 6-methyl-b-BCH resembled b-BCH in its action on the

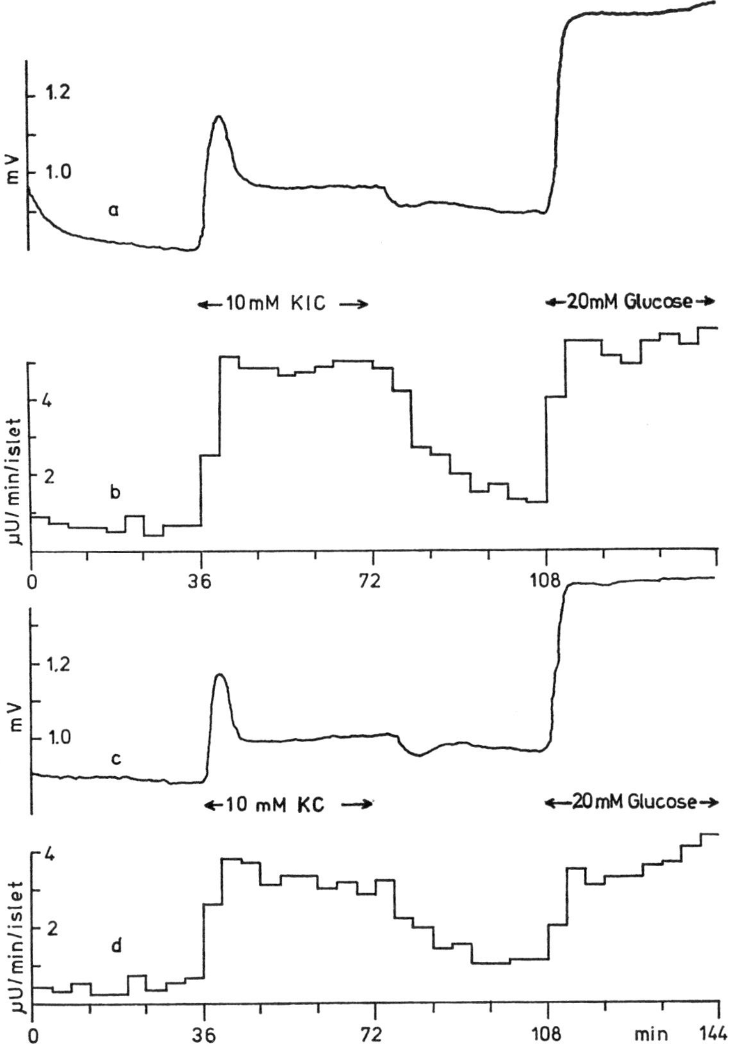

Fig. 3. a—d Effect of KIC or KC on NAD(P)H-fluorescence (curve a and c) and insulin release (curve b and d) from single perifused islets (longest diameter 0.30 mm). The islets were microdissected from obese-hyperglycemic mice. From min 0—36 and min 72—108 the media contained no substrates. An upward deflection of the traces (a and c) represents an increase of the fluorescence light (recorded as mV). (PANTEN, unpublished observations)

endocrine pancreas, a leucine conformation as shown in Fig. 4c appears to be active at its receptor site for insulin release. However the possibility exists that the leucine conformation corresponding to 7-methyl-b-BCH (Fig. 4b) is active too. The unchanged structure of its carbon chain is necessary to maintain the insulinotropic effect of L-leucine, since norleucine (TAGER and CHRISTENSEN, 1971b; PANTEN unpublished observations), norvaline (SCHÖNBORN *et al.*, 1973, 1974; ALBERTI and WHALLEY, 1973), and valine (FAJANS *et al.*, 1967; MALAISSE and MALAISSE-LAGAE, 1968; MILNER, 1970; PANTEN *et al.*, 1972) did not stimulate

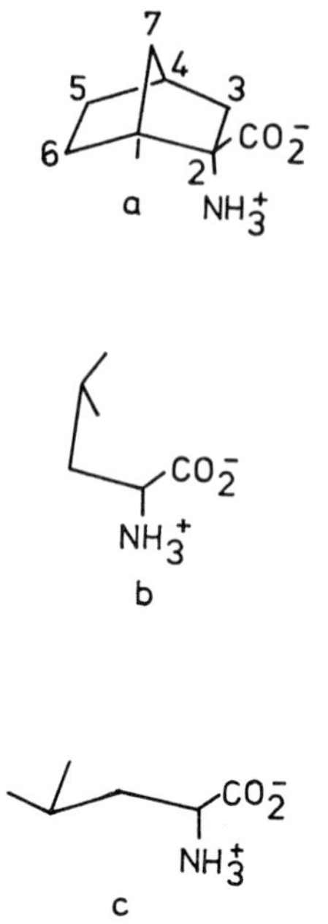

Fig. 4. a—c Conformations of L-leucine (b and c) allowing approximate superposition with (—)b-BCH(a)

insulin secretion. Isoleucine was less effective (MILNER, 1970; TAGER and CHRISTENSEN, 1971b) or ineffective (LERNMARK, 1972b), as compared to leucine. In addition to the above-mentioned amino acids, TAGER and CHRISTENSEN (1971a, b) tested the hypoglycemic activity of several other amino acids structurally related to leucine and BCH. With the exception of 2-methyl-1-aminocyclo-pentanecarboxylic acid, which decreased blood glucose slightly, none of these amino acids caused hypoglycemia.

Isocaproic acid or L-α-hydroxyisocaproic acid did not stimulate insulin release from isolated pancreatic islets (PANTEN *et al.*, 1973). KIC, however, released more insulin than L-leucine (PANTEN *et al.*, 1972; FERTEL *et al.*, 1972; SCHÖNBORN *et al.*, 1974).

Whether L-leucine and KIC act on different or on the same receptors is not clear. A search for competitive inhibitors of both substances may clarify the latter point.

c) Other Amino Acids

Alanine: In contrast to its insulin-releasing effect upon incubated cultured fetal rat pancreas (LAMBERT *et al.*, 1970), alanine (5 mM) did not stimulate insulin release from isolated mouse islets (LERNMARK, 1972a).

α-Aminoisobutyric acid: The insulinotropic effect of α-aminoisobutyric acid reported to occur in fetal rat pancreas (LAMBERT *et al.*, 1970) was not seen in isolated mouse islets (LERNMARK, 1972a).

Glutamate: Isolated islets from obese-hyperglycemic mice did not release insulin in response to glutamate (10 mM) (SEHLIN, 1972b).

Glycine: Glycine released insulin from incubated rat pancreas pieces (MALAISSE and MALAISSE-LAGAE, 1968) or from the perfused rat pancreas (ALSEVER *et al.*, 1970), but not from isolated mouse islets (SEHLIN, 1972a).

Histidine: In man histidine induced no significant insulin release (FAJANS *et al.*, 1967). In contrast to negative results from *in vitro* experiments (PFEIFFER and TELIB, 1968; MALAISSE and MALAISSE-LAGAE, 1968; MILNER, 1970), EDGAR *et al.* (1969) and LAMBERT *et al.* (1969) demonstrated a significant stimulatory activity of histidine (8.3 or 11 mM) on insulin secretion from rabbit pancreas pieces or cultured fetal rat pancreas.

Lysine: In man next arginine, L-lysine had the most potent insulinotropic effect (FAJANS *et al.*, 1967). Lysine (5—11 mM) induced insulin release from incubated pancreas tissue from rats (MALAISSE and MALAISSE-LAGAE, 1968), rabbits (EDGAR *et al.*, 1969; MILNER, 1970), or cultured fetal rat pancreas (LAMBERT *et al.*, 1969).

Methionine: In man methionine-induced elevation of plasma insulin levels was smaller than after application of phenylalanine or leucine (FAJANS *et al.*, 1967). MILNER (1970) and MALAISSE and MALAISSE-LAGAE (1968) failed to demonstrate an insulinotropic effect of methionine (5 or 10 mM) on rabbit or rat pancreatic tissue, whereas PFEIFFER and TELIB (1968) found that methionine (6.7 or 67 mM) released insulin from rabbit pancreas.

Ornithine: In man intravenous infusion of ornithine caused a small increase of plasma insulin levels (FAJANS *et al.*, 1967).

Phenylalanine: Phenylalanine was shown to stimulate insulin release in man, approaching the potency of leucine (FAJANS *et al.*, 1967). *In vitro* phenylalanine (10—11 mM) enhanced insulin secretion from rat pancreas pieces (MALAISSE and MALAISSE-LAGAE, 1968) or from cultured fetal rat pancreas (LAMBERT *et al.*, 1969), but 5 mM phenylalanine inhibited insulin release from rabbit pancreas (MILNER, 1970).

Proline: 8.7 or 87 mM proline induced only a weak insulin release from incubated pieces of rabbit pancreas (PFEIFFER and TELIB, 1968).

Threonine: Threonine was as potent as tryptophan or methionine in causing insulin release in man (FLOYD *et al.*, 1966b). *In vitro* threonine was ineffective as insulin secretagogue (MILNER, 1970).

Tryptophan: In man tryptophan induced a small insulin release (FLOYD *et al.*, 1966a, b). Tryptophan (10 mM) released insulin from incubated rat pancreas pieces (MALAISSE and MALAISSE-LAGAE, 1968), whereas 5 mM tryptophan had no insulinotropic effect on rabbit pancreas pieces (MILNER, 1970).

4. Conclusions

The experimental evidence summarized in this chapter demonstrates the direct stimulatory effect of single amino acids upon insulin release from pancreatic islets. The insulinotropic effect of arginine and leucine has been the subject of many studies. There is, however, a need for more detailed information on insulin secretion in response to other naturally occurring amino acids. The experimental data support the view that both arginine and leucine as such trigger insulin release by acting directly upon the β-cells. A definite proof of this hypothesis can be given by experiments with a pure β-cell preparation, which is not yet available. Pure β-cells also may be necessary to clarify whether amino acid-induced insulin release is mediated by cyclic AMP.

The finding that artificial nonmetabolized amino acids stimulated insulin release encourages the search for related substances which may represent new approaches to oral therapy of diabetes.

References

ALBERTI, K.G.M.M., WHALLEY, M.D.: Short chain analogues of arginine: Potent stimulators of insulin secretion. In: Proceedings VIII Congress of the International Diabetes Federation, p. 21. Amsterdam: Excerpta Medica 1973

ALSEVER, R.N., GEORG, R.H., SUSSMAN, K.E.: Stimulation of insulin secretion by guanidinoacetic acid and other guanidine derivatives. Endocrinology **86**, 332—336 (1970)

ASHCROFT, ST.J.H., WEERASINGHE, L.C.C., RANDLE, P.J.: Interrelationship of islet metabolism, adenosine triphosphate content and insulin release. Biochem. J. **132**, 223—231 (1973)

BASABE, J.C., LOPEZ, N.L., VIKTORA, J.K., WOLFF, F.W.: Insulin secretion studied in the perfused rat pancreas. I. Effect of tolbutamide, leucine and arginine; their interaction with diazoxide, and relation to glucose. Diabetes **20**, 449—456 (1971)

BRIEL, G., GYLFE, E., HELLMAN, B., NEUHOFF, V.: Microdetermination of free amino acids in pancreatic islets isolated from obese-hyperglycemic mice. Acta physiol. scand. **84**, 247—253 (1972)

CHESNEY, T.McC., SCHOFIELD, J.G.: Studies on the secretion of pancreatic glucagon. Diabetes **18**, 627—632 (1969)

CHRISTENSEN, H.N.: Nature and roles of receptor sites for amino acid transport. Advanc. Biochem. Psychopharm. **4**, 39—62 (1972)

CHRISTENSEN, H.N., CULLEN, A.M.: Behavior in the rat of a transport-specific, bicyclic amino acid. Hypoglycemic action. J. biol. Chem. **244**, 1521—1526 (1969)

CHRISTENSEN, H.N., HANDLOGTEN, M.E., LAM, J., TAGER, H.S., ZAND, R.: A bicyclic amino acid to improve discriminations among transport systems. J. biol. Chem. **244**, 1510—1520 (1969)

CHRISTENSEN, H.N., HELLMAN, B., LERNMARK, A., SEHLIN, J., TAGER, H.S., TÄLJEDAL, I.-B.: In vitro stimulation of insulin release by non-metabolizable, transport-specific amino acids. Biochim. biophys. Acta (Amst.) **241**, 341—348 (1971)

COORE, H.G., RANDLE, P.J., SIMON, E., KRAICER, P.F., SHELENSNYAK, M.C.: Block of insulin secretion from the pancreas by D-mannoheptulose. Nature (Lond.) **197**, 1264—1266 (1963)

CURTIS, D.R., WATKINS, J.C.: The pharmacology of amino acids related to gamma-aminobutyric acid. Pharmacol. Rev. **17**, 347—391 (1965)

DANIELSSON, A., HELLMAN, B., IDAHL, L.A.: Levels of ketoglutarate and glutamate in stimulated pancreatic cells. Horm. Metab. Res. **2**, 28—31 (1970)

EDGAR, P., RABINOWITZ, D., MERIMEE, T.J.: Effects of amino acids on insulin release from excised rabbit pancreas. Endocrinology **84**, 835—843 (1969)

EDWARDS, J.C., TAYLOR, K.W.: Fatty acids and the release of glucagon from isolated guinea-pig islets of Langerhans incubated in vitro. Biochim. biophys. Acta (Amst.) **215**, 310—315 (1970)

EFENDIC, S., CERASI, E., LUFT, R.: Role of glucose in arginine-induced insulin release in man. Metabolism **20**, 568—579 (1971)

FAJANS, S.S., KNOPF, R.F., FLOYD, J.C., POWES, L., CONN, J.W.: The experimental induction in man of sensitivity to leucine hypoglycemia. J. clin. Invest. **42**, 216—229 (1963)

FAJANS, S.S., FLOYD, J.C., JR., KNOPF, R.F., CONN, J.W.: A comparison of leucine- and acetoacetate-induced hypoglycemia in man. J. clin. Invest. **43**, 2003—2008 (1969)

FAJANS, S.S., FLOYD, J.C., JR., KNOPF, R.F., CONN, J.W.: Effect of amino acids and proteins on insulin secretion in man. Recent Progr. Hormone Res. **23**, 617—662 (1967)

FAJANS, S.S., FLOYD, J.C., JR., KNOPF, R.F., PEK, S., QUIBRERA, R., CONN, J.W.: Effects of amino acids on insulin release in vivo. In: 7th Congress of the International Diabetes Federation, Buenos Aires, pp. 123—136. Amsterdam: Excerpta Medica 1971

FAJANS, S.S., FLOYD, J.C., JR.: Stimulation of islet cell secretion by nutrients and by gastrointestinal hormones released during digestion. In: Handbook of Physiol. Section 7: Endocrinology, Vol. 1, pp. 473—493. Ed. by D.F. STEINER, N. FREINKEL. Baltimore: Williams and Wilkins 1972

FAJANS, S.S., FLOYD, J.C., JR., KNOPF, R.F., PEK, S., WEISSMAN, P., CONN, J.W.: Amino acids and insulin release in vivo. Israel J. med. Sci. **8**, 233—243 (1972)

FERTEL, R., KOTLER-BRAJTBURG, J., HOLOWACH-THURSTON, J., MATSCHINSKY, F.M.: Insulin secretion due to alpha-ketomonocarboxylic acids. Diabetes **21**, Suppl. 1, 359 (1972)

FLOYD, C.J., JR., FAJANS, S.S., CONN, J.W., KNOPF, R.F., RULL, J.: Insulin secretion in response to protein ingestion. J. clin. Invest. **45**, 1479—1486 (1966a)

FLOYD, J.C., JR., FAJANS, S.S., CONN, J.W., KNOPF, R.F., RULL, J.: Stimulation of insulin secretion by amino acids. J. clin. Invest. **45**, 1487—1502 (1966b)

FLOYD, J.C., JR., FAJANS, S.S., PEK, S., THIFFAULT, C.A., KNOPF, R.F., CONN, J.W.: Synergistic effect of essential amino acids and glucose upon insulin secretion in man. Diabetes **19**, 109—115 (1970)

FOA, P.P.: The secretion of glucagon. In: Handbook of Physiol. Section 7: Endocrinology, Vol. 1, pp. 261—277. Endocrine pancreas. Ed. by D.F. STEINER, N. FREINKEL, Baltimore: Williams and Wilkins 1972

FUSSGÄNGER, R.D., GRAJEDA, E., LAUBE, H., PFEIFFER, E.F.: Insulin und Glucagonsekretion des isoliert perfundierten Pankreas der Ratte nach verschiedenen Aminosäuren. Abstr. Congr. German Diabetes Association 7th., pp. 98—103. Copenhagen: Novo Documentation Service 1972

GEPTS, W., GREGOIRE, F., VAN ASSCHE, A., DE-GASPARO, M.: Quantitative enzyme pattern and insulin content of human islets of Langerhans. In: The structure and metabolism of the pancreatic islets, pp. 283—303. FALKMER, S., HELLMAN, B., TÄLJEDAL, I.-B. (Eds.). Oxford: Pergamon Press 1970

GREEN, I.C., TAYLOR, K.W.: Effects of pregnancy in the rat on the size and insulin secretory response of the islets of Langerhans. J. Endocr. **54**, 317—325 (1972)

GRODSKY, G.M.: Insulin and the pancreas. Vitam. and Horm. **28**, 37—101 (1970)

GYLFE, E., HELLMAN, B.: Free amino acids in mammalian pancreatic islets rich in β-cells. Diabetologia **8**, 363 (1972)

HALES, C.N., MILNER, R.D.G.: The role of sodium and potassium in insulin secretion from rabbit pancreas. J. Physiol. (Lond.) **194**, 725—743 (1968)

HEINZE, E., STEINKE, J.: Insulin secretion during development: Response of isolated pancreatic islets of fetal, newborn and adult rats to theophylline and arginine. Horm. Metab. Res. **4**, 234—236 (1972)

HELLERSTRÖM, C., HELLMAN, B.: Quantitative studies on isolated pancreatic islets of mammals. I. Peptidase activity in normal and obese-hyperglycaemic mice. Acta endocr. (Kbh.) **42**, 615—624 (1963)

HELLMAN, B.: Fluorometric assays of glutamic-pyruvic transaminase activity in microdissected pancreatic islets from obese-hyperglycemic mice. Acta physiol. scand. **65**, 357—363 (1965)

HELLMAN, B.: Islet morphology and glucose metabolism in relation to the specific function of the pancreatic β-cells. In: Proceedings of the sixth Congress of the International Diabetes Federation, ÖSTMANN, F., MILNER, P.D., (Eds.) Intern. Congr. Ser. 172, pp. 192—199. Amsterdam: Excerpta Medica 1969

HELLMAN, B., LARSSON, S.: The glucose metabolism in the islets of Langerhans. I. In vitro studies of the fate of uniformly ^{14}C-labelled glucose and fructose in cottus quadricornis L. Acta endocr. (Kbh.) **38**, 303—314 (1961)

HELLMAN, B., SEHLIN, J., TÄLJEDAL, I.-B.: Uptake of alanine, arginine and leucine by mammalian pancreatic β-cells. Endocrinology **89**, 1432—1439 (1971a)

HELLMAN, B., SEHLIN, J., TÄLJEDAL, I.-B.: Transport of α-amino-isobutyric acid in mammalian pancreatic β-cells. Diabetologia **7**, 256—265 (1971b)

HELLMAN, B., SEHLIN, J., TÄLJEDAL, I.-B.: Effects of glucose and other modifiers of insulin release on the oxidative metabolism of amino acids in micro-dissected pancreatic islets. Biochem. J. **123**, 513—521 (1971c)

HELLMAN, B., SEHLIN, J., TÄLJEDAL, I.-B.: Transport of L-leucine and D-leucine into pancreatic β-cells with reference to the mechanisms of amino acid-induced insulin release. Biochim. biophys. Acta (Amst.) **266**, 436—443 (1972)

HELLMAN, B., TÄLJEDAL, I.-B.: Histochemistry of the pancreatic islet cells. In: Handbook of Physiology, Section 7, Endocrinology, Vol. 1, pp. 91—110. Endocrine pancreas. Ed. by D.F. STEINER, N. FREINKEL. Baltimore: Williams and Wilkins 1972

HERTELENDY, F., MACHLIN, L.J., TAKAHASHI, Y., KIPNIS, D.M.: Insulin release from sheep pancreas in vitro. J. Endocr. **41**, 605—606 (1968)

HOWELL, S.L., MONTAGUE, W.: Adenylate cyclase activity in isolated rat islets of Langerhans. Effects of agents which alter rates of insulin secretion. Biochim. biophys. Acta (Amst.) **320**, 44—52 (1973)

HUMBEL, R.E., RENOLD, A.E.: Studies on isolated islets of Langerhans of teleost fishes. I. Metabolic activity in vitro. Biochim. biophys. Acta (Amst.) **74**, 84—95 (1963)

IDAHL, L.A., TÄLJEDAL, I.-B.: Leucyl-beta-naphthylamide-splitting enzymes in the mammalian endocrine pancreas. Biochem. J. **106**, 161—165 (1968)

IVERSEN, J.: Secretion of glucagon from the isolated, perfused canine pancreas. J. clin. Invest. **50**, 2123—2136 (1971)

JACOBSEN, J.G., SMITH, L.H., JR.: Biochemistry and physiology of taurine and taurine derivatives. Physiol. Rev. **48**, 424—511 (1968)

JOOST, J.G., HASSELBLATT, A.: Effects of bicyclic amino acids upon insulin release of the perfused rat pancreas. Naunyn-Schmiedebergs Arch. Pharmak. exp. Path. in press (1974)

KANETO, A., OSAKA, K.: Stimulation of glucagon secretion by arginine and histidine infused intrapancreatically. Endocrinology **88**, 1239—1245 (1971)

KANETO, A., KOSAKA, K.: Effects of leucine and isoleucine infused intrapancreatically on glucagon and insulin secretion. Endocrinology **91**, 691—695 (1972)

KISSANE, J.M., LACY, P.E., BROLIN, S.E., SMITH, C.H.: Quantitative histochemistry of the islets of Langerhans. In: The structure and metabolism of the pancreatic islets, pp. 281—287. BROLIN, S.E., HELLMAN, B., KNUTSEN, H., (Eds.). Oxford: Pergamon Press 1964

KIZER, J.S., BRESSLER, R.: Drugs and the mechanism of insulin secretion. Advanc. Pharmacol. **7**, 91—115 (1969)

KNOPF, R.F., FAJANS, S.S., FLOYD, J.C., JR., CONN, J.W.: Comparison of experimentally induced and naturally occurring sensitivity to leucine hypoglycemia. J. clin. Endocr. **23**, 579—587 (1963)

KUO, W.N., HODGINS, D.S., KUO, J.F.: Adenylate cyclase in islets of Langerhans. Isolation of islets and regulation of adenylate cyclase activity by various hormones and agents. J. biol. Chem. **248**, 2705—2711 (1973)

LAMBERT, A.E., JEANRENAUD, B., JUNOD, A., RENOLD, A.E.: Organ culture of fetal rat pancreas. II. Insulin release induced by amino and organic acids, by hormonal peptides, by cationic alterations of the medium and by other agents. Biochim. biophys. Acta (Amst.) **174**, 540—553 (1969)

LAMBERT, A.E., KANAZAWA, Y., ORCI, L., CHRISTENSEN, H.N.: Stimulation of insulin release by natural amino acids and their non-metabolized analogues. Diabetologia **6**, 635 (1970)

LANDGRAF, R., LANDGRAF-LEURS, M., SCRIBA, P., SCHWARZ, K.: Opposite kinetics of L-leucine and L-phenylalanine induced insulin release studied with the perfused rat pancreas. Diabetes **21**, Suppl. 1, 369 (1972)

LERNMARK, A.: Effects of neutral and dibasic amino acids on the in vitro release of insulin. Hormones **3**, 22—30 (1972a)

LERNMARK, A.: Specificity of leucine stimulation of insulin release. Hormones **3**, 14—21 (1972b)

LEVEY, G.S., SCHMIDT, W.M., MINTZ, D.H.: Activation of adenyl cyclase in a pancreatic islet cell adenoma by glucagon and tolbutamide. Metabolism **21**, 93—98 (1972)

LEVIN, S.R., GRODSKY, G.M., HAGURA, R., SMITH, D.F., FORSHAM, R.H.: Relationships between arginine and glucose in the induction of insulin secretion from the isolated, perfused rat pancreas. Endocrinology **90**, 624—631 (1972)

LEVIN, S.R., KARAM, J.H., HANE, S., GRODSKY, G.M., FORSHAM, P.H.: Enhancement of arginine-induced insulin secretion in man by prior administration of glucose. Diabetes **20**, 171—176 (1971)

LUCKE, C., KAGAN, A., ADELMAN, N., GLICK, S.M.: Effect of 2-deoxy-d-glucose and mannoheptulose on the insulin response to amino acids in rabbits. Diabetes **21**, 1—5 (1972)

MALAISSE, W.J.: Hormonal and environmental modification of islet activity. In: Handbook of Physiology, Section 7, Endocrinology Vol. 1, Endocrine pancreas, pp. 237—260. Ed. by D.F. STEINER, N. FREINKEL. Baltimore: Williams and Wilkins 1972

MALAISSE, W.J., MALAISSE-LAGAE, F.: Stimulation of insulin secretion by noncarbohydrate metabolites. J. Lab. clin. Med. **72**, 438—448 (1968)

MALAISSE, W.J., MALAISSE-LAGAE, F.: Biochemical, pharmacological and physiological aspects of the beta-cell's adenylcyclase-phosphodiesterase system. In: The Structure and Metabolism of the Pancreatic Islets, pp. 435—443. Ed. by S. FALKMER, B. HELLMAN, I.-B. TÄLJEDAL. Oxford: Pergamon Press 1970

MALAISSE-LAGAE, F., BRISSON, G.R., MALAISSE, W.J.: The stimulus-secretion coupling of glucose-induced insulin release. VI. Analogy between the insulinotropic mechanisms of sugars and amino acids. Horm. Metab. Res. **3**, 374—378 (1971)

MARKS, V., SAMOLS, E.: Intestinal factors in the regulation of insulin secretion. Advanc. Metab. Disord. **4**, 1—38 (1970)

MAYHEW, D.A., WRIGHT, P.H., ASHMORE, J.: Regulation of Insulin secretion. Pharmacol. Rev. **21**, 183—212 (1969)

MCGIVAN, J.D., BRADFORD, N.M., CROMPTON, M., CHAPPELL, J.B.: Effect of L-leucine on the nitrogen metabolism of isolated rat liver mitochondria. Biochem. J. **134**, 209—215 (1973)

MILNER, R.D.: The secretion of insulin from foetal and postnatal rabbit pancreas in vitro in response to various substances. J. Endocr. **44**, 267—272 (1969)

MILNER, R.D.: The stimulation of insulin release by essential amino acids from rabbit pancreas in vitro. J. Endocr. **47**, 347—356 (1970)

MILNER, R.D., ASHWORTH, M.A., BARSON, A.J.: Insulin release from human foetal pancreas in response to glucose, leucine and arginine. J. Endocr. **52**, 497—505 (1972)

MILNER, R.D., HALES, C.N.: The interaction of various inhibitors and stimuli of insulin release studied with rabbit pancreas in vitro. Biochem. J. **113**, 473—479 (1969)

MONTAGUE, W., HOWELL, S.L.: The mode of action of adenosine 3′:5′-cyclic monophosphate in mammalian islets of Langerhans. Biochem. J. **134**, 321—327 (1973)

OHNEDA, A., PARADA, E., EISENTRAUT, A.M., UNGER, R.H.: Characterization of response of circulating glucagon to intraduodenal and intravenous administration of amino acids. J. clin. Invest. **47**, 2305—2322 (1968)

OXENDER, D.L., CHRISTENSEN, H.N.: Distinct mediating systems for the transport of neutral amino acids by the Ehrlich cell. J. biol. Chem. **238**, 3686—3699 (1963)

PANTEN, U., CHRISTIANS, J.: Effects of 2-endo-aminonorbornane-2-carboxylic acid upon insulin secretion and fluorescence of reduced pyridine nucleotides of isolated perifused pancreatic islets. Naunyn-Schmiedebergs Arch. Pharmak. exp. Path. **276**, 55—62 (1973)

PANTEN, U., CHRISTIANS, J., VON KRIEGSTEIN, E., POSER, W., HASSELBLATT, A.: Studies on the mechanism of L-leucine- and α-ketoisocaproic acid-induced insulin release from perifused isolated pancreatic islets. Diabetologia in press (1973)

PANTEN, U., VON KRIEGSTEIN, E., POSER, W., SCHÖNBORN, J., HASSELBLATT, A.: Effects of L-leucine and α-ketoisocaproic acid upon insulin secretion and metabolism of isolated pancreatic islets. FEBS Letters **20**, 225—228 (1972)

PFEIFFER, E.F., RAPTIS, S., FUSSGÄNGER, R.: Gastrointestinal hormones and islet function. In: Handbuch der experimentellen Pharmakologie, Vol. 34, pp. 259—310. Berlin-Heidelberg-New York: Springer 1973

PFEIFFER, E.F., TELIB, M.: Insulin secretion in vitro: Studies in amphibians and mammalians. Acta diabet. lat. **5**, Suppl. 1, 30—63 (1968)

RABINOWITZ, D., MERIMEE, T.J., MAFFEZZOLI, R., BURGESS, J.A.: Patterns of hormonal release after glucose, protein, and glucose plus protein. Lancet **1966II**, 454—456

RAPTIS, S., DOLLINGER, H.C., SCHROEDER, K.E., SCHLEYER, M., ROTHENBUCHNER, G., PFEIFFER, E.F.: Differences in insulin, growth hormone and pancreatic enzyme secretion after intravenous and intraduodenal administration of mixed amino acids in man. New Engl. J. Med. **288**, 1199—1202 (1973)

ROCHA, D.M., FALOONA, G.R., UNGER, R.H.: Glucagon-stimulating activity of 20 amino acids in dogs. J. clin. Invest. **51**, 2346—2351 (1972)

SAMOLS, E., TYLER, J.M., MARKS, V.: Glucagon-insulin interrelationship In: Glucagon, pp. 151—173. LEFEBVRE, P.J., UNGER, R.H. (Eds.). Oxford: Pergamon Press 1972

SAMS, D.J., MONTAGUE, W.: The role of adenosine 3′:5′-cyclic monophosphate in the regulation of insulin release. Properties of islet-cell adenosine 3′:5′-cyclic monophosphate phosphodiesterase. Biochem. J. **129**, 945—952 (1972)

SCHÖNBORN, J., WESTPHAL, P., PANTEN, U.: Insulin release from the isolated perfused rat pancreas in the presence of L-leucine, 2-aminonorbornane-2-carboxylic acid, L-norvaline, and α-ketoisocaproic acid. Diabetologia **9**, 88 (1973a)

SCHÖNBORN, J., PANTEN, U., WESTPHAL, P.: Insulin release from the isolated perfused rat pancreas induced by L-leucine, 2-aminonorbornane-2-carboxylic acid and α-ketoisocaproic acid. Horm. Metab. Res., submitted for publication (1974)

SEHLIN, J.: Transport and oxidation of glycine in mammalian pancreatic islets with reference to the mechanism of amino acid-induced insulin release. Hormones **3**, 144—155 (1972a)

SEHLIN, J.: Uptake and oxidation of glutamic acid in mammalian pancreatic islets. Hormones **3**, 156—166 (1972b)

SELAWRY, H., MARCKS, C., FINK, G., LAVINE, R., CRESTO, J., RECANT, L.: A mechanism for glucose-induced insulin release. Diabetes **22**, Suppl. 1, 295 (1973)

STORK, H., HELLERSTRÖM, C., WESTMAN, S.: Respiration of the β-cells in the presence of sulfonylureas. In: The structure and metabolism of the pancreatic islets, pp. 331—336. FALKMER, S., HELLMAN, B., TÄLJEDAL, I.-B. (Eds.). Oxford: Pergamon Press 1970

SUSSMAN, K.E., STJERNHOLM, M., VAUGHAN, G.D.: Tolbutamide and its effect upon insulin secretion in the isolated perfused rat pancreas. In: Tolbutamide after ten years, pp. 22—31. Amsterdam: Excerpta Medica 1967

TAGER, H.S., CHRISTENSEN, H.N.: Transport of the four isomers of 2-aminonorbornane-2-carboxylic acid in selected mammalian systems and in Escherichia coli. J. biol. Chem. **246**, 7572—7580 (1971a)

TAGER, H.S., CHRISTENSEN, H.N.: Hypoglycemic action of 2-amino-norbornane-2-carboxylic acid in the rat. Biochem. biophys. Res. Commun. **44**, 185—191 (1971b)

TURTLE, J.R., KIPNIS, D.M.: An adrenergic receptor mechanism for the control of cyclic 3′5′ adenosine monophosphate synthesis in tissues. Biochem. biophys. Res. Commun. **28**, 797—802 (1967)

YALOW, R.S., BERSON, S.A.: Immunoassay of plasma insulin in man. J. clin. Invest. **39**, 1157—1175 (1960)

IV. Participation of the Adenylate Cyclase System

WILLY J. MALAISSE

1. Introduction

The idea that adenosine-3′,5′-cyclic monophosphate (cAMP) may play a role in the regulation of insulin secretion by the pancreatic B-cell was probably first raised when SAMOLS *et al.* (1965) reported that glucagon stimulated insulin release in man. Indeed, because the effect of glucagon in a variety of biological systems is apparently mediated by cellular accumulation of cAMP, the discovery of the insulinotropic action of glucagon was rapidly followed by a series of investigations on the effect upon insulin release of various agents known or thought to affect cAMP synthesis and breakdown. The inhibitory effect of catecholamines on insulin release, first disclosed by COORE and RANDLE (1964), was also soon considered in connection with the concept that cAMP played a significant role in the regulation of insulin secretion by the B-cell. Within the general framework of this concept, a tremendous number of investigations has been carried out over the last few years in order to elucidate the regulation of cAMP metabolism in insular tissue, the precise site of action of cAMP in the insulin secretory sequence, and the physiological significance of the B-cell adenylate cyclase system. As these topics have been reviewed on other occasions (MALAISSE and MALAISSE-LAGAE, 1970a; MALAISSE, 1972), emphasis will here be given to the most recent contributions in this field.

2. The Regulation of cAMP Metabolism in the B-cell

TURTLE and KIPNIS (1967) were the first to measure cAMP in insular tissue. Based on their own and subsequent work, the following picture was gained concerning the factors regulating the level of cAMP in the B-cell.

a) Membrane Receptors in the B-cell

According to current concepts, activation of adenylcyclase in a variety of biological systems is the consequence of the binding of a given hormone (or first messenger) to a receptor system located at the cell membrane. Recently, GOLDFINE *et al.* (1972) reported on the binding of glucagon and enteroglucagon to subcellular fractions obtained from a transplantable insular tumor of the Syrian Hamster. Incidentally, it has also been postulated that the membrane of the B-cell is equipped with a receptor molecule for glucose; at present, this concept remains entirely speculative. The binding of other insulinotropic agents, especially sulfonylureas, to the B-cell plasma membrane is also under active investigation (HELLMAN *et al.*, 1973).

b) Insular Adenylate Cyclase

According to cytochemical studies (HOWELL and WHITFIELD, 1972a), the adenylate cyclase activity is localized specifically at the B-cell membrane and can be stimulated by either NaF or glucagon. The enzyme is said to display a K_m for ATP of about 2.10^{-4}M (DAVIS and LAZARUS, 1972). The regulation of adenylate cyclase activity in islets of Langerhans was extensively examined by KUO *et al.* (1973). The most marked stimulation was obtained by NaF, which is supposed to activate adenylate cyclase only in acellular systems and not in the intact cell. The enzyme was also activated by polypeptide hormones (glucagon, ACTH, pancreozymin, secretin), β-adrenergic agonists (isoproterenol, or the combination of epinephrine or norepinephrine with an α-adrenergic blocking agent), prostaglandins, acetylcholine, tolbutamide, ethanol, EGTA, and both GTP and GDP. The calcium-chelating agent EGTA and GDP potentiated the glucagon-induced activation of adenylate cyclase. Insulin inhibited both basal and ACTH-stimulated adenylate cyclase activity. Epinephrine, norepinephrine, arginine, and other amino acids also inhibited the enzyme; whereas glucose, leucine, and phenformin failed to cause any significant effect. Some of these findings confirm previous observations. For instance, in an islet cell tumor of the Syrian Hamster, ROSEN *et al.* (1971) observed that the adenylate cyclase recovered in the material sedimented at 20,000 *g* (30 min) was indeed activated by NaF and glucagon and inhibited by Ca^{++}, but failed to detect any effect of glucose, arginine, catecholamines, PGE_1, ACTH, insulin, secretin, or ethanol. DAVIS and LAZARUS (1972) again found stimulation by NaF, glucagon, pancreozymin, and secretin; inhibition by calcium; and no effect of glucose and galactose. Using a pancreatic islet cell adenoma, LEVEY *et al.* (1972) where also unable to detect any obvious effect of glucose, arginine, or leucine on the tumor adenylate cyclase, which could be stimulated, however, by NaF, glucagon, and tolbutamide. HOWELL and MONTAGUE (1973) reported stimulation of adenylate cyclase by NaF, glucagon, PGE_1 or PGE_2, GTP; inhibition by catecholamines and its reversal in the presence of phenoxybenzamine; and no effect of glucose, glibenclamide, xylitol, leucine, arginine, or potassium. The results of other studies will be considered in the section devoted to the regulation of cAMP levels in the B-cell (see section 2.d.).

c) Insular Phosphodiesterase

Cyclic AMP phosphodiesterase activity in insular material has been characterized by different investigators (ROSEN *et al.*, 1971; GOLDFINE *et al.*, 1971; SAMS and MONTAGUE, 1972; KUO *et al.*, 1973). The enzymatic activity is apparently localized in areas of the cytoplasm close to secretory granules (HOWELL and WHITFIELD, 1972b). There appear to be two enzyme systems with K_m values for cAMP of 2—9 μM and 30 μM or more, respectively (GOLDFINE *et al.*, 1971; SAMS and MONTAGUE, 1972; BOWEN and LAZARUS, 1972). Optimal pH is in the range of 8.2—8.5 (SAMS and MONTAGUE, 1972; BOWEN and LAZARUS, 1972). The apparent molecular weight of the enzyme is 200000 (SAMS and MONTAGUE, 1972). About 70% of the total insular activity is found in the postmicrosomal supernatant, "particulate" activity also being present (ROSEN *et al.*, 1971; SAMS and MONTAGUE, 1972).

Most studies on the regulation of phosphodiesterase deal with the low K_m enzyme. Most investigators agree that the enzyme is, as expected from studies in other tissues, inhibited by theophylline, caffeine, 3-isobutyl-1-methylxanthine, sulfonylureas (glibenclamide, chlorpropamide, tolbutamide), and activated by imidazole. Glucose and glucose-6-phosphate, as well as diazoxide, do not seem to affect the activity of phosphodiesterase. Inhibition of the enzyme by xylitol and leucine and its activation by arginine (SAMS and MONTAGUE, 1972) are unexpected findings which require confirmation. Thus, according to ROSEN *et al.* (1971) and KUO *et al.* (1973), most amino acids including arginine fail to affect insular phosphodiesterase.

d) The Level of cAMP in the B-cell

The regulation of cAMP concentration is generally thought to depend on the respective activities of adenylate cyclase and phosphodiesterase. In addition to determinations on the separate activity of these two enzymes, it is thus also important to perform direct measurements on the cellular level of cAMP. In dealing with the results of such measurements, a distinction ought to be made between immediate and delayed (or chronic) regulation of cAMP concentration in the B-cell.

α) Immediate regulation of cAMP concentration in the B-cell

The present section aims at summarizing actually available experimental data concerning the immediate regulation of cAMP concentration in the B-cell. The effect of glucose and other nutrients, that of hormonal factors, and that of pharmacological agents will be considered.

One of the crucial issues in the regulation of cAMP level in the B-cell concerns the possible effect of glucose. Most of the available data suggest that glucose does not affect cAMP concentration in insular tissue. There are, however, three recent reports which suggest that glucose provokes cAMP accumulation in the B-cell.

MASHITER *et al.* (1972) in a preliminary account first reported on a glucose-induced increase in cAMP level in one out of two human islet cell adenomas studied for this purpose. Also, CHARLES *et al.* (1973), using a protein-binding radiodisplacement method for the assay of cAMP, found that glucose increases within 2 min, and for at least 20 min, cAMP levels in rat isolated islets. More recently, GRILL and CERASI (1973) observed that glucose (5.0 mg/ml) increases within 3 min the incorporation of ^{3}H-adenine into insular cAMP. As pointed out by the authors themselves, this increase could be mediated by changes in specific radioactivity of the precursor ATP pool.

In contrast with these three "positive" reports, other publications conclude that glucose has no significant effect on the insular level of cAMP. KIPNIS (1970), in a few preliminary studies, was unable to detect any change in the level of immunoassayable cAMP in islets incubated for 60 min at two different glucose levels. MONTAGUE and COOK (1971) reported that glucose (0.9—3.6 mg/ml) failed to affect the level of cAMP in both rat-isolated islets and the surrounding incubation medium over 5—30 min incubation at 37° C. Using a method for the assay of cAMP involving activation of inactive liver phosphorylase, they observed that various methylxanthine derivates provoked cAMP accumulation in both the islets and the incubation medium, whereas adrenaline and diazoxide lowered the cAMP concentration, whether in the presence or absence of 3-isobutyl-1-methylxanthine. MILLER *et al.* (1972) reported that glucose (0—3.0 mg/ml) failed to affect basal or glucagon-stimulated synthesis of cAMP, as judged by the incorporation of adenosine-8-^{14}C into cAMP in rat-isolated islets incubated for 15 min at 37° C in a buffer containing $MgCl_2$ (1.4 mM) and theophylline (5 mM). The failure of glucose in this system contrasts with the effects of glucagon (5—15 μg/ml), ACTH (1.2 U/ml), and isoproterenol (10^{-4}M), which all markedly stimulated cAMP formation. Also COOPER *et al.* (1973) were unable to detect any effect of glucose (0.6—3.6 mg/ml) on the level of cAMP in incubated mouse islets and medium or in perifused islets, measurements being performed between the 30th s and 60th min after the addition of glucose, whereas both caffeine and 3-isobutyl-1-methylxanthine markedly increased the concentration of nucleotide, whether at low or high glucose concentration. The initial studies of TURTLE and KIPNIS (1967) had already indicated that glucagon and theophylline acted synergistically in causing cAMP accumulation in islets. Epinephrine inhibits the theophylline-induced accumulation of cAMP, the effect of the catecholamine being reversed by phentolamine but unaffected by propranolol.

It would thus appear that, although a possible stimulant effect of glucose on the level of cAMP in the B-cell remains an open question, the accumulation of cAMP in response to either hormones known to activate the B-cell adenylate cyclase or inhibitors of phosphodiesterase has been much more convincingly documented.

β) Long-term regulation of cAMP concentration in the B-cell

The influence of a number of environmental factors known to affect the secretory activity of the B-cell in a chronic process could also be mediated, in part at least, by changes in the insular level of cAMP. For instance, SELAWRY *et al.* (1973) reported that fasting for 48—72 h reduced the cAMP level in isolated islets. The changes in insular function during the neonatal period may also be due, in part, to changes in the insular level of cAMP and phosphodiesterase activity (MINTZ *et al.*, 1973). This chronic regulation of cAMP metabolism, which could be mediated by induction or repression of adenylate cyclase and phosphodiesterase, should be further investigated within the framework of the so-called chronic regulation of insulin secretion by hormonal, nutritional, and ontogenic factors (MALAISSE, 1973a).

e) Conclusion

Although some discrepancy and much ignorance actually remain in this field, it can be concluded from the above-mentioned observations that the pancreatic B-cell is indeed equipped to synthesize and catabolize cAMP and that the level of this nucleotide in the B-cell is indeed the object of rapid and marked fluctuations under certain experimental conditions. Therefore, the next obvious question to be dealt with is that of the effect of cAMP upon various parameters of islet function. The influence of cAMP on insulin release will be considered first, not only because it is the best documented effect of cAMP in insular tissue, but also because insulin release teleologically represents the ultimate goal for the presence of B-cells in pluricellular organisms.

3. The Effect of cAMP Upon Insulin Release

a) The Insulinotropic Action of cAMP

The insulinotropic effect of cAMP was first reported by SUSSMAN and VAUGHAN (1967) in the isolated perfused rat pancreas. High concentrations of cAMP, in the range of 1.0—10.0 mM, are required to stimulate insulin release. This is generally ascribed to the fact that cAMP does not easily cross the cell membrane. Because of the high concentration of cAMP used in these experiments, the question of specificity should not be overlooked. Indeed, a number of other nucleotides when used at such high concentrations also provoke insulin release. For instance, stimulation of insulin secretion has been observed with ATP or 5′-AMP (LEVINE *et al.*, 1970). In order to overcome this problem of specificity, it seems advisable to use the dibutyryl derivative of cAMP (db-cAMP), which is thought to enter the cell more easily.

That the cellular accumulation of cAMP indeed stimulates insulin release is supported by the fact that a series of agents known or thought to either activate adenylate cyclase (e.g. isoproterenol, glucagon, enteroglucagon, ACTH, TSH) or inhibit phosphodiesterase (e.g. theophylline, caffeine) does indeed display insulinotropic potency (MALAISSE, 1972).

We now wish to define in greater detail the influence of other insulinotropic or inhibitory agents upon the magnitude of the secretory response to cAMP.

At this point, it should be underlined that throughout the following text, we will often refer to cAMP; whereas, actually, the agents under study are either activators of adenylate cyclase (especially glucagon), or db-cAMP, or inhibitors of phosphodiesterase (especially theophylline). We will thus assume, throughout this presentation, that all these agents affect islet function solely by an accumulation of cAMP in the B-cell. It should be kept in mind, however, that such an assumption might be incorrect. For instance, it is conceivable that methylxanthines (theophylline, caffeine) affect certain parameters of islet function independently of their effect on the level of cAMP in the B-cell. To our knowledge, however, there is as yet no evidence to imply the existence of such "side" effects in the B-cell.

b) Combined Effects of cAMP and Other Insulinotropic Agents

Although modest and/or short-lived stimulation of insulin release by cAMP in the absence of glucose has been reported, it is generally accepted that the effect of cAMP (as well as that of db-cAMP, isoproterenol, glucagon, enteroglucagon, ACTH, TSH, theophylline, and caffeine) on insulin release is indeed small and transient if not negligible in the absence of glucose; whereas all these agents enhance insulin secretion more efficiently in the presence of a sufficient amount of glucose, and exert their most marked enhancing action at the highest glucose concentrations (MALAISSE *et al.*, 1967).

In the presence of sulfonylureas and certain amino acids (leucine, glycine, but not arginine), cAMP is also able to cause sustained enhancement of insulin release (MALAISSE and MALAISSE-LAGAE, 1970a; MALAISSE *et al.*, 1972).

Although the significance of these combined effects of cAMP and other insulinotropic agents will be discussed later in this report (see section 4), we wish already to rule out two possible explanations for the failure of cAMP to cause sustained insulin release in the absence of glucose or any other insulinotropic compound.

On one hand, it could be postulated that, in the absence of glucose, the amount of ATP in the B-cell is not sufficient to allow for the synthesis of cAMP. The following observations suggest that such is not the case. First, db-cAMP itself fails to cause sustained release of insulin in the absence of glucose (Malaisse *et al.*, 1970). Second, theophylline indeed provokes cAMP accumulation in the B-cell, even in the absence of glucose (see section 2).

On the other hand, it is also theoretically conceivable that a sufficient amount of ATP is required in order to allow cAMP to stimulate insulin release. Indeed it is well documented that the release of insulin represents an energy-dependent process (Malaisse, 1969). Nevertheless, we feel that this ATP-dependency of the secretory process does not account for the fact that the accumulation of cAMP in the B-cell fails to provoke *per se* sustained insulin release. This belief is based on the following two series of observations. Firstly, metabolites such as pyruvate, which are able to increase ATP availability in the B-cell, cannot replace glucose, at least in adult if not in fetal insular tissue, as a substrate supporting the insulinotropic action of theophylline (Brisson *et al.*, 1972). Secondly, and conversely, sulfonylureas, which are indeed able to support the insulinotropic action of cAMP, are said to lower rather than to increase ATP concentration in isolated islets (Ashcroft *et al.*, 1973).

c) Combined Effects of cAMP and Inhibitory Agents

A better understanding of the precise mode of action of cAMP on insulin release might be gained by investigating the influence on its insulinotropic effect of various inhibitors of insulin release. The interpretation of this type of investigation may be uneasy for the following reason. As we have already mentioned, the accumulation of cAMP in the B-cell is unable to cause sustained insulin release in the absence of any other insulinotropic agent. Therefore, most experiments were carried out in the simultaneous presence of cAMP and glucose. Under these conditions, it might be difficult to assess whether a given inhibitory agent primarily affects the insulinotropic action of cAMP or indirectly modifies such an action through a primary effect on glucose-induced release. For instance, inhibitors of glucose metabolism, such as mannoheptulose and 2-deoxyglucose, modulate the insulinotropic effect of cAMP indirectly by their effect on glucose-induced release (Malaisse *et al.*, 1967).

Epinephrine and to a lesser extent norepinephrine suppress the stimulant action of glucose, leucine, and sulfonylurea on insulin release. This inhibitory effect of catecholamines is thought to be mediated by activation of the B-cell α-adrenergic receptors. Although epinephrine lowers the level of cAMP in the B-cell, there are reasons to believe that the inhibitory effect of epinephrine on insulin release is not solely due to such a change in cAMP concentration. Thus, epinephrine, which abolishes insulin secretion in response to glucose alone, also suppresses the higher rate of secretion evoked by the combination of glucose and db-cAMP (Malaisse *et al.*, 1970). The latter results indicate that flooding the B-cell with exogenous db-cAMP does not abolish the inhibitory effect of epinephrine. Epinephrine, in addition to lowering cAMP level, may thus affect some other metabolic event involved in the secretory sequence. A recent study on the effect of epinephrine on calcium-45 efflux from isolated islets will be later quoted in support of this idea (see section 4.e.).

Imidazole is known to be a phosphodiesterase activator and to increase the breakdown of cAMP to 5′-AMP. The insulinotropic action of glucagon, and even that of theophylline, has been found to be more sensitive to inhibition by imidazole than that of glucose (Malaisse *et al.*, 1968). These findings only afford nuanced informations concerning the role of cAMP in glucose-induced insulin release. On the one hand, the suppression of the enhancing action of glucagon by imidazole at a concentration of the drug which fails to affect glucose-induced insulin release would suggest that glucose may provoke release independently of cAMP. On the other hand, the fact that imidazole at a higher concentration also partially inhibits glucose-induced insulin release, might indicate, assuming a specific effect of imidazole on phosphodiesterase, that cAMP plays, at least, a permissive role in the insulinotropic action of the sugar.

Diazoxide concomitantly inhibits glucose-induced insulin release and the enhancing effect of theophylline (MALAISSE and MALAISSE-LAGAE, 1970b).

Lastly, it should be mentioned that a possible inhibitory effect of insulin on glucose-induced insulin secretion has also been considered as a tool in evaluating the consequence of a low level of cAMP upon B-cell secretory activity (SODOYEZ *et al.*, 1970).

4. The Mode of Action of cAMP in the B-cell

The intimate mode of action of cAMP in the B-cell is as yet poorly understood. At least, a working hypothesis can now be presented which seems to be able to account for all experimental data so far available.

a) Effects of cAMP on Glucose Metabolism in the B-cell

One possible explanation for the insulinotropic action of cAMP could be that this nucleotide facilitates glucose metabolism in the B-cell. However, it is unlikely that such a process would also account for the cAMP-induced enhancement of insulin release evoked by leucine or sulfonylurea, as the latter results were obtained in the absence of extracellular glucose. Moreover, the available data do not suggest that cAMP exerts a marked influence upon glucose metabolism in the B-cell, especially at high glucose concentrations, namely under those conditions where cAMP displays its more marked insulinotropic action (BRISSON *et al.*, 1972).

HELLERSTRÖM and GUNNARSSON (1970) have shown that, whereas glucose (16.7 mM) increases by about 50% the endogenous respiration of isolated islets, both glucagon and db-cAMP slightly depress the oxygen uptake of islets incubated in the presence of glucose (11.1 mM). ASHCROFT and RANDLE (1969) and RANDLE and ASHCROFT (1970) reported that, in the presence of glucose (7.4 mM), glucagon produces a slight fall in the rate of glucose oxidation by mouse islets and does not change their glucose-6-phosphate concentration. According to HELLMAN and IDAHL (1969), glucose increases the ATP content of isolated islets, whereas the level of ATP remains unaltered when the B-cell is stimulated by db-cAMP. Glucagon, theophylline, or db-cAMP have been found to decrease the glycogen content of mouse islets, whereas epinephrine may increase such a content (HELLMAN and IDAHL, 1970). Glucagon and theophylline might also increase the 6-phosphogluconate content of rat islets (MONTAGUE and TAYLOR, 1970), epinephrine causing an opposite change. However, these changes, which badly require confirmation, cannot be attributed to any change induced by db-cAMP in the islet level of citrate (HELLMAN and IDAHL, 1972) as initially suggested by MONTAGUE and TAYLOR (1970).

In conclusion, a stimulant action of cAMP upon glucose metabolism, especially a glycogenolytic effect, should not be overlooked. However, it should be kept in mind that such an effect is likely to lower the "K_m" but not to increase the "V_{max}" of the sigmoidal relationship between insulin release and the extracellular glucose concentration (MALAISSE, 1973b); whereas cAMP, which actually causes a modest lowering of the "K_m", also markedly enhances the "V_{max}" of such a relationship (BRISSON *et al.*, 1972).

b) Effects of cAMP on Insulin Biosynthesis

The stimulant effect of glucose on insulin biosynthesis is known to be dependent on the integrity of glucose metabolism in the B-cell (PIPELEERS *et al.*, 1973). Although it is obvious that the immediate insulinotropic action of cAMP could not be accounted for by effects of the nucleotide on insular biosynthetic activity, it is nevertheless worthwhile to examine such a process in order to reach a better understanding of the mode of action of cAMP in the B-cell. Potentiation of glucose-induced insulin biosynthesis by cAMP has been reported by various authors (see LIN and HAIST, 1973). From the results of SCHATZ *et al.* (1973) and MALAISSE *et al.* (unpublished observations), it would appear that this effect, which could be due in part to an overall stimulation of protein synthesis including that of noninsulinic compounds, also represents, to a limited extent, a glucose-like effect with preferential stimulation of (pro)insulin biosynthesis, especially at intermediate glucose levels (0.75—1.50 mg/ml). The latter finding is consistent with the view that cAMP facilitates glucose metabolism at glucose concentrations close to the threshold value for the insulinotropic action of the sugar.

c) Effects of cAMP on Islet-cell Protein Phosphokinase

MONTAGUE and HOWELL (1972, 1973) have characterized an islet-cell cAMP-dependent protein kinase. This kinase, which is found in the postmicrosomal supernatant, has a molecular weight of about 180000. It contains both a cAMP-binding subunit (MW 90000) and a catalytic subunit (MW 75000). The enzyme is Mg^{++} dependent and inhibited by Ca^{++}. Its K_m for cAMP is about 10^{-8}M. Since the level of cAMP in the islets is in the 0.5—1.0 μM range, the regulation of the protein kinase by lower levels of cAMP may imply the compartmentation of cAMP in the islets among a free and metabolically active pool and a bound and inert pool. The enzyme is unaffected by glucose, arginine, leucine, or xylitol; inhibited by adrenaline, diazoxide, and imidazole; and stimulated by theophylline, caffeine, 3-isobutyl-1-methylxanthine, glucagon, glibenclamide, and tolbutamide. The effect of methylxanthines is present whether at low or high glucose levels.

It is also important to underline that the postmicrosomal supernatant contains an endogenous substrate for the protein kinase (MONTAGUE and HOWELL, 1972; DODS and BURDOWSKI, 1973). The nature of such a substrate remains to be elucidated.

Incidentally, when insular proteins are exposed to [γ—^{32}P] ATP, a slow decline in phosphoprotein activity is observed after the initial 30 or 60 s of phosphorylation, suggesting the presence in the insular extract of phosphoprotein phosphatase activity (DODS and BURDOWSKI, 1973). The combined activities of a cAMP-dependent protein kinase and a phosphoprotein phosphatase would provide an enzymatic mechanism for rapid variations in the phosphorylation of cellular components, including possibly the microtubular-microfilamentous system of the B-cell.

d) Effects of cAMP on Tubulin Metabolism in the B-cell

If the effects of cAMP were to be mediated by activation of protein kinase, one should consider which protein might, by becoming phosphorylated, cause enhanced insulin release. Because a microtubular-microfilamentous system is known to participate in insulin release (see MALAISSE, 1973b) and because the microtubular protein might indeed serve as a substrate for a cAMP-dependent protein kinase (GOODMAN *et al.*, 1970), it has been suggested that the insulinotropic action of cAMP could be mediated by phosphorylation of the insular tubulin.

The postmicrosomal supernatant in insular homogenate contains 80% of the colchicine-binding proteins, and colchicine inhibits the cAMP-dependent phosphorylation of endogenous insular proteins (MONTAGUE and HOWELL, 1972).

On the other hand, it was found that theophylline does not interfere with the deleterious effect of colchicine upon glucose-induced insulin release, and that the impairment of the microtubular system induced by either colchicine or vincristine does not preferentially affect the respective insulinotropic actions of either glucose or theophylline. These data do not suggest, although they do not entirely rule out, a primary effect of cAMP on the microtubular protein (BRISSON *et al.*, 1972).

We would rather suggest that the cAMP-dependent phosphorylation of insular protein might lead (i) to alteration in the activity of enzymes involved in the control of glucose metabolism and (ii) to alteration in the subcellular distribution of calcium, the latter process being, in our view, the major pathway for cAMP-induced enhancement of insulin release.

e) Effects of cAMP on Calcium Handling by the B-cell

The net accumulation of calcium-45 in isolated islets is stimulated by glucose, a process dependent on the integrity of glucose metabolism within the B-cell. If cAMP were to enhance insulin release by accelerating glucose metabolism, one would expect cAMP also to enhance glucose-induced net uptake of calcium-45 by isolated islets. Such an enhancement was indeed observed at a 5.6 mM glucose concentration, suggesting once again that the lowering of the "K_m" for glucose-induced insulin release is due, in part at least, to a facilitation of glucose metabolism at glucose concentrations close to the threshold value for stimulation of insulin secretion. However, no enhancement of glucose-induced calcium-45 net uptake by isolated islets was provoked by theophylline or db-cAMP at high glucose concentrations, namely under conditions associated with the most marked potentiation of insulin release (BRISSON *et al.*, 1972).

It is nevertheless conceivable that, at high glucose concentration, insulin release is still under the control of the cytosolic concentration of Ca^{++}, and that cAMP increases such a concentration by causing an intracellular translocation of Ca^{++} from an organelle-bound pool, e.g. the vacuolar pool of Ca^{++}, into the cytosol. Obviously, the ability of the B-cell to maintain the translocated load of Ca^{++} intracellularly will depend on the balance between Ca^{++} inward and outward movements across the cell membrane. Since insulinotropic agents such as glucose, leucine, and sulfonylurea are known to stimulate ^{45}Ca net uptake, probably through inhibition of outward calcium transport (MALAISSE *et al.*, 1972 and 1973), these agents might indeed allow cAMP to cause a sustained increase in the cytosolic level of Ca^{++} and, hence, a sustained increase in insulin release.

In favour of such a concept, it was shown that, at low extracellular concentration of Ca^{++}, theophylline or db-cAMP partially restored the insulinotropic action of glucose and leucine; that theophylline provoked an immediate and sustained increase in calcium-45 efflux from perifused islets, suggesting a sudden enrichment of a pool of Ca^{++} readily available for outward transport (BRISSON *et al.*, 1972); and that glucose tended to minimize the theophylline-induced increase in calcium-45 efflux (BRISSON *et al.*, 1973). Epinephrine antagonizes the effect of both glucose and theophylline on calcium handling by the B-cell, thus suggesting a double mode of action (see section 3.c.).

Whether the cAMP-induced translocation of Ca^{++} in the B-cell is indeed the result of a cAMP-dependent phosphorylation of cellular proteins involved in the subcellular distribution of cations, as here suggested, remains at present a purely speculative concept.

5. Physiological Significance of the B-cell Adenylate Cyclase System

From the data so far discussed in the present account, it is obvious that cAMP could play a role in the regulation of insulin release in response to a variety of metabolic, humoral, and pharmacological agents. However, it is also obvious that the best documented changes in the insular level of cAMP, apart from the effect of pharmacological agents, relate to the influence of certain hormones. Hence, we believe that, as in other systems, the insular adenylate cyclase mainly represents a pathway for the hormonal modulation of physiological events in target cells, namely for the hormonal regulation of insulin secretion by the B-cell. More precisely, we wish to suggest that the activity of the adenylcyclase system is normally under the control of hormones which are able to modify the insulinotropic action of circulating nutrients. This view, which is unlikely to be unanimously shared, has been thoroughly examined in previous reports (MALAISSE and MALAISSE-LAGAE, 1970a; MALAISSE, 1972) and will here only shortly be dealt with. The main point to be discussed will be the participation of gastrointestinal hormones and catecholamines in the physiological regulation of insulin release. We will deliberately ignore those hormonal effects which, although well documented, may represent pharmacological rather than physiological responses of the B-cell.

a) Insulinotropic Action of Hormonal Polypeptides and the Entero-Insular Axis

A number of recent and documented reviews (CREUTZFELDT *et al.*, 1970; MALAISSE, 1972; PFEIFFER *et al.*, 1972) have emphasized the existence of an entero-insular axis in which hormones (gastrin, pancreozymin, secretin, enteroglucagon) released by the gastrointestinal tract after food intake cause a stimulation of insulin secretion. The existence of such an axis is thought to be responsible for the higher insulin response evoked by oral rather than intravenous administration of nutrients. Such a hormonal stimulation of the B-cell adenylate cyclase is likely to cause more marked enhancement of insulin release at a time of concomitant post-prandial hyperglycemia and hyperaminoacidemia than in the basal state (MOODY *et al.*, 1970). Teleologically, the dependency on a sufficient concentration of hexoses or amino acids for cAMP-induced insulin release offers certain advantages. For instance, such a dependency is likely to protect the organism against excessive insulin secretion which could otherwise result from the release of pancreatic glucagon in glucopenic situations (BRISSON *et al.*, 1972).

b) Inhibition of Insulin Release by Catecholamines During Stress and Exercise

Inhibition of insulin release during stress and exercise and the suppression of such an inhibition by phentolamine have been documented in rats (WRIGHT and MALAISSE, 1968; BRISSON *et al.*, 1971) and confirmed in other species (see MALAISSE, 1972). This phenomenon, taken together with the concomitant stimulation of glucagon release by catecholamines (LECLERCQ-MEYER *et al.*, 1971), is thought to ensure maximal mobilization of glucose from the liver and free fatty acids from the adipocyte at a time characterized by an increased need for metabolic substrates.

More recently, ROBERTSON and PORTE (1973) have provided data to suggest that basal insulin secretion in man is also submitted to adrenergic modulation. Serotonin, like catecholamines, when secreted in excessive amounts, inhibits insulin release (FELDMAN *et al.*, 1972a, b). Lastly, the role of pancreatic monoamines in the regulation of insulin secretion should also duly be considered (FELDMAN *et al.*, 1973; CHRISTENSEN and IVERSEN, 1973).

6. Concluding Remark

The present review represents an attempt to summarize the present knowledge concerning the role of cAMP in the regulation of β-insular function. Because of the recent development of sensitive methods for the assay of cAMP, adenylate cyclase, and phosphodiesterase in biological material, it is our firm belief that a wealth of experimental data on the same topic is to be expected in the coming months and, therefore, that the present review will soon become badly outdated.

References*

ASHCROFT, S.J.H., RANDLE, P.J.: Metabolism and insulin secretion in isolated islets. Acta diabet. lat. **6**, Suppl. 1, 538—553 (1969)

ASHCROFT, S.J.H., WEERASINGHE, L.C.C., RANDLE, P.J.: Interrelationship of islet metabolism, adenosine triphosphate content and insulin release. Biochem. J. **132**, 223—231 (1973)

BRISSON, G.R., MALAISSE-LAGAE, F., MALAISSE, W.J.: Effect of phentolamine upon insulin secretion during exercise. Diabetologia **7**, 223—226 (1971)

BRISSON, G.R., MALAISSE-LAGAE, F., MALAISSE, W.J.: The stimulus-secretion coupling of glucose-induced insulin release. VII. A proposed site of action for adenosine-3′,5′-cyclic monophosphate. J. clin. Invest. **51**, 232—241 (1972)

BRISSON, G.R., MALAISSE, W.J.: The stimulus-secretion coupling of glucose-induced insulin release. XI. Effects of theophylline and epinephrine on ^{45}Ca efflux from perifused islets. Metabolism **22**, 455—465 (1973)

BOWEN, V., LAZARUS, N.R.: Glucose-mediated insulin release from mouse islets of Langerhans: cyclic nucleotide phosphodiesterase. Biochem. J. **128**, 97P (1972)

CHARLES, M.A., FANSKA, R., SCHMID, F.G., FORSHAM, P.H., GRODSKY, G.M.: Adenosine 3′:5′-monophosphate in pancreatic islets: glucose-induced insulin release. Science **179**, 569—571 (1973)

CHRISTENSEN, N.J., IVERSEN, J.: Release of large amounts of noradrenaline from the isolated perfused canine pancreas during glucose deprivation. Diabetologia **9**, 396—399 (1973)

COOPER, R.H., ASHCROFT, S.J.H., RANDLE, P.J.: Concentration of adenosine 3′:5′-cyclic monophosphate in mouse pancreatic islets measured by a protein-binding radioassay. Biochem. J. **134**, 599—605 (1973)

COORE, H.G., RANDLE, P.J.: Regulation of insulin secretion studied with pieces of rabbit pancreas incubated *in vitro*. Biochem. J. **93**, 66—78 (1964)

CREUTZFELDT, W., FEURLE, G., KETTERER, H.: Current concept: effect of gastrointestinal hormones on insulin and glucagon secretion. New Engl. J. Med. **282**, 1139—1141 (1970)

DAVIS, B., LAZARUS, N.R.: Glucose-mediated insulin release from mouse islets of Langerhans: adenylate cyclase. Biochem. J. **128**, 96P—97P (1972)

DODS, R.F., BURDOWSKI, A.: Adenosine 3′,5′-cyclic monophosphate dependent protein kinase and phosphoprotein phosphatase activities in rat islets of Langerhans. Biochem. biophys. Res. Commun. **51**, 421—427 (1973)

FELDMAN, J.M., MARECEK, R.L., QUICKEL, K.E., JR., LEBOVITZ, H.E.: Glucose metabolism and insulin secretion in the carcinoid syndrome. J. clin. Endocr. **35**, 307—311 (1972a)

FELDMAN, J.M., QUICKEL, K.E., JR., LEBOVITZ, H.E.: Potentiation of insulin secretion in vitro by serotonin antagonists. Diabetes **21**, 779—788 (1972b)

FELDMAN, J.M., LEBOVITZ, H.E., BOMAN, J.: Role of pancreatic monoamines in the impaired insulin secretion of the fasting state. Endocrinology **92**, 1469—1474 (1973)

GOLDFINE, I.D., PERLMAN, R., ROTH, J.: Inhibition of cyclic 3′,5′-AMP phosphodiesterase in islet cells and other tissues by tolbutamide. Nature (Lond.) **234**, 295—297 (1971)

GOLDFINE, D., ROTH, J., BIRNBAUMER, L.: Glucagon receptors in β-cells. Binding of ^{125}I-glucagon and activation of adenylate cyclase. J. biol. Chem. **247**, 1211—1218 (1972)

GOODMAN, D.B.P., RASMUSSEN, H., DIBELLA, F., GUTHROW, C.E., JR.: Cyclic adenosine 3′:5′-monophosphate-stimulated phosphorylation of isolated neurotubule subunits. Proc. nat. Acad. Sci. (Wash.) **67**, 652—659 (1970)

GRILL, V., CERASI, E.: Activation by glucose of adenyl cyclase in pancreatic islets of the rat. FEBS Letters **33**, 311—314 (1973)

HELLERSTRÖM, C., GUNNARSSON, R.: Bioenergetics of islet function: oxygen utilization and oxidative metabolism in the β-cells. Acta diabet. lat. **7**, Suppl. 1, 127—151 (1970)

* The review of the literature was completed in September 1973.

HELLMAN, B., IDAHL, L.-A.: Control of ATP levels in stimulated pancreatic B-cells. Acta diabet. lat. **6**, Suppl. 1, 597—611 (1969)
HELLMAN, B., IDAHL, L.-A.: On the functional significance of the pancreatic β-cell glycogen. Wenner-Gren International Symposium Series **16**, 253—261 (1970)
HELLMAN, B., IDAHL, L.-A.: Pancreatic islet levels of citrate under conditions of stimulated and inhibited insulin release. Diabetes **21**, 999—1002 (1972)
HELLMAN, B., LERNMARK, A., SEHLIN, J., TÄLJEDAL, I.-B.: The pancreatic β-cell recognition of insulin secretagogues. Inhibitory effects of a membrane probe on the islet uptake and insulin-releasing action of glibenclamide. FEBS Letters **34**, 347—349 (1973)
HOWELL, S. L., MONTAGUE, W.: Adenylate cyclase activity in isolated rat islets of Langerhans. Effects of agents which alter rates of insulin secretion. Biochim. biophys. Acta (Amst.) **320**, 44—52 (1973)
HOWELL, S. L., WHITFIELD, M.: Cytochemical localization of adenyl cyclase activity in rat islets of Langerhans. J. Histochem. Cytochem. **20**, 873—879 (1972a)
HOWELL, S. L., WHITFIELD, M.: Cytochemical localization of adenyl cyclase and cyclic AMP phosphodiesterase in rat islets of Langerhans. Diabetes **21**, 328 (1972b)
KIPNIS, D. M.: Studies on insulin secretion: radioimmunoassay of cyclic nucleotides and the role of cyclic AMP. Acta diabet. lat. **7**, Suppl. 1, 314—334 (1970)
KUO, W.-N., HODGINS, D. S., KUO, J. F.: Adenylate cyclase in islets of Langerhans. Isolation of islets and regulation of adenylate cyclase activity by various hormones and agents. J. biol. Chem. **248**, 2705—2711 (1973)
LECLERCQ-MEYER, V., BRISSON, G. R., MALAISSE, W. J.: Effect of adrenaline and glucose on release of glucagon and insulin *in vitro*. Nature (New Biology) **231**, 248—249 (1971)
LEVEY, G. S., SCHMIDT, W. M. I., MINTZ, D. H.: Activation of adenyl cyclase in a pancreatic islet cell adenoma by glucagon and tolbutamide. Metabolism **21**, 93—98 (1972)
LEVINE, R. A., OYAMA, S., KAGAN, A., GLICK, S. M.: Stimulation of insulin and growth hormone secretion by adenine nucleotides in primates. J. Lab. clin. Med. **75**, 30—36 (1970)
LIN, B. J., HAIST, R. E.: Effects of some modifiers of insulin secretion on insulin biosynthesis. Endocrinology **92**, 735—741 (1973)
MALAISSE, W. J.: Etude de la sécrétion insulinique in vitro. Paris: Maloine 1969
MALAISSE, W. J.: Hormonal and environmental modification of islet activity. In: STEINER, D. F., FREINKEL, N. (Eds.) Endocrine pancreas. Washington: The American Physiological Society 1972
MALAISSE, W. J.: La régulation de la sécrétion insulinique. In: Hormones et régulations métaboliques. Paris: Masson 1973a
MALAISSE, W. J.: Insulin secretion: multifactorial regulation for a single process of release. The Minkowski Award Lecture. Diabetologia **9**, 167—173 (1973b)
MALAISSE, W. J., MALAISSE-LAGAE, F., MAYHEW, D.: A possible role for the adenylcyclase system in insulin secretion. J. clin. Invest. **46**, 1724—1734 (1967)
MALAISSE, W. J., MALAISSE-LAGAE, F., KING, S.: Effects of neutral red and imidazole upon insulin secretion. Diabetologia **4**, 370—374 (1968)
MALAISSE, W. J., MALAISSE-LAGAE, F.: Biochemical, pharmacological and physiological aspects of the adenylcyclase-phosphodiesterase system in the pancreatic β-cells. Wenner-Gren International Symposium Series **16**, 435—443 (1970a)
MALAISSE, W. J., MALAISSE-LAGAE, F.: Effects of glycodiazin and glybenclamide upon insulin secretion in vitro. Europ. J. Pharmacol. **9**, 93—98 (1970b)
MALAISSE, W. J., BRISSON, G., MALAISSE-LAGAE, F.: The stimulus-secretion coupling of glucose-induced insulin release. I. Interaction of epinephrine and alkaline earth cations. J. Lab. clin. Med. **76**, 895—902 (1970)
MALAISSE, W. J., MAHY, M., BRISSON, G. R., MALAISSE-LAGAE, F.: The stimulus-secretion coupling of glucose-induced insulin release. VIII. Combined effects of glucose and sylfonylureas. Europ. J. clin. Invest. **2**, 85—90 (1972)
MALAISSE, W. J., BRISSON, G. R., BAIRD, L. E.: Stimulus-secretion coupling of glucose-induced insulin release. X. Effect of glucose on ^{45}Ca efflux from perifused islets. Amer. J. Physiol. **224**, 389—394 (1973)
MASHITER, K., ZOR, U., BLOOM, G., FIELD, J. B.: Effects of glucose, glucagon, tolbutamide and theophylline on the cyclic AMP content and insulin release of slices of human islet cell adenomas. Diabetes **21**, 346—347 (1972)
MILLER, E. A., WRIGHT, P. H., ALLEN, D. O.: Effect of hormones on accumulation of cyclic AMP-^{14}C in isolated pancreatic islets of rats. Endocrinology **91**, 1117—1119 (1972)
MINTZ, D. H., LEVEY, G. S., SCHENK, A.: Adenosine 3′,5′-cyclic monophosphate and phosphodiesterase activities in isolated fetal and neonatal rat pancreatic islets. Endocrinology **92**, 614—617 (1973)
MONTAGUE, W., COOK, J. R.: The role of adenosine 3′:5′-cyclic monophosphate in the regulation of insulin release by isolated rat islets of Langerhans. Biochem. J. **122**, 115—120 (1971)

MONTAGUE, W., HOWELL, S.L.: The mode of action of adenosine 3′:5′-cyclic monophosphate in mammalian islets of Langerhans. Preparation and properties of islet-cell protein phosphokinase. Biochem. J. **129**, 551—560 (1972)

MONTAGUE, W., HOWELL, S.L.: The mode of action of adenosine 3′:5′-cyclic monophosphate in mammalian islets of Langerhans. Effects of insulin secretagogues on islet-cell protein kinase activity. Biochem. J. **134**, 321—327 (1973)

MONTAGUE, W., TAYLOR, K.W.: The role of the pentose phosphate pathway in insulin secretion. Wenner-Gren International Symposium Series **16**, 263—271 (1970)

MOODY, A.J., MARKUSSEN, J., SCHAICH-FRIES, A., STEENSTRUP, C., SUNDBY, F., MALAISSE, W. J., MALAISSE-LAGAE, F.: The insulin releasing activities of extracts of pork intestine. Diabetologia **6**, 135—140 (1970)

PFEIFFER, E.F., FUSSGÄNGER, R., RAPTIS, S.: Gastro-intestinal hormones and islet function. Acta diabet. lat. **9**, Suppl. 1, 233—273 (1972)

PIPELEERS, D.G., MARICHAL, M., MALAISSE, W.J.: The stimulus-secretion coupling of glucose-induced insulin release. XIV. Glucose regulation of insular biosynthetic activity. Endocrinology **93**, 1001—1011 (1973)

RANDLE, P.J., ASHCROFT, S.J.H.: Bioenergetics of islet function: islet glucose metabolism. Acta diabet. lat. **7**, Suppl. 1, 159—175 (1970)

ROBERTSON, R.P., PORTE, D., JR.: Adrenergic modulation of basal insulin secretion in men. Diabetes **22**, 1—8 (1973)

ROSEN, O.M., HIRSCH, A.H., GOREN, E.N.: Factors which influence cyclic AMP formation and degradation in an islet cell tumor of the Syrian Hamster. Arch. Biochem. **146**, 600—603 (1971)

SAMOLS, E., MARRI, G., MARKS, V.: Promotion of insulin secretion by glucagon. Lancet **1965 II**, 415—416

SAMS, D.J., MONTAGUE, W.: The role of adenosine 3′:5′-cyclic monophosphate in the regulation of insulin release. Properties of islet-cell adenosine 3′:5′-cyclic monophosphate phosphodiesterase. Biochem. J. **129**, 945—952 (1972)

SCHATZ, H., MAIER, V., HINZ, M., NIERLE, C., PFEIFFER, E.F.: Stimulation of H-3-leucine incorporation into the proinsulin and insulin fraction of isolated pancreatic mouse islets in the presence of glucagon, theophylline and cyclic AMP. Diabetes **22**, 433—441 (1973)

SELAWRY, H., GUTMAN, R., FINK, G., RECANT, L.: The effect of starvation on tissue adenosine 3′-5′ monophosphate levels. Biochem. biophys. Res. Commun. **51**, 198—204 (1973)

SODOYEZ, J.-C., SODOYEZ-GOFFAUX, F., FOA, P.P.: Feedback regulation of insulin secretion by insulin: role of 3′,5′-cyclic AMP. Wenner-Gren International Symposium Series **16**, 445—450 (1970)

SUSSMAN, K.E., VAUGHAN, G.D.: Insulin release after ACTH, glucagon, and adenosine-3′,5′-phosphate (cyclic AMP) in the perfused isolated rat pancreas. Diabetes **16**, 449—454 (1967)

TURTLE, J.R., KIPNIS, D.M.: An adrenergic receptor mechanism for the control of cyclic 3′,5′-adenosine monophosphate synthesis in tissues. Biochem. biophys. Res. Commun. **28**, 797—802 (1967)

WRIGHT, P.H., MALAISSE, W.J.: Effects of epinephrine, stress and exercise on insulin secretion by the rat. Amer. J. Physiol. **214**, 1031—1034 (1968)

V. Role of Cations

Willy J. Malaisse

With 1 Figure

1. Introduction

The pilot and independent studies led by Grodsky *et al.* (Grodsky and Bennett, 1966; Curry *et al.*, 1968a; Bennett *et al.*, 1969) and Hales and Milner (1968a, b; Milner and Hales, 1967, 1969) first drew attention to the participation of cations in the process of insulin release. Most of the fundamental information emerging from their work has been confirmed and extended in subsequent studies from other laboratories. For the sake of clarity, we will in the following review concentrate mainly on a simplified and still hypothetical model concerning the role of cations in the insulin secretory process.

2. Calcium

a) Effect of Calcium Upon Insulin Release

The omission of extracellular calcium abolishes the release of insulin evoked *in vitro* by glucose and a variety of other insulinotropic agents (Milner and Hales, 1967). More or less severe depletion of the pericellular and, hence, cellular calcium capital might be required to suppress secretion, depending on the agent or association of agents used to stimulate the B-cell. To our knowledge, there are only two apparent exceptions to such a calcium dependency. The first exception concerns the insulinotropic effect of barium, which will be discussed later in this chapter (see section 3). The second exception is observed when the B-cell is simultaneously exposed to agents known to increase the cellular level, of adenosine-3′,5′-cyclic monophosphate (cAMP) and to an insulinotropic metabolite, such as glucose or leucine; the significance of the latter finding is considered in full detail in another chapter of this volume (Malaisse, 1974).

Although the dependency of the releasing process on a sufficient amount of extracellular calcium is an universally accepted concept, there is no agreement as to the exact relationship between the rate of insulin release evoked by glucose and the concentration of calcium in the interstitial fluid bathing the B-cell. According to Curry *et al.* (1968b) and Malaisse *et al.* (1970), glucose-induced insulin release occurs at an almost invariable rate, once the calcium concentration exceeds a value of approximately 2 mEq/l. Milner and Hales (1967) found that the stimulant action of glucose increases as the level of calcium is raised from 0—5.4 mEq/l, but is reduced at higher calcium concentrations.

Incidentally, fluctuations in the level of ionized calcium *in vivo*, within the pathophysiological range, are also susceptible to alter the insulin secretory response of the B-cell (Laron and Rosenberg, 1970; Littledike *et al.*, 1968).

b) The Handling of Calcium by the B-cell

Most of our present knowledge concerning the handling of calcium by the B-cell is derived from radioisotopic measurements of calcium-45 net uptake, subcellular distribution, and efflux in isolated islets. The limitations of these three types of measurements have recently been emphasized (Malaisse and Pipeleers, 1974).

The net uptake of calcium-45 by islets is a static measurement performed after a fixed period of incubation followed by extensive washing in order to remove the extracellular radioactivity. This method does not allow of studying the dynamics of calcium handling, of distinguishing between increased influx or decreased efflux across the cell membrane, and of differentiating between changes in either the net uptake of calcium by the B-cell or the preferent accumulation of calcium in a particular pool less rapidly depleted of its content during the washing procedure (Hellman *et al.*, 1971).

The subcellular distribution of calcium-45 is also open to severe criticism in view of both the tendency of calcium binding on different structures and the lability of certain cell organelles.

The measurement of calcium-45 efflux from islets which have been loaded with the radioactive cation prior to perifusion affords a dynamic view of calcium outward transport across the cell membrane. However, in order to distinguish between true outward transport and emiocytotic release of calcium-45 presumably enclosed within the secretory granules (Malaisse *et al.*, 1973a), it is necessary to perform experiments under conditions known to abolish insulin release and yet supposed not to interfere with calcium handling by the B-cell.

With these limitations in mind, the experimental data have led us to postulate the following working hypotheses.

(i) Calcium is distributed in the B-cell among at least two pools: the first pool represents the calcium present in the cytosol; the second pool is likely to be heterogeneous and to correspond to the calcium taken up by or bound to various organelles: it is here quoted as the vacuolar pool. The rate of insulin release is controlled by the concentration of calcium in the cytosol of the B-cell, whatever agent is used to either stimulate or inhibit the secretory process (Malaisse, 1972, 1973). The relationship between the calcium content of the B-cell and the rate of insulin release is characterized by a threshold value for the stimulant action of calcium in insulin release; once the calcium concentration exceeds such a threshold value, output of insulin appears to be proportional to the extra amount of calcium accumulated in the B-cell.

(ii) Glucose and those agents which stimulate its insulinotropic modality (e.g. mannose and leucine) increase the cytosolic concentration of calcium by enhancing the net uptake of calcium by the B-cell (Malaisse-Lagae and Malaisse, 1971; Malaisse-Lagae *et al.*, 1971). In the case of glucose, the increased net uptake appears to be due mostly if not exclusively to reduced outward transport of calcium across the cell membrane (MALAISSE *et al.*, 1973a). The effect of glucose upon calcium handling is thought to represent an energy-consuming process dependent on the integrity of glucose metabolism in the B-cell. Incidentally, increased net uptake of calcium should theoretically lead to increased concentrations of calcium in both the cytosolic and vacuolar pools.

(iii) Agents such as theophylline and the dibutyryl derivative of adenosine-3′,5′-cyclic monophosphate (db-cAMP), which are thought to cause an accumulation of cAMP in the B-cell, provoke a glucose-independent intracellular translocation of calcium from the vacuolar system into the cytosol (BRISSON *et al.*, 1972; BRISSON and MALAISSE, 1973). By the term "glucose-independent" we mean that the effect of theophylline on calcium distribution in the B-cell does not require the presence of glucose. It is not meant to imply that the fate of the load of calcium initially translocated in the cytosol is not ultimately affected by the concentration of glucose either. As a matter of fact, we have obtained data to suggest that glucose, by inhibiting the outward transport of calcium, minimizes the theophylline-induced outflow of this cation (BRISSON and MALAISSE, 1973).

(iv) Sulfonylureas could exert a dual effect upon calcium handling by the B-cell, analogous to that of both glucose and theophylline (MALAISSE *et al.*, 1973b). Epinephrine antagonizes the effect of insulinotropic agents by facilitating both outward transport and vacuolar uptake of calcium (BRISSON and MALAISSE, 1973).

New approaches to the study of calcium handling by the B-cell, such as semi-quantitative measurement and localization of calcium at the ultrastructural level (HERMAN *et al.*, 1973), are likely to afford further knowledge in this field.

c) The Mode of Action of Calcium in the B-cell

Since insulin release appears to be triggered and controlled by the level of calcium in the cytosol of the B-cell, the question should be raised as to the mode of action of this cation in the secretory sequence.

Various lines of evidence suggest that the effect of calcium is not mediated through changes in glucose metabolism. Thus, even at calcium concentrations low enough to abolish glucose-induced insulin release, the stimulant action of glucose upon calcium-45 net uptake by isolated islets is markedly inhibited by mannoheptulose, indicating that glucose is still recognized by the B-cell and, as later demonstrated, still able to inhibit the outward transport of calcium-45 (MALAISSE-LAGAE and MALAISSE, 1971; MALAISSE *et al.*, 1973a). Moreover, glucose-induced insulin biosynthesis, a process quite sensitive to changes in glucose metabolism, is not reduced but actually slightly increased in calcium-depleted media (PIPELEERS *et al.*, 1973). Likewise, glucose oxidation by isolated islets is slightly increased in the absence of calcium (ASHCROFT and RANDLE, 1969). HELLMAN (1970), however, claims that omission of calcium inhibits glycolysis in the B-cell.

It is also unlikely that calcium affects insulin release through changes in synthesis, breakdown, or metabolic effect of adenosine-3′,5′-cyclic monophosphate (cAMP). Indeed, according to DAVIS and LAZARUS (1972), calcium (0.3 mM) inhibits insular adenylate cyclase, an effect which would cause inhibition rather than stimulation of insulin secretion. MONTAGUE and HOWELL (1972) have reported that increasing concentrations of calcium up to 10 mM cause a dose-related inhibition of histone phosphorylation by purified islet-cell protein phosphokinase, both in the absence or presence of cAMP, an inhibitory effect which could hardly account for the stimulant action of calcium on insulin release.

Basing their reasoning on the analogy between excitation-contraction coupling in muscle and stimulus-secretion coupling in the B-cell, MALAISSE and MALAISSE-LAGAE (1970) were the first to suggest that calcium accumulation in the B-cell triggers insulin release by activating a primitive contractile system, composed of microtubules and microfilaments, and involved in the migration and extrusion of secretory granules in the process of exocytosis. First postulated by LACY *et al.* (1968), the participation of this system in insulin release has been documented by a series of ultrastructural and biochemical studies reviewed in detail elsewhere (LACY and MALAISSE, 1973; MALAISSE *et al.*, 1973c). It should be noted, however, that no direct evidence is yet available to indicate that calcium indeed causes the microtubular-microfilamentous system of the B-cell to undergo contraction or a change in physical conformation resulting in both the transport of granules to the cell membrane and their release by emiocytosis. Nevertheless, the present concept is supported by the observation that agents known to alter the microtubular-microfilamentous system modify insulin release, without altering the effect of glucose or sulfonylurea on calcium-45 handling by the B-cell (MALAISSE *et al.*, 1971b, 1972a, b, 1973a, b).

As an alternative hypothesis, MATTHEWS (1970) has indicated that calcium, by collapsing the potential energy barrier to granule/membrane interaction, may facilitate the fusion with the cell membrane of granules translocated to the periphery of the cell by a stochastic or diffusive process.

3. Barium

Barium (2—6 mEq/l) apparently does not affect glucose-induced insulin release at normal calcium concentrations. In the absence of calcium but presence of barium, such a release also occurs at a normal rate (MALAISSE *et al.*, 1970). Incidentally, strontium, but not beryllium, can also substitute for calcium in such a process (HALES, 1970). These findings would suggest that barium can replace calcium as the key alkaline-earth cation in the insulin-releasing process. However, certain observations indicate that barium cannot be considered merely as a substitute for calcium. First, barium *per se* is able to promote insulin release (MILNER and HALES, 1969). This insulinotropic effect of barium, which is an immediate but rapidly fading-out process (MALAISSE *et al.*, 1973a), is observed in the absence of calcium but does not occur at normal calcium concentrations (HALES and MILNER, 1968b). Second, glucose-induced insulin biosynthesis, as well as the synthesis of other insular proteins, is abolished in calcium-depleted media enriched with barium (PIPELEERS *et al.*, 1973).

We are forced, therefore, to conclude that the precise mode of action of barium in the release of insulin remains to be elucidated. For instance, the reciprocal influence of calcium and barium upon their respective uptake and further handling by insular tissue should be thoroughly investigated.

4. Magnesium

The stimulant action of glucose and other insulinotropic agents is slightly enhanced in the absence of extracellular magnesium and markedly depressed at abnormally high magnesium concentrations. The latter inhibitory effect of magnesium is accentuated at subnormal calcium concentration, and it might be overcome at higher than normal calcium concentrations (BENNETT *et al.*, 1969; MALAISSE *et al.*, 1970). These findings have led to the concept that magnesium acts as a competitive inhibitor of calcium transport in the B-cell, possibly through competition for a common carrier system. This interpretation is supported by the facts that, (i) at high magnesium concentration glucose-induced calcium-45 uptake by the B-cell is indeed inhibited (MALAISSE-LAGAE and MALAISSE, 1971) and (ii) glucose-induced insulin synthesis is unaffected, thus suggesting that the influence of magnesium upon insular function results from alterations in calcium uptake rather than glucose recognition by the B-cell (PIPELEERS *et al.*, 1973). Incidentally, magnesium deficiency is reported to depress glucose-induced insulin biosynthesis, possibly by altering the interaction of ribosomes, mRNA and tRNA (LIN and HAIST, 1973).

5. Sodium

a) Effect of Sodium on Islet Function

In the present section we intend to present two different hypotheses concerning the possible role of sodium and other monovalent cations in insulin release.

The first and still best documented hypothesis is schematically depicted in Fig. 1. According to this first model, the outward and presumably active transport of sodium across the cell membrane from the cytosol into the interstitial fluid is mediated by two different pumps. The first one is a potassium-dependent and ouabain-sensitive sodium pump. The second one is a calcium-dependent and ouabain-insensitive sodium pump. In this second cationic pump, calcium and sodium are thought to compete for the same carrier system, in such a way that either low extracellular sodium or high intracellular sodium concentrations are likely to cause an increased net uptake of calcium and, subsequently, an increased release of insulin by the B-cell (HALES and MILNER, 1968a, b).

The model would explain why those factors known to cause a cellular accumulation of sodium indeed initiate or, at least enhance insulin release. Such would be the case when the first potassium-dependent pump is inhibited by either ouabain, the absence of extracellular potassium, or on the contrary, higher than normal potassium concentrations likely to cause cell depolarization. Conversely,

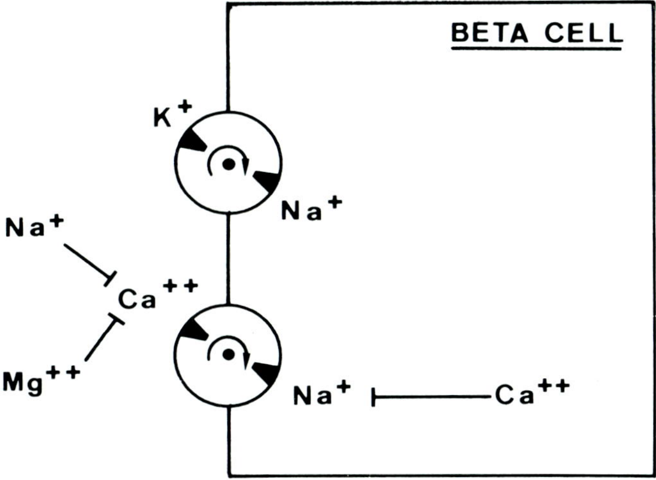

Fig. 1. Model for the movement of cations across the B-cell membrane. The potassium-dependent and calcium-dependent sodium pumps are shown together with the sites of competition between cations for the same carrier (T-shaped bars)

a cellular depletion in sodium due to either diphenylhydantoin or the replacement of large amounts of extracellular sodium by lithium, tris-(hydroxymethyl)-aminomethane, potassium, and possibly choline would inhibit release in response to a variety of insulinotropic agents. Incidentally, on replacement of sodium by other cations, an initial enhancement of insulin release might occur due to the facilitation of calcium inward transport, since extracellular sodium and calcium might indeed compete for the same carrier system. Such a mechanism may well explain certain apparent discrepancies between the immediate effect of monovalent cations (e.g. choline or potassium in subnormal concentrations), as investigated in experimental designs suitable to scrutinize the minute-by-minute dynamics of insulin release (LAMBERT *et al.*, 1974), and the integrated changes in insulin release evoked by the same cations, as measured over prolonged periods of incubation of 60—90 min.

Most of the available experimental data support the above-mentioned model. Stimulation of insulin release or enhancement of glucose-induced insulin release by ouabain has been observed both *in vivo* (TRINER *et al.*, 1968; LEFEBVRE and LUYCKX, 1972) and *in vitro* (HALES and MILNER, 1968a; MALAISSE *et al.*, 1971a; LAMBERT, 1971). Inhibition of insulin release by diphenylhydantoin (KIZER *et al.*, 1970) or on replacement of large amounts of sodium by other monovalent cations has also repeatedly been reported, although somewhat conflicting data were obtained when choline was used as the replacing cation (HALES and MILNER, 1968a, b; MALAISSE *et al.*, 1971a).

The model would also account for the multiple effects of potassium on insulin release (GRODSKY and BENNETT, 1966; HALES and MILNER, 1968a, b; MALAISSE *et al.*, 1971a; LAMBERT, 1971; GOMEZ and CURRY, 1973). In the complete absence of extracellular potassium, increased release of insulin is to be expected as a result of the inactivation of the potassium-dependent sodium pump. On the contrary, at low potassium levels (1.0 mEq/l) the secretory response is apparently very low (HOWELL and TAYLOR, 1968). As the potassium concentration is increased to normal or higher than normal values, a dose-related increase of insulin release would be due to the progressive depolarization of the cell membrane and resulting permeabilization of the cell membrane to sodium or/and calcium. Lastly, when larger amounts of sodium are replaced by potassium, the cellular sodium depletion might become the rate-limiting phenomenon responsible for depressed insulin release.

All these findings indeed support the model illustrated in Fig. 1 and suggest that the major effect of monovalent cations takes place at the level of the cell membrane and is mediated through concomitant changes in calcium transport. Further support in favour of such a concept is found in the fact that, at low extracellular calcium concentrations, the release of insulin evoked by the omission of potassium, ouabain, or high potassium concentrations is markedly reduced (HALES and MILNER, 1968b; MILNER and HALES, 1969; LAMBERT, 1971; MALAISSE *et al.*, 1971a).

Over the last few years, a second hypothesis has been put forward to account for the effect of monovalent cations on glucose-induced insulin release. Thus, it was claimed that the recognition of glucose by the B-cell might involve a sodium-dependent step of glucose transport and/or further metabolism in this cell (RANDLE, 1971; PIPELEERS *et al.*, 1973). In support of such a hypothesis, it was shown that metabolic events thought to be little sensitive to changes in calcium handling by the B-cell are markedly affected by sodium and other monovalent cations. For instance, glucose-induced insulin biosynthesis is slightly enhanced when sodium is partially replaced by potassium and inhibited on replacement of sodium by lithium, tris-(hydroxymethyl)-aminomethane, choline, and larger amounts of potassium. The latter inhibition of insular biosynthetic activity mimics both quantitatively and qualitatively the reduction of glucose-induced insulin biosynthesis by metabolic inhibitors such as mannoheptulose, and is paralleled by a concomitant inhibition of glucose-induced calcium uptake and subsequent insulin release (PIPELEERS *et al.*, 1973). Sodium replacement by other cations is also associated with a reduced utilization and oxidation of glucose (ASHROFT *et al.*, 1972), as well as with reduced glycolysis in isolated islets (MATSCHINSKY and ELLERMAN, 1973). These converging findings suggest that sodium indeed participates in the process of glucose recognition by the pancreatic B-cell.

It is our opinion that more information is required in order to establish the link between the two above-mentioned hypotheses concerning the role of monovalent cations in islet function.

b) Insular Handling of Sodium

To our knowledge, only one study is presently available in which the accumulation of sodium-22 by isolated islets has been investigated. The net uptake of sodium-22 in the presence of glucose (11.1 mM) was inhibited by diphenylhydantoin (KIZER *et al.*, 1970). In view of the important role of sodium in islet function, it would appear that there is a need for an extensive investigation of sodium handling by insular tissue.

6. Potassium

a) Effect of Potassium on Islet Function

The role of potassium in insulin release has already been discussed in the preceding part of this chapter (see section 5), where we have assumed that most of the effects of potassium could be accounted for by concomitant changes in sodium net uptake by the B-cell. Therefore, only some limited and more specific aspects of the relation between potassium and islet function will be discussed in the present section.

Whereas most of the experimental data on the effects of cations upon insulin release are relevant to our understanding of the intimate mechanism of the secretory process but have no obvious physiopathological counterpart, the influence of potassium on islet function, as studied with *in vitro* systems, is also encountered in clinical situations. Moreover, in view of the known role of insulin on potassium homeostasis in the intact organism, the influence of potassium on insulin release might be visualized as part of a feedback regulatory process.

A recent study by SANTEUSANIO *et al.* (1973) has emphasized the latter concept. Briefly, these authors observed that potassium infusion stimulates both insulin and glucagon release in normal dogs. If kaligenous insulin release is prevented by prior alloxanization, evidence of potassium intolerance appears. If, on the other hand, kaligenous glucagon release is prevented by prior hyperglycemia, tolerance to potassium remains normal but a fall in glycemia is noticed. These findings suggest that hyperkalemia is normally self-corrected, kaligenous insulin-release increasing potassium tolerance, and concomitant kaligenous glucagon-release providing enough glucose to prevent hypoglycemia.

Conversely, hypokalemia appears to be associated with low and delayed insulin responses to glucose. The low rate of insulin release found in the hypokalemic state is also characterized by an abnormally high proportion of circulating proinsulin to insulin. Both of these abnormalities are likely to contribute to the glucose intolerance often found in potassium deficiency (MONDON *et al.*, 1968; GORDEN *et al.*, 1972).

b) Insular Handling of Potassium

In the only available study on potassium handling by isolated islets (Howell and Taylor, 1968), ouabain was found, as expected, to inhibit the net uptake of potassium-42; whereas glucose, but not tolbutamide, increased such an uptake. The authors concluded that fluxes of potassium in the islets do not appear to be important in the initiation of insulin secretion.

7. pH

a) Effect of pH on Islet Function

Glucose-induced insulin biosynthesis and release are enhanced in alkalotic media and inhibited at low extracellular pH (Malaisse *et al.*, 1971a; Pipeleers *et al.*, 1973). Because of the possible role of glycolysis in glucose-induced insulin biosynthesis and release, and because of the well-known influence of pH on glycolysis in other tissues, it is likely that these effects are mediated by changes in the intracellular pH of the B-cell leading to subsequent changes in the rate of glycolysis. In our view, this process would result in enhanced or decreased production of the metabolite or cofactor serving as a common signal for both insulin biosynthesis and calcium uptake by the B-cell. This interpretation is consistent with the facts that (i) the inhibition of glucose-induced insulin release in acidotic media is apparently mediated by a decreased net uptake of calcium-45 by the islets and is not overcome either at high calcium concentrations or in the presence of barium, and (ii) the enhanced rate of glucose-induced insulin release observed at high pH is associated with increased uptake of calcium-45 and is markedly reduced when calcium is omitted from the incubation medium (Malaisse *et al.*, 1971a; Malaisse-Lagae and Malaisse, 1971; Pipeleers *et al.*, 1973). It is also possible that there exists some more direct influence of extracellular pH on calcium transport across the cell membrane and/or the subcellular distribution of calcium in the B-cell. However, such a process would not account for changes in the rate of insulin biosynthesis, since the latter phenomenon is apparently little affected by the movements of calcium in the B-cell.

At this point, it should be mentioned that by combining various cationic manipulations known to facilitate calcium uptake and subsequent insulin release (extracellular alkalosis, absence of magnesium, high potassium concentration), it is possible to cause a sustained stimulation of insulin release, even in the absence of any metabolic substrate (Malaisse *et al.*, 1971c). This finding supports the view that cations play a key role in triggering insulin release by the pancreatic B-cell.

b) Intracellular pH of Insular Tissue

Hellman *et al.* (1972) have recently measured the intracellular pH in isolated islets. They recorded values of about 7.05. The insular cellular pH was not affected by glucose, epinephrine, diazoxide, or anoxia.

8. Cations and Secretory Granules

Although somewhat beyond the purpose of the present review, we wish to recall that, among other factors, the pH and cationic compositon of the surrounding medium markedly affect the stability of isolated insulin secretory granules. According to Howell *et al.* (1969), optimal stability is observed at high potassium concentrations (160 mEq/l or more), low sodium levels, and low pH (6.0). Calcium apparently does not affect the stability of the granules. Since some of the cationic conditions required for optimal stability of isolated secretory granules are also characteristic of the composition of the intracellular milieu, it is conceivable that the disruption and rapid solubilization of secretory granules at the time of exocytosis is somehow related to the different cationic composition of the intracellular and interstitial fluid respectively.

9. Conclusion

This review underlines the fact that cations are intimately involved in the process of insulin biosynthesis and release by the B-cell. Our present knowledge in this field can be summarized in a simplified manner by the following two working hypotheses: (i) a sodium-dependent step of glucose handling is apparently involved in the recognition of this hexose by the B-cell, and (ii) calcium accumulation in the cytosol of the B-cell apparently triggers insulin release by activating a microtubular-microfilamentous system, itself involved in the migration and extrusion of secretory granules.

References*

Ashcroft, S.J.H., Bassett, J.M., Randle, P.J.: Insulin secretion mechanisms and glucose metabolism in isolated islets. Diabetes **21**, 538—545 (1972)

Ashcroft, S.J.H., Randle, P.J.: Metabolism and insulin secretion in isolated islets. Acta diabet. lat. **6**, Suppl. 1, 538—553 (1969)

Bennett, L.L., Curry, D.L., Grodsky, G.M.: Calcium-magnesium antagonism in insulin secretion by the perfused rat pancreas. Endocrinology **85**, 594—596 (1969)

Brisson, G.R., Malaisse-Lagae, F., Malaisse, W.J.: The stimulus-secretion coupling of glucose-induced insulin release. VII. A proposed site of action for adenosine-3′,5′-cyclic monophosphate. J. clin. Invest. **51**, 232—241 (1972)

Brisson, G.R., Malaisse, W.J.: The stimulus-secretion coupling of glucose-induced insulin release. XI. Effects of theophylline and epinephrine on ^{45}Ca efflux from perifused islets. Metabolism **22**, 455—465 (1973)

Curry, D.L., Bennett, L.L., Grodsky, G.M.: Requirement for calcium ion in insulin secretion by the perfused rat pancreas. Amer. J. Physiol. **214**, 174—178 (1968a)

Curry, D.L., Bennett, L.L., Grodsky, G.M.: Dynamics of insulin secretion by the perfused rat pancreas. Endocrinology **83**, 572—584 (1968b)

Davis, B., Lazarus, N.R.: Glucose-mediated insulin release from mouse islets of Langerhans: adenylate cyclase. Biochem. J. **128**, 96P—97P (1972)

Gomez, M., Curry, D.L.: Potassium stimulation of insulin release by the perfused pancreas. Endocrinology **92**, 1126—1134 (1973)

Gorden, P., Sherman, B.M., Simopoulos, A.P.: Glucose intolerance with hypokalemia: an increased proportion of circulating proinsulin-like component. J. clin. Endocr. **34**, 235—240 (1972)

Grodsky, G.M., Bennett, L.L.: Cation requirements for insulin secretion in the isolated perfused pancreas. Diabetes **15**, 910—913 (1966)

Hales, C.N.: Ion fluxes and membrane function in β-cells and adipocytes. Acta diabet. lat. **7**, Suppl. 1, 64—75 (1970)

Hales, C.N., Milner, R.D.G.: The role of sodium and potassium in insulin secretion from rabbit pancreas. J. Physiol. (Lond.) **194**, 725—743 (1968a)

Hales, C.N., Milner, R.D.G.: Cations and the secretion of insulin from rabbit pancreas in vitro. J. Physiol. (Lond.) **199**, 177—187 (1968b)

Hellman, B.: Methodological approaches to studies of the pancreatic islets. The Minkowski Award Lecture. Diabetologia **6**, 110—120 (1970)

Hellman, B., Sehlin, J., Täljedal, I.-B.: Calcium uptake by pancreatic β-cells as measured with the aid of ^{45}Ca and mannitol-^{3}H. Amer. J. Physiol. **221**, 1795—1801 (1971)

Hellman, B., Sehlin, J., Täljedal, I.-B.: The intracellular pH of mammalian pancreatic β-cells. Endocrinology **90**, 335—337 (1972)

* The review of the literature was completed in September 1973.

Herman, L., Sato, T., Hales, C.N.: The electron microscopic localization of cations to pancreatic islets of Langerhans and their possible role in insulin secretion. J. Ultrastruct. Res. **42**, 298—311 (1973)

Howell, S.L., Taylor, K.W.: Potassium ions and the secretion of insulin by islets of Langerhans incubated in vitro. Biochem. J. **108**, 17—24 (1968)

Howell, S.L., Young, D.A., Lacy, P.E.: Isolation and properties of secretory granules from rat islets of Langerhans. III. Studies of the stability of the isolated beta granules. J. Cell Biol. **41**, 167—176 (1969)

Kizer, S.J., Vargas-Cordon, M., Brendel, K., Bressler, R.: The in vitro inhibition of insulin secretion by diphenylhydantoin. J. clin. Invest. **49**, 1942—1948 (1970)

Lacy, P.E., Howell, S.L., Young, D.A., Fink, C.J.: New hypothesis of insulin secretion. Nature (Lond.) **219**, 1177—1179 (1968)

Lacy, P.E., Malaisse, W.J.: Microtubules and beta cell secretion. Recent Progr. Hormone Res. **29**, 199—221 (1973)

Lambert, A.E.: Biochemical and morphological studies of cultured fetal rat pancreas. Thesis (1971)

Lambert, A.E., Henquin, J.-C., Orci, L.: Role of beta cell membrane in insulin secretion. Amsterdam: Excerpta Medica, ICS **312**, 79—94 (1974)

Laron, Z., Rosenberg, T.: Inhibition of insulin release and stimulation of growth hormone release by hypocalcemia in a boy. Horm. Metab. Res. **2**, 121—122 (1970)

Lefebvre, P.J., Luyckx, A.S.: Effect of ouabain on insulin secretion in the anesthetized dog. Biochem. Pharmacol. **21**, 339—345 (1972)

Lin, B.J., Haist, R.E.: Effects of some modifiers of insulin secretion on insulin biosynthesis. Endocrinology **92**, 735—742 (1973)

Littledike, E.T., Witzel, D.A., Whipp, S.C.: Insulin: evidence for inhibition of release in spontaneous hypocalcemia. Proc. Soc. exp. Biol. (N.Y.) **129**, 135—139 (1968)

Malaisse, W.J.: Role of calcium in insulin secretion. Israel J. med. Sci. **8**, 244—251 (1972)

Malaisse, W.J.: Insulin secretion: multifactorial regulation for a single process of release. The Minkowski Award Lecture. Diabetologia **9**, 167—173 (1973)

Malaisse, W.J.: Participation of the adenylate cyclase system. This volume, 1974

Malaisse, W.J., Malaisse-Lagae, F.: A possible role for calcium in the stimulus-secretion coupling for glucose-induced insulin secretion. Acta diabet. lat. **7**, Suppl. 1, 264—275 (1970)

Malaisse, W.J., Brisson, G., Malaisse-Lagae, F.: The stimulus-secretion coupling of glucose-induced insulin release. I. Interaction of epinephrine and alkaline earth cations. J. Lab. clin. Med. **76**, 895—902 (1970)

Malaisse, W.J., Malaisse-Lagae, F., Brisson, G.: The stimulus-secretion coupling of glucose-induced insulin release. II. Interaction of alkali and alkaline earth cations. Horm. Metab. Res. **3**, 65—70 (1971a)

Malaisse, W.J., Malaisse-Lagae, F., Walker, M.O., Lacy, P.E.: The stimulus-secretion coupling of glucose-induced insulin release. V. The participation of a microtubular-microfilamentous system. Diabetes **20**, 257—265 (1971b)

Malaisse, W.J., Brisson, G.R., Malaisse-Lagae, F.: Effet insulinotrope du calcium. Ann. Endocr. (Paris) **32**, 621—622 (1971c)

Malaisse, W.J., Mahy, M., Brisson, G.R., Malaisse-Lagae, F.: The stimulus-secretion coupling of glucose-induced insulin release. VIII. Combined effects of glucose and sulfonylureas. Europ. J. clin. Invest. **2**, 85—90 (1972a)

Malaisse, W.J., Hager, D.L., Orci, L.: The stimulus-secretion coupling of glucose-induced insulin release. IX. The participation of the beta cell web. Diabetes **21**, 594—604 (1972b)

Malaisse, W.J., Brisson, G.R., Baird, L.E.: Stimulus-secretion coupling of glucose-induced insulin release. X. Effect of glucose on ^{45}Ca efflux from perifused islets. Amer. J. Physiol. **224**, 389—394 (1973a)

Malaisse, W.J., Pipeleers, D.G., Mahy, M.: The stimulus-secretion coupling of glucose-induced insulin release. XII. Effects of diazoxide and gliclazide upon ^{45}calcium efflux from perifused islets. Diabetologia **9**, 1—5 (1973b)

Malaisse, W.J., Malaisse-Lagae, F., Van Obberghen, E., Somers, G., Devis, G., Orci, L.: The microtubular-microfilamentous system of the pancreatic beta cell. Amsterdam: Excerpta Medica, ICS **273**, 282—287 (1973c)

Malaisse, W.J., Pipeleers, D.G.: The role of cations in insulin synthesis and release. Amsterdam: Excerpta Medica, ICS **312**, 95—103 (1974)

Malaisse-Lagae, F., Malaisse, W.J.: Stimulus-secretion coupling of glucose-induced insulin release. III. Uptake of ^{45}calcium by isolated islets of Langerhans. Endocrinology **88**, 72—80 (1971)

Malaisse-Lagae, F., Brisson, G.R., Malaisse, W.J.: The stimulus-secretion coupling of glucose-induced insulin release. VI. Analogy between the insulinotropic mechanisms of sugars and amino acids. Horm. Metab. Res. **3**, 374—378 (1971)

Matschinsky, F.M., Ellerman, J.: Dissociation of the insulin releasing and the metabolic functions of hexoses in islets of Langerhans. Biochem. biophys. Res. Commun. **50**, 193—199 (1973)

Matthews, E.K.: Electrical activity in islet cells and insulin secretion. Acta diabet. lat. **7**, Suppl. 1, 83—89 (1970)

Milner, R.D.G., Hales, C.N.: The role of calcium and magnesium in insulin secretion from rabbit pancreas studied in vitro. Diabetologia **3**, 47—49 (1967)

Milner, R.D.G., Hales, C.N.: The interaction of various inhibitors and stimuli of insulin release studied with rabbit pancreas in vitro. Biochem. J. **113**, 473—479 (1969)

Mondon, C.E., Burton, S.D., Grodsky, G.M., Ishida, T.: Glucose tolerance and insulin response of potassium-deficient rat and isolated liver. Amer. J. Physiol. **215**, 779—787 (1968)

Montague, W., Howell, S.L.: The mode of action of adenosine 3′:5′-cyclic monophosphate in mammalian islets of Langerhans. Preparation and properties of islet-cell protein phosphokinase. Biochem. J. **129**, 551—560 (1972)

Pipeleers, D.G., Marichal, M., Malaisse, W.J.: The stimulus-secretion coupling of glucose-induced insulin release. XV. Participation of cations in the recognition of glucose by the beta cell. Endocrinology **93**, 1012—1018 (1973)

Randle, P.J.: Islet metabolism and insulin secretion. Excerpta Medica **231**, 232—239 (1971)

Santeusanio, F., Faloona, G.R., Knochel, J.P., Unger, R.H.: Evidence for a role of endogenous insulin and glucagon in the regulation of potassium homeostasis. J. Lab. clin. Med. **81**, 809—817 (1973)

Triner, L., Killiam, P., Nahas, G.G.: Ouabain hypoglycemia: insulin mediation. Science **162**, 560—561 (1968)

VI. The Bioelectrical Activity of the Islet Cell Membrane

E. K. MATTHEWS, P. M. DEAN and Y. SAKAMOTO

With 12 Figures

1. Introduction

The exploration of islet-cell function and insulin release has involved the development of a wide variety of experimental technics, ranging from use of the whole pancreas for perfusion studies (e.g. GRODSKY *et al.*, 1970) to isolated islets for more specific biochemical determinations (e.g. HELLERSTRÖM, 1964). Even in the latter case, however, the measured net response remains a collective one involving many cells, each perhaps with a differing sensitivity to an imposed stimulus.

With the introduction of the microelectrode as an intracellular probe of islet activity (DEAN and MATTHEWS, 1968, 1970a, b) it became possible for the first time to study the membrane responsiveness of individual islet cells to stimulants of insulin secretion. Thus measurements of membrane bioelectrical activity can be made in single cells for prolonged periods or, alternatively, a statistical profile can be constructed of islet-cell response under various conditions. Each approach yields important information about the sensitivity of islet cells to stimulant or inhibitory molecules and this is described here together with the evidence which serves to emphasize the close correlation between islet-cell bioelectrical activity and insulin release. The nature of the stimulus-secretion coupling process in islet β-cells is also discussed in particular as it relates to the mode of action of the insulin-releasing hexoses, amino acids, and sulfonylureas.

2. Measurement of Electrical Properties of Islet Cells

In the electrophysiological studies, segments of pancreas excised from albino mice were secured to a small platform, mounted in a tissue bath (Fig. 1) and superfused with Krebs-Henseleit solution at 37° C.

Islets of Langerhans were exposed by microdissection after the technic of HELLERSTRÖM (1964) and cellular transmembrane potentials recorded with glass microelectrodes filled with K-citrate and having a tip resistance of about 100 MΩ (MATTHEWS, 1967; DEAN and MATTHEWS, 1970a, b). The microelectrode was inserted into cells with a micromanipulator and the potential measured across the cell membrane between the tip of the microelectrode (Fig. 1; E_1) and an indifferent electrode of low resistance placed in the bathing solution (Fig. 1; E_2). The electrical signals are amplified and displayed on an oscilloscope and pen recorder as indicated.

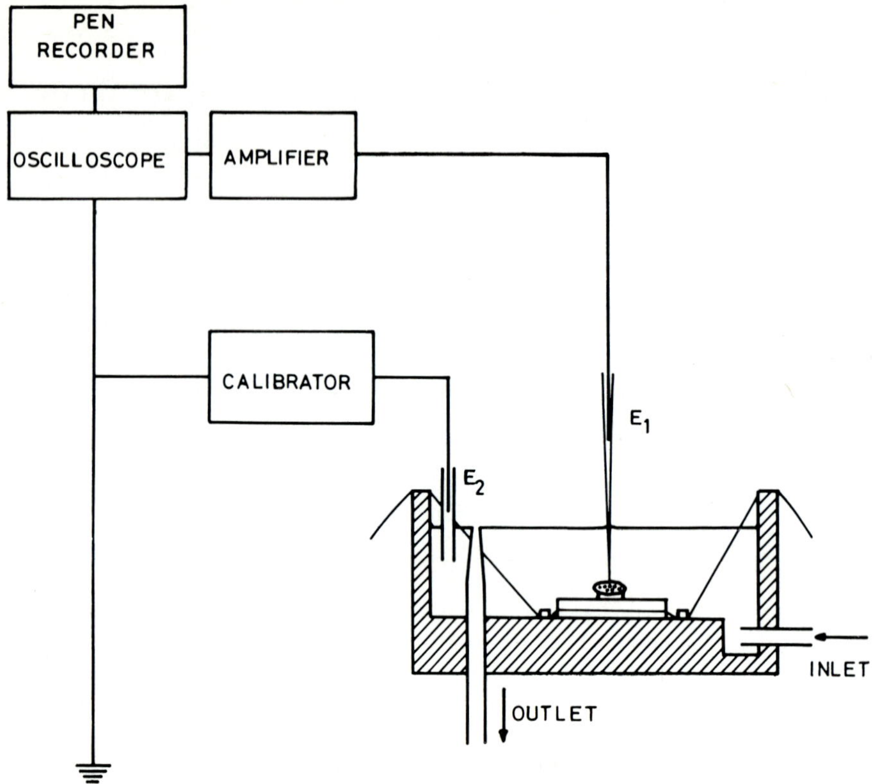

Fig. 1. Diagram of the apparatus used to measure the membrane potential in cells of the pancreas. A segment of pancreas is mounted on the plastic platform within the tissue bath; the islets are exposed by microdissection. E_1 = microelectrode. E_2 = indifferent electrode. (Modified from MATTHEWS and DEAN, 1970a)

A particular advantage of mouse islets of Langerhans for electrophysiological study is that not only may they be readily desegregated from the acinar parenchyma by microdissection but the α-cells, which constitute only about 10% of the islet cell population, are anatomically distributed as a mantle around the islet and so can be avoided by sampling only those cells, i.e. β-cells, located well within the islet.

Acinar cells have a mean membrane potential of about —41 mV and islet cells a mean potential of —20 mV (DEAN and MATTHEWS, 1970a, b). Relative frequency distributions are illustrated in Fig. 2a. Whereas acinar cell membrane potentials were not affected by alteration of the D-glucose concentration, the islet β-cells depolarized in 28 mM glucose (i.e. frequency distribution shifted to the left) and hyperpolarized in zero D-glucose (i.e. distribution shifted to higher potentials) as shown in Fig. 2b.

3. Electrical Activity Induced by Islet Stimulants

A further important distinction between acinar cells and islet cells becomes apparent when the extracellular D-glucose concentration is increased. As the D-glucose concentration is raised from 0—28 mM rapid fluctuations in membrane potential or 'action potentials' are seen in islet but not in acinar cells. The threshold for this effect appears to be about 3—4 mM. The action potentials tended to occur in bursts with lower concentrations of glucose (Fig. 3) but the discharge became continuous with higher concentrations. Thus the frequency rather than the magnitude of action-potential discharge appeared dependent on extracellular D-glucose (or D-mannose) concentration, our original finding (DEAN and MATTHEWS, 1970a) since being confirmed by others (PACE and PRICE, 1972).

Table 1. *Glucose Analogues and Other Sugars which do not Produce Action Potentials (Three or More Expts. for Each Compound)*

	mM		mM
L-Glucose	16.6	Sodium n-octoate	10
D-Galactose	50	D-Xylitol	50
D-Glucosamine	20	D-Ribose	20
2-Deoxy-D-glucose	20	D-Fructose	50
3-0-Methyl a D-glucose	25	D-Mannoheptulose	24

(From MATTHEWS and DEAN, 1970a).

D-mannose also elicited an action-potential discharge from islet cells but many other glucose analogues, including the glucose enantiomer, L-glucose, did not (Table 1). On the other hand, L-leucine, 10 mM (Fig. 3) and the hypoglycemic sulfonylureas tolbutamide, chlorpropamide, and glibenclamide (Figs. 3 and 4) all rapidly induced electrical activity (MATTHEWS and DEAN, 1970b). In fact, activity generated by L-leucine, D-glucose, and D-mannose appeared similar in that all three substances induced action potentials with a duration of about 50 m sec (Fig. 3) compared with about 300 m sec for the sulfonylureas (Figs. 3 and 4).

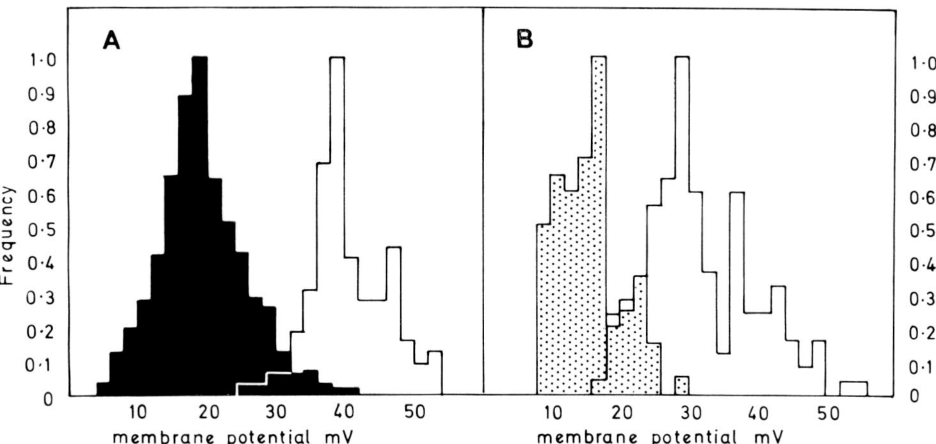

Fig. 2. Relative frequency distribution of membrane potentials recorded from cells of the mouse pancreas. A. Islet cells, filled columns; acinar cells, open columns; measurements in D-glucose 2.8 mM. B. Islet cells exposed to D-glucose 27.7 mM, stippled columns; and zero glucose, open columns. (From DEAN and MATTHEWS, 1970a)

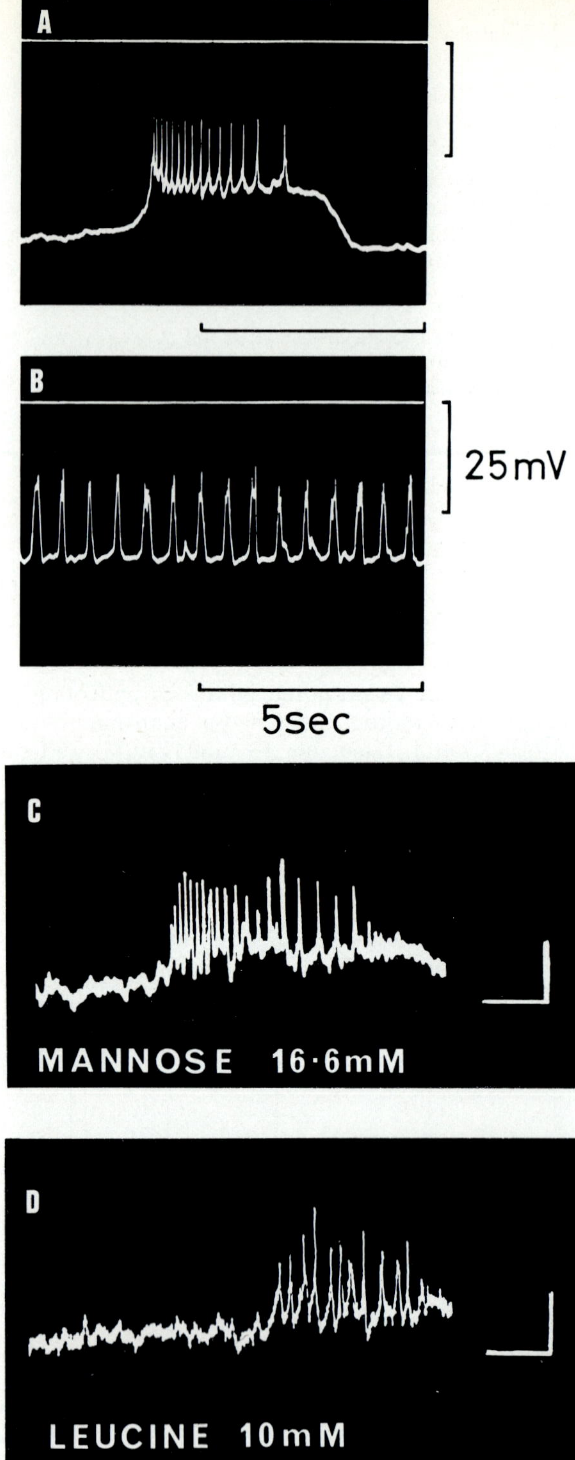

Fig. 3. Electrical activity induced in pancreatic islet cells by A, D-glucose 11.2 mM (after 20 min exposure); and B, tolbutamide 0.7 mM (after 20 min exposure). A and B are oscilloscopic recordings from two different cells in the same islet. (From MATTHEWS *et al.*, 1973). Effect of C, D-mannose 16.6 mM and D, L-leucine, 10 mM. Vertical calibration = 2 mV; horizontal calibration = 0.5 sec. (From MATTHEWS and DEAN, 1970a)

HB 419 2x10^{-5}M
0
mV
30
CHLORPROPAMIDE 6·7x10^{-4}M
0
mV
30
2s

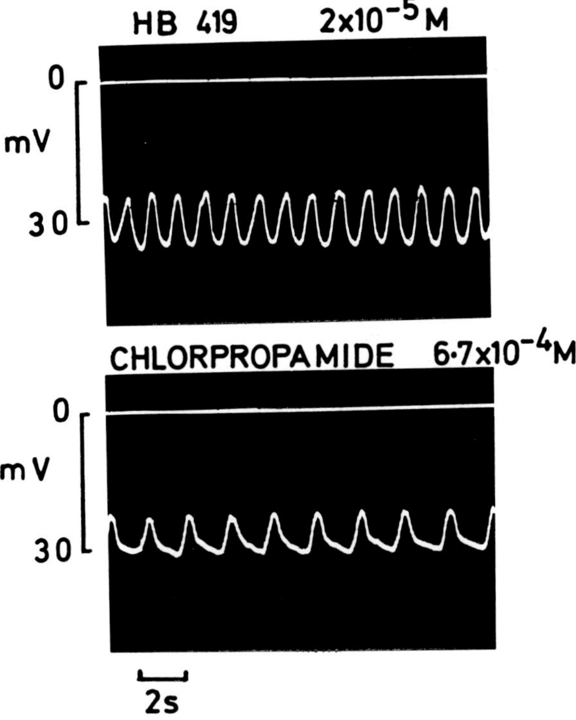

Fig. 4a. Action potentials induced in islet cells by glibenclamide and chlorpropamide. (From MATTHEWS and DEAN, 1970b)

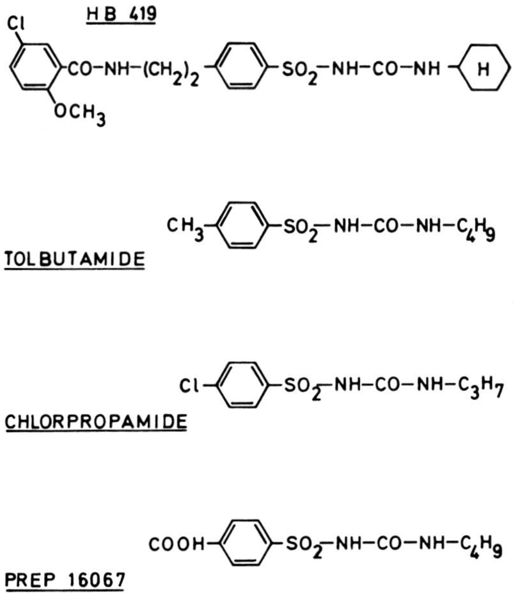

HB 419
Cl
CO–NH–$(CH_2)_2$
SO_2–NH–CO–NH
H
OCH_3
TOLBUTAMIDE
CH_3
SO_2–NH–CO–NH–C_4H_9
CHLORPROPAMIDE
Cl
SO_2–NH–CO–NH–C_3H_7
PREP 16067
COOH
SO_2–NH–CO–NH–C_4H_9

Fig. 4b. Sulfonylurea structure

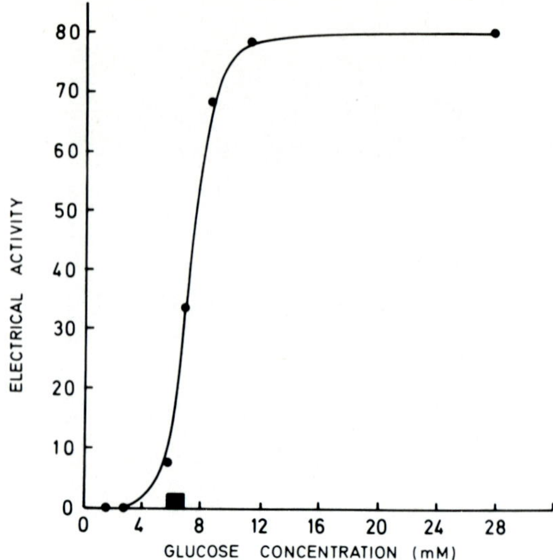

Fig. 5a. Relationship between glucose concentration and electrical activity of islet cells. Electrical activity expressed as the percentage of impaled cells which show action-potential discharge. The black bar indicates the normal range of blood glucose concentration in the mouse. (From MATTHEWS, 1970)

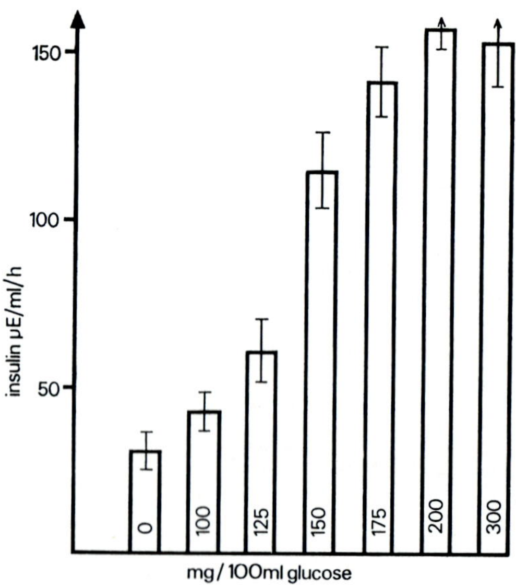

Fig. 5b. Insulin secretion in relation to the glucose concentration in the incubation medium, n = 6; mean ± S.D. (From WEINGES, 1970)

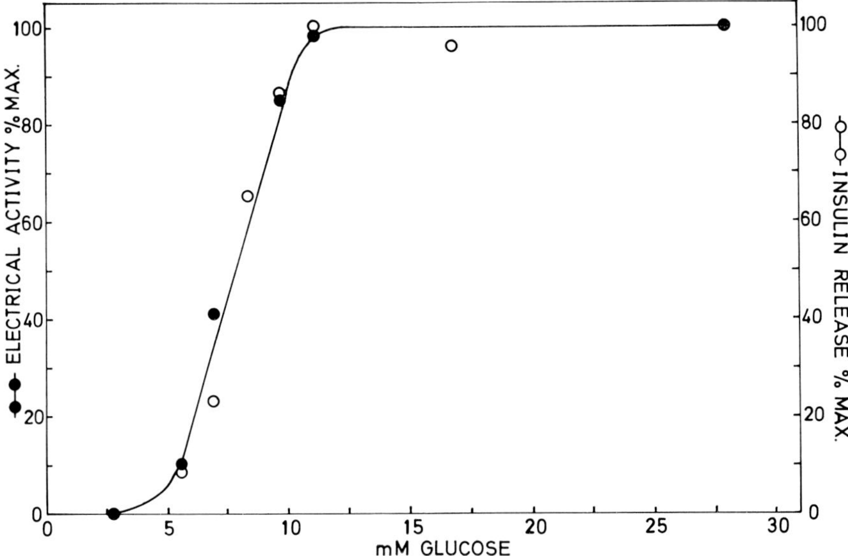

Fig. 5c. Dose-response relationships in a and b replotted and expressed as a percentage of the maximal response in each case. Electrical activity (●), and insulin release (○)

4. Relationship Between Electrical Activity and Insulin Release

It is particularly striking that as the extracellular D-glucose concentration is raised, so the incidence of electrical activity correspondingly increases. This fact first prompted us to examine a possible functional relationship between the appearance of glucose-induced electrical activity and insulin release (MATTHEWS and DEAN, 1970a).

Figure 5a and b illustrate for mouse islets the dose dependence of the glucose-induced electrical activity (DEAN and MATTHEWS, 1970a) and insulin release (WEINGES, 1970) respectively. The correlation between these phenomena is clearly emphasized by the remarkable coincidence of the regressions replotted in Fig. 5c. The profile of ability to induce electrical activity correlates well with capacity to evoke insulin release in the case of D-glucose, D-mannose, L-leucine, and the anti-diabetic sulfonylureas. Significantly, the failure of many other monosaccharides and glucose analogues to release insulin is paralleled by their inability to elicit electrical activity (Table 1). This structural specificity for both electrical activity and secretion is also borne out by the failure of the 0-dealkylated analogue of tolbutamide, (N-(4-carboxy-benzol-sulfonyl)-(n-butyl) urea (i.e. Prep 16067 in Fig. 4B) to evoke either a hypoglycemic response (VON DORFMULLER, 1956) or electrical activity (MATTHEWS and DEAN, 1970b).

5. Effect of Ions on Glucose-Induced Electrical Activity

In view of the demonstration by HALES and MILNER (1968a, b) that insulin release is critically dependent on extracellular cations it seemed likely that a study of the effects of changes in the ionic environment upon action potentials induced by glucose might yield useful information about their nature and functional significance (DEAN and MATTHEWS, 1970a, b).

a) Monovalent Ions

Potassium: raising the external potassium concentration, $[K]_0$, from 4.7 mM to 47 mM depolarized the islet cells but did not elicit action-potential discharge in 2.8 mM glucose. A tenfold increase in $[K]_0$ decreased the membrane potential by 13 mV but zero $[K]_0$ did not hyperpolarize the cells.

Chloride: replacement of NaCl with Na isethionate, so reducing the external chloride concentration, $[Cl]_0$, from 114 to 12 mM was without effect on the islet membrane potential or electrical activity generated by glucose.

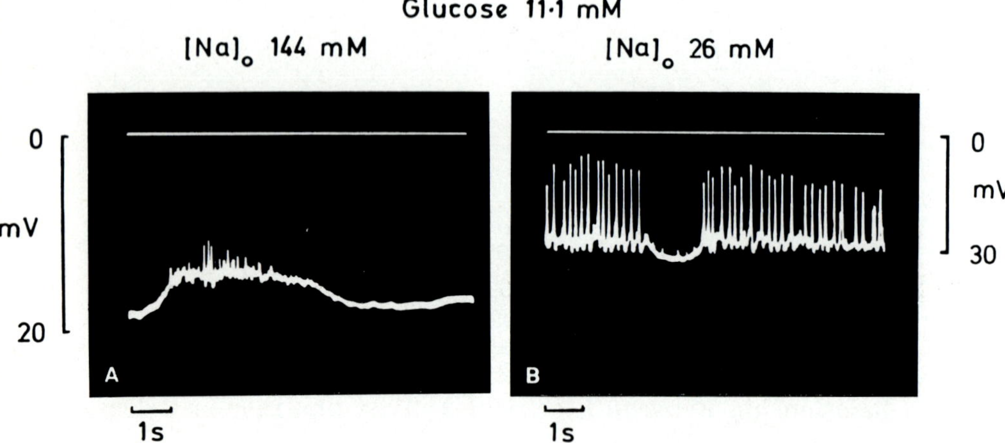

Fig. 6a. Effect of external sodium concentration on electrical activity induced by glucose, 11.1 mM. A) Action potentials induced by glucose in normal sodium medium $[Na]_0$ 144 mM. B) Action potentials induced by glucose 11.1 mM 55 min after exposure to low sodium medium $[Na]_0$ 25 mM. The records are from different experiments. (From Matthews and Dean, 1970b)

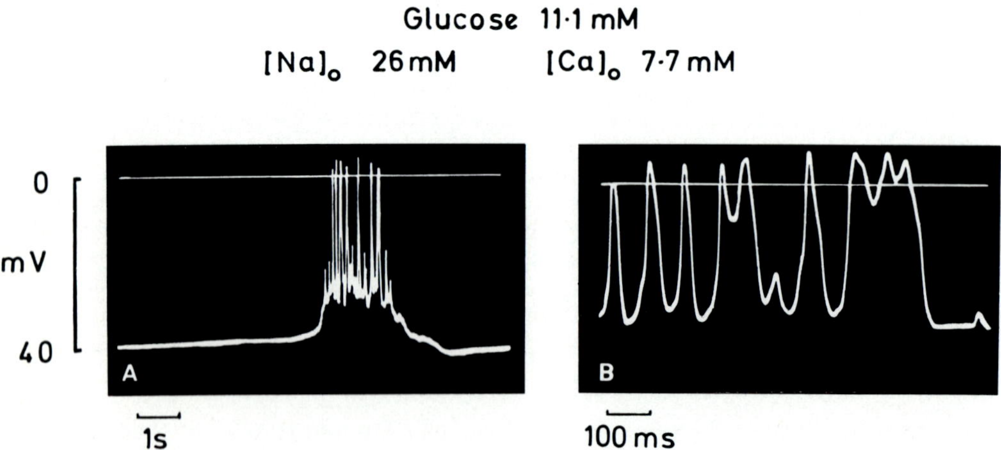

Fig. 6b. Effect of low sodium ($[Na]_0$ 26 mM) and high calcium ($[Ca]_0$ 7.7 mM) on the action potentials induced by glucose, 11.1 mM. A). A single burst of activity with action-potential overshoot. B). Increased time base amplification to show plateaux of action potential during a burst of activity. (From Dean and Matthews, 1970b)

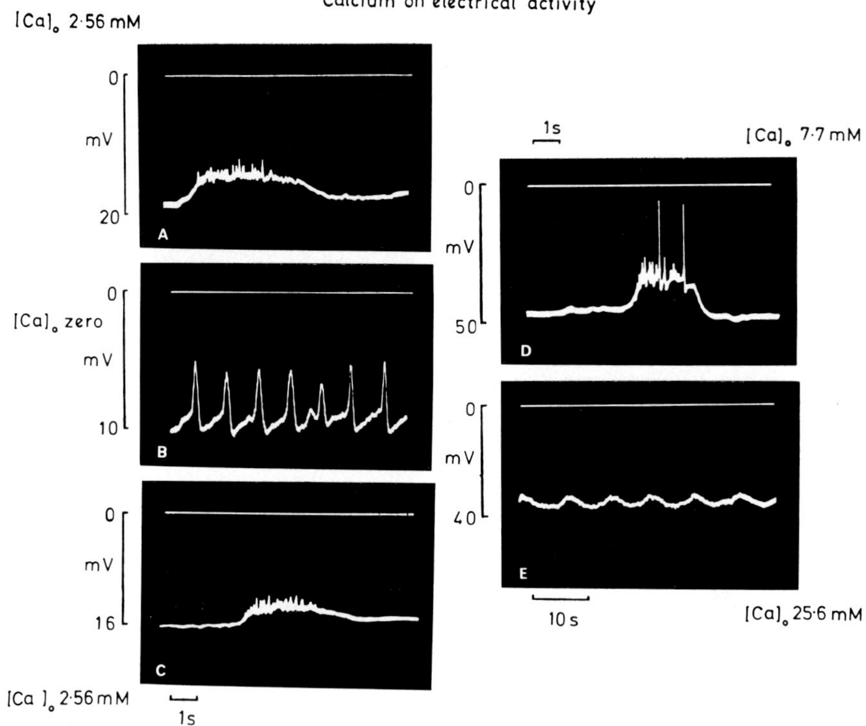

Fig. 7. Effect of external calcium concentration on action potentials induced in islet cells by glucose. A. A normal burst of action potentials induced by glucose, 11.1 mM $[Ca]_0$ 2.56 mM. B. Continuous firing of action potentials (200 ms duration) in zero $[Ca]_0$, glucose 11.1 mM. C. Return to a normal burst of action potentials on reintroduction of calcium 2.56 mM following continuous firing of action potentials in zero $[Ca]_0$, glucose 11.1 mM. D. Action potentials in $[Ca]_0$ 7.7 mM, glucose 11.1 mM. E. Slow-wave depolarizations induced by glucose 16.6 mM with an external calcium concentration of 25.6 mM. B and C are records from the same preparation; other records from different experiments. (From DEAN and MATTHEWS, 1970b)

Sodium: reduction of external sodium, $[Na]_0$, to 26 mM (from 144 mM) caused a considerable increase in the amplitude of glucose-induced action potentials (Fig. 6a). This potentiating effect was also seen initially in zero $[Na]_0$ but prolonged exposure to a Na^+-free environment eventually caused a complete block of electrical activity.

b) Divalent Cations

Calcium: removal of extracellular Ca^{2+}, $[Ca]_0$, in the presence of ongoing glucose-induced electrical activity caused a transition of firing pattern from burst-type to continuous activity (Fig. 7). Increasing $[Ca]_0$ threefold to 7.7 mM, hyperpolarized the cells and increased the amplitude of the action potentials especially in the presence of a low $[Na]_0$ (Fig. 6b). Higher concentrations of $[Ca]_0$ completely blocked activity (Fig. 7C).

Strontium: after replacing $[Ca]_0$ by strontium, islet cells responded with a normal pattern of firing to D-glucose. Thus, as in many other cells Sr^{2+} acts as an effective substitute for Ca^{2+}, presumably by virtue of its similar ionic characteristics (i.e. charge, size, and ionic potential).

Magnesium: neither the islet-cell membrane potential or glucose-induced action potentials were affected by the omission of magnesium, $[Mg]_0$; insulin secretion is similarly unaffected (HALES and MILNER, 1968b). Increasing $[Mg]_0$ tenfold, to 11.3 mM, did not entirely prevent the subsequent production of electrical activity by glucose although under these conditions a block of insulin release occurs (HALES and MILNER, 1968b). This may indicate a means by which electrical activity can be uncoupled from secretory activity.

Manganese: addition of 2 mM manganese rapidly blocked ongoing electrical activity in islet cells. In other tissues, for example, smooth muscle (BULBRING and TOMITA, 1969), manganese blocks action potentials which are dependent primarily on Ca^{2+} influx.

The results of these ionic manipulations are compatible with the hypothesis that the action potentials evoked in β-cells by glucose are due predominantly to calcium entry and that sodium ions tend normally to repress this calcium influx (see DEAN and MATTHEWS, 1970a, b). We have recently obtained further experimental evidence which substantiates this idea (MATTHEWS and SAKAMOTO, unpublished). The results with magnesium suggest that this ion may compete with the calcium ion at the β-cell membrane, even acting at least in part as a carrier of membrane current, but subsequently inhibiting intracellularly the calcium-activated stimulus-secretion coupling mechanism.

6. Effects of Inhibitors and Anoxia on Electrical Activity

Mannoheptulose, a 7-carbon glucose analogue, blocks the metabolism of glucose and inhibits insulin release (COORE and RANDLE, 1964). It is, therefore, of particular interest that in islet cells electrical activity induced by 28 mM D-glucose was rapidly antagonized by mannoheptulose 20 mM which also caused the cells to hyperpolarize (MATTHEWS and SAKAMOTO, 1973); these effects were reversible on removal of mannoheptulose (Fig. 8).

Whereas mannoheptulose blocks the metabolism of glucose, phlorizin prevents glucose uptake into the β-cells (HELLMAN *et al.*, 1972). We have found that it also inhibits glucose-induced electrical activity (MATTHEWS and SAKAMOTO, 1973). Thus ongoing electrical activity in response to 28 mM glucose activity was blocked within 30 min following exposure to 10 mM phlorizin. Alternatively, if the cells were exposed to phlorizin before D-glucose no electrical activity was generated.

In cells rendered anoxic by superfusing them with Krebs solution equilibrated with N_2:CO_2 rather than O_2:CO_2 the electrical activity induced by 28 mM glucose was progressively inhibited; these effects were reversed by O_2 (MATTHEWS *et al.*, 1973). If the cells were made anoxic for 60 min before exposure to D-glucose, the appearance of electrical activity and depolarization was completely prevented (Fig. 9a). On the other hand, the bioelectrical effects of the sulfonylureas tolbutamide and glibenclamide were not blocked by anoxia (Fig. 9b).

A further point of interest in Fig. 9 is that at the concentrations used both glucose and tolbutamide generate a 'phasic-tonic' receptor response in terms of discharge frequency, i.e. an initial peak frequency which quickly declines to a lower but maintained level. In view of the bi- and monophasic release of insulin induced by glucose and tolbutamide, respectively (GRODSKY *et al.*, 1970), this suggests that at a time when insulin release is maximal, action-potential frequency is also maximal (i.e. 0—10 min). Subsequently, despite a maintained (but lower) frequency of electrical activity (Fig. 9) insulin release declines (GRODSKY *et al.*,

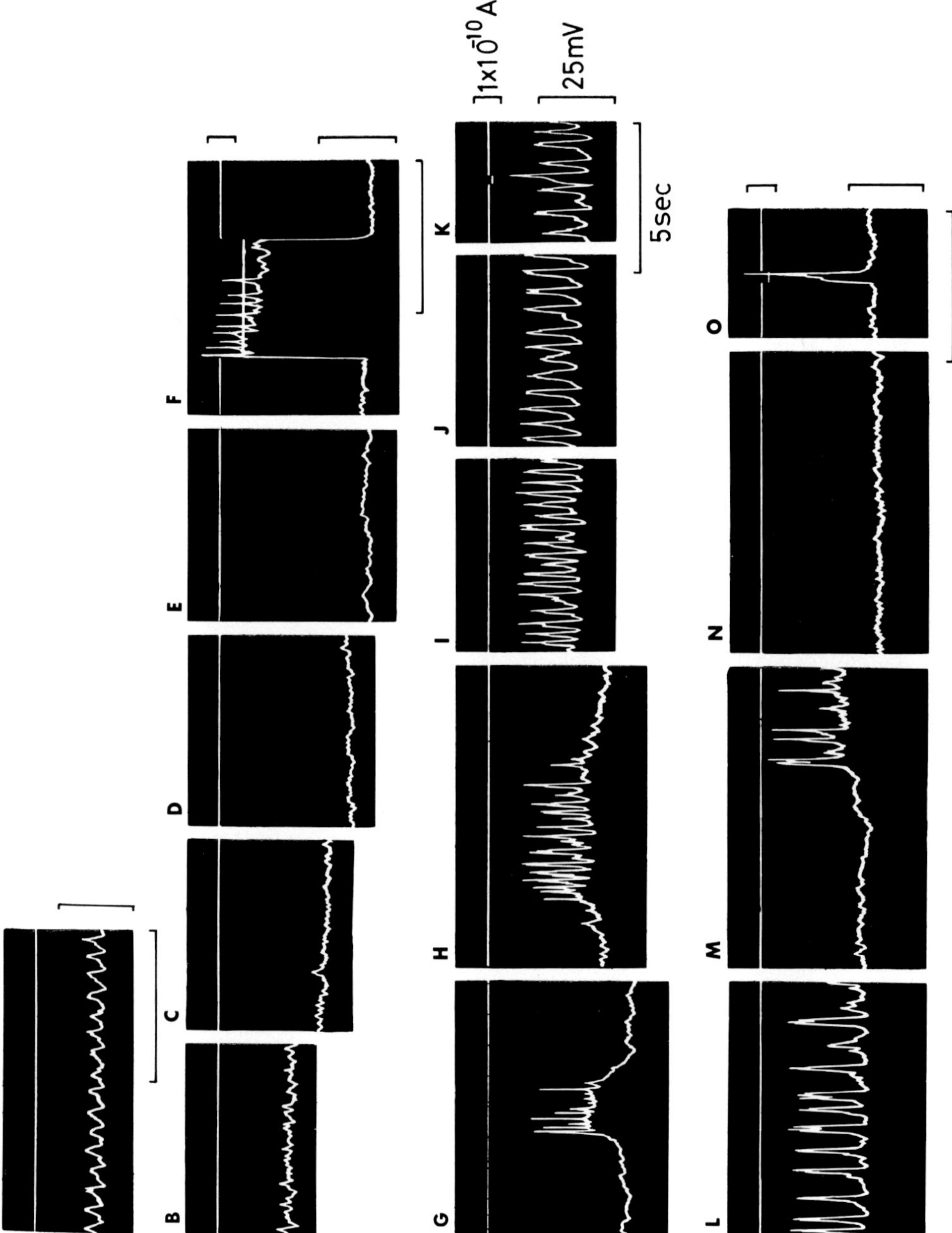

Fig. 8. The effect of mannoheptulose on glucose-induced electrical activity in a pancreatic islet cell. Intracellular records, all from the same cell; the horizontal white line indicates the zero potential. Records A to K in presence of D-glucose, 28 mM, and L to O in Krebs solution. Records B to F, 5, 15, 20, 30, and 35 min after addition of mannoheptulose, 20 mM; G to K, 18, 35, 45, 60, and 60 min following its removal; L to O, 20, 30, 60, and 60 min after changing to Krebs solution alone. Depolarizing current injected through the recording microelectrode in F, K, and O; current duration and magnitude indicated by deflection on zero potential level. (From MATTHEWS and SAKAMOTO, 1973)

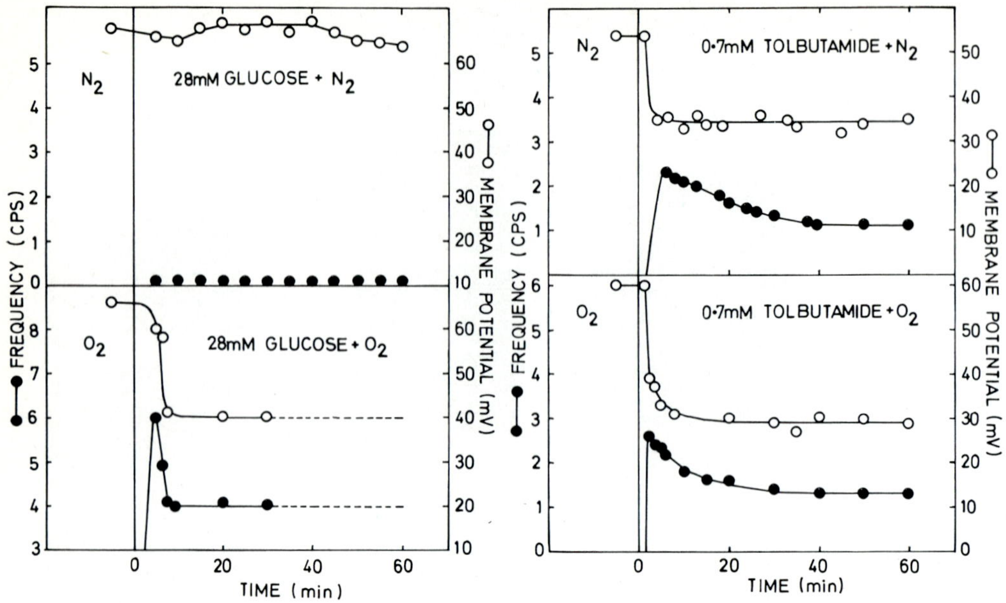

Fig. 9. Effect of anoxia on the electrical responses of pancreatic islet cells to A, D-glucose 28 mM or B, tolbutamide 0.7 mM. Membrane potential (○) and action potential frequency (●). Each panel shows the result of a single experiment (see text for further details). (From MATTHEWS et al., 1973)

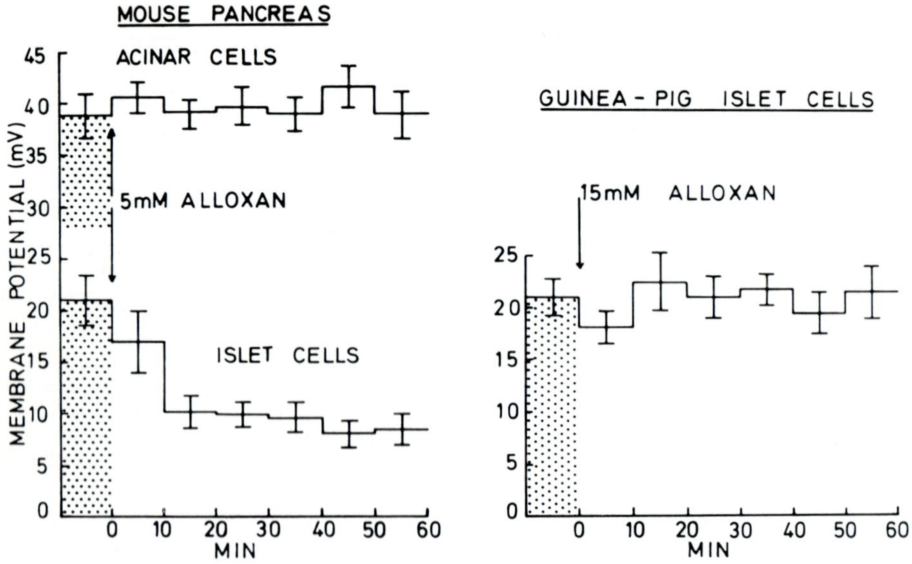

Fig. 10. The effect of alloxan on islet and acinar cells from mouse pancreas and on islet cells from guinea-pig pancreas. The stippled columns show the mean membrane potential obtained during the 60 min period before addition of alloxan, concentration as shown. SE of mean indicated by vertical bars. (From MATTHEWS and DEAN, 1970a)

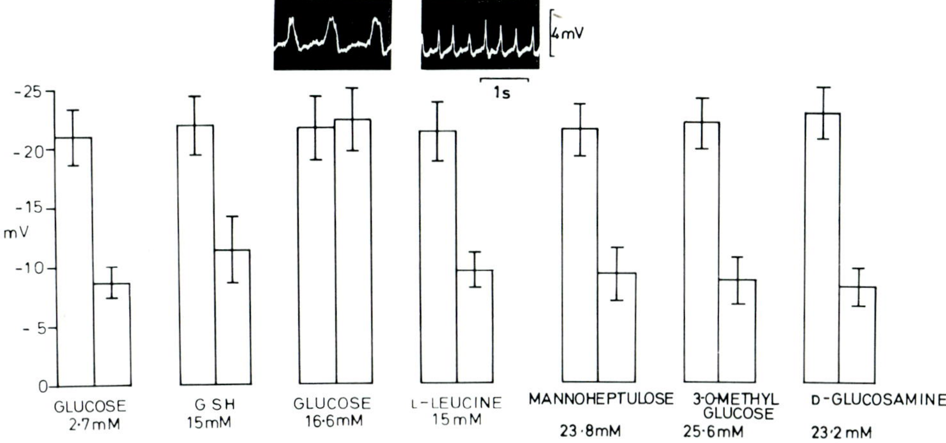

Fig. 11. The histograms show the effect of preincubation of islet cells for 15 min with various compounds, indicated beneath each histogram. The 1st column shows the mean membrane potential in normal solution, the 2nd column shows the effect of alloxan 5 mM after preincubation with a possible protective compound, the membrane potentials being measured during the 30—60 min period after alloxan. The inset oscilloscope traces show electrical activity during the preincubation period with glucose 16.6 mM and L-leucine 15 mM. (From DEAN and MATTHEWS, 1972)

1970); thus although a gated Ca^{2+} entry may still persist (see below) the insulin-release process displays partial inactivation.

7. Effect of Diabetogenic Agents

Experimentally, a diabetic state can be induced in an animal with the substances alloxan and streptozotocin; each agent damages the islet cells but apparently by a different mechanism. Alloxan depolarized the islet cells rapidly (MATTHEWS and DEAN, 1970a) but did not affect the acinar cells (Fig. 10). The guinea pig is relatively resistant to the diabetogenic action of alloxan (MASKE and WEINGES, 1957) and the islet cells from this species were not affected by concentrations of alloxan up to 15 mM, as shown in Fig. 10. A number of substances were tested for a possible protective effect against the action of alloxan on mouse islet cells but only D-glucose conferred protection (DEAN and MATTHEWS, 1972). This is not likely to be due simply to the induction of electrical activity since L-leucine, which also evoked electrical activity, exerted no protective effect (Fig. 11).

In contrast to alloxan, pretreatment with the potent diabetogenic antibiotic streptozotocin did not depolarize the islet cells yet completely blocked the electrical activity induced by D-glucose, D-mannose, D-glyceraldehyde, and L-leucine (DEAN and MATTHEWS, 1972). The alkylating moiety of streptozotocin, namely N-methyl N-nitroso urea, produced similar inhibitory effects (Table 2). Yet interestingly enough, tolbutamide-induced electrical activity persisted, indicating in this instance a marked resistance to streptozotocin action. Finally, exposure to nicotinamide conferred protection against the inhibition by streptozotocin of glucose action (Table 2), an effect not apparently dependent upon simple chemical inactivation of the streptozotocin molecule (DEAN and MATTHEWS, 1972).

Table 2. *The Effect of Pretreatment of Islet Cells with Streptozotocin on the Induction of Action Potentials by Various Compounds*

Compound inducing action potentials	concentration	% of cells induced to fire action potentials by the compound without pretreatment with streptozotocin	% of cells induced to fire action potentials by the compound after pretreatment with streptozotocin	n
D-glucose	11.1 mM	78%	0%	4
D-mannose	16.6 mM	84%	0%	4
L-leucine	10 mM	53%	0%	4
D-glyceraldehyde	11 mM	67%	0%	7
Tolbutamide	7×10^{-4}M	70%	67.5%	5
Nicotinamide pretreatment, followed by D-glucose	11.1 mM	78%	83%	6
Compound inducing action potentials	**concentration**	**% of cells induced to fire action potentials by the compound without pretreatment with N-nitroso N-methyl urea**	**% of cells induced to fire action potentials by the compound after pretreatment with N-nitroso N-methyl urea**	n
D-glucose	11.1 mM	78%	3.5%	7
Tolbutamide	7×10^{-4}M	70%	50%	6

n = number of experiments.
(From DEAN and MATTHEWS, 1972).

8. Discussion

There now seems little doubt that the islet β-cell membrane is vitally involved both in the recognition of stimulant molecules and in the dynamic control of insulin release. In fact, one of the fundamental questions about the islet cell concerns its molecular discriminator or receptor capacity since the cell recognizes a diversity of molecular signals yet responds with a single output, insulin. Thus, the cell may possess distinct receptor sites for each molecular signal, e.g. hexose, amino acid, sulfonylurea, or less sophisticated sites with broad-spectrum specificity (MATTHEWS *et al.*, 1973). It is, therefore, of prime importance to establish not only the precise location but also the specificity of the initial receptor site responsible for actuating insulin release, especially since the molecular defect of diabetes could well be located at an early stage in the stimulus-secretion coupling process. Measurements of insulin release alone, i.e. the final output stage, are unlikely to provide the information needed to build up a detailed picture of the initial molecular events associated with receptor activation, i.e. generation of the input signal.

On the other hand, one great advantage of the microelectrode as an intracellular probe is that it gives instant access to important information about permeability changes occurring at the β-cell membrane. It is, therefore, possible to subject to analysis the action of secretory stimulants at an early phase in the activation of the release process, that is at the cell membrane itself. Figure 5c shows clearly that the kinetics of glucose-induced insulin release and electrical activity (i.e. gated permeability changes) are closely related.

Now under normal circumstances, the glucose molecule constitutes the primary stimulus for insulin release, and it is at once apparent that the islet cell must possess a hexose receptor of quite considerable stereospecificity since only D-glu-

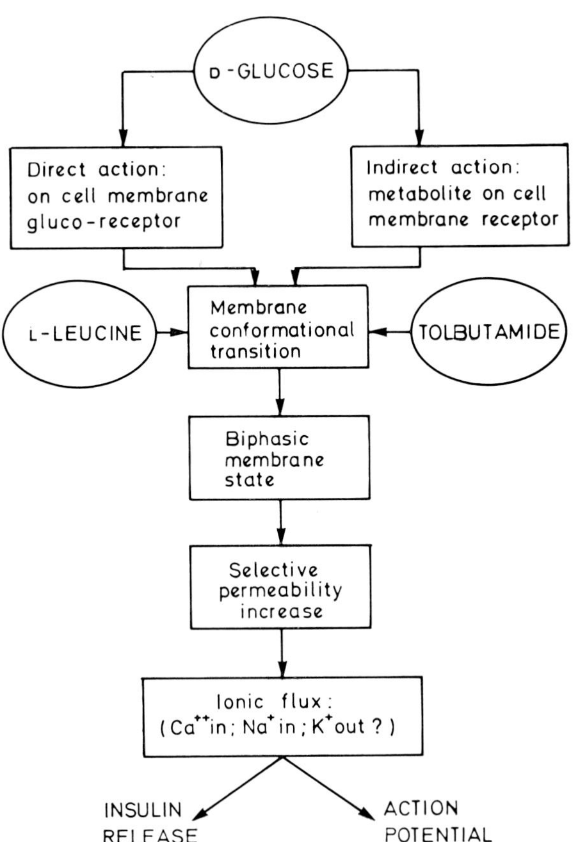

Fig. 12. A possible scheme by which action-potential incidence might be correlated with insulin secretion. (From MATTHEWS and DEAN, 1970a)

cose and D-mannose are recognized. L-glucose, glucose analogues, and other monosaccharides fail to evoke insulin release or elicit electrical activity (see Table 1); it is also perhaps not without significance that very few, if any, of these latter compounds are metabolized to any appreciable extent in β-cells. Whether this receptor specificity extends to compounds other than hexoses and monosaccharides is an important question.

In fact, the electrophysiological evidence already suggests, on the basis of inhibition by streptozotocin and anoxia of glucose-, but not sulfonylurea- induced electrical activity, an operational and perhaps functional distinction between the glucose- and sulfonylurea-receptor (MATTHEWS *et al.*, 1973). This follows if it is assumed that the stimulant molecule, whether glucose or sulfonylurea, interacts directly with some membrane-located receptor. If, on the other hand, a metabolite of glucose is responsible for initiating insulin release and electrical activity by interacting with a common membrane site, i.e. one accessible to both metabolite and sulfonylurea, it may simply be that streptozotocin, anoxia (and phlorizin or mannoheptulose), inhibit glucose uptake and/or metabolism and so cut off the supply of active metabolite. However, taken together with the fact that glyceraldehyde-induced electrical activity is also inhibited by streptozotocin (DEAN and MATTHEWS, 1972) but not by anoxia (MATTHEWS and SAKAMOTO, unpublished), the evidence favours the idea of a metabolite of glucose being responsible for inducing electrical activity (and probably also insulin release) and points to the metabolite being either glyceraldehyde-3-phosphate itself or a glycolytic intermediate located between glyceraldehyde-3-phosphate and pyruvate (a similar conclusion being drawn on different grounds by HELLMAN, 1970).

It turns out that leucine-induced electrical activity is also blocked by streptozotocin (DEAN and MATTHEWS, 1972) but not by anoxia (MATTHEWS and SAKAMOTO, unpublished). Our original model (MATTHEWS and DEAN, 1970) correlating electrical activity and insulin secretion seems therefore still perfectly applicable (Fig. 12), but with more recent evidence enabling some finer distinctions to be drawn:

(i) a metabolite of glucose or the glucose molecule itself activates a membrane receptor, conceivably via a membrane-located enzyme.

(ii) the leucine receptor shares some common properties with the receptor involved in (i).

(iii) the sulfonylureas appear to interact with a membrane site operationally distinct from (i) and (ii).

Just as in many secretory cells involving granule discharge, the release of insulin from the β-cell is Ca^{2+}-sensitive (CURRY *et al.*, 1968; HALES and MILNER, 1968b). Ca^{2+} entry appears to play a vital role in the exocytosis process (see MATTHEWS, 1970; MATTHEWS *et al.*, 1972, for earlier references and more detailed discussion). From Section 5. above, it is evident that the action potentials elicited by glucose in islet cells are primarily Ca^{2+}-dependent. If then Ca^{2+} is the main ion carrying depolarizing current, it should be possible to calculate the amount of Ca^{2+} entering an islet cell during each spike. Thus for an action potential of 20 mV and an assumed membrane capacitance of 1 $\mu F/cm^{-2}$ the quantity of calcium ntering per spike would be about 0.1 $pmole/cm^{-2}$. Now the volume of the mouse β-cell is 1434 μ^3 and its surface area 972 μ^2 (DEAN 1973). This corresponds to a cube of mean side-length 12 μ. Making the simplifying assumption that the Ca^{2+} carrying depolarizing current enters mainly through one face of a cuboidal cell (of 12 μ side-length) and penetrates inward a distance approximating to one secretory-granule diameter, e.g. 300 mμ, then the increase in cytoplasmic calcium concentration, Δ $[Ca]_i$, in this region of the cell is equal to 3.33 μM per action potential. Thus in 28 mM D-glucose it would require 750 action potentials or only 125 sec* to raise $[Ca]_i$ from its low resting level (say, 10^{-6}M) to 2.5 mM, i.e. equal to $[Ca]_0$; the accompanying passive depolarization may provide an additional inflow. Of course, calcium efflux is probably also stimulated, so reducing the net calcium inflow, but it is nonetheless evident that with a high extracellular concentration of glucose (and consequently a fast spike-discharge rate) the amount of calcium entering the β-cell is considerable, and its concentration, especially in the strategic region immediately below the cell membrane, is likely to be entirely adequate to facilitate granule-cell membrane adhesion and insulin release. It also follows that if action-potential incidence and frequency are concentration-dependent (DEAN and MATTHEWS, 1970a) then Ca^{2+} entry (and hence insulin release) will likewise display similar stimulant-concentration time-dependent characteristics. The gated entry of calcium initiated by glucose (or a metabolite), and possibly also by amino acids and sulfonylureas, would thus play a crucial role

* If the critical volume is reduced to 1/10th (i.e. by reducing the submembrane distance from 300 to 30 mμ), Δ $[Ca]_i$ increases tenfold per action potential and the time required for $[Ca]_i$ to equal $[Ca]_0$ decreases from 125 to 12.5 s. It is interesting to note that the peak insulin output evoked from either perfused pancreas or isolated islets occurs within 2—3 min after exposure to D-glucose (GRODSKY *et al.*, 1970; IDAHL, 1972).

in the stimulus-secretion coupling process. Future electrophysiological studies can be expected to yield further important information on the intricate function of this system.

References

Bulbring, E., Tomita, T.: Effect of calcium, barium and manganese on the action of adrenaline in the smooth muscle of the guinea-pig taenia coli. Proc. roy. Soc. B **172**, 112—136 (1969)

Coore, H.G., Randle, P.J.: Regulation of insulin secretion studied with pieces of rabbit pancreas incubated *in vitro*. Biochem. J. **93**, 66—78 (1964)

Curry, D.L., Bennett, L.L., Grodsky, G.M.: Requirement for calcium ion in insulin secretion by the perfused rat pancreas. Amer. J. Physiol. **214**, 174—178 (1968)

Dean, P.M.: Ultrastructural morphometry of the pancreatic β-cell. Diabetologia **9**, 115—119 (1973)

Dean, P.M., Matthews, E.K.: Electrical activity in pancreatic islet cells. Nature (Lond.) **219**, 389—390 (1968)

Dean, P.M., Matthews, E.K.: Glucose-induced electrical activity in pancreatic islet cells. J. Physiol. (Lond.) **210**, 255—264 (1970a)

Dean, P.M., Matthews, E.K.: Electrical activity in pancreatic islet cells; effect of ions. J. Physiol. (Lond.) **210**, 265—275 (1970b)

Dean, P.M., Matthews, E.K.: The biophysical properties of pancreatic islet cells; effect of diabetogenic agents. Diabetologia **8**, 173—178 (1972)

Dorfmuller, von T.: Nachweis und Isolierung der Ausscheidungsprodukte von D860. Dtsch. med. Wschr. **81**, 888 (1956)

Grodsky, G., Landahl, H., Curry, D., Bennett, L.: In vitro studies suggesting a two-compartmental model for insulin secretion. In: The Structure and Metabolism of the Pancreatic Islets. Ed. by Falkmer, S., Hellman, B., Täljedal, I.-B. London: Pergamon Press 1970

Hales, C.N., Milner, R.D.G.: The role of sodium and potassium in insulin secretion from rabbit pancreas. J. Physiol. (Lond.) **194**, 725—743 (1968a)

Hales, C.N., Milner, R.D.G.: Cations and the secretion of insulin from rabbit pancreas *in vitro*. J. Physiol. (Lond.) **199**, 177—187 (1968b)

Hellerström, C.: A method for the micro-dissection of intact pancreatic islets of mammals. Acta endocr. (Kbh.) **45**, 122—132 (1964)

Hellman, B.: Methodological approaches to studies on the pancreatic islets. Diabetologia **6**, 110 (1970)

Hellman, B., Lernmark, A., Sehlin, J., Täljedal, I.-B.: Effects of phlorizin on metabolism and function of pancreatic β-cells. Metabolism **21**, 60—66 (1972)

Idahl, L.A.: A micro-perifusion device for pancreatic islets allowing concomitant recordings of intermediate metabolites and insulin release. Analyt. Biochem. **50**, 386—398 (1972)

Maske, H., Weinges, K.: Untersuchungen über das Verhalten der Meerschweinchen gegenüber verschiedenen diabetogen Noxen: Alloxan under Dithizon. Arch. exp. Path. Pharmakol. **230**, 406 (1957)

Matthews, E.K.: Membrane potential measurement in cells of the adrenal gland. J. Physiol. (Lond.) **189**, 139—148 (1967)

Matthews, E.K.: Calcium and hormone release. In: Calcium and Cellular Function. Ed. by Cuthbert, A.W. London: Macmillan 1970

Matthews, E.K., Dean, P.M.: Electrical activity in islet cells. In: The Structure and Metabolism of the Pancreatic Islets. Ed. by Falkmer, S., Hellman, B., Täljedal, I.-B. Oxford: Pergamon Press 1970a

Matthews, E.K., Dean, P.M.: The biophysical effects of insulin-releasing agents on islet cells. Postgrad. med. J. Suppl. 21—33 (1970b)

Matthews, E.K., Dean, P.M., Sakamoto, Y.: Biophysical effects of sulphonylureas on islet cells. Proceedings of 5th International Congress of Pharmacology. Basel: Karger; **3**, 221—229 (1973)

Matthews, E.K., Evans, R.J., Dean, P.M.: The ionogenic nature of the secretory-granule membrane. Electrokinetic properties of isolated chromaffin granules. Biochem. J. **130**, 825—832 (1972)

Matthews, E.K., Sakamoto, Y.: Inhibition of glucose-induced electrical activity in pancreatic islet cells by phloridzin, mannoheptulose and anoxia. J. Physiol. (Lond.) **230**, 38 (1973)

Pace, C.S., Price, S.: Electrical responses of pancreatic islet cells to secretory stimuli. Biochem. biophys. Res. Commun. **46**, 1557—1563 (1972)

Weinges, K.F.: Comparative studies of the effects of glibenclamide and tolbutamide on insulin release from isolated rat islets in vitro. Postgrad. med. J. Suppl. 32—35 (1970)

D. Effects of Sulfonylurea Derivatives on Pancreatic ß-Cells*

Bo. Hellman and Inge-Bert Täljedal

With 5 Figures

I. Introduction

Sulfonylurea derivatives are known to affect several processes in a variety of tissues. In relation to their hypoglycemic action, particular attention has been paid to the effects on pancreatic islets. Loubatières (1946) early suggested that sulfonylureas stimulate insulin release. The validity of this proposal has since been established in humans as well as in laboratory animals. It is generally believed that the drugs owe their therapeutic value mainly to this particular capacity, although the significance of extrapancreatic effects has also been considered (Feldman and Lebowitz, 1969). Because of the clinical importance of sulfonylurea-induced insulin release, considerable efforts are being devoted to explaining in precise molecular terms how sulfonylureas act as insulin secretagogues. It is the purpose of this article to review these efforts by selecting from a rapidly growing literature representative illustrations of current concepts and trends. Various aspects of the subject have been dealt with in previous surveys, which the reader may wish to consult for further information (Creutzfeldt and Söling, 1960; Butterfield and van Westering, 1967; Loubatiéres and Renold, 1969; Pfeiffer *et al.*, 1969; Grodsky, 1970; Dubach and Bückert, 1971; Maske, 1971; Panten, 1972; Steiner and Freinkel, 1972).

II. Descriptive Aspects of Insulin Release, Insulin Biosynthesis, and ß-Cell Morphology

1. Acute Effects on Insulin Release

As shown with the aid of perfused pancreas preparations, sulfonylureas cause a prompt release of insulin (Mariani, 1969; Grodsky *et al.*, 1969, 1971). The secretory response to these drugs has been reported to start even earlier than the almost instantaneous response to glucose (Curry, 1971; Gabbay and Tze, 1972).

* The authors acknowledge the support of the Swedish Medical Research Council (12 × — 562 and 12 × — 2288), which made possible studies in our laboratory referred to in this review. The literature survey was completed in December 1972.

Apart from the prompt onset of insulin release, the dynamic pattern of response differs somewhat between individual drugs. For example, in the absence of glucose, tolbutamide causes a characteristic transient peak of insulin release followed by a moderate elevation of the release rate above basal values (GRODSKY *et al.*, 1969; LOUBATIÉRES, 1969). The effect of glibenclamide requires lower concentrations and is more persistent (GRODSKY *et al.*, 1969, 1971; PFEIFFER, 1969). Glibornuride resembles glibenclamide in having a high activity on a per mole basis but more closely resembles tolbutamide with respect to the qualitative appearance of the dynamic release pattern (GRODSKY *et al.*, 1971). None of the sulfonylureas seems to produce the secondary phase of increasing insulin release which is typical of the response to glucose (GRODSKY *et al.*, 1971). This does not mean that the sulfonylureas act by a mechanism that is totally unrelated to the mechanism of physiological insulin release. Sulfonylureas can potentiate the effect of glucose (CERASI *et al.*, 1969; MARIANI, 1969; GRODSKY *et al.*, 1971; MALAISSE *et al.*, 1972; WIDSTRÖM and CERASI, 1973a), which suggests that these secretagogues interact at some stage in the normal release process. Although 12—16-week-old human fetuses release insulin in response to glucagon, they respond neither to tolbutamide nor to glucose (ESPINOSA DE LOS MONTEROS *et al.*, 1970).

Like the insulin-releasing effect of glucose that of sulfonylureas is inhibited by calcium deficiency (CURRY *et al.*, 1968; MALAISSE *et al.*, 1972), as well as by adrenaline (MILNER and HALES, 1969; BRISSON and MALAISSE, 1971), diazoxide (MILNER and HALES, 1969; BRISSON and MALAISSE, 1971), iodoacetate (GEORG *et al.*, 1971; KANAZAWA *et al.*, 1971), antimycin A (GEORG *et al.*, 1971), oligomycin (KANAZAWA *et al.*, 1971), anoxia (MILNER and HALES, 1969), and hypothermia (CURRY and CURRY, 1970). However, the inhibitory effect of diazoxide is much less pronounced with sulfonylureas than with glucose as the stimulating agent. In fact, the sulfonylureas are able to protect glucose-induced insulin secretion from the inhibitory influence of diazoxide (SELTZER and CROUT, 1968; LOUBATIÉRES, 1969; BRISSON and MALAISSE, 1971). This may be the reason why pretreatment with diazoxide can paradoxically potentiate the insulin-releasing action of sulfonylureas *in vivo* (GULBENKIAN *et al.*, 1972).

Both glucose-induced and sulfonylurea-induced insulin release can be potentiated by methylxanthines (RENOLD *et al.*, 1971; MALAISSE *et al.*, 1972), glucagon (GRODSKY *et al.*, 1969; WIDSTRÖM and CERASI, 1973b), and α-adrenergic blocking agents (SIREK *et al.*, 1969). In relation to the possible role of cyclic AMP in sulfonylurea-induced insulin release (see below, 'Increase of cyclic AMP') it is notable that aminophylline did not potentiate the effect of tolbutamide in humans (WIDSTRÖM and CERASI, 1973b).

In marked contrast to the insulin-releasing effect of glucose, that of sulfonylureas is not inhibited by mannoheptulose (COORE and RANDLE, 1964a; MILNER and HALES, 1969; BRISSON and MALAISSE, 1971). However, since glucose potentiates the effect of sulfonylureas, mannoheptulose may seem to affect sulfonylurea-induced insulin release when glucose is present. Because the synergism between glucose and sulfonylureas is most pronounced at submaximally stimulating glucose concentrations, mannoheptulose can even produce a virtual enhancement of the sulfonylurea effect at high glucose concentrations (BRISSON and MALAISSE, 1971). This effect of mannoheptulose should be distinguished from a more direct interaction between mannoheptulose and the sulfonylureas. Some evidence for such a direct interaction has been obtained with a cultivated fetal pancreas preparation, which under certain conditions released more insulin in response to tolbutamide plus mannoheptulose than to tolbutamide alone (KANAZAWA *et al.*, 1971).

Somewhat diverging results have been reported concerning the sensitivity of sulfonylurea-induced insulin release to compounds which may interfere with the function of microtubules in the β-cells. Whereas colchicine was found to have no effect (GABBAY and TZE, 1972; LACY *et al.*, 1972), a significant inhibition was obtained with vinblastine and D_2O (LACY *et al.*, 1972; MALAISSE *et al.*, 1972).

2. Insulin Biosynthesis and Long-term Effects on Insulin Secretion

Sulfonylureas differ markedly from glucose in being poor or ineffective stimuli of insulin biosynthesis (TAYLOR and PARRY, 1967; MORRIS and KORNER, 1970; TANESE *et al.*, 1970; NIKI *et al.*, 1972; STEINER *et al.*, 1972; SCHATZ *et al.*, 1972). The observations that sulfonylureas may even inhibit RNA (PUCHINGER and WACHER, 1972) and insulin (MORRIS and KORNER, 1970; TANESE *et al.*, 1970; NIKI *et al.*, 1972; SCHATZ *et al.*, 1972) biosynthesis raise the question whether these drugs can promote insulin secretion for a long time. MALAISSE (1969) found that prolonged administration of tolbutamide to rats had no effect on the subsequent secretory response to glucose. In contrast, SODOYEZ *et al.* (1970) reported that treatment of hamsters or rats with tolbutamide or glibenclamide for 40—50 days significantly decreased the insulin-releasing capacity of the islets. Similarly, conflicting results have been reported concerning the chronic effect of sulfonylureas on insulin secretion in man. LAUVAUX *et al.* (1972) suggested that these discrepancies might in part be due to differences in body weight and initial blood insulin levels among the various groups of patients investigated. These authors concluded that at least in non-obese maturity-onset diabetics with poor insulin secretion, chronic treatment with tolbutamide results in a persisting improvement of the insulin response to glucose.

3. β-Cell Morphology

Changes of β-cell fine structure have been observed as early as 1—2 h after *in vitro* exposure to sulfonylureas. These changes include dilatations of the granule sacs (ORCI *et al.*, 1969), enlargement of the Golgi apparatus, and signs of increased granule and lysosome formation (GRODSKY *et al.*, 1971). Cultivation of fetal rat pancreas in the presence of sulfonylurea resulted in a striking development of the rough endoplasmic reticulum and Golgi complex as well as in a reduction of the electron density of the insulin secretory granules (ORCI *et al.*, 1969). Since there was no evidence of increased emiocytosis in these experiments, ORCI *et al.* (1969) suggested that sulfonylurea-induced insulin release primarily occurs through intragranular solubilization of insulin with subsequent transfer of the solubilized hormone out of the cell.

The morphology of insulin release has been more extensively studied after *in vivo* administration of sulfonylureas to mature animals. In a recent review LACY (1971) evaluated the available information and concluded that like glucose, the sulfonylureas stimulate emiocytosis, i. e. the extrusion of granule-stored insulin after the fusion of the granule sac with β-cell plasma membrane. Thus the mature β-cell may behave differently from the fetal ones studied by ORCI *et al.* (1969). On the other hand, CREUTZFELDT *et al.* (1970) suggested that insulin release from mature β-cells may not exclusively occur by emiocytosis; in addition to intracellular dissolution of the granules there may be a direct route not involving granules at all. As one of the arguments in favour of this view, the last-mentioned authors pointed out that the β-cells can release substantial amounts of insulin even after extensive degranulation. The statistical problems involved in evaluating the electron microscopic picture of insulin secretion have been considered by FINDLAY *et al.* (1968). By counting a large number of granule profiles these authors tried to determine the incidence of emiocytotic configurations after stimulation with tolbutamide. No evidence was obtained for an increased number of contacts between marginally disposed granules and the plasma membrane. However, this negative result does not disprove the emiocytosis hypothesis. As pointed out by FINDLAY *et al.* (1968), only a very small proportion of the granules need be engaged in emiocytosis to explain completely the observed rates of insulin release.

Whatever the discharge mechanism might be, *in vivo* treatment with sulfonylureas undoubtedly causes a marked degranulation of the β-cells (CREUTZFELDT *et al.* 1957; BÄNDER, 1959; WILLIAMSON *et al.*, 1961; BÄNDER *et al.*, 1969; ENGELBART *et al.*, 1969; KERN and KERN, 1969) that can be observed as early as 90 min after commencing the treatment (PFEIFFER *et al.*, 1957). The disappearance of the Gomori-positive β-granules is associated with a concurrent loss of histochemically demonstrable zinc (BÄNDER *et al.*, 1969). Proliferative changes of the rough endoplasmic reticulum were reported as occurring a few hours after the administration of glibenclamide to rats (ENGELBART *et al.*, 1969). More extensive signs of hyperactivity in the endoplasmic reticulum as well as in the Golgi complex and mitochondria were noted in rabbits receiving large dosages of tolazamide for several months (VOLK and LAZARUS, 1964). As further morphological evidence for increased β-cell function, several authors have observed that sulfonylureas induce an enlargement of the β-cell nuclei (CREUTZFELDT *et al.*, 1957; KRACHT *et al.*, 1957; PFEIFFER *et al.*, 1957).

Whether the sulfonylureas can promote not only the function of individual β-cells but also their mitotic activity is a matter of some controversy. LOUBATIÉRES has long argued in favour of the so-called 'β-cytotrophic effect' of sulfonylureas. By this concept he means a stimulation of islet growth due to multiplication of β-cells as well as their neoformation from ductular epithelium (for detailed references, see LOUBATIÉRES, 1969). It has been suggested that the β-cytotrophic effect contributes significantly to the value of sulfonylureas in the management of diabetes (LOUBATIÉRES, 1969). The validity of these ideas is supported by estimates of mitotic activity (JORES and KRACHT, 1959; BUNNAG *et al.*, 1966) and islet volume in experimental animals (ASHWORTH and HAIST, 1956; GEPTS, 1957; DAVIDSON and HAIST, 1962; LOUBATIÉRES, 1969) and in humans (BLOODWORTH, 1963). On the other hand, CREUTZFELDT *et al.* (1957) and LAZAROW *et al.* (1962) were unable to demonstrate a significant increase of the islet and β-cell volumes after prolonged administration of tolbutamide to rats.

III. Explanatory Hypotheses Concerning the Insulin-Releasing Action of Sulfonylureas

Generally speaking, secretory control can be envisaged as depending on three major mechanisms: a recognition system which identifies and measures the stimulus; a coupling device that provides a causal link between the recognition system and the mechanism for hormone output; and a discharge mechanism responsible for the transport of hormone out of the cell. Although these concepts are somewhat vague, they serve the useful purpose of facilitating the analysis of the various hypotheses that have been proposed to explain sulfonylurea-induced insulin release. Starting with those ideas which assume the greatest similarity between the actions of glucose and sulfonylureas, we shall proceed via less monolithic concepts to some which do not specify any similarity at all. All hypotheses will be discussed from the perspective that sulfonylureas stimulate insulin release through a direct effect on the β-cells themselves. This basic postulate seems to be well justified for reasons of theoretical simplicity. Another reason is that sulfonylureas have been reported to inhibit the release of glucagon, the other well-known islet hormone (LAUBE *et al.*, 1971; SAMOLS *et al.*, 1971). Since glucagon is a stimulus of insulin release (see below, 'Increase of cyclic AMP') these reports are against the assumption that sulfonylureas affect the β-cells only indirectly through effects on the α_2-cells. However, the principle we have adopted should not obscure the possibility that the ultimate analysis of islet function must consider interactions between the islet cells as well as their significance for sulfonylurea-induced insulin release.

1. Enhanced Glucose Recognition

Since glucose is the major physiological stimulus of insulin secretion, it has been natural to conjecture that sulfonylureas act by modifying the glucose recognition in the β-cells. As early as 1959 BÄNDER suggested that the β-cells are equipped with some glucose receptor whose sensitivity to glucose is increased by sulfonylureas. This hypothesis was based on histological studies of the β-cell degranulation at various time intervals after the administration of sulfonylureas to rats (BÄNDER, 1959). It is amply supported by more recent *in vitro* studies which show that the insulin-releasing effect of sulfonylureas depends on the accompanying concentration of glucose (MARIANI, 1969; GRODSKY *et al.*, 1971; MALAISSE *et al.*, 1972). A

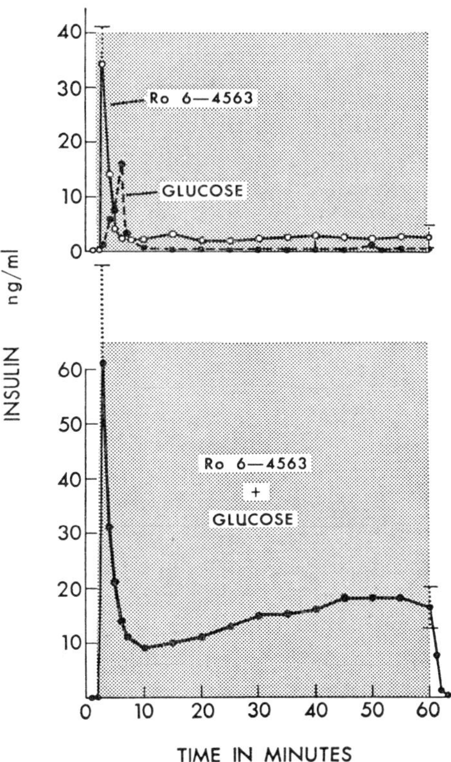

Fig. 1. Potentiation of glucose-stimulated insulin release with sulfonylurea. Upper figure shows the dynamics of insulin release from rat pancreas continuously perfused with either 1 mg/ml glucose or 20 μg/ml glibornuride (Ro 6-4563). Lower figure shows the dynamic response when the same concentrations of glucose and glibornuride were combined in the perfusion medium. Shaded areas indicate periods of perfusion. (From GRODSKY *et al.*, 1971)

particularly succinct demonstration of the interaction between glucose and sulfonylurea was presented by Grodsky *et al.* (1971), who studied the dynamics of insulin release from the perfused rat pancreas. As shown in Fig. 1, low concentrations of either glibornuride or glucose elicited only a transient peak of insulin release. In contrast, the combination of the same concentrations of glibornuride and glucose produced the initial peak as well as a pronounced secondary phase of increasing insulin release. This secondary phase is typical of glucose stimulation and cannot be produced with sulfonylureas alone. Grodsky *et al.* (1971) therefore concluded that the sulfonylureas potentiate the effect of glucose, as opposed to the less appropriate notion that glucose potentiates the effect of sulfonylureas. That sulfonylureas might somehow increase the effectiveness of the glucose stimulus in humans also is suggested by an altered dose-response relationship between blood glucose and plasma insulin (Widström and Cerasi, 1972a).

Lundquist (1971) has put forward a hypothesis which assumes the maximum similarity between the actions of sulfonylureas and glucose; without specifying the nature of glucose recognition this hypothesis proposes that sulfonylureas act by providing more glucose to be sensed by the physiological recognition system. Lundquist (1971) observed that the glibenclamide-induced insulin release in mice was increased by prior treatment with acid amyloglucosidase or with progesterone, a labilizer of lysosomes. In contrast, dexamethasone, a lysosome stabilizer, inhibited glibenclamide-induced insulin release. On the basis of these and related findings it was suggested that sulfonylureas labilize the β-cell lysosomes, resulting in an increase of the activity of 'free' acid amyloglucosidase in the β-cells. Since this enzyme splits glycogen to glucose, it would tend to raise the intracellular glucose concentration, which in turn controls insulin release. Although it remains to be tested whether exogenous amyloglucosidase is in fact incorporated into β-cell lysosomes as assumed by Lundquist (1971), some objections to this hypothesis arise from what is already known about sulfonylurea-induced insulin release. If the sulfonylureas were to act by providing more glucose to be sensed by the physiological trigger, the secretory response to these drugs would be expected to occur somewhat later than that to glucose. This is contradictory to reports that sulfonylureas act more promptly as insulin secretagogues than does glucose (Curry, 1971; Gabbay and Tze, 1972). Furthermore, the idea that the effect of sulfonylureas is mediated by glucose molecules seems to require that this effect should resemble that of glucose with regard to inhibition by other compounds. This requirement is in marked conflict with the well-documented failure of mannoheptulose to inhibit sulfonylurea-induced insulin release, although mannoheptulose is a potent inhibitor of the response to glucose (Coore and Randle, 1964a, Milner and Hales, 1969; Brisson and Malaisse, 1971).

In line with the idea that glucose is recognized as an insulin secretagogue by virtue of its metabolism, there are several suggestions as to how sulfonylureas could modify glucose degradation. The early proposal that sulfonylureas might prevent the waste of glucose-6-phosphate through cleavage by glucose-6-phosphatase (Lazarus, 1959; Coore and Randle, 1964b) was not supported by quantitative studies of the islet enzyme (Ashcroft and Randle, 1970; Täljedal, 1970). Direct measurments of glucose-6-phosphate in pancreatic islets have yielded conflicting results. Whereas Montague and Taylor (1969) reported that tolbutamide increased the concentration of glucose-6-phosphate and 6-phosphogluconate in rat islets, glibenclamide caused a small but significant depression of glucose-6-phosphate (Idahl, 1971) and had no effect on 6-phosphogluconate (Idahl *et al.*, 1971) in the β-cell-rich islets from *obob*-mice.

Another suggestion is that sulfonylureas might stimulate glycogenolysis and glycolysis by altering the phosphate potential in the β-cells (HELLMAN, 1970). This idea is consistent with the findings that sulfonylureas effectively mobilize glycogen (HELLMAN *et al.*, 1969) and enhance lactate formation (ASHCROFT *et al.*, 1970) in isolated islets. Since sulfonylureas have been found to uncouple oxidative phosphorylation in liver and diaphragm (PENTTILÄ, 1966; DE BEER and DE SCHEPPER, 1967), they might do so in the β-cells also and thereby decrease the ratio of ATP to ADP, AMP, and inorganic phosphate. Such a modification of the phosphate potential is known to stimulate glycolytic flux in other cells. The degree of coupling in oxidative phosphorylation has not been directly measured in sulfonylurea-exposed β-cells, but it has been observed that sulfonylureas reduce the islet content of ATP (HELLMAN *et al.*, 1969; ASHCROFT *et al.*, 1973) and stimulate the oxygen uptake (STORK *et al.*, 1969). The essential weaknesses of this particular hypothesis are that sulfonylureas have not been found to reduce islet ATP in all studies (KRZANOWSKI *et al.*, 1971), and that an uncoupling effect of the sulfonylureas would presumably require that they enter the β-cells in significant amounts. As will be discussed below ('Binding to plasma membrane'), the latter condition does not seem to be fulfilled. Furthermore, although tolbutamide stimulated lactate production and glucose oxidation (ASHCROFT *et al.*, 1970), neither tolbutamide nor glibenclamide had any demonstrable effect on glucose utilization in a subsequent study (ASHCROFT *et al.*, 1972b).

The above hypotheses do not specify the nature of stimulus-secretion coupling or the mode of insulin discharge. Attempts have been made to go a step further and define precisely how glucose metabolism might govern the release process. Assuming that insulin release requires intracellular dissolution of the β-granules, MASKE (1957) early suggested that this may be achieved through the chelation of granule-zinc by increased concentrations of citrate in the β-cells. In line with this idea, WALLENFELS *et al.* (1957) discussed the possibility that sulfonylureas can raise the β-cell content of citrate. However, apart from the fact that insulin discharge may involve emiocytosis rather than intracellular granulolysis (see above, 'β-Cell morphology'), glibenclamide was not found to increase the content of citrate in micro-dissected islets of *obob*-mice (HELLMAN and IDAHL, 1972).

That sulfonylureas seem to have relatively small effects on various metabolic parameters is a criticism that may be generalized to all hypotheses which envisage the insulin-releasing action of these drugs as a consequence of modified glucose metabolism. This criticism is emphasized by the failure of tolbutamide to induce measurable changes in the fluorescence of reduced pyridine nucleotides within intact islet cells (PANTEN, 1972). Similarly, the effects of glibenclamide on glucose metabolism are apparently too small to alter measurably leucine oxidation in the β-cells, although glucose has a marked inhibitory effect (HELLMAN *et al.*, 1971a). For these reasons it can well be questioned whether sulfonylureas stimulate insulin release by modifying glucose metabolism in the β-cells. It may be that the observed effects on ATP and other metabolic parameters are irrelevant side effects or are explicable as the consequences rather than as the cause of stimulated secretion. This does not exclude the possibility that the decrease of ATP might contribute to the inhibitory effect of sulfonylureas on insulin biosynthesis (MORRIS and KORNER, 1970; TANESE *et al.*, 1970; NIKI *et al.*, 1972; SCHATZ *et al.*, 1972).

2. Enhanced Recognition of Amino Acids

Like glucose, leucine is able to stimulate insulin release on its own. Several other amino acids are also insulin secretagogues, although they may require the presence of glucose or leucine in order to be fully active (MILNER, 1970). The possibility has therefore been considered that sulfonylureas act by modulating the β-cell content of amino acids. Since sulfonylureas can potentiate the insulin-releasing effect of leucine (FAJANS *et al.*, 1967), it is interesting that tolbutamide inhibited the production of $^{14}CO_2$ from islets incubated with ^{14}C-1-leucine (STORK *et al.*, 1970). However, there is the discordant finding that glibenclamide had no effect on the oxidation of uniformly ^{14}C-labeled leucine in the same type of microdissected islets (HELLMAN *et al.*, 1971a).

Stimulation of the reductive amination of α-ketoglutarate represents another mechanism by which sulfonylureas might theoretically increase the β-cell content of amino acids. Such stimulation has been observed in crude islet homogenates (HELLMAN, 1967). Carbutamide increased the activity of glutamate dehydrogenase whereas therapeutically inactive analogues had no effect. However, measurements of α-ketoglutarate and glutamate in whole islets exposed to sulfonylurea did not show any significant increase of amino acid (DANIELSSON *et al.*, 1970). This difference between results obtained with homogenized and intact islets is not surprising in view of more recent data on the penetration of sulfonylureas into β-cells (see below, 'Binding to plasma membrane'). These data make it seem unlikely that the sulfonylureas enter the β-cells in amounts that would be sufficient to produce the activating conformational change of the glutamate dehydrogenase molecule. Finally, the likelihood that sulfonylureas stimulate insulin release by altering the β-cell content of free amino acids was considerably reduced by recent microdeterminations of several amino acids in isolated islets exposed to glibenclamide (Table 1).

Table 1. *Islet contents of free amino acids*

Amino acid	Concentration in islets (mmoles/kg dry weight)	
	Control	Glibenclamide
Aspartic acid	7.9 ± 0.7 (6)	7.2 ± 1.0 (6)
GABA	3.1 ± 0.4 (6)	2.6 ± 0.3 (6)
Glutamic acid	19.1 ± 1.1 (6)	17.8 ± 1.6 (6)
Glycine	8.1 ± 0.8 (6)	7.9 ± 1.0 (6)
Leucine	9.0 ± 0.4 (6)	8.9 ± 1.1 (5)

Microdissected islets of *obob*-mice were incubated at 37°C for 2 h in Krebs-Ringer bicarbonate buffer containing 5 mM glucose (control) or 5 mM glucose plus 0.1 mM glibenclamide. Free amino acids were then extracted, dansylated and separated by microchromatography on polyamide sheets. Results are given as mean values $\pm$ S.E.M. for the numbers of animals stated within parentheses. Unpublished results of E. GYLFE, Department of Histology, Umeå.

It has been suggested that amino acids are recognized as insulin secretagogues through their binding to specific transport molecules in the β-cell plasma membrane (CHRISTENSEN and CULLEN, 1969; CHRISTENSEN *et al.*, 1971). The effect of sulfonylureas on amino acid transport has therefore been investigated in the β-cell-rich islets of *obob*-mice. Glibenclamide had no effect on the islet uptake of leucine (HELLMAN *et al.*, 1971b, 1972) but slightly inhibited the uptake of alanine, arginine, and α-aminoisobutyric acid (HELLMAN *et al.*, 1971b, c). These results do not indicate that sulfonylureas stimulate insulin release by increasing the transport of amino acids into the β-cells.

3. Increase of Cyclic AMP

Methylxanthines inhibit the activity of cyclic nucleotide phosphodiesterase in pancreatic islet extracts (ASHCROFT *et al.*, 1972a; SAMS and MONTAGUE, 1972). The marked synergism between glucose and methylxanthines as insulin secretago-

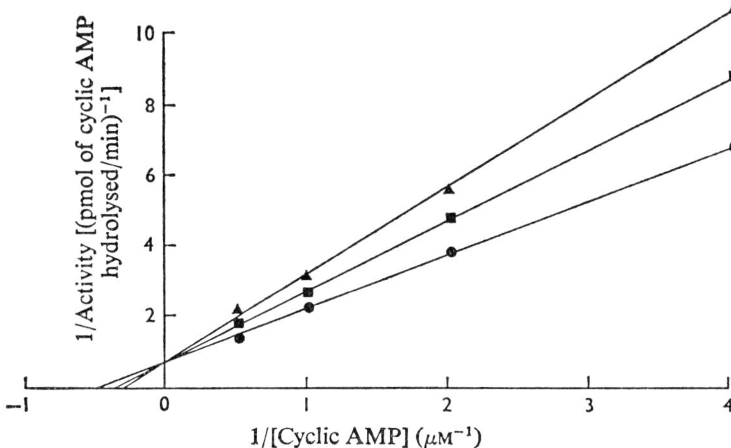

Fig. 2. Sulfonylurea-induced inhibition of cyclic nucleotide phosphodiesterase activity in extracts of guinea-pig islets incubated with cyclic AMP as substrate. Results are presented as a double-reciprocal plot, each point being the mean of three observations in the absence of sulfonylurea (●), or in the presence of 20 μM glibenclamide (▲), or 2.5 mM tolbutamide (■). (From SAMS and MONTAGUE, 1972)

gues is therefore consistent with the assumption that cyclic AMP modulates the secretagogic signal aroused by glucose (BURR *et al.*, 1970; MALAISSE *et al.*, 1971). However, the effects of methylxanthines on intact cells should not necessarily be equated with those of intracellular cyclic AMP. Insulin release is highly dependent on calcium (see below, 'Redistribution of ions'), and it is notable that caffeine has been reported to affect the uptake of calcium by muscle through a mechanism that might not involve cyclic AMP (WEBER, 1968).

Since sulfonylureas have been found to inhibit cyclic nucleotide phosphodiesterase in islet extracts (ASHCROFT *et al.*, 1972a; SAMS and MONTAGUE, 1972; Fig. 2), the question arises whether the sulfonylureas stimulate insulin release and potentiate the effect of glucose by increasing the β-cell content of cyclic AMP. This question is reinforced by the report that sulfonylurea also stimulates the activity of adenylate cyclase in human islet adenomas (LEVEY *et al.*, 1972). So far there seem to be no published data on the content of cyclic AMP in sulfonylurea-treated islets, but tolbutamide was reported to raise the content of cyclic AMP in human islet adenomas (MASHITER *et al.*, 1972). MONTAGUE and HOWELL (1973) observed that glibenclamide and tolbutamide stimulated the activity of a cyclic-AMP-dependent protein phosphokinase in isolated rat islets. Notwithstanding the indirect nature of this piece of evidence, the protein phosphokinase data have the attraction of signifying changes of a functionally important pool of cyclic AMP in intact β-cells.

The idea that the action of sulfonylureas is mediated by cyclic AMP is only partly consistent with the kinetics of sulfonylurea-induced insulin release, if it is assumed that the methylxanthines act by this mechanism. Both sulfonylureas and methylxanthines are poor insulin secretagogues in the absence of exogenous substrates, under which condition they elicit a brief initial peak of insulin release followed by a slight elevation of the secretory rate above basal values (BURR *et al.*, 1970; GRODSKY *et al.*, 1971). Another similarity is that sulfonylureas as well as methylxanthines act in synergism with glucose. However, this similarity may be superficial and deceptive. Whereas the methylxanthines undoubtedly increase the

V_{max} of sustained glucose-stimulated insulin release with little or no effect on the apparent K_m for glucose (MALAISSE *et al.*, 1971; ASHCROFT *et al.*, 1972b), the sulfonylureas have a less pronounced effect on V_{max} but lower the apparent K_m for glucose (GRODSKY, 1970; MALAISSE *et al.*, 1971; WIDSTRÖM and CERASI, 1973a).

Against this background the role of cyclic AMP as a mediator of the action of sulfonylureas appears unclear and perhaps even doubtful. The uncertainty is emphasized by the capacities of glucagon and methylxanthines to modulate the effect of sulfonylureas. Glucagon potentiates sulfonylurea-induced insulin release *in vitro* (CURRY, 1970) as well as *in vivo* (WIDSTRÖM and CERASI, 1973b), which would conform with the interpretation that sulfonylureas primarily act as phosphodiesterase inhibitors. However, this interpretation is complicated by several reports that methylxanthines can also enhance the insulin-releasing effect of sulfonylureas (RENOLD *et al.*, 1971; MALAISSE *et al.*, 1972), although aminophylline had no such effect in man (WIDSTRÖM and CERASI, 1972b). It may be pointed out that the inhibitory effect of sulfonylureas on cyclic nucleotide phosphodiesterase in islet extracts (ASHCROFT *et al.*, 1972a; SAMS and MONTAGUE, 1972) does not prove that a similar effect occurs in intact β-cells. Sulfonylureas appear to have a limited ability, if any, to enter these cells (see below, 'Binding to plasma membrane'), and it is questionable whether there is any cyclic nucleotide phosphodiesterase in the β-cell plasma membrane (HOWELL and WHITFIELD, 1972).

4. Redistribution of Metal Ions

MILNER and HALES (1970) proposed that glucose somehow stimulated the transport of calcium into the β-cells, resulting in a rise of intracellular calcium ion, which in turn causes insulin release. MALAISSE *et al.* (1972) suggested rather that glucose as well as sulfonylureas inhibit the efflux of calcium and thereby increase the concentration of this ion in the β-cells. According to the latter authors, calcium ion causes insulin release by inducing a contraction of β-cell microtubules, to which the secretory granules are attached (MALAISSE, 1972; MALAISSE *et al.*, 1972). None of these hypotheses claims to specify the detailed molecular mechanism by which sulfonylureas and other insulin secretagogues could alter the transport of calcium across the β-cell plasma membrane. They explain, however, the obligatory requirement for calcium in sustained insulin release, and, in the case of MALAISSE *et al.* (1972), suggest that the stimulus-secretion coupling and discharge mechanisms are the same in physiological and sulfonylurea-stimulated insulin release.

As part of the experimental evidence, MALAISSE *et al.* (1971, 1972) showed that there is an almost perfect correlation between the rate of sulfonylurea-induced insulin release and the radioactivity retained by islets after incubation with ^{45}Ca followed by extensive washing. Since calcium binds to several structures in the β-cells, it is exceedingly difficult to draw conclusions specifically about the calcium transport system from studies on ^{45}Ca uptake or loss. This difficulty is disturbing, whether the islets are extensively washed (MALAISSE *et al.*, 1972) or correction for extracellular label is attempted by using nonpermeating space markers (HELLMAN *et al.*, 1971d). Nevertheless, it might be inferred that sulfonylurea-stimulated insulin release is associated with a striking increase in a pool of calcium which is relatively firmly bound in the β-cells (Fig. 3). That the sulfonylureas do indeed alter the flux of ions across the β-cell plasma membrane is strongly suggested by the electrophysiological data of MATTHEWS and DEAN (1970a, b) and PACE and PRICE (1972). Although there were certain differences between individual sulfonylureas and other insulin secretagogues with respect to the pattern of β-cell depolarization, the sulfonylureas induced regular changes of membrane potential indicative of altered ionic fluxes.

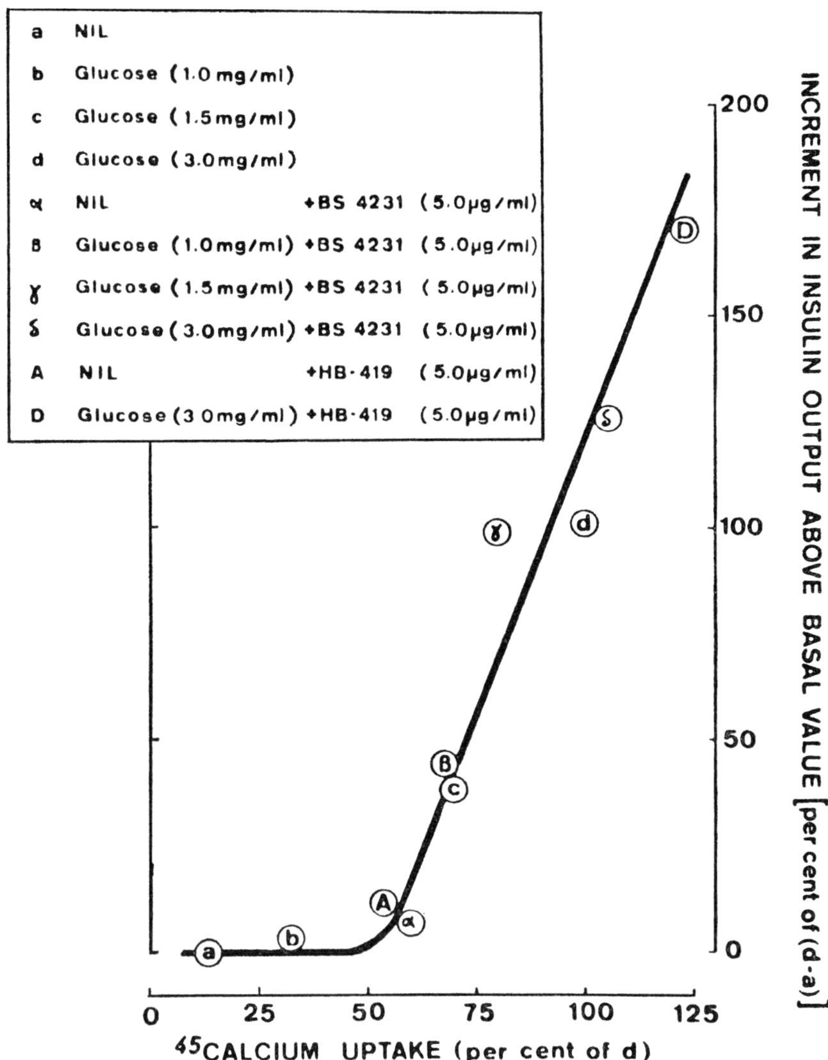

Fig. 3. Relationship between sulfonylurea-induced insulin release and the 'calcium uptake' by rat islets. Increments of insulin release above basal values are plotted against the radioactivity retained by the islets after incubation with ^{45}Ca followed by extensive washing. Various combinations of glibenclamide (HB 419), glisoxepide (BS 4231), and glucose were used as explained in the inset. (From MALAISSE *et al.*, 1971)

As to the nature of ionic fluxes in the β-cells, not only calcium but also sodium and potassium may be of critical importance for the regulation of insulin release. Thus it has been reported that the secretory response to sulfonylureas as well as to other stimuli depends on the concentration of sodium (MILNER and HALES, 1970) and potassium (HOWELL and TAYLOR, 1968) in the incubation medium. MILNER and HALES (1970) suggested that calcium entry is stimulated by increased concentrations of sodium within the β-cells but is inhibited by the extracellular sodium ions. This idea received some indirect support from the observation that tolbutamide-induced insulin release is markedly inhibited by diphenylhydantoin (KIZER *et al.*, 1970), an activator of that membrane-located adenosine triphosphatase which is assumed to catalyze the extrusion of sodium. Measurements of ^{22}Na uptake by isolated islets supported the interpretation that the effect of diphenylhydantoin was mediated by a reduction of intracellular sodium concentration (KIZER *et al.*, 1970).

5. Binding to Plasma Membrane

Observing that tolbutamide and glibenclamide decreased the osmotic resistance of red blood cells, ARIENS (1969) suggested that sulfonylureas might exert a direct action on the β-cell plasma membrane. MATTHEWS and DEAN (1970a, b) proposed that the sulfonylureas somehow react with the β-cell plasma membrane to induce a membrane conformation characterized by increased ion permeability. This hypothesis is attractively simple in not requiring that the sulfonylureas are recognized as insulin secretagogues through effects on glucose or amino acid metabolism or on any other intracellular process or structure. Furthermore, it is immediately linked with the idea that physiological stimulus-secretion coupling involves the redistribution of ions across the β-cell plasma membrane. However, the testing of this theoretically simple hypothesis might well entail considerable experimental difficulties. Since sulfonylureas can bind quite strongly to various proteins, cor-

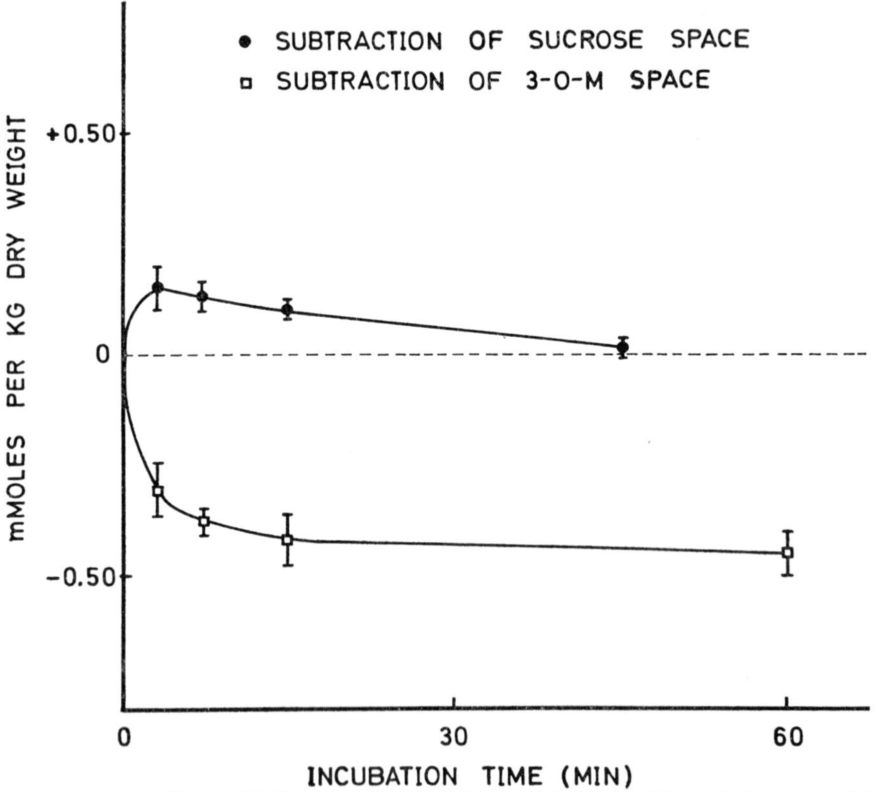

Fig. 4. Uptake of tolbutamide by microdissected islets of *obob*-mice. The points represent islet content of ^{35}S-labeled tolbutamide corrected for ^{35}S in the islet spaces occupied by sucrose or 3-*O*-methyl-D-glucose. The concentration of tolbutamide used was 0.3 mM. Mean values ± S.E.M. for 5—7 experiments. (Data from HELLMAN *et al.*, 1971e)

roboration of the hypothesis would require some means of testing the specificity of binding to the β-cells in relation to the recognition of sulfonylureas as insulin secretagogues. Such specificity studies have not yet been reported on. However, investigations on the distribution of sulfonylureas in pancreatic islets have yielded some indirect support for the idea that these drugs act primarily on the ß-cell plasma membrane.

Islets rich in β-cells were microdissected from *obob*-mice and were incubated with radioactively labeled sulfonylureas in the presence of space markers labeled with another radioisotope. The distribution volume of either tolbutamide or glibenclamide was determined in relation to that of sucrose or 3-*O*-methyl-D-glucose. Whereas sucrose is restricted to the extracellular space, 3-*O*-methyl-D-glucose equilibrates in the total islet water. As shown in Fig. 4, the tolbutamide space was equal to that of sucrose but considerably smaller than that of 3-*O*-methyl-D-glucose. This and related experiments indicate that tolbutamide does not enter the β-cells to any measurable extent (HELLMAN *et al.*, 1971e). In the absence of serum albumin, glibenclamide was taken up in amounts exceeding the 3-*O*-methyl-D-glucose space as if glibenclamide was bound to the β-cells (HELLMAN *et al.*, 1973a). HOWELL and LACY (1969) reported that glibenclamide does not behave as a typical extracellular space marker in rat islets either. The uptake of glibenclamide by islets of *obob*-mice (HELLMAN *et al.*, 1973a) was quickly reversed upon withdrawal of the drug and was inhibited by serum albumin. To test the idea that glibenclamide was bound predominantly to the surface of β-cells, the uptake of glibenclamide was examined in islets treated with chloromercuribenzene-*p*-sulfonic acid, antimycin A, or chlorpromazine. Under the conditions used, the three last-mentioned compounds increase the permeability of the β-cell plasma membrane. They also markedly stimulate the uptake of glibenclamide in whole islets (Fig. 5) but have no effect on the uptake in subcellular particles from disintegrated islets. The simplest interpretation of these observations is that glibenclamide, like tolbutamide, is mainly restricted to the outside of intact β-cells (HELLMAN *et al.* 1971e, 1973a). Glibenclamide seems, however, to have a stronger affinity for the β-cell surface than has tolbutamide. At least a fraction of the glibenclamide binding appears to occur at a site that is also occupied by glibornuride (HELLMAN, SEHLIN and TÄLJEDAL, unpublished data). When islets were incubated for 15 min with 20 μM ^{3}H-labeled glibornuride, the uptake of this drug in excess of the extracellular (sucrose) space was 0.16 ± 0.01 mmoles/kg dry weight of islets (mean value $\pm$ S.E.M. for 8 experiments). The addition of 100 μM glibenclamide to the medium resulted in a decrease of the glibornuride uptake to 0.12 ± 0.01 mmoles/kg dry weight, the difference between paired test and control incubations being statistically significant ($P < 0.005$).

Although the above studies support the idea that sulfonylureas act on the β-cell plasma membrane, they do not give any indication as to what kind of chemical reaction might lead to insulin release. On the whole, few studies have been directed to the chemistry of β-cell plasma membrane, which means that hypotheses on this point must be highly tentative and provisional. The possibility that sulfonylureas might modify the activity of some membrane-located enzyme was discussed above with specific reference to adenylate cyclase (see, 'Increase of cyclic AMP'). It has recently been shown that insulin release can be triggered by sulphydryl reagents, most probably by blocking of relatively superficial thiol groups in the β-cell plasma membrane (BLOOM *et al.*, 1972; HELLMAN *et al.*, 1973b, c). The precise role of these thiol groups is not yet fully understood. It seems worth considering the possibility of interactions between sulfonylureas and thiol groups leading to an altered ion permeability of the membrane.

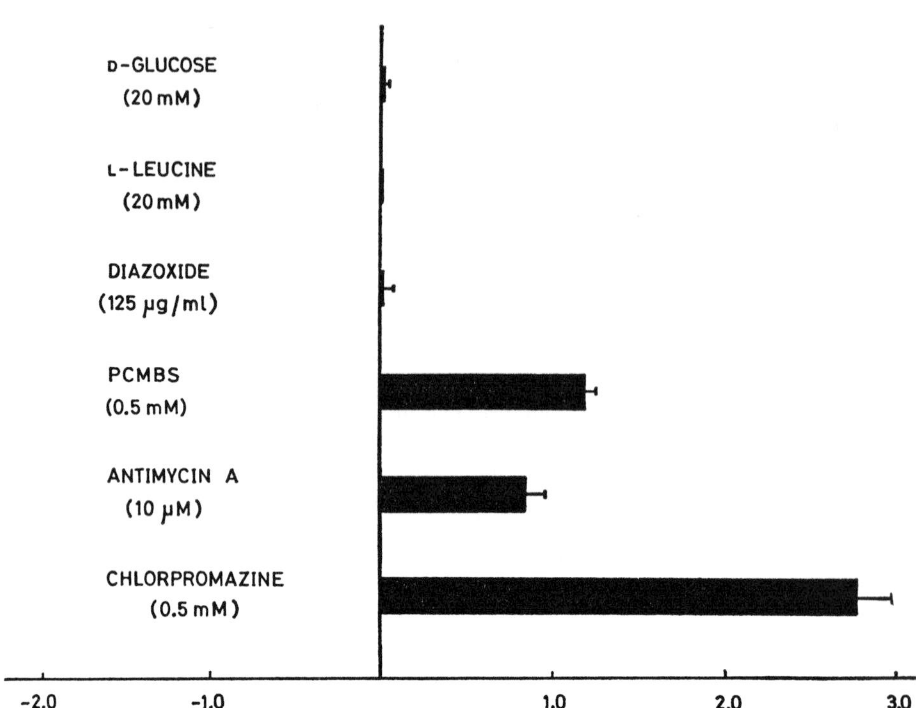

Fig. 5. Effects of various compounds on the uptake of glibenclamide by microdissected islets of *obob*-mice. Islets were incubated with 20 μM ^{14}C-labeled glibenclamide and 1.3 μM 3-*O*-methyl-D-glucose for 60 min. The uptake of glibenclamide in excess of the 3-*O*-methyl-D-glucose space was then calculated as mmoles glibenclamide per kg dry weight of islets. The effects of the listed compounds on this parameter are given as changes from controls. Mean values ± S.E.M. for 7—8 experiments. (Data from Hellman *et al.*, 1973a)

6. Direct Effects on Insulin Storage

The possibility has been considered that sulfonylureas exert a direct effect on the storage of insulin by competing for zinc (Wallenfels *et al.*, 1962; Yoshinaga and Yamamoto, 1966) or insulin-binding proteins (Bretschneider, 1971) in the β-cells. These hypotheses presuppose that the permeability of the β-cell plasma membrane is sufficient to permit significant intracellular concentrations of sulfonylurea. Since most of the insulin is stored in the form of secretory granules, it is notable that tolbutamide and glibenclamide have been found not to release insulin from isolated β-granules in suspension (Coore *et al.*, 1969; Howell *et al.*, 1969; Howell and Lacy, 1969).

IV. Concluding Remarks

It should be evident from the present survey of loosely-related hypotheses that there is as yet little experimental justification for strongly favouring one particular view on how sulfonylureas act as insulin secretagogues. The further exploration of this field will probably benefit from continued work along widely different lines.

To express our own personal bias, however, there seems to be no compelling reason for not assuming that insulin is discharged by the same mechanism, whether the stimulus is a sulfonylurea derivative or glucose. Similarly, the stimulus-secretion coupling might in both cases involve the redistribution of ions, although not necessarily in accordance with those hypotheses which have mostly been considered so far. There is a need to explain not only the movement of secretory granules within the β-cell but, perhaps more important, the nature of interaction between granule sac and cell membrane. As pointed out by MATTHEWS (1970), a divalent cation such as calcium might regulate this process by diminishing a potential energy barrier arising from fixed anions on the membrane. The possibility that fluxes of Na^+ and K^+ could affect the distribution of intracellular calcium may also be considered in this context.

The specific problem of insulin release in response to sulfonylureas might then be to explain how these particular stimuli are recognized. The idea that the sulfonylureas act directly on the plasma membrane to alter its ion permeability is not only theoretically simple but is also supported by some experimental results. It should be emphasized that a sulfonylurea-induced conformational change of β-cell plasma membrane need not be exactly the one induced by glucose. In fact it is rather more tempting to assume that the sulfonylurea-induced conformation represents some metastable intermediate between that of a resting β-cell and that of a cell exposed to high glucose concentrations. Such an assumption might help to explain the transient character of insulin release in response to sulfonylurea alone as well as the potentiating effect of sulfonylureas on glucose-stimulated insulin release. The results of GRODSKY *et al.* (1971) seem particularly important in this respect, for they show that potentiation of the glucose stimulus with sulfonylureas apparently results in a dynamic release pattern that is typical of a glucose-induced response. This suggests that the proposed metastable membrane conformation induced by sulfonylureas might well represent a transitory state in the physiological stimulation of insulin release, although the recognition of glucose is probably quite different from that of the sulfonylureas.

References

ARIENS, E.J.: Oral antidiabetics. Dose, plasma concentration and effect. Acta diabet. lat. **6**, Suppl. 1, 143—176 (1969)

ASHCROFT, S.J.H., HEDESKOV, C.J., RANDLE, P.J.: Glucose metabolism in mouse pancreatic islets. Biochem. J. **118**, 143—154 (1970)

ASHCROFT, S.J.H., RANDLE, P.J.: Enzymes of glucose metabolism in normal mouse pancreatic islets. Biochem. J. **119**, 5—15 (1970)

ASHCROFT, S.J.H., RANDLE, P.J., TÄLJEDAL, I.-B.: Cyclic nucleotide phosphodiesterase activity in normal mouse pancreatic islets. FEBS Letters **20**, 263—266 (1972a)

ASHCROFT, S.J.H., WEERASINGHE, L.C.C., BASSETT, J.M., RANDLE, P.J.: The pentose cycle and insulin release in mouse pancreatic islets. Biochem. J. **126**, 525—532 (1972b)

ASHCROFT, S.J.H., WEERASINGHE, L.C.C., RANDLE, P.J.: Interrelationships of islet metabolism, ATP content and insulin release. Biochem. J. **132**, 223—231 (1973)

ASHWORTH, M.A., HAIST, R.E.: Some effects of BZ-55 (carbutamide) on the growth of the islets of Langerhans. Canad. med. Ass. J. **74**, 975—976 (1956)

BÄNDER, A.: Zum Wirkungsmechanismus blutzuckersenkender Sulfonylharnstoffe D 860 und BZ 55. Dtsch. med. Wschr. **84**, 996—1002 (1959)

BÄNDER, A., PFAFF, W., SCHESMER, G.: Lichtoptisch-morphologische Untersuchungen an der B-Zelle der Langerhans'schen Insel nach Verabreichung von HB 419. Arzneimittel-Forsch. **19**, 1448—1451 (1969)

BLOODWORTH, J.M.B., JR.: Morphologic changes associated with sulfonylurea therapy. Metabolism **12**, 287—301 (1963)

BLOOM, G.D., HELLMAN, B., IDAHL, L.-Å., LERNMARK, Å., SEHLIN, J., TÄLJEDAL, I.-B.: Effects of organic mercurials on mammalian pancreatic B-cells. Insulin release, glucose transport, glucose oxidation, membrane permeability and ultrastructure. Biochem. J. **129**, 241—254 (1972)

Bretschneider, H.: Oral antidiabetics. In: Recent hypoglycemic sulfonylureas. Mechanisms of action and clinical indications, pp. 22—32 (Dubach, U.C., Bückert, A., eds.). Bern: Huber 1971

Brisson, G.R., Malaisse, W.: Insulinotropic effect and possible mode of action of a new potent sulfonylurea. Canad. J. Physiol. Pharmacol. **49**, 536—544 (1971)

Bunnag, S.C., Warner, N.E., Bunnag, S.: Effect of tolbutamide on postnatal neogenesis of the islet of Langerhans in mouse. Diabetes **15**, 597—603 (1966)

Burr, I.M., Balant, L., Stauffacher, W., Renold, A.E.: Perifusion of rat pancreatic tissue in vitro: substrate modification of theophylline-induced biphasic insulin release. J. clin. Invest. **49**, 2097—2105 (1970)

Butterfield, W.J.H., Van Westering, V. (eds.): Tolbutamide after ten years. Internat. Congress. Series, vol. 149. Amsterdam: Excerpta Medica 1967

Cerasi, E., Chowers, I., Luft, R., Widström, A.: The significance of the blood glucose level for plasma insulin response to intravenously administered tolbutamide in healthy subjects. Diabetologia **5**, 343—348 (1969)

Christensen, H.N., Cullen, A.M.: Behaviour in the rat of a transport specific, bicyclic amino acid. Hypoglycemic action. J. biol. Chem. **244**, 1521—1526 (1969)

Christensen, H.N., Hellman, B., Lernmark, Å., Sehlin, J., Tager, H.S., Täljedal, I.-B.: *In vitro* stimulation of insulin release by non-metabolizable, transport-specific amino acids. Biochim. biophys. Acta (Amst.) **241**, 341—348 (1971)

Coore, H.G., Hellman, B., Pihl, E., Täljedal, I.-B.: Physicochemical characteristics of insulin secretion granules. Biochem. J. **111**, 107—113 (1969)

Coore, H.G., Randle, P.J.: Regulation of insulin secretion studied with pieces of rabbit pancreas incubated *in vitro*. Biochem. J. **93**, 66—78 (1964a)

Coore, H.G., Randle, P.J.: Insulin secretion from rabbit pancreas *in vitro*. In: The structure and metabolism of the pancreatic islets, pp. 295—307 (Brolin, S.E., Hellman, B., Knutson, H. eds.). Oxford: Pergamon Press 1964b

Creutzfeldt, W., Creutzfeldt, C., Frerichs, H.: Evidence for different modes of insulin secretion. In: The structure and metabolism of the pancreatic islets, pp. 181—196. Falkmer, S., Hellman, B., Täljedal, I.-B. (Eds.). Oxford: Pergamon Press 1970

Creutzfeldt, W., Detering, L., Welte, O.: Das B-Zellsystem von normalen und hypophysektomierten Ratten sowie von Kaninchen unter D 860 und diabetogenen Hormonen. Dtsch. med. Wschr. 82, 1564—1568 (1957)

Creutzfeldt, W., Söling, D.: Orale Diabetestherapie und ihre experimentellen Grundlagen. Ergebn. inn. Med. Kinderheilk. N.F. **15**, 1—213 (1960)

Curry, D.L.: Glucagon potentiation of insulin secretion by the perfused rat pancreas. Diabetes **19**, 420—428 (1970)

Curry, D.L.: Is there a common beta cell insulin compartment stimulated by glucose and tolbutamide? Amer. J. Physiol. **220**, 319—323 (1971)

Curry, D.L., Bennett, L.L., Grodsky, G.M.: Requirement for calcium ion in insulin secretion by the perfused rat pancreas. Amer. J. Physiol. **214**, 174—178 (1968)

Curry, D.L., Curry, K.P.: Hypothermia and insulin secretion. Endocrinology **87**, 750—755 (1970)

Danielsson, Å., Hellman, B., Idahl, L.-Å.: Levels of α-ketoglutarate and glutamate in stimulated pancreatic B-cells. Horm. Metab. Res. **2**, 28—31 (1970)

Davidson, J.K., Haist, R.E.: Islet weight studies in rats treated with tolbutamide. Diabetes **11**, Suppl., 115—120 (1962)

De Beer, L., De Schepper, P.J.: Metabolic effects of hypoglycemic sulfonylureas. In vitro effect of sulfonylureas on cell-free protein synthesis and energy metabolism in rat tissues. Biochem. Pharmacol. **16**, 2355—2367 (1967)

Dubach, U.C., Bückert, A.: Recent hypoglycemic sulfonylureas. Mechanisms of action and clinical indications. Bern: Huber 1971

Engelbart, K., Bähr, H., Kief, H.: Ultrastruktur der B-Zellen des Ratten-Pankreas nach ein- und mehrmaliger Gabe von HB 419. Arzneimittel-Forsch. **19**, 1456—1463 (1969)

Espinosa de los Monteros, A., Driscoll, S.G., Steinke, J.: Insulin release from isolated human fetal pancreatic islets. Science **168**, 1111—1112 (1970)

Fajans, S.S., Floyd, J.C., Jr., Knopf, R.F., Guntsche, E.M., Rull, J., Thiffault, C.A., Conn, J.W.: A difference in mechanism by which leucine and other amino acids induce insulin release. J. clin. Endocr. **27**, 1600—1606 (1967)

Feldman, J.M., Lebovitz, H.E.: Appraisal of the extrapancreatic actions of sulfonylureas. Arch. intern. Med. **123**, 314—322 (1969)

Findlay, J.A., Gill, J.R., Irvine, G., Lever, J.D., Randle, P.J.: Cytology of B-cells in rabbit pancreas pieces incubated *in vitro*: Effects of glucose and tolbutamide. Diabetologia **4**, 150—160 (1968)

GABBAY, K.H., TZE, W.J.: Inhibition of glucose-induced release of insulin by aldose reductase inhibitors. Proc. nat. Acad. Sci. (Wash.) **69**, 1435—1439 (1972)

GEORG, R.H., SUSMAN, K.E., LEITNER, J.W., KIRSCH, W.M.: Inhibition of glucose and tolbutamide-induced insulin release by iodoacetate and antimycin A. Endocrinology **89**, 169—176 (1971)

GEPTS, W.: Etude histologique de l'effet des sulfamides hypoglycémiants sur les îlots de Langerhans du rat. Ann. endocr. (Paris) **18**, 204—217 (1957)

GRODSKY, G.M.: Insulin and the pancreas. Vitam. and Horm. **28**, 37—101 (1970)

GRODSKY, G.M., CURRY, D., LANDAHL, H., BENNETT, L.: Further studies on the dynamic aspects of insulin release in vitro with evidence for a two-compartmental storage system. Acta diabet. lat. **6**, Suppl. 1, 554—579 (1969)

GRODSKY, G.M., LEE, J., FANSKA, R., SMITH, D.: Insulin secretion from the *in vitro* perfused pancreas of the rat: Effect of Ro-4563 and other sulfonylureas. In: Recent hypoglycemic sulfonylureas. Mechanisms of action and clinical indications, pp. 83—94. DUBACH, U.C., BÜCKERT, A., eds.). Bern: Huber 1971

GULBENKIAN, A., ORNSTEIN, L., TABACHNICK, I.I.A.: The use of diazoxide inhibition of insulin secretion as a tool to investigate insulin stimulation by other agents. Horm. Metab. Res. **4**, 57—58 (1972)

HELLMAN, B.: Carbutamide stimulation of glutamic dehydrogenase activity in the pancreatic β-cells from obese-hyperglycemic mice. Metabolism **16**, 1059—1063 (1967)

HELLMAN, B.: Methodological approaches to studies on the pancreatic islets. Diabetologia **6**, 110—120 (1970)

HELLMAN, B., IDAHL, L.-Å.: Pancreatic islet levels of citrate under conditions of stimulated and inhibited insulin release. Diabetes **21**, 999—1002 (1972)

HELLMAN, B., IDAHL, L.-Å., DANIELSSON, Å.: Adenosine triphosphate level of mammalian pancreatic B cells after stimulation with glucose and hypoglycemic sulfonylureas. Diabetes **18**, 509—516 (1969)

HELLMAN, B., IDAHL, L.-Å., LERNMARK, Å., SEHLIN, J., TÄLJEDAL, I.-B.: Iodoacetamide-induced sensitization of the pancreatic B-cells to glucose stimulation. Biochem. J. **132**, 775—789 (1973b)

HELLMAN, B., IDAHL, L.-Å., LERNMARK, Å., SEHLIN, J., TÄLJEDAL, I.-B.: Role of thiol groups in insulin release: Studies with poorly permeating disulphides. Molec. Pharmacol. **9**, 792—801 (1973c)

HELLMAN, B., SEHLIN, J., TÄLJEDAL, I.-B.: Effects of glucose and other modifiers of insulin release on the oxidative metabolism of amino acids in micro-dissected pancreatic islets. Biochem. J. **123**, 513—521 (1971a)

HELLMAN, B., SEHLIN, J., TÄLJEDAL, I.-B.: Uptake of alanine, arginine, and leucine by mammalian pancreatic B-cells. Endocrinology **89**, 1432—1439 (1971b)

HELLMAN, B., SEHLIN, J., TÄLJEDAL, I.-B.: Transport of α-aminoisobutyric acid in mammalian pancreatic B-cells. Diabetologia **7**, 256—265 (1971c)

HELLMAN, B., SEHLIN, J., TÄLJEDAL, I.-B.: Calcium uptake by pancreatic β-cells as measured with the aid of ^{45}Ca and mannitol-^{3}H. Amer. J. Physiol. **221**, 1795—1801 (1971d)

HELLMAN, B., SEHLIN, J., TÄLJEDAL, I.-B.: The pancreatic B-cell recognition of insulin secretagogues. II. Site of action of tolbutamide. Biochem. biophys. Res. Commun. **45**, 1384—1388 (1971e)

HELLMAN, B., SEHLIN, J., TÄLJEDAL, I.-B.: Transport of L-leucine and D-leucine into pancreatic B-cells with reference to the mechanisms of amino acid-induced insulin release. Biochim. biophys. Acta (Amst.) **266**, 436—443 (1972)

HELLMAN, B., SEHLIN, J., TÄLJEDAL, I.-B.: The pancreatic B-cell recognition of insulin secretagogues. IV. Uptake of sulfonylureas by islet tissue. Diabetologia **9**, 210—216 (1973a)

HOWELL, S.L., LACY, P.E.: Studies on the effect of HB 419 (Glibenclamide) on isolated islets and granules. Horm. Metab. Res. **1**, Suppl., 45—47 (1969)

HOWELL, S.L., TAYLOR, K.W.: Potassium ions and the secretion of insulin by islets of Langerhans incubated *in vitro*. Biochem. J. **108**, 17—24 (1968)

HOWELL, S.L., WHITFIELD, M.: Cytochemical localization of adenyl cyclase and cyclic AMP phosphodiesterase in rat islets of Langerhans. Diabetes **21**, 328 (1972)

HOWELL, S.L., YOUNG, D.A., LACY, P.E.: Isolation and properties of secretory granules from rat islets of Langerhans. III. Studies of the stability of the isolated beta granules. J. Cell Biol. **41**, 167—176 (1969)

IDAHL, L.-Å.: Glucose-6-phosphate content in mammalian pancreatic β-cells. Hormones **2**, 371—377 (1971)

IDAHL, L.-Å., HURME, P., WAHLQUIST, Y., HELLMAN, B.: Pancreatic β-cell function and content of 6-phosphogluconate. Horm. Metab. Res. **3**, 141—144 (1971)

JORES, J., KRACHT, J.: Wirkung von Sulfonylharnstoffverbindungen auf die Mitosenfrequenz der insulären B-Zellen. Acta endocr. (Kbh.) **32**, 243—254 (1959)

Kanazawa, Y., Orci, L., Lambert, A.E.: Organ culture of fetal rat pancreas. IV. Effects of metabolic inhibitors on insulin release. Endocrinology **89**, 576—583 (1971)

Kern, H.F., Kern, D.: Die Feinstruktur der Langerhans'schen Inseln der Ratte nach Einwirkung von HB 419. Arzneimittel-Forsch. **19**, 1452—1456 (1969)

Kizer, J.S., Vargas-Cordon, M., Brendel, K., Bressler, R.: The in vitro inhibition of insulin secretion by diphenylhydantoin. J. clin. Invest. **49**, 1942—1948 (1970)

Kracht, J., Holt, C., Holt, L.: Morphologische Befunde zur Wirkungsweise oraler Antidiabetika. Endokrinologie **34**, 129—146 (1957)

Krzanowski, J.J., Fertel, R., Matschinsky, F.M.: Energy metabolism in pancreatic islets of rats. Studies with tolbutamide and hypoxia. Diabetes **20**, 598—606 (1971)

Lacy, P.E.: Light microscopic and electron microscopic changes and *in vitro* effects of sulfonylureas. Handbuch der experimentellen Pharmakologie, vol. 29, pp. 427—437 (Maske, H., ed.). Berlin-Heidelberg-New York: Springer 1971

Lacy, P.E., Walker, M.M., Fink, C.J.: Perifusion of isolated rat islets in vitro. Participation of the microtubular system in the biphasic release of insulin. Diabetes **21**, 987—998 (1972)

Laube, H., Fussgänger, R., Goberna, R., Schröder, K., Straub, K., Sussman, K., Pfeiffer, E.F.: Effects of tolbutamide on insulin and glucagon secretion of the isolated perfused rat pancreas. Horm. Metab. Res. **3**, 238—242 (1971)

Lauvaux, J.P., Mandart, G., Heymans, G., Ooms, H. A.: Effect of long-term tolbutamide treatment on glucose tolerance and insulin secretion in maturity-onset diabetes without obesity. Horm. Metab. Res. **4**, 58—62 (1972)

Lazarow, A., Carpenter, A.-M., Morgan, C., Wright, D.: Effects of long-term administration of tolbutamide in normal, subdiabetic and diabetic rats. Diabetes **11**, Suppl., 103—115 (1962)

Lazarus, S.S.: Acid and glucose-6-phosphatase activity of pancreatic B-cells after cortisone and sulfonylureas. Proc. Soc. exp. Biol. (N.Y.) **102**, 303—306 (1959)

Levey, G.S., Schmidt, W.M.I., Mintz, D.H.: Activation of adenylcyclase in a pancreatic islet cell adenoma by glucagon and tolbutamide. Metabolism **21**, 93—98 (1972)

Loubatières, A.: Etude physiologique et pharmacodynamique de certains dérivés sulfamidés hypoglycémiants. Arch. int. Physiol. (Paris) **54**, 174—177 (1946)

Loubatières, A.: Physiological and pharmacological aspects of the central role of the pancreas in the mode of action of hypoglycemic sulfonamides. Acta diabet. lat. **6**, Suppl. 1, 216—255 (1969)

Loubatières, A., Renold, A.E.: Pharmacokinetics and mode of action of oral hypoglycemic agents. Acta diabet. lat. **6**, Suppl. 1 (1969)

Lundquist, I.: Insulin secretion. Its regulation by monoamines and acid amyloglucosidase. Acta physiol. scand. Suppl. **327** (1971)

Malaisse, W.: Étude de la sécrétion insulinique in vitro, pp. 182—191. Bruxelles: Editions Arscia 1969

Malaisse, W.J.: Role of calcium in insulin secretion. Israel J. med. Sci. **8**, 244—251 (1972)

Malaisse, W.J., Mahy, M., Brisson, G.R., Malaisse-Lagae, F.: The stimulus-secretion coupling of glucose-induced insulin release. VIII. Combined effects of glucose and sulfonylureas. Europ. J. clin. Invest. **2**, 85—90 (1972)

Malaisse, W.J., Malaisse-Lagae, F., Brisson, G.: Combined effects of glucose and sulfonylureas on insulin secretion by the rat pancreas *in vitro*. In: Recent hypoglycemic sulfonylureas. Mechanisms of action and clinical indications, pp. 114—126 (Dubach, U.C., Bückert, A., eds.). Bern: Huber 1971

Mariani, M.-M.: The action of sulfonylureas on the insulin secretion of the perfused rat pancreas. Acta diabet. lat. **6**, Suppl. 1, 256—270 (1969)

Mashiter, K., Zor, U., Bloom, G., Field, J.B.: Effects of glucose, glucagon, tolbutamide and theophylline on the cyclic AMP content and insulin release of slices of human islet cell adenomas. Diabetes **21**, 346—347 (1972)

Maske, H.: Interaction between insulin and zinc in the islets of Langerhans. Diabetes **6**, 335—341 (1957)

Maske, H. (ed.): Oral wirksame Antidiabetika. Handbuch der experimentellen Pharmakologie, vol. 29. Berlin-Heidelberg-New York: Springer 1971

Matthews, E.K.: Electrical activity in islet cells and insulin secretion. Acta diabet. lat. **7**, Suppl. 1, 83—89 (1970)

Matthews, E.K., Dean, P.M.: Electrical activity in islet cells. In: The structure and metabolism of the pancreatic islets, pp. 305—312 (Falkmer, S., Hellman, B., Täljedal, I.-B., eds.). Oxford: Pergamon Press 1970a

Matthews, E.K., Dean, P.M.: The biophysical effects of insulin-releasing agents on islet cells. Postgrad. med. J. **3**, December Suppl., 21—23 (1970b)

Milner, R.D.G.: The stimulation of insulin release by essential amino acids from rabbit pancreas *in vitro*. J. Endocr. **47**, 347—356 (1970)

MILNER, R.D.G., HALES, C.N.: The interaction of various inhibitors and stimuli of insulin release studied with rabbit pancreas *in vitro*. Biochem. J. **113**, 473—479 (1969)

MILNER, R.D.G., HALES, C.N.: Ionic mechanisms in the regulation of insulin secretion. In: The structure and metabolism of the pancreatic islets, pp. 489—493 (FALKMER, S., HELLMAN, B., TÄLJEDAL, I.-B., eds.). Oxford: Pergamon Press 1970

MONTAGUE, W., HOWELL, S.L.: The mode of action of adenosine 3′, 5′-cyclic monophosphate in mammalian islets of Langerhans. Effects of insulin secretagogues on islet-cell protein kinase activity. Biochem. J. **134**, 321—327 (1973)

MONTAGUE, W., TAYLOR, K.W.: Islet-cell metabolism during insulin release. Effects of glucose, citrate, octanoate, tolbutamide, glucagon and theophylline. Biochem. J. **115**, 257—262 (1969)

MORRIS, G.E., KORNER, A.: The effect of glucose on insulin biosynthesis by isolated islets of Langerhans of the rat. Biochim. biophys. Acta (Amst.) **208**, 404—413 (1970)

NIKI, A., NIKI, H., KOIDE, T., LIN, B.J.: Insulin biosynthesis: effects of oral hypoglycemic agents. Abstr. 8th Congr. Europ. Assoc. Diabetes. Madrid: Novo Service 1972

ORCI, L., STAUFFACHER, W., BEAVEN, D., LAMBERT, A.E., RENOLD, A.E., ROUILLER, C.: Ultrastructural events associated with the action of tolbutamide and glibenclamide on pancreatic B-cells in vivo and in vitro. Acta diabet. lat. **6**, Suppl. 1, 271—374 (1969)

PACE, S.C., PRICE, S.: Electrical activity of islet cells in response to leucine and tolbutamide. Diabetes **21**, 345 (1972)

PANTEN, U.: Biochemical events in pancreatic islets as caused by sulfonylurea derivatives. Proc. 5th intl. Congr. Pharmacol. San Francisco 1972

PENTTILÄ, L.M.: Effect of insulin, chloropropamide and tolbutamide on the metabolism of branched chain amino acids. Ann. Med. exp. Fenn. **44**, Suppl. 11 (1966)

PFEIFFER, E.F.: Current pathophysiological and clinical aspects of the mode of action of blood glucose lowering sulfonamides. Acta diabet. lat. **6**, Suppl. 1, 477—504 (1969)

PFEIFFER, E.F., SCHÖFFLING, K., DITSCHUNEIT, H.: Der Wirkungsmechanismus der oralen Antidiabetica. In: Handbuch des Diabetes Mellitus, vol. 1, pp. 637—684 (PFEIFFER, E.F., ed.). München: J.F. Lehmanns Verlag 1969

PFEIFFER, E.F., STEIGERWALD, H., SANDRITTER, W., BÄNDER, A., MAGER, A., BECKER, U., RETIENE, K.: Vergleichende Untersuchungen von Morphologie und Hormongehalt des Kälberpankreas nach Sulfonylharnstoffen (D 860). Dtsch. med. Wschr. **82**, 1568—1574 (1957)

PUCHINGER, H., WACKER, A.: Effect of glucose and tolbutamide on RNA synthesis in isolated islets of Langerhans from rat pancreas. FEBS Letters **21**, 14—16 (1972)

RENOLD, A.E., LAMBERT, A.E., BURR, I.M., STAUFFACHER, W.: Effects *in vitro* of sulfonylurea derivatives on fetal and adult rat pancreas. In: Recent hypoglycemic sulfonylureas. Mechanisms of action and clinical indications, pp. 70—79 (DUBACH, U.C., BÜCKERT, A., eds.). Bern: Huber 1971

SAMOLS, E., TYLER, J.M., KAJINUMA, H.: Influence of the sulfonamides on pancreatic humoral secretion and evidence for an insulin-glucagon feedback system. Proceedings of the 7th Congress of the International Diabetes Federation, pp. 636—655. Internat. Congr. Series No. 231, Amsterdam: Excerpta Medica 1971

SAMS, D.J., MONTAGUE, W.: The role of adenosine 3′:5′-cyclic monophosphate in the regulation of insulin release. Properties of islet-cell adenosine 3′:5′-cyclic monophosphate phosphodiesterase. Biochem. J. **129**, 945—952 (1972)

SCHATZ, H., MAIER, V., HINZ, M., NIERLE, C., PFEIFFER, E.F.: The effect of tolbutamide and glibenclamide on the incorporation of (^{3}H)leucine and on the conversion of proinsulin to insulin in isolated pancreatic islets. FEBS Letters **26**, 237—240 (1972)

SELTZER, H.S., CROUT, J.R.: Insulin secretory blockade by benzothiadiazines and catecholamines: reversal by sulfonylureas. Ann N. Y. Acad. Sci. **150**, 309—321 (1968)

SIREK, O.V., VIGAS, M., NIKI, A., NIKI, H., SIREK, A.: Beta-adrenergic stimulation of insulin release in dogs following HB 419. Diabetologia **5**, 207—210 (1969)

SODOYEZ, J.-C., SODOYEZ-GOFFAUX, F., DUNBAR, J.C., FOA, P.P.: Reduction in the activity of the pancreatic islets induced in normal rodents by prolonged treatment with derivatives of sulfonylurea. Diabetes **19**, 603—609 (1970)

STEINER, D.F., FREINKEL, N. (eds.): Endocrine pancreas. Handbook of Physiology, section **7**, vol. 1. Baltimore: Williams and Wilkins 1972

STEINER, D.F., KEMMLER, W., CLARK, J.L., OYER, P.E., RUBENSTEIN, A.H.: The biosynthesis of insulin. In: Endocrine pancreas. Handbook of Physiology, section 7, vol. 1, pp. 175—198 (STEINER, D.F., FREINKEL, N., eds.). Baltimore: Williams and Wilkins 1972

STORK, H., SCHMIDT, F.H., HELLERSTRÖM, C., WESTMAN, S.: Respiration of the β-cells in the presence of sulfonylureas. In: The structure and metabolism of the pancreatic islets, pp. 331—336 (FALKMER, S., HELLMAN, B., TÄLJEDAL, I.-B., eds.). Oxford: Pergamon Press 1970

STORK, H., SCHMIDT, F.H., WESTMAN, S., HELLERSTRÖM, C.: Action of some hypoglycaemic sulphonylureas on the oxygen consumption of isolated pancreatic islets of mice. Diabetologia **5**, 279—283 (1969)

TÄLJEDAL, I.-B.: Glucose-6-phosphatase in pancreatic β-cell metabolism. In: The structure and metabolism of the pancreatic islets, pp. 233—244 (FALKMER, S., HELLMAN, B., TÄLJEDAL, I.-B., eds.). Oxford: Pergamon Press 1970

TANESE, T.N., LAZARUS, N.R., DEVRIM, S., RECANT, L.: Synthesis and release of proinsulin and insulin by isolated rat islets of Langerhans. J. clin. Invest. **49**, 1394—1404 (1970)

TAYLOR, K.W., PARRY, D.G.: Tolbutamide and the incorporation of (^{3}H)-leucine into insulin in vitro. J. Endocr. **39**, 457—458 (1967)

VOLK, B.W., LAZARUS, S.S.: B-cell hyperfunction after long-term sulfonylurea treatment. Arch. Path. **78**, 114—126 (1964)

WALLENFELS, K., SUMM, H.D., CREUTZFELDT, W.: Enzymatische Untersuchungen zum Wirkungsmechanismus der blutzuckersenkenden Medikamente. Dtsch. med. Wschr. **82**, 1581—1585 (1957)

WALLENFELS, K., SUND, H., BURCHARD, W.: Über den Einfluß von BZ 55 auf die Aggregation des Insulins in Gegenwart von Zinkionen. Biochem. Z. **335**, 315—324 (1962)

WEBER, A.: The mechanism of the action of caffeine on sarcoplasmic reticulum. J. gen. Physiol. **52**, 760—772 (1968)

WIDSTRÖM, A., CERASI, E.: Modulation of glucose-induced insulin release by tolbutamide in man. Acta endocr. (Kbh.) **72**, 519—531 (1973a)

WIDSTRÖM, A., CERASI, E.: Interaction of tolbutamide with glucagon, aminophylline, and arginine in stimulating insulin response in man. Acta endocr. (Kbh.) **72**, 532—544 (1973b)

WILIAMSON, J.R., LACY, P.E., GRISHAM, J.W.: Ultrastructural changes in islets of the rat produced by tolbutamide. Diabetes **10**, 460—469 (1961)

YOSHINAGA, T., YAMAMOTO, Y.: Über Beziehungen zwischen Sulfonylharnstoffen und einigen Metallionen. Endokrinologie **50**, 87—93 (1966)

Pharmacokinetics of Insulin

A. Distribution in the Organism

JOSEPH L. IZZO

With 13 Figures

I. Introduction

The development of methods for labelling of insulin with radioactive iodine and for measurement of insulin levels in body fluids by immunoassay technics has greatly expanded our knowledge on insulin distribution and the dynamics and kinetics involved. With respect to use of labelled insulin the physiological relevance of such data is dependent upon the assumption that the disposition of the labelled hormone is similar to, if not identical with, that of the native hormone from a quantitative as well as qualitative standpoint. Specifically, it is required that: a) labelled insulin retains biological activity; b) the nature and rate of the degradative processes for the unlabelled and labelled hormone are similar if not identical and c) removal of the radioactive iodine label from insulin occurs only as a result of physiological degradative processes and not deiodination. Finally, in order to fulfill the requirements of a tracer the total amount of injected insulin should be less than that present in the circulation or at least it should not raise concentration of insulin in plasma above physiological levels. The extent to which the individual studies fulfill these requirements will be discussed.

The insulin distribution studies have been grouped into two main categories i.e. studies which have been concerned not only with plasma disappearance but also with experimentally determined distribution to various organs and tissues and studies which have been concerned primarily with the kinetics of insulin distribution based on analysis of plasma disappearance. Dynamic processes involved with insulin distribution have been considered separately.

Distribution of Insulin in Body Compartments, Organs and Tissues

1. Early Distribution Studies

Rose and Nelson, 1954, were among the first to study the disappearance rate of radioiodinated insulin from the blood and its uptake by various tissues in the rat. At 10 min after the rapid intravenous injection of 2 units of ^{131}I labelled insulin the percent of injected trichloroacetic acid precipitable radioactivity in blood, liver, kidneys and muscle mass was: 28.0, 10.2, 14.7, and 14.5 respectively. Protein bound radioactivity declined progressively in blood and tissues over an 8 h period but the rate of decline was more rapid in blood and kidney than in liver and muscle. During the first hour less than 1% of the injected dose was excreted in the urine. Of particular interest was the absence of protein bound radioactivity in the brain. When ^{131}I insulin was administered by continuous infusion via the portal vein the concentration of protein bound radioactivity in the arterial blood was 16% lower, the portal blood 25% and liver 50% higher than when the same dose was infused continuously into the inferior vena cava. In 1954 Elgee *et al.*, also reported studies on the distribution and degradation of intravenous injections of ^{131}I-labelled insulin in rats within the range of 0.2—0.8 units. The time courses showed that insulin (as determined by trichloroacetic acid precipitable radioactivity) concentration reached a peak in liver, kidney and muscle in from 5—15 min and then fell rapidly paralleling that in blood. After 1 h the fall in insulin concentration was slight. Trichoroacetic acid soluble radioactivity appeared within the first few minutes after ^{131}I insulin injection and increased in concentration in tissues and blood in the first 15 min. At later times appreciable quantities of radioactivity were excreted in the urine in a non-precipitable form. At 15 min after injection 21% of the injected radioactivity was found in kidneys, 19% in skeletal muscle, 11% in liver, 10% in blood and 39% in other tissues. The greatest concentration of radioactivity was found in the kidney, with progressively decreasing concentration in the thyroid, liver, stomach, plasma, spleen, lung, salivary glands, skin, thymus, diaphragm, heart, skeletal muscle, fat, urine, adrenals, pituitary, small intestine, large intestine, bone, breast and testes. Little, if any, was in the brain or red blood cells. Perfusion and radio-autography studies showed that the renal radioactivity was bound in the convoluted tubules. Distribution studies in terminally ill humans showed many similarities to those in the rat.

In the studies of Elgee *et al.* (1954) as well as those of Rose and Nelson (1954) discussed above the total quantity of insulin injected intravenously was in the pharmacological range. Stein and Gross (1959) were the first to investigate the effects of decreasing doses of intravenously injected ^{131}I-labelled insulin from 5.0—0.025 μg/100 gm b.w. on the distribution of ^{131}I-insulin in various organs and tissues in the rat. At 10 min after injection of 0.025—0.05 μg of ^{131}I insulin the mean percent of ^{131}I insulin (measured as trichloroacetic acid precipitable radioactivity) in terms of injected dose/gm wet tissue in skeletal muscle was 0.26—0.29, in heart 0.75—0.75, in liver 2.1—1.9 and in kidney 10.4—11.8. As the dose was increased the concentration in kidney rose while the concentration in muscles fell somewhat. No changes in concentration of trichloroacetic acid precipitable radioactivity were noted in liver or heart. Since they found that with increasing dosage the ratio of insulin concentration in the excretory organs (kidney) and target organs (muscle) tended to increase, the minimum in this ratio was taken as indication of "tracer dosage". On this basis, the dose of insulin approaching tracer dose was found to lie in the range of 0.025—0.05 μg/100 gm b.w. Since the dose increment in the kidney between administered doses of 0.05 and 5 μg/100 gm was balanced by a corresponding decrease in dose found in the muscle mass it was concluded that the kidneys and muscles were the main regulators of the fate of injected insulin. Conversely, the role of the liver was considered of less importance in this connection since no clear relation between the injected dose and the liver concentration was noted in 10 min.

2. Specificity of Distribution Pattern of ^{131}I-labelled Insulin

The distribution pattern of ^{131}I insulin in the rat was shown to be different from that of ^{131}I-labelled prolactin (Rose and Nelson, 1954), ^{131}I labelled serum albumin (Rose and Nelson, 1954; Elgee *et al.*, 1954) or Na ^{131}I (Elgee *et al.*, 1954). Furthermore, Elgee and Williams (1955) found that the degradation *in vivo* of insulin, labelled with radioactive iodine, as measured by the appearance of trichloroacetic acid supernatant radioactivity in tissues of the rat, was depressed, and to the same extent, with increasing loads of either ^{131}I labelled or non-labelled insulin, implying that both types of insulin competed equally well for the degration system. Furthermore, degradation of ^{131}I labelled insulin was not depressed by the addition of corticotropin, ribonuclease or lactalbumin. From these observations it was concluded that the degradation system exhibited a certain degree of specificity, did not distinguish between labelled and unlabelled insulin, and that, therefore measurement of the degradation of ^{131}I insulin was probably representative of the degradation of nonlabelled insulin. However, it was pointed out that the type of distribution and degradation pattern of ^{131}I insulin was not dependent on its hormonal character, since a very similar pattern of distribution was observed with ^{131}I-labelled ribonuclease. The validity of these comparisons was compromised by the fact that the test substances which were used differed so fundamentally from the protein of interest. Lee (1959) attempted to correct this by comparing the distribution patterns of intravenous injections of ^{131}I-insulin possessing full hypoglycemic activity with that of ^{131}I-insulin which had been totally inactivated either by treatment with dilute NaOH at 32° or by heavy iodine substitution (5.6 atoms/molecule). In the case of active ^{131}I-insulin the dose ranged from 2.7×10^{-2} to 7.0×10^{-2} units (1.0—2.6 μg) while in the case of the inactivated preparation the dose ranged from (6.5—11.3 μg). Comparisons were made at 5 min after injection. Results showed that inactivation was associated with a marked reduction in concentration of total ^{131}I in liver and kidney as well as the fraction considered to represent the intact molecule, namely, the fraction precipitated by trichloroacetic acid. Furthermore, binding to liver was less firm and the amount and distribution of that bound to intracellular structures were changed. Lastly, the degradation by liver and kidney was altered. From these observations, it was concluded that the fate and distribution of ^{131}I insulin in the rat are characteristic and specific for the functionally intact molecule. Direct deiodination of ^{131}I insulin was not considered to be a significant problem for studies lasting only a few hours, and the appearance of radioiodide in biological systems was coincident with inactivation and degradation of the insulin molecule.

3. Limitations of Early Distribution Studies

Although the ^{131}I-labelled insulin used in the above mentioned studies appeared to possess at least some of the attributes of a tracer i.e. it appeared to retain biological activity, to compete for the same transport and degradative systems as unlabelled insulin and appeared not to be deiodinated except as a result of physiological degradation of the molecule, the physiological significance or interpretation of the early distribution studies may be questioned on several grounds. The first objection relates to the amount of exogenous insulin injected intravenously.

Rose and Nelson (1954) and Elgee *et al.* (1954) injected quantities of insulin in the pharmacological range. While such large doses may provide information on the behavior of the injected insulin they do not necessarily reflect the behavior of endogenous insulin in physiological concentrations. As pointed out above, Stein and Gross (1959) attempted to resolve the problem by determining the tracer dose on the basis of the ratios of ^{131}I-insulin in target and excretory organs. However, it should be pointed out that although the dose employed, i.e. approximately 1250 μU/100 gm b.w. was considered to approach the tracer level, the amount of insulin injected was still substantial compared to the level of insulin in the rat plasma. The concentration of endogenous insulin in rats which had been fasted for 18 h was reported to be approximately 60—70 μU (relative) per ml of plasma (Izzo *et al.*, 1967). The second objection is concerned with the waiting period of 5—10 min after intravenous injection before initial observations were made. The purpose for this presumably was to allow for sufficient mixing and equilibration of insulin between the plasma and the extracellular fluid compartments. This assumes that during the period of rapid plasma clearance reaction processes are not a factor; but, as will be shown below this is far from the case. The third objection has to do with the functional and structural integrity of the ^{131}I-labelled insulin. The statement that the labelled insulin possessed full biological activity is not sufficient to insure integrity of the labelled molecule, if indeed as was claimed the preparations were lightly iodinated and contained much less than an average of one atom of iodine per molecule. If only a small proportion of the total insulin molecules were iodinated it would be difficult to ascertain the biological activity of the labelled molecules, in view of the sensitivity of the biological assays available. The last objection is that no attempt was made to remove or correct for blood in the organs or tissues under consideration. Rose and Nelson (1954) stated that only a small fraction of protein bound radioactivity in muscle, liver and kidney could be recovered by perfusing the animal with Ringer's solution but no information was provided on the effect of perfusion on the non-protein bound radioactivity.

To a large extent, the limitations of the early disposition studies reflected the limitation in the available technics for iodinating insulin. The methods for iodinating insulin at the time utilized either iodine in potassium chloride solution (Hughes and Strassle, 1950), iodide oxidized to a reactive state with nitrous acid (Pressman and Eisen, 1950), or iodine liberated from a mixture of iodide and iodate with acid (Francis *et al.*, 1951). These methods were inefficient in the use of ^{131}I, were prone to considerable damage or structural alteration of iodine and frequently resulted in the incorporation of unknown amounts of iodine, especially when attempts were made to achieve preparations of higher specific-activity (Izzo *et al.*, 1962). Reexamination of the distribution of insulin was made possible by the development of a procedure by Izzo *et al.* (1962, 1964a) for preparing ^{131}I-insulin of high specific activity with little or no damage to the hormone, which was efficient in the use of starting ^{131}I and which permitted precise control of the total amount of iodine attached to the hormone and which was suitable for metabolic studies. The procedure was based on iodination of proteins with iodine monochloride (McFarlane, 1958). At about the same time a method for iodinating peptide hormones involving oxidation with chloramine-T (Banerjee and Gibson, 1962; Greenwood *et al.*, 1963) was also introduced. Although the chloramine-T method is efficient in the use of ^{131}I and can result in higher specific activities, it can also result in considerable oxidative damage to the protein and repurification procedures are usually necessary to render the preparation sufficiently pure for use in immunoassay of peptide hormones. Furthermore, in iodinations with iodine monochloride, the use of a fixed quantity of this reagent automatically maintains the iodine substitution at a known value which is dependent only upon the ratio of ICl to insulin used and is independent of the contribution of iodide carrier in the isotope preparation, or of iodine from any other source. This is not the case with chloramine-T iodination unless the total quantity of iodine in the isotope preparation is carefully determined. Hence, the ICl method has clear advantages when the degree of iodination has to be carefully controlled (GLOVER *et al.*, 1967).

The relationship between degree of iodination of insulin and its biological, immunological and electrophoretic properties was examined by IZZO *et al.* (1964b). Their studies showed that the biological activity of iodoinsulin was markedly influenced by the number of iodine atoms that were attached to the hormone. On the other hand, the immunological and electrophoretic properties on paper were influenced to a much lesser extent. As assayed by the mouse convulsion, rat diaphragm or epididymal fat pad methods, full biological activity was preserved only if the iodine content did not exceed on the average one atom per molecule of insulin (MW 6000). With increasing iodination the activity fell off sharply and progressively. ROSA *et al.* (1967), and BRUNFELDT *et al.* (1968) obtained essentially the same results. However, ARQUILLA *et al.* (1968) reported a markedly attenuated biological activity in purified iodoinsulin fractions of insulin preparations containing one atom or less of iodine per molecule, using the fat pad technic. On the other hand, FREYCHET, ROTH and NEVILLE (1971) showed more recently that purified iodoinsulin fractions of minimally iodinated insulin retained full biological activity as measured by the fat pad technic.

4. Reinvestigation of Distribution of ^{131}I-labelled Insulin in the Rat

In the light of the above considerations IZZO *et al.* (1967) reinvestigated the distribution of ^{131}I-labelled insulin in the rat with the aid of a structurally and functionally intact ^{131}I-insulin of high specific activity which would permit the injection of truly tracer of physiological doses as well as large pharmacological doses of the hormone. In these studies, the time courses of plasma disappearance and distribution and degradation in various body compartments, of single bolus intravenous injections of biologically active ^{131}I-labelled insulin of high specific activity containing an average of 0.8 atom of total iodine per molecule of insulin were compared at two dose levels: tracer of physiological levels (50—100 μU/100 gm b.w.) and large or pharmacological levels (10^5 μU/100 gm b.w.). Similar comparisons at the same dose levels were also carried out with ^{131}I-labelled biologically inactive insulin containing on the average 6 atoms of iodine per molecule. Initial observations were started at 1 min or less after the intravenous injection of insulin. Furthermore, each animal that was killed at times greater than 1 min after injection was subjected to a "two-way" whole body perfusion with normal saline solution before the tissues were removed in an attempt to remove residual blood and also any radioactivity in the extracellular compartments of the various tissues examined. In those animals that were killed at 1 min or less after injection perfusions were not performed but appropriate corrections were made for residual blood in liver and kidney. Trichloroacetic acid precipitable radioactivity was considered to represent intact ^{131}I insulin and trichloroacetic acid soluble radioactivity was considered to represent ^{131}I labelled insulin degradation products. BERSON *et al.* (1956) had observed differences in plasma disappearance of ^{131}I insulin when measured by paper chromatoelectrophoresis of ^{131}I radioactivity in plasma and by trichloroacetic acid precipitability in plasma. However, in these studies (Fig. 1)

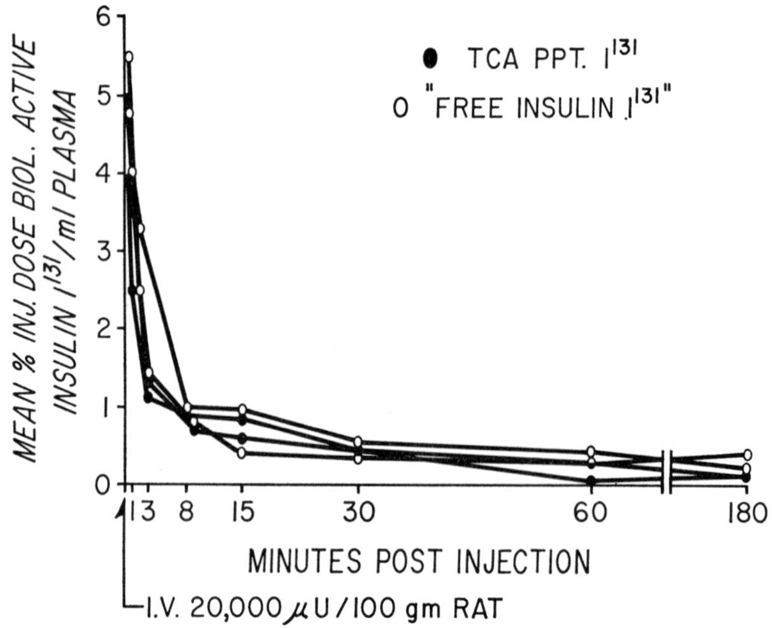

Fig. 1. Comparison of rates of disappearance from plasma of intravenously injected single doses (20,000 microunits/100 g rat body weight) of biologically active ^{131}I insulin in the rat as measured by trichloroacetic acid precipitable ^{131}I in plasma and as measured by isolation of ^{131}I insulin in plasma by means of paper chromatoelectrophoresis. Values are expressed as percentage of injected radioactivity per ml of plasma; μU, microunits. (From Izzo *et al.*, 1967)

no significant differences were noted in rate of disappearance of biologically active ^{131}I insulin in plasma as measured by either method.

The results showed that at 50—100 μU/100 gm b.w. ^{131}I insulin (0.8 I/mol) caused a slight transient lowering of blood sugar lasting about 8 min whereas at a dose level of .1 U (10^5 μU) profound and protracted hypoglycemia was observed with maximal lowering at 30—60 min and duration of action beyond the 3 h interval of study. In contrast the heavily iodinated insulin manifested little or no hypoglycemia activity at similar dose levels.

In the ensuing discussion, attention has been directed to results for plasma (Fig. 2), liver (Fig. 3), kidney (Fig. 4), and skeletal muscle mass (represented by the gastrocnemius) (Fig. 5) since these portions of the body contained or affected most or nearly all of the accountable fraction of the injected dose. Plasma clearance of 50—100 μU of ^{131}I insulin (0.8 I/mole) was very rapid. At 1 min after injection only 15.5% of injected radioactivity (13.3% trichloroacetic acid precipitable and 2.2% trichloroacetic acid soluble) was present in plasma. However, 31.2% of injected radioactivity was found in liver (18.6% precipitable, and 12.6% trichloroacetic acid soluble) 6.9% in kidney (4.2% trichloroacetic acid precipitable and 2.7% trichloroacetic acid soluble), 9.2% in skeletal muscle mass (5.9% trichloroacetic acid precipitable and 3.3% trichloroacetic acid soluble) and 6.6% in skin. Trichloroacetic acid precipitable radioactivity in plasma declined progressively; at 15 min only 3.4% of injected insulin remained in plasma. In contrast trichloroacetic acid soluble radioactivity increased in plasma for the first 15 min and then declined slowly during the 3 h period of observation. In the liver however, both

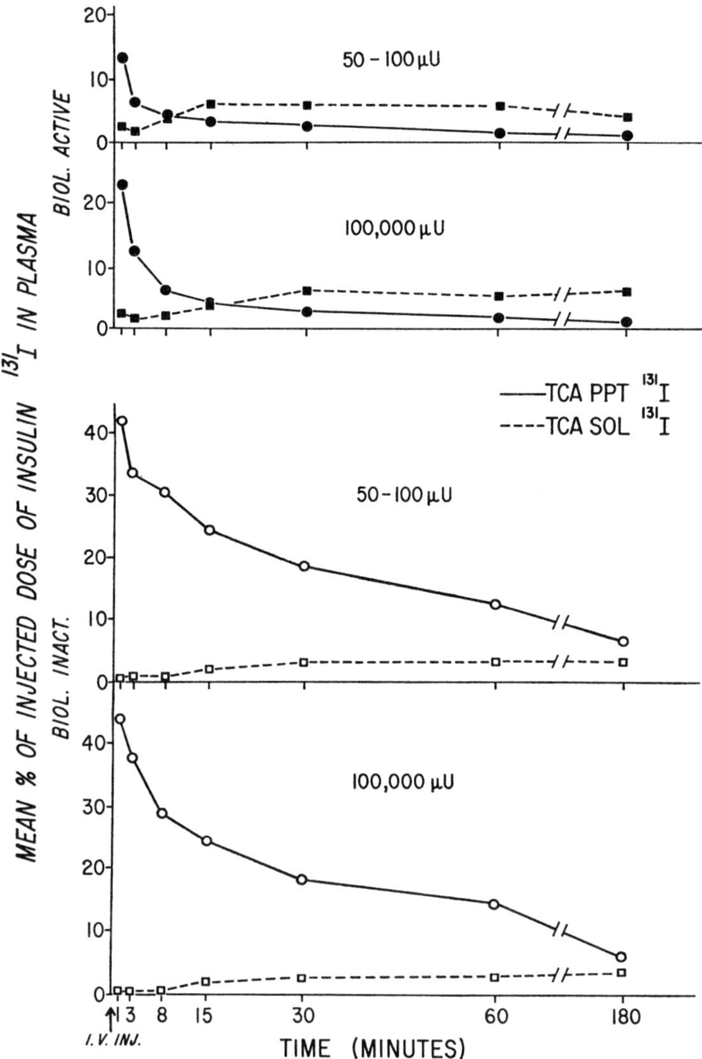

Fig. 2. Variations in concentration of trichloroacetic acid precipitable ^{131}I and trichloroacetic acid soluble ^{131}I in plasma with time after intravenous injections of 50—100 μU or 10^5 μU doses of either of biologically active or biologically inactive ^{131}I insulin. Concentration is expressed as mean percentage of the injected dose. (Adapted from Izzo *et al.*, 1967)

types of radioactivity declined progressively and at a faster rate than in plasma. In the kidneys, both trichloracetic acid precipitable and trichloroacetic acid soluble radioactivities reached peaks of 5.6% and 5.0% respectively at 8 min after ^{131}I insulin injection and both declined progressively thereafter. In the skeletal muscle mass, trichloroacetic acid precipitable radioactivity declined gradually after the first minute while trichloroacetic acid soluble radioactivity increased progressively reaching maximal levels of 11.3% at 30 min and then decreased slowly. Total radioactivity in skin increased slowly and progressively to a level of

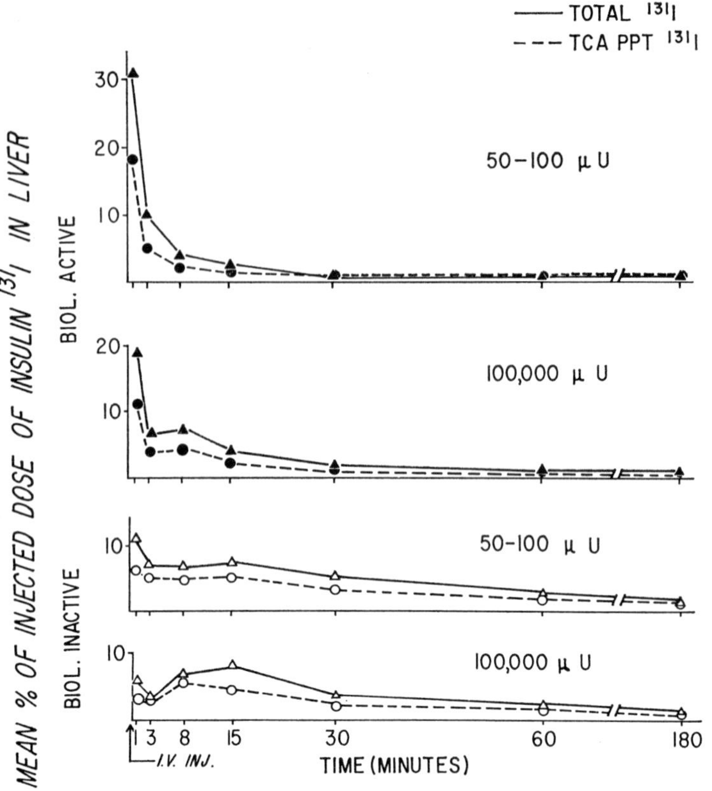

Fig. 3. Variations in concentration of trichloroacetic acid precipitable ^{131}I and total ^{131}I (trichloroacetic acid precipitable + trichloroacetic acid soluble) in liver with time after intravenous injections of 50—100 μU or 10^5 μU doses of either biologically active or biologically inactive ^{131}I insulin. (Adapted from Izzo *et al.*, 1967)

25.3% of injected radioactivity at 180 min. ^{131}I radioactivity most of which was trichloroacetic acid soluble was excreted very slowly in urine. At the end of 60 min 11.1% of injected radioactivity appeared in urine (1.2% trichloroacetic acid precipitable and 9.9% trichloroacetic acid soluble).

The time courses of plasma clearance, tissue distribution and degradation of large doses of ^{131}I insulin (0.8 I/mole) were in general similar to those of the tracer doses. However certain noteworthy quantitative differences were observed. During the first 15 min percent trichloroacetic acid precipitable radioactivity in plasma was higher and trichloroacetic acid soluble radioactivity lower than following injection of small doses. Peak distribution to liver was less and to kidneys greater than after injection of small doses. At 1 min after injection of large doses 25.4% of injected radioactivity remained in plasma (23.0% trichloroacetic acid precipitable and 2.4% trichloroacetic acid soluble) while 20.5% of injected dose was found in liver, of which 13.0% was trichloroacetic acid precipitable and 7.5% trichloroacetic acid soluble. Peak accumulation of radioactivity in kidneys at 8 min after injection of large doses was 16.4% (8.7% trichloroacetic acid precipitable and 7.7% trichloroacetic acid soluble).

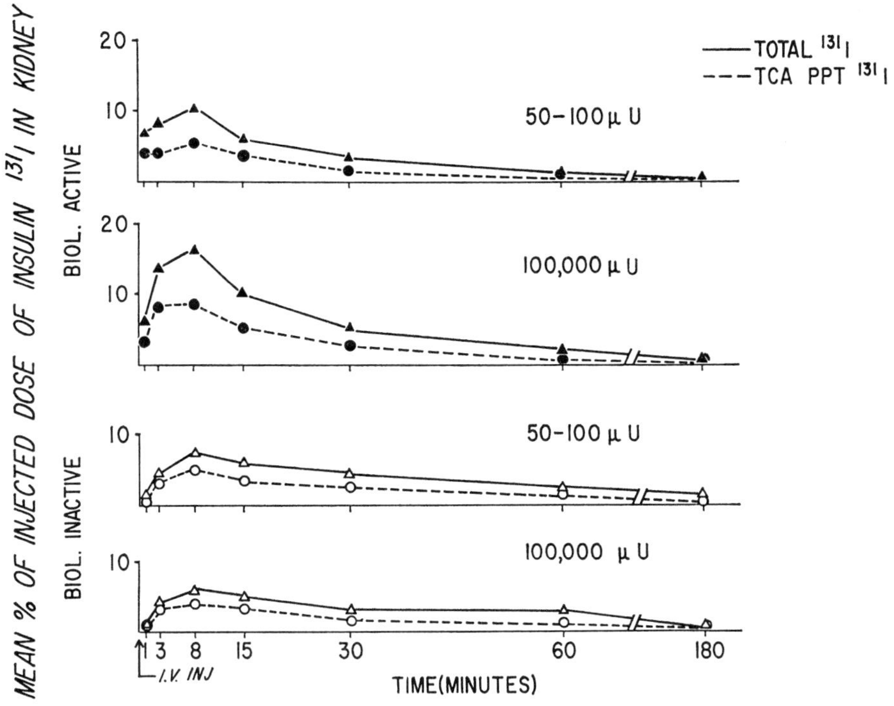

Fig. 4. Variations in concentration of trichloroacetic acid precipitable ^{131}I and otal ^{131}I (trichloroacetic acid precipitable + trichloroacetic acid soluble) in kidney with time after intravenous injections of 50—100 μU or 10^5 μU doses of either biologically active or biologically inactive ^{131}I insulin. (Adapted from Izzo *et al.*, 1967)

The patterns of disposition of small and large doses of biologically inactive ^{131}I insulin (6.0 I/mole) were strikingly different from the patterns of disposition of small and large doses of biologically active ^{131}I insulin (0.8 I/mole). No differences were noted in plasma clearance, tissue distribution and degradation between small and large doses of biologically inactive insulin. Concentrations of trichloroacetic acid precipitable radioactivity were much higher while concentrations of trichloroacetic acid soluble radioactivity were much lower in plasma throughout the entire 180 min period of observation. Furthermore, maximal concentrations of trichloroacetic acid precipitable radioactivity in liver were lower, decline was more gradual and ratios of trichloroacetic acid precipitable to trichloroacetic acid soluble radioactivity were and remained considerably higher than was observed after injection of biologically active ^{131}I insulin.

The data indicated that the level of iodination profoundly affected the disposition of ^{131}I insulin. The plasma clearance, tissue distribution and degradation of biologically active ^{131}I insulin involved dose-dependent processes and at physiological levels the liver seemed to dominate the rapid phase of plasma clearance and tissue degradation of ^{131}I insulin. The remarkable influence of the liver on plasma clearance is clearly shown in Figs. 6 and 7. Although the radioiodinated insulin was introduced directly into the systemic circulation the amount of trichloroacetic acid precipitable radioactivity in the liver at 1 min (Fig. 6) after injection exceeded that in plasma but thereafter declined at a faster rate than in plasma.

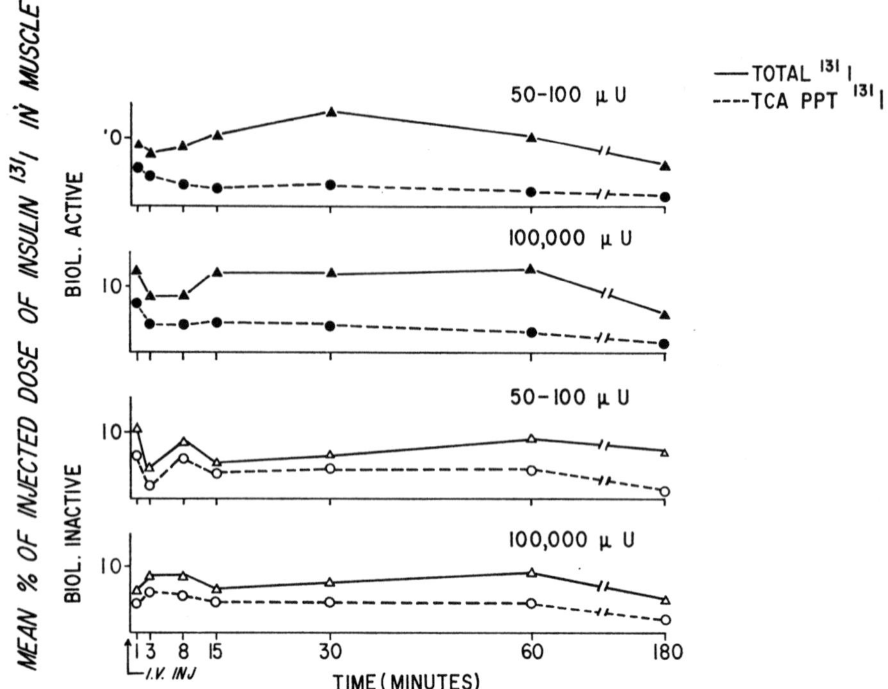

Fig. 5. Variations in concentration of trichloroacetic acid precipitable ^{131}I and total ^{131}I (trichloroacetic acid precipitable + trichloroacetic acid soluble) in muscle with time after intravenous injections of 50—100 μU or 10^5 μU doses of either biologically active or biologically inactive ^{131}I insulin. (Adapted from Izzo *et al.*, 1967)

In Fig. 7 the time scale is greatly expanded so that the peak in liver concentration which occurs in less than 1 min after injection may be clearly demonstrated. The peak in kidney concentration that is evident in Fig. 6 therefore appears as a plateau in Fig. 7. The rapid rise and fall in trichloroacetic acid soluble radioactivity in liver preceeded the rise in plasma suggesting that the liver rapidly degraded insulin and was largely responsible for the early appearance of ^{131}I-labelled insulin degradation products in plasma. The slower uptake of both physiological and pharmacological doses of biologically active ^{131}I insulin by the kidney compared to the liver and the greater percent uptake of pharmacological versus physiological doses by the kidney suggest that the kidney occupies a secondary role in insulin disposition which is inversely related to that of the liver, the process in the liver being relatively saturable and the process in the kidney relatively unsaturable. The decline in radioactivity in the kidney prior to accumulation of radioactivity in urine suggests that the ^{131}I insulin degradation products in liver and kidney were released to plasma, transported to muscle and skin and subsequently released and excreted in the urine. Furthermore, the marked difference in plasma clearance, tissue distribution and degradation of heavily iodinated biologically inactive versus biologically active ^{131}I insulin are in agreement with the conclusion of Lee (1959) that the fate and distribution of ^{131}I insulin in the rat are characteristic and specific for the functionally intact molecule.

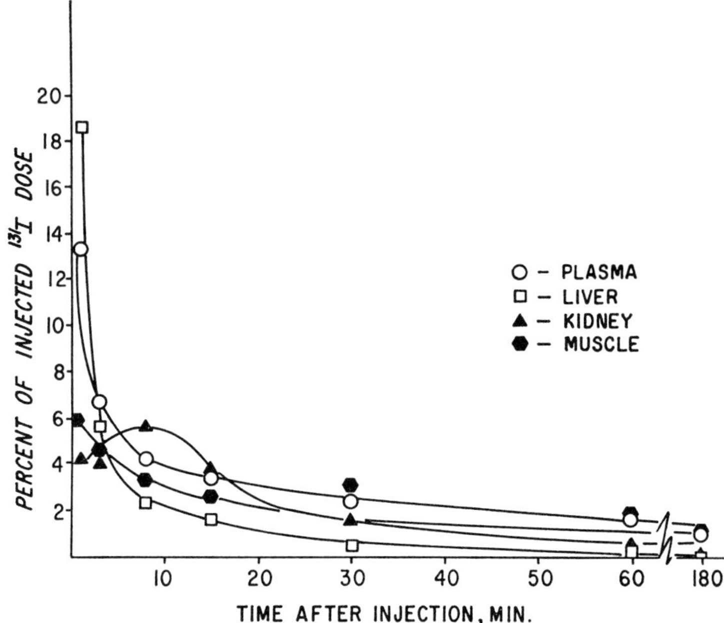

Fig. 6. Variation in concentrations of trichloroacetic acid precipitable ^{131}I in plasma, liver, kidney, and muscle with time after intravenous injection of 50—100 microunits of biologically active ^{131}I insulin. Concentration is expressed as percentage of the injected dose. (From Izzo *et al.*, 1967)

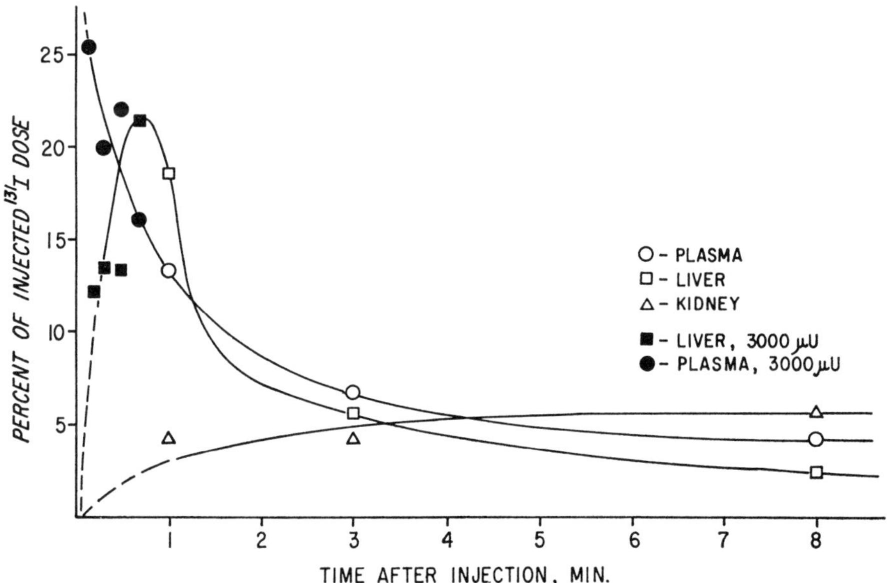

Fig. 7. Variation in concentrations of trichloroacetic acid precipitable ^{131}I in plasma, liver, and kidney for short times after intravenous injection of biologically active ^{131}I insulin. The peak in kidney concentration shown in Fig. 6 appears as a plateau. (From Izzo *et al.*, 1967)

The seemingly greater role of the kidneys than the liver in the disposition of ^{131}I insulin which was indicated by previous studies can be explained in several ways. First of all, as noted above, in previous studies a delay period of several (5—15) min after intravenous injection was permitted in order to insure thorough mixing and equilibration of the ^{131}I insulin between plasma and extracellular fluids. However, by the time the initial observations were made the influence of the liver had probably largely dissipated and hence could easily have been missed. Secondly, since larger doses of insulin were used the distribution to kidneys was greater than if tracer doses had been used. Lastly, the methods which had been utilized to radioiodinate insulin did not easily permit precise control of the amount of iodine attached to insulin and could easily have led to over-iodination or structural alteration of insulin (Izzo *et al.*, 1964a).

5. Role of the Liver and Kidneys in the Distribution and Degradation of Insulin

The major role of the liver in the plasma clearance and degradation of insulin established by the studies of Izzo *et al.* (1967) is in agreement with other studies on hepatic uptake of ^{131}I insulin. Madison *et al.* (1959) injected rapidly into the portal vein of 12 human subjects without liver or pancreatic disease a solution containing 0.55 U of ^{131}I labelled insulin and a known amount of inulin. Ten sec later a brachial arterial blood sample was collected over a 10—15 sec period. The concentration of inulin and ^{131}I insulin were then determined and the volumes of distribution were calculated and compared. Control studies were performed in 8 subjects by injecting the solution of inulin and ^{131}I insulin into the antecubital vein and collecting the arterial blood sample at precisely the same time as after portal injection. In the control sample the volumes of distribution of labelled insulin (2058 ml) and inulin (1989 ml) were almost identical. In contrast, after portal injection the volume of distribution of the labelled insulin (5581 ml) was more than twice as large as than of inulin (2584 ml) indicating to the authors that 52% of the insulin was bound to the human liver in a single transhepatic circulation.

Mortimore *et al.* (1959) investigated the uptake and degradation of ^{131}I insulin by isolated cyclically perfused rat liver and hind limb preparations by following with time the changing distribution of radioactivity among the plasma trichloroacetic acid soluble, trichloroacetic acid precipitable and cellular fractions of the whole blood perfusates. The initial concentration of iodoinsulin was 0.02 μg (500 μU)/ml of blood. A rapid decline in trichloroacetic acid precipitable radioactivity was observed, reaching a mean level of 29.4% by 60 min. However, the rate of appearance of plasma trichloroacetic acid soluble activity was initially slow and by 7.5 min there was only a negligible rise. The delay in appearance of degraded product in the perfusate raises the question of the integrity of the ^{131}I insulin which was utilized or the functional capacity of the isolated organ. Nevertheless the rate constant for the disappearance of plasma trichloroacetic acid precipitable radioactivity was calculable to be about 3 ml/min and on the basis of a hepatic flow rate of 7.0 ml/min it was calculated that approximately 40% of the ^{131}I insulin presented to the isolated perfused liver was removed during any single passage. The rate of ^{131}I insulin uptake by perfused hind limb preparations was far less than that of similarly perfused livers. A progressive decrease in the rate of degradation of ^{131}I insulin concomitant with increasing dilution by native insulin was observed, indicating substrate competition for one or more rate limiting steps.

In further studies (which were published in an abstract) Kaplan and Madison (1959) stated that progressive stimulation of endogenous insulin secretion resulted in a progressive alteration in the magnitude of distribution of insulin between hepatic and peripheral tissues. Studies were conducted in humans undergoing laparotomy by the previously reported method (see above). Endogenous insulin secretion was stimulated to varying degrees by altering the duration of a 5% glucose infusion. In 15 subjects who did not receive glucose prior to intraportal injection, 54% of the labelled insulin was bound to liver during initial transhepatic circulation. In 13 subjects who received 9 gms of glucose over 17 min, hepatic insulin binding fell to 38%. In 12 subjects who received 52 gm of glucose over 165 min, only 7.8% of the labelled insulin was bound to the liver. These results are in essential agreement with the studies of Izzo *et al.* (1967) in rats reported above which showed that the ratio of uptake of ^{131}I insulin by the liver and kidney was greater following intravenous injection of small doses of ^{131}I insulin compared to injection of large doses. However, SAMOLS and RYDER (1961) noted that the proportion of insulin taken up by liver before and during insulin infusion in patients with liver disease and portacaval anastomoses or extrahepatic portal blocks remained relatively constant. The results showed that the liver was capable of removing 20—50% of the insulin passing through it for a period of over 1 h. The hepatic uptake of endogenous insulin in each patient was relatively constant over a period of 60 min. During beef insulin infusion the mechanism for beef insulin capture in the liver behaved as though governed by a first-order system, and was not saturated by arterial plasma beef insulin levels of 250 μU per ml. Since a portal systemic shunt or liver disease was present in most of the patients the relevance of these findings to normals is open to question.

In more recent studies utilizing fasting anesthetized dogs, KADEN *et al.* (1971) have suggested that the hepatic extraction of insulin (HEI) may be directly rather than inversely related to concentration of insulin in the portal vein and that the liver plays a dynamic and important role in regulating peripheral insulin concentration. Blood was obtained frequently from the femoral artery, portal vein and mixed hepatic venous blood by using appropriately placed catheters. The inferior vena cava was ligated below the inflow of hepatic veins. After a control period, glucose (50 gm) was introduced into the duodenum (12 dogs) or increasing amounts of insulin were infused into the portal vein (5 dogs). In both instances, portal vein insulin levels were similar thus making it possible to separate the effects of increasing levels of insulin from hyperglycemia as a determinant of HEI. During the control period HEI was found to be 43 ± 2.7% of the 10 ± 4 mμ/min of insulin presented to the liver, a value in good agreement with the earlier studies of MADISON *et al.* (1959) and MORTIMORE *et al.* (1959). However, 30 min after glucose, HEI rose significantly to 70 ± 7% of the 100 ± 65 mμ/min of insulin presented to the liver. As insulin input fell, HEI returned toward control values. In five dogs infused with insulin, increasing infusion rates increased HEI to 65 ± 1%. Peak HEI coincided with maximal levels of insulin in the blood. Decreasing insulin input by reducing the infusion rate returned HEI toward control values. Insulin infusion lowered blood glucose from 90 to 56 mg/100 ml. The basis for the differences between the findings of KADEN *et al.* and previously mentioned studies is not clear but may possibly reflect species differences.

The role of the kidneys in regulating the concentration of insulin in the peripheral circulation has been fairly extensively investigated. RECORDIER and ANDRAC (1935) noted that bilateral nephrectomy resulted in the persistence up to 100 min of the action of 2 units of insulin injected intravenously, whereas in the same rabbits before nephrectomy, its action was over by then. GOADBY and RICHARDSON (1940) demonstrated a blood sugar lowering effect in the circulation of rabbits after the injection of 40 units intravenously into rabbits, by transfusing the blood in other fasted rabbits; the hypoglycemic effect gradually disappeared over a period of about 90 min. The rate of disappearance was not affected by excluding the liver from the circulation whereas excluding the kidneys from the circulation resulted in a persistence of the insulin action. DRURY *et al.* (1958) showed that ^{131}I insulin degradation, as measured by trichloroacetic acid solubility, was equally as rapid in the eviscerated rabbit with intact kidneys as in the intact rabbit but was relatively slow in the eviscerated-nephrectomized preparation.

PALMER and BOLINGER (1961) investigated the effect of nephrectomy and splanchnicectomy in plasma clearance and consumption of ^{131}I insulin in the rabbit, starting at 10 min after intravenous injection. The rate of insulin consumption was defined as $R = k_1SC$ where R is the consumption of insulin/milliunits/min/kg, k_1 is a first order rate constant for disappearance of labelled insulin from the plasma (min^{-1}), S is the space of distribution of the labelled insulin (ml/kg) and C is the concentration of insulin in the plasma as determined by biological assay (milliunits/ml) and assumed to be constant for each animal. The product k S expressed the volume of body fluid (per kg) which was cleared of labelled material per minute. Nephrectomy resulted in a decrease in plasma insulin clearance from 8.5—4.2 ml/min and a fall in insulin consumption from 7.04—3.64 mU/min/kg. On the other hand, although splanchnicectomy resulted in a fall in insulin clearance to only 2.1 ml/min, insulin consumption was unaffected 10.57×10^{-3}U/min/kg. The data were interpreted to indicate that both renal and splanchnic circulation can function in the degradation of insulin but that at a higher level of plasma insulin concentration the renal circulation can assume all this function, in spite of a decreased insulin clearance.

ZAHARKO *et al.* (1966) utilized a more direct approach in evaluating the role of the kidneys in removing insulin from plasma. Insulin concentration in each sample of dog urine, carotid artery plasma, or renal vein plasma was estimated following the infusion of bovine ^{131}I insulin, unlabelled bovine insulin or glucose. Insulin was estimated by immunoassay and by trichloroacetic acid insoluble radioactivity. Unlabelled insulin solutions were infused for approximately 15 min at the rate of 0.3 μg per kg per min and labelled insulin solutions at the rate of 0.3 mCi per kg per min. The V/A ratio of exogenously infused insulin over 50 min was 55% by immunoassay and 80% for insulin estimated as trichloroacetic acid activity. Assuming that 45% represented an average removal of exogenous insulin and that the blood flow to the kidneys was 25% of the cardiac output per min, it was calculated that the kidneys removed 11% of the circulating insulin per min. Data from experiments in which radioactive insulin was bound to guinea pig anti-insulin serum prior to infusion and from experiments in which ureteral ligation was performed prior to infusion indicated to the authors that the kidney removed insulin primarily by glomerular filtration but that direct absorption also played a role. These observations are in accord with the studies of CHAMBERLAIN and STIMMLER (1967) who investigated the renal handling of insulin by insulin immunoassay of arterial blood, renal venous blood, and urine of fasting patients with normal renal function and in peripheral venous blood and urine of normal subjects and patients with renal disease before and after an oral glucose load. A renal arteriovenous insulin concentration difference of approximately 29% was observed. Assuming a mean serum insulin throughout the day of 14 μU per ml (the midpoint of their normal fasting range, and a normal renal plasma flow of 650 ml per min), it was estimated that the basal daily renal consumption of insulin was approximately 4 units. The insulin excreted in the urine of normal individuals at no time exceeded 1.5% of the load filtered at the glomerulus. In contrast the urinary insulin clearance in patients with severely impaired renal tubular function approached glomerular filtration rate. It was suggested that insulin is normally filtered at the glomerulus and then almost completely reabsorbed or destroyed in the proximal tubule. It was further suggested that if reabsorption occurs, as seems more likely, reabsorbed insulin does not return to the renal vein and is presumably utilized in renal metabolism together with insulin taken up directly from the blood. This is in accord with the conclusions of Izzo *et al.* (1967). Caution was advised in the use of urinary insulin concentration or excretion as an index of serum insulin level or secretion because a very small and variable proportion of filtered insulin appears in the urine in normal subjects and major changes in urinary insulin secretion may arise as a result of minor tubular defects.

The effects of nephrectomy on the disappearance of insulin from plasma are in agreement with observations that have been made in patients with severe renal disease undergoing transplantation (O'Brien and Sharpe, 1967). A significant delay in the second phase of the curve of disappearance of ^{131}I insulin was noted in the uremic state. After transplantation the slope of the ^{131}I insulin disappearance curve approximated that seen in the normal patients (donors). No difference was noted in the slopes of ^{131}I insulin disappearance curves in the normal donors before or after unilateral nephrectomy. In more recent studies, Corvilain *et al.* (1971) have reported a marked reduction of the metabolic clearance rate (MCR) in patients with chronic renal insufficiency and in anephric patients, both of whom had been treated for several months by renal dialysis. Furthermore, the extent of the reduction was comparable in these two groups of patients. The methodology involved the constant infusion (23 μg/kg/min) of mildly iodinated (mean iodination degree less than 0.2 atom/molecule) ^{125}I insulin, the estimation of the plasma content of labelled insulin by chromatoelectrophoresis, and the use of an analog and a digital computer for the calculation of the MCR. The retardation in insulin clearance brought out by nephrectomy or severe renal disease is consistent with and may explain at least in part the amelioration of diabetes and reduction in insulin requirements that have been noted with the onset of the nephrotic syndrome in diabetics (Zubrod *et al.*, 1951; Runyan *et al.*, 1955; and Epstein and Zupa, 1956), in that with severe renal disease insulin clearance by the kidney is reduced and hence insulin remains in the blood stream for a longer period of time. However, Runyan *et al.* (1955) have attributed the amelioration of diabetes and reduction in insulin requirements in the late stages of Kimmelstiel-Wilson syndrome to a large part to anorexia and diminished food intake.

6. Intracellular Distribution of Insulin

On the basis of ultracentrifugation studies Lee and Williams postulated that ^{131}I insulin, which was concentrated in the liver following intravenous injection in rats, penetrated the cell wall, entered the cytoplasm and became fixed to the various cytoplasmic structures and to the nucleus. When ^{131}I insulin was added to homogenate of liver a much smaller amount became fixed to the intracellular components than when it was administered *in vivo*, thereby demonstrating the importance of cellular integrity for the concentration of the hormone. The concentration of insulin in kidney nuclei, mitochondria and residual fraction was greater than that in corresponding fractions of liver, but the concentration in the microsomes was less in the kidney. The concentration in all the elements of muscle was considerably less than in the liver and kidney.

The validity of differential centrifugation procedures in problems of intracellular distribution of insulin is open to criticism on the grounds that tissue fractionation involves marked perturbation of the subcellular components which may lead to their disruption or alteration and hence the observed distribution of radioactivity under these conditions may not reflect the physiological situation. Also, it is possible that insulin in the extracellular fluid might be adsorbed to the subcellular fractions during preparation. However, utilizing a different approach, Stein and Gross (1959) also came to the conclusion that insulin penetrated cells. Ten min after intravenous injection, ^{131}I insulin was shown to be distributed in a volume of about 19% of the volume of muscle. This was in excess of the extracellular space volume and was interpreted as indicating that there is either an intracellular distribution or a concentration of the hormone on the sarcolemma membrane. However, after subcellular fractionation of muscle cells, not only was a concentration in the soluble protein fractions observed but autoradiographically this localization of ^{131}I was shown to be evenly distributed throughout the muscle fibre, without any evidence of sarcolemmal concentration. On the basis of autoradiographic distribution an intracellular distribution was also found in heart muscle, liver and lungs. In the diaphragm, following *in vitro* incubations with ^{131}I insulin the hormone was shown to localize mainly on the fascia covering the muscle.

In more recent studies Brush and Kitabchi (1970) investigated the rate of uptake and release of physiological levels of biologically active ^{131}I insulin from subcellular components of isolated intact rat diaphragm, which was incubated with insulin for 30 min. They also found the largest amount of radioactivity in the soluble fraction i.e. the 100,000 × g supernatant solution, of which more than 70% was degraded insulin. Of the particulate fractions the cell debris sedimenting at 700 × g incorporated 5 times the radioactivity of the mitochondria and 25 times that of the microsomes. The incorporation of radioactivity from ^{131}I insulin into the 100,000 × g supernatant fraction, precipitable with 60% saturated $(NH_4)_2SO_4$, was the only fraction of those studied that was significantly suppressed by the addition of unlabelled insulin. Sephadex G 50 filtration of the fraction demonstrated components of higher molecular weight than insulin, suggesting the presence of an insulin-specific binding component in the fraction.

II. Dynamics of Insulin Distribution

In their studies on the disposition of ^{131}I insulin in the rat Izzo and Bartlett (1967, 1969) directed their attention as much as possible at determination of the role of fundamental processes such as diffusion, mechanisms of chemical reaction and transport of species in the distribution of ^{131}I insulin and its reaction products in the bodies of the rats. A plot of the measured plasma concentrations of trichloroacetic acid precipitable ^{131}I in plasma as a function of the reciprocal of the square root of time after injection of 50—100 and 100,000 μU of biologically active ^{131}I insulin injected intravenously was linear in the low concentration range (Fig. 8). The linearity of the relationship for the data obtained with the 50—100-microunit dose is, with this representation of the data, strongly suggestive of diffusion controlled dispersion from the plasma to other body compartments. Further indication of diffusion-controlled dispersion was obtained through consideration of plasma concentrations for times less than 1 min after injection. The data for times of 1 through 180 min after injection were plotted on log-log paper, and the resulting linear curve was extrapolated back through several decades on the time scale to the point at which 100% plasma concentration (i.e. the injection dose) was predicted to exist (Fig. 9). As seen in Fig. 9 the predicted time is about 0.6 sec and the data obtained for times less than 1 min after injection were found to fall in this extrapolated curve within the limits of experimental error. Thus, diffusion controlled dispersion of trichloroacetic acid precipitable ^{131}I insulin is

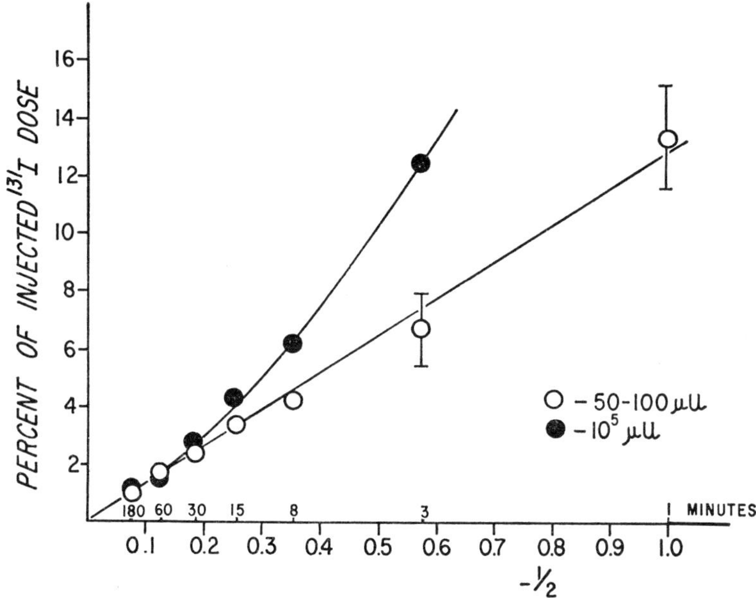

Fig. 8. Variation in concentration of trichloroacetic acid precipitable ^{131}I in plasma as a function of the reciprocal of the square root of time after injection, for 50- to 100-microunit and for 10^5-microunit doses of biologically active ^{131}I insulin injected intravenously. (From Izzo *et al.*, 1967)

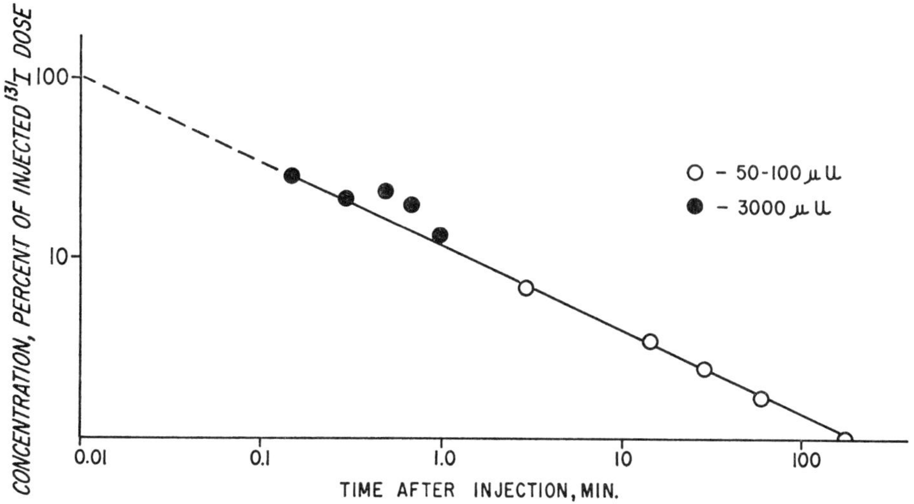

Fig. 9. Variation in concentration of trichloroacetic acid precipitable ^{131}I in plasma as a function of time after intravenous injection, in log-log coordinates. 50—100 microunits of biologically active ^{131}I insulin; 3000 microunits of biologically active ^{131}I insulin. The linear correlation has a slope of —0.5. (From Izzo *et al.*, 1967)

indicated for the 50—100 microunit dose, throughout the entire time interval studied.

Diffusion-controlled dispersion was not clearly indicated for the 10^5 microunit dose of biologically active ^{131}I insulin (Fig. 7). Rather, for times up to about 30 min, higher plasma concentrations and more rapid rate of concentration decrease were observed relative to the 50—100 microunit dose. After 30 min the percent concentrations in respect to injected dose and rate of change appeared to be comparable to those for the 50—100 microunit dose. These differences were believed due to the influence of the peripheral clearance mechanism (reaction rate capacity of the liver and kidney) on plasma concentrations with the 10^5 microunit dose. In brief the observed changes in plasma concentration of the 10^5 microunit dose could be explained qualitatively by assuming that there was so much reactant (i.e. intact ^{131}I insulin) available, that the rate at which it could be handled by reaction sites was severely limited. High concentrations of intact ^{131}I insulin were present in the liver and kidney, the concentration gradient for diffusion was correspondingly diminished or eliminated, and concentrations in plasma were actually governed by mechanisms associated with the reaction process.

The plasma clearance of low and high doses of heavily iodinated biologically inactive insulin also appeared to be a diffusion controlled process as indicated by the shape of the curves which were obtained by plotting the variation in concentration of trichloroacetic acid precipitable ^{131}I in plasma as a function of the reciprocal of the square root of time after the intravenous injection of 50—100 microunit and 10^5 microunit doses (Fig. 10). The sluggish clearance of biologically inactive ^{131}I insulin was attributed to lack of degradation presumably in liver and kidney. Subsequent studies *in vitro* (Izzo *et al.*, 1972) showed that liver homogenates were capable of degrading heavily iodinated insulin but at a much slower

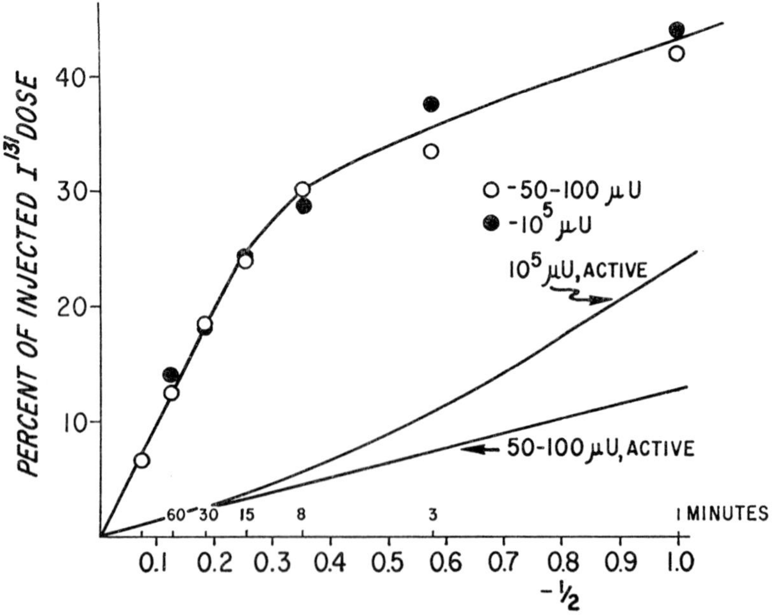

Fig. 10. Variation in concentration of trichloroacetic acid precipitable ^{131}I in plasma as a function of the reciprocal of the square root of time after injection, for 50- to 100-microunit and for 10^5-microunit doses of biologically inactive ^{131}I insulin injected intravenously. Correlations for biologically active ^{131}I insulin, given in Fig. 8 are shown for comparison. (From Izzo *et al.*, 1967)

rate than lightly iodinated insulin. Failure of the studies *in vivo* to indicate degradation of heavily iodinated insulin by liver and kidney was explained on the basis that degradation processes in these organs were so slow that they were overwhelmed by transport or flow processes. Further evidence of the relationships between biological activity, ^{131}I insulin degradation and *in vivo* plasma clearance was demonstrated by comparing the clearance rates for ^{131}I insulin and inert iodide containing ^{131}I. As shown in Fig. 11 rate of clearance for the biologically inactive ^{131}I insulin and the inert iodide were identical and much lower than the clearance rate for the biologically active ^{131}I insulin. In the figure actual concentrations of intact biologically inactive ^{131}I insulin were divided by 3.13 to bring concentrations at 1 min after injection to the same level.

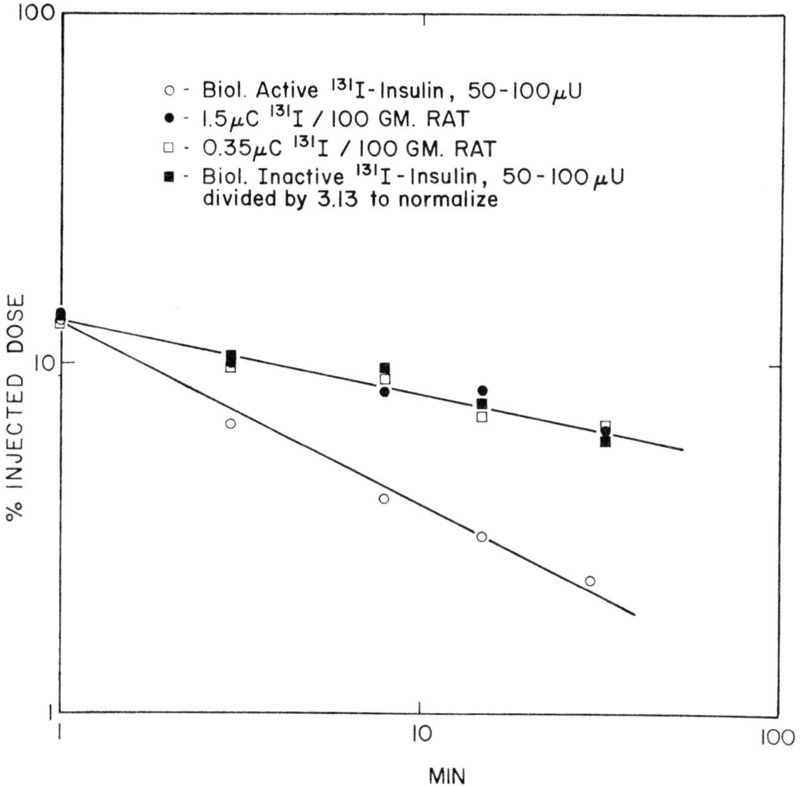

Fig. 11. Clearance of biologically active and biologically inactive ^{131}I insulins and sodium ^{131}I from the plasma of the rat. (From Izzo and Bartlett, 1969)

It was concluded that ^{131}I insulin species seem to be exchanged between the plasma and various body compartments by unsteady-state molecular diffusion processes in which the body compartments behave as semi-infinite homogenous media. Superimposed on the diffusional processes are chemical reaction processes in the liver and kidney, with both organs behaving as semibatch reactors. The existence of peak concentrations of ^{131}I insulin in liver and kidneys suggested that a "critical volumetric capacity" must be achieved before significant reaction occurs, of about 3.7% of the injected ^{131}I dose per gm of organ. Analysis of the degradative process in liver and kidneys indicated that degradation of ^{131}I insulin appeared to occur by a reaction which was second order with respect to reactant species. The major muscle mass appeared to behave as a capacitor which accepts ^{131}I insulin from the plasma when the concentrations are high and rejects material to the plasma, for transport to other organs and tissues, when plasma concentrations are low. The existence of degradation reactions in the muscle mass was neither confirmed nor denied by the experimental data.

III. Kinetics of Insulin Distribution

1. Rate of Plasma Insulin Disappearance (Half-Life Concept)

Berson *et al.* (1956) attempted to derive information on the biological half-life of insulin in humans by analysis of the curve of plasma disappearance of intravenously injected ^{131}I labelled insulin in the range of 0.1—7.0 U. In this type of analysis the initial rapid disappearance phase of the curve is attributed to mixing of the radioactive tracer throughout its volume of distribution and subsequent slower phase of disappearance to its metabolic removal. The late portion of the curve is extrapolated to time zero and the resulting straight line is then analyzed. Plasma ^{131}I insulin was isolated by a paper electrophoresis technic in which the labelled insulin is adsorbed to the paper at the site of application thus permitting separation from plasma protein bound radioactivity. On this basis the half time of disappearance from plasma of adsorbed radioactivity (^{131}I insulin) after distribution in body fluids was of the order of 40 min which was found to be in good agreement with the rate of degradation of ^{131}I insulin as estimated from the rate of appearance of non-precipitable radioactivity in the plasma. ^{131}I insulin was distributed into an apparent volume averaging about 37% of body weight. In diabetic subjects who had been treated with insulin for months to years the plasma disappearance of ^{131}I insulin was much slower than in subjects never treated with insulin or treated with insulin for 2—3 months. The persistence of relatively high concentrations of ^{131}I insulin in the plasma of insulin-treated subjects was shown to be due to binding of ^{131}I insulin by an acquired globulin which satisfied the criteria for an antibody. The insulin-insulin binding antibody complex migrated in the front running γ globulin region on paper or starch block electrophoresis at pH 7.3 or 8.6. The binding of insulin to circulating globulin in insulin-treated diabetics was confirmed by ultracentrifugation studies in which it was observed that ^{131}I insulin in the serum of these subjects sedimented with the globulins while in normal subjects the radioinsulin sedimented at a slower rate than serum albumin.

Orskov and Christensen (1966) observed in the course of studies of human forearm metabolism that the half-life of insulin after its injection was much shorter than had been reported by Berson *et al.* (1956). The decrease in serum insulin concentrations in arterial and venous blood at 3 min intervals after injection of 8 units of exogenous unlabelled human insulin was followed. Insulin was determined by immunoassay. Fasting serum insulin values were subtracted from the observed values which were plotted on a logarithmic scale on the ordinate, against time. Half-life was determined from the slope of disappearance in insulin concentration after the first 15 min. Assuming that the pancreatic output of insulin did not change during the experiment, they calculated in 5 patients, investigated in this manner, that the insulin half-life was between 5 and 15 min. In contrast to the results of BERSON *et al.* the volume of distribution was calculated to be only about 20 % of body-weight when the arterial curves were used for calculation. SAMOLS and MARKS (1966) arrived at a similar conclusion in their studies of half-life of endogenous insulin in plasma. The latter found that endogenous plasma insulin, measured by immunoassay, decreased with a half-time of 7—15 min in healthy volunteers after discontinuing prolonged intravenous infusions of a combination of glucose (12 g/min) and glucagon (30 μg/min). The infusions were used to produce a relative plateau of very high endogenous insulin levels ca. 500 μU/min for at least 60 min so that the rate of decline would represent metabolic turnover of insulin rather than its distribution into extravascular spaces. WILLIAMS *et al.* (1968) estimated the half-life of endogenous serum insulin following the end of prolonged glucose infusions in actual subjects who achieved peak levels of glucose between 131—221 mg %. The estimates were 16 min if pancreatic insulin production was assumed to cease following the end of glucose infusion or 9 min if basal insulin secretion was assumed to continue following the end of the glucose infusion. The t 1/2 values were calculated by simple regression analysis of the decline in serum IRI. The calculations included only those values at consecutive time intervals where the decline following the cessation of glucose perfusion best fit a single exponential.

Similar results were also reported by two other groups of investigators utilizing unlabelled insulin and immunoassay procedures. TOMASI *et al.* (1967) utilizing the second slope of the plasma disappearance curve, that is, the portion of the curve between 10 and 35 min after injection, calculated a t 1/2 of 6.5—9.0 min in normal subjects who received 2 units of unlabelled insulin intravenously. HORTON *et al.* (1968) estimated an average half-life of 13 min in normals and a longer half-life in uremic subjects following intravenous injection of 0.1 unit of beef insulin per kg b.w. On the other hand MARTIN *et al.* (1967) observed a plasma half-life of only 3—7 min with a mean of 4.9 min in healthy human volunteers. In their studies, 0.1 unit per kg of glucagon-free insulin (obtained from Eli Lilly) was injected into a vein, blood samples were taken at 5 min intervals and insulin determined by immunoassay. The half-time of disappearance of plasma insulin was calculated by plotting the values on a semi-logarithmic scale and extrapolating from the line of best fit. When they recalculated the data of ORSKOV and CHRISTENSEN (1966), according to their method, an approximate half-time of disappearance of $6^1/_2$ min was obtained. Based on calculations from the known rate of removal of insulin from the circulation by the liver, and kidney at "tracer levels" STIMMLER (1966) estimated a half-life of 3—$3^1/_2$ min. Both of the latter investigators utilized the initial steeper portion of the curve to calculate plasma half-life of insulin. In a subsequent study ORSKOV and CHRISTENSEN (1969) analyzed the curves of disappearance of intravenously injected unlabelled exogenous insulin, as measured by immunoassay in several ways. Four different calculations were made on the basis of the individual curve plotted on semilog paper: a) half-life obtained from the linear portion of the graph after 20 min (t 1/2), b) the half-life calculated on the basis of the linear part of the curve as in a) but in this case after subtraction of the fasting insulin concentration (t 1/2 — sub), c) the time before the graph became linear and d) the initial half-life obtained after retropolation and subtraction of the linear part of the curve from the initial steep part (t 1/2 initial). The values (in min) $\pm$S.D.M. in younger non-diabetic subjects were: a) 10.6$\pm$1.9, b) 7.6$\pm$0.9, c) 20.6$\pm$1.9 and d) 2.9$\pm$0.7. In older nondiabetic subjects the values were: a) 13.0$\pm$2.5, b) 9.0$\pm$1.4, c) 20.3$\pm$4.1 and d) 3.5$\pm$0.9.

No significant differences were noted by ORSKOV and CHRISTENSEN (1969) in the disappearance rates of intravenously-injected unlabelled insulin between non-diabetics and adult-onset diabetics who had never been treated with insulin on the basis of any of the four different methods of calculation that were employed to estimate disappearance rate. Tomasi *et al.* (1967) and Martin *et al.* (1967) also found no significant difference in disappearance rates of non-diabetics and diabetics who had not been treated with insulin. However, Stimmler (1967) reported significantly lower rates of disappearance in adult-onset diabetics, t 1/2 of 4.8 min versus a t 1/2 of 3.3 min in normals. On the basis of their own observations that the t 1/2 of their older subjects was slightly longer than that of younger subjects whether they were diabetic or not, Orskov and Christensen attributed Stimmler's findings to age differences since in the latter studies the mean age of the diabetics was 56 ± 9 years versus 41 ± 16 years for the controls. However, Stimmler noted no significant differences between rate constant for insulin disappearance and age or weight, and in the diabetic group there was also no significant correlation with duration of diabetes.

Bolinger *et al.* (1964) investigated the curves of disappearance of ^{131}I-labelled insulin from plasma as a guide to management of diabetes. Intravenous injections of 25 mCi of ^{131}I-labelled insulin containing less than 0.5 unit of insulin were administered to diabetic patients who had never received insulin (Group 1), insulin-treated patients who were easily regulated (Group 2) and insulin-treated patients with excessive lability characterized by frequent insulin reactions alternating with periods of hyperglycemia and ketoacidosis (Group 3). Serum specimens were collected at intervals of 10 min for 60 min after injection. A logarithmic plot of serum trichloroacetic acid precipitable radioactivity was interpreted as showing an initial rapid component, linear 10—20 min, and a slower component reaching linearity after 30 min. The mean half-life (t 1/2) of ^{131}I insulin disappearance based on the rapid component (10—20 min) for the Group 1 patients was 14.6 min, for Group 2 patients 23.5 min and for Group 3 patients 58.6 min. It was found that patients with the longest half-life for disappearance of labelled insulin (740 min) obtained optimal regulation on regular insulin alone whereas those with a half-life in the range of 20—40 min were best regulated with mixtures of isophane insulin and regular insulin. Those with an insulin half-life of less than 20 min were best regulated on isophane insulin alone.

McAdams *et al.* (1967) also investigated the "rapid-phase" disappearance curve following intravenous injections of radioinsulin in 43 cases of diabetes, grouped according to the criteria of Bolinger *et al.* (1964). However, although in all but four of 30 patients who had received insulin prior to the test the t 1/2 was definitely prolonged as compared with those patients who had not taken insulin, no difference was noted between the groups who were considered to be easily regulated on one dose of insulin a day and those who were difficult to manage. The half-time disappearance of intravenously-injected ^{131}I insulin based on slopes obtained from serum samples between 10 and 20 min were 13.9, 34.1 and 31.0 min for Group I, II and III respectively and 11.1, 31.4 and 32.3 min respectively based on slopes between 10 and 15 min samples. An inverse relationship between the t 1/2 values and the percent of unbound insulin in the serum was observed. An inverse relationship was also noted between the percent of unbound insulin in the serum and the percent of total radioactivity in the gamma globulin fraction of the serum protein.

2. Limitations of Plasma Half-Life Estimates

A major problem in estimation of metabolic or, more strictly speaking, plasma half-life of insulin on the basis of decline of intravenously-injected doses of labelled or unlabelled insulin utilizing extrapolation technics such as described above is that such technics may be useful only when mixing is rapid relative to metabolic removal or degradation. However, where both processes proceed at rapid rates, a smoothly curvilinear junction is obtained which shows no definite break to indicate the point at which distribution and mixing is complete and metabolic removal has begun. Under these conditions the decision as to where the break occurs is arbitrary and the half-life will depend upon which portion of the curve is "linearized". The rapid removal of insulin mainly by the liver during the initial phase of distribution has been clearly demonstrated in the studies of Izzo *et al.* (1967). The latter also noted that the plasma disappearance of biologically active ^{131}I insulin was a non-linear process, as shown by the curvilinearity of the data when plotted on semilog paper, and that the data could not be validly described by a simple exponential relationship. Furthermore, the disappearance curve was influenced by the amount of insulin injected and this sensitivity was related to chemical rate processes in the liver and kidney. The non-linearity of the ^{131}I plasma disappearance curve was also pointed out by ARNOULD *et al.* in dogs (1967) and by STERN *et al.* in humans (1969). The plasma disappearance curve of unlabelled insulin also appears to be non-linear when plotted on semilog paper (ORSKOV and CHRISTENSEN (1966), SAMOLS and MARKS (1966), and TOMASI *et al.* (1967)). However, by subtracting the equilibrium levels which were reached following the intravenous injection of insulin, from each of the plasma insulin levels at each time interval, STIMMLER (1967) reported that the natural logarithm of the resultant values plotted against time demonstrated a negative linear relationship.

ARNOULD *et al.* (1967) studied the kinetics of plasma disappearance of intravenous injections of lightly iodinated biologically active ^{131}I insulin in dogs in an effort to obtain a precise mathematical expression governing the whole of the disappearance curve. This involved the administration of large doses of radioactivity, the use of specific techniques for the determination of plasma insulin and the assistance of computers to analyze the experimental data. The analysis was performed in a compartmental perspective and was directed at determining the minimal number of exponentials which might account for the kinetics of the labelled compound. The plasma disappearance curve of labelled insulin was found to correspond to a multiexponential function comprising at least 3 exponentials and one constant. The formula was confirmed by studying curves obtained by continuous infusions which represented the integrals of disappearance curves. On the basis of the results after analysis the authors felt obliged to reject a catenary model and to accept for the kinetics of labelled insulin a mamillary model with feedback of the labelled compound from the peripheral compartments towards the plasmatic compartment. A catenary model, which had previously been accepted to study kinetics of insulin disappearance, assumed that after diffusion within the extracellular fluids, insulin definitely disappeared from the fluid compartments by tissue degradation and urine excretion. In such a system, after the stage of diffusion, the disappearance curve should be expressed by a single exponential, the slope of which would represent the sum of the rate constants of the various elimination processes. It was further pointed out that with a multiexponential function each exponential term cannot be the direct expression of the unique physiological process but represents the results of the various movements of the labelled compound to and from the plasmatic compartment. It was concluded that this consequence precludes the use of *any part* or *component* of the curve for the direct calculation of a so-called "half-life" of radioinsulin.

3. Alternative Methods of Analysis of Plasma Insulin Disappearance

In view of the shortcomings of utilizing first order concepts to analyze the curves of disappearance of ^{131}I insulin from plasma, Stern *et al.* (1968) analyzed the plasma disappearance curves of immunoprecipitable radioactive insulin in alternative ways. In the first approach removal of ^{131}I insulin from plasma was studied in normal and diabetic subjects with both single injection and continuous infusion of isotope technics. Patients were studied either in the fasting state or during steady-state hyperglycemia produced by a continuous intravenous glucose infusion. Steady-state plasma insulin concentration during these studies ranged from 10—264 μU/ml. Labelled insulin specific activity time curves consisted of more than one exponential indicating that a multicompartmental system for insulin metabolism existed. A mathematical technic which was considered applicable to non-first order processes was utilized to calculate the rate at which insulin was lost irreversibly from the plasma pool. In this procedure the disappearance curve of plasma immunoprecipitable radioactivity was plotted on graph paper with ordinary coordinates, the area under the circumscribed curve, which was estimated by planimetry, was divided into the dose of administered tracer, and the quotient, under appropriate conditions was considered to represent the *fractional irreversible loss rate of insulin from plasma*. Irreversible loss rate of insulin from plasma ranged from 1200—10,455 μU/min (0.02—0.63 U/hour) for the fasting studies and from 3320—37,818 μU/min (1.20—2.27 U/hour) for the glucose infusion studies. The observed linearity was considered to imply lack of saturability of the insulin removal mechanisms. Since the plasma insulin pool was in a steady state during these studies, it was assumed that insulin irreversible loss rate was equal to the rate at which newly secreted insulin was being delivered to the general circulation. The results were interpreted to indicate that changes in plasma insulin concentration resulted from parallel changes in the rate of insulin delivery and not from changes in the opposite direction of the rate of insulin removal. The wide range of insulin delivery rates among patients with similar plasma glucose relationships suggested that the responsiveness to endogenous insulin among these patients was quite variable.

In an effort to begin construction of a more sophisticated model of insulin kinetics, Silvers *et al.* (1969), extended their studies of plasma disappearance of ^{131}I insulin to include patients with terminal renal failure, in view of the earlier studies suggesting that the kidneys played an important role in plasma decrease and degradation of insulin. ^{131}I insulin in doses of 0.25 mCi/kg b.w. (approximately ca. 4500 μU/kg) was injected intravenously to normal subjects, to patients with maturity-onset diabetes and normal renal function, and to non-diabetic patients with renal failure. Typical ^{131}I insulin plasma disappearance curve for each group is shown in Fig. 12. The plasma disappearance curves of immunoprecipitable radioactive insulin were analyzed in three increasingly complex ways. In the first approach, fractional irreversible loss rates of insulin from plasma were calculated as previously described and were found to be greatly decreased in patients with renal failure ($t\,1/2 = 39$ min), as compared to normals ($t\,1/2 = 15$ min) and diabetics ($t\,1/2 = 12$ min). Although the method appeared to provide quantitative data which clearly distinguished patients with renal failure from those with renal function, it failed to provide any description of the predicted multicompartmental system of insulin disposition. Hence, a second and more complicated quantitative method was utilized based upon resolution of plasma ^{131}I insulin disappearance into various numbers of components by the method of "peeling". The plasma

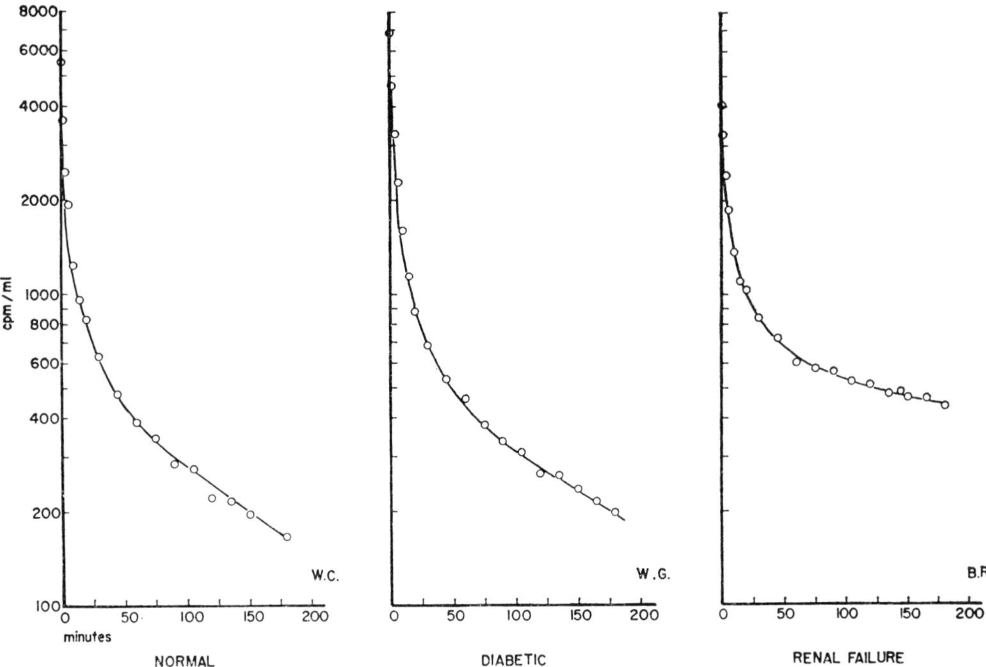

Fig. 12. Typical insulin-^{131}I plasma disappearance curves for each patient group. (From SILVERS *et al.*, 1969)

^{131}I insulin disappearance curves were resolved into sums of three exponentials and the values for the resultant three slopes and half-lives were determined. Diabetic patients with normal renal function had slightly lower half-lives for all three components (Table 1) while patients with renal failure displayed a marked prolongation of the half-life of the third component to 275 min (approximately twice normal).

Finally, recognizing that the results of the second type of analysis, although capable of generating the most meaningful data, were not necessarily relevant to any biological system a three pool model was formulated to describe the kinetics of plasma insulin disappearance in man (Fig. 13). The first pool was considered to represent plasma, the second interstitial fluid volume and the third all those

Table 1. *Half Life of Component Slopes (t 1/2)**

	Three component case		
	First component[a]	Second component[a]	Third component[a]
Normal	2.411 ± 0.192	14.114 ± 0.623	132.80 ± 11.88
Diabetic	1.875 ± 0.260	8.281 ± 0.497	101.18 ± 7.40
Renal failure	1.557 ± 0.217	10.400 ± 1.272	275.54 ± 31.30

* t 1/2 was obtained from the component slopes using the formula $t\,1/2 = \frac{0.693}{\text{slope}}$ and is expressed in minutes.

[a] Mean ± SE.

From SILVERS *et al.* (1969).

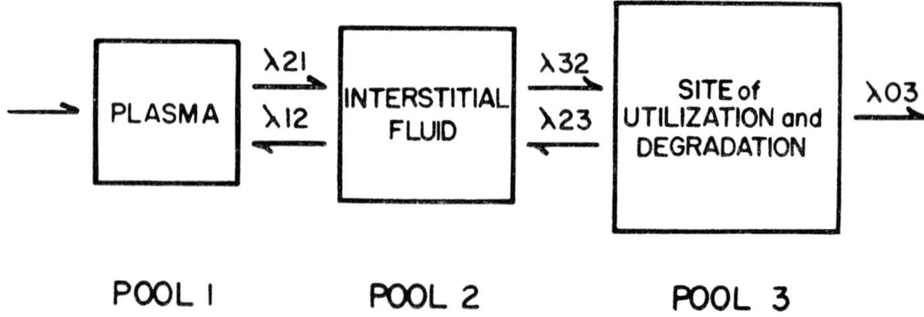

Fig. 13. A three compartment model describing ^{131}I-insulin plasma disappearance. (From SILVERS *et al.*, 1969)

tissues which utilize and degrade insulin. The third pool is not clearly homogenous and is considered to represent at least muscle, adipose tissue, kidney and liver. The proposed model provided an excellent fit for the experimental data obtained in all three groups of patients. Furthermore, volumes (percent of body weight) of postulated pool 1 (4.04) and pool 2 (10.11), calculated on the basis of the model and the experimental data, corresponded very closely to estimates of these pool sizes obtained by different technics. The model also demonstrated that patients with renal failure were characterized by a decreased removal rate of insulin from pool 3 and an increased recycling rate of insulin from pool 3 to pool 2.

KRISHNA RAM *et al.* (1972) investigated the fractional insulin clearance rates (metabolic clearance rate of TAIT, 1963) in 7 controls and 19 patients with different types of diabetes mellitus on the basis of the plasma ^{131}I insulin disappearance curves, following rapid intravenous injection of 0.75 mCi (1.8—2.5 milliunit) per kg b.w. of ^{131}I beef insulin into a peripheral vein. In these studies the data were plotted on semilog paper and theoretical zero time radioactivity was calculated by interpolating the 5 and 15 min values. These values were then plotted on ordinary coordinates and areas under these radioactivity time curves determined by planimetry after extrapolating the terminal portion of the time curve. Fractional clearance rate of insulin was calculated as follows:

$$\begin{matrix}\text{FCRI} \\ \text{or} \\ \text{MCR}\end{matrix} = \frac{\text{R}}{\int_0^{\infty} x' \, dt} \qquad \text{TAIT (1963)}$$

where FCRI represents the fractional clearance rate of insulin (metabolic clearance rate of TAIT, 1963) R the injected dose and $\int_0^{\infty} x' \, dt$ the integral of plasma radioactive concentrations, determined by planimetry. The FCRI obtained in μCi was converted into μU of insulin, using appropriate factors obtained from each batch of iodinated insulin used. The biological half-lives were also calculated for the second and third components of curve obtained on semilog paper.

Excluding the first component on the assumption that it represented predominantly the distribution phase of insulin, the biological half-lives of the second and third component of the experimental curves did not show any statistically significant variation in the control or diabetic groups. The fractional insulin clearance rates (Table 2) from plasma did not significantly differ in the various groups studied. From these data they concluded that the higher plasma insulin concentrations, they had reported earlier (KRISHNA RAM and AHUJA, 1970) in young

Table 2. *Fractional insulin clearance rates (μU/min/unit concentration in plasma) from plasma of control and various diabetic groups*

Number of subjects	Control	Young ketosis prone diabetics (5)	Young ketosis resistant diabetics (7)	Maturity onset diabetics (7)
1	14230	2754	1470	3494
2	2720	2774	5616	4158
3	2831	3666	5828	3426
4	2970	5160	17216	925
5	8068	6283	11483	1415
6	5204	—	2890	9541
7	5911	—	17635	10314
Mean	5990.6	4127.4	8862.6	4753.3
Median	5204.0	3666.0	5828.0	3494.0

$x^2 = 1.7$ $p = 0.63693$

From Krishna Ram *et al.* (1972).

ketosis resistant diabetics and maturity onset diabetics were probably achieved by higher secretion rates in these groups than in the control or ketosis prone groups. They stated that the t 1/2 obtained for the second and third components, which in time sequence corresponded with the tissue phase of Silvers *et al.* (1969) were much longer than those reported by the latter, possibly related to different methods which were employed in isolating and quantitating the ^{131}I insulin.

Since the method of Stern *et al.* (1968) for calculating insulin delivery rate did not apply to "non-steady state" situations and were not suitable for assessing changes in the rate of hormonal delivery Turner *et al.* (1971) have recently reported a method in which the disappearance rate of an intravenous injection of insulin is used to interpret plasma insulin levels so that rapid changes in the rate at which insulin enters the systemic circulation can be estimated. Plasma insulin levels were examined in relation to the "non-steady state" disappearance rate measured following an intravenous infusion of human monocomponent insulin μg/kg (i.e. 0.025 U/kg) into six normal non-obese subjects. Plasma insulin levels were determined by immunoassay. The plasma insulin disappearance rate was obtained from the declining plasma insulin levels following the peak insulin value which occurred at the end of the 1-min infusion. The insulin delivery rates were calculated on the basis of the difference between the measured insulin levels and the insulin levels which were calculated from the insulin disappearance rate, assuming that no more insulin had entered the circulation since last measurement of plasma insulin concentration. The insulin delivery rate in response to intravenous glucose (35 gm) was determined. The previously-reported biphasic insulin secretory response to intravenous glucose (Cerasi and Luft, 1963; and Porte and Pupo, 1969) was confirmed. The basal rate of insulin delivery to the systemic circulation in the six subjects studied was 0.007—0.016 U/min. In the first phase (taken as the first 6 min) after intravenous glucose 0.23—1.53 U of insulin entered the general circulation and 1.2—3.3 U in the subsequent 54 min.

Recently Genuth (1972) also investigated the metabolic clearance of insulin in man under conditions of acutely and chronically altered endogenous plasma insulin utilizing ^{131}I bovine insulin as tracer and the technic of constant infusion to equilibrium. In addition, clearances of unlabelled porcine insulin were also measured simultaneously with that of radioiodinated insulin in order to determine the quantitative accuracy of the latter. Metabolic clearance of ^{131}I bovine insulin was calculated from the infusion rate divided by plasma level (according to Tait, 1963). Metabolic clearance of unlabelled porcine insulin was calculated from the same equation. The results showed that compared to normal subjects clearance of radioiodinated insulin (measured as immunoprecipitable radioactivity) was unaffected by diabetes, but was increased 25% in obese subjects with hyperinsulinemia and did not change when their plasma insulin was reduced by 7 day fasting. Acute elevations of plasma endogenous insulin of 50—200 μU/ml above basal levels by glucose or tolbutamide injections to normal and obese subjects also failed to change clearance of iodinated insulin. The data were interpreted to support the assumption that alterations of plasma insulin in such circumstances reflected largely alterations in insulin secretion. However, simultaneous clearance of unlabelled insulin and radioiodinated insulin in both normal and diabetic subjects produced disparate results. The mean values were as follows: in normals: unlabelled insulin 860 ml/min, radioiodinated insulin 227 ml/min; in diabetics: unlabelled insulin 788/ml, radioiodinated insulin 202 ml/min. The ratio of unlabelled to radioiodinated insulin clearance was 3.8 (normals), 4.1 (diabetics).

Sherwin *et al.* (1972) have utilized the SAAM computer program to calculate insulin's metabolic clearance rate (MCR), basal systemic delivery rate (BSD) and parameters of a multicompartmental model in young (mean = 28 years) and older (mean = 66 years) male volunteers. The studies were undertaken to determine whether difference in kinetics of the distribution and destruction of insulin may contribute to the decreased carbohydrate tolerance of aging. Native porcine insulin was administered intravenously either as a single pulse (25 mU/kg) or as a primed continuous infusion (1 or 2 mU/kg/min) for 80 min. The arterial blood glucose concentration was maintained at basal levels for 10 h by a periodically adjusted infusion of intravenous glucose (glucose clamp technic). The amount of infused glucose was used as an index of glucose utilization. The MCR and BSD (451 ± 18 ml/min/M^2 and $5{,}000 \pm 341$ μU/min/M^2 of young subjects did not differ significantly from the MCR and BSD of older subjects (422 ± 7 ml/min/M^2 and $4{,}520 \pm 511$ μU/min/M^2 (mean$\pm$SEM)). A three compartmental model which is somewhat at variance with that proposed by Silvers *et al.* (1969) was found necessary to fit the data from the different protocols: compartment 1 (plasma) in rapid equilibrium with compartment 2 (interstitial fluid) and in slow equilibrium with compartment 3 (interstitial fluid beds of large size and low blood flow, i.e. muscle and adipose tissue). Model parameters were not significantly different for young and old subjects. The time course of glucose utilization did not correlate with the time course of plasma insulin concentration but closely paralleled the computed insulin concentration in compartment 3.

In very recent studies Palumbo *et al.* (1972) compared the "relative disappearance curves" of both radioiodinated and unlabelled bovine insulin from plasma in normals as well as in stable and unstable diabetics. In this study initial serum samples were collected at 5 min after injection and measured insulin concentrations beyond 5 min were all replaced by relative concentrations defined as the ratio of a concentration to the one measured at 5 min (expressed as a percentage). Bovine unlabelled insulin in plasma was measured by immunoassay and radioiodinated insulin was determined by measuring total radioactivity in the plasma. The mean height of the disappearance curve from 5—60 min plotted on semilog paper was selected as a practical measure of insulin disappearance curve characteristics. Mean height was measured as the area under the relative disappearance curve divided by the time span, 55 min. A mixture of 10 μCi of ^{131}I labelled bovine insulin which contained less than 0.1 unit of biologically active insulin and three units of unlabelled crystalline unmodified insulin was injected intravenously in all 30 patients studied. A significant negative association was found between the disappearance of bovine insulin from plasma and the insulin binding level of circulating insulin antibodies in patients taking insulin. The mean heights (± SEM) of disappearance curves of radioiodinated (RII) and immunoreactive insulin (IRI) (% of 5 min concentration) were respectively 56.7±1.7 and 33.9±2.2 in insulin taking diabetics with <5% insulin-binding, 64.2±2.5 and 48.3±5.4 in diabetics with 5—25% insulin binding and 87.5±0 and 106.0±27.8 in these patients with >25% insulin-binding (insulin resistant). No significant differences were noted in the mean heights (± SEM) of disappearance of RII and IRI, 43.3±1.3 and 15.8±1.3 in normal subjects and diabetics not taking insulin 46.9±2.0 and 18.5±1.4. In contrast to studies of Bolinger *et al.* (1964) and in agreement with the results of McAdams *et al.* (1967) no evidence was found that patients with unstable diabetes had a slower disappearance of bovine insulin than did patients with stable diabetes. The overall difference in bovine insulin disappearance in the two groups could be accounted for by differences in the number of patients in each group with insulin antibody binding of 5% or more. Chronic diabetic complications had no effect on the plasma disappearance of insulin. However, a small (but not statistically significant) delay was observed in the disappearance of bovine insulin from plasma in diabetic patients who were not on insulin treatment and demonstrated no insulin-binding antibodies. The authors concluded that immunologic determination of unlabelled insulin for the evaluation of the insulin disappearance from plasma seemed to be preferable to the use of radioiodinated insulin because of the delay in disappearance of the latter. However, it should be pointed out that radioiodinated insulin disappearance was based on total radioactivity in plasma. This is not a valid measure of radioiodinated insulin disappearance since total radioactivity measures both radioiodinated insulin and radioiodinated degradation products in plasma and since as shown in studies in rats (Izzo *et al.*, 1967) the fall in plasma radioiodinated insulin is accompanied by a parallel rise in ^{131}I labelled degradation products in plasma.

4. Limitations of Estimation of Metabolic Clearance Rates or Fractional Loss Rates of Insulin from Plasma

The studies of Genuth (1972) suggesting that radioiodinated insulin is cleared from plasma more slowly than unlabelled insulin cast some doubts on the validity of utilizing radioiodinated insulin as a tracer. Ooms *et al.* (1968) had arrived at a similar conclusion in their studies of the effect of degree of iodination on metabolic clearance of insulin. ^{125}I or ^{131}I pork insulin preparation containing an average of 0.2—4.9 iodine atoms per molecule of insulin were prepared by either an electrolytic or elementary iodine oxidation method. Normal anesthetized dogs which were maintained in normoglycemia by glucose infusion were infused with mixtures of crystalline and labelled insulins or with two differently labelled insulins (^{125}I and ^{131}I). Total metabolic clearance rates were determined by infusion to equilibrium technic. Crystalline insulin was determined by immunoprecipitation. Their results showed that metabolic clearance of insulin was reduced by radioiodination in direct proportion to the average amount of iodine incorporated into the molecule. Furthermore, for a similar level of iodination the impairment in metabolic clearance was of smaller magnitude with ^{125} than with ^{131} labelling. However, ^{125}I insulin containing 0.2 atom I/mol had a catabolic (clearance) rate which averaged 70% of that for crystalline insulin. In addition direct competition with unlabelled insulin could be demonstrated and the slope expressing the decrease in catabolic rate in relation to the increase in plasma level was similar to the corresponding slope for crystalline insulin.

The studies of Ooms *et al.* (1968) suggest that under proper conditions radioiodinated insulin can serve as a valid tracer of insulin. In their studies only ^{125}I insulin (0.2 atom I/mol) exhibited a behavior approaching that of crystalline insulin. The progressive impairment in clearance with increasing iodination was attributed to probable increase in the fraction of insulin molecules containing diiodotyrosines. Preparations containing 0.2 I/mol or less were said to be more homogeneous and contained 97% of the attached iodine as monoiodotyrosine. The greater impairment in metabolic clearance of ^{131}I versus ^{125}I labelled preparation was attributed to probable damage to the insulin molecule produced by β-radiations from the ^{131}I isotope. It should be pointed out however, that the restrictions of Ooms *et al.* are not necessarily applicable when other methods of iodination are utilized. The studies of Izzo *et al.* (1962) revealed little or no damage to ^{131}I insulin preparation i.e. $<5\%$ prepared by the iodine monochloride method when properly protected by albumin. Furthermore, in studies involving degradation of ^{131}I labelled insulin by rat liver homogenates, most, if not all, of the ^{131}I attached to insulin was recovered as ^{131}I labelled monoiodotyrosine upon completion of degradation of ^{131}I insulin containing an average of 0.8 atom of iodine per molecule. Thus, it would seem that the method of iodination as well as the amount of iodine attached to insulin has to be considered. In view of the rigid specifications required for preparing radioiodinated insulin for use in metabolic studies it is doubtful that the specifications have been always met in commercial preparations of radioiodinated insulin and may account for some of the discrepancies that have been reported.

The problems inherent in the use of radioiodinated insulin in the study of insulin distribution and kinetics are not completely resolved by the use of unlabelled insulin. The use of labelled insulin permits an accurate calculation of the MCR or fractional insulin clearance rate since it relates only to radioactive insulin activity (inflow rate and plasma level) and since it is not altered by the unknown secretion rate of endogenous insulin. As pointed out by Corvilain *et al.* (1971): "This type of measurement cannot be made with cold insulin or cannot include endogenous insulin since the inhibitive action of the administration of insulin upon the pancreatic release of the hormone is still controversial". Finally, estimations of metabolic clearance rates, fractional insulin removal rate or systemic plasma delivery rates are compromised by the fact that in these studies only insulin delivered into the general circulation is considered. Physiologically, insulin is secreted by the pancreatic β-cells into the portal vein and must traverse the liver before entering the systemic circulation. Since a large fraction of insulin is removed from the blood in a single transhepatic passage and since the amount extracted can be influenced by the level of insulin in plasma a meaningful description of insulin distribution and clearance must include the role of the liver.

IV. Summary and Conclusions

^{131}I labelled insulin injected intravenously in rats is widely distributed in various organs and tissues in the body. Less than 1.5% of injected dose is excreted in urine in unaltered form. At tracer levels lightly iodinated biologically active ^{131}I insulin is very rapidly removed from plasma in rats; accumulation is most rapid and greatest in liver and slower and lesser in kidneys. With pharmacological doses plasma clearance is slower and accumulation in liver is less and in kidneys greater than after injection of tracer doses. Biological inactivation of insulin either by heavy iodination (5—6 I/mol) or alkali treatment results in its slower removal from plasma, reduced concentrations in liver and kidneys and alterations in binding to intracellular structures, suggesting that the fate and distribution of ^{131}I insulin in the rat are characteristic and specific for the functionally intact molecule. Competition between ^{131}I labelled insulins and unlabelled insulin for reactive sites, and simularities in patterns of plasma decrease and uptake by liver and kidneys suggest that under proper conditions the distribution and metabolic fate of ^{131}I labelled insulin are probably similar if not identical with that of the native hormone.

The liver dominates the rapid plasma insulin clearance processes by virtue of its anatomical position and its large capacity to remove and degrade insulin. Studies in humans and laboratory animals indicate that approximately 40—50% of either labelled or unlabelled insulin is removed by the liver in a single trans-hepatic passage. The extraction process, at least in rats, appears to be saturable at high doses but studies on the relationships between hepatic extraction and plasma insulin concentration in man and in animals have yielded contradictory data. The kidney removes about 30% of insulin in the systemic circulation. The basal insulin consumption by the kidneys in fasted man has been calculated to be about 4—6 units per 24 h. However, the extraction process in the kidneys appears to be relatively unsaturable and at higher plasma insulin concentrations the kidneys are capable of assuming the functions of the liver in extracting insulin from the plasma. Insulin is cleared from plasma by the kidney primarily by glomerular filtration but also by direct absorption. The insulin in the glomerular filtrate is then almost completely reabsorbed or destroyed in the proximal tubule. Nephrectomy and severe renal disease have been shown to cause a delay in disappearance of insulin from plasma. This suggests a slower turnover and may account at least in part for the reduced insulin requirements in some diabetic patients with severe renal disease.

Studies based on distribution patterns of ^{131}I labelled insulin in subcellular fractions of liver, muscle and kidneys as well as studies on volume of distribution of ^{131}I labelled insulin in muscle and distribution of radioactivity in tissue cross sections suggest but do not establish that insulin penetrates muscle and other cells as well as liver and kidney. If this is so, the process governing intracellular transport could play an important role in regulating plasma insulin concentration.

Studies have been carried out in rats which have been directed as much as possible at determining the role of fundamental processes such as diffusion, mechanism of chemical reaction and transport of species in the distribution of ^{131}I insulin and its reaction products in the body of the rat. The data have been interpreted as indicating that ^{131}I insulin species are exchanged between the plasma and various body compartments by unsteady state molecular diffusion processes in which the body compartments behave as semi-infinite homogenous media. Superimposed on the diffusional processes are chemical reaction processes occurring in the liver and kidneys. The degradation of ^{131}I species in the liver and kidneys appeare to occur by a reaction which is second order with respect to ^{131}I insulin. The major muscle mass is indicated to behave as a capacitor which accepts ^{131}I insulin species from the plasma when plasma concentrations are high and rejects material to the plasma when concentrations are low. The existence of degradation reactions in the muscle mass are neither confirmed nor denied by the data.

Based on rates of disappearance of intravenous injections of insulin, plasma half-life estimation by different investigators have ranged from 11.1—40 min for ^{131}I labelled insulin, 3—13 min for unlabelled insulin and 7—15 min for endogenous plasma insulin following cessation of intravenous glucose and glucagon. The data on rates of disappearance of intravenously injected insulin in non-insulin treated diabetics and normals is contradictory. In diabetic subjects treated with insulin for months to years plasma disappearance of ^{131}I insulin is much slower due to binding of ^{131}I insulin by an acquired specific antibody to the injected insulin. The rate of disappearance seems to be negatively correlated with the level of circulating antibody.

In estimating half-life of insulin in plasma following intravenous injections of the hormone, the assumption is made that the curve of disappearance can be mathematically expressed as a simple exponential after the initial period of mixing. However, disappearance of insulin has been shown to involve a non-linear, multiexponential function which precludes the use of any part or component of the disappearance curve for direct calculation of so called "half-life" of insulin. Hence, the physiological relevance or usefulness of such estimations is open to question. In recognition of this problem alternative methods of analysis of nonlinear functions have been devised. Metabolic clearance rates and fractional irreversible loss rate of insulin from plasma, utilizing both single injection and continuous infusion to equilibrium technics of either ^{131}I insulin or unlabelled insulin have been calculated in normal humans and in patients with diabetes, obesity or chronic renal disease both under steady state conditions or after administration of glucose loads. The values for clearance rates of labelled insulin as well as the rate between labelled and unlabelled insulin have varied among investigators. Two somewhat different three compartment mathematical models have been proposed to describe clearance of insulin in the systemic circulation. The problem with all the models thus far is that they do not adequately account for the role of the liver in insulin disposition. Since the liver has a large capacity to remove insulin from the circulation and since insulin is secreted into the portal vein and traverses the liver before entering the systemic circulation a physiologically relevant model of insulin distribution must include the full role of the liver.

References

Arnould, Y., Cantraine, F., Ooms, H.A., Delcroix, C., Franckson, J.R.M.: Kinetics of plasma disappearance of labelled iodoinsulins following intravenous injection. Arch. int. Pharmacodyn. **166**, 225—237 (1967)

Arquilla, E.R., Ooms, H., Mercola, K.: Immunological and Biological Properties of iodoinsulin labeled with one or less atoms of iodine per molecule. J. clin. Invest. **47**, 474—487 (1968)

Banerjee, R.N., Gibson, K.: Preparation and Purification of High Specific activity insulin-^{131} iodine. J. Endocr. **25**, 145—146 (1962)

Berson, S.A., Yalow, R.S., Bauman, A., Rothschild, M.A., Newerly, K.: Insulin-I^{131} metabolism in human subjects: Demonstration of insulin binding globulin in the circulation of insulin treated subjects. J. clin. Invest. **35**, 170—190 (1956)

Bolinger, R.E., Morris, J.H., McKnight, F.G., Diederich, D.A.: Disappearance of I^{131}-labeled insulin from plasma as a guide to management of diabetes. New Engl. J. Med. **270**, 767—770 (1964)

Brunfeldt, K., Hansen, B.A., Jorgensen, K.R.: The immunological reactivity and biological activity of iodinated insulin. Acta endocr. (Kbh.) **57**, 307—329 (1968)

Brush, J.S., Kitabchi, A.E.: Metabolic disposition of ^{131}I iodoinsulin within the rat diaphragm. Biochim. biophys. Acta (Amst.) **215**, 134—144 (1970)

Cerasi, E., Luft, R.: Plasma insulin response to sustained hyperglycaemia induced by glucose infusion in human subjects. Lancet **2**, 1359—1361 (1963)

Chamberlain, M.J., Stimmler, L.: The renal handling of insulin. J. clin. Invest. **46**, 911—919 (1967)

Corvilain, J., Brauman, H., Delcroix, C., Toussaint, C., Vereerstraeten, P., Franckson, J.R.M.: Labeled insulin catabolism in chronic renal failure and in the anephric state. Diabetes **20**, 7, 467—475 (1971)

DRURY, D.R., KARASEK, M.A., BRITTON, R., WICK, A.N.: Metabolism of insulin I^{131} in the extrahepatic tissues. Amer. J. Physiol. **192**, 501—505 (1968)

ELGEE, N.J., WILLIAMS, R.H., LEE, N.D.: Distribution and degradation studies with insulin-I^{131}. J. clin. Invest. **33**, 1252—1260 (1954)

ELGEE, N.J., WILLIAMS, R.H.: Specificity of insulin degradation reaction. Diabetes **4**, 87—91 (1955)

EPSTEIN, F.H., ZUPA, V.J.: Clinical correlates of the Kimmelstiel-Wilson lesion. New Engl. J. Med. **254**, 896—900 (1956)

FRANCIS, G.E., MULLIGAN, W., WORMALL, A.: Labelling of proteins with iodine-^{131} sulfur 3S and phosphorus-32. Nature (Lond.) **167**, 748—751 (1951)

FREYCHET, P., ROTH, J., NEVILLE, D.M., JR.: Monoiodoinsulin: demonstration of its biological activity and binding to fat cells and liver membranes. Biochem. biophys. Res. Commun. **43**, 400—408 (1971)

GENUTH, S.M.: Metabolic clearance of insulin in man. Diabetes **21**, 1003—1012 (1972)

GLOVER, J.S., SALTER, D.N., SHEPHERD, B.P.: A study of some factors that influence the iodination of ox insulin. Biochem. J. **103**, 120—128 (1967)

GOADBY, H.K., RICHARDSON, J.S.: On the disappearance from the blood of intravenously injected insulin. J. Physiol. (Lond.) **97**, 417—428 (1940)

GREENWOOD, F.C., HUNTER, W.M., GLOVER, J.S.: The preparation of ^{131}I-labelled human growth hormone of high specific radioactivity. Biochem. J. **89**, 114—123 (1963)

HORTON, E.S., JOHNSON, C., LEBOWITZ, H.E.: Carbohydrate metabolism in uremia. Ann. intern. Med. **68**, 63—74 (1968)

HUGHES, W.L., JR., STRAESSLE, R.: Preparation and properties of serum and plasma proteins. XXIV. Iodination of human serum albumin. J. Amer. chem. Soc. **72**, 452—457 (1950)

IZZO, J.L., BALE, W.F., IZZO, M.J., RONCONE, A.: High specific activity labeling of insulin with I^{131}. Fed. Proc. **21**, 204 (1962)

IZZO, J.L., BALE, W.F., IZZO, M.J., RONCONE, A.: High specific activity labeling of insulin with ^{131}I. J. biol. Chem. **239**, 3743—3748 (1964a)

IZZO, J.L., RONCONE, A., IZZO, M.J., BALE, W.F.: Relationship between degree of iodination of insulin and its biological, electrophoretic, and immunochemical properties. J. biol. Chem. **239**, 3749—3754 (1964b)

IZZO, J.L., BARTLETT, J.W., RONCONE, A., IZZO, M.J., BALE, W.F.: Physiological processes and dynamics in the disposition of small and large doses of biologically active and inactive ^{131}I-insulins in the rat. J. biol. Chem. **242**, 2343—2355 (1967)

IZZO, J.L., BARTLETT, J.W.: Insulin-glucose dispersion and interaction system. Arch. intern. Med. **123**, 272—283 (1969)

IZZO, J.L., RONCONE, A., IZZO, M.J., FOLEY, R., BARTLETT, J.W.: Degradation of ^{131}I-insulins by rat liver. J. biol. Chem. **247**, 1219—1226 (1972)

KAPLAN, N., MADISON, L.L.: The effect of endogenous insulin secretion upon the magnitude of hepatic binding of labeled insulin during a single transhepatic circulation in human subjects. Clin. Res. **7**, 145 (1959)

KADEN, M., CURTIN, R., CAREY, L., TAYLOR, F., FIELD, J.B.: Evaluation of factors regulating hepatic extraction of insulin. Diabetes **20**, Suppl. 1, 341 (1971)

KRISHNA RAM, B.K., AHUJA, M.M.S.: A study of intermediary metabolism in different clinical types of diabetes mellitus in India (with special reference to pyruvate, lactate, glycerol and plasma insulin). Indian J. med. Res. **58**, 456—467 (1970)

KRISHNA RAM, B.K., AHUJA, M.M.S., GARG, V.K.: A study of fractional insulin clearance rates from plasma in control and different clinical types of diabetes mellitus. Indian J. med. Res. **60**, 114—122 (1972)

LEE, N.D.: The specificity of the interaction of insulin-I^{131} with tissue. Endocrinology **65**, 347—355 (1959)

MADISON, L.L., COMBES, B., UNGER, R.H., KAPLAN, N.: The relationship between the mechanism of action of the sulfonylureas and the secretion of insulin into the portal circulation. Ann. N.Y. Acad. Sci. **74**, 548—556 (1959)

MARTIN, F.I.R., STOCKS, A.E., PEARSON, M.J.: Significance of disappearance-rate of injected insulin. Lancet **1**, 619—620 (1967)

MCADAMS, G.B., KNOX, K.R., WILCOX, D.S.: The initial, rapid-phase disappearance of intravenous radioinsulin in diabetes. J. nucl. Med. **8**, 173—178 (1967)

MCFARLANE, A.S.: Efficient trace labelling of proteins with iodine. Nature (Lond.) **182**, 53 (1958)

MORTIMORE, G.E., TIETZE, F., STETTEN, D.: Metabolism of insulin-I^{131} studies in isolated perfused rat liver and hind-limb preparations. Diabetes **8**, 307—314 (1959)

O'BRIEN, J.P., SHARPE, A.R., JR.: The influence of renal disease on the insulin I^{131}disappearance curve in man. Metabolism **16**, 76—83 (1967)

Ooms, H.A., Arnould, Y., Rosa, U., Pennisi, G.F., Franckson, J.R.M.: Clearances metaboliques globales de l'insuline cristalline et d'insulines substituees au radioiode. Path. et Biol. **16**, 241—245 (1968)
Orskov, H.C., Christensen, N.J.: Disappearance rate of exogenous human insulin. Lancet **2**, 701 (1966)
Orskov, H.C., Christensen, N.J.: Plasma disappearance rate of injected human insulin in juvenile diabetic, maturity-onset diabetic and non-diabetic subjects. Diabetes **18**, 653—659 (1969)
Palmer, D.L., Bolinger, R.E.: Effect of nephrectomy and splanchnicectomy on plasma disappearance of labeled insulin in the rabbit. Proc. Soc. exp. Biol. (N.Y.) **107**, 809—812 (1961)
Palumbo, P.J., Taylor, W.F., Molnar, G.D., Tauxe, W.N.: Disappearance of bovine insulin from plasma in diabetic and normal subjects. Metabolism **21**, 787—798 (1972)
Porte, D., Pupo, A.A.: Insulin responses to glucose: Evidence for a two pool system in man. J. clin. Invest. **48**, 2309—2319 (1969)
Pressman, D., Eisen, H.N.: The zone of localization of antibodies. V. An attempt to saturate antibody-binding sites in mouse kidney. J. Immunol. **64**, 273—279 (1950)
Recordier, M., Andrac, M.: Recherches sur la reaction de l'animal a l'insuline avant et apres nephrectomie. Marseille-méd. **72**, 741 (1935)
Rosa, U., Massaglia, A., Pennisi, G.F., Cozzani, I., Rossi, C.A.: Effect of the insulin iodination on the reactivity of the inter-chain disulphide bonds towards sodium sulphite. Biochem. J. **103**, 407—412 (1967)
Rose, S., Nelson, J.: Studies with radio-iodinated insulin. Austral. J. exp. Biol. **32**, 429—436 (1954)
Runyan, J.W., Jr., Hurwitz, D., Robbins, S.L.: Effect of Kimmelstiel-Wilson syndrome on insulin requirements in diabetes. New Engl. J. Med. **252**, 388—391 (1955)
Samols, E., Ryder, J.A.: Studies on tissue uptake of insulin in man using a differential immunoassay for endogenous and exogenous insulin. J. clin. Invest. **40**, 2092—2102 (1961)
Samols, E., Marks, V.: Disappearance-rate of endogenous insulin in man. Lancet **1**, 700 (1966)
Sherwin, R.S., Insel, P.A., Tobin, J.D., Liljenquist, J.E., Andres, R., Berman, M.: Computer modeling: An aid to understanding insulin action. Diabetes **21**, Suppl. 1, 347 (1972)
Silvers, A., Swenson, R.S., Farquhar, J.W., Reaven, G.M.: Derivation of a three compartment model describing disappearance of plasma insulin-^{131}I in man. J. clin. Invest. **48**, 1461—1469 (1969)
Stein, O., Gross, J.: The localization and metabolism of ^{131}I insulin in the muscle and some other tissues of the rat. Endocrinology **65**, 707—716 (1959)
Stern, M.P., Farquhar, J.W., Silvers, A., Reaven, G.M.: Insulin delivery rate into plasma in normal and diabetic subjects. J. clin. Invest. **47**, 1947—1957 (1968)
Stimmler, L.: Disappearance-rate of insulin. Lancet **2**, 1078 (1966)
Stimmler, L.: Disappearance of immunoreactive insulin in normal and adult-onset diabetic subjects. Diabetes **16**, 652—655 (1967)
Tait, J.F.: Review: The use of isotopic steroids for the measurement of production rate *in vivo*. J. clin. Endocr. **23**, 1285—1297 (1963)
Tomasi, T., Sledz, D., Wales, J.K., Recant, L.: Insulin half-life in normal and diabetic subjects. Proc. Soc. exp. Biol. (N.Y.) **126**, 315—317 (1967)
Turner, R.C., Grayburn, J.A., Newman, G.B., Nabarro, J.D.N.: Measurement of the insulin delivery rate in man. J. clin. Endocr. **33**, 279—286 (1971)
Williams, R.F., Heason, R.E., Soeldner, J.S.: The half-life of endogenous serum immunoreactive insulin in man. Metabolism **17**, 1025—1029 (1968)
Zaharko, D.S., Beck, L.V., Blankenbaker, R.: Role of the kidney in the disposal of radioiodinated and nonradioiodinated insulin in dogs. Diabetes **15**, 680—685 (1966)
Zubrod, C.G., Eversole, S.L., Dena, G.W.: Amelioration of diabetes and rarity of acidosis in patients' with Kimmelstiel-Wilson lesions. New Engl. J. Med. **245**, 518—525 (1951)

B. Degradation of Insulin

Joseph L. Izzo

I. Qualitative Aspects of Inactivation of Insulin

1. Inactivation of Insulin by Tissue Brei and Extracts

In 1929, Schmidt and Saachian reported that breis prepared from several rabbit tissues were able to inactivate insulin, presumably by proteolytic activity, which was believed to be present in their preparation. Liver brei was most active in this respect. Almost a decade later, Lehmann and Schlossman (1938) reported in an abstract that cell-free extracts of rabbit muscle contained two principles that could inactivate insulin. Each was capable of acting separately. The first principle was a heat-stable diffusible factor and was considered to be a sulfhydryl compound, probably glutathione or cysteine, both of which are known to occur in muscle. The second principle was heat-labile and non-dialyzable through semipermeable membranes. It was proposed that both factors inactivated insulin by reduction and cleavage of disulfide linkages. The inactivation of insulin by cysteine and glutathione at neutral pH, by reducing its —SS— groups, had already been demonstrated by Du Vigneaud *et al.* (1931) and Wintersteiner (1933). The hormone was found to be inactive when only one third of the disulfide linkages were reduced Wintersteiner (1933), Fraenkel-Conrat and Fraenkel-Conrat (1950).

The findings of Schmidt and Saachian were confirmed by Mirsky and Brohkahn (1949). Extracts from various tissues were prepared and analyzed for their ability to inactivate insulin during incubation *in vitro*. Systems capable of inactivating insulin at pH 7.5 were found to be widely distributed. In the rat the greatest activity per gram of tissue was found in liver extracts. Extracts prepared from kidney and muscle were found to contain progressively less activity, while whole blood, plasma, the washed or hemolyzed cellular constituents of blood, and brain extracts were relatively inactive. The livers of rabbit, steer, chicken, and man (obtained both from biopsy and autopsy sources) were also found to be rich in the insulin-inactivating system. Furthermore, the system appeared to have the properties of an enzyme that was dependent upon the participation of a sulfhydryl group and it was tentatively designated "insulinase." The activity was inhibited by inorganic metals such as copper and organic compounds such as iodoacilate.

2. ^{131}I-Insulin Degradation by Tissue Extracts, Slices and Homogenates

In the early studies, insulin destruction was measured by a semiquantitative technique in which the hypoglycemic response of rabbits to the intravenous injection of an incubation mixture containing insulin was determined, before and after a designated period of incubation. Although the procedure was sufficiently quantitative to demonstrate the insulin inactivation capacity of various tissues, the method was not suitable for studies of the nature and specificity of insulin degradation. With the availability of ^{131}I, it became possible to label insulin and to trace the fate of the insulin molecule *in vivo* and *in vitro*. The release of ^{131}I-labeled fragments into the nonprotein, trichloroacetic acid-soluble fraction of an extract was utilized as a measure of the quantity of labeled hormone that was degraded during a designated period (Mirsky *et al.*, 1954). After demonstrating that the inactivation of insulin as measured by bioassay paralleled the degradation of the insulin molecule as measured by the increase of radioactivity in the nonprotein fraction of the incubation mixture, Mirsky and his associates reinvestigated the degradation of insulin by liver homogenates and extracts with ^{131}I-labeled insulin as tracer. By the use of both the bioassay procedure and the release of labeled trichloroacetic acid-soluble fragments, it was demonstrated that "insulinase" was present in the liver of rat, mouse, guinea pig, rabbit, cow, chicken, duck, monkey, and man. However, the concentration of "insulinase" appeared to vary from species to species (Mirsky and Perisutti, 1951; Mirsky *et al.*, 1954; Mirsky *et al.*, 1955). Liver slices were also capable of destroying insulin *in vitro*, but the activity was much less than that of an equivalent amount of liver homogenate (Mirsky and Perisutti, 1953; Mirsky *et al.*, 1954). As with liver extracts, the activity of liver slices was dependent upon the quantity of liver, pH, temperature, and other properties characteristic of an enzyme system. Finally, insulin degradation was demonstrated *in vivo* by measuring the percentage of total radioactivity that appeared in the nonprotein fraction of homogenates of intact mice prepared at intervals after the intraperitoneal injection of various concentrations of labeled insulin (Mirsky *et al.*, 1955). The data showed that, like liver homogenates, extracts, and slices, the intact mouse destroyed insulin very rapidly by a reaction which, at high doses, appeared to follow first-order kinetics. It was found that, in order to measure the rate of destruction accurately, as much as 40 units of ^{131}I-insulin had to be injected intraperitoneally to saturate the enzyme system.

The studies of Williams *et al.* (1959) were essentially in agreement with those of Mirsky reported above. Most of the homogenates of different rat tissue caused some degradation of ^{131}I-insulin. Among the more active tissues were liver, pancreas, kidney, and testes. Plasma and washed red blood cells had little or no activity. The activity of brain, diaphragm, gastrocnemius, and lymph node was relatively small. In the case of muscle, however, the total activity was quite significant, because muscle mass comprises a large fraction of the total body mass. Tissue homogenates degraded insulin much faster than tissue slices.

3. Specificity of ^{131}I-Insulin Degradation by Tissue Extracts and Homogenates

On the basis of several lines of evidence, Mirsky and his coworkers concluded that the system they designated as "insulinase" was specific for insulin inactivation by tissue extracts, slices, or homogenates. The fact that tissues like brain and erythrocytes—which are rich in proteinases and peptidases—were found to be poor in "insulinase" activity first suggested to MIRSKY (1953) that "insulinase" was relatively specific. In supoort of this, he presented evidence indicating that long after the "insulinase" activity of an aged liver extract had been lost, the catheptic activity persisted. Further data on the relative specificity of "insulinase" were obtained by comparing the effects of a liver extract on ^{131}I-labeled insulin with the effects on similarly labeled ribonuclease, pepsin, prolactin, lysozyme, chymotrypsin, and human serum albumin (MIRSKY, 1955). The results showed that, whereas there was no significant effect of the extract on the labeled lysozyme, chymotrypsin, and human serum albumin, an appreciable degradation of labeled ribonuclease, pepsin, and to a lesser degree prolactin, was observed. Nevertheless, on the basis of the effect of different concentrations of these proteins on the velocity of their degradation by liver extract, the authors concluded that the system responsible for the destruction of insulin was different from that responsible for the destruction of the other proteins. Studies which revealed that the addition of various proteins to the incubation mixture containing labeled insulin did not influence the degradation of various concentrations of insulin were submitted as further evidence of the specificity of the system.

TOMIZAWA and WILLIAMS (1955) also reported that the insulin-inactivating system of liver extracts had some degree of specificity since ^{131}I-labeled human serum albumin, bovine serum albumin, α-lactalbumin, and ribonuclease did not influence the percentage of radioactivity of the trichloroacetic acid soluble fraction. However, they cautioned against the use of the term "insulinase" since other substances, such as α-corticotropin, casein, glucagon, and growth hormone, could also be substrates for this system. They suggested that whether a substance is or is not a substrate may depend not only upon the presence of given peptide bonds, but also on their accessibility to the enzyme (or enzymes): "Bonds which conform to the specificity of the enzyme system would probably be easily accessible in the case of smaller compounds such as insulin, α-corticotropin, and glucagon, whereas, with larger substances such as casein, accessibility may depend on prior denaturation or partial degradation. With insulin, the possibility has not been eliminated that prior cleavage of disulfide bonds may be involved."

In subsequent studies, MIRSKY and PERISUTTI (1957) reported that extracts of rat liver that catalyzed the degradation of ^{131}I-labeled insulin also catalyzed the degradation of casein, ribonuclease, corticotropin, growth hormone, and glucagon under identical conditions. However, the demonstration that aging and dialysis decreased and the presence of citrate ions increased the activity of liver extract in the degradation of insulin whereas such measures did not influence the degradation of other proteins, was interpreted as indicating the relative specificity of the system responsible for the destruction of insulin, i.e. "insulinase." Three-hour acid hydrolysates of insulin, glucagon, corticotropin, growth hormones, ribonuclease, and casein were found to contain peptides capable of inhibiting the destruction of insulin by liver extracts. Since these proteins were destroyed by liver extracts, MIRSKY argued that it was quite probably that their hydrolytic products, like those of acid hydrolysates, could act as inhibitors of "insulinase." Thus, the observation of TOMIZAWA and WILLIAMS (1955), that the degradation of insulin was inhibited in the presence of the above proteins, may not have been due to competition between insulin and the protein for the enzyme system but to inhibition of "insulinase" by some hydrolytic products of the added protein.

4. Further Studies on the Nature, Specificity, and Localization of Enzymatic Degradation Processes for Insulin

a) Evidence for Reductive Cleavage of S-S Bonds in Insulin

Rall and Lehninger (1952) reported the presence in rat liver of an enzyme, glutathione reductase, which catalyzed the reduction of GSSG. The reduction of disulfide compounds, including insulin, by a crude liver preparation to which DPN and a hydrogen donor system had been added was described by Racker (1953). Narahara and Williams (1959) reported that a second enzyme system in extracts prepared from rat-liver acetone powder activated the reduction of insulin by GSH. Unlike GSSG reductase, the second enzyme system did not require TPN and appeared to act directly upon insulin. Furthermore, partial separation from GSSG reductase was achieved by acid fractionation of liver extract. On the basis of the data available, they proposed that reduction of insulin by GSH and liver extract was enhanced by two separate enzyme systems and could be represented by the following reactions:

$$\text{Insulin} + 2\ \text{GSH} \xrightarrow{\text{dialyzed liver enzyme}} \text{reduced insulin} + \text{GSSG}$$

$$\text{GSSG} + \text{TPNH} + \text{H}^{+} \xrightarrow{\text{glutathione reductase}} 2\ \text{GSH} + \text{TPN}^{+}$$

Of the several possibilities considered, the hypothesis that the second enzyme system catalyzed the transfer of hydrogen from GSH to insulin appeared to these authors to be that most compatible with the experimental data.

In a subsequent study Tomizawa and Halsey (1959) isolated a beef-liver enzyme which degraded insulin in the presence of sulfhydryl compounds of low molecular weight such as reduced glutathione or 2-mercaptoethanol. Several observations suggested to Tomizawa (1962) that this purified enzyme was similar in its action to the enzyme system in rat-liver extracts reported by Narahara and Williams (1959). The A chain was identified as the only trichloroacetic acid-soluble product from insulin catalyzed by this purified beef-liver enzyme (Tomizawa, 1962).

Katzen and Stetten (1962) proposed the name glutathione-insulin transhydrogenase (GIT) for the hepatic insulin-degrading enzyme described by Tomizawa and Halsey (1959). Hydrolysis of peptide bonds by this enzyme could not be detected. However, reductive cleavage of disulfide bonds in the presence of reduced glutathione was strongly catalyzed. Both of the interchain disulfide linkages were reptured in the course of the reaction, since the phenylalanyl and glycyl chains were separable. Direct evidence was lacking for reduction of the cyclic disulfide bridge between half-cystines in positions 6 and 11 in the glycyl chain. However, since both vasopressin and oxytocin also served as substrate for reduction, it was inferred by analogy that the latter bond is also susceptible of cleavage. Cystine, homocystine, lipoic acid, and ribonuclease could not replace insulin in the reaction; the purified enzyme was readily coupled with purified glutathione reductase. Under these circumstances insulin was shown to readily oxidize triphosphopyridine nucleotide in the presence of glutathione. Kinetic studies revealed a Km for insulin of 4.3×10^{-5}M.

In further studies (Katzen *et al.*, 1963) all three disulfide bonds of insulin were found to be susceptible to cleavage by hepatic glutathione-insulin transhydrogenase. The Km for reduced glutathione was 8.9×10^{-3}M. The products of insulin reduction, which were physiologically inactive, were subjected to reoxidation by oxidized glutathione in the presence and absence of transhydrogenase. Approximately 20 times as much insulin-like activity was recovered in the presence of GIT as in its absence, when assayed by the effect on the metabolism of adipose tissue. Furthermore, approximately five times as much immunological activity corresponding to insulin was recovered when GIT was present. From these observations, the authors inferred that the presence of GIT favors the reconstitution of the naturally occurring disulfide bonds of insulin. However, further inquiry into the observed role of glutathione-insulin transhydrogenase in the formation of insulin-like protein from chemically reduced precursors (KATZEN and TIETZE, 1966) revealed that, although GIT exerted a significant effect on the rate on insulin reconstruction, the data did not indicate any capacity of the enzyme to direct specifically the preferential reestablishment of the native configuration.

KATZEN and TIETZE (1966) proceeded to examine further the specificity and mode of action of glutathione-insulin transhydrogenase. By coupling reactions catalyzed by GIT to that of glutathione reductase, they indicated that during the course of enzyme action GIT undergoes reduction by GSH and that the reduced enzyme is autooxidizable. It was inferred that this reduced form is an active intermediate during GIT-catalyzed reduction of disulfide substrates. Under conditions of limited spontaneous air oxidation of protein sulfhydryls, GIT was shown also to promote the net oxidation of such thiols as the reduced forms of insulin and RNase. It was also observed that, during the process of reoxidation of reduced forms of insulin and RNase, GIT was capable of enhancing the rates of regeneration of the native proteins from their reduced precursors, as determined by their immunologic and enzymic properties, respectively. In addition, GIT was able to promote the reconstitution of the native activity from a reduced form of RNase, which had already been extensively oxidized by dehydroascorbate. A mechanism involving a series of disulfide-interchange reactions was proposed to explain the aforementioned reaction catalyzed by GIT. Substrate-specificity studies were also carried out with several chemically modified and proteolytically degraded forms of insulin, such as zinc insulin, zinc-free insulin, deoctapeptide insulin, acetyl insulin, dealanyl-deasparaginyl insulin, and dealanyl insulins. None of these modifications interfered with the capacity of GIT to reduce the disulfide bonds of insulin. This indicated to the authors that neither biological activity nor native structure is a prerequisite for activity as substrate for GIT-catalyzed reduction.

KATZEN and TIETZE (1966) also examined the possible relationships of glutathione-insulin transhydrogenase with other known proteins possessing similar catalytic properties. Of particular interest was the RNase-reactivity enzyme that had been isolated by ANFINSEN and his associates (GIVOL *et al.*, 1964; GOLDBERGER *et al.*, 1964; GIVOL *et al.*, 1965). This enzyme was found to accelerate the rate of regeneration of native RNase and other proteases during the oxidation of their fully or partially reduced and "scrambled" forms. Apart from their similarities with respect to RNase regeneration, the two enzymes mentioned above displayed other remarkable similarities. Both activities were found in mammalian liver (TOMIZAWA and HALSEY, 1959; NARAHARA and WILLIAMS, 1959; KATZEN and STETTEN, 1962; GIVOL *et al.*, 1964) and pancreas (VENETIANER and STRAUB, 1965; TOMIZAWA, 1965, KOTOULAS *et al.*, 1965). The purified liver enzymes were reported to possess similar sedimentation coefficients (TOMIZAWA and HALSEY, 1959; KATZEN and STETTEN, 1962; GIVOL *et al.*, 1964). Also both enzymes were capable, in the presence of small amounts of thiol, of catalyzing the transformation of insulin into similar soluble and insoluble products TOMIZAWA and HALSEY, 1959; KATZEN and STETTEN, 1962; TOMIZAWA, 1962, GIVOL *et al.*, 1965). Finally, the RNase-reactivating enzyme, like GIT, was inactivated by iodoacetate following pre-treatment of the purified enzyme with mercaptoethanol. The remarkable similarities in the two enzymes raised the possibility that they were one and the same. Also, of interest was the isolation from *Escherichia coli* (LAURENT *et al.*, 1964) of a highly purified acidic protein named thioredoxin, which was capable of being reversibly oxidized and reduced by virtue of a single reactive cystine residue. Reduced thioredoxin, formed chemically or enzymatically, was shown to serve as a reactive intermediate in the complete reduction of insulin (MOORE *et al.*, 1964), as well as in a system involved in the reduction of ribonucleotides to deoxyribonucleotides. Thioredoxin was also shown to be present in rat hepatoma (MOORE and REICHARD, 1964). BLACK *et al.* (1960) had described what appeared to be a completely analogous system in yeast.

In view of the aforementioned possibilities of similarity or identity among the several insulin-reducing systems found in mammalian and other tissue, KATZEN and TIETZE (1966) suggested that further studies would be required before assigning to glutathione-insulin transhydrogenase a role in the synthesis, function, or metabolism of insulin. Furthermore, in view of the enzymic activity displayed by GIT toward other thioldisulfide pairs, the authors suggested that a broader designation, e.g. thiol: protein disulfide oxidoreductase, might be more appropriate for this enzyme.

VARANDANI *et al.* (1972) studied the nature of the products formed when ^{125}I-insulin was incubated with rat liver homogenate in the presence of glutathione (1 mM). The products were examined by chromatography in a Sephadex G-75 column with 50% acetic acid as eluant. Two products were initially formed when insulin was incubated with reduced glutathione and liver protein. One of the products was identified as the A chain, which was further broken down to low-molecular-weight components. Since the liver homogenates from which insulin transhydrogenase had been specifically removed by precipitation were almost completely devoid of insulin-degrading activity, the data were interpreted to indicate that insulin is degraded in sequential order: first, insulin is split into A and B chains by the transhydrogenase, then the resulting polypeptides are proteolyzed to small-molecular-weight compounds.

The physical and enzymatic properties of purified glutathione-insulin transhydrogenase from rat liver, beef liver, beef pancreas, human liver, and kidney were shown to be similar (VARANDANI, 1972). Immunological data obtained with the use of three antisera—one against beef-pancreas GIT, the second against human-liver GIT, and the third against rat-liver GIT—indicated that there was considerable similarity in the structure of the five enzymes. The homologous enzyme reacted most strongly with each antibody but the heterologous enzymes also cross-reacted to an appreciable extent. Rat GIT differed immunologically to a greater extent from human than from bovine enzyme, while the bovine enzyme differed less from human than from rat enzyme.

Insulin-degrading activity dependent upon the presence of reduced glutathione was found in all rat-tissue extracts examined by CHANDLER and VARANDANI (1972). ^{125}I-insulin degradation by tissue extracts prepared in potassium phosphate-EDTA buffer was determined by the trichloroacetic-acid precipitation technique. In the presence of 1 mM glutathione, insulin-degrading activity was detected in all of the tissues examined. The relative activities (per mg of tissue protein) were found to be in the order: pancreas > liver > intestine > spleen > kidney, testes, thymus, fat, lung > brain > heart, diaphragm, skeletal muscle. Prior dialysis of the tissue extract and omission of glutathione from the assay buffer eliminated nearly all insulin degradation. Omission of glutathione from the assay buffer when nondialyzed tissue extracts were used yielded low levels of insulin degradation. The addition of N-ethylmaleimide was found to completely block all insulin degradation under these conditions. On the basis of these findings, it was concluded that the small amounts of insulin-degrading activity found in the absence of added glutathione were due to the presence of endogenous thiol compounds. Furthermore, the presence of glutathione-insulin transhydrogenase was demonstrated in all tissue extracts by double immuno diffusion with antibody to purified GIT. In the case of brain, testes, fat, and diaphragm extracts, which had been found to contain insulin-degrading activity of intermediate order, it was found necessary to concentrate the extract to demonstrate the precipitin in liver. In the case of heart and muscle, whose extracts contained the lowest concentrations of insulin-degrading activity, a precipitin band was demonstrable with each only when a concentrated extract of an acetone powder of these tissues was employed. The authors concluded from these studies that most or all of the insulin-degrading activity observed under the experimental conditions used was due to the presence of GIT, and that GIT may be responsible for the major insulin-degrading activity in the animal.

b) Evidence for Proteolytic Degradation of Insulin

On the basis of studies showing an increase in nonprotein nitrogen in liver extracts that had been incubated with insulin, TOMIZAWA *et al.* (1955) concluded that insulin was probably proteolytically inactivated by rat-liver extract at pH 7.5. The splitting of disulfide bonds, however, was not excluded. In fact, in subsequent studies, TOMIZAWA did indeed isolate from liver an enzyme that reduced the S-S bonds of insulin (see previous section). However, the relationships and physiological significance were not established for any of these processes. A parallel rise in nonprotein nitrogen or ninhydrin color in the TCA supernatant as inactivation or degradation of insulin by liver extract proceeded was also noted by VAUGHAN (1954). Moreover, autoradiography of the incubation mixture containing ^{131}I-insulin revealed that the products included small fragments of the original peptide (MIRSKY *et al.*, 1955; BERSON, YALOW and VOLK, 1957).

KENNY (1958) studied the proteolysis at pH 7.4 of insulin as well as of fractions A and B from oxidized insulin by a dilute supernatant fraction of a rat-liver homogenate. Proteolysis was assessed in a semiquantitative manner by the intensity of the ninhydrin-stained spots after paper chromatography of the reactive mixtures. No significant proteolysis of the intact molecule was found under these experimental conditions unless incubation was prolonged (17 h) or the concentration of the enzyme preparation was increased severalfold. However, in spite of the stability of the intact insulin molecule, the two oxidized chains were readily attacked, fraction B more extensively than fraction A. Complete inhibition was obtained with *p*-chloromercuribenzoate.

In further experiments the products obtained by incubation of fraction A with the liver preparation were isolated and identified. All the fractions that were identified and attributed to the protolysis of the oxidized fraction A proved to be single amino acids. No peptides were found. The amino acids identified were glycine, isoleucine, valine, glutamic acid, and glutamine. Only traces of cysteic acid, alanine, and serine were found. Since the N-terminal sequence of fraction A from oxidized insulin is as follows: Gly Ile Val Glu Glu NH_2 $CySO_3H$ Ala Ser Val (RYLE *et al.*, 1955), the results of the experiments were considered to be consistent with the action of an aminopeptidase that sequentially hydrolyzed single residues from the N terminus of the peptide. The cysteic acid residues were thought to have limited the rate of progress beyond that point in the chain. Similar experiments in which fraction B of oxidized insulin and glucagon were utilized as substrates also indicated that free amino acids and not peptides were the products of the liver enzyme system. Although the findings supported the view that an exopeptidase was present in the enzyme system, a clear choice between an aminopeptidase and a carboxypeptidase could not be made in view of the large number of amino acids identified.

Although KENNY demonstrated proteolysis of the A and B chains of insulin by dilute supernatant fraction of rat liver extract, he concluded that proteolysis was not the primary event in the degradation of insulin but was probably secondary to reductive cleavage of the S-S bonds. On the other hand, DI GIROLAMO *et al.* (1965) and RUDMAN *et al.* (1966) demonstrated the presence of a primary proteolytic insulin-degrading system in the insoluble fractions of homogenized adipose tissue of rat and hamster, but not rabbit or guinea pig, that cleaved and inactivated bovine insulin into numerous fragments soluble in 5% trichloroacetic acid. Studies involving incubation of the insoluble fraction derived from rat adipose tissue with bovine insulin indicated that disulfide and acid amide groups of insulin remained intact while internal and terminal peptide bonds were hydrolyzed. From their analysis of the cleavage products, RUDMAN *et al.* (1966) concluded that the initial event was hydrolysis of internal bonds in the region of A 13—14, A 18—19, B 11—12, B 15—16, B 24—25, and B 25—26. The 5 or 6 peptides thus formed then underwent stepwise removal of terminal residues from both N and C terminals. The insulin-cleaving enzyme system also hydrolyzed synthetic dipeptides which are susceptible to aminopeptidase or carboxypeptidase action, thus confirming the presence of two nonspecific exopeptidase activities in the insoluble fraction of rat adipose tissue. However, a variety of endopeptidase substrates other than insulin were not hydrolyzed, which suggested to the authors that the tissue enzyme that performed the initial internal hydrolysis might be specific for insulin.

More recently, BRUSH (1971) has reported the presence of a soluble protease from rat muscle with a high degree of specificity for insulin. On the basis of loss of immunoreactivity BRUSH conclude that the partially purified enzyme from rat muscle attacked proinsulin and proinsulin intermediates at only 3% and 10%, respectively, of the rate at which it attacked insulin. Proinsulin competitively inhibited insulin degradation (as determined by loss of immunoreactivity) with an inhibition constant of 0.28 μM, whereas the K_m for insulin was 0.18 μM. Insulin derivatives with amino or carboxyl terminal residues removed were attacked with K_m's about five times greater. However, removal of an octapeptide from the B chain of insulin resulted in a K_m which did not differ from that of insulin. The enzyme was found to be inhibited by the sulfhydryl reagent, N-ethylmaleimide, and *p*-hydroxymercuribenzoate, but not by an inhibitor of pancreatic proteases, phenylmethylsulfomyl fluoride. The enzymatic activity as measured by loss of immunoactivity was not inhibited by a large excess of A or B chains of insulin, bovine serum albumin, globin, glucagon, or human growth hormone. Proteolytic activity of the enzyme was established by demonstration of release of ninhydrin-positive material in mixtures of insulin and purified enzyme which had been incubated at 37° for 16 h.

The presence of a proteolytic enzyme which was designated "insulin-specific protease" was also reported in muscle, fat, liver, kidney, and pancreas (BURGHEN *et al.*, 1971). In fractionated liver homogenate the 100,000 *g* supernatant was found to contain 96% of the total insulin-degrading activity. The remaining 4% was distributed in the debris, mitochondrial, and microsomal fractions (BURGHEN *et al.*, 1972). The enzyme which was isolated from the 100,000 *g* supernatant of rat liver and purified 97-fold by ultracentrifugation, $Ca_3(PO_4)_2$ gel adsorption-elution, Sephadex G-200 filtration and DEAE-Sephadex A-50 chromatographys was estimated to have a mol. wt. of 80,000 from its behavior on Sephadex G-200. The K_m for insulin degradation was found to be 0.10 μM. The enzyme exhibited a relatively narrow pH range with optimal activity at pH 7.6. Marked specificity of the purified enzyme was indicated by a 15-fold greater rate of destruction of insulin compared to the insulin precursor proinsulin. Other proteolytic exzymes (trypsin, chymotrypsin, and papain) did not show any preferential degradation of insulin over proinsulin. Human growth hormone was not appreciably degraded by the purified enzyme. Mercaptoethanol and glutathione were found to slightly stimulate enzyme activity, whereas N-ethylmaleimide and *p*-hydroxy-mercuribenzoate were shown to be potent inhibitors of enzyme activity, suggesting that a sulfhydryl group in the enzyme molecule was necessary for its activity. Tolbutamide and phenformin were found to inhibit the enzyme by a complex type of noncompetitive inhibition.

In the above studies insulin destruction was measured either by loss of immunoreactivity or in the case of ^{125}I-labeled insulin, by appearance of TCA-soluble radioactivity in the incubation mixtures. In determining if the enzyme was a protease with specificity for insulin, Burghen *et al.* (1972) evaluated the ability of the calcium phosphate gel-purified enzyme to convert globin, bovine serum albumin, and casein as well as insulin to ninhydrin-reactive material. Bovine serum albumin was not attacked, whereas destruction of globin was 40% and of casein 11% of that of insulin. However, strangely enough, the total proteolytic activity of the preparation was quite low, the experiment requiring 22 h to obtain an appreciable accumulation of ninhydrin-reactive material. In the case of insulin, the total yield of ninhydrin-reactive material was 0.713 ± 0.019 μmol of leucine equivalents. Since insulin contains 51 amino acids, the complete proteolysis of 1.5 mg of insulin (0.28 μmol) as used in the experiment should have yielded 12.75 μmol of leucine equivalents. Hence the production of 0.713 μmol of leucine equivalent represented only 5.59% degradation of insulin after 22 h incubation.

II. Subcellular Localization of Insulin Degradation

In the studies of Mirsky (1953, 1957), Vaughan (1954), Narahara *et al.* (1955), Kenny (1960), and Burghen *et al.* (1971) insulin-degrading activity was reported to be localized predominantly in the cytosol fraction of liver cells. These results were obtained without activation of the hormone-degrading enzymes. In 1968, however, Morgan and Spahn reported that considerable insulin-degrading activity was detectable in the 450,000 *g* fraction, referred to as mitochondrial (and lysosomal) fraction, when incubation weres carried out with 5 mM mercaptoethanol at pH 7.4 (2.5 mM EDTA) as effector. From these results they concluded that the mitochondrial (and lysosomal) fraction plays an important role in degradation of insulin.

Utilizing radioiodinated hormones, Ansorge *et al.* (1971) studied the intracellular localization of enzyme systems involved in the degradation of insulin and glucagon in rat liver under conditions of SH activation by glutathione. The breakdown of ^{131}I-labeled hormones was determined by measuring the increase of trichloroacetic acid-soluble radioactivity during incubation of various cell fractions with radioiodinated hormones at neutral and acidic pH. Glucagon was degraded at pH 7.0 mainly by the cytosol fraction, with or without addition of glutathione and EDTA. Without effectors, insulin breakdown also occurred predominantly in the cytosol fraction at pH 7.0 .However, it was observed that the distribution pattern of insulin breakdown at pH 7.0 was completely different in the presence of 1 mM GSH and 5 mM EDTA. Under these conditions about 90%

of the insulin-degrading activity was located in the microsomal fraction, and only about 10% in the cytosol fraction. Moreover, the pattern of insulin breakdown in the presence of GSH and EDTA was very similar to that of glucose-6-phosphatase, a marker for microsomes. In contrast to glucose-6-phosphatase, the insulin-degrading activity was soluble after deoxycholate treatment of microsomes. By subsequent centrifugation at 200,000 *g* for some hours the insulin-degrading activities in the supernatant were purified about 10- to 24-fold as compared to the homogenate. The specific activity of this supernatant was found to be 20 to 48 times higher than that of the cytosol fraction. At acidic pH both glucagon and insulin were degraded predominantly by the lysosomal fractions of rat liver.

From their results Ansorge *et al.* (1971) concluded that the microsomal fraction of rat liver, especially the membrane-bound enzyme systems, represents the potentially highest capacity of insulin-degrading activity of liver at physiological pH. In view of the relatively high glutathione concentration in liver tissues (5 mM) (Jocclyn, 1959) and its localization in the post-mitochondrial fraction (Rall and Lehninger, 1952), it was suggested that GSH acts as an important factor for the insulin-degrading system at physiological pH. The findings of Ansorge *et al.* (1971) were in agreement with the observation of Jacques and Wattiaux-Deconinck (1969) who examined the intracellular distribution of radioactivity in rat livers after intravenous injection of radioiodinated insulin. The latter authors noted that minutes after the administration of ^{131}I-labeled insulin the distribution of acid-insoluble radioactivity was similar to that of glucose-6-phosphatase, whereas after a longer period the distribution pattern of acid-insoluble radioactivity became very similar to that of 2-glycero-phosphatase. Ansorge *et al.* (1971) found no evidence for a mitochondrial enzyme system possessing the activity and capacity reported by Morgan and Spahn. They also noted that an appreciable portion of insulin-degrading activity was spun down together with the mitochondria (32,000 *g*), but this was found to be due to microsomal contamination of the mitochondrial fraction, as shown by the content of glucose-6-phosphatase.

In further studies Ansorge *et al.* (1973) isolated and purified from microsomes of rat liver an enzyme that catalyzed the reductive breakdown of insulin. Its properties strongly resembled those of glutathione-insulin transhydrogenase (thiol-protein disulfide oxidoreductase) from bovine liver, human liver, bovine pancreas, and human kidney. The enzyme was separated from microsomes by deoxycholate and purified by gel filtration on Sephadex G-75 and subsequent chromatography on DEAE-Sephadex A-50. Disc electrophoresis of highly purified fresh enzyme preparations revealed only two enzymatically active proteins, forming one main band and a faint band, without further visible contaminants. The mol. wt. of the microsomal transhydrogenase as determined by gel filtration in Sephadex G-75 was 50,000 to 55,000. By means of disc electrophoresis in sodium dodecyl sulfate-containing gels a molecular weight of 60,000 was estimated for the main component and 121,000 for the slower-migrating band of the enzyme. The content of glutathione-insulin transhydrogenase in rat liver was estimated at about 0.5—1% of total liver proteins as calculated from the purification factor. The Michaelis-Menten constants for insulin and glutathione (in the presence of EDTA) were 31 μM (mol. wt. 6000) and 1.43 mM, respectively. Maximal breakdown of insulin occurred at pH 7.3. The authors concluded that their transhydrogenase from rat-liver microsomes was probably identical or very similar to the enzyme catalyzing the reactivation of "randomly oxidized" ribonuclease (Anfinsen), as had been previously suggested by Katzen and Tietze (1966).

Freychet *et al.* (1972) have reported recently that ^{125}I-insulin is rapidly degraded upon exposure to purified liver membranes. After 10 min of exposure to purified liver membranes (1.7 mg/ml) approximately 40% of the ^{125}I-insulin was found to be "degraded" as measured by binding to anti-insulin antibodies or binding to fresh liver membranes. Degradation was increased to 70—80% by 90 min. Degradation was also demonstrated by talc absorption and trichloroacetic-acid precipitation but these methods were less sensitive. Degradation of ^{125}I-insulin was reduced to less than 15% after 90 min at 1°. In contrast, significant specific binding of insulin to liver membranes was observed at this temperature. The nature of the degradation products was studied by gel filtration on Sephadex G-50 of ^{131}I-insulin after exposure to liver membranes for 90 min at 30°. No significant deiodination was associated with the degradation. The gel filtration patterns indicated that ^{125}I-insulin degradation products were composed mainly of small peptide fragments, suggesting that degradation had been achieved primarily by proteolysis. On the other hand, the authors were unable to detect any significant glutathione-insulin transhydrogenase activity.

FREYCHET *et al.* (1972) also considered that degradation of ^{125}I-insulin upon exposure to the purified membranes and specific binding of the hormone to its receptor in the same membranes were largely independent phenomena. This conclusion was suggested by a comparison of the degradation of insulin analogs manifesting varying degrees of affinity to the insulin receptor. ^{125}I-desalanine-des-asparagine insulin, whose affinity for receptors is only 2% that of insulin, was degraded to almost the same extent as ^{125}I-insulin. No relationship was found between the bioactivity of an insulin analogue and its ability to prevent the degradation of ^{125}I-insulin. The apparent K_m for insulin degradation as measured by TCA precipitation was 1.7×10^{-7}M, which is 40 times more than the concentration of insulin that produces half-maximal inhibition of specific binding of ^{125}I-insulin to receptors in the liver membrane. An insulin-degrading activity of fat cells and fat-cell fractions was also observed; this was of about the same order of magnitude as that of purified liver membranes in amounts having comparable specific binding capacity. Proinsulin was degraded very slowly by the liver membranes but appeared to act as a competitive inhibitor of insulin degradation.

Plasma membranes from rat epididymal fat cells and soluble extracts from the plasma membranes as well as intact fat cells have also been reported by CROFFORD *et al.* (1972) to contain a highly active insulin-degrading system. Furthermore, both the capacity of the plasma membranes to bind ^{125}I-insulin and the ^{125}I-insulin-degrading activity of the membrane extract could be inhibited by the addition of unlabeled insulin to the incubation medium, even though albumin was present in excess. The degraded products were not characterized, but on the basis of solubility in 10% trichoroacetic acid, nonreactivity with anti-insulin guinea-pig serum and nonadsorbability to a ^{125}I-adsorbing resin were considered to represent fragments of the insulin molecule. Since plasma membranes from trypsin-treated fat cells were found to have a reduced capacity to bind insulin and the insulin-degrading system of the membranes (or in soluble extracts from the membrane) was inactive, it was concluded that both the insulin receptor and the insulin-degrading system are located on the external surface of the plasma membrane of the fat cells. It was also postulated that an insulin-degrading system of the plasma membrane may be one of the physiological mechanisms for terminating the response of the fat cells to insulin.

III. Regulation of Insulin-Degrading Activity

BROH-KAHN and MIRSKY (1949) observed that fasting for 48—162 h produced a marked reduction in the "insulinase" activity of rat liver but that the activity was fully restored by feeding a balanced diet. Williams *et al.* (1959) also reported that starvation caused a decrease in total liver ^{131}I-insulin degrading activity. However, insulin, prednisolone injections hypophysectomy, adrenalectomy, alloxan diabetes, phlorizinization, and diets high in carbohydrate, fat, or protein produced relatively few changes. Doisy (1965) observed that the livers of rats fed a diet low in sulfur amino acids had a reduced insulin-degrading activity, which was associated with decreased glutathione levels. More recently, Morgan and Wiesman (1968) noted that rat "insulinase" activity was greatly reduced not only in fasted but also in alloxan-diabetic rats. The reduced "insulinase" activity was associated with low levels of plasma insulin. The association of markedly lowered insulin levels and "insulinase" activity in the fasted and alloxan-treated rat suggested the possibility that insulin is an inducer of "insulinase" activity.

The question of an autoregulatory system of insulin degradation in liver was more extensively studied by Uete and Tsuchikura (1972), who investigated the adaptive capacity of the liver to metabolize ^{131}I-insulin in response to fluctuations of blood level of insulin in normally fed, fasted, and alloxan-diabetic rats. They also noted that the degradation of insulin by liver homogenates of fasted or alloxan-diabetic rats was less than that by livers of normally fed control rats. However, the capacity of liver homogenate to hydrolyze casein, α-N-benzoyl-DL-arginine-β-naphthylamide and L-leucyl-β-naphthylamide was unchanged under the same conditions of fasting or alloxan diabetes. This suggested that degradation of insulin was specific and dependent upon changes in the concentration of insulin in the blood. Furthermore, the rate of insulin degradation in the liver correlated well with the level of reduced glutathione in the liver. Yet, when the decreased level of reduced glutathione in diabetic liver was restored to the control value by adding crystalline reduced glutathione to the incubation mixture, the degradation of insulin did not return to the control value. On the other hand, degradation of insulin was restored to the control level in the diabetic rat by administration of insulin. Also, increasing the insulin concentration in incubation media (human sera) enhanced the insulin degradation in liver slices and homogenates. Uete and Tsuchikura (1972) stated that a specific insulin-degradation system is responsible not only for the decreased insulin degradation in insulin deficiency states but also for the enhanced insulin degradation with increased levels of insulin in the body. They suggested that the liver possesses an autoregulatory mechanism for the control of insulin degradation in which the rate of insulin degradation is governed by the level of insulin in the blood. Such a mechanism would serve to supplement regulation of insulin secretion by controlling the concentration of blood insulin. ^{131}I-insulin degradation in these studies was measured by precipitability of the labeled insulin by trichloroacetic acid. These studies failed to determine whether the enzyme system responsible for this regulatory system of insulin degradation was "proteolytic insulinase" or glutathione-insulin transhydrogenase, or both. The recent studies of Varandani *et al.* (1974) suggest that the latter enzyme system is responsible.

Rat-liver homogenates from which GIT had been specifically removed by precipitating it with antibody were almost completely devoid of insulin-degrading activity. Immunochemical titration showed that the GIT content per unit DNA in livers of fed, diabetic rats 40—60 days after alloxan administration was 62% that of normal fed rats. Upon insulin treatment over a 50-hour period, the hepatic GIT content increased to 29% of that of untreated diabetic rats and to 182% of that of normal rats. Neither A nor B chain had any effect when administered in the same manner to diabetic rats, either alone or in combination with insulin. The hepatic GIT content is low in diabetes and starvation, where insulin is known to occur in low amounts, and the GIT content high in insulin-treated diabetic animals. These facts indicated to the authors that insulin functions as an inducer for the synthesis of GIT and that this could be a physiologically important feedback mechanism to regulate the levels of insulin.

VARANDANI *et al.* have reported that the insulin-mediated increase of GIT in diabetic rats was abolished by the concomitant administration of either actinomycin D (an inhibitor of RNA synthesis) or cycloheximide (an inhibitor of protein synthesis), suggesting that insulin induces synthesis of GIT protein via RNA synthesis.

IV. Quantitative and Kinetic Aspects of Proteolytic Degradation of ^{131}I-Insulin

None of the reported studies on proteolytic degradation of radioiodinated insulin has provided a reliable quantitative estimate of the nature and extent of the proteolytic degradation of insulin in terms of specific metabolites. In fact, the studies *in vitro* in which degradation (presumably proteolytic) of ^{131}I-insulin was investigated by means of accumulation of trichloroacetic acid-soluble radioactivity in the medium have all seemed to indicate that degradation did not go to completion but instead reached a plateau after a period of time (MIRSKY *et al.*, 1955; TOMIZAWA *et al.*, 1955; TOMIZAWA, 1962; SUMNER and DOISY, 1970). As indicated in the foregoing discussions, the trichloroacetic-acid method is a relatively simple technique for measuring ^{131}I-insulin degradation and has been widely used by numerous investigators to measure degradation of labeled insulin both *in vivo* and *in vitro*. However, the validity of the method for studying the mechanisms and kinetics of degradation of radioiodinated insulin *in vitro* was questioned by IZZO *et al.* (1972). Studies in which degradation of ^{131}I-insulin by supernatant fractions of rat-liver homogenates was investigated by both the trichloroacetic-acid method and by isolation and quantitation of ^{131}I-insulin and ^{131}I-labeled degradation products through the use of paper electrophoresis, showed that the trichloroacetic-acid method has serious limitations as a method for studying insulin-degradation kinetics *in vitro*.

In confirmation of the results of others mentioned above, the studies of IZZO *et al.* (1972) showed that, as measured by the trichloroacetic-acid method, degradation of ^{131}I-insulin containing 0.8 atom of total iodine per molecule, appeared to reach a plateau when approximately 60% of the insulin had been degraded. However, in striking contrast, degradation, as measured by the electrophoretic method, proceeded rapidly to completion. The discrepancy was shown to be the result of partial coprecipitation of degraded products, i.e. iodotyrosines, along with protein in the incubation mixtures by trichloroacetic acid, in direct proportion to the amount of protein present. With the electrophoretic method, the ^{131}I-insulin-degradation products migrated as a single major peak toward the cathode at a slower rate than ^{131}I-insulin. The major constituent of the peak was identified as ^{131}I-monoiodotyrosine. Upon completion of degradation, most, if not all, of the ^{131}I attached to insulin was recovered as ^{131}I-monoiodotyrosine.

The recent results of IZZO *et al.* (1972) have shown for the first time that in physiological concentrations ^{131}I-insulins are rapidly and extensively, if not completely, degraded by rat liver by proteolysis to simple amino acid constituents. This finding is in agreement with the work of KENNY (1960) showing that single amino acids rather than peptides were the end products of degradation of A and B chains of insulin by supernatant fractions of rat liver homogenate. Furthermore, neither ^{131}I-labeled A chain nor ^{131}I-labeled B chain was identified at any time during the entire course of degradation. However, this did not exclude the possibility of reductive cleavage of insulin into A and B chains as the primary event in insulin degradation by the liver, since it was considered possible under the conditions of the study that, if reduction of insulin had indeed occurred as a primary event, then either the degradation of the chains was so rapid that chains did not accumulate in sufficient quantities to be detected, or that cleavage of only one interchain -S-S bond was required for proteolytic attack of the insulin molecule.

Izzo *et al.* (1972) indicated that the rate and extent of degradation of ^{131}I-insulins were inversely proportional to the amount of iodine incorporated into the insulin molecule. The rate constants of iodoinsulins containing less than 1 atom of iodine per molecule were found to be almost 10 times greater than the rate constant of iodoinsulin containing 6 atoms of iodine per molecule. Yet, despite the difference in rates of degradation, all of the iodoinsulin studied seem to display second-order degradation kinetics according to the electrophoretic method. Interestingly, no correspondence to any specific reaction order could be shown for any of the iodoinsulins by the trichloroacetic-acid method. The studies *in vitro* confirmed and extended previous studies *in vivo* (Izzo *et al.*, 1967) suggesting that ^{131}I-insulin was degraded in liver and kidney by reaction kinetics that appeared to be second-order with respect to intact ^{131}I-insulin. Second-order reaction kinetics have been confirmed by Varandani *et al.* (1972) in the course of investigating degradation of labeled insulin by rat-tissue homogenates.

Second-order reaction was interpreted to indicate a bimolecular reaction in which two molecules of ^{131}I-insulin combine simultaneously with the catalyzing enzyme in each degradation event. It was indicated by Izzo and Bartlett (1969) that the consistency of a second-order reaction curve favors a sequence of events with only one step, which is rate-controlling, as opposed to the simultaneous action of multiple reaction mechanisms. If one step is to be rate-controlling, the orderly cleavage of the insulin molecule by glutathione as catalyzed by glutathione-insulin transhydrogenase is overwhelmingly more acceptable as a second-order process than the random splitting of the molecule by proteolytic enzymes. Thus, second-order degradation kinetics is consistent with a degradation process that involves reductive cleavage of the insulin molecule as the first step.

V. Comments

It is apparent from the foregoing discussion that, despite numerous studies on the nature, specificity, and site of insulin degradation, it is not yet clear precisely how and where insulin is destroyed in the body. The physiological significance or interrelationships of the processes that have been described for insulin degradation—namely, reductive cleavage of insulin by GIT followed by proteolysis of the two chains, and direct proteolysis of insulin by an insulin-specific protease—remains to be clarified. The physiological significance of the first process rests mainly on the studies of Varandani *et al.*, who showed not only that liver homogenates from which GIT had been specifically removed by precipitation with antibody were almost devoid of insulin-degrading activity, but also that GIT synthesis in the liver was induced by insulin. These studies have not yet been confirmed. However, indirect evidence in support of the first process was also provided by the kinetic studies of Izzo *et al.* (1967, 1972) on insulin disposition *in vivo* and degradation *in vitro*, indicating that ^{131}I-insulin was degraded according to second-order kinetics. The interpretation was that the consistency of a second-order reaction curve favors a sequence of events with only one step, which is rate-limiting, and that, if this be the case, then the orderly cleavage of the insulin molecule by reduced glutathione as catalyzed by GIT is overwhelmingly more acceptable as a second-order process than the ramdon splitting of the molecule by proteolytic enzymes. In the second process, insulin is said to undergo direct proteolytic attack by an "insulin-specific protease" without prior reduction of S-S bonds (Brush *et al.*, 1971). These studies have also not been confirmed as yet. Furthermore, evidence for the proteolytic nature of the enzyme is based primarily on the relatively small accumulation of ninhydrin-reactive material, expressed as leucine equivalents at the end of 22 hours' incubation of insulin with a calcium phosphate-gel purified enzyme.

Both glutathione-insulin transhydrogenase and insulin-specific protease (ISP) have been reported to be widely distributed in body tissus, with high concentrations in liver and kidney, and both have a narrow pH range of activity with an optimum at 7.3—7.6. GIT has been shown to have an activity toward other thiol-disulfide pairs, and in view of this a broader designation (e.g. thiol: protein disulfide oxidoreductase) was proposed as a more appropriate term. In fact, the studies of Ansorge (1973) suggest that this enzyme may be identical with the enzyme catalyzing the reactivation of "randomly oxidized" ribonuclease (Haber and Anfinsen, 1962; Givol *et al.*, 1964). On the other hand, ISP was reported to have a high specificity for insulin although it did exhibit some activity toward globin, and to a lesser extent casein, but not to albumin. Neither glucagon nor A and B chains were said to have any inhibiting effect on degradation of insulin by ISP. However, in the latest report from the same laboratory (Duckworth and Kitabchi, 1973) ISP was also stated to be capable of rapidly degrading glucagon. Hence, the degree of specificity of the enzyme remains to be established.

Since GIT seems to be located primarily in the microsomal fraction and ISP resides in the cytosol fraction, degradation of insulin by either of these two enzymes would require entry of insulin into the cell. This is of particular interest in liver and kidney, which are the major organs concerned with insulin destruction in the body. In this respect the findings of Freychet *et al.* (1972) are of interest, since they raise the intriguing possibility that it may not be necessary for insulin to penetrate the cell interior for degradation. They have reported the presence in purified liver-cell membranes of a protease capable of degrading insulin in concentrations equal to those present in portal blood. This, if true, would minimize the importance of reductive cleavage of insulin in the physiological degradation of insulin. However, it is not clear whether the enzyme is located on the outer or inner surface of the plasma membrane, whether it is similar to the "insulin-specific" protease in the cytosol, or whether it possesses sufficient activity and is present in sufficient concentration to account for the extremely rapid removal and degradation of ^{131}I-insulin by the liver reported by Izzo *et al.* (1967). Furthermore, the studies of Izzo *et al.* suggest that insulin does penetrate the liver and kidneys. In their studies, accumulation of both TCA-soluble and TCA-precipitable radioactivity was shown in both liver and kidneys following intravenous injection of biologically active ^{131}I-insulin into rats. Prior to homogenization of these tissues for assay of TCA-precipitable and TCA-soluble radioactivity, the animals were thoroughly perfused with ice-cold normal saline to remove not only residual blood but any residual radioactivity in the extracellular fluid spaces. Under these conditions it is very unlikely that the TCA-soluble radioactivity would have an extracellular source. This is further substantiated by the fact that intravenous administration of Na^{131}I did not result in any accumulation of radioactivity in the liver.

There is other evidence for intracellular penetration and degradation of insulin. On the basis of differences in the distribution of radioactivity among the intracellular components of liver and muscle, following intravenous injection of ^{131}I-insulin in rats and following incubation of ^{131}I-insulin in homogenates of liver, kidney, and muscle, LEE and WISEMAN (1959) concluded that insulin penetrated the cell wall, entered the cytoplasm and became fixed to the various cytoplasmic structures and to the nucleus. When ^{131}I-insulin was added to homogenate of liver, a much smaller amount became fixed to the intracellular components than when it was administered *in vivo*, demonstrating the importance of cellular integrity for the concentration of the hormone. It has been argued that, in the intact animal, radioiodine might actually be concentrated at or in extracellular liver and kidney structures, and that it is found at higher concentrations in mitochondrial and microsomal structures only because of redistribution following homogenization. This suggestion was refuted by LEE and WISEMAN (1959). They demonstrated that the ^{131}I of ^{131}I-insulin added to rat liver homogenates was rapidly transformed from TCA-insoluble to TCA-soluble radioactivity and was not accumulated to any great extent by the mitochondria and microsomes. On the other hand, such accumulation did occur when the ^{131}I-insulin was administered intravenously. The concentration of ^{131}I-insulin in the microsomal fraction was later confirmed by the findings of JACQUES and WATTIAUX-DECONINCK (1969), who examined the intracellular distribution of radioactivity in rat livers after intravenous injection of insulin. They found that very soon after the administration of ^{131}I-insulin the distribution of acid-insoluble radioactivity was similar to that of glucose-6-phosphatase whereas after a longer period the distribution pattern of acid-insoluble radioactivity became very similar to that of 2-glycerophosphatase. The argument that TCA-insoluble radioiodine, which was found to be concentrated in human and rat liver after ^{131}I-insulin administration, might not represent any significant amount of intact insulin was dispelled by the studies of BECK *et al.* (1966). These authors noted that, after radioiodoinsulin administration, mouse liver and kidney contained not only TCA-insoluble radioiodine but also roughly equivalent amounts of insulin, as estimated by immunoassay.

Additional support for the hypothesis that intact insulin molecules penetrate into and accumulate in significant amounts in mammalian liver cells was provided by the work of KALLEE (1965). Perfusion of rat liver with ^{131}I-insulin was followed by human anti-insulin serum to wash out any molecules that might been present in the extracellular fluids or attached to the cell surface. The isolated mitochondrial and microsomal fractions contained high concentrations of ^{131}I. Furthermore, much of this ^{131}I could be separated from the subcellular particles by incubating them with human anti-insulin serum. This ^{131}I was then shown to move electrophoretically in the same manner as the ^{131}I of ^{131}I-insulin which had been reacted directly with this anti-insulin serum.

VI. Summary and Conclusions

Degradation of insulin by slices, homogenates, and extracts of various mammalian organs and tissues has been rather extensively investigated in the past 20—25 years, mostly with the aid of radioiodinated insulin as a tracer. However, despite these numerous studies, precisely how and where insulin is destroyed in the body remains to be clarified.

While most tissues have been shown to have some capacity to degrade insulin, the greatest activity has been found in liver and kidney, whereas little or no activity has been found in brain and erythrocytes. Two different enzyme systems have been isolated from liver and other tissues that are capable of degrading insulin. The first system involves a sequential degradation of insulin whereby insulin first undergoes reductive cleavage of the -S-S- bonds, and the resultant chains are then proteolytically degraded to simple amino acids. The first step is enhanced by an enzyme designated glutathione-insulin transhydrogenase, while proteolysis of the chains is probably enhanced by an exopeptidase. The second enzyme system involves direct proteolytic attack of the insulin molecule without prior reductive cleavage by an "insulin-specific protease."

GIT seems to reside primarily in the microsomal fraction, especially the membrane-bound enzyme systems, whereas "ISP" is located principally in the cytosol fraction. GIT shows activity toward other thiol disulfide pairs and for this reason a broader designation (e.g. thiol: protein disulfide oxidoreductase) has been suggested. The enzyme also appears to be identical or very similar to the enzyme catalyzing the reactivation of "randomly oxidized" ribonuclease (Haber and Anfinsen, 1962; Givol *et al.*, 1964). "ISP" has been reported to be highly specific for insulin in that neither a large excess of A or B chains of insulin, bovine serum albumin, globin, glucagon, nor growth hormone inhibited the activity of the enzyme. On the other hand, ISP attacked proinsulin and proinsulin intermediates at only 3 and 10%, respectively, of the rate at which it attacked insulin. Subsequent studies, however, have indicated that "ISP" or a similar enzyme readily attacks glucagon also.

The interrelationships, if any, and the importance of GIT and "ISP" in the physiological degradation of insulin remain to be clarified. The inability of liver homogenates from which GIT had been removed by precipitation with specific antibody to degrade insulin suggests that the enzyme is important in the physiological degradation of insulin. Both enzyme systems are located intracellularly and would require penetration of insulin into the cell. Several lines of evidence support an intracellular penetration of insulin, at least in liver and kidney. This would raise serious questions concerning the physiological significance of "specific binding" of insulin to plasma membranes of organs such as liver. However, purified liver plasma membranes have been shown to have proteolytic activity for insulin, suggesting that perhaps intracellular penetration is not necessary for degradation of insulin by the liver.

The rate of insulin degradation by liver homogenates has been shown to be directly proportional to the level of plasma insulin, suggesting that the liver possesses an autoregulatory mechanism for the control of insulin degradation in which the rate of insulin degradation is governed by the level of insulin in plasma.

Information concerning the kinetics of radioiodinated insulin degradation, based on studies *in vitro* utilizing trichloroacetic-acid precipitability as an index of degradation, may have limited significance in view of the fact that it has recently been shown that degraded products such as iodotyrosine can be partially coprecipitated along with proteins in the mixture. Studies utilizing a paper-electrophoretic technique for separating labeled insulin from products of degradation have indicated that in physiological concentration insulin is extensively, if not completely, degraded to simple amino acids by rat liver homogenates, and that the reaction appears to follow second-order kinetics.

References

Ansorge, S., Bohley, P., Kirschke, H., Langner, J., Hanson, H.: Metabolism of insulin and glucagon breakdown of radioiodinated insulin and glucagon in rat liver cell fractions. Europ. J. Biochem. **19**, 283 (1971)

Ansorge, S., Bohley, P., Kirschke, H., Langner, J., Wiederanders, B., Hanson, H.: Metabolism of insulin and glucagon glutathione — insulin transhydrogenase from microsomes of rat liver. Europ. J. Biochem. **32**, 27 (1973)

Beck, L.V., Roberts, N., Blankenbaker, R., King, C.: On insulin immunologic activity in livers and kidneys of mice injected with beef insulin. Proc. Soc. exp. Biol. (N.Y.) **122**, 768—774 (1966)

Berson, S.A., Yalow, R.S., Volk, B.W.: *In vivo* and *in vitro* metabolism of ^{131}I-insulin and ^{131}I-glucagon in normal and cortisone treated rabbits. J. Lab. clin. Med. **49**, 331—342 (1957)

Black, S., Harte, E.M., Hudson, B., Wartofsky, L.: A specific enzymatic reduction of L (—) methionine sulfoxide and a related non-specific reduction of disulfides. J. biol. Chem. **235**, 2910—2916 (1960)

Broh-Kahn, R.H., Mirsky, I.A.: The inactivation of insulin by tissue extracts. II. The effect of fasting on the insulinase content of rat liver. Arch. Biochem. **20**, 10—14 (1949)

Brush, J.S.: Purification and characterization of a protease with specificity for insulin from rat muscle. Diabetes **20**, 140 (1971)

Burghen, G.A., Brush, J.S., Solomon, S.S., Etteldorf, J.N., Kitabchi, A.E.: Inhibition of insulin degradation by extracts of human plasma. Diabetes **20**, Suppl. 1, 342 (1971)

Burghen, G.A., Kitabchi, A.E., Brush, J.S.: Characterization of a rat liver protease with specificity for insulin. Endocrinology **91**, 633—642 (1972)

Chandler, M.L., Varandani, P.T.: Insulin degradation. II. The widespread distribution of glutathione-insulin transhydrogenase in the tissues of the rat. Biochim. biophys. Acta (Amst.) **286**, 136—145 (1972)

Crofford, O.B., Rogers, N.L., Russell, W.G.: The effect of insulin on fat cells. An insulin-degrading system extracted from plasma membranes of insulin-responsive cells. Diabetes **21**, Suppl. 2, 403—413 (1972)

Di Girolamo, M., Rudman, D., Malkin, M.F., Garcia, L.: Inactivation of insulin by adipose tissue. Diabetes **14**, 87—92 (1965)

Doisy, R.: Effect of diet on hepatic and serum inactivation of insulin. Endocrinology **77**, 49—59 (1965)

Duckworth, W.C., Kitabchi, A.E.: Insulin and glucagon degradation by a single enzyme. Diabetes **22**, 58 (1973)

Du Vignaud, V., Fitch, A., Pekarek, E., Wayne-Lockwood, W.: Inactivation of crystalline insulin by cysteine and glutathione. J. biol. Chem. **94**, 233—242 (1931)

Fraenkel-Conrat, J., Fraenkel-Conrat, H.: The essential groups of insulin. Biochim. biophys. Acta (Amst.) **5**, 89—97 (1950)

Freychet, P., Kahn, R., Roth, J., Neville, D.M., Jr.: Insulin interactions with liver plasma membranes. Independence of insulin binding and degradation. J. biol. Chem. **247**, 3953—3961 (1972)

Givol, D., Goldberger, R.F., Anfinsen, C.B.: Oxidation and disulfide interchange in the reactivation of reduced ribonuclease. J. biol. Chem. **239**, PC 3114 (1964)

Givol, D., Delorenzo, F., Goldberger, R.F., Anfinsen, C.B.: Disulfide interchange and the three-dimensional structure of proteins. Proc. nat. Acad. Sci. (Wash.) **53**, 676—684 (1965)

Goldberger, R.F., Epstein, C.J., Anfinsen, C.B.: Purification and properties of a microsomal enzyme system catalyzing the reactivation of reduced ribonuclease and lysozyme. J. biol. Chem. **239**, 1406—1410 (1964)

Haber, E., Anfinsen, C.B.: Side-chain interactions governing the pairing of half-cystine residues in ribonuclease. J. biol. Chem. **237**, 1839—1844 (1962)

Izzo, J.L., Bartlett, J.W., Roncone, A., Izzo, M.J., Bale, W.F.: Physiological processes and dynamics in the disposition of small and large doses of biologically active and inactive ^{131}I-insulin in the rat. J. biol. Chem. **242**, 2343—2355 (1967)

Izzo, J.L., Bartlett, J.W.: Insulin glucose dispersion and interaction system. Arch. intern. Med. **123**, 272—283 (1969)

Izzo, J.L., Roncone, A., Izzo, M.J., Foley, R., Bartlett, J.W.: Degradation of ^{131}I-insulin by rat liver. J. biol. Chem. **247**, 1219—1226 (1972)

Jacques, P.J., Wattiaux-Deconinck, S.: Abstr. Commun. 6th Meet. Fed. Europ. Biochem. Soc. **279**, (1969)

Jocelyn, P.C.: Glutathione metabolism in animals. In: Glutathione (ed. E.M. Crook). Biochem. Soc. Symp. **17**, 43—65 (Feb. 1958). Cambridge: University Press 1959

Kallee, E.: Naturforschung **196**, 357 (1965)

Katzen, H.M., Stetten, D., Jr.: Hepatic glutathione-insulin transhydrogenase. Diabetes **11**, 271—280 (1962)

Katzen, H.M., Tietze, F., Stetten, D.: Further studies on the properties of hepatic glutathione-insulin transhydrogenase. J. biol. Chem. **238**, 1006—1011 (1963)

Katzen, H.M., Tietze, F.: Studies on the specificity and mechanism of action of hepatic glutathione-insulin transhydrogenase. J. biol. Chem. **241**, 3561—3570 (1966)

KENNY, A.J.: The proteolysis of glucagon and other peptides by rat liver *in vitro*. Biochem. J. **69**, 32—33 (1958)

KENNY, A.J.: Metabolism of peptide hormones. Brit. med. Bull. **16**, 202—208 (1960)

KOTOULAS, O.B., MORRISON, G.R., RECANT, L.: Glutathione-insulin transhydrogenase activity in pancreatic islets. Biochim. biophys. Acta (Amst.) **97**, 350—353 (1965)

LAURENT, T.C., MOORE, E.C., REICHARD, P.: Enzymatic synthesis of deoxy-ribonucleotides. IV. Isolation and characterization of thioredoxin, the hydrogen donor from *Escherichia coli B*. J. biol. Chem. **239**, 3436—3444 (1964)

LEE, N.D., WISEMAN, R., JR.: The significance of the binding of ^{131}I-insulin to cytostructural elements of rat liver. Endocrinology **65**, 442—450 (1959)

LEHMANN, H., SCHLOSSMAN, H.: The action of cell-free muscle extract on insulin. Proc. physiol. Soc. **15P** (1938)

MIRSKY, A., BROH-KAHN, R.H.: The inactivation of insulin by tissue extracts. I. The distribution and properties of insulin-inactivating extracts (insulinase). Arch. Biochem. **20**, 1—9 (1949)

MIRSKY, I.A.: Ciba Found. Colloq. Endocrinology **6**, 263 (1953)

MIRSKY, I.A., PERISUTTI, G.: Abs. Am. Chem. Soc. 120th Mtg., N.Y.C., 1951

MIRSKY, I.A., PERISUTTI, G.: The inactivation of insulin by liver slices of the rat. Endocrinology **52**, 698 (1953)

MIRSKY, I.A., PERISUTTI, G., DIXON, F.J.: Destruction of ^{131}I-labeled insulin by liver slices. Proc. Soc. exp. Biol. (N.Y.) **86**, 228—230 (1954)

MIRSKY, I.A., PERISUTTI, G., DIXON, F.J.: The destruction of ^{131}I-labeled insulin by rat liver extracts. J. biol. Chem. **214**, 397—408 (1955)

MIRSKY, I.A., PERISUTTI, G.: The relative specificity of the insulinase activity of rat liver extracts. J. biol. Chem. **228**, 77 (1957)

MOORE, E.C., REICHARD, P.: Enzymatic synthesis of deoxy-ribonucleotides. VI. The cytidine diphosphate reductase system from Novikoff hepatoma. J. biol. Chem. **239**, 3453—3456 (1964)

MORGAN, C.R., SPAHN, J., FRAZIER, V., FLEITZ, S.: Relative insulinase activity in the liver and kidney of the rat. Proc. Soc. exp. Biol. (N.Y.) **128**, 485—488 (1968)

MORGAN, C.R., WIESMAN, H.J.: Liver insulinase activity in insulin-deficient rats. Proc. Soc. exp. Biol. (N.Y.) **127**, 763—765 (1968)

NARAHARA, H.T., TOMIZAWA, H.H., MILLER, R., WILLIAMS, R.H.: Mode of inactivation of insulin by rat liver extracts. J. biol. Chem. **214**, 285—294 (1955)

NARAHARA, H.T., WILLIAMS, R.H.: Reduction of insulin by extracts of rat liver. J. biol. Chem. **234**, 71—77 (1959)

RACKER, E.: Metabolism of thiolesters of glutathione. Fed. Proc. **12**, 711—715 (1953)

RALL, T.W., LEHNINGER, A.L.: Glutathione reductase of animal tissues. J. biol. Chem. **194**, 119—130 (1952)

RUDMAN, D., GARCIA, L.A., DI GIROLAMO, M., SHANK, P.W.: Cleavage of bovine insulin by rat adipose tissue. Endocrinology **78**, 169—185 (1966)

RYLE, A.P., SANGER, F., SMITH, L.F., KITAI, R.: The disulphide bonds of insulin. Biochem. J. **60**, 541—556 (1955)

SCHMIDT, A.A., SAACHIAN, R.L.: Zh. exptl. biol. Med. **11**, 42 (1929)

SUMNER, K., DOISY, R.J.: Degradation of insulin by a particulate fraction from adipose tissue. Biochem. J. **116**, 825—831 (1970)

TOMIZAWA, H.H., WILLIAMS, R.H.: Studies on the specificity of an insulin-inactivating system of the liver. J. biol. Chem. **217**, 685—694 (1955)

TOMIZAWA, H.H., HALSEY, Y.D.: Isolation of an insulin-degrading enzyme from beef liver. J. biol. Chem. **234**, 307—310 (1959)

TOMIZAWA, H.H.: Mode of action of an insulin-degrading enzyme from beef liver. J. biol. Chem. **237**, 428—431 (1962)

TOMIZAWA, H.H.: An insulin-reducing transhydrogenase of beef pancreas. Fed. Proc. **24**, 577 (1965)

UETE, T., TSUCHIKURA, H.: Autoregulatory system of insulin degradation in liver. J. Biochem. **72**, 157—163 (1972)

VARANDANI, P.T., NAFTZ, M.A., SHROYER, L.A.: Glutathione-insulin transhydrogenase: evidence for a key role in insulin metabolism. Diabetes **20**, Suppl. 1, 342 (1971)

VARANDANI, P.T., SHROYER, L.A., NAFTZ, M.A.: Sequential degradation of insulin by rat liver homogenates. Proc. nat. Acad. Sci. (Wash.) **69**, 1681—1684 (1972)

VARANDANI, P.T.: Insulin degradation. I. Purification and properties of glutathione-insulin transhydrogenase of rat liver. Biochim. biophys. Acta (Amst.) **286**, 126—135 (1972)

VARANDANI, P.T.: VI. Feedback control by insulin of liver glutathione-insulin transhydrogenase in rat. Diabetes **23**, 117—125 (1974)

Vaughan, M.: Inactivation of insulin by an enzyme from rat liver. Biochim. biophys. Acta (Amst.) **15**, 432—433 (1954)
Venetianer, P., Straub, F.B.: Studies on the mechanism of action of the ribonuclease-reactivating enzyme. Acta physiol. Acad. Sci. hung. **27**, 303—315 (1965)
Williams, R.H., Martin, F.B., Henley, E.D., Swanson, H.E.: Inhibitors of insulin degradation. Metabolism **8**, 99—113 (1959)
Wintersteiner, O.: The action of sulfhydryl compounds on insulin. J. biol. Chem. **102**, 473—488 (1933)

Effects of Insulin and Proinsulin

A. Insulin Receptor Interactions and the Action of Insulin

GUY P.E. TELL, FOLKER KRUG, PEDRO CUATRECASAS

I. Introduction

In the past a great many studies have been directed primarily to studying the nature of the metabolic and biological effects of insulin. A wide variety of metabolic events are clearly altered by insulin, and many of these have been studied in detail. In recent years attention has been directed to the earliest events in the action of insulin with the expectation that a common early process could be discovered which would explain all the subsequent effects of the hormone. The search for a common biochemical intermediate seemed logical on the basis that the vast array of biological effects were unlikely to be mediated by an equally large number of biological receptors. The concept of a receptor for insulin, as well as for other peptide hormones, is based on the belief of the existence of highly specific structures in the cell which are capable of recognizing the hormone with a high degree of selectivity and affinity. In addition, interaction with this receptor must lead to biologically significant events. The possibility of multiple kinds of receptors in a single cell is generally regarded as unlikely. There is no precedence for such processes, there is no compelling reason to believe that this should be different for insulin, and it is difficult conceptually to visualize how hormonal control can be

Supported by grants from National Institute of Arthritis and Metabolic Diseases (AM14956), The American Cancer Society (BC-63), National Science Foundation (GB-34300), and The Kroc Foundation.

P. CUATRECASAS is the recipient of a United States Public Health Service Research Career Development Award AM31464.

properly effected by having different kinds of receptors for a single hormone on a given cell.

As with other hormones, attempts to recognize and identify receptors for insulin are based on the demonstration of binding of the hormone to target tissues. The first evidence of binding of insulin was obtained by indirect measurements. Addition of radioactively labelled insulin to the incubation medium resulted in an increase in glycogen synthesis in isolated rat diaphragms. After a brief incubation period, the content of radioactivity in the muscle was determined after removal of insulin from the medium by washing procedures (Stadie *et al.*, 1949). Similar observations were made with epididymal fat pads (Haugaard and Marsh, 1952) and with the lactating mammary gland (Hills and Stadie, 1952). Binding studies of this hormone to striated muscle and adipose tissue by these and other authors were hindered by the very low specific activity of the hormone, which was labeled with sulfur or with iodine (Stadie *et al.*, 1952; Wolthmann and Narahara, 1966). Because of the necessity of using intact tissues, these workers were hindered by the inability to discriminate between specific binding and nonspecific physical adsorption to tissue structures other than specific hormone receptors. The early insulin binding studies have recently been reviewed in detail (Narahara, 1972). In the past few years considerable progress has been made in the study of hormone receptor interactions by measuring the binding of biologically active iodoinsulin to intact cells which lack basement membranes (isolated fat cells), or to isolated membrane preparations. Insulin derivatives labeled with ^{125}I have been obtained which have specific activities ranging from 500 to 2,000 Curies per mmole.

II. Insulin Receptors

1. Binding of Iodoinsulin to Receptors

Binding of iodoinsulin and the correlation between the binding process and the biological response to insulin can best be demonstrated in intact fat cells (Cuatrecasas, 1971a, b; Kono and Barham, 1971; El-Allawy and Gliemann, 1972) or in broken cell preparations from hepatocytes and adipocytes (House and Weidemann, 1970; Cuatrecasas, 1971d; Freychet *et al.*, 1971, Freychet *et al.*, 1972a). The process of iodination of insulin which is used in these comparative studies requires extreme care, and the iodinated hormone must be rigorously purified (Cuatrecasas, 1971a, b, c). Minimal criteria which should be met are that the insulin be more than 95% precipitable by 5% trichloroacetic acid and more than 95% adsorbable to talc or microfine silica (Cuatrecasas, 1971a, b). It has been shown that under certain conditions the biological potency and the specificity of the binding of iodoinsulin to fat cells is unaffected by varying the iodine content between 0.1 and 0.8 atoms of ^{125}I per molecule of insulin (Cuatrecasas, 1972a). If the biological integrity of the radiohormone depended on the amount of substituted iodine a corresponding fall in activity should be observed with increasing amounts of substitution with iodine. Although the exact position of the substituted iodine on the insulin molecule is not known and the preparation cannot be described as monosubstituted, the apparent lack in the variability of biological behavior of iodoinsulin proves its usefulness of tracer studies in membrane systems. Many experiments demonstrate that the biological activity and the binding properties of labeled insulin correlate extremely well (Cuatrecasas, 1971a). In one study, monoiodoinsulin was purified by ion exchange chromatography and shown to be biologically active (Freychet *et al.*, 1971). The tendency of insulin to aggregate at higher concentrations complicates the large scale preparation of radiohormone (CUATRECASAS, 1971a; HUNTER and GREENWOOD, 1962; YALOW and BERSON, 1966) in quantities sufficient to perform chemical identification for comparative purpose. The results of such studies must be interpreted with great care since the pattern of iodine substitution may depend on the actual insulin concentration and on its state of aggregation during the iodination procedure.

The simple demonstration of binding of radioactive hormones to cells or to membrane preparations does not by itself constitute proof that such binding is occurring to biologically significant receptors, even if binding occurs at extremely low concentrations of the hormone. It is known that insulin, as many other peptide hormones, has a great propensity for nonspecific adsorption to a variety of organic and inorganic surfaces (such as glass, nylon, etc.). Such binding also can occur with proteins such as albumin and it is not unreasonable that this binding may also occur with a variety of cellular structures. One of the more important features of nonspecific binding processes in general is the relative unsaturability of the process. This, of course, is true only within reasonable limits. For this reason, it is very important to demonstrate experimentally that the receptor binding process being measured is a saturable process with respect to insulin over reasonably low concentrations of the hormone. In previous studies (CUATRECASAS, 1971a) the nonspecific binding has been corrected by making identical measurements in which the radioactive hormone is added to the cells or to the membranes after a short preincubation of the tissues with the native hormone. It is presumed in these kinds of experiments that a finite number of receptors exists which are saturated by such prelabeling with nonradioactive hormone. Another very important general feature of nonspecific adsorptive processes is that the binding is directly proportional to the concentration of hormone in the medium. This, of course, would not be expected for the binding to a biological receptor. These considerations imply that with increasing concentrations of hormone in the medium the nonspecific adsorptive processes will continually increase and will make detection of specific receptor interactions most difficult at the higher concentrations of the hormone. For example (CUATRECASAS, 1971a) at high concentrations of hormone, where the receptor is nearly saturated, the nonspecific binding component will be considerable. Furthermore, the proportion of the radioactive hormone which nonspecifically binds to the membranes is very critically dependent on the quality of the radioactive hormone which is used. In this laboratory preparations of the hormone made with tracer-free ^{125}I which is not extremely fresh will lead to iodoinsulin which has great nonspecific adsorptive properties. In addition, iodinated insulin will progressively deteriorate with time, and the most sensitive indicator of this deterioration is a large increase which occurs in the nonspecific binding to membranes or to cells. In view of the above considerations, it is apparent that examination of specific interactions at high concentrations of the hormone is most difficult. It has been reported that cells and membranes contain a second class of low affinity receptors (HAMMOND *et al.*, 1972). These have been based on Scatchard plots which extrapolate to a finite number of receptors with a given affinity. The direct demonstration of saturability of this low affinity binding system has not been demonstrated experimentally. The significance of this latter class or type of binding is not clear, and may not reflect biologically significant interactions. The specificity of this type of binding has not been demonstrated since its displacement by varying concentrations of native hormone as well as the ability of hormone analogs to displace it have not been studied; these have been performed only with the higher affinity binding, at lower concentrations of hormone. It must be remembered that even if saturation were demonstrable with the use of extremely high concentrations of the hormone it would not necessarily mean that these are biologically significant receptors since the "unsaturability" of nonspecific binding must be considered as being relative and is only one of the criteria which must be studied. It is unreasonable to expect that a very small quantity of material would have an infinite number of binding sites, even if these are nonspecific. Until proof to the contrary is available, it must be considered that the insulin receptors are a unique class which corresponds to the measurements which are performed with physiological concentrations of the hormone and which demonstrate saturability and an affinity consistent with that which would be expected from biological data.

Considerable evidence now exists that the high-affinity binding which is observed with physiological concentrations of iodoinsulin reflects interaction of the hormone with structural components of the membrane which are of physiological significance. The principal points which corroborate this include: 1) The similarity between the concentration dependence of binding of iodoinsulin to membranes and cells with the concentration dependence of biological responses to the same iodoinsulin or to the native hormone. 2) The similarity between the apparent insulin-cell dissociation constant (about 10^{-10}M) which results from metabolic studies and from binding studies. 3) The ability of native insulin but not of a variety of other peptide hormones, even at a concentration 20,000 times greater than that of iodoinsulin, to compete with binding. 4) The exact correspondence (measured by affinity) between the relative ability of insulin analogs to initiate the biological response and to compete with iodoinsulin for binding. Desalanine insulin is indistiguishable from native insulin (CUATRECASAS, 1971a). Proinsulin binds to the receptor with an affinity which is about 20 times less than that of native insulin (CUATRECASAS, 1972b). A decrease of corresponding magnitude in the effect of proinsulin on glucose oxidation is observed as well. Desalanine-desasparagine-insulin and desoctapeptide-insulin show a further decrease in activity. Reduced insulin, S-sulfonated and carboxymethylated insulins do not compete for binding and do not elicit metabolic effects. 5) The parallelism between binding and biological effectiveness of insulins derived from various species (FREYCHET *et al.*, 1971). 6) The similarity between the relative ability of ^{125}I-insulin to bind to cells and of native insulin to evoke a biological response when these cells have been modified by proteolytic digestion (CUATRECASAS, 1971b). Tryptic digestion, for example, decreases the affinity of ^{125}I-insulin for binding to the same extent when the ability of native insulin to enhance glucose transport is measured. 7) The ability of certain plant lectins to bind to the insulin receptor, to displace insulin, and to initiate an insulin-like biological response (CUATRECASAS and TELL, 1973; CUATRECASAS, 1973a).

Structures which are capable of specifically binding iodoinsulin have been detected in isolated fat cells (CUATRECASAS, 1971a; KONO and BARHAM, 1971), fat cell membranes (CUATRECASAS, 1971d), liver cell membranes (FREYCHET *et al.*, 1971; FREYCHET *et al.*, 1972; CUATRECASAS *et al.*, 1971), and in circulating blood cells (GAVIN *et al.*, 1972; KRUG *et al.*, 1972). Human lymphocytes transformed *in vitro* with plant lectins also are capable of binding insulin. No significant binding has been observed to purified, resting, untransformed human lymphocytes (KRUG *et al.*, 1972) or to human erythrocytes. Binding has also been described with thymocytes (GOLDFINE *et al.*, 1972; GOLDFINE and SHERLINE, 1972). The human placenta has recently been found to possess a very large number of insulin receptors (unpublished). The detailed properties of the insulin receptor interaction will be considered in a later section of this chapter.

2. Localization of Receptors

a) Localization of Receptors to Cell Surfaces

For some years there have been theoretical grounds for postulating that the cell membrane is the primary site of insulin action (LEVIN, 1965). The localization of insulin receptors to the cell surface was suggested by the loss of insulin responsiveness of fat cells by digestion with trypsin (KONO, 1969a, b; FAIN and LOKEN, 1969). However, it could not be excluded that trypsin, which is not much larger than insulin, could not itself penetrate the cell and thus act intracellulary.

More convincing evidence has been presented by using insoluble and bulky derivatives of insulin prepared by the covalent attachment of the hormone to agarose beads through the α-amino group of the N-terminal residue of the B-chain, or through the ε-amino group of the lysyl residue. These insulin-agarose derivatives (but not unsubstituted agarose) effectively increase the utilization of glucose, inhibit hormone stimulated lipolysis (CUATRECASAS, 1969), stimulate α-amino isobutyric acid accumulation in isolated mammary cells (OKA and TOPPER, 1971, 1972), and activate glycogen synthetase in liver (BLATT and KIM, 1971). Although the exact mechanism of action of these insulin agarose beads does not seem to be identical to that of native insulin (CUATRECASAS, 1973b), these studies indicate that interaction of insulin with superficial membrane structures alone may suffice to initiate transport as well as other metabolic processes. It is equally significant that soluble polymers (dextran) containing covalently-bound insulin are also biologically active (ARMSTRONG *et al.*, 1972; SUZUKI *et al.*, 1972).

The ability to simulate insulin-like biological effects by perturbation of the cell surface does not exclude the possibility that additional insulin receptors exist inside of the cell. It has been demonstrated that the insulin-binding activity of intact fat cells is quantitatively recovered in the microsomal fraction of the cell homogenate (CUATRECASAS, 1971a). However, it is still possible that during homogenization some surface receptors are destroyed which are compensated by the appearance of some new intracellular binding structures. This eventuality was examined (CUATRECASAS, 1971b) by treating fat cells with a trypsin-agarose derivative (large complex which cannot enter the cell) before homogenization. The virtually complete loss of insulin binding (when tested with low concentrations of insulin) after digestion is not altered by homogenization, indicating that there are no significant quantities of intracellular structures which are capable of binding insulin. In addition, no specific binding of insulin can be detected in the mitochondrial and nuclear fractions prepared by differential centrifugation, and the soluble cellular fraction does not compete for the binding of insulin by the cytoplasmic membranes (CUATRECASAS, 1971a).

Independent studies have also been performed with intact fat cells which are labeled by incubating with ^{125}I-insulin and subsequently homogenized to study the localization of radioactivity in subcellular fractions by sucrose gradient centrifugation (CHANG *et al.*, 1974). In these studies the radioactivity migrates almost exclusively with the cytoplasmic membrane fractions.

A number of studies have indicated that the properties of the insulin receptor interaction in the isolated membrane preparations are almost identical to those observed with intact cells. Therefore, given the quantitative and qualitative assurances that the binding being measured in the isolated membranes is the same as that observed in the intact cells in which the interaction is closely correlated with the biological response to insulin, the groundwork is set for the further characterization and purification of receptors with the use of isolated membrane preparations.

b) Assymetric Positioning of the Insulin Receptor in the Membrane

A stable external orientation of the insulin receptor has been demonstrated in a membrane preparation from isolated rat fat cells which contains inside-out plasma membrane vesicle (Bennett and Cuatrecasas, 1973). Insulin, which is first bound to the external receptors, is subsequently trapped inside of such inverted vesicles. In contrast to insulin bound to normally-oriented membrane vesicles, the labeled hormone in the inside-out vesicles is released into the medium at a negligible rate. This finding indicates that physical inversion of the normal inside-outside organization of the plasma membrane is not accompanied by a major reorientation or flip-flopping of the receptor-insulin complex. These observations are consistent with the fluid mosaic model of membranes (Singer and Nicolson, 1972) which predicts only lateral movements of membrane proteins, since a high energy barrier prevents any rotation of polar molecules through the phospholipid bilayers.

3. Insulin Receptor Interaction

a) Properties of the Insulin Receptor Interaction

The half maximal saturation of insulin binding occurs at a concentration of about 10^{-10}M insulin (Cuatrecasas, 1971a, 1971d; Cuatrecasas *et al.*, 1971). A maximum of about 10,000 molecules of insulin can be bound per fat cell (Cuatrecasas, 1971a), and about 0.1 pg of the hormone is bound per mg of liver cell membrane (Cuatrecasas *et al.*, 1971).

The binding of insulin to the receptor can be reversed with acid, and the hormone released from this complex is similar to previously unbound insulin with respect to several physical properties. It interacts with insulin antiserum, it can bind again to membrane receptors, and its ability to stimulate glucose transport in isolated fat cells (Cuatrecasas, 1971a, d; Freychet *et al.*, 1972a) is similar to that of unused hormone. Addition of a large excess of antiserum to the insulin-cell complex results in complete dissociation of the bound insulin. The subsequent insulin-binding capacity of the cells from which the insulin was dissociated is not significantly reduced or altered (Cuatrecasas, 1971a).

Insulin inactivation has been clearly demonstrated in preparations of liver membranes obtained by the technique of Neville (Freychet *et al.*, 1972a). Careful studies by these investigators, however, indicate that the inactivation observed is unrelated to the binding to biologically significant receptors. Furthermore, it has been demonstrated independently that binding equilibrium can be obtained with other liver cell membranes as well as with intact fat cells and fat cell membranes in the absence of significant inactivation. The demonstration that binding of a biologically significant nature can occur without significant inactivation of the insulin in the medium indicates quite strongly that when inactivation is observed it probably is unrelated to the activation of biological receptors. Furthermore, it is unlikely that inactivation is related at all to insulin receptor binding.

The rate constants of insulin-membrane association (8.5×10^6 mole^{-1} sec^{-1}) and dissociation (4.2×10^{-4} mole^{-1} sec^{-1}) have been measured independently and the dissociation constant calculated from these rate constants (about 10^{-10}M) closely approximates the dissociation constant calculated from equilibrium data (Cuatrecasas, 1971c). Binding of insulin is much tighter at lower temperature because the decrease in the dissociation rate is greater than the decrease in the association rate.

It appears quite clear that the interaction of insulin with receptors occurs by relatively classical and predictable reversible processes which follow the law of mass action. The insulin receptor interaction does not appear to involve the formation of stable covalent intermediates and the binding is not associated with activities which result in destruction of either the insulin or the receptor.

The presence of heavy metals or metal complexing agents do not affect the binding of insulin to fat cells (CUATRECASAS, 1971c). The optimum pH for binding occurs sharply at about pH 7.5. An abrupt thermal transition occurs with a midpoint at 53° C. Binding of insulin to fat cell membranes is greatly enhanced by high ionic strength buffers (CUATRECASAS, 1971c). Increasing concentrations of NaCl up to 2 M increase insulin binding up to 6-fold. This is probably the result of the appearance (unmasking) of new receptor structures. These binding sites are kinetically indistinguishable from the receptors normally exposed. These effects of NaCl appear to be similar to those observed after digestion of membranes with phospholipase C, which will be described shortly.

Chemical modification of cell membranes with several protein modifying reagents suggests that the histidyl residues play an important role in the binding of insulin to membrane structures (CUATRECASAS, 1971c). The properties of the interaction of insulin with isolated liver cell membranes (CUATRECASAS and ILLIANO, 1971; HOUSE and WEIDEMANN, 1970; CUATRECASAS, 1971d) resembles very closely that observed in fat cell membranes. On the basis of these data a close structural similarity between the insulin receptor in both tissues has been postulated.

b) Effect of Enzymatic Digestions

α) Neuraminidase

Neuraminidase is a glycosidase which selectively cleaves exposed, terminal sialic acid residues of membrane glycoprotein structures. Digestion of isolated fat cells with very low concentrations of neuraminidase (10—20 mμg per ml for 15 min at 37° C) results in an enhancement of glucose transport which can be nearly as great as the one observed with insulin in untreated cells (CUATRECASAS and ILLIANO, 1971). The effect of insulin is unaffected by such concentrations of neuraminidase; no further increase is observed provided maximal concentrations of insulin are used. This suggests that these two apparently different stimuli may have similar effects on the cell membrane. Moderately greater digestion with this enzyme (1 μg per ml) results in the abolition of the effect described above and in the loss of responsiveness to insulin. Such treatment has little or no detectable effect on glucose transport and lipolysis induced by various hormones (epinephrine, ACTH, glucagon), but it prevents any further alteration of these processes by insulin. However, such digestion does not induce a selective destruction of the insulin receptor since the binding capacity remains intact even after drastic digestion of cells. It thus appears that moderate digestion by neuraminidase is responsible for a dissociation of the biological and the receptor-binding properties of insulin in isolated fat cells. This uncoupling effect suggests that sialic acid, which is released into the medium during the digestion with neuraminidase, may be present on the insulin receptor and that it is involved not in insulin recognition and binding but in conveying the information of binding.

β) Proteases

The binding process itself may be affected by other types of enzymic digestion, suggesting that other molecules are specifically involved in the attachment of insulin to the membrane receptors. Very mild digestion of fat cells with trypsin is responsible for a selective fall in the affinity of the receptors for insulin (CUATRECASAS, 1971b); correspondingly, there is a loss in the responsiveness of glucose transport to low concentrations of insulin. This fall in affinity of the insulin-cell complex appears to be nearly the same whether it is measured by insulin binding or by the effect of insulin on glucose oxidation. Under such conditions the maximal insulin response (glucose oxidation) as well as the total amount of receptor remain unaffected. Precisely the same maximal effects as in untreated cells can be obtained using sufficiently high concentrations of insulin. More drastic tryptic digestion, however, results in a severe loss of both insulin responsiveness (Fain and Loken, 1969) and insulin binding (Cuatrecasas, 1971b; Kono and Barham, 1971). Such digestion may affect more critical regions of the receptor, and in addition it may alter the ability of the insulin-receptor complex to convey signals to the glucose transport mechanism of the cell membrane. It is important, however, that regardless of the specific mechanisms involved the trypsin effects appear to be due to interaction of this enzyme with superficial structures of the cell surface. This has been demonstrated by using trypsin-agarose derivatives which cannot enter the cell and which do not release free trypsin; such derivatives can reproduce the same effects as those observed with soluble trypsin (Cuatrecasas, 1971b).

γ) Galactosidases

Although very mild digestion of fat cells by β-galactosidase does not affect the binding of insulin, the effect of this enzyme is profound when the digestion is performed on cells predigested by neuraminidase or when it is used simultaneously with neuraminidase (Cuatrecasas, 1971b, 1972a). Since neuraminidase digestion does not affect insulin binding by itself, it can be surmised that the covalent removal of sialic acid residues exposes galactose groups which are susceptible to hydrolysis by β-galactosidase. The loss of binding after the hydrolysis of galactose groups suggests that galactose may contribute to the binding function and may be a constituent of the receptor. Further evidence that the insulin receptor is a glycoprotein will be presented in a later section.

δ) Phospholipases

Digestion of fat and liver cell membranes with phospholipase A or C but not phospholipase D leads to a substantial increase (3 to 6 fold) in the specific binding of insulin to these membranes (Cuatrecasas, 1971c). This effect reflects an increase in the total quantity of binding sites without affecting the affinity of the insulin-receptor complex. Kinetic data indicate that the newly exposed or "unmasked" binding-sites in phospholipase C-treated cells have the same characteristics as those normally exposed to the medium. The effect of phospholipase digestion can be mimicked by extraction of membrane lipids with organic solvents, and it is partially reversed by the addition of extracted lipids or certain purified phospholipids. This indicates that phospholipase effect may be due to the removal or displacement of membrane phospholipids.

The normally "buried" insulin binding sites are inaccessible to macromolecules other than insulin itself since phospholipase digestion still has a major effect on fat cells which have first been digested with trypsin. On the other hand, digestion with phospholipase greatly increases the susceptibility of the receptors to low concentration of trypsin. Thus, after removal of membrane phospholipids, mild digestion with trypsin appears to severely destroy insulin binding by damaging more critical regions of the insulin receptor.

The unmasking of new insulin binding sites by phospholipase digestion appears to be very similar to the effects described earlier for exposure of membranes to high ionic strength. The effects of sodium chloride are completely reversible by simply washing the membranes. This suggests that the polar heads of the phospholipids are involved in the masking of these insulin-binding sites. As described above, the "buried" nature of the receptors is relative to the kind of probe which is used to measure the receptor. Whereas these binding sites are not normally accessible to insulin or to trypsin, they are readily destroyed and thus accessible, to a small reagent such as tetranitromethane. The significance of these cryptic sites is not yet understood. It is not known whether these binding sites represent totally new and separate molecular structures in the membrane or whether they might represent duplication of binding sites within the same micromolecular complex. The biological significance is not understood. It has recently been demonstrated that membranes obtained from livers of very young rats have an equally large amount of masked binding capacity compared to the livers of much larger animals (BENNETT and CUATRECASAS, unpublished). Thus, the possibility that these binding sites may represent receptors which were significant and required during earlier stages of development appears to be very unlikely.

c) Effects of Insulin-Agarose Derivatives

One of the single most dramatic demonstrations that insulin affects cellular metabolism by interacting with structures located in the plasma membrane comes from the demonstration that insulin coupled to large agarose beads is biologically active and stimulates glucose oxidation in fat cells (BLATT and KIM, 1971; CUATRECASAS, 1969; TURKINGTON, 1970). The reversible binding of fat cell ghosts (CUATRECASAS, 1971e; SODERMAN *et al.*, 1973) and insulin binding macromolecules (CUATRECASAS, 1972c) further strengthens the evidence of a specific polymer-receptor interaction.

Although native insulin and the polymer-insolubilized hormone compete for the same specific insulin receptor in the membrane, there is reason to believe that the agarose-bound insulin elicits its biologic effect on the cells by mechanisms which are different from those which are activated by the native hormone. Maximal responses to insulin should require the binding of about 10,000 molecules of the hormone per fat cell. However, for steric reasons it is very difficult to imagine how this number of insulin molecules coupled to agarose beads can simultaneously interact with a single fat cell to achieve a maximal response.

OKA and TOPPER (1971, 1972) have shown that immature mammary gland explant cells do not respond to native insulin but do respond to insulin-agarose. Native insulin, which cannot elicit a biological response in these cells, can block the activation by the polymer (OKA and TOPPER, 1971, 1972). These findings clearly indicate that properly prepared insulin-agarose can be used in such studies under conditions that do not release free insulin into the medium from the polymer. These studies indicate further that insulin-agarose derivatives activate cells by somewhat different mechanisms since they are able to affect responses that are not possible (in some cells) with native insulin. The actions of these derivatives of course depend on the existence of insulin receptors since the effect is blocked by native insulin.

One possible explanation of this unusual effect of insulin-agarose is that in addition to the binding of the insulin moiety of the polymer to the specific insulin receptor the closeness of a large foreign surface to the cell surface (in the region of the receptor) perturbs the plasma membrane in such a way that a biological response is initiated nonspecifically. The small size of the insulin molecule and the effectiveness of preparations in which insulin is directly linked to the agarose backbone without the interposition of a hydrocarbon chain strongly supports this interpretation. It has been observed that insulin attached to agarose by relatively long arms (25—50 Å) is less effective in activating glucose transport in fat cells but is more effective in specifically adsorbing soluble insulin-binding molecules derived from cell membranes.

It is also quite important that insulin linked to soluble polymers, such as dextran derivatives, are also quite potent in activating biological responses (ARMSTRONG *et al.*, 1972; SUZUKI *et al.*, 1972). With such soluble polymeric derivatives of insulin, it has been possible to demonstrate biological activity *in vivo*. Administration of such polymers to animals produces profound hypoglycemia. It is quite interesting that the effects appear to be more protracted than with native insulin. This may indicate a greater effectiveness of the polymeric insulin, or it may represent protection of such derivatives from degradative processes.

The demonstration of the retention of biological activity by insulin covalently bound to large, polymeric matrixes provides evidence that the biological activity of native insulin resides in the monomeric species rather than in the insulin dimer (CUATRECASAS, 1969). Since the linkage of insulin to the agarose backbone is followed by extensive washing with guanidine and with HCl, and several derivatives are prepared in the presence of these denaturants, it appears very likely that insulin is coupled to the matrix as a monomer.

d) Insulin Receptors and Plant Lectins

Concanavalin A and wheat germ agglutinin are two plant proteins which can bind to specific carbohydrate determinants of mammalian cell surfaces; they can agglutinate various normal and neoplastic animal cells and can alter the metabolism of leucocytes. In addition, concanavalin A and wheat germ agglutinin have been shown to have potent insulin like effects on glucose transport and on epinephrine-stimulated lipolysis in isolated adipocytes (CUATRECASAS and TELL, 1973; CZECH and LYNN, 1973). It has been shown that both lectins alter the binding of insulin to the membrane receptors (CUATRECASAS, 1973a). Low concentrations of wheat germ agglutinin enhance the binding of insulin to fat cells and to liver membranes. Higher concentrations of this plant lectin, as well as concanavalin A, displace the binding of iodinated insulin to the receptor structures of the intact tissues as well as to the solubilized insulin-binding protein of the membranes. Addition of simple, specific sugars reverses all the effects of the lectins as well as the adsorption of solubilized insulin-binding protein to agarose derivatives of the plant lectins. These findings strongly suggest that concanavalin A and wheat germ agglutinin can interact directly with insulin receptors. The existence of this interaction is consistent with the studies of neuraminidase and β-galactosidase digestion (described in earlier section) which suggested that the insulin receptor structures may be glycoproteins. It is possible that some of the biological effects of the plant lectins in various tissues might be explained on the basis of the insulin-like properties of these proteins (CUATRECASAS and TELL, 1973).

e) Insulin-Resistant States

The possible alteration of insulin receptors in metabolic states characterized by insulin resistance has been examined. There are no changes in the total insulin-binding capacity per cell or in the affinity of the insulin-cell complex in adipocytes obtained from starved, prednisone-treated, and diabetic rats and in various species showing insulin resistance (BENNETT and CUATRECASAS, 1972). Adipose cells from obese rats share the same binding capacity and affinity for insulin as normal rats (LIVINGSTON *et al.*, 1972). The basic glucose transport mechanisms of these obese cells appear to be intact, a fact that suggests that the defect lies at the level of the receptor or in the processes that couple the receptor to the transport mechanisms. Although the insulin receptor density appears to be much lower in the large cells it is not clear whether this difference is sufficient to explain the insulin resistance in obesity since in certain cases large adipocytes obtained from large rats are still quite sensitive to insulin. It has been suggested that the principal metabolic defect lies in coupling the binding interaction signal to the adjacent membrane structures responsible for hormonal response (CUATRECASAS, 1973b), perhaps in a way analogous to the alteration observed after neuraminidase digestion (CUATRECASAS and ILLIANO, 1971).

It is pertinent that liver membranes and adipocytes from mice with the obese-hyperglycemic syndrome, a recessively inherited trait, appear to have greatly reduced insulin-binding sites (KAHN *et al.*, 1973; FREYCHET *et al.*, 1972b). This decreased binding correlates well with the insulin resistance in these animals, suggesting that at least in this case faulty receptor structures may play an important role in insulin resistance.

The ability of insulin to inhibit adenylate cyclase activity in subcellular membranes (ILLIANO and CUATRECASAS, 1972; HEPP, 1972; HEPP and RENNER, 1972) raises the possibility that in certain cases insulin resistance may be based on defects in the function of this enzyme such that this inhibition does not occur properly. It is interesting in this respect that the sensitivity of liver adenylate cyclase to glucagon is greatly increased in streptozotocin-induced diabetes in rats (HEPP, 1972).

4. Solubilization and Isolation of the Insulin Receptor

Comparative qualitative and quantitative aspects of insulin binding in intact cells and in membrane preparations indicate that the receptors in membranes are not seriously altered during breakage of the cells. Since the kinetic properties of the insulin receptor are unaffected by homogenization the use of membranes for further characterization of the receptor seems justified.

The insulin binding structures are "integral" components of the membrane (SINGER and NICOLSON, 1972) since they can only be extracted in high yield by very vigorous conditions (CUATRECASAS, 1972c, d) which involve dissolution of the membrane. Quantitative extraction of the binding protein is possible with nonionic detergents such as Triton X-100.

It has been shown that the presence of these detergents in higher concentrations (above 0.5% v/v, Triton X-100; and above 0.2% w/v, Lubrol PX) decreases the binding of insulin to the water-soluble insulin receptor (CUATRECASAS, 1972c). However, dialysis or dilution of these preparations to decrease the detergent concentration results in restoration of insulin-binding activity. Dialysis of a Triton-treated cell extract against detergent-free buffers leads to the formation of aggregates in which the insulin-binding capacity present before such treatment is quantitatively recovered.

Several commonly used protein denaturants such as urea, guanidine hydrochloride, and sodium dodecylsulfate markedly decrease insulin-binding activity. Glycerol in concentrations greater than 20% (v/v) similarly interferes with the insulin-receptor interaction. Although 0.16% dodecyl sulfate, 3 M urea, and 20% glycerol cause a severe or nearly total suppression of binding, the effects are reversed by decreasing the concentration of the reagent 10-fold. Exposure of the insulin receptor to higher concentrations of these reagents results in apparent irreversible denaturation.

The dissociation constant of insulin binding to the soluble receptor protein (CUATRECASAS, 1972d) shows the same high affinity observed in the binding of insulin to membranes not exposed to detergents (k_d 10^{-10}M). The hormone is not degraded or damaged during binding to the soluble protein.

Agarose filtration of the insulin binding protein shows that it has a large molecular size. Addition of native insulin during this procedure nearly completely prevents the binding of ^{125}I-insulin in these experiments. The reversibility of the hormone interaction with the soluble protein has been demonstrated by gel-filtration over Sephadex G-50 (CUATRECASAS, 1972d). Similar experiments with Triton X-100 of red blood cell ghosts do not result in significant radioactivity which is displaceable by native insulin. The elution position of the soluble receptor in gel filtration experiments (K_{AV}) is highly reproducible and no difference is detected between proteins extracted from fat cells or liver cell membranes.

The molecular weight of the insulin binding protein cannot be determined by gel filtration alone since it is apparent that the migration of proteins during elution correlates with the Stokes radius rather than with the molecular weight. A Stokes radius of about 70 Å has been calculated for the insulin receptor (CUATRECASAS, 1972d). To prevent aggregation of the insulin-binding protein its sedimentation behavior was studied in the presence of detergents. By comparing the sedimentation patterns of several standard proteins on 5—20% sucrose gradients containing 0.2% (v/v) Triton X-100 it could be established that linear sedimentation relationships exist under these conditions, and are not affected by the presence of detergents in the gradient buffers. A sedimentation constant of 11 S was determined. The sedimentation coefficient is unaltered by phospholipase digestion or organic solvent extraction of the membranes before solubilization with Triton X-100. These parameters are identical for receptor proteins isolated from fat cell and liver cell membranes and are unaffected by NaCl or Triton concentrations provided that the detergent concentration is sufficiently high to prevent aggregation of the protein.

It has been calculated that the molecular weight of the binding protein is about 300,000, that the frictional coefficient is about 1.53 (neglecting solvation) and the axial ratio is about 9 (neglecting solvation). These values are calculated with the assumption that the partial volume (v) of the protein is 0.734. This assumption is based on several determinations of the sedimentation rate in cesium chloride concentrations of varying density. These data, however, must be interpreted with caution since until now the amount of detergent bound to the insulin receptor under these conditions has not been determined.

At present the data suggest that the insulin binding protein is not grossly a lipoprotein, that lipids are not required or involved in the binding of insulin, and that the protein is a large, asymmetric macromolecule. The proper assembly of this protein into the membrane, however, very likely requires specific lipid-protein interactions. It is very interesting that the recently solubilized (MEUNIER *et al.*, 1972) bungarotoxin-binding membrane protein from *Electrophorus electricus* shares many of the physicochemical and binding properties of the insulin receptor.

A relatively simple and rapid assay has been devised to study the kinetic properties of the insulin receptor (CUATRECASAS, 1972c, d). The same binding behavior and degree of competition of insulin analogs is observed in the soluble and in the particulate (intact cells or membranes) binding reactions. Association and dissociation rates determined in the soluble binding protein are similar to those of the particulate receptor. As expected from the studies performed with the particulate fractions, complex formation of insulin with the soluble receptor is unaffected by 2 M NaCl and neuraminidase or phospholipase digestion. Treatment with trypsin, however, completely destroys insulin binding to the soluble protein at concentrations which do not affect the binding of the hormone to intact cells or membranes but which do decrease the binding to phospholipase-treated membranes. On the basis of these findings it seems very likely that the soluble insulin binding structures are the same as those observed in intact cells.

Purification of the receptor in amounts needed for further structural analysis is hindered by the extreme scarcity of the receptors in the tissues studied so far and by the necessity for continual presence of detergents during isolation. It has been estimated that the receptor represents only about $10^{-4}\%$ of the protein of a rat liver homogenate (CUATRECASAS, 1972e).

A combination of conventional purification procedures such as ammonium sulfate fractionation and DEAE-cellulose chromatography (CUATRECASAS, 1972e), and affinity chromatography (CUATRECASAS *et al.*, 1968; CUATRECASAS, 1970; CUATRECASAS and ANFINSEN, 1971; CUATRECASAS, 1972e) results in about 2.5×10^{-5} fold purification of the receptor protein from Triton X-100 extracts (CUATRECASAS, 1972e). This approaches theoretical purity on the basis of the binding of one insulin molecule per receptor molecule of 300,000 MW. At present large scale purification has not been possible due to the limited capacity of affinity chromatography columns. It has not been possible to disaggregate the large (MW 300,000) insulin-binding complex into smaller sub-units which retain high affinity for insulin, and it is not yet known whether these large complexes can bind other peptide hormones or whether they contain specific enzymic activities.

III. Mechanism of Insulin Action

It has not yet been possible to explain all of the biologic effects of insulin by a single, defined mediator. Since most of the activities modulated by insulin, such as lipolysis, glycogen synthesis and protein metabolism are anabolic processes and are thus the reverse of those mediated by adenosine-3′-5′-monophosphate (cyclic AMP) a fundamental effect of insulin may be the control of the intracellular concentrations of this metabolite.

It has been shown that under certain conditions insulin can decrease the cyclic AMP concentration in adipose tissue (BUTCHER *et al.*, 1956; JUNGAS, 1966; MANGANIELLO *et al.*, 1971; BUTCHER *et al.*, 1968) and in liver cells (JEFFERSON *et al.*, 1968; EXTON *et al.*, 1971). At physiological concentrations (10^{-11} to 10^{-10}M) insulin can inhibit adenylate cyclase activity in partially purified membranes prepared from isolated fat and liver cells (ILLIANO and CUATRECASAS, 1972; RAY *et al.*, 1970; HEPP, 1971). The inhibitory activity of insulin is apparently independent of the manner by which the enzyme is stimulated. Inhibition by insulin can be observed in the enzyme stimulated by epinephrine, glucagon, ACTH, and sodium fluoride as well as in the unstimulated enzyme. Unphysiological concentrations of the hormone (10^{-9}M) can cause a paradoxical effect and increase the activity of the enzyme. It has recently been shown that insulin can profoundly inhibit the baseline and stimulated activities of adenylate cyclase in purified membrane preparations from *Neurospora crassa* (TORRES, 1973).

It is also pertinent that treatment of intact tissues can result in an increase in the activity of cyclic AMP phosphodiesterase (LOTEN and SNEYD, 1970; VAUGHAN, 1972). Since it has not yet been possible to demonstrate these effects in subcellular systems, this effect may be mediated indirectly; nevertheless, it may contribute to the fall in the levels of cyclic AMP observed after exposing intact cells to insulin.

At present it is not possible to make conclusions on the nature of the relationship between the inhibition of adenylate cyclase activity and the action of insulin. Three different alternatives seem possible:

1) Insulin can directly modulate the activity of adenylate cyclase. Under these circumstances the hormone-binding and the catalytic units might be contiguous or connected by some other closely interposed subunits. This model would require that all of the effects of insulin be mediated by cyclic AMP or by this and other processes which are inherent parts (yet unrecognized) of this receptor-enzyme system.

2) Insulin initiates the formation of an unknown chemical mediator, "X", which then can independently modify various insulin-sensitive activities. There is as yet no clear evidence for the existence of such a mediator. Such a compound, however, might best be found in the rather simple isolated membrane systems in which insulin has recently been shown to affect adenylate cyclase activity. This substance would likely be an endogenous compound of the membrane (e.g., prostaglandins or phospholipid derivatives).

3) Insulin causes a major conformational change in the membrane, and this change then alters simultaneously various processes which are not physically contiguous or functionally related. Just as seen with adenylate cyclase, other enzymes might be regulated by insulin if studied by appropriate techniques. The recent demonstration (HADDEN *et al.*, 1972) that insulin can stimulate the activity of ATPase in membrane suspensions from lymphocytes is an intriguing observation in this context.

It has recently been demonstrated (ILLIANO *et al.*, 1973) that insulin causes a marked and prompt elevation in the intracellular levels of cyclic GMP which are analogous to the changes which certain hormones (epinephrine, glucagon) cause in the levels of cyclic AMP. The interesting possibility has been raised that changes in the concentrations of cyclic AMP and cyclic GMP can occur in concert by modifying a single membrane localized enzyme, and that the biological effects of various hormones may result from the relative concentrations of these cyclic nucleotides. It is thus possible that cyclic GMP can modulate or assist in the modification of certain insulin-sensitive biological responses. These observations are most consistent with model 1) described above.

References

ARMSTRONG, K.J., WOALL, M.W., STOUFFER, J.E.: Dextran-linked insulin: a soluble high molecular weight derivative with biological activity *in vivo* and *in vitro*. Biochem. biophys. Res. Commun. **47**, 354—360 (1972)

BENNETT, G.V., CUATRECASAS, P.: Insulin receptor of fat cells in insulin resistant states. Science **176**, 805—806 (1972)

BENNETT, V., CUATRECASAS, P.: Preparation of inverted plasma membrane vesicles from isolated adipocytes. Biochim. biophys. Acta (Amst.) **311**, 362—380 (1973)

BLATT, L.M., KIM, K.H.: Regulation of hepatic glycogen synthetase. J. biol. Chem. **241**, 4895—4898 (1971)

BUTCHER, R.W., SNEYD, J.G.T., PARK, C.R., SUTHERLAND, E.W.: Effect of insulin on adenosine 3′-5′-monophosphate in the rat epididymal fat pad. J. biol. Chem. **241**, 1651—1653 (1956)

BUTCHER, R.W., BAIRD, C.E., SUTHERLAND, E.W.: Effects of lipolytic and antilypolitic substances on adenosine 3′-5′-monophosphate levels in isolated fat cells. J. biol. Chem. **243**, 1705—1712 (1968)

CHANG, K.-J., BENNETT, V., CUATRECASAS, P.: Membrane receptors as general markers for plasma membrane isolation procedures. The use of ^{125}I-labelled wheat germ agglutinin, insulin and cholera toxin. J. biol. Chem. in press (1974)

CUATRECASAS, P.: Interaction of insulin with the cell membrane: the primary action of insulin. Proc. nat. Acad. Sci. (Wash.) **63**, 450—457 (1969)

CUATRECASAS, P.: Derivatization of agarose and polyacrilamide beads. J. biol. Chem. **245**, 3059—3065 (1970)

CUATRECASAS, P.: Insulin receptor interaction in adipose tissue cells: direct measurement and properties. Proc. nat. Acad. Sci. (Wash.) **68**, 1264—1268 (1971a)

Cuatrecasas, P.: Perturbation of the insulin receptor of isolated fat cells with proteolytic enzymes: direct measurement of insulin-receptor interactions. J. biol. Chem. **246**, 6522—6531 (1971b)
Cuatrecasas, P.: Unmasking of insulin receptors in fat cells and fat cell membranes: Perturbation of membrane lipids. J. biol. Chem. **246**, 6532—6542 (1971c)
Cuatrecasas, P.: Properties of the insulin receptor of isolated fat cell membranes. J. biol. Chem. **246**, 7265—7274 (1971d)
Cuatrecasas, P.: Selective adsorbents based on biochemical specificity. In: Biochemical aspects of reactions on solid supports. London-New York: Academic Press 1971e
Cuatrecasas, P.: The nature of insulin-receptor interactions. In: Insulin action. London-New York: Academic Press 1972a
Cuatrecasas, P.: The insulin receptor. Diabetes **21**, Suppl. 2, 396—402 (1972b)
Cuatrecasas, P.: Isolation of the insulin receptor of liver and fat cell membranes. Proc. nat. Acad. Sci. (Wash.) **69**, 318—322 (1972c)
Cuatrecasas, P.: Properties of the insulin receptor isolated from liver and fat cell membranes. J. biol. Chem. **247**, 1980—1991 (1972d)
Cuatrecasas, P.: Affinity chromatography and purification of the insulin receptor of liver cell membranes. Proc. nat. Acad. Sci. (Wash.) **69**, 1277—1281 (1972e)
Cuatrecasas, P.: Interaction of concanavalin A and wheat germ agglutinin with the insulin receptor of fat cells and liver. J. biol. Chem. **248**, 3528—3534 (1973a)
Cuatrecasas, P.: The insulin receptor of liver and fat cell membranes. Fed. Proc. **32**, 1838—1846 (1973b)
Cuatrecasas, P., Anfinsen, C.B.: Affinity chromatography. In: Annual Review of Biochemistry 40. Palo Alto, California: Annual Reviews 1971
Cuatrecasas, P., Desbuquois, B., Krug, F.: Insulin-receptor interaction in liver cell membranes. Biochem. biophys. Res. Commun. **44**, 333—339 (1971)
Cuatrecasas, P., Illiano, G.: Membrane sialic acid and the mechanism of insulin action in adipose tissue cells — effect of digestion with neuraminidase. J. biol. Chem. **246**, 4938—4946 (1971)
Cuatrecasas, P., Tell, G.P.E.: Insulin-like activity of concanavalin A and wheat germ agglutinin — direct interactions with insulin receptors. Proc. nat. Acad. Sci. (Wash.) **70**, 485—489 (1973)
Cuatrecasas, P., Wilchek, M., Anfinsen, C.B.: Selective enzyme purification by affinity chromatography. Proc. nat. Acad. Sci. (Wash.) **61**, 636—643 (1968)
Czech, M.P., Lynn, W.S.: Stimulation of glucose metabolism by lectins in isolated white fat cells. Biochem. biophys. Res. Commun. **297**, 368—377 (1973)
Exton, J.H., Lewis, S.B., Ho, R.J., Robinson, G.A., Park, C.R.: Role of cyclic AMP in interaction of glucagon and insulin in control of liver metabolism. Ann. N.Y. Acad. Sci. **185**, 85—100 (1971)
El-Allawy, R.M.M., Gliemann, J.: Trypsin treatment of adipocytes: effect on sensitivity to insulin. Biochem. biophys. Res. Commun. **273**, 97—109 (1972)
Fain, J.N., Loken, S.C.: Response of trypsin-treated brown and white fat cells to hormones. J. biol. Chem. **244**, 3500—3506 (1969)
Freychet, P., Roth, J., Neville, D.M.: Insulin receptor in the liver: specific binding of [^{125}I]-insulin to the plasma membrane and its relation to insulin bioactivity. Proc. nat. Acad. Sci. (Wash.) **68**, 1833—1837 (1971)
Freychet, P., Kahn, R., Roth, J., Neville, D.M.: Insulin interactions with liver plasma membranes — independence of binding of the hormone and its degradation. J. biol. Chem. **247**, 3953—3961 (1972a)
Freychet, P., Laudat, M.H., Laudat, P., Rosselin, G., Kahn, C.R., Gorden, P., Roth, J.: Impairment of insulin binding to the fat cell plasma membrane in the obese hyperglycemic mouse. FEBS Letters **25**, 239—242 (1972b)
Gavin, J.R. III, Roth, J., Jen, P., Freychet, P.: Insulin receptors in human circulating cells and fibroblasts. Proc. nat. Acad. Sci. (Wash.) **69**, 747—751 (1972)
Goldfine, I.D., Sherline, P.: Insulin action in isolated rat thymocytes, II. J. biol. Chem. **247**, 6927—6931 (1972)
Goldfine, I.D., Gardner, J.D., Neville, D.M., Jr.: Insulin action in isolated rat thymocytes, I. J. biol. Chem. **247**, 6919—6929 (1972)
Hadden, J.W., Hadden, E.M., Wilson, E.E., Good, R.A., Coffey, R.G.: Direct action of insulin of plasma membrane ATPase activity in human lymphocytes. Nature New Biol. **235**, 174—176 (1972)
Hammond, J.M., Jarret, L., Mariz, I.K., Daughaday, W.H.: Heterogeneity of insulin receptors on fat cell membranes. Biochem. biophys. Res. Commun. **49**, 1122—1128 (1972)

Haugaard, N., Marsh, J.B.: Effect of insulin on the metabolism of adipose tissue from normal rats. J. biol. Chem. **194**, 33—34 (1952)

Hepp, K.D.: Inhibition of glucagon stimulated adenylate cyclase by insulin. FEBS Letters **12**, 263—266 (1971)

Hepp, K.D.: Adenylate cyclase and insulin action. Europ. J. Biochem. **31**, 266—276 (1972)

Hepp, K.D., Renner, K.: Insulin action and the adenylate cyclase system: antagonism to activation by lipolytic hormones. FEBS Letters **20**, 191—194 (1972)

Hills, A.G., Stadie, W.C.: The effect of combined insulin upon the metabolism of the lactating mammary gland of the rat. J. biol. Chem. **194**, 25—31 (1952)

House, P.D.R., Weidemann, M.J.: Characterization of an [^{125}I]-insulin binding plasma membrane fraction from rat liver. Biochem. biophys. Res. Commun. **41**, 541—548 (1970)

Hunter, W.M., Greenwood, F.C.: Preparation of iodine ^{131}-labelled human growth hormone of high specific activity. Nature (Lond.) **194**, 495—496 (1962)

Illiano, G., Cuatrecasas, P.: Modulation of adenylate cyclase activity in liver and fat cell membranes by insulin. Science **175**, 906—908 (1972)

Illiano, G., Tell, G.P.E., Siegel, M.I., Cuatrecasas, P.: Guanosine 3′:5′-cyclic monophosphate and the action of insulin and acetylcholine. Proc. nat. Acad. Sci. (Wash.) **70**, 2443—2447 (1973)

Jefferson, L.S., Exton, J.H., Butcher, R.W., Sutherland, E.W., Park, C.R.: Role of adenosine 3′-5′ monophosphate in the effects of insulin and anti-insulin serum and liver metabolism. J. biol. Chem. **243**, 1031—1038 (1968)

Jungas, R.L.: Role of cyclic 3′-5′ AMP in the response of adipose tissue to insulin. Proc. nat. Acad. Sci. (Wash.) **56**, 757—763 (1966)

Kahn, C.R., Neville, D.M., Roth, J.: Insulin-receptor interaction in the obese-hyperglycemic mouse. J. biol. Chem. **248**, 244—250 (1973)

Kono, T.: Destruction of insulin effector system of adipose tissue cells by proteolytic enzymes. J. biol. Chem. **244**, 1772—1777 (1969a)

Kono, T.: Destruction and restoration of the insulin effector system of isolated fat cells. J. biol. Chem. **244**, 5777—5784 (1969b)

Kono, T., Barham, T.W.: The relationships between the insulin binding capacity of fat cells and the cellular response to insulin. J. biol. Chem. **246**, 6210—6216 (1971)

Krug, U., Krug, F., Cuatrecasas, P.: Emergence of insulin receptors of human lymphocytes during *in vitro* transformation. Proc. nat. Acad. Sci. (Wash.) **69**, 2604—2608 (1972)

Levine, R.: Cell membrane as a primary site of insulin action. Fed. Proc. **24**, 1071—1073 (1965)

Livingston, J.N., Cuatrecasas, P., Lockwood, D.H.: Insulin insensitivity of large fat cells. Science **177**, 626—628 (1972)

Loten, E.G., Sneyd, J.G.T.: An effect of insulin on adipose-tissue adenosine 3′:5′-cyclic monophosphate phosphodiesterase. Biochem. J. **120**, 187—193 (1970)

Manganiello, V.C., Murad, F., Vaughan, M.: Effects of lipolytic and antilipolytic agents on cyclic 3′-5′ adenosine monophosphate in fat cells. J. biol. Chem. **246**, 2195—2202 (1971)

Meunier, J.C., Oslen, R.W., Menez, A., Fromageot, P., Boquet, P., Changeux, J.-P.: Some physical properties of the cholinergic receptor protein from Electrophorus electricus revealed by a tritiated α-toxin from Naja nigricallis venom. Biochemistry **11**, 1200—1210 (1972)

Narahara, H.T.: Binding of insulin to tissues in relation to biological action of the hormone. In: Handbook of Physiology-Endocrinology I. Baltimore: Waverly Press 1972

Oka, T., Topper, Y.J.: Insulin sepharose and the dynamic of insulin binding. Proc. nat. Acad. Sci. (Wash.) **68**, 2066—2068 (1971)

Oka, T., Topper, Y.J.: Dynamics of insulin action on mammary epithelium. Nature New Biol. **239**, 216—217 (1972)

Ray, T.K., Tomasi, V., Marinetti, G.V.: Hormone action at the membrane level. I. Properties of adenyl cyclase in isolated plasma membranes. Biochim. biophys. Acta (Amst.) **211**, 20—30 (1970)

Singer, S.J., Nicolson, G.L.: The fluid mosaic model of the structure of cell membranes. Science **175**, 720—731 (1972)

Soderman, D.D., Germershausen, J., Katzen, H.H.: Affinity binding of intact fat cells and their ghosts to immobilized insulin. Proc. nat. Acad. Sci. (Wash.) **70**, 792—796 (1973)

Stadie, W.C., Haugaard, N., Marsh, J.B., Hills, A.G.: The chemical combination of insulin with muscle (diaphragm) of normal rat. Amer. J. med. Sci. **218**, 265—274 (1949)

Stadie, W.C., Haugaard, N., Vaughan, M.: Studies of insulin binding with isotopically labelled insulin. J. biol. Chem. **199**, 729—739 (1952)

SUZUKI, F., DAIKUHARA, Y., ONO, M., TAKEDA, Y.: Studies on the mode of action of insulin: properties and biological activity of an insulin-dextran complex. Endocrinology **90**, 1220—1230 (1972)

TURKINGTON, R.W.: Stimulation of RNA synthesis in isolated mammary cells by insulin and prolactin bound to sepharose. Biochem. biophys. Res. Commun. **41**, 1362—1367 (1970)

VAUGHAN, M.: The role of insulin in regulation of cyclic AMP metabolism. In: Insulin action. London-New York: Academic Press 1972

WOLTHMANN, H.J., NARAHARA, H.T.: Binding of iodine ^{131}-insulin by isolated fragment sartorius muscle — relationship to changes in permeability to sugar caused by insulin. J. biol. Chem. **241**, 4931—4939 (1966)

YALOW, R.S., BERSON, S.A.: Purification of ^{131}I-parathyroid hormone with microfine granules of precipitated silica. Nature (Lond.) **212**, 357—358 (1966)

B. Effects of Insulin on Cellular Protein Synthesis*

IRA G. WOOL

With 15 Figures

* This review is dedicated to DIETER ROT who see every thing, and to OSWALD WIENER who tells us the meaning.

I. Introduction

Diabetic animals are unable to regulate their protein metabolism in a normal manner, although their response — an acceleration of protein catabolism and a severe restriction of protein synthesis — is appropriate to their precarious metabolic state. The diabetic animal needs calories, and especially it needs glucose, so it is appropriate for the animal to sacrifice protein to satisfy its requirements. The diabetic syndrome includes then a negative nitrogen balance and wasting of muscle as reflections of the alterations of protein metabolism. In ordinary circumstances insulin dampens protein breakdown and stimulates its synthesis. The mechanism by which the hormone does so is not known. Indeed, insulin mechanism of action is a common enemy against whom scientists have for decades been mounting search and destroy missions with no more success than so many General Westmorelands.

The problems that have engaged our attention are: first, the nature of the regulation of protein synthesis in animal cells, particularly the structure and function of ribosomes; second, the mechanisms of action of insulin, especially the means whereby insulin affects the synthesis of protein. Superficially the problems seem to complement each other, indeed, appear as facets of a single problem. However, there is no evidence for a direct effect of insulin on the ribosome or any of its functional appendages. In an experiment, the importance of which cannot be overestimated, CUATRACASAS (1969) has shown that insulin need not enter the adipocyte in order to accelerate glucose transport into the cell. If his results are applicable to all cells and all the biological actions of the hormone, then an analysis of the effect of insulin on ribosome function is not likely to yield information on its primary action. But what has been shown is that insulin need not enter the adipose cell to mediate the membrane (or transport) actions of the hormone. Still to be determined is whether the anabolic effects of insulin (the synthesis of macro-molecules) can occur without its entry into the cell. If insulin does not enter the muscle cell then it must generate some intermediate that acts as its deputy in the modulation of protein synthesis. The identification of that intermediate is a hot problem — certainly that is where a good deal of the action is going to be in the near future. But no matter the outcome insulin has proven an important tool in analyzing the regulation of protein synthesis in animal cells (just as it was useful in studying the details of the biochemistry and the regulation of carbohydrate metabolism).

In this chapter I shall review mainly the action of insulin on protein synthesis in muscle. I shall not consider in detail the effects of insulin on protein metabolism in liver and in other cells and tissues, since the changes have not been shown to be the result of a direct action of insulin (not even in the limited sense that the hormone acts directly on protein synthesis in muscle). Moreover the changes caused by insulin in protein synthesis in liver and muscle seem to differ in a fundamental way [for example, the effect in liver requires the synthesis of RNA (SALAS *et al.*, 1963; SCHIMKE, 1966)]. The action of insulin on protein breakdown is not discussed here, although there is increasing evidence that modulation of the process is an important aspect of the control of protein metabolism in animal cells (BROSTROM and JEFFAY, 1970; SCHIMKE, 1962, 1966) and perhaps a significant part of insulin action (MORTIMER and MONDON, 1970). Finally, this review is mainly of our own work. Our last comprehensive review was published in 1972 (WOOL *et al.*, 1972). The present chapter should be read in conjunction with and as a sequel to earlier reviews (WOOL, 1964, 1965, 1968; WOOL and SCHARFF, 1968; WOOL *et al.*, 1968a, 1972).

One of the prominent effects of insulin is to increase the transport of glucose and of other substrates into the cell's interior (LEVINE and GOLDSTEIN, 1955). It is nonetheless a melancholy fact that the influence of insulin on substrate transport cannot account for all of the hormone's biological actions; for example, the increase in synthesis of protein in muscle can be shown to occur apart from the influence of the hormone on glucose (WOOL, 1964) or amino acid transport (WOOL, 1965, 1968; WOOL and SCHARFF, 1968). The evidence is simple: insulin will increase protein synthesis in muscle in situations where there is no extracellular substrate, hence where no effect of the hormone on substrate transport could have occurred. The work reviewed rests then on two assumptions: 1) insulin's stimulatory effect on protein synthesis in muscle and its influence on glucose transport are independent phenomena; and 2) insulin increases amino acid transport in muscle, but the stimulation of protein synthesis is independent of that effect also. The experimental data we believe to support those assumptions have been reviewed (WOOL, 1964, 1965, 1968; WOOL and SCHARFF, 1968). We understand not everyone accepts the second proposition (HIDER *et al.*, 1969, 1971a, 1971b; HIDER and MEADE, 1972) so the demur will be discussed below.

II. Insulin and Amino Acid Transport in Muscle Reconsidered

1. Relation of Insulin Action on Protein Synthesis to the Action of the Hormone on Amino Acid Transport

It is possible that insulin brings about an increase in protein synthesis by accelerating the rate of entry of amino acids into the cell. Under physiological circumstances the first step in protein biosynthesis must of necessity be concerned with logistics, with providing a supply of amino acids for the manufacture of protein and transporting them to the site of synthesis. Since the intracellular pool of most amino acids appears to be relatively large with respect to the concentration of amino acids in the extracellular fluid (SCHARFF and WOOL, 1964, 1965; MORGAN *et al.*, 1971a), it is possible that protein synthesis can proceed for a time without requiring additional amounts of amino acids. That seems to be so in isolated rat diaphragm (WOOL and KRAHL, 1959a) where amino acid incorporation is not appreciably increased over that observed in Krebs bicarbonate buffer by addition of a complete amino acid mixture (i.e., plasma). Nonetheless, at some point the intracellular amino acid pool must be replenished, and transport of amino acid from the extracellular compartment into the cell interior is required. Insulin causes a decrease in the concentration of amino acids in the plasma of intact animals (LUCK *et al.*, 1928) and suppresses the rate of rise of plasma amino acids after evisceration (RUSSEL, 1955). The amino acids disappear in the same ratio as they exist in muscle protein (LOTSPEICH, 1949). Those observations support the idea that insulin increases amino acids transport into the cell *pari passu* with an increase in protein synthesis; one cannot, of course, decide from that information alone whether the increase in amino acid uptake is secondary to increased intracellular utilization of amino acids for protein synthesis, or if the increase in protein synthesis is secondary to an increase in the availability of amino acids. The second possibility was given substance by the demonstration by KIPNIS and NOALL (1958) that insulin increased the rate and final magnitude of accumulation in isolated 'intact' diaphragm of ^{14}C-labeled aminoisobutyric acid, a non-utilized model amino acid. Since aminoisobutyric acid is not utilized by muscle, its rate of penetration can be isolated from its subsequent metabolism.

The finding that insulin stimulated aminoisobutyric acid transport created great excitement, for it once again gave a unity to the effect of insulin on carbohydrate and protein metabolism, in both cases insulin was presumed to act to enhance substrate transfer. Obviously the possibility that accelerated transport was responsible for the insulin-mediated stimulation of amino acid incorporation into protein had to be tested, and tested it was (WOOL and KRAHL, 1959b). The strategy adopted was to divorce penetration and incorporation by effecting amino acid accumulation before adding insulin. To accomplish this the ^{14}C-labeled amino acid, instead of being added *in vitro*, was injected into diaphragm donors. In those experiments, insulin added *in vitro* increased amino acid incorporation into protein despite accumulation having been effected before insulin was added, and despite the absence of added glucose in the medium.

A second and more elegant approach to the same problem was made by MANCHESTER and KRAHL (1959). Taking advantage of the observation by MANCHESTER and YOUNG (1959) that ^{14}C of pyruvate, ketoglutarate, and bicarbonate can be incorporated by isolated diaphragm into certain amino acids (mainly alanine, glutamic, and aspartic) of its protein, MANCHESTER and KRAHL (1959) incubated diaphragm with a variety of ^{14}C-labeled carboxylic acids and bicarbonate in the presence or absence of insulin. They reckoned, that if insulin stimulated amino acid incorporation into protein solely by accelerating the rate of entry of amino acids into the cell, then the hormone should be without effect on incorporation into protein of radioactivity from the various precursors for, in those circumstances, the amino acids are presumed to be synthesized intracellularly. Yet in each instance insulin increased the incorporation into muscle protein of radioactivity from the several amino acid precursors. Moreover, the magnitude of the stimulation of incorporation produced by insulin was in all cases of the same order as had been found with amino acids. Finally, it was possible to rule out enhanced accumulation of the radioactive precursor as a prerequisite for the effect of insulin on incorporation.

Those two experiments taken together seem, at first, to provide convincing evidence, that, whether or not insulin influences amino acid accumulation, it must accelerate protein synthesis by acting at a site distal to the transport process, presumably on an aspect of the intracellular biochemical machinery for protein synthesis. However, both experiments suffer from at least one defect. There is no assurance that the amino acids preaccumulated, or those formed intracellularly, did not leak out of the muscle (a not unlikely prospect since 'cut' hemidiaphragm was used in both experiments) and were then more rapidly pumped back into the muscle cell under the influence of insulin. This possibility was tested too (WOOL and KRAHL, 1964) by incubating diaphragm with ^{14}C-pyruvate and high concentrations of ^{12}C-alanine, -glutamic, and -aspartic acids (the amino acids formed from pyruvate) so as to trap radioactive amino acids that might leak out of the cell and thereby reduce the possibility of their being reaccumulated. It needs to be pointed out that HIDER and MEADE (1972) have argued that the precautions were not sufficient. Nonetheless, in those circumstances insulin still stimulated incorporation of radioactivity from pyruvate into muscle protein. Most notably at a concentration of 10^{-2} M the ^{12}C-amino acids diluted the incorporation of radioactivity from pyruvate to 43% of the control value but did not diminish the magnitude of the insulin effect. There remains an alternate interpretation of the experimental data (not likely in my opinion but nonetheless possible) that needs to be ruled out. The possibility is that insulin increases the entry into muscle of all amino acids, but that it is the increase in the transport of only one (or a few) that is relevant, i.e., that one (or a few) amino acid(s) serves as a pacemaker with respect to protein synthesis — an increase in the intracellular concentration of that amino acid leading to an increase in the utilization of all for protein synthesis. The possibility could have been tested if we had incubated our diaphragms (in the experiment described above) with ^{14}C-pyruvate and high concentrations of all twenty ^{12}C-amino acids.

An extremely important discovery with respect to the mechanism and the means of regulation of amino acid transport has been made by KIPNIS and PARRISH (1965). They found that the isoosmotic replacement of sodium by choline depressed the basal penetration into isolated rat diaphragm of amino-isobutyric acid and abolished the increase in the active transport of the amino acid that ordinarily follows on addition of insulin. KOSTYO (1964) was quick to see the use to which the discovery could be put: that the stimulation by hormones of protein synthesis might be studied in the absence of an effect on amino acid transport. When diaphragm was incubated in a sodium-free medium, the basal accumulation of glycine was reduced and the stimulation of transport by insulin was abolished; what is more, the intracellular concentration of the amino acid was never greater than that in the medium — that is to say muscle was no longer capable of active transport of glycine. In the absence of sodium, the synthesis of protein in diaphragm muscle was also reduced (about 45%), but synthesis could be reduced still further by dinitrophenol or puromycin. The decisive observation, however, was that insulin stimulated glycine incorporation into protein even when no sodium was present in the medium — a clear demonstration that insulin can stimulate protein synthesis by a mechanism that does not require an increase in amino acid transport.

2. Insulin and Amino Acid Transport in Muscle

a) Accumulation of Individual Natural Amino Acids

One might ask if insulin does in fact increase the transport of natural amino acids. In circumstances similar to those in which it increases the incorporation of labeled amino acids into protein of isolated rat diaphragm, insulin also enhances the accumulation of six of the natural, utilized amino acids (glycine, proline, hydroxyproline, serine, methionine, and threonine) but not of 13 others (cysteine has not yet been tested) — See WOOL (1964), for references. There is nothing of the structure, or the metabolism, of the six natural amino acids responsive to insulin, or of the mechanism of amino acid transport in muscle, that allows systematic sense to be made of the findings.

It is important to bear in mind that, with but rare exception, what had been examined to then was the ratio of radioactivity in the tissue water to that in the medium after incubating diaphragm, or perfusing heart, with a single, radioactive amino acid. So in reality what had been studied was the accumulation of radioactivity rather than amino acids and there is no assurance that the ratio so determined accurately reflects the concentration ratio for the unlabeled amino acids. Obviously, what is required for a proper study of the regulation by insulin of amino acid penetration into muscle is a chemical determination of the exact amount of each amino acid in intracellular water in circumstances reflecting as faithfully as is possible those found physiologically (SCHARFF and WOOL, 1965a).

Rat heart was perfused with medium containing: a mixture of amino acids in the same concentration as they are found in plasma; pyruvate (an energy substrate whose utilization is not influenced by insulin); and albumin. The effect of insulin on the concentration of amino acids and like material in the medium and in the intracellular water of the heart was then determined after perfusion for different periods of time.

The concentration of amino acids in the medium, in general, remained constant during the course of 60 min of perfusion of heart in control experiments, and was not sensibly changed by the addition of insulin (Scharff and Wool, 1965a). The concentration of amino acids in the intracellular water of perfused heart evinced a certain amount of variability. The total amino acid concentration tended to decrease as a function of time: the decrease could be accounted for by a relatively large fall in the concentration of aspartic acid, glutamic acid, and alanine (amino acids that are readily transaminated in muscle); the concentration of most of the other amino acids, especially leucine, tyrosine, phenylalanine, ornithine, lysine, histidine, tryptophan, and arginine, however, increased during the course of perfusion. The addition of insulin to the perfusion medium did not produce a significant change in the total concentration of amino acids in heart muscle. Examination of the concentration of individual amino acids in heart muscle revealed no clearer, or more meaningful, pattern. The concentration of most amino acids tended to be reduced in the presence of insulin; the only certain exceptions were aspartic acid, proline, serine, and threonine (the latter two were significantly increased).

Most frequently then insulin was without effect on the concentration of amino acids in either the medium or the intracellular water of perfused heart; such changes as were induced by the hormone were quantitatively small, both positive and negative, and, finally, provided no clearly meaningful pattern. It is important to bear in mind that this was true despite the fact that insulin significantly increased the accumulation, in each of the very same hearts, of radioactivity from ^{14}C-aminoisobutyric acid.

b) Amino Acid Transport in the Absence of Protein Synthesis

And then we struck on an approach that has at least allowed a partial reconciliation of the paradox. The tacit assumption has always been made in studying accumulation of ^{14}C-labeled amino acid that because the amount of amino acid incorporated into protein is a small fraction of that added to the medium, it might, therefore, safely be ignored. A calculation testing that assumption was made. In the circumstances of one experiment 12.1% of the radioactivity (from ^{14}C-phenylalanine) added to the medium was found after 2 h to be present in protein; the fraction was increased to 18.9% by insulin (Wool, Castles and Moyer 1955).

There is, then, significant utilization for the synthesis of protein of ^{14}C-amino acid added to the medium in the circumstances commonly used to study accumulation alone. Obviously, account must be taken of the fact. One way of dealing with the complication is to block protein synthesis, and a convenient way of doing that is with the antibiotic puromycin. Fritz and Knobil (1963) had shown that the accumulation of ^{14}C-aminoisobutyric acid by intact rat diaphragm was not affected by puromycin in concentrations that completely abolish amino acid incorporation into protein; nor was the stimulation by insulin of accumulation influenced.

It was found that in the presence of sufficient puromycin to suppress protein synthesis, the accumulation of radioactivity from five amino acids (histidine, leucine, phenylalanine, tyrosine, and alanine), not ordinarily responsive to insulin, was increased by the hormone (Castles and Wool, 1964).

The results provide at least a partial solution to the problem of why insulin increased accumulation of some utilized amino acids and not others. Apparently, in the presence of insulin the increase in the rate of incorporation into protein of most, but not all, amino acids is sufficient to prevent their accumulation to a concentration greater than that which occurs in the absence of the hormone, even when transport too is stimulated. Puromycin blocks amino acid incorporation into protein and thereby uncovers the insulin stimulation of amino acid transport. The antibiotic would seem then to be a valuable tool in the study of the mechanism and the means of regulation of amino acid transport.

If the foregoing proposal as to the means whereby puromycin makes manifest the effect of insulin on amino acid transport is correct, it follows that insulin should decrease the concentration of the radioactive amino acid in the incubation medium, and, inasmuch as the concentration ratio for the radioactive amino acid does not change, the hormone should also decrease the intracellular concentration of the radioactive amino acid. The prediction was tested (Wool *et al.*, 1965). Intact diaphragm was incubated in buffer containing a single radioactive amino acid and, at the conclusion of the incubation, the concentration of radioactivity in the medium and in the intracellular water of diaphragm muscle determined. In each instance the disappearance of radioactivity from the medium was increased by insulin and this was true whether puromycin was present or not. The decrease in concentration of radioactivity in the medium due to insulin appeared to be slightly less in the presence of puromycin. Despite the insulin-mediated increase in uptake of ^{14}C-amino acid from the medium less radioactivity was present in the intracellular water of muscle and as a result the concentration ratio was not appreciably altered. That this is so implies, of course, that insulin is stimulating transport and incorporation into protein of amino acids, but that the stimulation of incorporation is greater than that of transport. When puromycin is added to the medium the situation is altered; insulin still increases the uptake of amino acid, albeit perhaps to a slightly lesser degree, but since there is no stimulation of incorporation by the hormone the amino acid taken up accumulates in the intracellular water to a greater concentration than in the absence of insulin.

Armed now with the results of the puromycin experiments we returned to an examination of the effect of insulin on the concentration of amino acids in the perfused rat heart (Scharff and Wool, 1965b). In the presence of sufficient puromycin to all but completely suppress protein synthesis insulin increased the total intracellular concentration of amino acids as well as the concentration gradient between the intracellular water and the medium. The concentration in heart muscle of almost all the individual amino acids was increased by insulin, when puromycin was present, and, inasmuch as there were only small changes in concentration of amino acids in the medium (the changes that did occur were in accord with an effect of the hormone to increase transfer of the amino acids from the medium to cell water of the heart) the concentration ratio for the amino acids was also increased.

The results of the studies with puromycin support the conclusion that insulin acts on muscle to accelerate the transfer of most, if not all, amino acids from the extracellular space into the cell interior. The results are not to be interpreted, however, as proving that insulin increases protein synthesis in muscle solely by an influence on amino acid accumulation.

3. The Nature of the Effect of Insulin on Amino Acid Transport

There is much circumstantial evidence to support the notion that transport of amino acids into microbial and mammalian cells is carrier-mediated. Since the kinetics of the process are closely analogous to those of enzyme-catalyzed reactions is it not unreasonable to believe that the carrier molecules are proteins —

either enzymes or structural proteins contained in, or closely associated with, the cell's membrane. Studies on the chemistry and genetics of substrate (sugar and amino acid) transport in microorganisms (Fox and Kennedy, 1965; Heppel, 1967) have made the postulate increasingly more likely. Most germane to the problem at hand, there is now at least indirect evidence that protein(s) participate in the active transmembrane transport of amino acids in animal cells. Adamson *et al.* (1966) and Kostyo and Redmond (1966) discovered at about the same time that puromycin would inhibit amino acid uptake, in embryonic bone and in diaphragm respectively, provided only that the tissue was incubated with the antibiotic for a sufficiently long time. Elsas and Rosenberg (1967) using rat kidney cortex slices have added considerably to our knowledge of the details of the process. The three groups seem agreed on the following general features: Puromycin inhibits the transport of a number of amino acids (α-aminoisobutyric acid, glycine, 1-aminocyclopentane-1-carboxylic acid, proline, and leucine). Protein synthesis is inhibited within 10 min by puromycin, but transport of amino acids is significantly impaired only after approximately 2 h of preincubation with the antibiotic. Because of the delay in the inhibition of amino acid transport by puromycin there is no conflict between the results described here and our findings (Wool *et al.*, 1965; Castles and Wool, 1964; Scharff and Wool, 1965b) referred to above; in the latter experiments incubation with puromycin and measurement of amino acid transport never exceeded two hours and frequently was for 1 h or less. Puromycin does not affect oxygen consumption, tissue water spaces, or tissue cation concentration — thus the action of the antibiotic on amino acid transport is not the indirect result of non-specific tissue injury — or an alteration in tissue metabolism or cell permeability. Puromycin reduced α-aminoisobutyric acid accumulation by slowing influx; efflux is not altered, nor is the apparent affinity of the amino acid for the membrane-carrier. One interpretation of the data is that the selective, active, mediated, inward transport of amino acids in muscle and in other mammalian tissues requires the participation of one or more proteins. The half-life of the protein(s), calculated from the impairment of transport by puromycin (assuming the antibiotic inhibits synthesis of that particular protein), is about three and one-half hours. (*N.B.*: The half-life of the protein(s) is sufficiently long so as to have concealed the inhibitory effect in our experiments.)

Elsas *et al.* (1967) sought to determine the relation of the putative membrane protein to the insulin-mediated enhancement of amino acid entry into muscle. Aware that the inhibition of the synthesis of new protein by puromycin did not impair the stimulatory effect of the hormone on amino acid transport in experiments of shorter duration (i.e., 2 h or less) they preincubated diaphragm for three hours with the antibiotic before adding ^{14}C-α-aminoisobutyric acid and insulin. Puromycin not only inhibited basal uptake of α-aminoisobutyric acid but also impaired insulin's stimulation of the process. The results suggest that insulin accelerates amino acid transport in muscle by an influence on the putative membrane protein, since the effect of the hormone is reduced when the amount of that protein is reduced. It is important to recognize, however, that the stimulation of transport by insulin does not require the synthesis of new membrane protein, for the hormone can increase amino acid uptake when protein synthesis is inhibited by puromycin — provided only that the inhibition has not been for so long as to reduce significantly the amount of the putative membrane protein (bear in mind it has a half-life of approximately three and one-half hours). The distinction between the effects of puromycin over a short (2 h or less) and over a long period, on the response to insulin is absolutely critical. Since it is not the synthesis of the postulated carrier protein that accounts for insulin's stimulation of amino acid transport in muscle it must be its efficiency (perhaps its mobility) that is increased by the hormone. Insulin, or some intermediate generated by the hormone, may alter the conformation of the carrier protein. Whatever the proper interpretation there can be little doubt that the experiments with puromycin, once their meaning is fathomed, must provide an important insight into the mechanism and mode of regulation of amino acid transport in muscle.

4. Does Availability of Amino Acids Limit Protein Synthesis in Muscle

It is important to know if the concentration of amino acids in cells ever limits protein synthesis. The most detailed and meticulous study of that question has been carried out by Morgan and his colleagues (Morgan *et al.*, 1971a, 1971b). In carefully controlled experiments, rat hearts were perfused with buffer containing glucose and various amino acid mixtures. There is a progressive decline in the rate of protein synthesis in isolated rat hearts, however, the decline was mitigated by addition of amino acids to the perfusion medium. For example, the synthesis of whole heart protein and myosin was increased 40% when the concentration of amino acids was raised to five times that present in plasma. The intracellular concentrations of amino acids were also increased, thus it seems that in this case availability of amino acids was decisive in limiting protein synthesis. It need be kept in mind that the conditions of the experiments are less than physiological and there must be some doubt if the same holds in more normal circumstances.

Morgan and associates (Morgan *et al.*, 1971b) have also shown that an excess of amino acids (five times the normal plasma concentration) would increase the initiation of the synthesis of peptide chains in perfused rat hearts — deduced from a decrease in the number of ribosome subunits. Insulin increased the synthesis of protein in heart muscle; the increase occurred when the concentration of amino acids was the same as in plasma. The effect of insulin was no greater (if anything it was less) when the amino acid concentration in the perfusate was five times the plasma level, which suggests again that insulin has an effect on protein synthesis over and above its influence on amino acid transport.

5. The Dilemma of the Functional Heterogeneity of the Intracellular Amino Acid Pool

a) Evidence for Compartmentalization

An important question with respect to protein synthesis is the precise source of the amino acids. It was assumed originally that the amino acids that served as precursors for the synthesis of protein were drawn from the general intracellular pool. There is now a good deal of evidence, albeit mostly circumstantial or indirect, that the assumption may not be correct (Kipnis *et al.*, 1961; Hider *et al.*, 1969, 1971a, 1971b; Rosenberg *et al.*, 1963; Guidotti *et al.*, 1964, Kostyo, 1964); that the actual physiological situation may be more complex.

The doubts have arisen from experiments in which the kinetics of the entry of an amino acid into the free intracellular pool have been compared with the kinetics of incorporation of the same amino acid into cellular protein. In general, when tissues are incubated with a radioactive amino acid, the specific activity of that amino acid in the intracellular pool increases exponentially until a constant specific activity is achieved — no matter the amino acid there is a finite (usually appreciable) delay before the steady state is reached. The incorporation of the very same amino acid into protein, on the other hand, is frequently linear and constant from the beginning. The latter observation suggests that the amino acids used in the synthesis of protein do not equilibrate with the entire free intracellular pool, for if they did one would have expected that incorporation would not become linear until the specific activity of the amino acid in the intracellular pool had become constant. The anomaly has led to the proposal that the intracellular pool of amino acids is functionally compartmentalized; moreover, it is necessary to postulate that the protein precursor is in a pool that is small and perforce equilibrates rapidly with extracellular amino acids. There is by no means universal agreement that the data requires postulating separate amino acid pools, at least not for all amino acids (Manchester and Wool, 1963; Morgan *et al.*, 1971a).

b) Possible Organization of Amino Acid Pools

If there are separate pools the amino acids might be physically or structurally compartmentalized: that is, some portion of the pool may be sequestered in the mitochondria, endoplasmic reticulum, nuclei, or at some other morphological site, or that discrete noncommunicating pools exist in each of these sites. It is at least equally possible that some portion or even all of the pool is chemically sequestered. Amino acids could be bound by covalent linkage, hydrogen bonds, or van der Waals forces to various intracellular molecules: to amino acid-activating enzymes; to transfer RNA as aminoacyl-tRNA; to ribosomes; or, perhaps most important, in amino acid-lipid complexes. The existence of complexes and compounds between amino acids and lipids is found in a number of tissues. The amino acids in lipoidal complexes are in a dynamic state and may be causally related to protein synthesis (Hendler, 1962a). Lipid-rich cellular membranes may provide structural orientation for the many complex steps in protein synthesis, including amino acid transport as well as incorporation into protein (Hendler, 1962b). It has been suggested that amino acids are actually incorporated into protein directly from the extracellular pool (Hider *et al.*, 1969). Any one of these possible compartments might be the one on the direct line to protein synthesis. Obviously, decisive experiments are needed to characterize the intracellular amino acid pool.

c) Amino Acid Pools and the Measurement of Protein Synthesis

The importance, for our purposes, of the possibility of the existence of separate amino acid pools is the uncertainty it casts on conjectures concerning the nature of the mechanism by which insulin increase protein synthesis. It is possible that insulin changes the specific activity of amino acids in a small pool that is used directly for protein synthesis. An increase in the rate of incorporation might then seem to have occurred without an actual change in rate of peptide synthesis, since the amino acid being used for protein synthesis would be drawn from a pool of higher specific activity. But even those who are the most ardent advocates of separate pools (Hider *et al.*, 1969) would seem to agree that, "... it is unlikely that the insulin effect on amino acid incorporation results from any increase in the specific radioactivity of amino acid entering protein; but rather, there is a true increase in the rate of protein synthesis" (Hider *et al.*, 1971b). It is also possible that an increase in the concentration of amino acids in a distinct pool might in some way increase the synthesis of protein; perhaps by accelerating the initiation of protein synthesis (Morgan *et al.*, 1971b); perhaps by some other mechanism. Insulin does increase the specific radioactivity of aminoacyl-tRNA in heart muscle perfused with ^{3}H-labeled amino acids (Davey and Manchester, 1969); and Germanyuk and Mironenko (1969) have suggested that diabetes impairs the formation of aminoacyl-tRNA in liver.

Obviously, one way to resolve the problem is to devise a means of determining the actual specific activity of the amino acid used for the synthesis of protein and compare it with the specific activity of the amino acid in the free intracellular pool. That has not been done yet. I should like to propose a strategy: namely to determine the specific activity of an amino acid in nascent peptide, for it must provide the specific activity of the amino acid used for protein synthesis. If one then compares the specific activity of an amino acid in nascent peptide with the specific activity of the same amino acid in the free intracellular pool, it should be possible to decide whether there are separate intracellular compartments: if the specific activities are the same then it follows that amino acids are drawn from the free intracellular pool for protein synthesis. The same thing might be accomplished by measuring the specific activity of an amino acid in aminoacyl-tRNA.

The technique might then be used to resolve the dilemma of whether insulin increases protein synthesis by a direct effect on the synthetic machinery or whether the influence of the hormone on protein metabolism is the secondary result of an acceleration of amino acid transport. One could determine the specific activity of an amino acid in nascent protein from insulin treated and control tissues: if insulin increases the synthesis of protein without altering the specific activity of that amino acid in nascent protein, it must have an effect over and above that on transport.

III. Insulin, Diabetes and the Function of Muscle Ribosomes

1. Muscle Ribosomes from Diabetic Animals Catalyze Protein Synthesis Less Effectively than do Ribosomes from Normal Animals

Our analysis of the mechanism whereby insulin increases protein synthesis has been helped by the discovery (Wool and Cavicchi, 1967) that ribosomes from the muscle of alloxan-diabetic rats incorporate decreased amounts of amino acid into protein (Table 1). The decrease in protein synthesis is due to insulin deficiency rather than to a toxic action of the alloxan, for the same defect occurs when the animals are depancreatized or made acutely diabetic by administration of anti-insulin serum (Wool and Cavicchi, 1967). The difference in the function of normal and diabetic ribosomes is evident even if the source of the soluble fraction (which contains the enzymes and cofactors needed to support protein synthesis) is an indifferent one, as for example, the liver of normal animals (Wool *et al.*, 1968a).

Table 1. *Incorporation into Protein of Radioactivity from ^{14}C-Phe-tRNA by Skeletal Muscle Ribosomes*

Source of Ribosomes	Incorporation into Protein, counts/min	Change, %
Normal	2,730	
Diabetic	980	— 64
Diabetic + Insulin	2,810	+287

The method of assaying protein synthesis by skeletal muscle ribosomes is to be found in Wool and Cavicchi (1967). The insulin (0.1 unit) was administered 5 min before the animals were killed.

2. Small Amounts of Insulin Administered to Diabetic Animals Rapidly Increase the Synthesis of Protein by Ribosomes

When diabetic animals are treated with insulin before they are killed, the synthesis of protein by muscle ribosomes is restored to normal (Table 1). As little as 0.1 unit (or 4 μg) of the hormone per animal produces a full response within 5 min (Wool and Cavicchi, 1967). For insulin to be effective it must be administered to the animal (or added *in vitro* to intact muscle tissue); when added directly to the reaction mixture it does not affect ribosome function. Nonetheless the speed and the specificity with which insulin acts when administered to diabetic animals is remarkable: we know of no other agent or circumstance that can more rapidly stimulate the synthesis of protein in a mammalian tissue.

Experiments were carried out using aminoacyl-tRNA (AA-tRNA) as substrate and in circumstances where all the cofactors required for the synthesis of protein were added in amounts that were optimal or excessive — thus protein synthesis was directly proportional to the concentration of ribosomes. We compared equal numbers of ribosomes from normal, from diabetic, and from diabetic animals treated with insulin. Hence the differences between the groups are due solely to the effectiveness with which individual ribosomes translate messenger RNA (mRNA). The findings are uncomplicated by effects of diabetes on the density of the population of ribosomes, independent of the level of endogenous transfer-RNA, or the amount or activity of the aminoacyl synthetases — all of which parameters are secondarily affected by diabetes (Wool *et al.*, 1968a, 1968b). We reiterate because the point is important: our concern is with the effectiveness of the function of individual ribosomes.

3. Insulin Increases the Synthesis of all Muscle Proteins

We sought to determine the identity of the proteins whose synthesis was increased by insulin. To that end, diaphragm muscle from diabetic animals was incubated with a radioactive amino acid and with or without insulin (Kurihara and Wool, 1968). At the end of the period of incubation (generally 1 h) the sarcoplasmic and ribosomal proteins were fractionated by electrophoresis on discontinuous polyacrylamide gels. The synthesis of all the protein fractions was decreased to approximately the same extent by diabetes, and all were restored to normal by insulin. It appears that all muscle proteins continue to be synthesized, albeit in reduced amounts, in the absence of insulin. Thus the hormone's effect is general rather than selective. Although there is still a possibility that insulin causes a disproportionate increase in the synthesis of one or a few proteins, the predominant effect is to facilitate the translation of messenger RNA for all muscle proteins.

4. Diabetes Reduces the Number of Active Ribosomes in Muscle

What is the nature of the population of diabetic ribosomes? Is it composed of ribosomes all of which are one-half as effective as the normal, or is it made up of ribosomes, half of which are fully active and half of which are without activity? We decided to take advantage of the properties of puromycin in an attempt to solve the problem (Wool and Kurihara, 1967). We reasoned that puromycin would inhibit protein synthesis, but each active ribosome would make one peptide bond, and the nascent protein bound by a covalent bond to puromycin would be released. If we used tritium-labeled puromycin, then the nascent peptide would be radioactive. From the radioactivity of the ^{3}H-labeled peptidyl-puromycin we could calculate the number of peptide bonds formed and hence the number of active ribosomes. Finally, parallel determinations with preparations of normal and diabetic ribosomes should, in theory, give an answer to our question.

If the formation of peptidyl-puromycin was to serve as a measure of the number of active ribosomes, it would be necessary to ensure that each active particle formed one, and only one, peptide bond. We accomplished that by omitting supernatant protein and AA-tRNA from the reaction mixture. Those two components are not necessary for the puromycin reaction; both are essential if the ribosomes are to make more than one peptide bond.

The ^{3}H-labeled peptidyl-puromycin formed by normal and diabetic ribosomes was separated from the ^{3}H-puromycin itself by filtration on Sephadex G-10 after equilibration with 8 M urea in Tris buffer (Fig. 1). Diabetes reduces the number of ribosomes capable of forming a single peptide bond (WOOL and KURIHARA, 1967). From the results of a large number of experiments we estimated the number of active ribosomes in a preparation. On the average, about 25% of the ribosomes from normal muscle are active; diabetes reduces the average to less than 10% (Table 2). What is more, there is a close correspondence between the decrease in protein synthesis caused by diabetes and the decrease in the number of active ribosomes. Insulin, in 5 min, increases the number of active ribosomes by 150% and at one and the same time restores protein synthesis to normal.

From the percentage of active ribosomes and from the moles of amino acid incorporated into protein by ribosomes in the same preparation, we have calculated the number of peptide bonds formed by each active particle (WOOL and KURIHARA, 1967). In one experiment each active normal ribosome made 27 peptide bonds; each active (and we emphasize active) diabetic ribosome made 26. The results are decisive in resolving the problem posed in the beginning. They establish that the difference in the capacity of preparations of normal and diabetic ribosomes to synthesize protein is due to the diabetic ribosomes having a smaller proportion of active particles, rather than each diabetic ribosome being less efficient than normal.

Table 2. *Synthesis of Protein and Formation of Peptidyl-Puromycin by Ribosomes from Skeletal Muscle*

Source of Ribosomes	Protein Synthesis, counts/min	Formation of Peptidyl-Puromycin, counts/min	Active Ribosomes, %
Normal	4,092	3,505	22.1
Diabetic	1,611 (—61%)	1,242 (—65%)	7.8 (—65%)
Diabetic + Insulin	4,072 (+153%)	3,099 (+150%)	19.5 (+150%)

Ribosomes were assayed for their ability to synthesize protein (WOOL and CAVICCHI, 1967) and to form peptidyl-puromycin (WOOL and KURIHARA, 1967). The insulin (0.1 unit) was administered 5 min before rats were killed.

5. Preparatios of Ribosomes from the Muscle of Diabetic Animals Contain Fewer Polysomes and More Monomers than Normal

It has been our fond hope that a study of the chemical and physical properties of the ribosome would provide a clue to the nature of the putative change in the particle that occurs in diabetes. One change that results from a lack of insulin is in the sedimentation of the ribosomes (STIREWALT *et al.*, 1967; RANNELS *et al.*,

1970; Morgan *et al.*, 1971b). Diabetes reduces the number of larger aggregates or polysomes and causes a corresponding increase in the number of the smaller particles or monosomes (Fig. 2). Insulin rapidly reverses the effect of diabetes (Stirewalt *et al.*, 1967); the hormone causes the reaggregation of the smaller particles to form polysomes, and it does so in 5 min (Fig. 2). Insulin also decreases the number of ribosomal subunits (Morgan *et al.*, 1971b). The speed with which insulin acts to recruit ribosomes to form large assemblies is once again worth remarking.

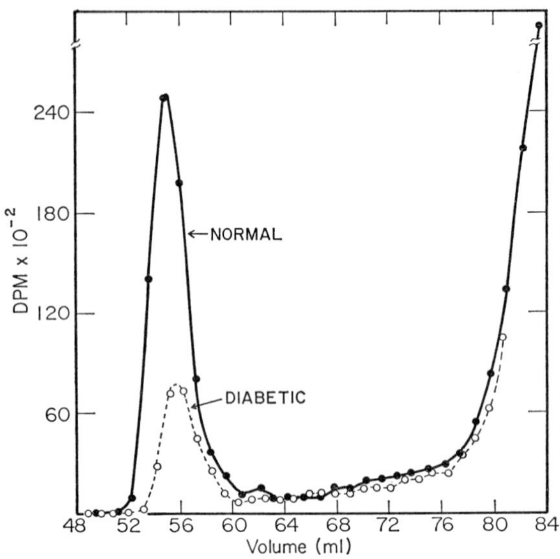

Fig. 1. Separation of ^{3}H-peptidyl puromycin by chromatography on Sephadex G-10. The ^{3}H-peptidyl puromycin formed by normal and by diabetic ribosomes was separated from the ^{3}H-puromycin (fractions 75—84). (From Wool and Kurihara, 1967)

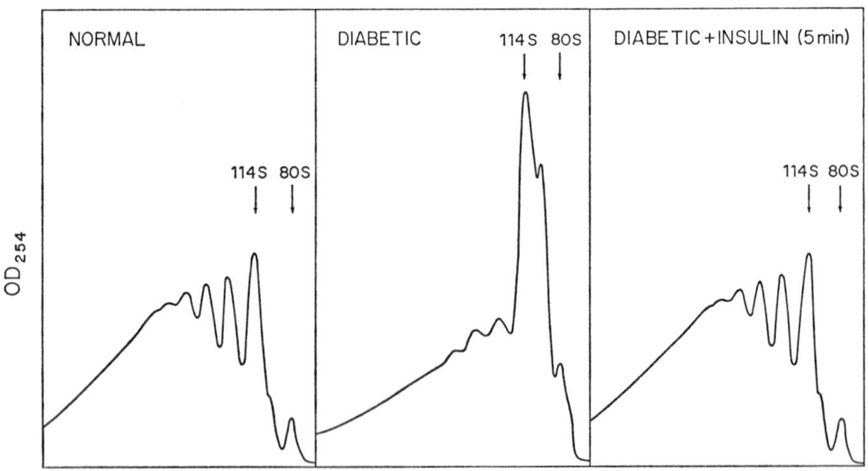

Fig. 2. Sedimentation of muscle ribosomes in linear sucrose gradients: effect of diabetes and insulin. One group of diabetic rats was given (intraperitoneally) 5 units of insulin 5 min before the ribosomes were isolated (From Wool *et al.*, 1972)

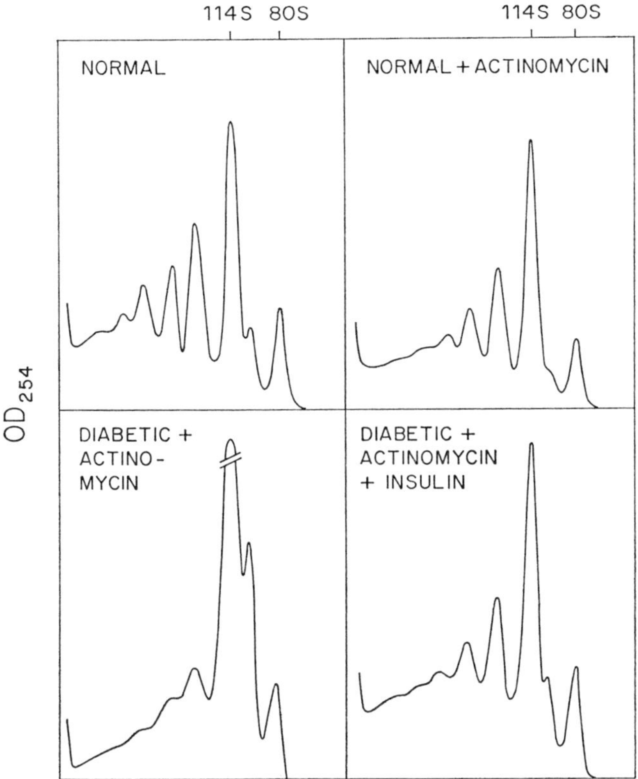

Fig. 3. Sedimentation of skeletal muscle ribosomes in linear sucrose gradients: effect of diabetes and insulin in the presence of actinomycin. The animals received (intraperitoneally) 1 mg of actinomycin, or an equal volume of 2% ethanol in saline and, 15 min later, 5 units of insulin (intraperitoneally) or an equal volume of saline. The animals were killed 75 min after the first injection (actinomycin or 2% ethanol in saline), 1 hr after the insulin (or saline), and the ribosomes were isolated. An aliquot of the ribosome preparation analyzed in each gradient was assayed for its ability to catalyze the transfer of radioactivity from ^{14}C-Phe-tRNA to protein. Results (in counts/min per 30 μg of ribosomal RNA): normal, 477; normal treated with actinomycin, 464; diabetic treated with actinomycin, 293; diabetic treated with actinomycin and insulin, 460. The sedimentation coefficients were calculated from schlieren patterns obtained in the analytical ultracentrifuge. (From Stirewalt *et al.*, 1967)

6. Insulin-Induced Formation of Polysomes and Increase in Protein Synthesis Do not Require the Synthesis of RNA

We sought, by pretreating animals with actinomycin (Stirewalt, 1967), to determine if the insulin-mediated assembly of polysomes required RNA synthesis. The antibiotic does not affect the sedimentation of muscle ribosomes (Fig. 3), at least not in 75 min (the duration of this experiment), a finding consonant with the surmise that mRNA in muscle is on the whole relatively stable. The crucial finding was that insulin induced the formation of polysomes (Fig. 3) and increased protein synthesis by ribosomes (see legend to Fig. 3) even in diabetic animals that had been pretreated with actinomycin — that is in the all but complete absence of DNA-dependent RNA synthesis. We interpret the results to mean the hormone acted in the absence of the formation of new ribosomes or of the synthesis of mRNA; there must be in the muscle of diabetic animals an unutilized reservoir of mRNA. We presume that insulin conditions the binding and translation of that preformed mRNA, accounting in that way for the assembly of polysomes and the increase in protein synthesis.

7. The Reduced Ability of Diabetic Ribosomes to Translate Messenger RNA is not Related to the Binding of the Template

We knew that RNA synthesis was not required for the effect of insulin on muscle ribosomes (Wool and Cavicchi, 1966) and that messenger RNA was present in the muscle of diabetic animals but was not being translated. Consideration of those observations led us to test the ability of diabetic ribosomes to bind template RNA. For technical reasons the best template to use is viral mRNA and the only radioactive viral mRNA available to us at the time was ^{32}P-labeled turnip-yellow mosaic virus (TYMV) RNA. The TYMV RNA we used was hydrolyzed with KOH under controlled conditions so that each polynucleotide chain contained no more than one ribosome binding site (Rolleston *et al.*, 1970).

Addition of TYMV RNA to muscle ribosomes stimulated protein synthesis; however, at each magnesium concentration diabetic ribosomes were subnormal in translation of TYMV RNA (Fig. 4). We reckoned that this might be due to a decrease in binding of the template, either because of a reduction in the number of diabetic ribosomes able to bind TYMV RNA or to a decrease in the affinity of all diabetic ribosomes for TYMV RNA. The fraction of ribosomes capable of binding TYMV RNA was measured in the presence of an excess of the polynucleotide and found not to be reduced by diabetes (Rolleston *et al.*, 1970), nor was there a difference in the equilibrium constant for the binding of TYMV

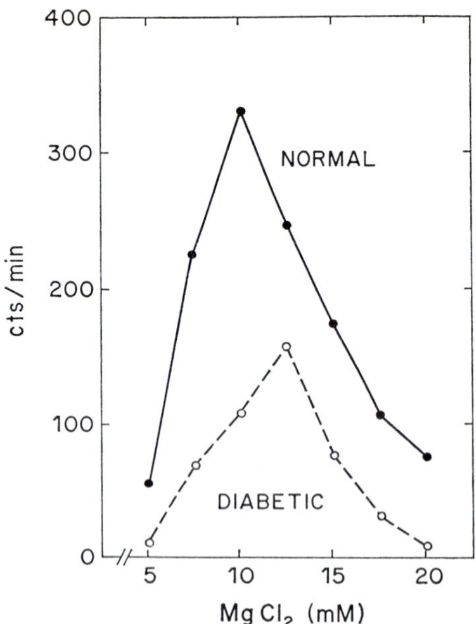

Fig. 4. Stimulation of protein synthesis by normal and diabetic muscle ribosomes due to addition of TYMV RNA. Only the stimulation over endogenous incorporation due to addition of TYMV RNA is plotted. (From Rolleston *et al.*, 1970)

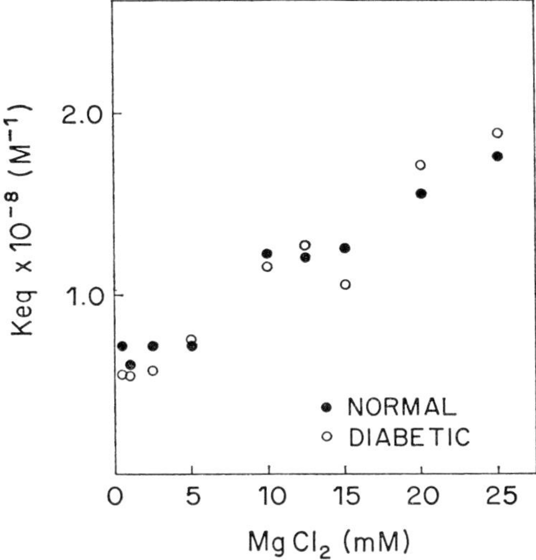

Fig. 5. Equilibrium constants for the binding of ^{32}P-TYMV RNA to normal and diabetic muscle ribosomes. (From ROLLESTON *et al.*, 1970)

RNA to an excess of normal and diabetic ribosomes (Fig. 5). It seemed then that the reduced ability of diabetic ribosomes to translate TYMV RNA was not related to binding of the template. However, the experiments suffer a weakness that militates against generalizing the results to the binding of mRNA in the cell. There is no assurance that the TYMV RNA was bound to the ribosome in the same manner as natural mRNA. Indeed, that process requires specific initiation factors that may not have been present in our assay. If insulin and diabetes influence the availability or use by the ribosome of a specific mRNA binding factor, the experiments would not reveal that effect.

8. Diabetic Ribosomes Are Less Effective than Normal in the Translation of Polyuridylic Acid at Lower Concentrations of Magnesium and More Effective at Higher Concentrations of the Cation

We had quite early on made an observation that proved important. Diabetic ribosomes were less active than normal ribosomes in the translation of endogenous mRNA at all concentrations of magnesium. However, the difference — and this is the crux of the matter — in the capacity of normal and diabetic ribosomes to synthesize polyphenylalanine (polyphe) in the presence of polyuridylic acid (poly U) was critically dependent on the magnesium concentration (WOOL *et al.*, 1968a). At high magnesium concentrations diabetic ribosomes synthesized more polyphe than normal, whereas at low concentrations the reverse was true (Fig. 6). The greater synthesis of polyphe we believe to be the secondary consequence of diabetic ribosomes having less mRNA and as a result being able to bind more poly U in the favorable circumstances provided by a high concentration of magnesium. If diabetic ribosomes bind more poly U they will synthesize more polyphe, all other things being equal. Therefore we focused attention on the results at low magnesium concentrations as more nearly reflecting the physiological condition.

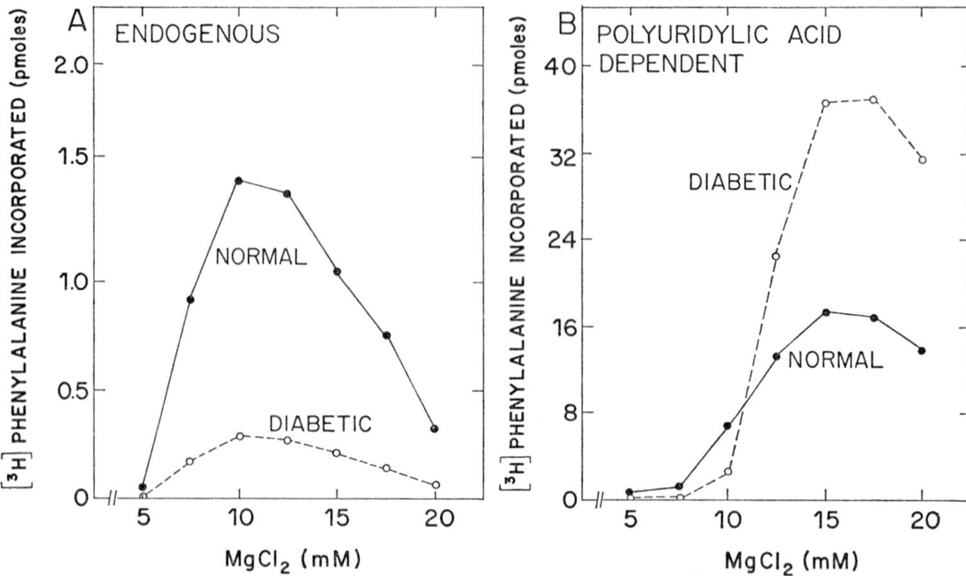

Fig. 6. Synthesis of protein by normal and diabetic ribosomes in the presence and absence of poly U: effect of the concentration of magnesium. A, endogenous incorporation; B, poly U-dependent protein synthesis, calculated by subtracting endogenous incorporation from that in the presence of poly U. (From Wool *et al.*, 1968a)

9. When Hybrid Ribosomes Containing a Normal and Diabetic Subunit Are Constructed, the Defect in Protein Synthesis Appears to Be Carried by the 60S Subunit

What is the nature of the insulin-mediated change in the ribosome that leads to an alteration in the ability of the particle to translate mRNA? We reckoned that the complexity of the problem would be reduced and our analysis simplified if a decision could be had as to whether the insulin-sensitive site is on the large or small ribosome subunit, for certain of the reactions of protein synthesis occur on one, or the other, of the two subunits. For example, binding of mRNA and of AA-tRNA is to the small subunit, whereas peptide bond formation is catalyzed by an enzyme that is a component of the large subunit. For those reasons we decided to try to determine which of the two subunits carries the diabetic defect. One way to reach a decision is to make hybrid ribosomes containing normal and diabetic subunits (Fig. 7 has a schematic portrayal of the strategy).

The first step was to devise a means of dissociating and reassociating ribosomes in a way that preserved their activity (Martin *et al.*, 1969). We achieved that by treating ribosomes with 0.8—1.0 M KCl at 25—30° in the presence of 10 mM β-mercaptoethanol (Fig. 8). The ribosomes dissociated into particles having sedimentation coefficients of 60 and 40 in a ratio of 2.5 : 1 (A_{254}). When the 40S and 60S ribosomal subunits were combined and dialyzed to remove the excess KCl they reassociated to form 80S particles (Fig. 8).

We were now able to undertake the hybridization experiment. But first it was necessary to show that the reassociated subunits were active. Little or no protein synthesis occurred in the absence of added template RNA (dissociation probably

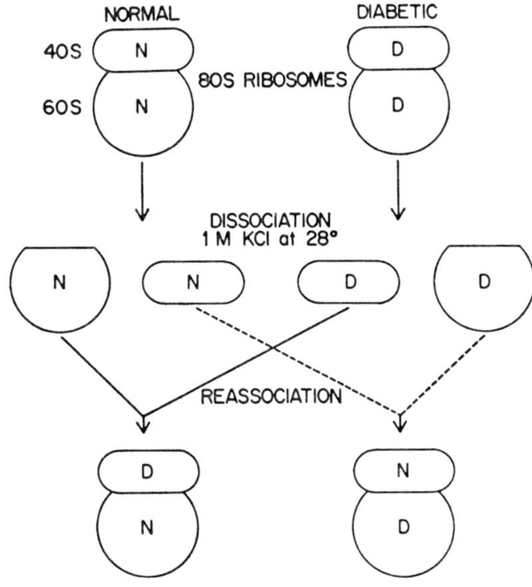

Fig. 7. Scheme for the formation of hybrid ribosomes containing a normal and a diabetic subunit. (From Wool *et al.*, 1972)

strips the ribosome of mRNA), and for that reason we assayed the synthesis of polyphe in the presence of poly U.

The 40S particle had little ability to catalyze the synthesis of polyphe — the 60S fraction had approximately 25% of the activity of the control, due to contamination with 40S subunits (Table 3). Combination of the subunits created particles that were fully active in poly U-directed synthesis of polyphe (Martin *et al.*, 1969).

We next prepared 40S and 60S subunits from ribosomes of normal and diabetic rats, made hybrid ribosomes from the subunits, and measured their ability to catalyze polypeptide synthesis. When the four combinations of normal and diabetic subunits (N40—N60; D40—D60; N40—D60; D40—N60) were assayed at

Table 3. *Synthesis of Polyphenylalanine by Hybrid 80S Ribosomes Formed from Normal and Diabetic Subunits*

Ribosomal Particles	Polyphenylalanine Synthesis, counts/min per 10 μg ribosomal RNA
Normal	1,292
Diabetic	388
Normal 40S (N40)	100
Diabetic 40S (D40)	4
Normal 60S (N60)	347
Diabetic 60S (D60)	174
N40+N60	1,370
D40+D60	658
N40+D60	654
D40+N60	1,124

The method for preparing subunits and for reassociating 80S ribosomes is to be found in Martin and Wool (1968). The assay of protein synthesis was as in Wool and Cavicchi (1967).

9 mM magnesium (Table 3), the diabetic defect appeared to reside entirely in the 60S subunit (Martin and Wool, 1968).

The results indicated that insulin had altered a function of the 60S particle. We now know a possible explanation of the apparent defect in the 60S subunit and discuss it below.

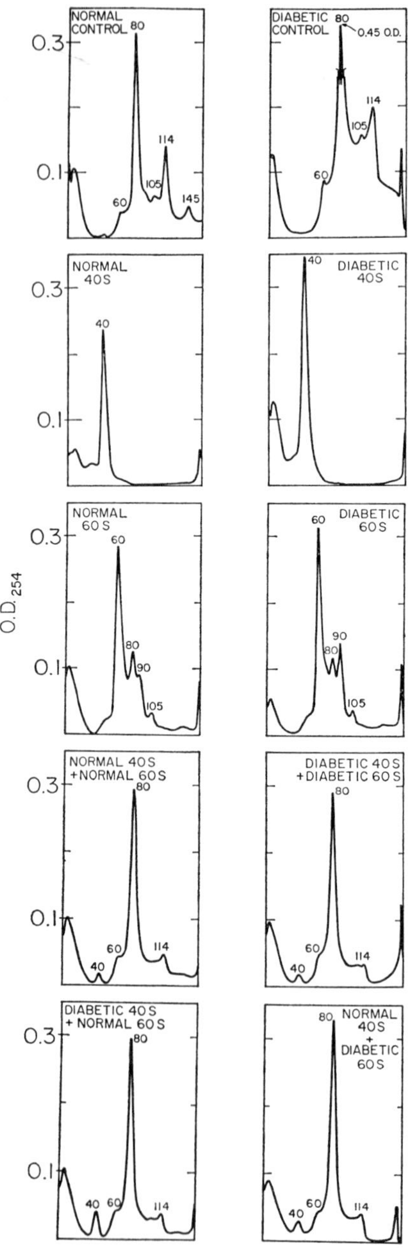

Fig. 8. Formation of subunits from normal and diabetic muscle ribosomes, their reassociation, and the formation of hybrid ribosomes. (From Martin *et al.*, 1969)

10. Diabetes Does not Alter the Peptidyl Transferase Activity of Ribosomes

Peptidyl transferase, the enzyme that catalyzes the formation of peptide bonds during protein synthesis, is a component of the large subunit of bacterial and animal ribosomes (MADEN *et al.*, 1968; MONRO, 1967; MONRO *et al.*, 1969; NETH *et al.*, 1970; VAZQUEZ *et al.*, 1969). Peptidyl transfer can be conveniently measured separate from other steps in protein synthesis in the fragment reaction devised by MONRO (1967). The substrates for the enzyme are puromycin and the CACCA-terminal portion of tRNA acylated with acetyl-leucine. Normal and diabetic ribosomes, and normal and diabetic 60S subunits (Fig. 9), had equal activity in

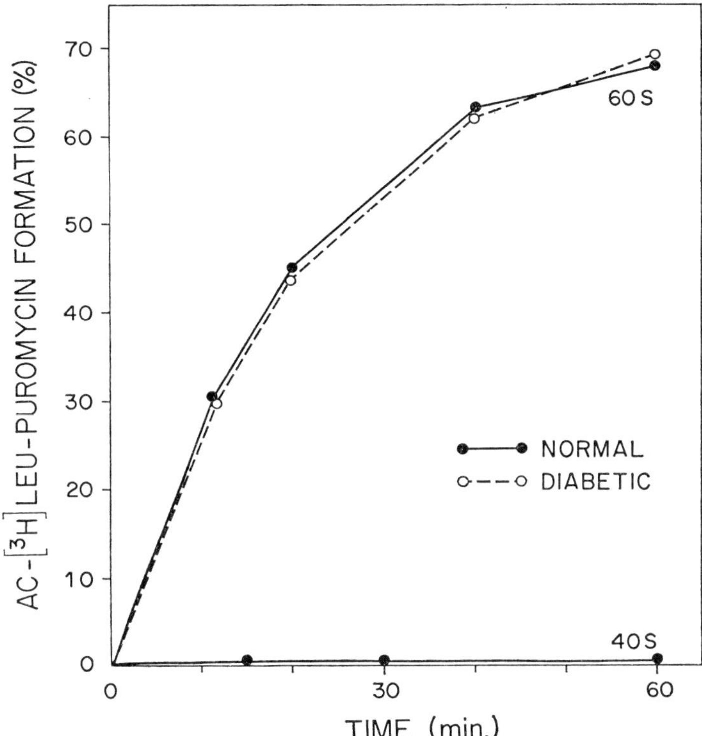

Fig. 9. Acetyl-^{3}H-leucyl-puromycin formation in the fragment reaction by 60S subunits of normal and diabetic muscle ribosomes. (From STIREWALT and WOOL, 1970)

the fragment reaction (STIREWALT and WOOL, 1970). Modulation of protein synthesis by insulin then is not likely to be mediated by an effect on peptidyl transferase. One reservation must be kept in mind: the alcohol used in the fragment reaction may generate maximum peptidyl transferase activity, whereas in physiological circumstances a portion of that activity may be restrained. If that is the case, there could be a difference in the peptidyl transferase activity of normal and diabetic ribosomes, which would not be revealed in the fragment reaction.

11. The Elongation Factor-2 Catalyzed Hydrolysis of GTP by Muscle Ribosomes is not Changed in Diabetes

We continued to seek to discover the nature of the diabetic defect by examining the ability of ribosomes to utilize elongation factor-2 (EF-2) to catalyze the hydrolysis of GTP (Leader *et al.*, 1970). On addition of each amino acid during the synthesis of protein there occurs a complex series of reactions including the movement of mRNA and the ribosome the length of a codon with respect to each other. The process, termed translocation, is catalyzed by elongation factors (probably EF-2) and in some complicated way uses the energy liberated when GTP is hydrolyzed. That activity can be assessed by measuring the ribosome dependent hydrolysis of GTP in the presence of EF-2.

There was no significant difference in the amount of EF-2 catalyzed hydrolysis of GTP with ribosomes from the muscle of normal or diabetic rats — the comparison was made at magnesium chloride concentrations of 2.5 and 10 mM. The same results were obtained whether the amount of EF-2 was limiting or saturating (Fig. 10).

We conclude that the decrease in the capacity of diabetic ribosomes to synthesize protein probably does not result from an inability to utilize EF-2, at least not for the hydrolysis of GTP.

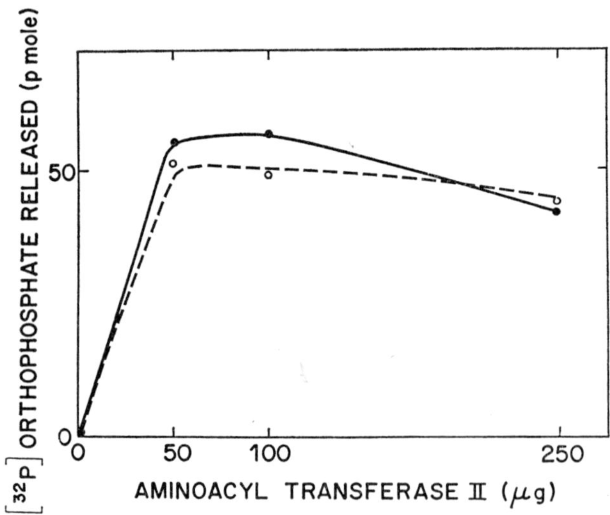

Fig. 10. Effect of EF-2 concentration on the hydrolysis of GTP by muscle ribosomes from normal and diabetic rats. (From Leader *et al.*, 1970)

12. Diabetic Ribosomes Bind Less Phe-tRNA than Normal at Low Concentrations of Magnesium and More at High Concentrations

The decreased capacity of diabetic ribosomes to translate poly U at low concentrations of magnesium might be due to decreased binding of Phe-tRNA. At least the possibility seemed worth testing. We compared the ability of normal and diabetic ribosomes to bind Phe-tRNA in the absence of enzyme (Castles *et al.*, 1971) and in the reaction catalyzed by elongation factor-1 (EF-1) (Leader *et al.*, 1971). At almost any magnesium concentration the amount of Phe-tRNA bound in the absence of EF-1 is trivial when compared with the enzyme-catalyzed reaction (Fig. 11). A more important finding was that diabetic ribosomes bound less Phe-tRNA than normal ribosomes at low concentrations of magnesium and more at high concentrations. Thus the binding of Phe-tRNA closely parallels the translation of poly U. What is more, the decreased binding of Phe-tRNA to diabetic ribosomes at low magnesium concentration persisted even with saturating amounts of EF-1 (Fig. 12). It seemed that diabetic ribosomes could not use EF-1 effectively.

The functional significance of binding of aminoacyl-tRNA to ribosomes can only be assessed when the product of the reaction is known (Castles and Wool, 1970; Leader *et al.*, 1970). For that reason we analyzed the radioactive material bound to ribosomes by isolating the particles, subjecting them to alkaline hydrolysis, and then analyzing the hydrolysate by paper chromatography. When ribosomes were incubated in 7.5 mM magnesium — the concentration at which the diabetic defect in binding of Phe-tRNA was seen — almost all of the radioactive material bound to the ribosome remained at the origin on paper chromatograms (Fig. 13). Little phenylalanine was recovered. What is more, the difference in the amount of origin material accounted for the difference in binding to normal and diabetic ribosomes. We recognized the importance of determining the nature of the origin material. In the chromatographic system that we used, homopolymers of phenylalanine with a chain length of 5 or greater will remain at the origin. However, our failure to detect di- or triphenylalanine made it unlikely the origin material was oligophenylalanine. But the ribosomes we used contain nascent peptide chains, that is peptidyl-tRNA; in addition the peptide bond-forming enzyme, peptidyl transferase, is a component of the ribosome. Thus it seemed possible that the radioactive Phe-tRNA bound to the ribosome was incorporated into the carboxyl-terminus of nascent chains. To test this possibility the origin material was subjected to hydrazinolysis (Castles *et al.*, 1971). (The heating of proteins in hydrazine causes transamidation of all peptide bonds to hydrazides; only the carboxyl-terminal amino acid is liberated as free α-amino-α carboxylic acid). Some 97% of the radioactivity of the origin material was recovered as free ^{14}C-Phe after hydrazinolysis, indicating that the origin material was nascent peptide with a single carboxyl-terminal ^{14}C-Phe (Castles *et al.*, 1971).

Apparently at low concentrations of magnesium, and in the absence of specific initiation factors, AA-tRNA is bound only to ribosomes that carry peptidyl-tRNA, and no initiation of protein synthesis occurs. Rather, AA-tRNA is bound to the acceptor site of those ribosomes that have peptidyl-tRNA in the donor site, a peptide bond is synthesized, and the nascent chain is elongated by one amino acid. The new peptide is transferred to the acceptor site, and no further binding can take place. A consideration of the observations provides us with a possible explanation for the difference in function of normal and diabetic ribosomes, namely, that preparations of normal ribosomes have more peptidyl-tRNA than diabetic ribosomes and that peptidyl-tRNA is necessary for the binding of AA-tRNA at low concentrations of magnesium. We knew from experiments with puromycin that a greater percentage of ribosomes in a normal preparation have peptidyl-tRNA bound to them (Fig. 1 and Table 2).

The observations also provide a possible explanation for the difference in function of normal and diabetic 60S subunits (see results of experiments with hybrid ribosomes, Table 3), namely, that normal 60S subunits have more peptidyl-tRNA than diabetic 60S subunits and that peptidyl-tRNA serves to initiate protein synthesis at low concentrations of magnesium. Some peptidyl-tRNA

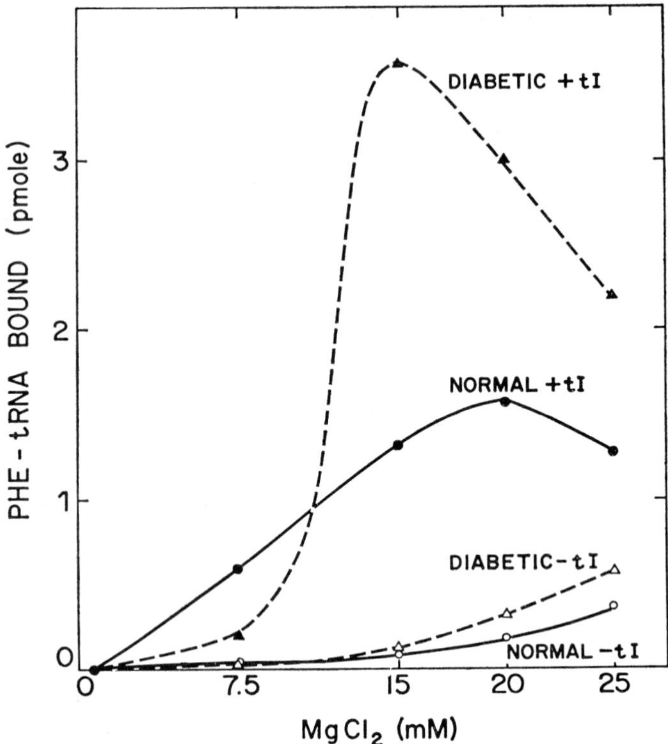

Fig. 11. EF-1 catalyzed and nonenzymatic binding of ^{3}H-Phe-tRNA to normal and diabetic muscle ribosomes as a function of magnesium concentration. (From Leader *et al.*, 1971)

does remain bound to the 60S subunit when ribosomes are dissociated (Stirewalt *et al.*, 1971). (We emphasize that while the explanation is plausible, we do not know that it is sufficient to account entirely for the difference in function of normal and diabetic ribosomes or normal and diabetic 60S subunits.)

The problem then is to account for the decrease in peptidyl-tRNA on diabetic ribosomes. It seems reasonable that it might result from a defect in muscle cells in the capacity for the initiation of endogenous protein synthesis, a possibility considerably reinforced by the finding of increased numbers of ribosome subunits in the muscle of diabetic animals (Rannels *et al.*, 1970; Morgan *et al.*, 1971b). The decisive question then is whether there is an intrinsic difference between normal and diabetic ribosomes or whether they are distinguished only by the amount of attached peptidyl-tRNA (indeed, one might say by the amount of peptidyl-tRNA with which they are contaminated).

13. Diabetic Ribosomes Are Less Effective than Normal in the Translation of Polyuridylic Acid and RNA Extracted from Encephalomyocarditis Virus (EMCV RNA)

In an attempt to abtain answers to the questions posed above, we have for a time been engaged in an effort to compare the capacity of normal and diabetic ribosomes to initiate the synthesis of proteins as distinct from the elongation of peptide chains actually started in the cell. We were aware, as are all those who work seriously on the problem, that the use of cell-free systems to study the control of protein synthesis is greatly facilitated when natural mRNA is available. One need only contemplate the magnificent progress that has come from the use of bacteriophage RNA. What is more, it is so obvious as to be trivial that the most economical way to regulate protein synthesis is to control the initiation of peptide chains. It makes far more sense than to cause queuing in the midst of the synthesis of a chain (as would occur if elongation were controlled), or to cause a hold-up at chain termination. Ideally, the study of initiation of protein synthesis would make use of natural (i.e., cellular) mRNA, but that is not so easy to come by. The next best alternative is viral mRNA. The RNA extracted from encephalomyocarditis virus when added to mammalian ribosomes will stimulate protein synthesis; moreover, the synthesis of virus-specific peptides is carried out with fidelity (MATHEWS, 1970; MATHEWS and KORNER, 1970). We have established that in strictly defined conditions, and I shall give those conditions in a moment, normal and diabetic muscle ribosomes will also translate EMCV RNA with fidelity, for the peptides synthesized *in vitro* correspond to the proteins synthesized in EMCV-infected cells.

Translation of EMCV RNA requires ribosomes. We have used ribosomes reconstituted from subunits. Ribosomal subunits are prepared by treating normal and diabetic ribosomes with puromycin in 0.8 M-KCl. The antibiotic removes nascent peptide from the ribosomes; the high concentrations of salts remove initiation factors. Thus we believe the subunits to be relatively pure (i.e., free of non-ribosomal contaminants). Ribosomes formed from subunits have no endogenous activity, that is to say they do not synthesize protein unless an exogenous template is added.

The translation of EMCV RNA also requires ascites cell supernatant. The cytosol from no other cell will do. The reason is that the supernatant from ascites cells contains all three initiation factors (EIF-1, EIF-2, and EIF-3); supernatant from other tissues has only EIF-1 (LEADER *et al.*, 1972). I might point out that ascites supernatant fraction (like that from other tissues) also contains the two elongation factors required for protein synthesis, EF-1 and EF-2.

The following are also required for assay of EMCV RNA translation: ATP, and an energy-generating system (creatine phosphate and creatine phosphokinase); twenty amino acids of which one is radioactive, [^{3}H] phenylalanine ([^{3}H] Phe); buffer; KCl; and, most critically, 5 mM magnesium, because at higher concentrations of the cation the need for initiation factors is obviated; and finally EMCV RNA. Actually, we have used a second template, poly U. At 5 mM magnesium, two of the three initiation factors, EIF-1 and EIF-2, are required for optimum synthesis of polyphe (SHAFRITZ and ANDERSON, 1970).

Diabetic ribosomes reconstituted from subunits are less efficient than normal in the translation of either poly U or EMCV RNA (Table 4). I wish to emphasize the following points: the experiments are carried out in circumstances where the synthesis of protein requires the initiation of new peptide chains; that EMCV RNA is translated with fidelity for virus-specific peptides are synthesized; and that the initiation factors are added to normal and diabetic ribosomes in equal amounts from an indifferent source (ascites cells). The results then would indicate that diabetic ribosomes suffer a defect that renders them less capable than normal of using factors to initiate the synthesis of proteins. But I hasten to submit a caveat. It remains still to be established that the difference I have just described is intrinsic to the ribosome rather than carried by some fortuitous contaminant unequally distributed between normal and diabetic ribosomal subunits — just as unequal amounts of peptidyl-tRNA on normal and diabetic ribosomal subunits account for the apparent difference in their ability to bind AA-tRNA.

Table 4. *Translation of Polyuridylic Acid and EMCV RNA by Normal and Diabetic Ribosomes Reconstituted from Subunits*

Template	[^{3}H]Phenylalanine Incorporated into Protein (pmole)	
	Normal	Diabetic
None	0.04	0.03
Poly U	89.4	46.4 (—48%)
EMCV RNA	0.86	0.52 (—40%)

EMCV RNA, RNA extracted from encephalamyocarditis virus; poly U, polyuridylic acid. (From Wool, 1972)

14. Formation of an Initiation Complex by Normal and Diabetic Ribosomes

There is a factor (40S binding factor or 40S BF) in the supernatant of muscle and liver cells which catalyses the binding of Phe-tRNA to 40S subunits (Leader *et al.*, 1970). It now seems likely that the 40S BF and EIF-1 are one and the same (Leader and Wool, 1972). We suspected from the beginning that the 40S BF would catalyse the formation of an initiation complex containing the 40S subunit, the template, AA-tRNA, and perhaps EIF-1 itself. What is more, it seemed likely that the initiation complex would be an obligatory intermediate in the reassociation of ribosomal subunits. Thus EIF-1 should catalyse the formation of 80S monomers from 40S and 60S ribosomal subunits. We tested those predictions by incubating subunits in buffer containing 3.5 mM $MgCl_2$ and 80 mM KCl, in which circumstances no reassociation ordinarily takes place (Wettenhall *et al.*, 1971). Addition of a preparation of EIF-1 along with the other components leads to formation of a considerable number of 80S monomers. We (Wettenhall and Wool, unpublished observations) have now tested the ability of normal and diabetic ribosomal subunits to participate in the reassociation reaction catalysed by the initiation factor preparation. Diabetic ribosomes are

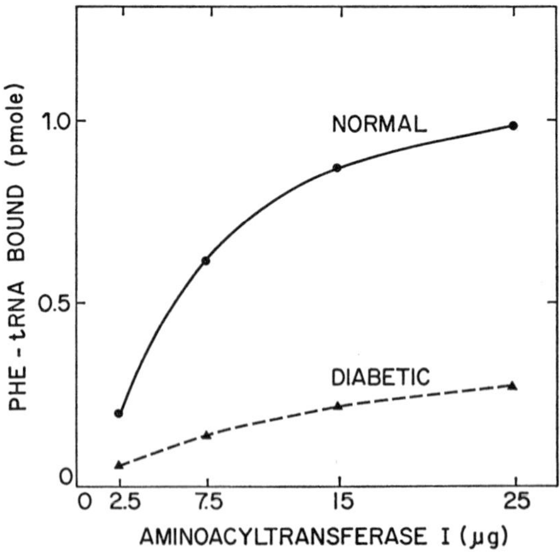

Fig. 12. Effect of EF-1 concentration on binding of ^{3}H-Phe-tRNA to normal and diabetic muscle ribosomes. The magnesium concentration was 7.5 mM. (From Leader *et al.*, 1971)

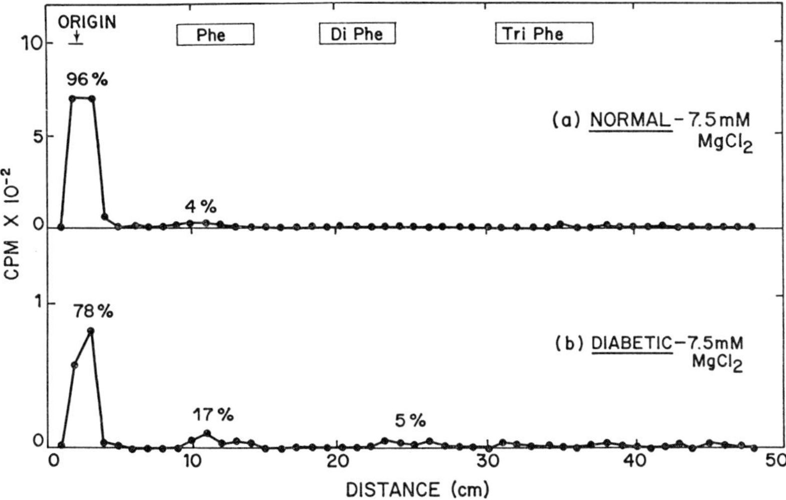

Fig. 13. The product formed as the result of binding of ^{14}C-Phe-tRNA in 7.5 mM $MgCl_2$ to normal and diabetic muscle ribosomes. Ribosomes were incubated with ^{14}C-Phe-tRNA in 7.5 mM $MgCl_2$ in the reaction mixture for the assay of binding. The bound radioactive material was isolated, hydrolyzed, and chromatographed. Locations of phenylalanine, diphenylalanine, and triphenylalanine standards are indicated on the chromatogram. (From LEADER *et al.*, 1971)

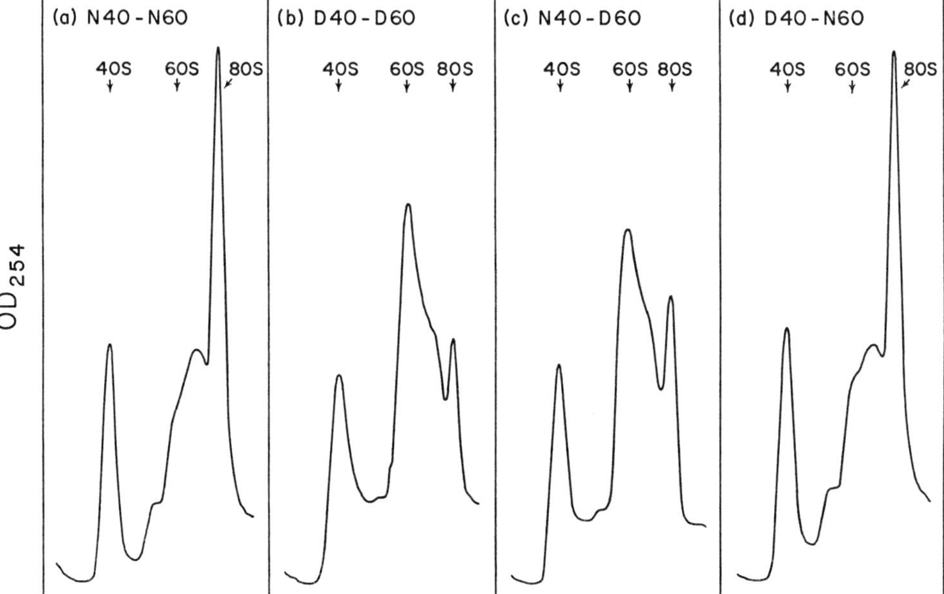

Fig. 14. Reassociation of normal and diabetic ribosomal subunits. The assay was carried out as described by WETTENHALL *et al.* (1971). N40, 40S ribosomal subunits from skeletal muscle of normal rats; N60, 60S ribosomal subunits from skeletal muscle of normal rats; D40, 40S ribosomal subunits from skeletal muscle of alloxan-diabetic rats; D60, 60S ribosomal subunits from skeletal muscle of alloxan-diabetic rats. (From WOOL, 1972)

less effective than normal in the reassociation reaction, and what is more, the defect is carried by the 60S subunit (Fig. 14). We find the observation exciting, but once again understand that caution is the prudent attitude.

IV. Insulin, Diabetes, and the Structure of Ribosomes

Normal and diabetic ribosomes differ in their ability to synthesize protein. However, we have not discovered the structural change in the particles responsible for the functional alteration.

The exact part played by ribosomes in protein synthesis remains to be discovered. There is an increasing suspicion that a great deal of the regulation of protein synthesis occurs on the ribosome. Ribosomes interact with messenger RNA, AA-tRNA, a specific chain-initiating tRNA (Met-tRNA$_f$), GTP, and a number of protein initiation, elongation, and termination factors. The initiation of protein synthesis, the polymerization of amino acids (catalyzed by ribosomal peptidyl transferase), movement of the ribosomes along messenger RNA, the hydrolysis of GTP, and the termination of the process all occur in an orderly and specific manner. The coordination of so complex a series of biochemical reactions may account for the large number of proteins contained in the ribosome. Progress in understanding the mechanism and means of regulation of protein synthesis would seem to be dependent on knowledge of the chemical structure and the biological function of ribosomal proteins.

1. No Difference Has Been Found in the Proteins of Normal and Diabetic Ribosomes

It seems likely from analysis of ribosomal protein by electrophoresis on discontinuous polyacrylamide gels (Low *et al.*, 1969; Gould, 1970; Sherton and Wool, 1972) and from chromatography on carboxymethylcellulose (Kanai *et al.*, 1969) that each eukaryotic ribosomal subunit has a unique set of proteins.

We have compared, by electrophoresis on one-dimensional discontinuous polyacrylamide gels, the proteins of the two subunits of normal and diabetic ribosomes (Low *et al.*, 1969). Sad to say we did not find a difference. However, there are severe limitations to the precision with which one can determine the exact quantities of individual proteins in each band of a one-dimensional polyacrylamide gel, and we may have missed a subtle change. The study should be repeated taking advantage of the far greater resolving power of two-dimensional gel electrophoresis (Sherton and Wool, 1972). In addition the analyses were done in 6 M urea, so that if the insulin-induced change was in the conformation of a protein it would have escaped our notice.

2. No Difference Has Been Found in the RNA of Normal and Diabetic Ribosomes, although Diabetes Does Decrease the Number of Ribosomes to Be Found in Muscle

Diabetes does not alter the relative proportions of 28 and 18S ribosomal RNA in muscle, nor the sedimentation coefficients, nor the base composition of the ribosomal RNA (Wool *et al.*, 1968b). However, in muscle of diabetic animals, the total amount of RNA and the ratio of RNA to DNA were reduced. Since the amount of RNA in muscle cells was decreased, and since there was no disproportionate reduction in the amount of transfer RNA, diabetes must have led to a decrease in the number of ribosomes. The decrease was, in part at least, due to a slowing of the rate of synthesis of ribosomal RNA.

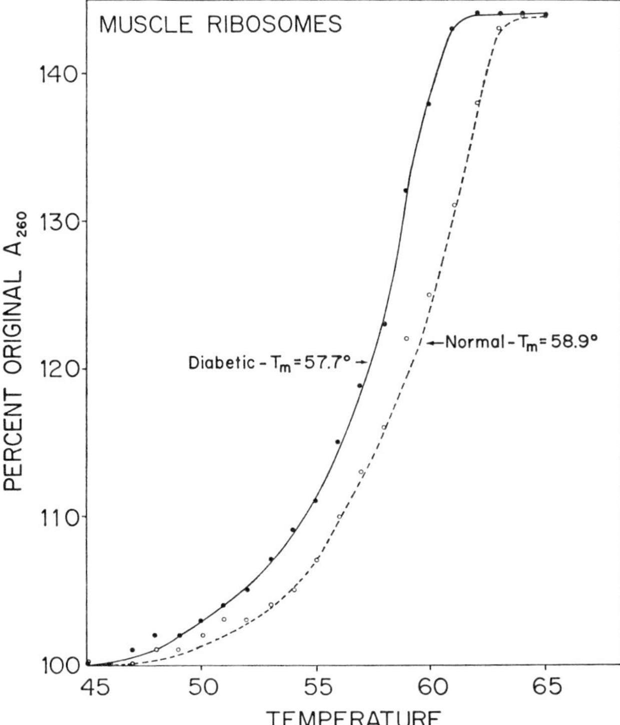

Fig. 15. Thermal denaturation of normal and diabetic muscle ribosomes. (From Wool *et al.*, 1972)

3. Diabetes Decreases the Melting Temperature of Ribosomes

Having failed to discover a change in the chemistry of the ribosomal RNA or protein, we have considered the possibility that the change is more subtle — perhaps, in the conformation of a ribosomal protein or in the internal order of the particle. The problem was to find a method to probe the fine structure of the ribosome. We chose to study the thermal denaturation of normal and diabetic ribosomes. The melting curve — the increase in chromicity with increase in temperature — of ribosomes differs substantially from that of ribosomal RNA; for example, the melting of ribosomes is over a narrower range of temperature (Tal, 1969). The difference in the thermal denaturation of ribosomes and of ribosomal RNA is believed to reflect the contribution of the proteins to the structure and order of the particle. We have found a difference in the melting temperature of normal and diabetic ribosomes (Wool and Fox, unpublished data). Diabetic ribosomes melt at a slightly lower temperature than normal ribosomes — indicating, perhaps, a loosening of ribosomal structure (Fig. 15). The difference is small, a little more than 1°, but is consistent and statistically significant when a large number of preparations are compared (Table 5). There is also a difference in the melting of normal and diabetic 40S subunits and normal and diabetic 60S subunits. There is, on the other hand, no difference in the melting of normal and diabetic 28 and 18S ribosomal RNA (Wool and Fox, unpublished observations). We do not know the exact meaning of the difference in the melting of normal and

Table 5. *Thermal Denaturation of Normal and Diabetic Ribosomes*

Ribosome Particle	T_m, degrees centigrade		Significance of the Difference, P
	Normal	Diabetic	
80S	58.3 ± 0.17 (45)	57.2 ± 0.19 (43)	< 0.001
60S	57.7 ± 0.34 (42)	56.3 ± 0.42 (42)	< 0.001
40S	53.0 ± 0.18 (35)	52.5 ± 0.20 (32)	< 0.02

The results are the mean ± the SEM of the number of observations (in parenthesis). (From Wool *et al.*, 1972)

diabetic ribosomes but think the results accord with the idea that diabetes leads to a change in the structure of the ribosome, which change may cause a decrease in the ability to initiate protein synthesis.

4. The Pleotypic Program and the Intracellular Mediator of Insulin Action

Tomkins and his associates (Hershko *et al.*, 1971; Mamont *et al.*, 1972; Kram *et al.*, 1973; Kram and Tomkins, 1973; see also Chapter C and G in Effects of insulin and proinsulin) have drawn attention to a set of biochemical reactions which respond coordinately when the environment in which mammalian cells are growing is altered. The processes affected include the transport into the cells of sugars (glucose and 2-deoxyglucose), amino acids and nucleotides; the synthesis of RNA and protein; and the degradation of protein. Because of the multiplicity and diversity of the reactions involved they refer to the response as the "pleotypic program" and distinguish between a positive (increase in substrate transport and macromolecular synthesis, and a decrease in protein degradation) and a negative pleotypic response.

The negative pleotypic response closely resembles stringent control in bacteria. In prokaryotes a decrease in the availability of required amino acids causes a decrease in the synthesis of RNA and protein, a decrease in polysome formation, protein degradation, and an inhibition of the uptake of glucose and nucleic acid precursors. That such closely analogous reactions occur in bacterial and animal cells suggests that the pleotypic response may be a universal biological phenomenon. But for our purposes it is perhaps most significant that the response of cells to insulin is congruent with the positive pleotypic reaction. In cultured hapatoma cells insulin will stimulate the synthesis of protein and induce the enzyme tyrosine aminotransferase (Gelehrter and Tomkins, 1969; Gelehrter and Tomkins, 1970), as well as the other reactions of the pleotypic program (Hershko *et al.*, 1971). Moreover, insulin can replace serum in support of the growth of chick fibroblasts (Schwartz and Amos, 1968). Hence insulin can be considered a pleotypic activator. What that suggests is that the intracellular mediator of the pleotypic response may also serve as the mediator of the action of insulin on macromolecule synthesis. Some of the reactions under pleotypic control (substrate transport, for example), like some of the biological effects of insulin, might result from an interaction of the activator with the cell membrane; but other of the responses, such as macromolecule synthesis, require that a "deputy" be formed as a consequence of the interaction of the activator with the cell membrane; the deputy is assumed to coordinate the intracellular reactions of the pleotypic response.

A critical problem is the identity of the intracellular mediator. In trying to understand the molecular basis of the pleotypic response, Tomkins and his colleagues (Mamont *et al.*, 1972) were attracted by the resemblance of the reaction in mammalian cells to the stringent response to amino acid starvation in bacteria. In that organism a novel nucleotide guanosine tetraphosphate (ppGpp) accumulates, and there is a great deal of evidence that the nucleotide mediates the stringent response (CASHEL, 1969; CASHEL and KALBACHER, 1970). Accordingly, a search was carried out for ppGpp in mammalian cells deprived of serum — serum deprival or "step-down" causes a negative pleotypic response in cultured cells. Predictions to the contrary they were unable to detect ppGpp (MAMONT *et al.*, 1972).

The burden of a large number of reports is that cyclic AMP participates in the regulation of the morphology and growth of cultured cells and that the nucleotide might be responsible for contact inhibition (BÜRK, 1971; JOHNSON *et al.*, 1971; HSIE *et al.*, 1971; OTTEN *et al.*, 1971). Those observations led to a test of whether cyclic AMP might not mediate the negative pleotypic response (KRAM *et al.*, 1973). In conformity with the prediction it was found that raising the intracellular concentration of cyclic AMP in fibroblasts in culture (by serum starvation, by treating them with prostaglandin E_1, or by adding dibutyryl cyclic AMP) caused a negative pleotypic effect: inhibition of the transport of sugars, amino acids, and nucleotides; slowing of the synthesis of RNA and protein; and stimulation of protein degradation. In parallel studies cyclic GMP was shown to counteract the negative pleotypic effects of cyclic AMP (KRAM and TOMKINS, 1973). Thus the expression of the pleotypic program may be conditioned by the relative concentrations of cyclic AMP ("negative mediator") and cyclic GMP ("positive mediator").

What significance do these results have for the mechanism of insulin action, especially for the mechanism by which the hormone controls protein synthesis? If the pleotypic response in cultured mammalian cells and the biological effects of insulin in animals have a common basis we would suppose the hormone acts either to decrease the intracellular concentration of cyclic AMP, raise the concentration of cyclic GMP, or both. There is, however, a grate deal of evidence that a decrease in intracellular cyclic AMP is not an essential element in insulin action (RODBELL, 1967; CRAIG *et al.*, 1969; PARK *et al.*, 1972). It is true that if the cyclic AMP level is initially high (as it is in the liver of diabetic animals, or in adipose tissue after epinephrine administration), then insulin will lower it at the same time that it exerts its biological actions. But in rat diaphragm muscle from normal donors the concentration of cyclic AMP is ordinarily very low and unaffected by addition of insulin (CRAIG *et al.*, 1969), although the hormone does of course increase substrate transport, protein and nucleic acid synthesis and decrease protein degradation. There are other instances where the effects of insulin are clearly divorced from, and independent of, alterations in cyclic AMP concentration (PARK *et al.*, 1972). Thus at least one aspect of the analogy breaks down: it is unlikely that the intracellular effects of insulin are due to a decrease in cyclic AMP. On the other hand it is possible that cyclic GMP is the intracellular deputy for insulin: that a result of the interaction of insulin with a receptor in the membrane is to generate cyclic GMP, that cyclic GMP in turn stimulates the synthesis of nucleic acids and protein as well as the synthesis of glycogen and lipid. That possibility remains to be tested. It is important to bear in mind that at the moment all that has been demonstrated is that cyclic GMP added to cultured fibroblasts will overcome the negative pleotypic effect of serum starvation, of prostaglandin E_1 and of dibutyryl cyclic AMP. It remains to be established that the intracellular concentration of cyclic GMP is actually elevated by addition of serum to cells (positive pleotypic effect), and even more important, that insulin increases the concentration of the nucleotide in muscle. The prospects are, nonetheless, most exciting.

V. Coda

There are two fundamental ways to increase synthesis of protein: by initiating the transcription of additional or new messenger RNA, or by accelerating the translation of stable messenger RNA. With regard to insulin action, it is most unlikely that it is on transcription so we may concentrate our attention on translation. Common wisdom has it that regulation of the translation of messenger RNA is most likely to be achieved by conditioning the availability or activity of initiation factors. We accept that likelihood. We propose an additional mechanism: its essence is a malleable or dynamic ribosome, a particle whose structure and hence function can be changed so as to moderate protein synthesis. One can imagine a number of ways in which the structure and function of ribosomes might be altered: by addition or deletion of proteins that are not essential for function but amplify ribosome activity (Kurland, 1970); by chemical modification of ribosomal proteins [as for example, by phosphorylation (Kabat, 1970) or acetylation]; by a change in the conformation of a ribosomal protein, or in the structure or order of the ribosome itself. Specifically we suggest that insulin and diabetes alter the structure of the ribosome in a way that changes the ability of the particle to initiate protein synthesis. The exact nature of the putative change in the particle and how it is effected by insulin are unsolved problems.

References

Adamson, L.F., Langeluttig, S.G., Anast, C.S.: Inhibition by puromycin of amino acid transport by embryonic chick bone. Biochim. biophys. Acta (Amst.) **115**, 355—360 (1966)

Brostrom, C.O., Jeffay, H.: Protein catabolism in rat liver homogenates. A re-evaluation of the energy requirement for protein catabolism. J. biol. Chem. **245**, 4001—4008 (1970)

Bürk, R.R.: Reduced adenyl cyclase activity in a polyoma virus transformed cell line. Nature (Lond.) **219**, 1272—1275 (1968)

Cashel, M.: The control of ribonucleic acid synthesis in *Escherichia coli*. IV. Relevance of unusual phosphorylated compounds from amino acid-starved stringent strains. J. biol. Chem. **244**, 3133—3141 (1969)

Cashel, M., Kalbacher, B.: The control of ribonucleic acid synthesis in *Escherichia coli*. V. Characterization of a nucleotide associated with the stringent response. J. biol. Chem. **245**, 2309—2318 (1970)

Castles, J.J., Rolleston, F.S., Wool, I.G.: Polyphenylalanine synthesis and binding of phenylalanyl-transfer ribonucleic acid by ribosomes from muscle of normal and diabetic rats. J. biol. Chem. **246**, 1799—1805 (1971)

Castles, J.J., Wool, I.G.: Effect of puromycin and insulin on amino acid accumulation by isolated intact rat diaphragm. Biochem. J. **91**, 11—12c (1964)

Castles, J.J., Wool, I.G.: Polyuridylic acid directed binding of phenylalanyl-transfer ribonucleic acid to mammalian 40S ribrosomal subunits. Biochemisty **9**, 1909—1916 (1970)

Craig, J.W., Rall, T.W., Larner, J.: The influence of insulin and epinephrine on adenosine 3′,5′-phosphate and glycogen transferase in muscle. Biochim. biophys. Acta (Amst.) **177**, 213—219 (1969)

Cuatracasas, P.: Interaction of insulin with the cell membrane: the primary action of insulin. Proc. nat. Acad. Sci. (Wash.) **63**, 450—457 (1969)

Davey, P., Manchester, K.L.: Isolation of labeled aminoacyl transfer RNA from muscle. Studies of the entry of labeled amino acids into acyl transfer RNA linkage *in situ* and its control by insulin. Biochim. biophys. Acta (Amst.) **182**, 85—97 (1969)

Elsas, L.J., Albrecht, I., Koehne, W., Rosenberg, L.E.: Effect of puromycin on insulin-stimulated amino-acid transport in muscle. Nature (Lond.) **214**, 916—917 (1967)

Elsas, L.J., Rosenberg, L.E.: Inhibition of amino acid transport in rat kidney cortex by puromycin. Proc. nat. Acad. Sci. (Wash.) **57**, 371—378 (1967)

Fox, C.F., Kennedy, E.P.: Specific labeling and partial purification of the M protein, a component of the β-galactoside transport system of *Escherichia coli*. Proc. nat. Acad. Sci. (Wash.) **54**, 891—899 (1965)

Fritz, C.R., Knobil, E.: *In vitro* stimulation by insulin of α-aminoisobutyric acid transport in the absence of protein synthesis. Nature (Lond.) **200**, 682 (1963)

GELEHRTER, T.D., TOMKINS, G.M.: Control of tyrosine aminotransferase synthesis in tissue culture by a factor in serum. Proc. nat. Acad. Sci. (Wash.) **64**, 723—730 (1969)

GELEHRTER, T.D., TOMKINS, G.M.: Posttranscriptional control of tyrosine aminotransferase synthesis by insulin. Proc. nat. Acad. Sci. (Wash.) **66**, 390—397 (1970)

GERMANYUK, Y.L., MIRONENKO, V.I.: Insulin and the attachment of amino-acids to the liver transfer RNAs. Nature (Lond.) **222**, 486—487 (1969)

GOULD, H.J.: Proteins of rabbit reticulocyte ribosomal subunits. Nature (Lond.) **227**, 1145—1147 (1970)

GUIDOTTI, G.G., RAGNOTTI, G., ROSSI, C.B.: Compartmentation of intracellular amino acid pool for protein synthesis in rat liver. Ital. J. Biochem. **13**, 145—156 (1964)

HENDLER, R.W.: Further characterization of an amino acid-lipid complex from hen oviduct. Biochim. biophys. Acta (Amst.) **60**, 90—97 (1962a)

HENDLER, R.W.: A model for protein synthesis. Nature (Lond.) **193**, 821—823 (1962b)

HEPPEL, L.A.: Selective release of enzymes from bacteria. Science **156**, 1451—1455 (1967)

HERSHKO, A., MAMONT, P., SHIELDS, R., TOMKINS, G.M.: Pleotypic response. Nature (Lond.) **232**, 206—211 (1971)

HIDER, R.C., FERN, E.B., LONDON, D.R.: Relationship between intracellular amino acids and protein synthesis in the extensor digitorum longus muscle of rats. Biochem. J. **114**, 171—178 (1969)

HIDER, R.C., FERN, E.B., LONDON, D.R.: Identification in skeletal muscle of a distinct extracellular pool of amino acids, and its role in protein synthesis. Biochem. J. **121**, 817—827 (1971a)

HIDER, R.C., FERN, E.B., LONDON, D.R.: The effect of insulin on free amino acid pools and protein synthesis in rat skeletal muscle *in vitro*. Biochem. J. **125**, 751—756 (1971b)

HIDER, R.C., MEADE, L.: The conversion of [1-^{14}C] pyruvate into [^{14}C] alanine in rat skeletal muscle: Its relevance to the effect of insulin on protein synthesis. Biochem. J. **128**, 165—167 (1972)

HSIE, A.W., JONES, C., PUCK, T.T.: Further changes in differentiation state accompanying the conversion of Chinese hamster cells to fibroblastic form by dibutyryl adenosine cyclic 3′:5′-monophosphate and hormones. Proc. nat. Acad. Sci. (Wash.) **68**, 1648—1652 (1971)

JOHNSON, G.S., FRIEDMAN, R.M., PASTAN, I.: Restoration of several morphological characteristics of normal fibroblasts in sarcoma cells treated with adenosine-3′:5′-cyclic monophosphate and its derivatives. Proc. nat. Acad. Sci. (Wash.) **68**, 425—429 (1971)

KABAT, D.: Phosphorylation of ribosomal proteins in rabbit reticulocytes. Characterization and regulatory aspects. Biochemistry **9**, 4160—4175 (1970)

KANAI, K., CASTLES, J.J., WOOL, I.G., STIREWALT, W.S., KANAI, A.: The proteins of liver and muscle ribosomal subunits: partial separation by carboxymethyl-cellulose column chromatography. FEBS Letters **5**, 68—72 (1969)

KIPNIS, D.M., NOALL, M.W.: Stimulation of amino acid transport by insulin in the isolated rat diaphragm. Biochim. biophys. Acta (Amst.) **28**, 226—227 (1958)

KIPNIS, D.M., PARRISH, J.E.: Role of Na^+ and K^+ on sugar (2-deoxyglucose) and amino acid (α-aminoisobutyric acid) transport in striated muscle. Fed. Proc. **24**, 1051—1059 (1965)

KIPNIS, D.M., REISS, E., HELMREICH, E.: Functional heterogeneity of the intracellular amino acid pool in mammalian cells. Biochim. biophys. Acta (Amst.) **51**, 519—524 (1961)

KOSTYO, J.L.: Separation of the effects of growth hormone on muscle amino acid transport and protein synthesis. Endocrinology **75**, 113—119 (1964)

KOSTYO, J.L., REDMOND, A.F.: Role of protein synthesis in the inhibitory action of adrenal steroid hormones on amino acid transport by muscle. Endocrinology **79**, 531—540 (1966)

KRAM, R., MAMONT, P., TOMKINS, G.M.: Pleotypic control by cyclic AMP: a model for growth control in animal cells. Proc. nat. Acad. Sci. (Wash.) **70**, 1432—1436 (1973)

KRAM, R., TOMKINS, G.M.: Pleotypic control by cyclic AMP. The interaction with cyclic GMP and the possible role of microtubules. Proc. nat. Acad. Sci. (Wash.) **70**, 1659—1663 (1973)

KURIHARA, K., WOOL, I.G.: Effect of insulin on the synthesis of sarcoplasmic and ribosomal proteins of muscle. Nature (Lond.) **219**, 721—724 (1968)

KURLAND, C.G.: Ribosome structure and function emergent. Science **169**, 1171—1177 (1970)

LEADER, D.P., KLEIN-BREMHAAR, H., WOOL, I.G., FOX, A.: Distribution of initiation factors in cell fractions from mammalian tissues. Biochem. biophys. Res. Commun. **46**, 215—224 (1972)

LEADER, D.P., WOOL, I.G.: Partial purification and characterization of an initiation factor from rat liver which promotes the binding of phenylalanyl-tRNA to 40S ribosomal subunits. Biochim. biophys. Acta (Amst.) **262**, 360—370 (1972)

LEADER, D.P., WOOL, I.G., CASTLES, J.J.: A factor for the binding of aminoacyl transfer RNA to mammalian 40S ribosomal subunits. Proc. nat. Acad. Sci. (Wash.) **67**, 523—528 (1970)

Leader, D.P., Wool, I.G., Castles, J.J.: Aminoacyltransferase I-catalyzed binding of phenylalanine-transfer ribonucleic acid to muscle ribosomes from normal and diabetic rats. Biochem. J. **124**, 537—541 (1971)

Leader, D.P., Wool, I.G., Leader, J.E.: Aminoacyltransferase II catalyzed hydrolysis of GTP by muscle ribosomes from normal and daibetic rats. Acta diabet. lat. **7**, 990—1003 (1970)

Levine, R., Goldstein, M.: On the mechanism of action of insulin. Recent Progr. Hormone Res. **11**, 343—375 (1955)

Lotspeich, W.D.: The role of insulin in the metabolism of amino acids. J. biol. Chem. **179**, 175—180 (1949)

Low, R.B., Wool, I.G., Martin, T.E.: Skeletal muscle ribosomal proteins: General characteristics and effect of diabetes. Biochim. biophys. Acta (Amst.) **194**, 190—202 (1969)

Luck, J.M., Morrison, G., Wilbur, L.F.: The effect of insulin on the amino acid content of blood. J. biol. Chem. **77**, 151—156 (1928)

Maden, B.E.H., Traut, R.R., Monro, R.E.: Ribosome-catalyzed peptidyl transfer: the polyphenylalanine system. J. molec. Biol. **35**, 333—345 (1968)

Mamont, P., Hershko, A., Kram, R., Schacter, L., Lust, J., Tomkins, G.M.: The pleotypic response in mammalia cells: search for an intracellular mediator. Biochem. biophys. Res. Commun. **48**, 1378—1384 (1972)

Manchester, K.L., Krahl, M.E.: Effect of insulin on the incorporation of C^{14} from C^{14}-labeled carboxylic acids and bicarbonate into the protein of isolated rat diaphragm. J. biol. Chem. **234**, 2938—2942 (1959)

Manchester, K.L., Wool, I.G.: Insulin and incorporation of amino acids into protein of muscle. II. Accumulation and incorporation studies with perfused rat heart. Biochem. J. **89**, 202—209 (1963)

Manchester, K.L., Young, F.G.: Location of ^{14}C in protein from isolated rat diaphragm incubated *in vitro* with [^{14}C] amino acids and with $^{14}CO_2$. Biochem. J. **72**, 136—141 (1959)

Martin, T.E., Rolleston, F.S., Low, R.B., Wool, I.G.: Dissociation and reassociation of skeletal muscle ribosomal. J. molec. Biol. **43**, 135—149 (1969)

Martin, T.E., Wool, I.G.: Formation of active hybrids from subunits of muscle ribosomes from normal and diabetic rats. Proc. nat. Acad. Sci. (Wash.) **60**, 569—574 (1968)

Mathews, M.B.: Tissue-specific factor required for the translation of a mammalian viral RNA. Nature (Lond.) **228**, 661—663 (1970)

Mathews, M.B., Korner, A.: Mammalian cell-free protein synthesis directed by viral ribonucleic acid. Europ. J. Biochem. **17**, 328—338 (1970)

Monro, R.E.: Catalysis of peptide bond formation by 50S ribosomal subunits from *E. Coli*. J. molec. Biol. **26**, 147—151 (1967)

Monro, R.E., Staehelin, T., Celma, M.L., Vazquez, D.: The peptidyl transferase activity of ribosomes. Cold Spr. Harb. Symp. quant. Biol. **34**, 357—368 (1969)

Morgan, H.E., Earl, D.C.N., Broadus, A., Wolpert, E.B., Geiger, K.E., Jefferson, L.S.: Regulation of protein synthesis in heart muscle. I. Effect of amino acid levels on protein synthesis. J. biol. Chem. **246**, 2152—2162 (1971a)

Morgan, H.E., Jefferson, L.S., Wolpert, E.B., Rannels, D.E.: Regulation of protein synthesis in heart muscle. II. Effect of amino acid levels on ribosomal aggregation. J. biol. Chem. **246**, 2163—2170 (1971b)

Mortimer, G.E., Mondon, C.E.: Inhibition by insulin of valine turnover in liver. Evidence for a general control of proteolysis. J. biol. Chem. **245**, 2375—2383 (1970)

Neth, R., Monro, R.E., Heller, G., Battaner, E., Vazques, D.: Catalysis of peptidyl transfer by human tonsil ribosomes and effects of some antibiotics. FEBS Letters **6**, 198—202 (1970)

Otten, J., Johnson, G.S., Pastan, I.: Cyclic AMP levels in fibroplats: relationship to growth rate and contact inhibition of growth. Biochem. biophys. Res. Commun. **44**, 1192—1198 (1971)

Park, C.R., Lewis, S.B., Exton, J.H.: Relationship of some hepatic actions of insulin to the intracellular level of cyclic adenylate. In: Insulin Action, p. 509—527 (ed. I. Fritz). New York: Academic Press 1972

Rannels, D.E., Jefferson, L.S., Hjalmarson, Å.C., Wolpert, E.B., Morgan, H.E.: Maintenance of protein synthesis in hearts of diabetic animals. Biochem. biophys. Res. Commun. **40**, 1110—1116 (1970)

Rodbell, M.: Metabolism of isolated fat cells. VI. The effects of insulin, lipolytic hormones, and theophylline on glucose transport and metabolism in "ghosts." J. biol. Chem. **242**, 5751—5756 (1967)

Rolleston, F.S., Wool, I.G., Martin, T.E.: Binding and translation of turnip-yellow-mosaic-virus ribonucleic acid by skeletal-muscle ribosomes from normal and diabetic rats. Biochem. J. **117**, 899—905 (1970)

ROSENBERG, L.E., BERMAN, M., SEGAL, S.: Studies of the kinetics of amino acid transport, incorporation into protein and oxidation in kidney-cortex slices. Biochim. biophys. Acta (Amst.) **71**, 664—675 (1963)

RUSSELL, J.A.: Hormonal control of amino-acid metabolism. Fed. Proc. **14**, 696—705 (1955)

SALAS, M., VIÑUELA, E., SOLS, A.: Insulin-dependent synthesis of liver glucokinase in the rat. J. biol. Chem. **238**, 3535—3538 (1963)

SCHARFF, R., WOOL, I.G.: Concentration of amino acids in rat muscle and plasma. Nature (Lond.) **202**, 603—604 (1964)

SCHARFF, R., WOOL, I.G.: Accumulation of amino acids in muscle of perfused rat heart: effect of insulin. Biochem. J. **97**, 257—271 (1965a)

SCHARFF, R., WOOL, I.G.: Accumulation of amino acids in muscle of perfused heart: effect of insulin in the presence of puromycin. Biochem. J. **97**, 272—276 (1965b)

SCHIMKE, R.T.: Adaptive characteristics of urea cycle enzymes in the rat. J. biol. Chem. **237**, 459—468 (1962)

SCHIMKE, R.T.: Studies on the roles of synthesis and degradation in the control of enzyme levels in animal tissues. Bull. Soc. Chim. biol. (Paris) **48**, 1009—1030 (1966)

SCHWARTZ, A.G., AMOS, H.: Insulin dependence of cells in primary culture: influence on ribosome integrity. Nature (Lond.) **219**, 1366—1367 (1968)

SHAFRITZ, D.A., ANDERSON, W.F.: Isolation and partial characterization of reticulocyte factors M_1 and M_2. J. biol. Chem. **245**, 5553—5559 (1970)

SHERTON, C.C., WOOL, I.G.: Determination of the number of proteins in liver ribosomes and ribosomal subunits by two-dimensional polyacrylamide gel electrophoresis. J. biol. Chem. **247**, 4460—4467 (1972)

STEINER, D.F.: Insulin and the regulation of hepatic biosynthetic activity. Vitam. and Horm. **24**, 1—61 (1966)

STIREWALT, W.S., CASTLES, J.J., WOOL, I.G.: Skeletal muscle ribosome subunits and petidyl-transfer ribonucleic acid. Biochemistry **10**, 1594—1598 (1971)

STIREWALT, W.S., WOOL, I.G.: Peptidyl-tRNA and peptidyl transferase activity of skeletal muscle ribosomes. Effect of diabetes. FEBS Letters **10**, 38—40 (1970)

STIREWALT, W.S., WOOL, I.G., CAVICCHI, P.: The relation of RNA and protein synthesis to the sedimentation of muscle ribosomes: effect of diabetes and insulin. Proc. nat. Acad. Sci. (Wash.) **57**, 1885—1892 (1967)

TAL, M.: Thermal denaturation of ribosomes. Biochemistry **8**, 424—435 (1969)

VAZQUEZ, D., BATTANER, E., NETH, R., HELLER, G., MONRO, R.E.: The function of 80S ribosomal subunits and effects of some antibiotics. Cold Spr. Harb. Symp. quant. Biol. **34**, 369—375 (1969)

WETTENHALL, R.E.H., LEADER, D.P., WOOL, I.G.: Initiation factor promoted reassociation of eukaryotic ribosomal subunits. Biochem. biophys. Res. Commun. **43**, 994—1000 (1971)

WOOL, I.G.: Effect of insulin on accumulation of radioactivity from amino acids by isolated intact rat diaphragm. Nature (Lond.) **202**, 196—197 (1964)

WOOL, I.G.: Insulin and protein biosynthesis. In: Action of Hormones on Molecular Processes p. 422—469. (ed G. LITWACK and D. KRITCHEVSKY). New York: Wiley 1964

WOOL, I.G.: Insulin and the regulation of protein synthesis in muscle. Proc. Nutr. Soc. **31**, 185—191 (1972)

WOOL, I.G.: Relation of effects of insulin on amino acid transport and on protein synthesis. Fed. Proc. **24**, 1060—1070 (1965)

WOOL, I.G.: Insulin and amino acid transport in muscle. In: Protein and Polypeptide Hormones, p. 285—295 (ed. M. MARGOULIES). Amsterdam: Excerpta Medica Foundation 1968

WOOL, I.G., CASTLES, J.J., LEADER, D.P., FOX, A.: Insulin and the function of muscle ribosomes. In: Handbook of Physiology, (ed. R. O. GREEP and F. B. ASTWOOD). Section 7: Endocrinology, Volume I, Endocrine Pancreas, (ed. D. F. STEINER and N. FREINKEL), p. 385—394. Washington: American Physiological Society

WOOL, I.G., CASTLES, J.J., MOYER, A.N.: Regulation of amino acid accumulation in isolated rat diaphragm: effect of puromycin and insulin. Biochim. biophys. Acta (Amst.) **107**, 333—345 (1965)

WOOL, I.G., CAVICCHI, P.: Insulin regulation of protein synthesis by muscle ribosomes: effect of the hormone on translation of messenger RNA for a regulatory protein. Proc. nat. Acad. Sci. (Wash.) **56**, 991—998 (1966)

WOOL, I.G., CAVICCHI, P.: Protein synthesis by skeletal muscle ribosomes. Effect of diabetes and insulin. Biochemistry **6**, 1231—1242 (1967)

WOOL, I.G., KRAHL, M.E.: Incorporation of C^{14}-amino acids into protein of isolated diaphragms: an effect of insulin independent of glucose entry. Amer. J. Physiol. **196**, 961—964 (1959a)

WOOL, I.G., KRAHL, M.E.: An effect of insulin on peptide synthesis independent of glucose or amino acid transport. Nature (Lond.) **183**, 1399—1400 (1959b)

Wool, I. G., Krahl, M. E.: Effect of insulin *in vitro* on incorporation of [14C] from pyruvate into protein of isolated diaphragm in the presence of [12C] aspartic acid, and [12C] glutamic acid. Biochim. biophys. Acta (Amst.) **82**, 606—608 (1964)
Wool, I. G., Kurihara, K.: Determination of the number of active muscle ribosomes: effect of diabetes and insulin. Proc. nat. Acad. Sci. (Wash.) **58**, 2401—2407 (1967)
Wool, I. G., Scharff, R.: Effect of insulin and diabetes on amino acid transport in muscle. In: Protein Nutrition and Free Amino Acid Patterns, p. 157—186 (ed. J. H. Leathem). New Brunswick, N. J.: Rutgers Univ. Press 1968
Wool, I. G., Stirewalt, W. S., Kurihara, K., Low, R. B., Bailey, P., Oyer, D.: Mode of action of insulin in the regultion of protein biosynthesis in muscle. Recent Progr. Hormone Res. **24**, 139—208 (1968a)
Wool, I. G., Stirewalt, W. S., Moyer, A. N.: Effect of diabetes and insulin on nucleic acid metabolism of heart muscle. Amer. J. Physiol. **214**, 825—831 (1968b)

C. Effects of Insulin on Nucleic Acids, Nucleotides and Cyclic AMP

PIERRE VOLFIN and JACQUES HANOUNE

With 8 Figures

I. Introduction

It is generally agreed that hormones can be divided into two categories, according to their mechanism of action. The hormones of the first category may be called "morphogenic hormones" since their action is characterized by an extended lag period and a sensitivity to inhibitors of protein and RNA biosynthesis. In contrast, the hormones of the second category act instantaneously and are insensitive to inhibitors of protein and RNA biosynthesis.

Insulin belongs to the second category even though some of its effects are of the first type and entail modification of RNA biosynthesis. The main effects of insulin on liver and on peripheral tissues (muscle: diaphragm, heart; adipose tissue) are of the second type and are reproducible in *in vitro* systems, as was first demonstrated for glucose uptake on isolated rat diaphragm by GEMMIL in 1940 (1). The use of simple *in vitro* systems has led in recent years to a considerable amount of research on the mechanism of action of insulin on muscle and adipose tissues. This work can be divided into two series:

— On one hand, it has been demonstrated that insulin directly affects cell permeability. Extensive work on glucose transport into the cell under the influence of insulin as well as on the metabolic consequences of this transport has been carried out in the eviscerated animal (LEVINE and GOLDSTEIN, 1955), the isolated rat diaphragm (KIPNIS and CORI, 1957), the isolated perfused heart (MORGAN *et al.*, 1961) and the isolated fat pad (WINEGRAD and RENOLD, 1958; BALL *et al.*,

1959). Insulin stimulation seems to involve not only an enhanced transport rate, but also an increased intracellular distribution space as measured with non-metabolizable sugars (Kipnis and Cori, 1957) and amino acids (Kipnis and Noall, 1958; Manchester and Young, 1960).

— On the other hand, investigations of the direct effect of insulin on metabolic parameters under conditions in which permeability phenomena and pile-up of precursors are most probably not implicated have been carried out. These include work on protein biosynthesis (Manchester and Young, 1958) and on glycogen metabolism (Beloff-Chain *et al.*, 1959).

We shall consider in this chapter the effects of insulin on nucleic acids, nucleotides and cyclic AMP and shall try to relate them to the general mechanism of action of the hormone.

II. Preliminary Considerations

Difficulties have been encountered in explaining the effect of insulin purely in terms of the direct stimulation of transport of sugar because insulin-induced stimulation has been clearly observed in the absence of extracellular or intracellular glucose. Two possible hypotheses have been considered for the mechanism of action of insulin:

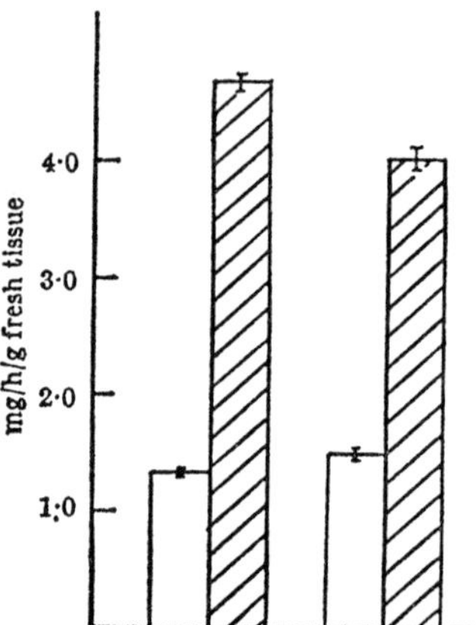

Fig. 1. Influence of puromycin on the uptake of glucose by the isolated diaphragm of the rat in absence (white) and presence (hatched) of insulin (10 μg/ml). Left, no puromycin (500 μg/ml). Standard error of the mean indicated at the top in each case. (From Eboué-Bonis *et al.*, 1963)

1. Insulin as an Inductor or Depressor

Evidence that insulin induces multiple metabolic modifications has led to the postulation of a unique mechanism for its primary action: if insulin induced the biosynthesis of a messenger RNA, the consequence would be an increase in the biosynthesis of enzymatic proteins, which themselves would be responsible for the modifications in carbohydrate and lipid metabolism as well as for changes in the permeability of cellular membranes. Changes in ^{32}P incorporation in free nucleotides would reflect these insulin-induced modifications.

In our laboratory, we made two sets of observations (Eboué-Bonis *et al.*, 1963) indicated in Tables 1, 2, 3, and Fig. 1.

a) Even when protein synthesis is inhibited by puromycin, insulin still enhances nucleotide turnover and glucose uptake.

b) Inhibition by actinomycin D of the biosynthesis of messenger RNA does not influence stimulation of protein biosynthesis, glucose uptake or nucleotide turnover by insulin.

These results, which ruled out the direct dependence of the metabolic effects of insulin on the stimulation of RNA or protein synthesis, were later confirmed by

Table 1. *Influence of actinomycin D on the insulin-induced stimulation of the biosynthesis of RNA and protein in the isolated rat diaphragm*

Actinomycin D (10 μg/ml)	0	0	+	+
Insulin (10 μg/ml)	0	+	0	+
A Biosynthesis of RNA from (8-^{14}C) adenine				
ATP (counts/μg)	201	212	207	280
RNA fraction (counts incorporated/100 mg tissue)	1.006	2.040	26	38
B Biosynthesis of proteins from (U-^{14}C) protein hydrolysate				
Extracellular amino-acid pool (counts/μg)	319	374	327	399
Intracellular amino-acid pool (counts/μg)	66	71	69	72
Proteins (counts/mg)	316	706	395	765

From Eboué-Bonis *et al.* (1963)

Table 2. *Influence of actinomycin D and puromycin on the insulin-induced stimulation of the labelling of phosphates in the isolated rat diaphragm*

Specific activity (percentage of extracellular or intracellular phosphorus)							
Actinomycin *D* (10 μg/ml)		0	0	+	+	0	0
Puromycin (500 μg/ml		0	0	0	0	+	+
Insulin (10 μg/ml)		0	+	0	+	0	+
Intracellular inorganic phosphorus	(*E*)	6.9	6.2	7.2	6.7	8.7	10.7
PC*	(*I*)	35.8	44.4	32.7	53.3	31.4	40.5
ATP	(*I*)	44.5	58.5	40.2	68.0	43.4	70.0
ADP	(*I*)	19.7	24.5	19.5	30.2	17.9	21.7
U+G†	(*I*)	24.4	37.9	26.2	51.5	16.7	32.5

(*E*) Percentage of extracellular inorganic phosphorus.
(*I*) Percentage of intracellular inorganic phosphorus.
* Phosphocreatine.
† Sum of uridine and guanosine phosphates.

From Eboué-Bonis *et al.* (1963)

Table 3. *Influence of puromycin on the insulin-induced stimulation of protein biosynthesis in isolated rat diaphragm*

A Precursor: U-^{14}C protein hydrolysate				
Puromycin (500 μg/ml)	0	0	+	+
Insulin (10 μg/ml)	0	+	0	+
Extracellular amino-acid pool (counts/μg)	940	740	545	518
Intracellular amino-acid pool (counts/μg)	115	120	152	131
Proteins (counts/mg)	750	1.371	24	11
B Precursor: D,L-1^{14}C Valine				
Incubation medium (counts/100 mg)	7.800	8.800	—	8.767
Intracellular medium (counts/100 mg)	6.300	5.745	—	6.352
Proteins (counts/mg)	166	213	—	1

From Eboué-Bonis *et al.* (1963)

four different laboratories: SØVIK and WALAAS (1964), WOOL and MOYER (1964), FRITZ and KNOBIL (1963) and MANCHESTER (1964). The stimulation of RNA synthesis by insulin, as will be discussed below, must be considered as an independent phenomenon.

2. Insulin as a Ligand Interacting with the Cell Membrane

One could also postulate that insulin interacts either with proteins or with lipoproteins of the cell membrane. Such interaction would lead to modifications of permeability phenomena and active transport and, as a consequence, to an increased turnover of phosphorylated intermediates.

An SH interchange between insulin and a membranous protein has been postulated as the primary hormone-receptor reaction. We tested this hypothesis with an SH reagent, N-ethyl maleimide (NEM), and, using the rat diaphragm *in vitro*, we observed:

a) Stimulation of the sugar transport system by insulin is totally suppressed by NEM, these results being in agreement with those of KAJI and PARK (1961) and of MIRSKY and PERISUTTI (1962)

b) In spite of this inhibition, stimulation by insulin of glycogen biosynthesis and increased incorporation of ^{32}P into free nucleotides (EBOUÉ-BONIS *et al.*, 1967) are always observed in the presence of NEM.

We concluded from these experiments that one or several SH groups located in the cell membrane are necessary for the stimulation of the sugar transport system by insulin. It is also possible that activation of the glucose transport system, glycogen synthetase and nucleotide turnover, respectively, are independent phenomena.

These examples of unrelated insulin-sensitive parameters do not signify that all the insulin sensitive metabolic events in a tissue are independent; rather, they indicate either the occurrence of multiple sites of insulin-receptor interactions, each one of them being specific, or a common transducer system for insulin action (CHAMBAUT *et al.*, 1969). We shall discuss later attempts which have been made to test the model for the action of insulin developed in recent years by SUTHERLAND and his associates (JEFFERSON *et al.*, 1968; SUTHERLAND and ROBINSON, 1969).

III. Action of Insulin on Nucleic Acids

Many research groups have demonstrated a rapid and selective effect by a hormone — and more specifically by insulin — on nucleic acid biosynthesis. The effect of insulin on nucleic acids is certainly the most controversial. We shall not try to resolve the controversy, but shall only report the conflicting results which have been obtained.

1. In Rat Diaphragm

Insulin seems to influence protein synthesis in muscle through an effect on some intracellular process, perhaps on the protein-synthesizing machinery itself. Nucleic acids play a predominant role in protein synthesis; soluble RNA is involved in the transport of activated amino-acid residues to the site of protein synthesis and at the site itself. Because the synthesis of new RNA seems obligatory for the activation of protein synthesis, WOOL (1960) investigated the effect of insulin on the incorporation of ^{14}C from various labelled precursors into the nucleic acid fraction of isolated rat diaphragm, having in mind the possibility that nucleic acid synthesis is the intracellular process on which insulin acts to stimulate protein biosynthesis.

Insulin *in vitro* enhances the incorporation of ^{14}C-labelled glucose, -adenine and -orotic acid into the nucleic acid fraction of isolated rat diaphragm. This effect can occur in the absence of added glucose and therefore is independent of the effect of the hormone on glucose transport. The incorporation of labelled thymine into diaphragm nucleic acids is minimal in comparison to the incorporation of adenine or orotic acid. Since thymine occurs in DNA but not in RNA, Wool concluded that insulin enhanced RNA biosynthesis but not DNA biosynthesis.

Assuming that a net synthesis of nucleic acids was effectively occurring, he investigated the effect of insulin both on the level of and on the specific activity of the nucleic acids present in muscle. Wool (1963) observed, in the presence of insulin, an increase in the amount of RNA extracted from insulin-stimulated muscle and — according to several experiments performed under various conditions — concluded that an increase both in the synthesis of messenger RNA and in the specific activity of ribosomal RNA was taking place (Wool and Munro, 1963). However, he gave up his claim that the primary effect of insulin was the synthesis of messenger RNA when, in agreement with our results (Eboué-Bonis *et al.*, 1963), he verified the effect of actinomycin D on his system (Wool and Moyer, 1964). One could also hypothesize that insulin produced an alteration at the ribosomal level. This action would lead to a modification in the translation of preformed messenger RNA (Wool *et al.*, 1966), or would make available some kind of initiation factor (Stirewald *et al.*, 1967).

Since the effects of insulin on protein synthesis in mammalian cells are independent of a rapid synthesis of RNA, an action of insulin on a pre-existing messenger RNA with slower turnover and greater stability has been considered. The conclusions concerning the rapid effect of insulin on RNA distribution patterns made several years ago by Kidson and Kirby (1964) have been contradicted by several authors (Jackson and Sells, 1968; Leader and Barry, 1967) as being due to artifacts in RNA preparations. Using heart muscle, Wool *et al.* (1968) showed that the RNA from diabetic animals did not differ qualitatively from that obtained from normal animals. The relative proportions of ribosomal (28 and 18 S) and transfer (4 S) RNA were not altered and the sedimentation values for the three varieties of RNA remained unchanged.

Based on these observations and the fact that insulin in muscle seems neither to alter the RNA pattern nor to stimulate the biosynthesis of a messenger RNA, can we reasonably affirm that in this tissue insulin really stimulates the rapid synthesis of another type of RNA ?

2. In Liver

An answer to this important question is unfortunately not to be found in data obtained from other tissues. For example in liver, insulin has been reported to increase (Steiner and King, 1966; Morgan and Bonner, 1970) as well as to decrease (Weber *et al.*, 1965) the over-all RNA synthesis.

3. Discussion

In our laboratory we confirmed, on isolated diaphragm, the rapidly increased incorporation of labelled precursors (^{14}C-adenine) in RNA under the influence of insulin (Eboué-Bonis *et al.*, 1963) and showed that this effect is not the reflection of an increased incorporation of ^{14}C adenine in ATP. However, we have been unable to show that insulin acts at the RNA level in the incubated diaphragm (Chambaut, 1969), which is contradictory to the findings of Wool (1963).

The interpretation of these results is challenged by Manchester (1967) who feels that, changes in the degree of extractability of nucleic acids can occur and may explain the effect of insulin observed on the incorporation of precursors. Further thorough experiments are needed. It is certain that insulin enhances protein synthesis very early, even in absence of newly synthetized RNA (experiments with actinomycin D), but it cannot be excluded that insulin may act at the translational level (Stirewalt *et al.*, 1967).

IV. Action of Insulin on the Incorporation of ^{32}P-Labelled Inorganic Phosphate into Mononucleotides in Rat Diaphragm and Adipose Tissue

Most metabolic changes in a tissue are likely to be reflected in modifications of the rates of phosphorylation and dephosphorylation of the nucleotide coenzymes. The first to be affected are the adenine nucleotides, the role of which in the activation of sugars, fatty acids and amino acids is well established. An increased catabolism of sugars should only be reflected in the accelerated turnover of the γ-phosphate of ATP which is the only one to be implicated in the phosphorylation of glucose and furthermore of fructose-6-phosphate. ATP is also involved in the activation of fatty acids and amino acids, but in this case the reaction which occurs is ATP→P—P+AMP. The rephosphorylation of the AMP formed during this reaction should equalize the specific radioactivities of the two labile phosphates of ATP. It is also possible to predict that an increased biosynthesis of glycogen would accelerate the turnover of the guanylic compounds. Consequently, it should be possible to detect very rapid metabolic changes induced by a hormone before any changes are detectable in other parameters such as glycogen or protein biosynthesis, glucose uptake or pile-up of non-metabolizable analogs.

For this reason, we thought that any primary metabolic changes taking place under the action of insulin would be reflected in the turnover of free mononucleotides and more specifically of adenosine nucleotides.

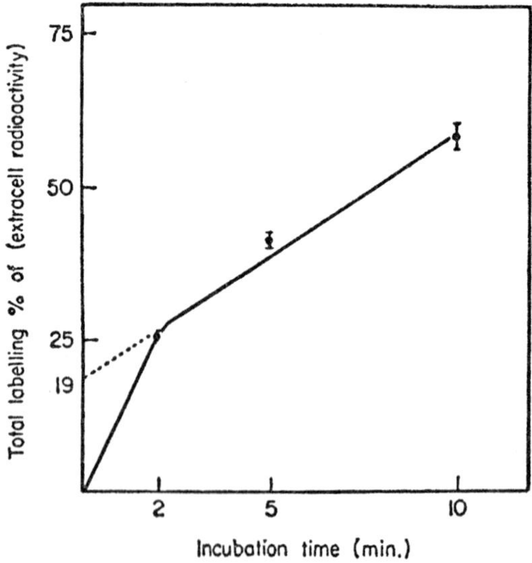

Fig. 2. Total labelling of rat diaphragm in percentage of the extracellular radioactive medium at different incubation times. The straight line has been plotted according to the method of least squares. By extrapolation to zero time an extracellular space of 19.0 ± 0.65% is calculated. (From Clauser *et al.*, 1962)

Table 4. *Influence of insulin on the labelling of phosphates n the isolated diaphragm of the normal rat in the absence of added substrate*

	µg P/100 mg fresh weight		Specific activity (% extracellular P)		Specific activity (% intracellular P)			Specific activity (% terminal P of ATP)		
					A. Incubation time: 10 min					
Insulin 10 µg/ml . . .	0	+	0	+	0	+	P[a]	0	+	P[a]
Number of experiments	4	4	3	3	3	3		4	4	
Intrac. I.P.	31.7 ± 3.3	33.3 ± 1.9	6.0 ± 1.0	5.0 ± 0.4	—	—	—	—	—	—
P.C.	16.1 ± 1.9	13.2 ± 2.9	2.63 ± 0.35	3.75 ± 0.73	43 ± 2.8	56 ± 6.8	0.001	104 ± 3.8	100 ± 3.6	—
ATP[b]	29.1 ± 2.8	28.5 ± 2.9	2.53 ± 0.34	3.03 ± 0.38	42 ± 4.8	56 ± 6.0		—	—	
ADP[c]	5.9 ± 0.6	6.1 ± 0.8	1.18 ± 0.12	1.80 ± 0.20	22 ± 1.7	37 ± 4.9	0.01	49 ± 7.9	51 ± 6.0	0.0
U + G[d]	2.6 ± 0.5	2.5 ± 0.5	1.94 ± 0.24	2.54 ± 0.36	30 ± 2.8	52 ± 1.4	0.05	77 ± 6.0	93 ± 12	—
"Residual" phosphorus	4.6 ± 1.0	4.8 ± 1.1	1.67 ± 0.22	2.10 ± 0.28	36 ± 5.7	45 ± 5.4	—	73 ± 5.5	63 ± 5.9	—
					B. Incubation time: 30 min					
Insulin 10 µg/lm . . .	0	+	0	+	0	+	P[a]	0	+	P[a]
Number of experiments	2	2	2	2	2	2		2	2	
Intrac. I.P.	35.8 ± 2.6	38.7 ± 0.1	19.6 ± 0.6	19.1 ± 4.5	—	—	—	—	—	—
P.C.	15 ± 1.5	14.4 ± 1	9.2 ± 1.2	12.0 ± 2.0	47 ± 4.5	64 ± 4.2	0.001	86 ± 10.8	86 ± 2.5	—
ATP[b]	27.8 ± 0.3	23.4 ± 0.4	11.1 ± 2.7	14.9 ± 2.0	56 ± 12.1	80 ± 8		—	—	—
ADP[c]	5.3 ± 0.0	5.3 ± 0.7	5.1 ± 1.6	9.8 ± 3.5	26 ± 7.3	50 ± 6	0.01	46 ± 7.3	64 ± 1.4	0.01
U + G[d]	2.1 ± 0.2	1.5 ± 0.1	9.9 ± 1.7	12.6	50 ± 7.5	—	—	91 ± 7	—	—
"Residual" phosphorus	4.8	4.6	—	—	—	—	—	—	—	—
Labile organic P (sum)	—	—	—	—	38 ± 5.3	58 ± 9.7	0.01			

[a] P refers to the sum of the experiments (10 min and 30 min incubation time). P values greater than 0.05 are not included.
[b] The specific activity refers to the terminal group of ATP.
[c] The specific activity refers to the terminal group of ADP.
[d] Sum of uridine and guanosine phosphates. The specific activity refers to the labile phosphate groups if only UTP and GTP were present.

From H. Clauser *et al.* (1962).

Table 5. *Influence of insulin on the labelling of phosphates in the isolated diaphragm of the normal rat in the presence of glucose (2 mg/ml)*

	µg P/100 mg fresh weight		Specifice activity (% extracellular P)		Specific activity (% intracellular P)			Specific activity (% terminal P of ATP)		
A. Incubation time: 10 min										
Insulin 10 µg/ml . . .	0	+	0	+	0	+	P[a]	0	+	P[a]
Number of experiments	3	3	2	2	2	2		3	3	
Intrac. I.P.	30.3 ± 2.7	38.4 ± 5.4	5.6 ± 0.6	4.6 ± 0.5	—	—	—	—	—	—
P.C.	15.5 ± 3.4	14.0 ± 2.1	3.1 ± 0.25	3.6 ± 0.15	49.0 ± 1.8	72 ± 2.5 }	0.001	93 ± 8.0	104 ± 1.0	—
ATP[b]	27.9 ± 3.4	20.6 ± 1.1	3.4 ± 0.25	3.4 ± 0.13	58 ± 1.0	70 ± 3.0 }		—	—	
ADP[c]	5.6 ± 0.4	5.6 ± 1.0	1.3 ± 0.06	1.8 ± 0.16	21 ± 2.0	39 ± 1.0	0.01	39 ± 2.8	54 ± 2.1	0.05
U + G[d]	1.9 ± 0.4	1.8 ± 0.4	2.9 ± 0.39	3.2 ± 0.02	47 ± 9.0	69 ± 5.8	—	75 ± 9	95 ± 2.9	—
"Residual" phosphorus	6.4 ± 1.3	7.3 ± 1.6	2.8 ± 0.26	3.0 ± 0.28	52 ± 10.4	65 ± 10.2	—	83 ± 11	89 ± 17	—
B. Incubation time: 30 min										
Insulin 10 µg/ml . . .	0	+	0	+	0	+	P[a]	0	+	P[a]
Number of experiments	2	2	2	2	2	2		2	2	
Intrac. I.P.	39.7 ± 0.6	35.4 ± 3.8	19.3	18.3 ± 4	—	—	—	—	—	—
P.C.	20 ± 3.6	17.9 ± 5.1	9 ± 1.7	15 ± 0.3	63 ± 7	84	0.001	79 ± 1.3	102	—
ATP[b]	28.5 ± 0.7	27.3 ± 1.6	11 ± 2.0	15 ± 2.7	80 ± 10	83 ± 6		—	—	
ADP[c]	5.8 ± 0.8	5.5 ± 1.1	7 ± 3.0	11 ± 2.7	46 ± 6.2	57 ± 2.0	0.01	59 ± 14.7	71 ± 5.3	0.05
U + G[d]	1.8 ± 0.4	2.4 ± 0.1	10 ± 3.0	13 ± 1.3	71 ± 1.0	75 ± 9	—	90 ± 10	92 ± 8	—
"Residual" phosphorus	6.1	6.8	—	—	—	—	—	—	—	—
Labile organic P (sum)	—	—	—	—	53 ± 2.1	70 ± 2.9	0.01			

[a] P refers to the sum of the experiments (10 min and 30 min incubation time). P values superior to 0.05 are not included.
[b] The specific activity refers to the terminal group of ATP.
[c] The specific activity refers to the terminal group of ADP.
[d] Sum of uridine and guanosine phosphates. The specific activity refers to the labile phosphate groups if only UTP and GTP were present.

From H. CLAUSER *et al.* (1962).

In 1961 we reported (VOLFIN *et al.*) an effect of insulin on the labelling of free mononucleotides in the isolated rat diaphragm in the controlled absence of extracellular glucose. In 1962, we investigated (CLAUSER *et al.*) the *in vitro* effect of insulin on both the penetration of inorganic phosphate and the labelling of organic phosphates in the excised diaphragm of rats in different physiological states.

We shall discuss these results and some more recent ones obtained by HEPP *et al.* (1968a) on isolated adipose tissue cells as well as those of WALAAS *et al.* (1969) on intact rat diaphragm.

1. Experimental Approach

The *in vitro* studies of ^{32}P incorporation into various tissues require, first of all, determination of the extracellular space of the incubated diaphragm as well as calculation of the specific radioactivities of various labelled intermediates. In our study, the value of the extracellular space of the incubated diaphragm was

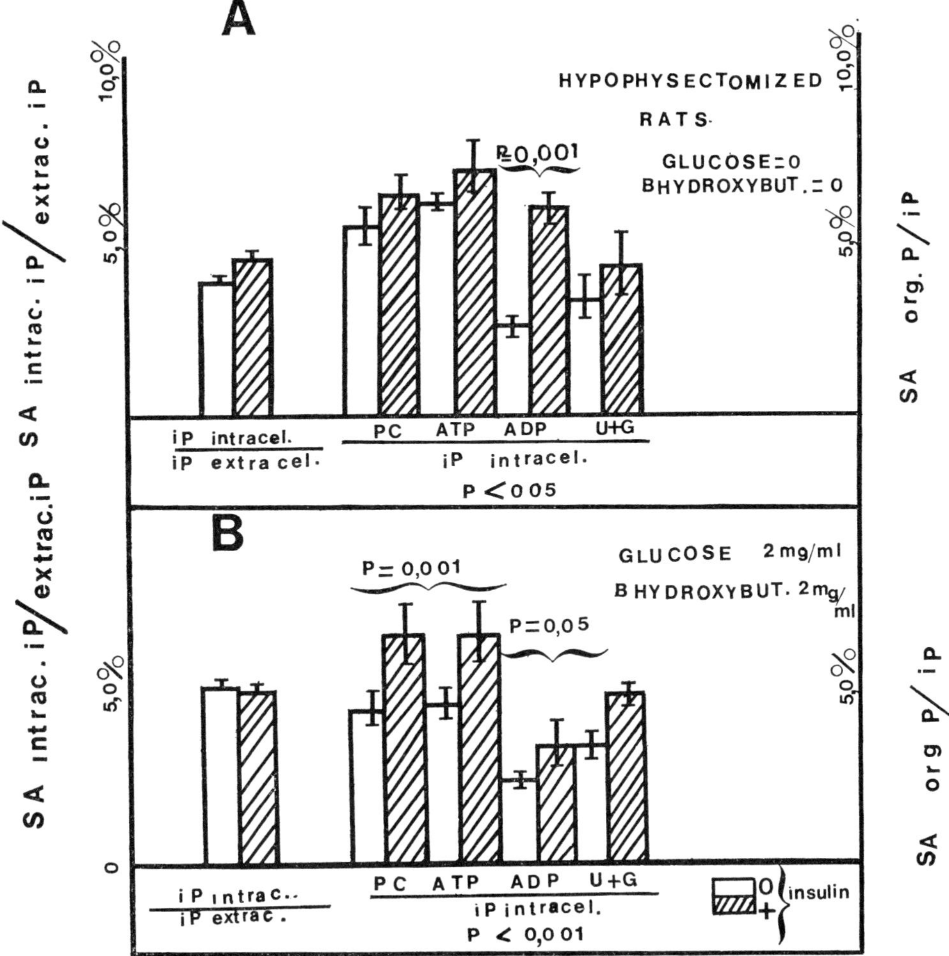

Fig. 3. Influence of insulin on the labelling of phosphates in the isolated diaphragm of the hypophysectomized rat with or without substrates. (From CLAUSER *et al.*, 1962)

established by extrapolating to 0 time the linear portion of the curve indicating the total labelling (*viz.* inorganic+organic phosphates) of the tissue. There is a slow phosphate penetration into the muscle and a rapid equilibration of the extracellular space; consequently, such a method seems reasonable (Fig. 2).

An extracellular space of 19% (±0.65) was found. This value is in close agreement with that established by KIPNIS and CORI in 1957 for the intact diaphragm (18%), which was the value used by WALAAS *et al.* (1969) in their calculations. No influence of insulin and glucose was found on this extracellular space. The amount and specific radioactivity of the intracellular phosphate were calculated from both the total inorganic phosphate and the specific activity of the medium (considered to be equal to that of the extracellular phosphate, assuming that the extracellular space was equal to 19% as indicated previously). No labelling of the ribose-*a* linked phosphate occurred within the limited incubation times used in this work.

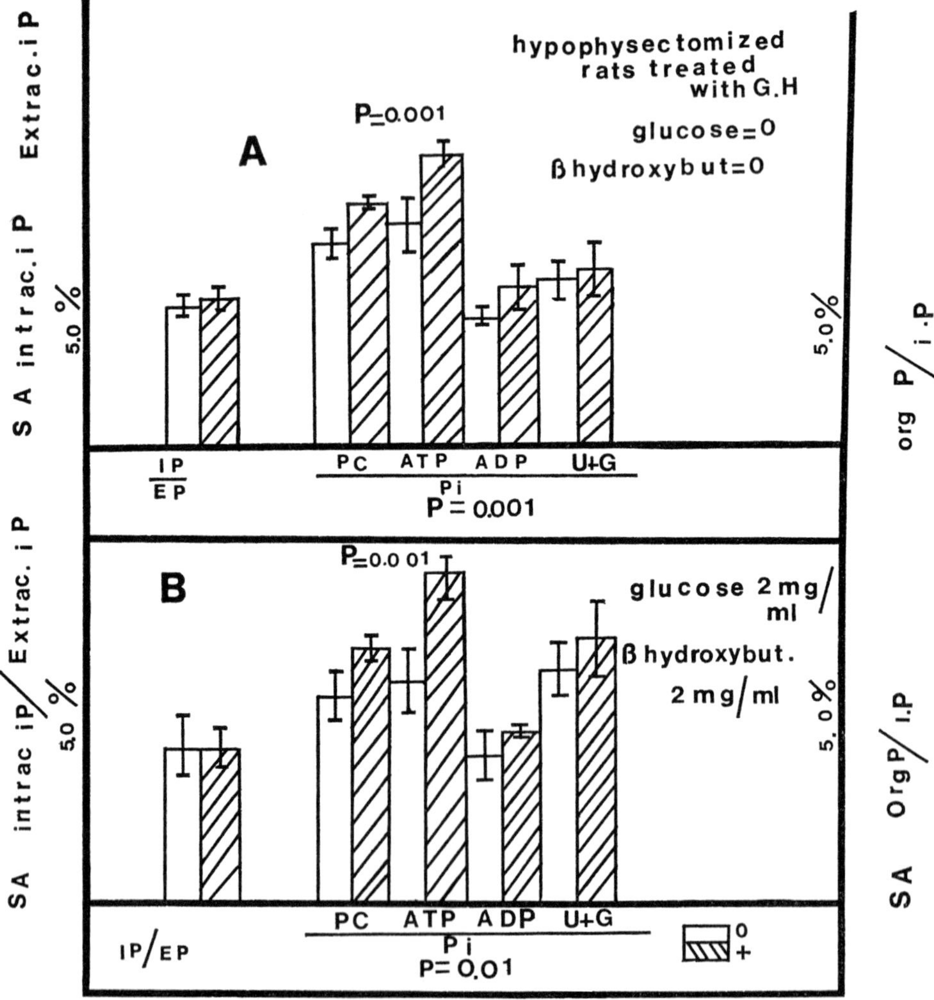

Fig. 4. Influence of insulin on the labelling of phosphates in the diaphragm of the Growth Hormone-treated hypophysectomized rat with or without added substrates (Growth Hormone 2×250 µg). (From CLAUSER *et al.*, 1962)

For this reason, labelling of ADP refers exclusively to the labile phosphate present in this compound. The specific activity of the γ-phosphate of ATP has been calculated, based on the assumption that the β-phosphate of ATP is in isotopic equilibrium with the terminal phosphate of ADP. The correctness of this assumption was founded on the work of FLECKENSTEIN and JANKE (1957) and that of HARTH and MANDEL (1961) who demonstrated that in all tissues studied, ADP isolated by column chromatography was almost exclusively an artifact arising from the limited breakdown of ATP during the handling of the tissue and the isolation procedure.

2. Phosphate Turnover in the Diaphragm of the Normal Rat

The level of the various phosphate fractions and the percentage labelling of the intracellular inorganic phosphate (IP), with respect to either the extracellular IP or the terminal phosphate of ATP in the incubated diaphragm of the normal rat, are shown in Table 4 (in the absence of substrate) and in Table 5 (in the presence of glucose). No differences were found between phosphate levels in diaphragms incubated for 10 and 30 min, nor was there any influence of insulin and glucose on these levels, except with regard to the "residual phosphate". The latter fraction consistently increased in the presence of glucose ($P < 0.01$ compared with controls without glucose), as may be expected if it consists mainly of glycolytic intermediates. Labelling of the total labile organic phosphates with respect to intracellular IP is always markedly augmented by insulin. This increase averages 55% in the absence of glucose and 32% in its presence. Over-all labelling in the presence of glucose was however, consistently higher than without substrate. Phosphocreatine is in isotopic equilibrium with the terminal group of ATP after 10 min incubation, which is the indication that homeostasis is maintained. However, equilibrium is not maintained when incubation is performed for 30 min or more. The effect of insulin on the labelling of both these labile groups averages 35—45% in the absence of glucose and 30—40% in the presence of glucose. The increase in the labelling of ADP under the influence of insulin amounts to 70—90% with or without glucose. It results in a marked randomization of labelling between both labile groups of ATP.

Because the uridine and guanosine fractions measured are extremely small, extensive scattering occurs when specific radioactivities are determined. It seems, however, that insulin enhances the labelling of the fractions.

3. Phosphate Turnover in the Diaphragm of the Hypophysectomized Rat Treated with or without Growth Hormone

The influences of hypophysectomy, treatment by growth hormone, presence or absence of glucose, on phosphate turnover in the isolated diaphragm are summarized in Fig. 3 and Fig. 4.

In the diaphragm of hypophysectomized rats in the absence of glucose (Fig. 3A), insulin stimulation of phosphate turnover involves almost exclusively the second phosphate of ATP (+130%), which nearly reaches isotopic equilibrium with the terminal phosphate. Stimulation of the turnover of all the other phosphates is limited (γP of ATP: +15%), but it must be kept in mind that the extra labelling of the second group of ATP derives compulsorily from the terminal ATP phosphate, so that any increased labelling of the second group is bound to reflect an increased turnover of the terminal phosphate. The addition of glucose (Fig. 3B) to these diaphragms almost completely reverses the effect of insulin. Specific labelling of the second group of ATP is no longer found, and the effect of insulin is reflected only by increased labelling of the terminal ATP phosphate.

Diaphragms from hypophysectomized, growth hormone-treated rats (Fig. 4A—B) no longer exhibit sensitivity to the presence of substrates, and the main insulin effect is observed on the terminal ATP phosphate.

4. Phosphate Turnover in Isolated Adipose Tissue Cells

In studies with adipose tissue of the rapid effects of insulin which are unrelated to glucose transport across the cell membrane, Hepp *et al.* (1968a) confirmed our observations made from the rat diaphragm and demonstrated that insulin stimulated the incorporation of ^{32}P from the incubation medium into the acid-soluble mononucleotides in fat cells. The fact that this reaction can be blocked by oligomycin indicates that the major portion of the incorporation of label is achieved via oxidative phosphorylation (Hepp *et al.*, 1968b). The incorporation of ^{32}P in the mononucleotides proceeds in a linear fashion over 60 minutes and is sharply enhanced by insulin.

The measured stimulation of 200% is independent of the presence of glucose and occurs with insulin concentrations as low as 10 μunits per ml.

5. Effects of Insulin on Phosphate Turnover

a) Discussion

The effect of insulin on mononucleotide labelling may be explained by two alternatives:

a) action of insulin on the transport of phosphate ions leading to an accelerated labelling of its metabolites, including ATP;

b) an increased turnover of mitochondrial mononucleotides in the presence of free diffusion of IP into the cell.

We have estimated phosphate penetration into the surviving tissue (Clauser *et al.*, 1962) by the percentage labelling of intracellular IP versus IP of the medium. Insulin or substrate dependence of this penetration has in no case been observed. Penetration of extracellular phosphate between 0 and 30 min seems to proceed at a fairly constant rate, and a small decrease in the labelling of intracellular IP seems to occur even under the influence of insulin.

This result is apparently contradictory to the data reported by Morgan *et al.* (1961), who found an increase of phosphate uptake in the isolated perfused rat heart under the influence of insulin, and by Walaas *et al.* (1969) who observed the same effect in the intact rat diaphragm. This lack of agreement may be explained by the difference existing between the intact muscle fibers of the heart or the diaphragm and the cut muscle fibers of the excised diaphragm. In our experiments, the specific activity of the intracellular IP was consistently higher than the specific activity of any organic fraction tested. The results obtained were consistent with the hypothesis that labelling of intracellular IP preceded labelling of the terminal phosphate of ATP which, in turn, acts as a precursor of all other organic phosphates.

Hepp *et al.* (1968a) were confronted with the same problem. In order to decide if their data, obtained from adipose tissue, were consistent with a direct effect of insulin on nucleotide turnover rather than on phosphorus transport, they performed short incubations of lipocytes with ^{32}P, and then washed the cells free of extracellular ^{32}P. Under these phosphate-free conditions, they observed an increase in the disappearance of radioactivity from mononucleotides under the influence of insulin, which indicates an increased turnover.

Similarly, Manchester (1963) reported that insulin stimulated the incorporation of ^{32}P and ^{14}C from acetate into lipid and protein of isolated diaphragm and concluded that insulin acted upon an energy-consuming process rather than on ^{14}C and ^{32}P uptake. These results agree with our conclusions concerning the stimulation by the hormone of the nucleotide turnover. Hence, we could justify the metabolic conclusions we had drawn, from the fact that according to the physiological state of the animal from which the diaphragm has been removed and the substrates added to the incubation medium — the action of insulin bears preferentially on a phosphorylated compound or a distinct labile phosphate.

As an example we can interpret one of these specific actions as a function of hormonal treatment and of the presence or absence of substrate. If the animal considered is hypophysectomized and its diaphragm is incubated in the absence of substrate, the action of insulin will result in a specific increase in the turnover of the labile phosphate of ADP. This may be a consequence of the stimulation of fatty acid catabolism under these physiological conditions, because this source of energy is the only metabolic alternative. The presence of substrate (glucose) or treatment by growth hormone (which results in an increase in glycogen) relieves the diaphragm from this emergency situation, and the action of insulin is reflected, as could be expected, in the phosphocreatine and the terminal phosphate of ATP. These results are in good agreement with physiological predictions and justify the use of this method to obtain a rapid "fingerprint" of the metabolism of a tissue and perhaps, in our case, to reveal an original primary action of insulin.

b) Significance

The interpretation of these results obtained in the presence of insulin has led to various speculations or attempts at elucidation. Among them, the possibility that insulin stimulates a metabolic parameter linked to the oxidative phosphorylations has been suggested. Effects of insulin on rat liver mitochondria have been reported by NEUBERT and LEHNINGER (1962) and HALL *et al.* (1960) but in both cases, the specificity of the insulin action has not been established. A systematic investigation of a possible action of insulin on pig heart sarcosomes by LEBLANC *et al.* (1968) indicated that there is absolutely no direct action of insulin on the metabolism of sarcosomes.

KLACHKO (1966) tried to explain the mechanism of action of insulin by its effect on nucleotide metabolism. Certain biosynthetic pathways require that energy be provided by specific nucleoside phosphates. Because the effects of insulin include the stimulation of many of these biosynthetic pathways, KLACHKO thought that insulin must act by accelerating the transfer of high energy phosphate from ATP to all the non-adenosine nucleoside diphosphates, thus causing a general increase in the rate of synthesis and of storage within the cell. A single site for this insulin action would be the enzyme nucleoside diphosphokinase.

In view of its action on nucleotide turnover, we also considered that insulin may act on an enzyme — adenylate kinase — which regulates adenine nucleotide levels within the cell (VOLFIN, 1970). ATP and AMP play important roles in the regulation of energy metabolism not only as substrates and products but also as regulators of enzymatic reactions. The relative concentrations of ATP and AMP in the tissue are particularly important: for example, glycolytic rates depend to a large extent on the activity of phosphofructokinase (NEWSHOLME and RANDLE, 1961); activation by IP, AMP, ADP and inhibition by ATP are thought to act as signals for this enzyme to speed up or slow down its activity in response to the demand for high energy phosphate compounds. We have investigated the ensuing relationships between the early effects of insulin on glycolysis rate (NEWSHOLME and RANDLE, 1961, 1964), on nucleotide labelling (VOLFIN *et al.*, 1961; CLAUSER *et al.*, 1962) and on adenylate kinase activity in subcellular fractions of previously incubated isolated rat diaphragm (VOLFIN, 1970). We observed in the presence of the hormone an inhibition of cytosol adenylate kinase activity (48%) and a parallel increase (+85%) in the rate of glycolysis in the absence of external glucose.

Similar conclusions were reached by BEITNER and KALANT (1971) from their studies on the effects of insulin on glycolysis in the rat diaphragm. They also concluded that insulin increases glycolysis independently of its effect on glucose transport. Stimulation by insulin of incorporation of ^{32}P into energy rich phosphates of the nucleotides may reflect these metabolic changes, particularly the activation of metabolites — especially glucose and sugar phosphates — which occurs during this process. Because the course of energy is controlled by the intracellular concentration of AMP, ADP and ATP, the immediate action of insulin on cytosol adenylate kinase activity may be related to this control system.

V. Interaction of Insulin with the Cyclic AMP System

In its three major target tissues (liver, muscle and adipose tissue), insulin exerts pleiotropic effects which are the exact opposite of the well-known effects of the adenosine 3′,5′-cyclic monophosphate (cAMP)-mediated hormones (glucagon and catecholamines): increased levels of cAMP are associated with lipolysis, gluconeogenesis, glycogenolysis, ureogenesis and ketogenesis whereas insulin administration leads to lipogenesis, glycolysis and glycogenogenesis.

This fact has led to the hypothesis that insulin could produce a lowering of the intracellular cAMP level and that this action on cAMP could explain all the effects of insulin (SUTHERLAND and ROBINSON, 1969; WILLIAMS *et al.*, 1971). So far, this attractive and simple scheme has not been sustained by conclusive experimental findings. The only clear exception to this scheme is the induction of liver tyrosine transaminase by both insulin and cAMP (BARNETT and WICKS, 1971; HANOUNE *et al.*, 1971).

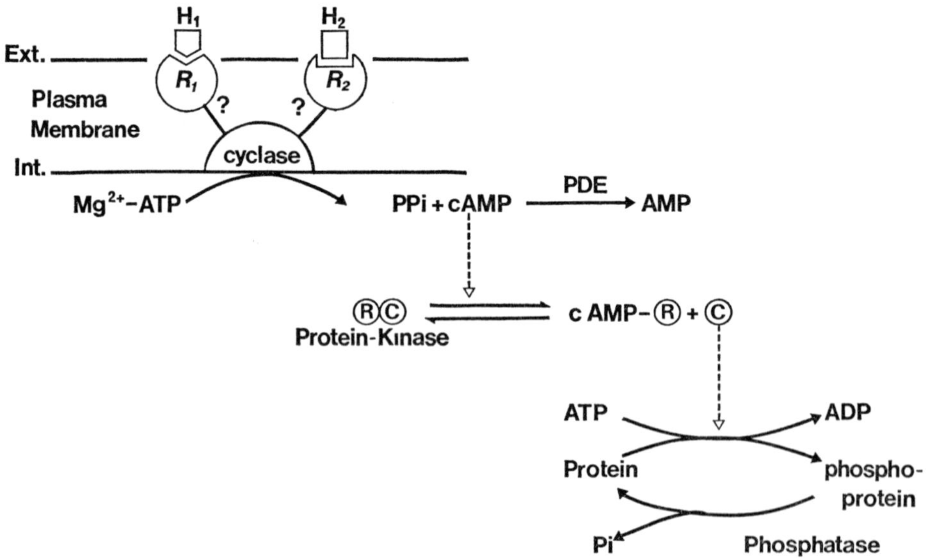

Fig. 5. *The cAMP system:* H_1, H_2: Activating hormones; R_1, R_2: Hormonal receptors; PPi: Inorganic pyrophosphate; PDE: cAMP-specific phosphodiesterase; R-C: inactive protein-kinase; R: Regulatory component; C: Catalytic subunit

Figure 5 summarizes the current status of knowledge concerning the cAMP system. Hormones (H_1, H_2 ...) bind to receptors (R_1, R_2 ...) thought to be located at the external face of the plasma membrane. Conformational changes within the receptors lead to an activation of the enzyme adenylate cyclase, thus enhancing the synthesis of cAMP from Mg^{2+}-ATP, with a parallel release of pyrophosphate. It is believed at present that the main effect of cAMP is to increase the activity of protein kinase(s) by binding to and removing an inhibitory component (R), thus releasing an active, free catalytic subunit (C).

Phosphorylation of various proteins (histones, ribosomal proteins, enzymes) represents the only mechanism of action of cAMP, even though other possibilities cannot be excluded. Finally, cAMP is transformed into inactive AMP by a specific degradative enzyme, the cAMP-phosphodiesterase.

This simple outline should be weighed with the following considerations, which may either underlie additional regulatory processes or modify the current hypothesis:

— All the components of the cyclase system are membrane-bound, which makes solubilization difficult. One can predict that progress in understanding cyclase activation at the molecular level will be slow.

— Hormonal binding sites in the plasma membrane usually reveal many features (kinetics and specificity of binding) which make them unlikely to be the "actual physiological receptors" (Birnbaumer and Pohl, 1973).

— The mode of transduction of the information from the receptor site to the catalytic site, within the membrane, is unknown. Guanine nucleotides probably play an important activating role (Rodbell *et al.*, 1971; Leray *et al.*, 1972, 1973). Prostaglandins are likely to play a modifying role. Other inhibitory factors have been described, which can also be subject to further subtle hormonal regulations.

— The "protein-kinase system" is at the same time complex (many regulatory and catalytic subunits) and seemingly too simple to account for all the specific effects of cAMP. A "protein-kinase inhibitor" has been described, the physiological role of which is unknown. The actual substrates for the kinase are usually unknown.

— Regulations of the phosphatase activity are unknown.

— The role of guanosine 3′,5′-monophosphate (cGMP) at each step is either unknown or complex.

We shall deal first with the over-all effect of insulin upon the cAMP level, then with the molecular mechanism of this phenomenon. Finally, we shall consider the uncertainties and difficulties of the proposed model.

1. The Action of Insulin upon the cAMP Level

The simple analysis of the effects of insulin and cAMP on a series of metabolic phenomena suggests that these phenomena may depend on a balance between agents which increase the level of cAMP — such as glucagon and catecholamines — and others which lower it, such as insulin. Table 6, from Park *et al.* (1972), contains some effects of elevated levels of cAMP (or of glucagon and epinephrine) on the liver. It is indicated in the table whether or not insulin antagonizes each effect in the cases which have been studied.

For Park *et al.* (1972), for example, liver glucose output is clearly modulated in this way: the level of cAMP increases in liver from unfed rats and from rats made diabetic by injection of alloxan. Moreover, Jefferson *et al.* (1968) demonstrated that the *in vivo* administration of anti-insulin serum increased the level of liver cAMP (Fig. 6). More recently, Park *et al.* (1972) demonstrated directly the antagonistic effect of glucagon and insulin upon the cAMP level in perfused liver and were able to correlate this effect with the variations of the glucose output (Fig. 7). In a similar way, BUTCHER *et al.* (1966) showed that insulin rapidly lowered the intracellular cAMP level in adipose tissue incubated with epinephrine or epinephrine plus caffeine. This effect was not due to increased escape of cAMP to the medium. The control level, without epinephrine, was not influenced by insulin (Fig. 8).

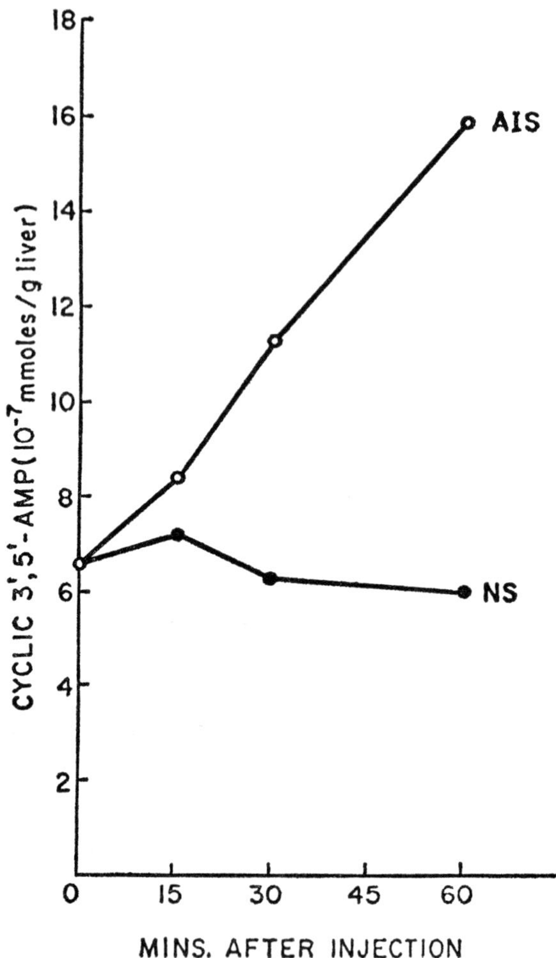

Fig. 6. Effect of anti-insulin serum (AIS) and normal serum (NS) on cyclic AMP levels in rat liver *in vivo*. Serum was injected intravenously into anesthetized rats and the livers exposed and rapidly frozen at the indicated times. (From JEFFERSON *et al.*, 1968)

In conclusion, it seems clear that the antagonistic effect of insulin in relation to glucagon and catecholamines is associated in liver and adipose tissue at least, with a decreased level of cAMP. Insulin does not decrease the level of cAMP which has not previously been elevated by glucagon or catecholamines nor does it seem to do so in diaphragm (GOLDBERG *et al.*, 1967).

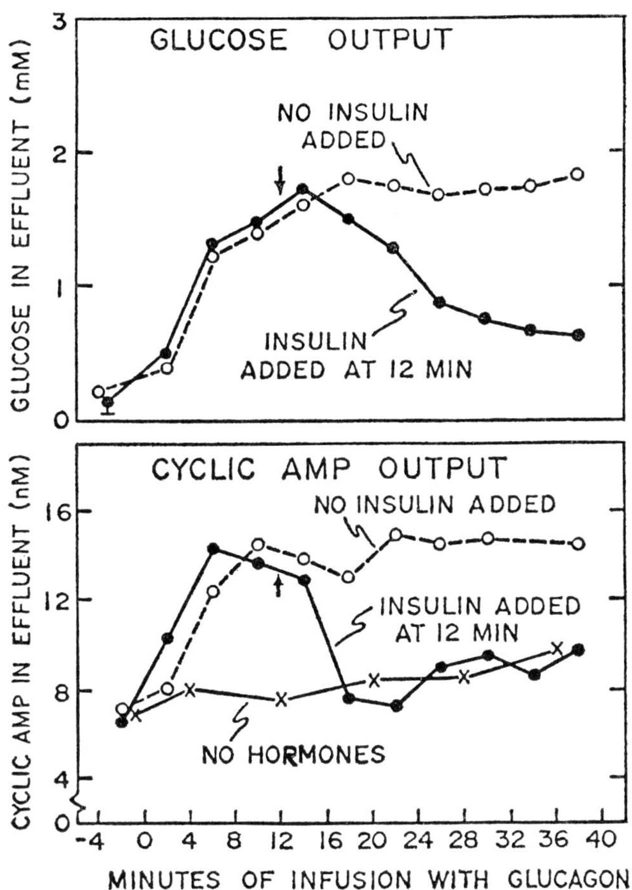

Fig. 7. Interaction of glucagon and insulin in the control of glucose output by the perfused rat liver. Livers of fed rats were perfused with recirculating media for a one-hour control period and then perfusion without recirculation was begun at —4 min. Glucagon infusion was maintained from O time (except for the curve shown by x's) at a steady rate well below that giving a maximal effect. Insulin infusion was superimposed on the glucagon infusion when indicated. (From Park *et al.*, 1972)

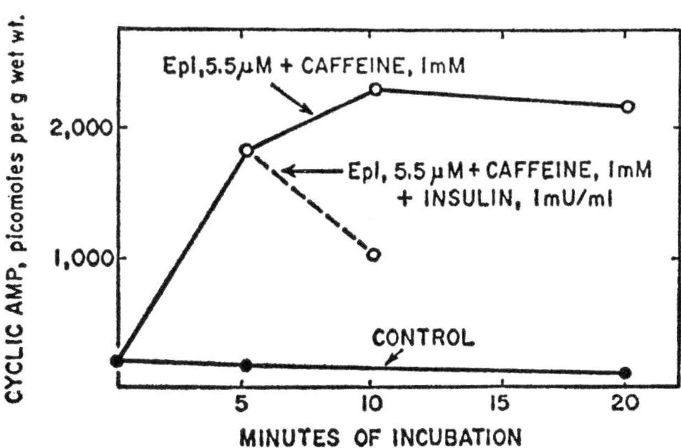

Fig. 8. Effect of insulin on cyclic AMP levels in rat epididymal fat pads incubated with epinephrine and caffeine. (From Butcher *et al.*, 1966)

Table 6. *Effects of cAMP (or glucagon or catecholamine) on the isolated rat liver, and the antagonistic action of insulin*

Effect	Agent	Antagonized by insulin
Stimulation of glycogenolysis or activation of phosphorylase	glucagon	+
	catecholamine	+
	cAMP	+
Stimulation of gluconeogenesis	glucagon	+
	catecholamine	not tested
	cAMP	+
Stimulation of ureogenesis	glucagon	+
	catecholamine	not tested
	cAMP	not tested
Stimulation of initial K uptake	glucagon	not tested
	catecholamine	not tested
	cAMP	not tested
Stimulation of K loss	glucagon	+
	cAMP	+
Stimulation of Ca flux	glucagon	not tested
	catecholamine	not tested
	cAMP	not tested
Stimulation of histone phosphorylation	glucagon	not tested
	cAMP	not tested
Stimulation of proteolysis (probably by lysosomal activation)	glucagon	+
Inhibition of lipoprotein release	glucagon	not tested
Induction of enzymes: tyrosine amino transferase	glucagon	
	cAMP	
phosphoenolpyruvate carboxykinase	glucagon	+
	catecholamine	+
	cAMP	+

From PARK *et al.* (1972)

2. Mechanisms of the Effect of Insulin upon the cAMP Level

Since cyclic AMP is synthesized from ATP by the enzyme adenylate cyclase and is degraded into inactive 5′ AMP by the enzyme cyclic AMP phosphodiesterase, two possible mechanisms for the action of insulin are offered:

a) Decrease in the Activity of Adenylate Cyclase

Since insulin is thought not to penetrate the target cell, the simplest explanation would be an inhibitory effect upon the adenylate cyclase which is located in the plasma membrane. First suggested by JUNGAS (1966) in experiments with intact fat cells, this effect has been described recently by HEPP (1971); HEPP and RENNER (1972), and ILLIANO and CUATRECASAS (1971). Both groups use a particulate fraction (not a purified plasma membrane preparation) from rat liver and adipose tissue as the source of enzymatic activity. In these systems, addition *in vitro* of a very low dose (50—100 μU/ml) of insulin results in decrease of the glucagon and the catecholamine activation of the cyclase. The effect of insulin upon the cyclase basal level is considerably less marked.

Similar results were obtained by DE ASUA *et al.* (1973) for adenylate cyclase activity from BHK fibroblasts. The generality of the insulin effect upon any cyclase system might be inferred from the experiments of FLAWIA and TORRES (1973) who showed that low concentrations of insulin (30—60 μU/ml) could also inhibit the adenylate cyclase activity of *Neurospora crassa*, at low concentration of the substrate Mn^{2+}-ATP.

An absolute requirement for this type of experiment seems to be the use of a very low concentration of insulin since a higher concentration (1 mU/ml) can actually lead to a stimulation of the cyclase. Whether or not insulin acts directly upon the cyclase system is still open to discussion since it has always been impossible to repeat this kind of experiment with a purified membrane preparation (Pohl *et al.*, 1971; Combret and Laudat, 1972; Rosselin and Freychet, 1973). We used a purified plasma membrane preparation from rat liver. The basal and the stimulated cyclase activities were insensitive to porcine insulin at concentrations from 2—60 ng/ml. Adding variable amounts of glucose or the supernatant from centrifugation at $105000 \times g$ to the incubation medium did not change the enzyme activities, whether or not GTP (an activator in our system) was present (Leray *et al.*, 1973). The possibility that a certain degree of cellular organization is needed for the effect of insulin upon the cyclase to show up, is worth considering.

b) Increase in the Activity of Cyclic AMP-Phosphodiesterase

Another possibility is therefore an effect of insulin at the level of the degrading enzyme phosphodiesterase. First described by Senft *et al.* (1968) with the liver enzyme, this effect was later denied by the work of Blecher *et al.* (1968), Müller-Oerlinghausen *et al.* (1968), Menahan and Wieland (1969), Menahan *et al.* (1969). More recently, the finding by Thompson and Appleman (1971) that phosphodiesterase could have two different Km's gave a new impetus to studies in this direction. Loten and Sneyd (1970) studied the phosphodiesterase from homogenates prepared from epididymal fat pad and isolated fat cells incubated in the absence and in the presence of insulin. Homogenates of insulin-treated tissues showed an increase in phosphodiesterase activity as compared to controls. Insulin raised the maximal velocity for the low Km-enzyme and lowered the Km of the higher Km-enzyme (Table 7). No effect of insulin was observed when the hormone was added directly to the homogenates. It is possible that the failure of the previous authors to detect such an effect was due to the use of a high substrate concentration, allowing the study of only the high Km-enzyme.

House *et al.* (1972) also showed that a plasma membrane subfraction from rat liver contained a specific low Km phosphodiesterase which was stimulated by insulin. The stimulation was already observed at the shortest time interval tested (30 sec). Unlike the experiments of Loten and Sneyd (1970) in which insulin was without effect if added to the preparation of adipocytes after the disruption of the intact epididymal fat pad, in the experiments of House *et al.*, insulin was active in an acellular system. The mechanism by which insulin increased the phosphodiesterase activity is not known. This effect is manifest within seconds,

Table 7. *Kinetic data for adipose tissue phosphodiesterase. Enzyme activity was measured in homogenates of isolated fat cells incubated for 10 min in the presence or absence of insulin (100 μU/ml). The values for the low-K_m enzyme were derived from measurements made at substrate concentrations below 1 μm, and those for the high-K_m enzyme from measurements made at substrate concentrations between 50 and 330 μm*

Addition	Low-K_m enzyme		High-K_m enzyme	
	K_m (μm)	V_{max} (pmol of adenosine formed/min per g dry wt.)	K_m (μm)	V_{max} (pmol of adenosine formed/min per g dry wt.)
None	0.88	1700	41	6800
Insulin	0.87	2640	27	6830

From Loten and Sneyd (1970)

which argues against induction of an enzyme. If a mere activation takes place, then the problem of how to determine the mechanism through which insulin acts directly upon the soluble form of the phosphodiesterase reappears.

More recently, THOMPSON *et al.* (1973a) showed that rat liver cAMP phosphodiesterase activity, which displayed negatively cooperative kinetic behavior and appeared bound to membranes particles, was uniquely sensitive to insulin. Thirty minutes after the injection of insulin (3 units/100 g) into streptozotocine diabetic rats, this membrane-bound phosphodiesterase was activated, but there was no effect on the cytosol phosphodiesterase (mostly cGMP phosphodiesterase). The activated phosphodiesterase retained negatively cooperative kinetic behavior and showed no change in the apparent Km value, but had increased apparent maximum velocity. However, insulin stimulation in normal rats was not consistent and was complicated by associated hypoglycemia. No effect of insulin *in vitro* could be demonstrated.

According to LOTEN and SNEYD (1970), although the effect on phosphodiesterase is small, it is probably sufficient to account for the decrease in cyclic AMP concentration in response to insulin. The rate of formation of cyclic AMP by adenylate cyclase in cells in the basal state is slow whereas the activity of phosphodiesterase is comparatively high. Consequently, only a small increase in the activity of the latter enzyme could significantly alter the amount of cyclic AMP present.

c) Is Insulin Acting at the Kinase Level?

It was emphasized previously that insulin does not lead to a decrease in the cAMP level in all tissues (more precisely in muscle, GOLDBERG *et al.*, 1967). This discrepancy led to the hypothesis that insulin could act at a later step, for example upon the kinase systems through which most cAMP effects are thought to take place. It has been suggested that insulin could alter directly the sensitivity of the various kinase systems without necessarily altering the level of cAMP, in muscle (SHEN *et al.*, 1970) as well as in liver (MILLER and LARNER, 1973). KHOO *et al.* (1973) showed also that in adipose tissue, the action of insulin was not correlated with the cyclic AMP level. However, these results are not in agreement with the data of SODERLING *et al.* (1973) which support the hypothesis that insulin and epinephrine do modify the "activation state" of the cAMP-dependent protein kinase in adipose tissue owing to changes in the cAMP concentration.

In conclusion, it is clear that no definitive answer as to whether insulin modifies the activity of cAMP without modifying the level, can be given. The "kinase-inhibitor factor" (ASHBY and WALSH, 1972) may represent another regulatory site which deserves thorough study.

3. Conclusion: The Search for "Another" Transducer Specific for Insulin

There is as yet no convincing evidence that insulin acts by decreasing the amount of intracellular cyclic AMP and that insulin depresses the adenylate cyclase, increases the phosphodiesterase or does both. This problem is still open to discussion. We have emphasized that the normal intracellular level of cyclic AMP without additional hormonal stimulation is high enough to completely activate all the kinases which are thought to be the target sites for cyclic AMP (CHAMBAUT *et al.*, 1971). The main issue seems therefore to be how the "activity", and not the level, of cyclic AMP, is normally kept under control — the two enzymes adenylate cyclase and phosphodiesterase, being perhaps not the only two key enzymes.

On the other hand, our studies (Chambaut *et al.*, 1969) on the metabolism of surviving diaphragm revealed antagonistic actions between dibutyryl cyclic AMP and insulin on a series of metabolic parameters (glucose, galactose, glucosamine uptake; turnover of phosphorylated compound; glycogen synthesis). This phenomenon could also be explained by the biosynthesis, under the influence of insulin, of a transducer, different from cyclic AMP, which could competitively antagonize the action of the latter compound in all the enzymatic systems involved in insulin action. There is no direct evidence for such a possibility and the nature of this "other" transducer is unknown. As possibilities, one should think of prostaglandins, of cyclic GMP and of the inhibitory factor of Mangianello *et al.* (1971) and Ho and Sutherland (1971). A pleiotypic mediator known in bacteria ppGpp, is probably absent in mammalian cells, or at least in the cell lines studied (Mamont *et al.*, 1972).

Among the foregoing possibilities, cGMP is the most studied at the present time. If cGMP were the "second messenger" responsible for the action of insulin, it should act as an insulin substitute for all effects of insulin; in turn, insulin should increase the cGMP level. Since guanylate cyclase is, in most tissues, a soluble enzyme, one should also demonstrate a mechanism by which insulin, in agreement with current knowledge, could regulate the guanylate cyclase from the external face of the plasma membrane. This hypothesis is being investigated in a number of laboratories, but the data published are so far sketchy. For example, Illiano *et al.* (1973) reported that low concentrations of insulin (120 μU/ml) and carbamyl choline (1 μM) increased cGMP content in isolated fat cells by 350%. The maximal amount of cGMP, achieved within 2 min after addition of insulin, fell rapidly thereafter. Insulin increased also the concentration of cGMP in rat liver slices by 400%. The data support the view that a close and reciprocal relationship may exist between the concentrations and actions of cAMP and cGMP, as well as between the enzymes responsible for the biosynthesis and degradation of these nucleotides.

However, Thompson *et al.* (1973 b) were unable to demonstrate any direct effect of insulin (1.8×10^{-8}M) upon the guanylate cyclase activity of the $18000\times g$ supernatant of rat liver homogenate. When tested directly in perfused liver at 2.10^{-5}M (Exton *et al.*, 1971), cGMP was 1/3 to 1/2 as potent as cAMP in stimulating glucose production, net glycogenolysis, gluconeogenesis from lactate and release of K^+; these data argue against antagonistic behavior of cAMP and cGMP in a physiological sense, at least at the concentration studied.

VI. General Conclusions

Pleiotropy is the principal characteristic of the insulin action, and the main issue at present is to decipher whether the multiple effects of insulin are unrelated or secondary to a common primary event. As have many others, we have attempted to search for such a correlation. It is clear that neither RNA synthesis nor increased ^{32}P incorporation into phosphorylated compounds can be "the" primary site of action of insulin. The model proposed by Sutherland constitutes an attractive alternative even though, as we have seen, direct evidence of the involvement of a second messenger in insulin action is still lacking.

References

Asua, L.J. de, Surian, E.S., Flawia, M.M., Torres, H.N.: Effect of insulin on the growth pattern and adenylate cyclase activity of BHK Fibroblasts. Proc. nat. Acad. Sci. (Wash.) **70**, 1388—1392 (1973)

Ashby, C.D., Walsh, D.A.: Assessment of the role of a protein inhibitor of cyclic AMP dependent protein kinases. Fed. Proc. **31**, 439 (1972)

BALL, E.G., MARTIN, D.B., COOPER, O.: Studies on the metabolism of adipose tissue. I. The effect of insulin on glucose utilization as measured by the manometric determination of carbon dioxide output. J. biol. Chem. **234**, 774—780 (1959)

BARNETT, C.A., WICKS, W.D.: Regulation of phosphoenol pyruvate carboxykinase and tyrosine transaminase in hepatoma cell culture. J. biol. Chem. **246**, 7201—7206 (1971)

BEITNER, R., KALANT, N.: Stimulation of glycolysis by insulin. J. biol. Chem. **246**, 500—503 (1971)

BELOFF-CHAIN, A., CATANZARO, R., CHAIN, E.B., LONGINOTTI, L., MASI, I., POCCHIARI, F.: Influence of anaerobiosis on glucose metabolism in the isolated rat diaphragm muscle. Selected Sci. Papers Inst. Super. Sanita. **2**, 139—149 (1959)

BIRNBAUMER, L., POHL, S.L.: Relation of glucagon specific binding sites to glucagon dependent stimulation of adenylyl cyclase activity in plasma membranes of rat liver. J. biol. Chem. **248**, 2056—2061 (1973)

BLECHER, M., MERLINO, N.S., RO'ANE, J.T.: Control of the metabolism and lipolytic effects of cyclic-3',5'-adenosine monophosphate in adipose tissue by insulin, methylxanthines, and nicotinic acid. J. biol. Chem. **243**, 3973—3977 (1968)

BUTCHER, R.W., SNEYD, J.G.T., PARK, C.R., SUTHERLAND, E.W.: Effect of insulin on adenosine-3',5'-monophosphate in the rat epididymal fat pad. J. biol. Chem. **241**, 1651—1653 (1966)

CHAMBAUT, A.M.: Stimulation du métabolisme du diaphragme et du tissu adipeux par l'insuline. Corrélation de ces stimulations avec l'action des nucléotides cycliques. Thèse Université de Paris (1969)

CHAMBAUT, A.M., EBOUÉ-BONIS, D., HANOUNE, J., CLAUSER, H.: Antagonistic actions between dibutyryl adenosine-3',5'-cyclic monophosphate and insulin on the metabolism of the surviving rat diaphragm. Biochem. biophys. Res. Commun. **34**, 283—290 (1969)

CHAMBAUT, A.M., LERAY, F., HANOUNE, J.: Relationship between cyclic AMP dependent protein kinase(s) and cyclic AMP binding protein(s) in rat liver. FEBS Letters **15**, 328—334 (1971)

CLAUSER, H., VOLFIN, P., EBOUÉ-BONIS, D.: Effect of insulin on the phosphorus-32 mononucleotide and phosphocreatine labelling in the isolated diaphragm of the normal, the hypophysectomized, and the hypophysectomized Growth-Hormone treated rat. Gen. comp. Endocr. **2**, 369—384 (1962)

COMBRET, Y., LAUDAT, P.: Adenyl cyclase activity in a plasma membrane fraction purified from "ghosts" of rat fat cells. FEBS Letters **21**, 45—49 (1972)

EBOUÉ-BONIS, D., CHAMBAUT, A.M., VOLFIN, P., CLAUSER, H.: Action of insulin on the isolated rat diaphragm in the presence of Actinomycin D and Puromycin. Nature (Lond.) **199**, 1183—1184 (1963)

EBOUÉ-BONIS, D., CHAMBAUT, A.M., VOLFIN, P., CLAUSER, H.: Action sélective de la N-éthylmaléimide sur la stimulation par l'insuline du métabolisme du diaphragm en survie. Bull. Soc. Chim. biol. (Paris) **49**, 415—425 (1967)

EXTON, J.H., HARDMAN, J.G., WILLIAMS, T.F., SUTHERLAND, E.W., PARK, C.R.: Effects of guanosine 3',5' monophosphate on the perfused rat liver. J. biol. Chem. **246**, 2658—2664 (1971)

FLAWIA, M.M., TORRES, H.N.: Adenylate cyclase activity in Neurospora Crassa. J. biol. Chem. **248**, 4517—4520 (1973)

FLECKENSTEIN, A., JANKE, J.: Der Austausch von radioaktivem ^{32}P-markierten Orthophosphat mit dem Py, Pα und Pβ von ATP und mit Kreatinphosphat bis Muskelruhe, Temperaturvariation und elektrischer Reizung. Pflügers Arch. ges. Physiol. **265**, 237—263 (1957)

FRITZ, G.R., KNOBIL, E.: *In vitro* stimulation by insulin of α-amino-isobutyric acid transport in the absence of protein synthesis. Nature (Lond.) **200**, 682—683 (1963)

GEMMIL, C.L.: Effect of insulin on glycogen content of muscles. Bull. Johns Hopk. Hosp. **66**, 232—236 (1940)

GOLDBERG, N.G., VILLAR-PALASI, C., SASKO, H., LARNER, J.: Effects of insulin treatment on muscle 3',5' cyclic adenylate levels *in vivo* and *in vitro*. Biochim. biophys. Acta (Amst.) **148**, 665—672 (1967)

HALL, J.C., SORDAHL, L.A., STEFKO, P.L.: The effect of insulin on oxidative phosphorylation in normal and diabetic mitochondria. J. biol. Chem. **235**, 1536—1539 (1960)

HANOUNE, J., CHAMBAUT, A.M., JOSIPOWICZ, A.: The glucose effect and the cortisone action upon rat liver metabolism. Biochim. biophys. Acta (Amst.) **244**, 338—348 (1971)

HARTH, S., MANDEL, P.: La répartition des nucléotides libres du cerveau chez diverses espèces de mammifères. Bull. Soc. Chim. biol. (Paris) **43**, 969—980 (1961)

HEPP, D., CHALLONER, D.R., WILLIAMS, R.H.: Studies on the action of insulin in isolated adipose tissue cells. J. biol. Chem. **243**, 4020—4026 (1968a)

HEPP, D., CHALLONER, D., WILLIAMS, R.H.: Respiration in isolated fat cells and the effects of epinephrine. J. biol. Chem. **243**, 2321—2327 (1968b)

HEPP, K.D.: Inhibition of glucagon stimulated adenyl cyclase by insulin. FEBS Letters **12**, 263—266 (1971)

HEPP, K.D., RENNER, R.: Insulin action on the adenyl cyclase system: antagonism to activation by lipolytic hormones. FEBS Letters **20**, 191—194 (1972)

HO, R.J., SUTHERLAND, E.W.: Formation and release of a hormone antagonist by rat adipocytes. J. biol. Chem. **246**, 6822—6827 (1971)

HOUSE, P.D.R., POULIS, P., WEIDEMANN, M.J.: Isolation of a plasma-membrane subfraction from rat liver containing an insulin-sensitive cyclic AMP phosphodiesterase. Europ. J. Biochem. **24**, 429—437 (1972)

ILLIANO, G., CUATRECASAS, P.: Modulation of adenylate cyclase activity in liver and fat cell membranes by insulin. Science **175**, 906—908 (1971)

ILLIANO, G., TELL, G.P.E., SIEGEL, M.I., CUATRECASAS, P.: Guanosine 3′,5′-cyclic monophosphate and the action of insulin and acetyl-choline. Proc. nat. Acad. Sci. (Wash.) **70**, 2443—2447 (1973)

JACKSON, C.D., SELLS, B.H.: Countercurrent distribution of RNA from rat liver: effect of Growth Hormone, thyroxine and hydrocortisone on distribution patterns. Biochim. biophys. Acta (Amst.) **155**, 417—423 (1968)

JEFFERSON, L.S., EXTON, J.H., BUTCHER, R.W., SUTHERLAND, E.W., PARK, C.R.: Role of adenosine 3′,5′-monophosphate in the effects of insulin and anti-insulin serum on liver metabolism. J. biol. Chem. **243**, 1031—1038 (1968)

JUNGAS, R.L.: Role of cyclic-3′,5′ AMP in the response of adipose tissue to insulin. Proc. nat. Acad. Sci. (Wash.) **56**, 757—763 (1966)

KAJI, H., PARK, C.R.: Stimulation of phosphate uptake by insulin and its relation to sugar transport in the perfused rat heart. Fed. Proc. **20**, 190 (1961)

KIDSON, C., KIRBY, K.S.: Selective alterations of mammalian messenger-RNA synthesis: Evidence for differential action of hormones on gene-transcription. Nature (Lond.) **203**, 559—560 (1964)

KIPNIS, D.M., CORI, C.F.: Studies of tissue permeability. III. The effect of insulin on pentose uptake by the diaphragm. J. biol. Chem. **224**, 681—693 (1957)

KIPNIS, D.M., NOALL, M.N.: Stimulation of amino acid transport by insulin in the isolated rat diaphragm. Biochim. biophys. Acta (Amst.) **28**, 226—227 (1958)

KLACHKO, D.M.: Regulation of intermediary metabolism by nucleotides the mechanism of action of insulin. J. theor. Biol. **12**, 266—272 (1966)

KHOO, J.C., STEINBERG, D., THOMPSON, B., MAYER, S.E.: Hormonal regulation of adipocyte enzymes. J. biol. Chem. **248**, 3823—3830 (1973)

LEADER, D.P., BARRY, J.M.: Counter-current distribution of radidly labelled RNA from rats treated with hormones. Nature (Lond.) **215**, 1374—1375 (1967)

LEBLANC, P., BOURDAIN, M., CLAUSER, H.: Etude des propriétés oxydophosphorylantes des sarcosomes de coeur de porc en présence et en absence d'insuline. Bull. Soc. Chim. biol. (Paris) **50**, 2091—2119 (1968)

LERAY, F., CHAMBAUT, A.M., HANOUNE, J.: Role of GTP in epinephrine and glucagon activation of adenyl cyclase of rat liver plasma membrane. Biochem. biophys. Res. Commun. **48**, 1385—1391 (1972)

LERAY, F., CHAMBAUT, A.M., PERRENOUD, M.L., HANOUNE, J.: Adenylate cyclase activity of rat liver Plasma membranes: Hormonal stimulations and effect of Adrenalectomy. Europ. J. Biochem. **38**, 185—192 (1973)

LEVINE, R., GOLDSTEIN, M.S.: On the mechanism of action of insulin. Recent Progr. Hormone Res. **11**, 343—380 (1955)

LOTEN, E.G., SNEYD, J.G.T.: An effect of insulin or adipose tissue adenosine 3′,5′-cyclic monophosphate phosphodiesterase. Biochem. J. **120**, 187—193 (1970)

MAMONT, P., HERSHKO, A., KRAM, R., SHACTER, L., LUST, J., TOMKINS, G.M.: The pleiotypic response in mammalian cells: search for an intracellular mediator. Biochem. biophys. Res. Commun. **48**, 1378—1384 (1972)

MANCHESTER, K.L., YOUNG, F.G.: The effect of insulin on incorporation of amino acids into protein of normal rat diaphragm *in vitro*. Biochem. J. **70**, 353—358 (1958)

MANCHESTER, K.L., YOUNG, F.G.: The effect of insulin *in vitro* on the accumulation of amino acids by isolated rat diaphragm. Biochem. J. **75**, 487—495 (1960)

MANCHESTER, K.L.: Stimulation by insulin of incorporation of (^{32}P) phosphate and ^{14}C from acetate into lipid and protein of isolated rat diaphragm. Biochim. biophys. Acta (Amst.) **70**, 208—210 (1963)

MANCHESTER, K.L.: The rate of turnover of messenger ribonucleic acid in rat diaphragm muscle. Biochem. J. **90**, 5c (1964)

Manchester, K.L.: Re-evaluation of the effect of insulin on nucleic acid synthesis in muscle. Biochem. J. **105**, 13c (1967)

Mianglianello, V.C., Murad, F., Vaughan, M.: Effects of lipolytic and anti-lipolytic agents on cyclic 3′,5′-adenosine monophosphate in fat cells. J. biol. Chem. **246**, 2195—2202 (1971)

Menahan, L.A., Wieland, O.: Interactions of glucagon and insulin on the metabolism of perfused livers from fasted rats. Europ. J. Biochem. **9**, 55—62 (1969)

Menahan, L.A., Hepp, K.D., Wieland, O.: Liver 3′,5′-nucleotide phosphodiesterase and its activity in rat livers perfused with insulin. Europ. J. Biochem. **8**, 435—443 (1969)

Miller, T.B., Larner, J.: Mechanism of control of hepatic glycogenesis by insulin. J. biol. Chem. **248**, 3483—3488 (1973)

Mirsky, I.A., Perisutti, G.: The inhibition of the action of insulin on rat epididymal adipose tissue by sulphydryl blocking agents. Biochim. biophys. Acta (Amst.) **62**, 490—496 (1962)

Morgan, H.E., Henderson, M.J., Regen, D.M., Park, C.R.: Regulation of glucose uptake in muscle. I. The effect of insulin and anoxia on glucose transport and phosphorylation in the isolated perfused heart of normal rats. J. biol. Chem. **236**, 253—261 (1961)

Morgan, C.R., Bonner, J.: Template activity of liver chromatin increased by *in vitro* administration of insulin. Proc. nat. Acad. Sci. (Wash.) **65**, 1077—1080 (1970)

Müller-Oerlinghausen, B., Schwabe, V., Hasselblatt, A., Schmidt, F.H.: Activity of A-3′,5′-Mp-PDE in liver and adipose tissue of normal and diabetic rats. Life Sci. **7**, 593—598 (1968)

Neubert, D., Lehninger, A.L.: The effect of thiols and disulfides on water uptake and extrusion by rat liver mitochondria. J. biol. Chem. **237**, 952—958 (1962)

Newsholme, A.E., Randle, P.J.: Regulation of glucose uptake by muscle. 5. Effects of anoxia, insulin, adrenaline and prolonged starving on concentrations of hexose phosphates in isolated rat diaphragm and perfused isolated rat heart. Biochem. J. **80**, 655—662 (1961)

Newsholme, A.E., Randle, P.J.: Regulation of glucose uptake by muscle. 7. Effects of fatty acids, ketone bodies and pyruvate, and of alloxan diabetes, starvation, hypophysectomy and adrenalectomy on the concentrations of hexose phosphates, nucleotides and inorganic phosphate in perfused rat heart. Biochem. J. **93**, 641—651 (1964)

Park, C.R., Lewis, S.B., Exton, J.H.: Relationship of some hepatic actions of insulin to the intracellular level of cyclic adenylate. Diabetes **21**, Suppl. 2, 439—446 (1972)

Pohl, S.L., Birnbaumer, L., Rodbell, M.: The glucagon sensitive adenyl cyclase system in plasma membranes of rat liver. I. Properties. J. biol. Chem. **246**, 1849—1856 (1971)

Rodbell, M., Birnbaumer, L., Pohl, S.L., Krans, H.M.J.: The glucagon-sensitive adenyl cyclase system in plasma membranes of rat liver. V. An obligatory role of guanyl nucleotide in glucagon action. J. biol. Chem. **246**, 1877—1882 (1971)

Rosselin, G., Freychet, P.: Basal and Hormone-stimulated Adenylate cyclase in liver plasma membranes: measurement by radioimmunoassay of cyclic AMP. Biochim. biophys. Acta (Amst.) **304**, 541—551 (1973)

Senft, G., Munske, K., Hoffman, M.: Influence of insulin on cyclic 3′,5′-AMP phosphodiesterase activity in liver, skeletal muscle, adipose tissue and kidney. Diabetologia **4**, 332—329 (1968)

Shen, L.C., Villar-Palasi, C., Larner, J.: Hormonal stimulation of protein kinase sensitivity to 3′,5′-cyclic AMP. Physiol. Chem. Physics **2**, 536—544 (1970)

Soderling, T.R., Corbin, J.D., Park, C.R.: Regulation of Adenosine 3′,5′-monophosphate dependent Protein kinase. J. biol. Chem. **248**, 1822—1829 (1973)

Søvik, O., Walaas, O.: Insulin stimulation of glycogen synthesis in the isolated rat diaphragm in the absence and in the presence of puromycin and actinomycin D. Nature (Lond.) **202**, 396—397 (1964)

Steiner, D.F., King, J.: Insulin-stimulated ribonucleic acid synthesis and RNA polymerase activity in alloxan-diabetic rat liver. Biochem. biophys. Acta (Amst.) **119**, 510—516 (1966)

Stirewalt, W.S., Wool, I.G., Cavicchi, P.: The relation of RNA and protein synthesis to the sedimentation of muscle ribosomes: effect of diabetes and insulin. Proc. nat. Acad. Sci. (Wash.) **57**, 1885—1892 (1967)

Sutherland, E.W., Robison, G.A.: The role of cyclic AMP in the control of carbohydrate metabolism. Diabetes **18**, 797—819 (1969)

Thompson, W.J., Appleman, M.M.: Multiple cyclic nucleotide phosphodiesterase activities from rat brain. Biochemistry **10**, 311—316 (1971)

Thompson, W.J., Little, S.A., Williams, R.H.: Effect of insulin and Growth Hormone on rat liver cyclic nucleotide phosphodiesterase. Biochemistry **12**, 1889—1894 (1973a)

Thompson, W.J., Williams, R.H., Little, S.A.: Activation of guanyl cyclase and adenyl cyclase by Secretin. Biochim. biophys. Acta (Amst.) **302**, 329—337 (1973b)

VOLFIN, P., EBOUÉ-BONIS, D., CLAUSER, H.: Effect of insulin on the phosphorus-32 mononucleotide labelling of the isolated rat diaphragm in the controlled absence of extracellular glucose. Nature (Lond.) **192**, 166—168 (1961)

VOLFIN, P.: Effect of insulin on adenylate kinase and glycolysis rate of the isolated rat diaphragm in the absence of added glucose. FEBS Letters **9**, 317—320 (1970)

WALAAS, O., WALAAS, E., WICK, A.N.: The stimulatory effect by insulin on the incorporation of ^{32}P radioactive inorganic phosphate. Adenine nucleotides and guanine nucleotides of the intact isolated rat diaphragm. Diabetologia **5**, 79—87 (1969)

WEBER, G., SINGHAL, R.L., SRIVASTAVA, S.K.: Insulin: suppressor of biosynthesis of hepatic gluconeogenic enzymes. Proc. nat. Acad. Sci. (Wash.) **53**, 96—104 (1965)

WILLIAMS, T.F., EXTON, J.H., FRIEDMANN, N., PARK, C.R.: Effects of insulin and adenosine 3′,5′-monophosphate on K^+ flux and glucose output in perfused rat liver. Amer. J. Physiol. **221**, 1654—1651 (1971)

WINEGRAD, A.I., RENOLD, A.E.: Studies on rat adipose tissue *in vitro*. I. Effects of insulin on the metabolism of glucose, pyruvate and acetate. J. biol. Chem. **233**, 265—272 (1958)

WOOL, I.G.: Insulin and incorporation of radioactivity into nucleic acid fraction of isolated diaphragm. Amer. J. Physiol. **199**, 719—721 (1960)

WOOL, I.G.: Effects of insulin on nucleic acid synthesis in isolated rat diaphragm. Biochim. biophys. Acta (Amst.) **68**, 28—33 (1963)

WOOL, I.G., MUNRO, A.J.: An influence of insulin on the synthesis of a rapidly labelled RNA by isolated rat diaphragm. Proc. nat. Acad. Sci. (Wash.) **50**, 918—923 (1963)

WOOL, I.G., MOYER, A.N.: Effect of actinomycin and insulin on the metabolism of isolated rat diaphragm. Biochim. biophys. Acta (Amst.) **91**, 248—256 (1964)

WOOL, I.G., RAMPERSAD, O.R., MOYER, A.N.: Effect of insulin and diabetes on protein synthesis by ribosomes from heart muscle. Amer. J. Physiol. **40**, 716—723 (1966)

WOOL, I.G., STIREWALT, W.S., MOYER, A.N.: Effect of diabetes and insulin on nucleic acid metabolism of heart muscle. Amer. J. Physiol. **214**, 825—831 (1968)

D. Metabolic Effects on Muscular Tissue

Torben Clausen

With 2 Figures

I. Introduction

Muscular tissues constitute the largest single volume of insulin-sensitive cells in the body. Due to metabolic activities and the selective permeability characteristics of the plasma membrane, the composition of this cytoplasmic reservoir differs markedly from that of its immediate surroundings. Therefore, the concentrations of metabolites and electrolytes in the extracellular milieu are to a significant extent controlled by the rates of transport and metabolism in muscle cells, and hence, the effects of insulin on these processes are of major importance also for the function of several other systems in the body. For the same reasons, the analysis of the over-all effects of insulin in the intact organism has often been based on studies with isolated preparations of muscular tissues. Thus, it is a natural purpose of this review to consider whether the results of such experiments may account for the observations made under *in vivo* conditions. Since the processes influenced by insulin are controlled by many factors, and since several conditions modify the response of muscle cells to the hormone, the effects of factors mimicking or interfering with insulin action have also been described, in particular when such studies yield information about basic mechanisms of control.

This survey is based on the literature available by the fall of 1972. Reviews pertaining to specific sections are referred to below, and several more general and comprehensive presentations of the earlier literature have been published (Krahl, 1961; Rieser, 1967; Dickens *et al.*, 1968; Litwack, 1970; Steiner and Freinkel, 1972).

II. Muscular Tissues Used for the Study of Insulin Action

Numerous preparations have been used for the characterization of the effects of insulin on muscle cells (Table 1a and b). In slices or homogenates of mammalian tissues, insulin has little or no effect, and in the diaphragm muscle, the response to the hormone has been shown to decrease in proportion to the number of fibres which have been cut (Liebecq, 1956; Kipnis and Cori, 1957). Even when this muscle is prepared with all its fibers intact, the stimulating effect of insulin on glycogen deposition is considerably less than that *in vivo* (Søvik, 1966).

The maintenance of optimum sensitivity to insulin is primarily a question of preserving the structural integrity of the cells, but since anoxia, contractile activity and disturbances in the normal distribution of electrolytes markedly modify the parameters influenced by the hormone, it is difficult to establish *in vitro* conditions which will allow comparison with observations made *in vivo*. Perfused tissues may maintain various cellular functions (including insulin responsiveness) better than isolated tissues incubated *in vitro*, but they are often less versatile, and sometimes not homogenous with respect to cell types and irrigation. Most skeletal muscles contain two or more fiber types, which may differ considerably with respect to structure (Needham, 1971) and metabolism (Bocek *et al.*, 1966). None of the preparations developed are entirely satisfactory, and in order to obtain a complete picture of the effects of insulin on muscle cells, the evidence obtained with one system will have to be supplemented with that gained in others.

The isolated perfused rat heart has the advantage of being able to maintain a considerable degree of functional integrity (Bleehen and Fisher, 1954; Morgan *et al.*, 1961a), and since it is easy to prepare for large series of experiments, it has been widely used for the study of insulin action (for review, see Morgan and Neely, 1972). The isolated rat diaphragm, which was first proposed by Meyerhof and Himwich in 1924, has become the classical choice for *in vitro* studies of insulin action (Gemmill, 1940). With the purpose of preserving the integrity of the muscle fibers, various modifications have been devised, in which the muscle is incubated with its attachments to the rib cage (Kipnis and Cori, 1957; Kono and Colowick, 1961; Creese and Northover, 1961; Creese, 1968). Whereas such "intact" diaphragm muscles have decisive advantages in studies of sugar and electrolyte uptake, the adhering central tendon, cartilage and cut intercostal fibers represent a major difficulty when such parameters as glucose uptake, the production of metabolites or the efflux of various solutes are to be evaluated. Because of these limitations together with the fact that the muscle is rythmically contracting up to the moment of its isolation, it is often desirable to consider alternative preparations, which are perhaps more representative of peripheral skeletal muscle. A variety of intact skeletal muscle preparations have been characterized (Table 1b) and seem to offer a number of advantages as compared to the diaphragm muscle.

Attempts to prepare intact isolated muscle cells by mechanical separation of fibers from large mammalian muscles have to some extent been successful, but not without appreciable loss of insulin-responsiveness (Beatty *et al.*, 1960). The

Table 1. *Basal and insulin-stimulated glucose consumption in some tissues used for the study of insulin action in muscle cells. The values are based upon measurements in the absence and the presence of a supramaximal concentration of the hormone*

a) Perfused preparations	Extracellular concentration of glucose (mM)	Glucose consumption (μmoles/g w.w./h) Basal	+insulin	References
1. Isolated heart (rabbit)	11.1	4.8	17.0	HEPBURN and LATCHFORD (1922)
Isolated heart (rabbit)	5.5	6.8	12.3	BODO and MARKS (1927)
Isolated heart (rat)	8.3	13.9	56.7	BLEEHEN and FISHER (1954)
Isolated heart (rat)	5.5	27.2	55.6	MORGAN *et al.* (1959)
Isolated heart (rat)	5.5	62.0	222.0	MORGAN *et al.* (1965)
2. Isolated rat diaphragm	5.6	28.9	32.2	BELOFF-CHAIN *et al.* (1971)
3. Eviscerated cat	12.0	2.3	4.0	BEST *et al.* (1926)
4. Hindquarter (rat)	5	1.9	4.5	MAHLER *et al.* (1968)
Hindquarter (rat)	5.5	1.0	14.6	RUDERMAN *et al.* (1971)
5. Hemicorpus (rat)	18.0	2.5	6.3	JEFFERSON *et al.* (1972)
6. Human forearm	5.0	0.4	4.1	ANDRES *et al.* (1962)
Human forearm	4.3	0.3	8.3	CHRISTENSEN and ØRSKOV (1968)
7. Human heart	5.3	8.1	26.8	RUDOLPH *et al.* (1969)

b) Preparations incubated *in vitro*	Extracellular concentration of glucose (mM)	Glucose consumption (μmoles/g/h) Basal	+insulin	References
1. Hemidiaphragm (rat)	11.1	10.0	18.9	GEMMILL (1940)
Hemidiaphragm (rat)	11.1	21.4	39.5	CLAUSEN (1968a)
Hemidiaphragm (rat)	7.8	27.8	43.3	LIEBECQ (1956)
Quarterdiaphragm (rat)	7.8	33.3	41.7	LIEBECQ (1956)
Hemidiaphragm (mouse)	5.5	37.1	45.1	OYAMA and GRANT (1959)
2. Intact diaphragm (rat) *o*) D-xylose	30[x])	11.2	30.4	KIPNIS and CORI (1957)
3. Soleus muscle (rat)	10.0	13.0	22.0	CHAUDRY and GOULD (1969)
Soleus muscle (rat)	1.0	0.7	3.1	CLAUSEN *et al.* (1973)
4. Extensor dig. long. (rat)	5.5	10.4	16.3	PAIN and MANCHESTER (1970)
5. M. levator ani + m. bulbocavernosus (rat)	13.9	7.9	13.7	ARVILL (1967)
6. Muscle fiber bundles (rat)	8.3	7.2	11.7	BEATTY *et al.* (1960)
Muscle fiber (macasus rhesus)	5.5	6.0	7.8	BOCEK and BEATTY (1969)
Muscle fiber (human)	8.3	5.0	5.0	HOLM and SCHERSTEN (1972)
7. Whole heart (fetal rat)				
15th day of gestation	7.0	22.2	25.0	CLARK (1971)
20th day of gestation	7.0	6.1	10.3	CLARK (1971)
Isolated heart cells (fetal rat)	7.0	1.5	3.2	CLARK (1971)
8. Whole hearts (chick)	8.0	10.5	15.5	GUIDOTTI *et al.* (1966)
9. Sartorius muscle (frog)	11.1	0.8	4.5	NARAHARA *et al.* (1960)
10. Taenia coli (guinea pig)	5.5	2.9	5.3	GROSSMANN and MANCHESTER (1966)
11. Bladder wall (toad)	5.5	0.5	0.8	BOWER and GRODSKY (1963)
12. Aorta (rabbit)	5.0	3.5	3.9	MULCAHY and WINEGRAD (1962)

digestion with collagenase, which has so successfully been used for the isolation of fat cells (RODBELL, 1964), has been tested in several laboratories, but still cannot be applied for the preparation of isolated muscle cells. By digesting hearts of newborn rats with trypsin and hyaluronidase, viable cells are obtained which can be cultivated and used for metabolic studies. However, these cells have a variable and modest responsiveness to insulin (DUNAND *et al.*, 1972; CLARK, 1971).

Much significant information about the effects of insulin on skeletal muscle and the heart in normals and diabetics has been obtained by simultaneous measurements of blood flow and the arterio-venous levels of metabolites and electrolytes in humans (ANDRES *et al.*, 1956; RUDOLPH *et al.*, 1969). With these techniques it has been possible in humans to confirm several of the observations made with isolated preparations of animal tissues.

III. Effects of Insulin on Transport Processes

1. Glucose and Other Sugars

a) Use of Sugars and Analogues

The prompt hypoglycemic effect of insulin is accounted for by a marked stimulation of glucose uptake in certain tissues, primarily skeletal muscle. In 1939, LUNDSGAARD showed that in the perfused hind limbs of the cat, the rate of glucose uptake approached saturation at high concentrations, and that the muscle cells contained no free glucose. This indicated that the diffusion of glucose from the blood plasma to the cells is not rate-limiting for its utilization, and it was suggested that the stimulating effect of insulin on glucose uptake was due to an action on the transport across the plasma membrane. Several other studies have shown that under basal conditions, little or no free glucose can be detected in the cytoplasm of skeletal or heart muscle cells, even at rather high extracellular levels (CORI *et al.*, 1933; BLEEHEN and FISHER, 1954; PARK *et al.*, 1955; PARK *et al.*, 1957; RANDLE and SMITH, 1958; KIPNIS, 1959; NARAHARA *et al.*, 1960; MORGAN *et al.*, 1961a). In the rat heart, free glucose accumulates in the cytoplasm only in the presence of insulin, and when the glucose concentration in the perfusate exceeds 5 mM (MORGAN *et al.*, 1961a). When the level of glucose-6-phosphate is increased by the administration of epinephrine, free glucose may be detected both *in vivo* and *in vitro* in the cytoplasm of skeletal muscle (KIPNIS, 1959). Under physiological conditions, transport of glucose seems to be rate-limiting for its utilization, but the capacity of the hexokinase may be exceeded.

A major argument for the idea that the action of insulin on glucose transport can be separated from the processes of phosphorylation was obtained by the demonstration that the hormone increases the space available to D-galactose, L-arabinose and D-xylose in the nephrectomized dog (LEVINE *et al.*, 1949). Since these sugars are only slowly metabolized under these conditions, it was concluded that insulin facilitates the transmembrane transport of sugars. This concept has been corroborated by numerous experiments with eviscerated animals, isolated muscles and perfused heart preparations, and non-metabolized sugars have become important tools in the characterization of insulin action (for reviews, see PARK *et al.*, 1959; LEVINE, 1965; PARK *et al.*, 1968; MORGAN and NEELY, 1972). In muscle cells, insulin increases the transport of several naturally occurring sugars — D-galactose (FISHER and LINDSAY, 1956; RESNICK and HECHTER, 1957; YOUNG, 1965), D-arabinose (CARLIN and HECHTER, 1961), L-arabinose (CARLIN and HECHTER, 1961; PARK *et al.*, 1961; FISHER and GILBERT, 1970), L-xylose (CARLIN and HECHTER, 1961), D-xylose (KIPNIS and CORI, 1957; FISHER and GILBERT, 1970), D-fructose (NAKADA, 1956), and D-glucosamine (NAKADA *et al.*, 1955; BELOFF-CHAIN *et al.*, 1970).

It seems likely that D-xylose and L-arabinose may share the glucose transport system, but their affinity is relatively low (Fisher and Lindsay, 1956; Battaglia and Randle, 1960). Studies with erythrocytes have shown that a C-1 chair conformation in the sugar molecule is the preferred structure for transport (LeFevre and Marshall, 1958), and this stereospecificity of the glucose transport system has led to the deliberate designing of synthetic glucose analogues (3-O-methylglucose and 2-deoxyglucose). These sugars have been found to have a high affinity for the glucose transport system, and their uptake is stimulated considerably by insulin (Kipnis, 1959; Narahara and Özand, 1963; Morgan *et al.*, 1964; Kipnis and Parrish, 1965; Kohn and Clausen, 1971). 3-O-methylglucose is not metabolized and causes no interference with carbohydrate metabolism in muscle (Csaky and Wilson, 1956; Narahara and Özand, 1963; Kohn and Clausen, 1971). Furthermore, its transport is not modified by labelling with ^{3}H or ^{14}C (Narahara and Özand, 1963).

b) Methodical Problems

One of the difficulties in evaluating results obtained with non-metabolized sugars is related to the fact that these compounds are readily released from the cytoplasm, and usually only the net result of influx and efflux is measured. Under basal conditions, the return of already accumulated sugar becomes a significant error when the intracellular concentration exceeds 16% of the extracellular (Narahara and Özand, 1963). Since an increase in influx is associated with a similar acceleration of efflux, the effect of stimuli to the sugar transport system may be considerably underestimated if only the net uptake is measured. Although these problems may partially be solved by reducing the incubation period, the time interval which ought to be used is often too short to allow an even distribution of the sugar in the extracellular space. In frog sartorius muscle and rat soleus muscle, the equilibration of mannitol and sucrose, respectively, was found to require from 40—60 min (Narahara and Özand, 1963; Law, 1967), and in the diaphragm and soleus muscles of the rat the concentration of glucose in the interstitual space was found to be lower than that of the incubation medium (Randle and Smith, 1958; Chaudry and Gould, 1969). Therefore, it is difficult to ascertain that all of the cells in a muscle preparation are exposed simultaneously to the sugar and that the concentration in the interstitial space is uniform.

The use of double-labelling for the simultaneous determination of the space available to a sugar and an extracellular marker of similar molecular weight has increased precision in the measurement of sugar uptake (Narahara and Özand, 1963; Bihler, 1968). However, the above-mentioned systematical sources of error have not been overcome, and the values obtained for kinetic constants (in particular in the presence of insulin) are as yet only of operational significance, and not a very reliable basis for models describing the effect of insulin on the properties of the glucose transport system.

Measurements of efflux from tissues which have been preloaded with a labelled non-metabolized sugar may yield values which over longer intervals of time are more representative of transport in mainly one direction (Morgan *et al.*, 1961b; Narahara and Özand, 1963; Young, 1965; Kohn and Clausen, 1971). Thus various stimuli for 3-O-methylglucose transport in soleus muscle of the rat were found to produce a considerably larger rise in the rate of efflux than in the rate of uptake. The same study provided some evidence that the individual cells in this muscle may differ considerably with respect to sugar permeability and insulin responsiveness — a conclusion also supported by studies of the incorporation of ^{14}C-labelled glucose into glycogen in muscle cells of the tongue (Coimbra, 1968).

c) Insulin Membrane Action and Degradation

It is generally assumed that the first step in the action of insulin consists of a contact or binding between the hormone and some specific receptor. Various muscle preparations can bind appreciable amounts of ^{131}I-labelled insulin (STADIE *et al.*, 1949; GARRATT *et al.*, 1966; WOHLTMANN and NARAHARA, 1966), but since it is rapidly degradated upon contact with this tissue, such studies have not yielded any precise information about the number of insulin receptors. In fact it is still not ascertained that the specific (displaceable) binding is related to the action of insulin and not merely the first step in the inactivation of the hormone (WOHLTMANN and NARAHARA, 1966). The recent demonstration that insulin bound to agarose particles stimulates glucose metabolism and amino acid transport (CUATRECASAS, 1969; OKA and TOPPER, 1972) indicates that the hormone need not enter the target cells to exert its action and that a very superficial and brief contact with the plasma membrane may be sufficient to elicit its effect.

During fetal life the basal rate of glucose uptake gradually decreases, and sensitivity towards insulin develops rather late, apparently coinciding with the appearance of insulin in the pancreas (GUIDOTTI *et al.*, 1961; CLARK, 1971; FELIX *et al.*, 1971).

In the perfused rat heart, the human forearm, and isolated rat soleus muscle, the stimulating effect of insulin on the transport of glucose and non-metabolized sugar can be detected within the time resolution of the systems used, i.e. less than 5 min after the first exposure to the hormone (BLEEHEN and FISHER, 1954; WILLIAMS, 1959; MORGAN *et al.*, 1961b; ANDRES *et al.*, 1962; MAHLER *et al.*, 1968; KOHN and CLAUSEN, 1971). Conversely, when a rat heart following exposure to insulin is perfused with insulin-free medium, the rate of glucose uptake returns to basal levels with the same speed as inulin is washed out ($T^1/_2$ of 3—5 min) (BLEEHEN and FISHER, 1954), indicating that the "resetting" of the glucose transport system can take place a few minutes after the removal of the hormone. In amphibian muscle, both the activation and the deactivation of the glucose transport system show a considerably longer time-lag. Thus, in the isolated frog sartorius muscle, stimulation of glucose uptake and 3-O-methylglucose transport could only be detected after 30 min of exposure to insulin (at 19°), and maximal rates were not achieved before 3 h later (NARAHARA *et al.*, 1960; NARAHARA and ÖZAND, 1963). The observation that the same preparation binds ^{131}I-insulin within 15 min indicates that the process of activation of the glucose transport system may be rate-limiting for the onset of insulin action (WOHLTMANN and NARAHARA, 1966). The same study showed that insulin-treated muscles maintain an increased sugar permeability during several hours of washing in insulin-free buffer.

The effect of insulin on glucose transport shows a definite dose-response relationship, but presumably due to degradation of the hormone or binding to glassware, the concentration range is often considerably higher than that prevailing in normal blood plasma. However, a stimulating effect of physiological levels of insulin on the transport of glucose and other sugars has repeatedly been demonstrated *in vitro*, allowing the use of this parameter for bioassay of serum insulin.

The response of smooth muscle cells to insulin is small and has so far only been detected with high concentrations of the hormone. Insulin stimulates glucose uptake in guinea pig taenia coli (GROSSMAN and MANCHESTER, 1966) and glycogen deposition in rabbit stomach muscle and bovine mesenteric arteries (LUNDHOLM and MOHME-LUNDHOLM, 1963). In the rat detrusor muscle, the facilitated transport of 3-O-methylglucose was reported to be insulin-sensitive (BIHLER *et al.*, 1971), and in the rat aorta, insulin was claimed to increase the incorporation of (1-^{14}C)-acetate into lipids (STOUT, 1971). Recently, a more systematic study has revealed that in the aorta of rabbits and rats, in rabbit colon and in bovine mesenteric arteries, insulin has a clear-cut, although delayed, stimulating effect on the transport of both glucose and non-metabolized sugars (ARNQUIST, 1973).

d) Kinetics

In muscle cells, the uptake of glucose takes place by a saturable process, and the demonstration of stereospecificity, competition by other sugars, and counterflow phenomena argue that the transfer across the plasma membrane is carrier-mediated. In order to obtain a more quantitative description of the mechanisms involved in the stimulation of the glucose transport system, the kinetic parameters of sugar permeation have been determined. On the basis of studies with erythrocytes and the formalism originally developped for the description of enzymatic processes, WILBRANDT and ROSENBERG (1961) proposed a series of mathematical expressions for the characterization of sugar transport. This approach requires that the cell population be homogeneous, that the sites capable of interacting with the sugar molecules are uniform with respect to affinity and accessability, and that unidirectional fluxes can be precisely determined. These requirements are almost certainly not met by the preparations of muscular tissues generally used, and there-

Table 2. *Kinetic constants for sugar uptake in various preparations of muscular tissue. The concentration of the sugars giving halfsaturation of the transport system (Apparent K_M) and the maximal transport rate (V_{max}) have been determined in the absence and the presence of a supramaximal concentration of insulin*

Preparation and sugar used for kinetic analysis (Reference)	Apparent K_M (mM)		V_{max} (μmoles/g/h)	
	Control	+Insulin	Control	+Insulin
Rat hemidiaphragm				
Glucose	22	9	46	46
(NORMAN *et al.*, 1959)				
Rat soleus				
Glucose	76	28	83	83
(CHAUDRY and GOULD, 1969)				
Perfused rat heart				
Glucose	9	28	102	500
(POST *et al.*, 1961)				
Perfused rat heart				
Glucose	11	27		
(MORGAN *et al.*, 1964)				
Perfused rat heart				
D-xylose	0.21	6.6		
L-arabinose	0.06	25.0		
(FISHER and ZACHARIAH, 1961)				
Perfused rat heart				
D-xylose	0.16	5.6	85	1440
L-arabinose	0.05	1.9	133	1580
(FISHER and GILBERT, 1970)				
CHICK heart				
Glucose	13	8	29	31
(GUIDOTTI *et al.*, 1966)				
Frog sartorius				
Glucose	6			
(NARAHARA *et al.*, 1960)				
Frog sartorius				
3-O-methylglucose	4.2	3.6	3.1	9.1
(NARAHARA and ÖZAND, 1963)				

fore, it is perhaps not so surprising that the effects of insulin on the apparent K_m and V_{max} for sugar transport obtained in various studies agree so poorly (Table 2).

Theoretically, insulin may stimulate sugar transport either by modifying the properties of the systems mediating the transfer of sugars under basal conditions, or by bringing new (and perhaps kinetically different) transport systems into function. The available information about kinetic constants does not allow any clear distinction between these general alternatives. The complex structure of muscle cells indicates that different areas of the plasma membrane (sarcolemma and T-tubules) separating the cytoplasm from the extracellular phase may participate to a variable extent in the exchange of sugars (KOHN and CLAUSEN, 1972) in analogy with what has already been suggested for the exchange of potassium and chloride (ALMERS, 1972).

These problems of heterogeneity together with those mentioned previously limit the value of kinetic analysis in the characterization of the action of insulin on sugar transport.

e) Inhibition of Insulin-Stimulated Sugar Transport

Phlorizin and phloretin are relatively specific inhibitors of sugar transport in a variety of tissues (CRANE, 1960). Several studies have indicated that phlorizin preferentially inhibits sugar transport in the presence of insulin, being ineffective under basal conditions (KELLER and LOTSPEICH, 1959; LOTSPEICH and WHEELER, 1962; BIHLER *et al.*, 1965). However, others have found an inhibitory effect on basal transport also (PARK *et al.*, 1959; WEIS and NARAHARA, 1969; KOHN and CLAUSEN, 1971), and it seems doubtful whether this compound (or phloretin) can be used as a tool for distinguishing different properties of the glucose transport system in the absence of and the presence of insulin.

Under basal conditions, the transport of 3-O-methylglucose and glucose in rat soleus muscle was not inhibited by high extracellular levels of K^+, hypotonicity or membrane stabilizers, all of which suppressed or abolished the stimulating effect of insulin (KOHN and CLAUSEN, 1972; CLAUSEN and KOHN, 1972; CLAUSEN *et al.*, 1973) (Fig. 1). However, also when 3-O-methylglucose transport was stimulated with trypsin, hyperosmolarity or 2,4-dinitrophenol, these factors caused considerable inhibition. Therefore, it seems likely that the glucose transport system (or systems) may exist in two alternative states, a basal and an active one. Insulin and a number of other factors may induce a reversible conversion of the former into the latter. A complete analysis of the insulin-induced signals eliciting this activation would require further experiments with inhibitors which allow a more detailed dissociation between the stimulating effect of insulin and that of other factors.

2. Electrolytes and Water

Ever since the first preparations of insulin became available, it has been known that the hormone besides its hypoglycemic effect also produces a prompt decrease in the concentration of potassium and phosphate in plasma (HARROP and BENEDICT, 1924; KERR, 1928). However, only recently, it has become clear that several of the effects on electrolyte metabolism can be dissociated from those on glucose transport (MANERY *et al.*, 1956; ZIERLER, 1959b; CREESE, 1968; WALAAS *et al.*, 1969). Thus, there are reasons to believe that the effects of insulin on the distribution of electrolytes and water can have a separate and specific significance — either in the regulation of electrolyte metabolism *per se* or by constituting signals modifying the processes of organic metabolism. A detailed review describing the effects of insulin on electrolytes and membrane potentials has recently appeared (ZIERLER, 1972).

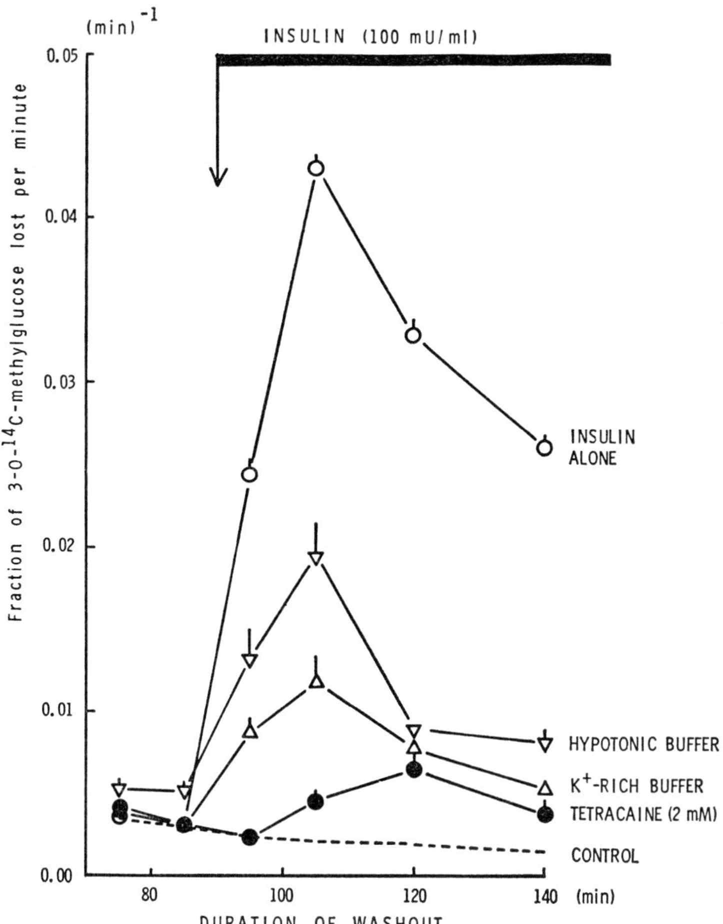

Fig. 1. Effect of insulin on 3-O-methylglucose transport in rat soleus muscle. Soleus muscles preloaded with 3-O-^{14}C-methylglucose were washed in a series of tubes containing Krebs-Ringer bicarbonate buffer without 3-O-methylglucose (for details, see KOHN and CLAUSEN, 1971). Control - - - - - -; Insulin (100 mU/ml) alone ○——○; Insulin (100 mU/ml) and tetracaine ●——●; Insulin (100 mU/ml), 100 mM NaCl replaced by 100 mM KCl △——△; Insulin (100 mU/ml), 80 mM NaCl omitted from the buffer ▽——▽. Insulin was added 90 min after the onset of washout; the other modifications or additions were introduced 10 min earlier. Each curve represents the mean of 3—11 observations with bars indicating S.E.M. (KOHN, P.G. and T. CLAUSEN, in preparation)

a) Monovalent Cations

α) Potassium

The hypokalemic effect of insulin seems to be the combined result of increased accumulation of K^+ in the cytoplasm of liver cells (MORTIMORE, 1961; WILLIAMS *et al.*, 1971), adipocytes (GOURLEY and BETHEA, 1964; PERRY and HALES, 1970), brain (ELLISON *et al.*, 1958) and (what probably accounts for the major part of the effect) in muscle cells (KAMMINGA *et al.*, 1950; ZIERLER, 1972). Several studies have shown that insulin produces an increase in the K^+-content of a variety of isolated preparations of muscular tissue. This effect is dose-dependent and can be detected with concentrations down to 10 μU/ml (KAMMINGA *et al.*, 1950). It is not affected by the omission of glucose from the incubation medium (ZIERLER, 1959b), but in frog muscle it seems to be associated with an increased metabolism of lactate (MANERY *et al.*, 1956). In the human forearm, infusion of insulin (200—700 μU/ml) into the brachial artery was found to increase the arterio-venous concentration difference for K^+ from —0.29 mM to +0.35 mM (ANDRES *et al.*, 1962), indicating that the effect of the hormone on K^+-exchange in muscle can be of major direct significance for the over-all K^+-distribution in humans. The augmented K^+-retention in peripheral muscle showed the same rate of onset as the rise in glucose consumption, but persisted at concentrations (38 μU/ml) where it was no longer possible to detect any change in the arterio-venous concentration difference for glucose (ZIERLER and RABINOWITZ, 1964). Also *in vitro*, insulin was found to cause a prompt decrease in K-efflux (ZIERLER, 1960).

Studies with the isolated extensor digitorum longus muscle of the rat indicate that the increased net accumulation of K^+ is the result of a decrease in K^+-efflux exceeding the decrease in K^+-influx, and it should be noted that only in muscles prepared from hypophysectomized rats, insulin produced a significant rise in the

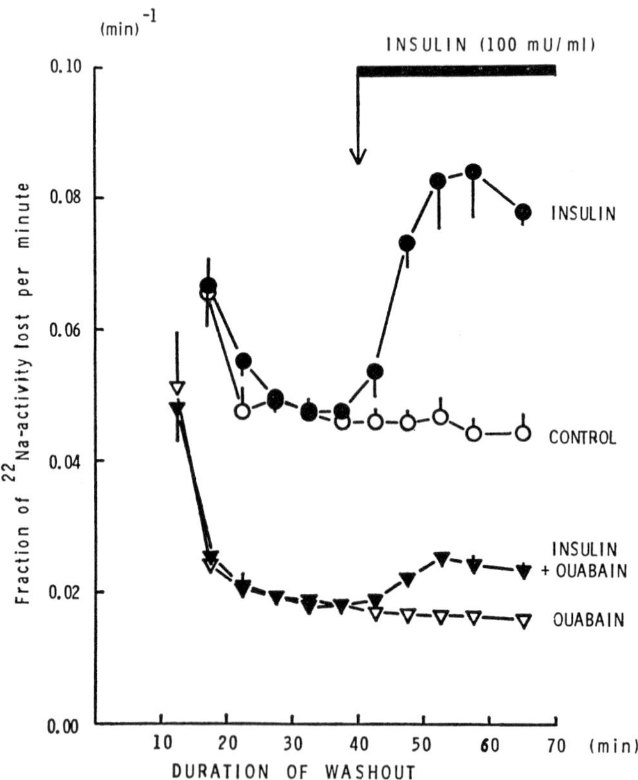

Fig. 2. Effects of insulin and ouabain on ^{22}Na-efflux from rat soleus muscle. Soleus muscles were preloaded with ^{22}Na for 60 min and washed in a series of tubes containing unlabdlled Krebs-Ringer bicarbonate buffer. Control ○——○; Ouabain (1 mM) present during loading and washout ▽——▽; Insulin (100 mU/ml) ●——●; Ouabain (1 mM) present during loading and washout, insulin (100 mU/ml) ▼——▼. Insulin was added 40 min after the onset of washout. Each curve represents the mean of 3 observations with bars indicating S.E.M. (KOHN, P.G. and T. CLAUSEN, in preparation)

intracellular concentration of K^+ (ZIERLER *et al.*, 1966). The alterations in K^+-exchange may be related to the concomitant rise in resting membrane potential, but the latter effect is almost certainly not the outcome of an increase in the concentration gradient for K^+ across the plasma membrane (ZIERLER, 1959a, 1972).

Insulin has never been found to produce more than a 10% increase in K^+-content (CREESE and NORTHOVER, 1961; GOURLEY, 1965), and because of the concomitant increase in cell volume, the increase in the intracellular K^+-concentration is very modest. Insulin has also been found to stimulate the accumulation of Rb^+ (HECHTER and LESTER, 1960).

β) Sodium

Studies with rat diaphragm indicate that the cytoplasmic concentration of Na^+ is much more markedly affected by insulin than is the K^+ level. CREESE and NORTHOVER (1961) found that following incubation for 2 h in the presence of insulin, the concentration of Na^+ in the fiber water was only one half that of the controls. This effect is probably accounted for by the observation that in the same tissue insulin accelerates the efflux of labelled Na^+ by 36% (CREESE, 1968). It was suggested that the hormone stimulates the active coupled transport of Na^+ and K^+, but according to unpublished findings, the efflux of labelled Na^+ from the extensor digitorum longus muscle was increased both in the absence and in the presence of ouabain (ZIERLER, 1966). Furthermore, the activity of Na-K-activated ATPase isolated from rat skeletal muscle is not significantly altered by insulin treatment, neither *in vivo* nor *in vitro* (ROGUS *et al.*, 1969).

From Fig. 2 it can be seen that insulin stimulates the release of ^{22}Na from isolated rat soleus muscle even when the active Na-K-transport is blocked by 1 mM ouabain. As already shown by CREESE (1968), this effect did not depend on the availability of glucose (or other metabolizable substrate) in the incubation medium. Phlorizin (5 mM) or tetracaine (0.5—1.0 mM) did not interfere with the effect, indicating that it is not related to sugar transport or the non-active flux of Na^+ (KOHN and CLAUSEN, in preparation). The stimulating effect of insulin on the release of both ^{22}Na and ^{14}C-labelled 3-O-methylglucose could be detected within 2 min after the onset of exposure to the hormone, and the time resolution of the method has not allowed any conclusion about dissociation in time (CLAUSEN, unpublished observations).

Insulin has also been found to decrease the Na^+-content in frog muscles (KERNAN, 1962; MOORE, 1965), and in the extensor digitorum longus muscle of hypophysectomized rats, insulin reduced both total and intracellular Na^+ to the level found in untreated muscles from normal animals (ZIERLER *et al.*, 1966). The true cytoplasmic concentration of Na^+ cannot be determined with satisfactory precision, and the recent suggestion that 95% of the fiber Na^+ is located in the sarcoplasmic reticulum would indicate that previous figures represent considerable overestimates (ZIERLER, 1972). It is still possible that the effect of insulin on Na^+-content is not the result of accelerated efflux across the sarcolemma, but rather related to changes in the Na^+-pool contained in the sarcoplasmic tubules.

In crab muscle, intracellular application of the hormone leads to acceleration of Na^+efflux (BITTAR, 1967). There is some indirect evidence that insulin may under certain conditions (in diaphragm muscle from K^+-depleted rats) stimulate the influx of Na^+ (OTSUKA and OHTSUKI, 1970).

It is still difficult to draw any conclusions about the over-all significance of the preceding effects. Thus, no reports have described the effect of physiological concentrations of the hormone on Na^+-transport, and since incubation with insulin *in vitro* does not reduce the Na^+ content to levels below those found in fresh muscle, it is impossible to assess the role of the hormone in the maintenance of Na^+ distribution *in vivo*. Insulin does not produce any detectable change in serum Na^+, but effects on Na-transport have been claimed to be of importance for the genesis of muscular failure in patients with hypokalemic periodic paralysis (OTSUKA and OHTSUKI, 1970). A paralyzing effect of insulin on diaphragm muscles from K^+-depleted animals has been related to the generalized paralysis of the extremities occasionally seen in patients treated for diabetic coma (OFFERIJNS *et al.*, 1958). It was recently reported that K^+-infusion leads to a rise in insulin-secretion and a transfer of K^+ to the intracellular fluid in dogs. In pancreatectomized animals, there was almost no net transfer of K^+ into the intracellular phase, and insulin normalized this defect. On this basis it was suggested that the hormone is of significance in the regulation of the extracellular K^+-level during episodes of hyperkaliemia (HIATT *et al.*, 1974).

b) Divalent Cations

The injection of insulin has been found to produce a small transient increase in the concentration of Ca in the blood plasma of rabbits (DAVIES *et al.*, 1926), dogs (BROUGHER, 1927) and humans (VALENCIA, 1954; HAMMARSTEN and SMITH, 1956). In dogs, hyperglycemia induced by intravenous administration of glucose led to a rise in serum Ca^{++} (COWAN and WRIGHT, 1932). Since changes in serum phosphate are often associated with inverse alterations in the Ca^{++} level, it was suggested that the hypercalcemic effect of insulin was related to the simultaneous decrease in serum phosphate (BROUGHER, 1927). Unfortunately, there are no reports on the effect of insulin on Ca-transport in muscle, but the hormone seems to influence the interaction between Ca and the plasma membrane. Thus insulin was found to inhibit the binding of Ca to isolated liver plasma membrane (MARINETTI *et al.*, 1972) and to a monolayer composed of monooctadecyl phosphate (KAFKA and PAK, 1969). This together with the observation that insulin stimulates the release of ^{45}Ca from preloaded epididymal fat pads (CLAUSEN, 1969) suggests that changes in Ca^{++} distribution may be a more direct and general part of insulin action.

Serum Mg has been reported to be increased (VALENCIA, 1954), unaltered (HAMMARSTEN and SMITH, 1956; AIKAWA, 1960) or decreased (Martin and WERTMAN, 1947; WHANG *et al.*, 1969) by insulin. A significant increase in the Mg content of skeletal muscle and the heart was observed in insulin-treated rabbits (AIKAWA, 1960). The relationship between Mg and carbohydrate metabolism has recently been reviewed (DURLACH, 1971).

c) Anions

It is an old observation that the administration of insulin to diabetics (HARROP and BENEDICT, 1924) and normals leads to a drop in the level of inorganic phosphate in serum or whole blood (WIGGLESWORTH *et al.*, 1922; KERR, 1928; CORI and CORI, 1931), and several studies with perfused hindlimbs (POLLACK *et al.*, 1934; LUNDSGAARD, 1938) and isolated muscles (CLAUSER *et al.*, 1962; WALAAS *et al.*, 1969) indicate that this may be related to a stimulation of the uptake of phosphate in muscle cells. Insulin was found to increase the incorporation of ^{32}P into organic phosphates in rat hemidiaphragm (CLAUSER *et al.*, 1962), and more recently, experiments with the intact diaphragm preparation demonstrated that this is the outcome of a stimulating effect on the uptake of inorganic phosphate (WALAAS *et al.*, 1969). Contrary to previous belief, the effect of insulin on phosphate transport was found to be unrelated to the phosphorylation of glucose. Both in the isolated diaphragm and in the perfused heart of rats, insulin was found to stimulate phosphate uptake or prevent the loss of phosphate in the absence of glucose (KAJI and PARK, 1961; SARKAR and OTTAWAY, 1962).

Since the effect of insulin on phosphate uptake was suppressed by ouabain or the omission of Na^+ from the incubation medium, it is possible that the hormone activates a component of phosphate transport which is related to the active Na-K-transport (WALAAS *et al.*, 1969). In muscle, inorganic phosphate must be transported into the cytoplasm against an electrochemical gradient, and in intact muscle preparations, this is a very slow process. The fact that insulin more than doubled the specific activity of cellular inorganic phosphate cannot be accounted for by a rise in the resting membrane potential, but suggests that the hormone stimulates an energy-requiring transport mechanism. See furthermore section C (article of Volfin + Hanoune).

Insulin was found to decrease the Cl^- content and the intracellular Cl^- concentration in extensor digitorum longus muscles from hypophysectomized rats (ZIERLER *et al.*, 1966).

d) Membrane Potential

ZIERLER (1957) first demonstrated that insulin increases the resting membrane potential in the extensor digitorum longus muscle of the rat. In frog skeletal muscle (DE MELLO, 1967; MOORE, 1965) and in the isolated diaphragm muscle a closely similar effect has been observed (BOLTE and LÜDERITZ, 1968; OTSUKA and OHTSUKI, 1970), but there is no direct evidence that the phenomenon occurs *in vivo*.

In the extensor digitorum longus muscle of the rat, insulin (100 mU/ml) was found to produce a progressive rise in the resting membrane potential, which could be detected within 10 min (ZIERLER, 1959). The average value was increased from 74—79 mV, the deeper fibers being more sensitive than the superficial. The same effect was obtained in the absence of glucose (ZIERLER, 1959). The dose-response relationships have not been reported, and it is not known whether the membrane potential is also elevated by physiological concentrations of insulin. Although the effect seems modest, it cannot be accounted for by the rise in K^+-content of the muscles, which was furthermore shown to occur much later (ZIERLER, 1959). The stimulating effect of insulin on Na-efflux may well contribute to the hyperpolarization, but much more complete bookkeeping is required before it will be possible to explain the effect of insulin on the membrane potential in terms of ionic fluxes.

It should be noted that insulin may also produce a depolarization of up to 20 mV when added to diaphragm muscles from K-deficient animals (OTSUKA and OHTSUKI, 1970; BOLTE and LÜDERITZ, 1968). Since this effect correlated with the extracellular concentration of Na^+, it was assumed to be the outcome of accelerated Na-influx. Low extracellular levels of K^+ were found to accentuate the effect, possibly because the K^+-permeability is lowered to a level where a rise in the efflux of K^+ is insufficient to produce a resetting of the membrane potential (OTSUKA and OHTSUKI, 1970).

e) Water

One of the difficulties in evaluating the relatively modest effects of insulin on electrolyte distribution arises from the fact that the hormone seems to cause a shift in cellular water. Both in the diaphragm and in the extensor digitorum longus muscle of the rat, insulin was found to induce a decrease in inulin space (RANDLE and SMITH, 1958; CREESE and NORTHOVER, 1961; FRITZ and KNOBIL, 1963; ZIERLER *et al.*, 1966; HIDER *et al.*, 1971). In mammalian muscle, this seems almost entirely to be accounted for by a corresponding rise in cell volume, but in frog sartorius, insulin was found to increase total wet weight (GOURLEY and KYU SUH, 1966). In the extensor digitorum longus muscle of the rat, it was suggested that the swelling effect of insulin is secondary to an increased uptake of glucose (ZIER-

LER *et al.*, 1966). However, insulin induced a gain in wet weight of frog sartorius also in the absence of glucose. It is interesting that when the extracellular space is measured using markers of lower molecular weight (raffinose, mannitol or sulfate), insulin seems to be without effect (RANDLE and SMITH, 1958; NARAHARA *et al.*, 1960; HIDER *et al.*, 1971).

3. Relationship Between the Transport of Glucose and Electrolytes

In cells capable of transporting glucose against a concentration gradient (in kidney and intestine), the accumulation of sugars has been shown to require Na^+ ions (RIKLIS and QUASTEL, 1958; KLEINZELLER and KOTYK, 1961) and to be inhibited by cardiac glycosides (CSAKY, 1963). In intestine, the concentration gradients for Na^+ and K^+ across the mucosal cell membrane seem to determine the capacity for cytoplasmic accumulation of sugars (CRANE, 1964), and sugars are co-transported with Na^+ ions (CURRAN, 1965). These findings have prompted a wealth of studies into the role of electrolytes in the transport of organic compounds (for review, see SCHULTZ and CURRAN, 1970; HEINZ, 1972). Although it has not been possible to demonstrate an active accumulation of sugars coupled to ionic gradients in muscle, electrolytes or the distribution of electrolytes across the plasma membrane may influence both basal and insulin-stimulated sugar transport quite markedly (CLAUSEN, 1972).

a) Extracellular Ionic Milieu

In muscle, the presence of Na^+ or K^+ in the extracellular milieu is not essential for the uptake or efflux of sugars or the stimulation of these processes by insulin (PARRISH and KIPNIS, 1964; KOHN and CLAUSEN, 1972; CLAUSEN, 1972). The isoosmolar replacement of NaCl by sucrose or LiCl leads to an increase in glucose uptake or in the influx and efflux of non-metabolized sugars (BHATTACHARYA, 1961, 1964; CLAUSEN, 1968b; ILSE and ONG, 1970; KOHN and CLAUSEN, 1972; CLAUSEN, 1972). However, when K^+ is used for the substitution of Na^+, the basal uptake of glucose, xylose and 3-O-methylglucose may be diminished (BHATTACHARYA, 1961; MENOZZI and POLLERI, 1961; CLAUSEN, 1968a; GOULD and CHAUDRY, 1970; BIHLER and SAWH, 1971b). Others found no effect of K^+-substitution on the basal permeability to glucose, 2-deoxyglucose or 3-O-methylglucose (KIPNIS and PARRISH, 1965; KOHN and CLAUSEN, 1972), but the stimulating effect of insulin on sugar transport was consistently found to be suppressed by K^+, even at concentrations as low as those used in the standard incubation media (6 mM) (GOULD and CHAUDRY, 1970; BIHLER and SAWH, 1971a). Since the stimulating effect of metabolic inhibitors, trypsin and hyperosmolarity is also suppressed by K^+-substitution, the phenomenon is not specifically related to the action of insulin, but is rather the result of interference with the function of the glucose transport system or its mechanisms of activation (KOHN and CLAUSEN, 1972).

This evidence is suggestive of some similarity with the process of sugar accumulation in kidney and intestine, where K^+ seems to exert a rather specific inhibitory action. On the other hand, the addition of up to 100 mM of KCl in excess of the other components of the incubation medium caused no change in the insulin-stimulated efflux of 3-O-methylglucose in rat soleus muscle (KOHN and CLAUSEN, 1972). Isoosmotic K^+-substitution may cause considerable swelling of muscle cells (KIPNIS and PARRISH, 1965; KOHN and CLAUSEN, 1972; CLAUSEN and KOHN, 1972). When swelling is induced merely by reducing the tonicity of the incubation medium, insulin-stimulated glucose uptake and 3-O-methylglucose transport are inhibited to about the same extent as they are in K^+-substituted media (Fig. 2).

This fact argues against any direct or specific effect of K^+ ions on the glucose transport system. Systematic studies on the effect of various cations and anions on basal and insulin-stimulated glucose uptake indicate that under certain conditions, Cl^- and Mg^{++} may be of importance for the effect of insulin (BHATTACHARYA, 1961; GOULD and CHAUDRY, 1970). Although it is difficult on the basis of the evidence available to identify any of the common extracellular ions as being essential for the processes of glucose transport and its activation by insulin there is no doubt that certain ions may have quite pronounced effects *per se*. In rat hemidiaphragm, Li^+ was found to promote glucose uptake at concentrations down to 5 mM (BHATTACHARYA, 1964; CLAUSEN, 1968b). Li^+-injection causes a decrease in blood glucose in rabbits and rats (BHATTACHARYA, 1964). The stimulating effect of Li^+ on glucose uptake and 3-O-methylglucose transport increased with the duration of exposure, suggesting an indirect mode of action, possibly developing *pari passu* with the intracellular accumulation of the ion (CLAUSEN, 1968b; KOHN and CLAUSEN, 1972). In frog rectus abdominis muscle, Li-substitution was found to increase the resting tension, indicating that factors eliciting the processes of muscle contraction may be of importance for the increased sugar permeability (IRWIN and OLIVER, 1970). A correlation between a stimulating effect of nitrate ions on twitch tension and 3-O-methylglucose transport in frog sartorius muscle has been considered as an argument for a similar contention (HOLLOSZY and NARAHARA, 1967b).

In the intact organism, acidosis has been shown to reduce glucose tolerance (HALDANE *et al.*, 1924), to produce hyperglycemia and to reduce the effects of insulin on the concentration of glucose, K^+ and phosphate in serum (MACKLER *et al.*, 1951; WALKER *et al.*, 1963). In the isolated rat diaphragm a lowering of the extracellular pH inhibited the uptake of glucose (GEVERS and DOWDLE, 1963) and its stimulation by insulin (WALKER *et al.*, 1963). In the perfused rat heart, glucose utilization increased with pH in the range from 6.7—7.7 (DELCHER and SHIPP, 1966). In rat soleus muscle, glucose uptake attained maximum values at a pH of 8, and was clearly increased by insulin in the whole range from 6.7—8.9 (CHAUDRY and GOULD, 1969). Since hydrogen ions have marked metabolic effects, it is difficult to draw any conclusion about their significance for the function of the glucose transport system without information about the transport of nonmetabolized sugars.

b) Intracellular Ionic Milieu

Inhibition of the active Na^+-K^+-transport with cardiac glycosides or by incubation in K^+-free buffer was found to stimulate glucose uptake (KYPSON *et al.*, 1968b) and 3-O-methylglucose transport in rat diaphragm muscle (BIHLER, 1968). This effect was correlated with the ensuing rise in the intracellular Na/K-ratio and was not the direct consequence of an inhibited active Na-K-transport (BIHLER and SAWH, 1971b). Others have not been able to detect any early effects of these compounds (or K^+-omission on the uptake of glucose, 2-deoxyglucose or galactose in diaphragm muscle (KIPNIS and PARRISH, 1965; CLAUSEN, 1965b, 1966) or the transport of 3-O-methylglucose in soleus muscle (KOHN and CLAUSEN, 1971, 1972).

The variability and time-lag of the insulin-like effect produced by reducing the Na^+-K^+gradients across the plasma membrane would suggest that other factors are involved. Similar conditions have been found to induce contractures in the rectus abdominis muscle of the frog (SHIGEI *et al.*, 1963; IRWIN and OLIVER, 1970), indicating a rise in the cytoplasmic level of Ca^{++}. In frog sartorius muscle, K^+-omission or ouabain was found to increase the uptake of labelled Ca, and the Ca-content was correlated to the Na^+ content (COSMOS and HARRIS, 1960). In nerve axon (BAKER, 1970), cardiac muscle (REUTER and SEITZ, 1968), aortic wall (REUTER *et al.*, 1973) and in adipose tissue (CLAUSEN, 1970), the transport of Ca^{++} across the plasma membrane seems to be linked to Na^+-transport. A rise in the intracellular Ca-content might be induced by an increase in the Na^+-level, and this would again depend on the rates of Na^+-fluxes and the exchangeability of the Ca accumulated in various cellular pools. HOLLOSZY and NARAHARA (1967a) were the first to suggest that Ca^{++} ions may be of importance in the activation of the sugar transport system.

In slices of heart muscle, cardiac glycosides were found to stimulate the metabolism of glucose (WOLLENBERGER, 1947). Digoxin (10^{-7} mole/kg) was reported to stimulate glucose utilization (KIEN and SHERROD, 1960) and galactose uptake in the heart of normal dogs (KIEN *et al.*, 1960). Studies with isolated perfused hearts from rats and guinea pigs have shown that ouabain increases glucose consumption and arabinose uptake (KREISBERG and WILLIAMSON, 1964; HOESCHEN, 1971; ELBRINK and BIHLER, 1973). This may be secondary to the inotropic effects of these drugs and may be related to a change in intracellular Ca^{++}. Toxic concentrations of ouabain, however, seemed to stimulate arabinose transport markedly, independently of contractile activity (ELBRINK and BIHLER, 1973). Ouabain has also been found to mimick the effect of insulin in reducing the blood sugar (TRINER *et al.*, 1968) and in accelerating the disappearance of intravenously injected ^{14}C-galactose (KIEN *et al.*, 1960). This may in part be the result of increased release of of insulin (MILNER and HALES, 1967), since it is not seen in pancreatectomized dogs.

Several studies have shown that K^+-depletion *in vivo* leads to decreased glucose tolerance (GARDNER *et al.*, 1950; FUHRMAN, 1951; SAGILD and ANDREASEN, 1961; BARTELHEIMER *et al.*, 1967; SPERGEL *et al.*, 1967; MONDON *et al.*, 1968; GORDEN *et al.*, 1972). In view of the complex compensatory phenomena associated with K^+-depletion in the intact organism, it is difficult to account for this effect, and unfortunately, there is no information available on basal permeability to glucose or the insulin-responsiveness in muscular tissues isolated from K^+-deficient animals.

c) Ionic Permeability of the Plasma Membrane

A wide variety of compounds have been found to suppress excitatory phenomena and reduce the permeability of the plasma membrane to ions (SHANES, 1958). Various categories of these so-called membrane stabilizers have been found to reduce the glucose tolerance, but it is difficult to determine whether this is due to peripheral effects or to disturbances in the secretion of the hormones controlling carbohydrate metabolism (AMDISEN, 1958; DUNDEE, 1956; JORI *et al.*, 1964; MENNEAR and MIYA, 1970; FARISS and LUTCHER, 1971; TREASURE and TOSELAND, 1971; DAVIDSON, 1971).

On the other hand, chlorpromazine and other phenothiazines were found to inhibit the uptake of glucose and galactose in rat hemidiaphragm (RAFAELSEN, 1961), and phenytoin was recently reported to diminish the permeability to 3-O-methylglucose in the intact rat diaphragm (BIHLER and SAWH, 1971c). HALES and PERRY (1970) showed that local anesthetics suppress the stimulating effect of insulin and epinephrine on glucose utilization in fat cells, and later, several categories of membrane stabilizers (tetracaine, lidocaine, thiomebumal, chlorpromazine and imipramine) have been found to diminish or abolish the effect of insulin on glucose uptake, glycogen deposition and 3-O-methylglucose transport in isolated rat soleus muscle (CLAUSEN *et al.*, 1973). These compounds did not inhibit basal sugar transport, but partly prevented the rise in 3-O-methylglucose permeability induced by trypsin and hyperosmolarity. The short time-lag of the effect suggests a rather direct action on the sugar transport system (Fig. 2). Lower concentrations of the membrane stabilizers, which clearly diminished the permeability to Na^+ and K^+, had no effect on sugar transport, and since there was no correlation between the change in K^+-content and the inhibition of 3-O-methylglucose transport, it seems reasonable to conclude that the latter is a separate manifestation of the phenomenon of membrane stabilization, not directly related to the transport or distribution of Na^+ and K^+ across the plasma membrane (CLAUSEN *et al.*, 1973).

IV. Effects of Insulin on Metabolic Processes

1. Sugar Phosphorylation

The first step in the metabolism of glucose is a phosphorylation catalyzed by hexokinase. In muscle extracts, at least 3 types of this enzyme can be isolated chromatographically. The K_m's of types I, II, and III (KATZEN and SCHIMKE, 1965) are, respectively, 2.4×10^{-5}M, 2×10^{-4}M and 5×10^{-6}M. However, in the intact tissue, the apparent K_m for glucose phosphorylation seems to be considerably higher (ÖZAND *et al.*, 1962; MORGAN *et al.*, 1961a), indicating that part of the cellular hexokinase is separated from its substrate. Indeed, up to 45% of the hexokinase activity in skeletal muscle was found to be associated with cell organelles (KATZEN *et al.*, 1970), and the reversibility of this binding (KARPATKIN and BRAUN, 1971) suggests that changes in the over-all phosporylating capacity may be regulated by redistribution of the enzyme among various pools.

The rate of phosporylation can be increased by anoxia (MORGAN *et al.*, 1959; ÖZAND *et al.*, 1962; KARPATKIN *et al.*, 1966), contractile activity (KARPATKIN *et al.*, 1966), and to some extent by insulin (MORGAN *et al.*, 1961a). Under all of these conditions (in particular in the presence of insulin), however, the rate of glucose penetration may exceed the phosphorylating capacity leading to accumulation of free glucose in the cytoplasm (KIPNIS *et al.*, 1959; NARAHARA *et al.*, 1960; MORGAN and NEELY, 1972). The phosphorylation of glucose may also be rate limiting for its utilization under other conditions, i.e. when the glucose-6-phosphate level is augmented by epinephrine (KIPNIS *et al.*, 1959; ÖZAND *et al.*, 1962).

Streptozotocin-induced diabetes is associated with a 30—40% decrease in the total activity of muscle hexokinase, probably primarily accounted for by an apparently selective suppression of type II. The administration of insulin leads to restoration of activity within a few hours, and even supranormal levels may be achieved (KATZEN *et al.*, 1970). This may explain the decreased phosphorylating capacity of muscular tissues isolated from diabetic animals (KIPNIS and CORI, 1960; PARK *et al.*, 1961).

It has been suggested that the membrane-associated hexokinases may have a role in sugar transport, possibly as carrier structures (KATZEN, 1969), but if this hypothesis should account for the transport of non-phosphorylated sugars also, more detailed information about the relative affinities of these compounds is required.

2. Glycogen Metabolism

a) Amount and Labelling Studies

The single metabolic process in muscle cells which is most markedly stimulated by insulin is the synthesis of glycogen. As early as 1926, BEST *et al.* demonstrated that in the eviscerated spinal cat, more than half of the extra glucose taken up in the presence of insulin could be accounted for as glycogen; and the effect of the hormone on glycogen metabolism has now been characterized in numerous studies with a large variety of preparations. The detailed information available has been described in recent reviews (WHELAN, 1968; VILLAR-PALASI, 1969; VILLAR-PALASI and LARNER, 1970; NUTTALL, 1972; ADOLFSSON, 1972), and here, only some major features of the phenomenon will be discussed.

Both *in vivo* and *in vitro*, insulin may bring about a net increase in the total glycogen content of diaphragm muscle (GEMMILL, 1940; STADIE and ZAPP, 1947; RAFAELSEN, 1964; WERMERS *et al.*, 1970), soleus muscle (MOORTHY and GOULD, 1969), the heart (EVANS, 1934; WILLIAMSON and KREBS, 1961; ADOLFSSON, 1972; ADOLFSSON *et al.*, 1972), and levator ani muscle of rats (ADOLFSSON, 1972); but experiments with intact diaphragm muscles *in vitro* indicate that the rate of incorporation of glucose and the turnover of glycogen may be markedly increased without major alterations in the glycogen content (SØVIK, 1966; BELOFF-CHAIN *et al.*, 1971). In patients with diabetes mellitus the muscle glycogen content is lowered and insulin treatment leads to a net increase (ROCH-NORLUND *et al.*, 1970). In perfused hearts and diaphragm muscles from diabetic rats, the incorporation of ^{14}C-labelled glucose into glycogen is suppressed both in the absence and in the presence of insulin (BELOFF-CHAIN *et al.*, 1971; CHAIN *et al.*, 1969). The same authors found that insulin causes a marked rise in the labelling of oligo-saccharides.

Since even very low concentrations of insulin increase the glycogen content, this parameter has been used in bioassay (JESSUP and WIBERG, 1961; RAFAELSEN, 1964), but measurements of the amount of ^{14}C-glucose incorporated into glycogen undoubtedly yields a much more sensitive means of evaluating changes in the rate of glycogen synthesis. The bioassay developed by RAFAELSEN *et al.* (1965) exemplifies the pronounced favoring of glycogen deposition induced by insulin. In rats or mice, the incorporation of ^{14}C-activity into diaphragm glycogen was increased up to 200-fold when ^{14}C-glucose was injected intraperitoneally along with the hormone (RAFAELSEN *et al.*, 1965; CLAUSEN, 1965a; STAUFFACHER and RENOLD, 1969; YOUNG and BALANT, 1972). These studies together with *in vitro* experiments show that the magnitude of the insulin effect depends on the integrity of the muscle preparation used (STADIE and ZAPP, 1947; SØVIK, 1966).

In vitro, the stimulating effect of insulin on the incorporation of labelled glucose into glycogen is most pronounced during the initial phase of incubation (CLAUSEN, 1968a; ADOLFSSON *et al.*, 1972), probably because the accumulation of glycogen leads to inhibition of further synthesis (DANFORTH, 1965).

In rat hemidiaphragms incubated for 10 min, 96% of the insulin-stimulated uptake of glucose could be accounted for as glycogen (LARNER *et al.*, 1959). Increased glycogen deposition may also be achieved by augmenting the glucose concentration, but this rise is considerably smaller than that seen with similar increases in glucose uptake produced by the addition of insulin (NORMAN *et al.*, 1959).

b) Glycogen Synthetase

The enzyme which catalyzes the transfer of glucose from uridine-diphosphoglucose into glycogen (LELOIR and CARDINI, 1957) has been shown to exist in two forms, synthetase D, which is phosphorylated and essentially only active in the presence of glucose-6-phosphate, and synthetase I, which is the dephosphorylated form of the same enzyme and active in the absence of glucose-6-phosphate (VILLAR-PALASI and LARNER, 1960; LARNER *et al.*, 1969). The synthetase is rate-limiting for the conversion of glucose into glycogen (VILLAR-PALASI and LARNER, 1961). It has been purified and seems to consist of 2—4 subunits with a molecular weight of 90,000 (SODERLING *et al.*, 1970; SMITH *et al.*, 1971). In the isolated rat hemidiaphragm it was shown that insulin (even in the absence of glucose) induced a prompt (within 10 min) increase in the ratio between the activities of synthetase

I and D (Villar-Palasi and Larner, 1960; Craig and Larner, 1964). This effect has later been detected in several other muscular tissues, both *in vitro* and *in vivo* (see review by Nuttall, 1972) as well as in muscle biopsies from diabetic patients (Roch-Norlund *et al.*, 1972). These observations led to the now generally accepted view that insulin specifically facilitates the conversion of glucose into glycogen by an action that is separate from and cannot be accounted for by its stimulating effect on glucose transport. The two effects of insulin can also be dissociated by inhibitors of protein synthesis (puromycin and actinomycin D) which diminish or abolish the effect of insulin on glycogen deposition and on the glycogen synthetase without causing any change in the action on glucose uptake (Søvik, 1965, 1967). Conversely, insulin stimulates glycogen synthesis and the D to I conversion of synthetase even when the effect on glucose uptake is considerably suppressed by N-ethylmaleimide (Eboué-Bonis *et al.*, 1967).

The D-form of the synthetase may not be able to catalyze the synthesis of glycogen at all under the conditions normally prevailing in the cytoplasm (Piras *et al.*, 1968), and a conversion into the I-form would therefore appear to account for the stimulation of glycogen synthesis produced by insulin.

However, although the incorporation of ^{14}C-glucose into glycogen of rat diaphragm showed a continued rise 30 or 120 min after an intraperitoneal injection of insulin, the ratio between the I- and the D-form of the synthetase was unaltered (Søvik, 1966; Adolfsson, 1972). Also in the isolated perfused rat heart 30 min of perfusion with insulin caused no change in the I/D ratio (Huijing *et al.*, 1969; Adolfsson et al., 1972). In the rat heart *in situ*, the effect of insulin on glycogen synthetase was detectable 1 min after the administration of the hormone (Williams and Mayer, 1966), and careful analysis of the time course indicates that the rise in I/D ratio is an initial phenomenon and that other factors may be of importance in maintaining the accelerated rate of glycogen synthesis both in the heart, the diaphragm, and levator ani muscle of rats (Adolfsson, 1972; Adolfsson *et al.*, 1972). The fact that insulin induces a rise in the glucose-6-phosphate content of muscle cells both *in vitro* and *in vivo* may well account for the continued stimulation of glycogen synthesis (Newsholme and Randle, 1961; Søvik, 1966; Adolfsson, 1972).

The conversion of glycogen synthetase D into the I-form occurs by a dephosphorylation catalyzed by glycogen synthetase D phosphatase. This enzyme is stimulated by glucose-6-phosphate and inhibited by physiological levels of ATP (Gilboe and Nuttall, 1972). The observation that this inhibition is enhanced by glycogen may account for the inverse relationship between glycogen content and the activity of synthetase I (Danforth, 1965; Huijing *et al.*, 1969). The synthesis of glycogen seems to be a self-limiting process (Daw and Berne, 1967) where the accumulation of product leads to gradual deactivation of synthetase. Insulin seems to increase the activity of synthetase D phosphatase in liver (Gold, 1970), but not in muscle (Shen *et al.*, 1970).

The I to D conversion occurs by a phosphorylation catalyzed by synthetase I kinase, which can be isolated from muscle (Whelan, 1968; Schlender *et al.*, 1969) and is probably identical with the protein kinase catalyzing the activation of phosphorylase kinase (Soderling *et al.*, 1970). It has been suggested that this kinase exists in two forms, one that is active in the absence of cyclic AMP, and another which is dependent on this compound. The cAMP independent synthetase I kinase was found to be inhibited by insulin in skeletal muscle (Shen *et al.*, 1970). This suggests a mechanism by which insulin might increase the I/D ratio of glycogen synthetase by preventing the conversion of the I into the D form, even when the cellular level of cAMP remains unaltered. In rat diaphragm muscle insulin was found to cause no change in the cAMP content except in the presence of epinephrine (GOLDBERG *et al.*, 1967; CRAIG *et al.*, 1969), and at the moment it seems unlikely that the stimulating effect of the hormone on glycogen synthesis can be secondary to changes in the cellular level of this nucleotide (NUTTALL, 1972; DRUMMOND *et al.*, 1972).

In diaphragm muscle, insulin has no effect on the degradation of glycogen (GEMMILL, 1940; Clausen, 1972) and the activity of phosphorylase (TORRES *et al.*, 1966; CRAIG *et al.*, 1969; ADOLFSSON, 1972).

In muscle, a major part of the glycogen particles seem to be located around the sarcoplasmic reticulum (WANSON and DROCHMANS, 1968), and the enzymes directly regulating the metabolism of glycogen are apparently closely associated with these structures (ANDERSSON, CEDERGREN and MUSCATELLO, 1963; MEYER *et al.*, 1970). Thus there is some structural basis for a separate route along which glucose may be made available for glycogen synthesis. It has been suggested that insulin may stimulate the uptake of glucose preferentially at a site where glycogen is synthetized (SIMS and LANDAU, 1966), and the „directive effect" of the hormone on glycogen synthesis may not solely be the consequence of increased activity of glycogen synthetase.

3. Glycolysis

Even in well-oxygenated muscles, a rather large proportion of the glucose taken up is converted into lactate, which may be released from the cells (SHAW and STADIE, 1959; BEATTY *et al.*, 1966; LANDAU and SIMS, 1967; DULLY *et al.*, 1969; CHAIN *et al.*, 1969; BELOFF-CHAIN *et al.*, 1971; CLAUSEN, 1972). In the human forearm, around 60% of the resting glucose uptake is accounted for by lactate production (ANDRES *et al.*, 1956).

SHAW and STADIE (1959) showed that in the isolated rat hemidiaphragm, insulin stimulates the conversion of labelled glucose into fructose-1,6-diphosphate and lactate. In a phosphate buffered medium without bicarbonate, this effect could not be detected, and glucose was never converted into fructose-1,6-diphosphate (SHAW and STADIE, 1957). This emphasizes the importance of including all the normal electrolytes of the extracellular phase in buffers used for the evaluation of metabolic effects of insulin *in vitro*.

Several others have demonstrated a stimulating effect of insulin on lactate production in diaphragm muscle (RAFAELSEN and CLAUSEN, 1961; CLAUSEN, 1966, 1968a, b; BELOFF-CHAIN *et al.*, 1971), isolated skeletal muscle fibers from the rat and macasus rhesus (DULLY *et al.*, 1969), in the perfused rat heart (CHAIN *et al.*, 1969) and in epinephrine-treated frog sartorius muscle (ÖZAND and NARAHARA, 1964). In several instances, this increase might be the outcome of accelerated glucose uptake, but in the perfused rat heart, insulin produced a larger rise in the conversion of glucose into lactate than that obtained by increasing the concentration of glucose (CHAIN *et al.*, 1969).

In the intact and the cut rat diaphragm and in the perfused rat heart, insulin was found to increase the concentration of glucose-6-phosphate, fructose-6-phosphate and fructose-1,6-diphosphate (NEWSHOLME and RANDLE, 1961), but under conditions where the glucose uptake could be kept constant, insulin was reported to increase only the concentrations of those glycolytic intermediates formed past the phosphofructokinase step (BEITNER and KALANT, 1971). In the isolated rat hemidiaphragm, the conversion of glucose or prelabelled glycogen into CO_2 was increased by around 50%, whereas when labelled lactate was used as substrate, only a modest rise in $^{14}CO_2$-production was obtained. This indicates that insulin stimulates glycolysis independent of an action on the glucose transport, probably by increasing the activity of phosphofructokinase (BEITNER and KALANT, 1971). In the heart of diabetic rats, the activity of this key enzyme is considerably reduced (GARLAND *et al.*, 1963; REGEN *et al.*, 1964), perhaps because of increased cellular levels of citrate or an accelerated fatty acid metabolism (NEWSHOLME and RANDLE, 1964).

A major difficulty in evaluating the effect of insulin on glycolysis is the existence of several pools (or pathways) for the metabolites of this process. SHAW and STADIE (1959) proposed that in rat diaphragm muscle, glucose may be metabolized via two separate pathways — one located intracellularly and forming lactate and glycogen by an insulin-sensitive process, another which was supposed to take place on the cell membrane and convert glucose (or glucose-6-phosphate) into lactate, but not glycogen. The latter did not respond to insulin. Several reinvestigations of this suggested compartmentalization have confirmed that both in cut and intact muscle cells of the rat and macasus rhesus, glucose-6-phosphate prevails in two pools with rather different accessability to endogenous or extraneous glucose and glucose-6-phosphate (SIMS and LANDAU, 1966; LANDAU and SIMS, 1967; DULLY *et al.*, 1969; ANTONY *et al.*, 1969; KALANT and BEITNER, 1971). In rat hemidiaphragms incubated for 2 h in the presence of ^{14}C-labelled glucose or pyruvate, the specific activities of glucose-6-phosphate and phosphoglyceric acid were much lower than those of the substrates and of their immediate precursors, but insulin had no detectable effect on the pattern of specific activities (KALANT and BEITNER, 1971). The other major, but perhaps less direct argument for compartmentalization is the observation that there is a considerably larger incorporation of label from ^{14}C-glucose than from ^{14}C-glucose-6-phosphate into glycogen (SIMS and LANDAU, 1966; DULLY *et al.*, 1969). The preferential incorporation of glucose was accentuated by insulin, and it is possible that glycogen is derived from a separate pool formed from glucose, but to which exogenous glucose-6-phosphate has limited access. The total output of end products and intermediates of glycolysis may be derived from at least two sources — the glucose directly entering the usual series of reactions in the Embden-Meyerhof pathway, and the glucose made available by degradation of the glycogen pool, which may be located in such a way as to allow a separate pathway for incorporation of glucose and for the first steps following the phosphorylase reaction. As described above, the enzymes of glycogen metabolism seem to be located in the sarcoplasmic reticulum, and there is histochemical evidence that the same structure contains high activities of lactic acid dehydrogenase, glyceraldehyde-3-phosphate dehydrogenase (FAHIMI and KARNOVSKY, 1966), and hexokinase (KARPATKIN and BRAUN, 1971). Thus, there seems to be some structural basis for a separate pathway for glycogen metabolism and glycolysis.

4. Oxidation of Glucose and Other Substrates

In 1938 KREBS and EGGLESTON found that in minced pigeon muscle, insulin stimulated the uptake of oxygen when citrate was used as substrate. In the following decade several workers confirmed this observation (see STADIE *et al.*, 1948), whereas in homogenates of mammalian muscle, no effect could be detected (STADIE *et al.*, 1940; SHORR and BARKER, 1939).

Experiments with intact skeletal muscles (GEMMILL, 1941; VILLEE and HASTINGS, 1949; BELOFF-CHAIN *et al.*, 1955; HALL, 1960), isolated perfused rat hearts (FISHER and WILLIAMSON, 1961), the human heart (RUDOLPH and HAUER, 1969), and forearm (ANDRES *et al.*, 1962) indicate that insulin produces either no change or a very modest stimulation (KERLY and OTTAWAY, 1954; HACKEL, 1960; BEATTY *et al.*, 1960) of oxygen uptake.

On the other hand, insulin deficiency may diminish oxygen consumption, and in various skeletal muscle or heart preparations from diabetic rats and dogs, insulin seems to restore the Qo_2 towards the normal level (VILLEE and HASTINGS, 1949; HALL, 1960; BEATTY *et al.*, 1960). Since this effect was also seen in the absence of extraneous substrate, insulin may influence mitochondrial function independently of any action on the transport of substrates across the plasma membrane (HALL, 1960).

In frog skeletal muscle, insulin stimulates oxygen uptake both in the absence and in the presence of extraneous substrate (GOURLEY and FISHER, 1954; for further references, see GOURLEY and BRUNTON, 1969). This effect is not suppressed by cardiac glycosides, indicating that it is not due to a stimulation of active Na-K-transport (GOURLEY, 1961).

Measurements of the conversion of various ^{14}C-labelled compounds into $^{14}CO_2$ indicate that insulin accelerates the oxidation of substrates in muscle cells. In the diaphragm and adductor muscles of the rat (FRITZ, 1960; BEATTY *et al.*, 1960; MORIWAKI and LANDAU, 1962; BEITNER and KALANT, 1971), and in fetal rhesus monkey muscle (BOCEK and BEATTY, 1969), insulin was found to stimulate the conversion of glucose into CO_2. This seems to be a relatively small effect, and it could not be detected in the isolated perfused rat diaphragm (BELOFF-CHAIN *et al.*, 1971). Since insulin has little or no effect on the conversion of extraneous pyruvate and acetate (VILLEE and HASTINGS, 1949; PEARSON *et al.*, 1949) or lactate (BEITNER and KALANT, 1971) into CO_2 in skeletal muscle, the increase may be secondary to stimulation of glucose uptake or of the activation of phosphofructokinase activity (BEITNER and KALANT, 1971).

In the isolated perfused rat heart, insulin clearly stimulates the conversion of ^{14}C-labelled glucose into CO_2 (CHAIN *et al.*, 1969), and in the human heart, CO_2-production, the uptake of glucose, pyruvate and lactate as well as their conversion into CO_2 increased markedly following the administration of insulin (RUDOLPH *et al.*, 1969).

Although the role of insulin in the control of substrate oxidation has been difficult to illustrate in studies with normal tissues, it is evident that in diabetes, the capacity of these processes is severely impaired. In the heart and diaphragm of diabetic rats, the oxidation of glucose or pyruvate into CO_2 may be markedly reduced and partly or totally restored by insulin (PEARSON *et al.*, 1949; VILLEE and HASTINGS, 1949; GARLAND *et al.*, 1962; GARLAND *et al.*, 1964).

The observation that insulin augments the activity of pyruvate dehydrogenase (COORE *et al.*, 1971) and that this enzyme is less active in the heart of diabetic rats (WIELAND *et al.*, 1971), indicates that mitochondrial function is controlled by insulin, perhaps via changes in ion distribution (MARTIN *et al.*, 1972).

5. Lipid Metabolism

Lipids may serve as an important energy source in muscle cells. In the isolated rat diaphragm, lipid metabolism seems to account for all of the oxygen utilization (GEMMILL, 1941; NEPTUNE *et al.*, 1959), and in the human forearm, the amount of free fatty acids taken up would account for 50% of the oxygen consumption (RABINOWITZ and ZIERLER, 1962). In the isolated rat heart, the oxidation of added palmitate could account for 60% of the carbon dioxide output (OPIE *et al.*, 1963).

The major effect of insulin seems to be a conversion of this pattern into one in which the metabolism of glucose dominates. Thus, insulin was found to have a sparing action on the oxidation of palmitate in rat diaphragm, but only in the presence of glucose (FRITZ and KAPLAN, 1960; BODEL *et al.*, 1962). Insulin produces a slight rise in the incorporation of palmitate into triglycerides (BODEL *et al.*, 1962). Both in the heart and in the diaphragm of rats, insulin augments the glycerol phosphate content, and the concomitant decrease in free fatty acid content and increase in glycerol output indicate that the esterification was increased. In contrast to adipose tissue, insulin apparently has no inhibitory effect on lipolysis in normal muscle cells (GARLAND and RANDLE, 1964). The incorporation of acetate into neutral fat and phospholipids is stimulated by insulin in the isolated rat hemidiaphragm (MANCHESTER, 1963).

Free fatty acids and ketone bodies inhibit basal and insulin-stimulated sugar transport and glucose metabolism in the heart (RANDLE *et al.*, 1966; RANDLE, 1970), but to a much lesser extent or not at all in skeletal muscle (JERVELL, 1965; SCHONFELD and KIPNIS, 1968; BEATTY and BOCEK, 1971; JEFFERSON *et al.*, 1972). The interaction between lipid and carbohydrate metabolism may be of importance for carbohydrate tolerance and insulin sensitivity (for review, see RUDERMAN *et al.*, 1969; RANDLE, 1970). Although it is difficult to demonstrate immediate effects *in vitro*, longer exposure to fatty acids or their degradation products may cause a more lasting reduction in insulin sensitivity. The composition of the lipids in the plasma membrane is important for its permeability characteristics, and in this connection it should be noted that fatty acids have been found to act as membrane stabilizors (SEEMAN and ROTH, 1971). The fact that several membrane stabilizers prevent the stimulating effect of insulin on glucose transport and glycogen deposition suggest that the over-all mobility of the lipid layer in the plasma membrane is important for the action of insulin (CLAUSEN *et al.*, 1973).

6. Electrolytes and Glucose Metabolism

The observation that insulin activates glycogen synthetase (and possibly phosphofructokinase) in the absence of metabolizable substrates suggests that electrolytes may be mediators — in analogy to their role in the metabolic control exerted by several other hormones (RASMUSSEN, 1970). Although new information about the ionic control of organic metabolism is rapidly accumulating (for review see BYGRAVE, 1967; CLAUSEN, 1972), it has not yet been possible to account for the action of insulin on glucose metabolism as secondary to effects on electrolyte distribution. On the other hand, the relatively specific effect of insulin on glycogen synthesis in diaphragm muscle may be mimicked by inhibition of the active Na-K-transport (CLAUSEN, 1965b, 1966). The stimulation of glycogen deposition (and inhibition of glycogenolysis and CO_2-production) produced by cardiac glycoside or by the omission of K^+ from the incubation medium is probably the outcome of reduced utilization of ATP for active Na-K-transport (KYPSON *et al.*, 1968a, b; CLAUSEN, 1972). Neither the active Na-K-transport nor the presence of Na^+ or K^+ in the extracellular milieu is essential for the stimulating effect of insulin on glycogen synthesis, but ouabain was found to abolish the stimulating effect of insulin on lactate production in rat hemidiaphragm (CLAUSEN, 1966).

Replacing extracellular Na^+ by K^+ inhibited the incorporation of glucose into glycogen in rat hemidiaphragm (STADIE and ZAPP, 1947; CLAUSEN, 1968a), and soleus muscle (MOORTHY and GOULD, 1969; KOHN and CLAUSEN, 1972), both in the absence and in the presence of insulin. This might in part be the result of decreased glucose uptake, but experiments with homogenates of pigeon breast muscle have shown that the incorporation of ^{14}C-glucose into glycogen is suppressed by high concentrations of K^+, maximum rates being obtained at 30 mM (TORRES *et al.*, 1966). Also the degradation of glycogen may directly or indirectly be influenced by K^+ ions. Exposure to K^+-rich media stimulates the degradation of glycogen in rat soleus muscle (MOORTHY and GOULD, 1969); and in frog sartorius muscle, DANFORTH and HELMREICH (1964) found that the activity of phosphorylase a is promptly increased by augmenting the extracellular concentration of K^+. This may be related to an increase in the cytoplasmic Ca^{++} level, although it may also be of significance that K^+-substitution leads to a marked rise in the cellular level of cAMP (LUNDHOLM *et al.*, 1967). Ca^{++} has been found to increase the activity of phosphorylase b kinase (OZAWA *et al.*, 1967) and to stimulate the I to D conversion of glycogen synthetase (BELOCOPITOW *et al.*, 1965), effects which both would favor the degradation of glycogen. The glycogenolysis seen during contractile activity, in the presence of metabolic poisons, and in a hyperosmolar medium (CLAUSEN, 1968a) may be the outcome of an increase in the concentration of Ca^{++} in the cytoplasm (ISAACSON, 1969).

Na^{+} ions have been shown to inhibit phosphorylase phosphatase (KAESS *et al.*, 1966), and the hyperglycemic effect of K^{+}-depletion (with increased intracellular Na^{+}-level) has been related to increased glycogenolysis (BARTELHEIMER *et al.*, 1967).

Li^{+} ions have been found to mimick the effect of insulin on glycogen deposition in muscle (CLAUSEN, 1968a; PLENGE *et al.*, 1970).

The phenomena described above may yet seem peripheral to the action of insulin, but they are relevant if the significance of the effects of insulin on electrolyte distribution should be analyzed further.

V. "Insulin-Like" Effects

A wide variety of conditions and compounds mimic the effect of insulin in stimulating the transport of glucose and other sugars across the plasma membrane in muscle cells (CAMPBELL, 1969).

Since some of the hypotheses for the mechanism of insulin action and the function of the glucose transport system are in part based upon studies of insulin-like effects, the major categories of stimuli for glucose transport will be commented upon and compared with insulin.

Apart from the extraneous control of sugar permeability exerted by insulin, muscle cells seem capable of regulating their sugar exchange by endogenous factors also. Thus, in situations where there is an increased demand for metabolizable substrate, the uptake of glucose (and non-metabolized sugars) is increased. This is seen in connection with contractile activity, increases in the permeability to actively transported ions and when energy-yielding processes are impaired by anoxia or metabolic poisons. It seems likely that the function of the glucose transport system is controlled by factors generated during the processes of muscle contraction and energy metabolism. Therefore, a number of insulin-like effects may be secondary to changes in conditions for energy production and contractile activity and not the direct outcome of an action on the glucose transport system.

Furthermore, the mechanism of insulin action has been studied using compounds with molecular structures similar to those of insulin and enzymes which might modify the configuration of the target for insulin action.

1. Contractile Activity

Exercise can lower the concentration of blood glucose in man (STRÄNDELL, 1934) and animals (INGLE *et al.*, 1950). The observation that exercise stimulates the penetration of non-metabolized sugars into the intracellular space of muscles in nephrectomized animals indicates that the increased consumption of glucose induced by contractile activity is associated with an activation of the glucose transport system in the plasma membrane (GOLDSTEIN *et al.*, 1953; HELMREICH and CORI, 1957). This insulin-like effect has later been demonstrated in a variety of isolated preparations of skeletal muscle (HOLLOSZY and NARAHARA, 1965; ARVILL, 1967; VASYANIN and SEREBRYAKOV, 1968; PAIN and MANCHESTER, 1970; KOHN and CLAUSEN, 1971; RUDERMAN, *et al.*, 1971), the heart (MORGAN *et al.*, 1965; NEELY *et al.*, 1967; OPIE *et al.*, 1971), as well as in muscles *in situ* (CHAPLER and STAINSBY, 1968), including the human forearm (GARRATT *et al.*, 1972; WAHREN, 1970; DIETERLE *et al.*, 1972) and leg (WAHREN *et al.*, 1971).

In the perfused hindquarter and the isolated soleus muscle of the rat, the stimulating effect of contractile activity is slightly smaller and somewhat later in onset than that of insulin (RUDERMAN *et al.*, 1971; KOHN and CLAUSEN, 1971).

In the isolated frog sartorius muscle, the uptake of 3-O-methylglucose was correlated with the frequency of stimulation, and maximum rates were not significantly different from those obtained by stimulation with insulin. At maximum levels of stimulation, the effects of insulin and electrical stimulation were not additive, and the kinetic constants showed the same change (increased V_{max} and unaltered apparent K_M). This indicates that the two stimuli act on the same glucose transport system, but at variance with the effect of insulin, electrical stimulation leads to a prompt rise in the uptake of 3-O-methylglucose which could be detected even at 0° (HOLLOSZY and NARAHARA, 1965).

Muscular work may lead to localized relative hypoxia or substrate depletion, but this cannot account for the rise in sugar permeability (HOLLOSZY and NARAHARA, 1965; NEELY *et al.*, 1967).

In frog sartorius muscle, there was no correlation between the rise in 3-O-methylglucose permeability and the amount of work performed or the rate of lactate production (HOLLOSZY and NARAHARA, 1965). On the other hand, in the isolated perfused rat heart, the uptake of glucose (and L-arabinose) increased in proportion to the mechanical activity even at constant frequencies of contraction (MORGAN *et al.*, 1965; NEELY *et al.*, 1967; OPIE *et al.*, 1971). When the perfusion takes place via the left atrium (so as to allow the performance of pressure work), the glucose uptake and insulin sensitivity are clearly higher than when LANGENDORFF's method of retrograde perfusion is used (NEELY *et al.*, 1967).

Among the processes eliciting contraction, the depolarization of the plasma membrane does not seem to play any essential role in the activation of the glucose transport system. Thus, caffeine, which may induce contractions without producing action potentials, accelerates the uptake of 3-O-methylglucose, an effect which has been related to an increase in the concentration of Ca^{++} in the myoplasm (HOLLOSZY and NARAHARA, 1967a) Contractions elicited by K^+-rich buffer lead to a stimulation of sugar transport which is dependent on the extracellular concentration of Ca^{++}, and when Ca-uptake was stimulated by incubation in a medium where Cl^- was replaced by NO_3^-, sartorius muscles showed an increase in the rate of 3-O-methylglucose uptake (HOLLOSZY and NARAHARA, 1967b). However, since the glucose transport system seems to remain activated for up to several hours after the cessation of contractile activity (and the re-establishment of a low cytoplasmic level of free Ca^{++}), the suggested role of Ca^{++} as a trigger for the activation of the glucose transport system may be indirect (HOLLOSZY and NARAHARA, 1965; GOULD and RAWLINSON, 1966a; ARVILL, 1967; CHAPLER and STAINSBY, 1968). During contraction, a variety of muscular tissues (including uterus and intestine) have been shown to release a labile humoral factor which stimulates the transport of glucose and other sugars in diaphragm and adipose tissue (GOLDSTEIN *et al.*, 1953; LEVINE and GOLDSTEIN, 1955; GOLDSTEIN, 1961; HAVIVI and WERTHEIMER, 1964; BIHLER *et al.*, 1970). This factor is non-dialyzable and precipitable with ammonium sulfate (HAVIVI and WERTHEIMER, 1964). It also differs from insulin immunologically (BIHLER *et al.*, 1970).

It is evident that the stimulating effect of contractile activity on sugar transport must be considered not only as an acute phenomenon, but as an outcome of a sometimes more persistent modification of the properties of the glucose transport system so as to enable the muscle cells to cover not only the immediate, but also the subsequent metabolic demands. Training was found to augment the response of the glucose transport system to the stimulus of exercise (GOULD and RAWLINSON, 1966b) and that of insulin (LIPMAN *et al.*, 1972). An analogous adaptation (in the reverse direction) is seen in tissues isolated from diabetic animals, where the diminished responsiveness to insulin may be related to a preceding period with diminished exposure to the hormone (RANDLE *et al.*, 1966).

2. Anoxia and Metabolic Poisons

RANDLE and SMITH (1958) demonstrated that in muscle cells, inhibition of energy production by exposure to anoxia or metabolic poisons leads to stimulation of sugar transport. Several others have described similar effects in rat diaphragm muscle (LOTSPEICH and WHEELER, 1962; KONO and COLOWICK, 1961; BIHLER, 1968), monkey sartorius muscle (BEATTY *et al.*, 1966), rat soleus muscle (CHAUDRY and GOULD, 1969; KOHN and CLAUSEN, 1971), the isolated perfused rat heart (MORGAN *et al.*, 1959; MORGAN *et al.*, 1961a and b) and the sartorius muscle of frogs (ÖZAND *et al.*, 1962; VINOGRADOVA *et al.*, 1968). The stimulation was found to be somewhat slower in onset than that induced by insulin, and it is difficult to compare the effects of the two stimuli with respect to absolute magnitude and to determine whether they are additive (ÖZAND *et al.*, 1962; KONO and COLOWICK, 1961; KOHN and CLAUSEN, 1971).

During inhibition of energy production, glucose uptake shows saturation kinetics (CHAUDRY and GOULD, 1969), and phlorizin suppress the increase in permeability to non-metabolized sugars (LOTSPEICH and WHEELER, 1962; KOHN and CLAUSEN, 1971), indicating that the effect is due to an activation of the glucose transport system and not a non-specific over-all increase in the permeability of the plasma membrane.

It has been suggested that ATP might control the permeability of the plasma membrane to glucose (SMITH *et al.*, 1961), but under conditions where the ATP-content was unaltered, anaerobiosis was found to produce a marked rise in glucose uptake (ÖZAND *et al.*, 1962; CHAUDRY and GOULD, 1970). Inhibition of energy production will change the cytoplasmic concentration of a considerable number of metabolites and electrolytes, and it is difficult to identify those which may be of significance in eliciting the rise in sugar transport. It seems likely that this effect is only induced when the energy production can no longer meet the metabolic demands of the cell. This is likely to occur earlier in mammalian muscles than in frog muscles, which may maintain a sufficient energetic level by glycolysis. It is interesting that muscles from winter frogs, which are more sparsely provided with endogenous energy sources, are more permeable to 3-O-methylglucose than muscles from summer frogs (NARAHARA and ÖZAND, 1963). Lack of metabolizable substrate in the perfusate was found to increase the permeability to pentoses in the heart (HENDERSON *et al.*, 1961; BIHLER *et al.*, 1965); and in rat soleus muscle, the basal rate of 3-O-methylglucose transport was almost doubled by 18 h of fasting (KOHN and CLAUSEN, 1971).

There is evidence that inhibition of energy production leads to a rise in the cytoplasmic concentration of Ca^{++} in a variety of tissues (PAUL, 1961; ROJAS and HIDALGO, 1968; BLAUSTEIN and HODGKIN, 1969; CLAUSEN, 1970; KOHN and CLAUSEN, 1971). However, it remains to be determined whether a redistribution of cellular Ca is of importance for the stimulation of glucose transport seen under these conditions.

3. Hyperosmolarity

KUZUYA *et al.* (1965) found that the addition of NaCl, sucrose or mannitol in the concentration range 50—200 mOsm caused a considerable increase in the uptake of glucose in rat hemidiaphragm. The addition of a rapidly penetrating solute, urea, produced no change. These observations were confirmed (CLAUSEN, 1968a), and in rat soleus muscle, hyperosmolarity was found to stimulate both the influx and the efflux of 3-O-methylglucose (CLAUSEN *et al.*, 1970; KOHN and CLAUSEN, 1971, 1972). Hyperosmolarity may stimulate glucose uptake and 3-O-methylglucose transport to approximately the same level as a supramaximal concentration of insulin, but with slightly slower rate of onset (CLAUSEN *et al.*, 1970). At variance with the effects of insulin, hyperosmolarity inhibits the incorporation of glucose into glycogen and markedly stimulates glycogenolysis and CO_2-production in the hemidiaphragm preparation (KUZUYA *et al.*, 1965; CLAUSEN, 1968a). The effect of hyperosmolarity on sugar transport is not affected by insulin antibody (KUZUYA *et al.*, 1965), but suppressed by factors which also interfere with the effect of insulin on sugar transport (phlorizin, high extracellular K^+ and membrane stabilizors) (CLAUSEN *et al.*, 1970; KOHN and CLAUSEN, 1972; CLAUSEN *et al.* 1973).

On the basis of the observation that both longitudinal and transverse sarcoplasmic tubules undergo considerable swelling in hypertonic media (FREYGANG *et al.*, 1964; VINOGRADOVA, 1968), it was suggested that the concomitant stimulation of sugar transport could in part be the outcome of an increase in the area available for solute exchange (KOHN and CLAUSEN, 1972). These intracellular structures are accessible to solutes from the extracellular phase, and there is some evidence that they participate in the exchange of amino acids (HIDER *et al.*, 1971), K^+ (ADRIAN and FREYGANG, 1962; HODGKIN and NAKAJIMA, 1972; ALMERS, 1972) and Na^+ (ZIERLER, 1972) between cytoplasm and the environment. It is not known whether the membranes lining the sarcoplasmic tubules are permeable to sugars, but since their area is several fold larger than that of the outer plasma membrane (sarcolemma), a major part of the transport may in fact take place via these structures. However, the observation that hyperosmolarity also accelerates sugar transport in adipocytes (KUZUYA *et al.*, 1965; CLAUSEN *et al.*, 1970) suggests more direct effects on the plasma membrane. The stimulating effect of hyperosmolarity on respiration and lactate production which is seen both *in vitro* and *in vivo* (KUZUYA *et al.*, 1965; CLAUSEN, 1968a; AINSWORTH and ALLISON, 1971) suggests that the increased sugar permeability is elicited by mechanisms similar to those operating during anoxia or in the presence of metabolic inhibitors. It may also be relevant that hyperosmolarity seems to induce a rise in the cytoplasmic level of Ca^{++} in muscle (ISAACSON, 1969).

4. Enzymes

Trypsin and chymotrypsin were found to stimulate the uptake of glucose and non-metabolized sugar as well as the glycogen deposition in rat diaphragm (RIESER and RIESER, 1964). In the alloxan-diabetic rat, the same enzymes were reported to produce hypoglycemia (RIESER, 1965). In frog sartorius muscle (WEIS and NARAHARA, 1969) and soleus muscle (KOHN and CLAUSEN, 1971), trypsin was found to stimulate the influx and the efflux of 3-O-methylglucose. This effect was not associated with any increase in the permeability to mannitol and it was abolished by soybean trypsin inhibitor and phlorizin, indicating that it is relatively specific and not the outcome of a general impairment of plasma membrane integrity. Like insulin, contractile activity and anaerobiosis, trypsin was found to increase the V_{max} of sugar transport without changing apparent K_M (WEIS and NARAHARA, 1969). The relatively slow onset and reversal of the effect suggest that it is related to a progressive modification of the plasma membrane. Since phospholipase C and neuraminidase have also been found to increase the permeability to glucose (in fat cells, RODBELL, 1966) and 3-O-methylglucose (WEIS and NARAHARA, 1969), it seems reasonable to assume that enzymatic cleavage of a variety of chemical bonds in the plasma membrane may diminish the rigidity of its structure so as to allow an increased mobility of the glucose transport system. Although this provides some basis for understanding a mechanism for the activation of the glucose transport system, the extremely weak proteolytic activity of insulin indicates that the hormone acts in a considerably more subtle way (see RIESER, 1967).

5. Compounds Structurally Related to Insulin

Another approach to the study of relationships between structure and function has been made by the evaluation of the insulin-like effects of compounds with molecular configurations similar to those of insulin. Proinsulin is a single chain polypeptide in which the middle portion, the C-peptide, links the A and the B chain of insulin (STEINER *et al.*, 1972). It produces the same pattern of metabolic effects as insulin in a variety of preparations, but with a potency ranging from 2—25% of that of insulin (RUBENSTEIN *et al.*, 1972). It has been suggested that its effect is anteceded by proteolytic conversion into insulin (SHAW and CHANCE, 1968; LAZARUS *et al.*, 1970), but other studies with muscle have not yielded any evidence in support of this mechanism, and it seems likely that proinsulin has a definite intrinsic biological activity (BRUSH, 1971; NARAHARA, 1972). The data are compatible with the idea that proinsulin interacts with the same receptor as insulin, but with a considerably lower affinity.

Like proinsulin, the A chain has been found to produce hypoglycemia (FENICHEL *et al.*, 1968) and to stimulate glucose uptake in the isolated rat diaphragm (VOLFIN *et al.*, 1964; SURMACZYNSKA and METZ, 1969). *In vitro*, the potency of A chain is about 1/1000 that of insulin, but since synthetic A chain has a similar activity, the stimulating effect of glucose uptake cannot be accounted for as due to contamination with insulin.

Although the isolated B chain does not stimulate glucose uptake in muscle (MAHLER *et al.*, 1968; SURMACZYNSKA and METZ, 1969), several derivatives of arginine (B_{22}) mimic the effect of insulin in augmenting glucose uptake and glycogen deposition in rat diaphragm, but only when present in very high concentrations (WEITZEL *et al.*, 1971).

The presence of disulfide bridges in the insulin molecule has given rise to some speculation that these structures might be of importance for the binding or biological action of the hormone. Sulfhydryl compounds have been found to stimulate glucose uptake in rat hemidiaphragm, but the late onset of the effect together with the simultaneous acceleration of glycogenolysis suggests a mechanism of action similar to that of metabolic inhibitors (HAUGAARD *et al.*, 1972).

The preceding results emphasize the specificity of the insulin receptor, and for a further analysis of the active components of the insulin molecule, comparisons between the biological activity and the affinity for binding to the insulin receptor seem required.

References

ADOLFSSON, S.: Regulation of glycogen synthesis in muscle. Thesis, University of Göteborg, 1972

ADOLFSSON, S., ISAKSSON, O., HJALMARSON, Å.: Effect of insulin on glycogen synthesis and synthetase enzyme activity in the perfused rat heart. Biochim. biophys. Acta (Amst.) **270**, 146 (1972)

ADRIAN, A.H., FREYGANG, W.H.: The potassium and chloride conductance of frog muscle membrane. J. Physiol. (Lond.) **163**, 61 (1962)

AIKAWA, J.K.: Effect of glucose and insulin on magnesium metabolism in rabbits. Proc. Soc. exp. Biol. (N.Y.) **103**, 363 (1960)

AINSWORTH, S.K., ALLISON, F.: Effects of hypertonic solutions infused intravenously in rabbits. I. Metabolic acidosis and lactic acidemia. J. Lab. clin. Med. **78**, 619 (1971)

ALMERS, W.: The decline of potassium permeability during extreme hyperpolarization in frog skeletal muscle. J. Physiol. (Lond.) **225**, 57 (1972)

AMDISEN, A.: Diabetes mellitus as a side effect of treatment with tricyclic neuroleptics. Acta psychiat. scand. Suppl. **180**, 411 (1964)

ANDERSSON-CEDERGREN, E., MUSCATELLO, U.: The participation of the sarcotubular system in glycogen metabolism. J. Ultrastruct. Res. **8**, 391 (1963)

ANDRES, R., CADER, G., ZIERLER, K.L.: The quantitatively minor role of carbohydrate in oxidative metabolism by skeletal muscle in intact man in the basal state. Measurements of oxygen and glucose uptake and carbon dioxide and lactate production in the forearm. J. clin. Invest. **35**, 671 (1956)

ANDRES, R., BALTZAN, M.A., CADER, G., ZIERLER, K.L.: Effect of insulin on carbohydrate metabolism and on potassium in the forearm of man. J. clin. Invest. **41**, 108 (1962)

ANTONY, G.J., SRINIVASAN, I., WILLIAMS, H.R., LANDAU, B.R.: Studies on the existence of a pathway in liver and muscle for the conversion of glucose into glycogen without glucose-6-phosphate as an intermediate. Biochem. J. **111**, 453 (1969)

ARNQUIST, H.: Metabolism in vascular and intestinal smooth muscle; action of insulin. Linköping University Medical Dissertation, No. 16 (1973)

ARVILL, A.: Relationship between the effects of contraction and insulin on the metabolism of the isolated levator ani muscle of the rat. Acta endocr. (Kbh.) **56**, Suppl. 122, 27 (1967)

ARVILL, A., AHREN, K.: Effects of insulin on the intact levator ani muscle of the rat. Acta endocr. (Kbh.) **56**, 279 (1967)

BAKER, P.F.: Sodium-calcium exchange across the nerve cell membrane. In: Calcium and cellular function, p. 96 (A.W. CUTHBERTH, ed.). London: Macmillan 1970

BARTELHEIMER, H.K., LOSERT, W., SENFT, G., SITT, R.: Störungen des Kohlenhydratstoffwechsels im Kaliummangel. Naunyn-Schmiedebergs Arch. Pharmak. exp. Path. **258**, 391 (1967)

BATTAGLIA, F.C., RANDLE, P.J.: Regulation of glucose uptake by muscle: 4. The specificity of monosaccharide-transport systems in rat diaphragm muscle. Biochem. J. **75**, 408 (1960)

BEATTY, C.H., PETERSON, R.D., BOCEK, R.M.: Effect of insulin on carbohydrate metabolism of skeletal muscle fibers and diaphragm from control and pancreatectomized rats. J. biol. Chem. **235**, 277 (1960)

BEATTY, C.H., PETERSON, R.D., BASINGER, G.M., BOCEK, R.M.: Major metabolic pathways for carbohydrate metabolism of voluntary skeletal muscle. Amer. J. Physiol. **210**, 404 (1966)

BEATTY, C.H., BOCEK, R.M.: Interrelation of carbohydrate and palmitate metabolism in skeletal muscle. Amer. J. Physiol. **220**, 1928 (1971)

BEITNER, R., KALANT, N.: Stimulation of glycolysis by insulin. J. biol. Chem. **246**, 500 (1971)

BELOCOPITOW, E., APPLEMAN, M.M., TORRES, H.N.: Factors affecting the activity of muscle glycogen synthetase. J. biol. Chem. **240**, 3473 (1965)

BELOFF-CHAIN, A., CATANZARO, R., CHAIN, E.B., MASI, I., POCCHIARI, F., ROSSI, C.: The influence of insulin on carbohydrate metabolism in the isolated diaphragm muscle of normal and alloxan diabetic rats. Proc. roy. Soc. B **143**, 481 (1955)

BELOFF-CHAIN, A., CHAIN, E.B., ROOKLEDGE, K.A.: The influence of insulin on the metabolism of glucosamine in the isolated rat diaphragm muscle. Biochem. J. **119**, 27 (1970)

BELOFF-CHAIN, A., CHAIN, E.B., ROOKLEDGE, K.A.: The influence of insulin and of contraction on glucose metabolism in the perfused diaphragm muscle from normal and streptozotocin-treated rats. Biochem. J. **125**, 97 (1971)

BEST, C.H., HOET, J.P., MARKS, H.P.: The fate of the sugar disappearing under the action of insulin. Proc. roy. Soc. B **100 B**, 32 (1926)

BHATTACHARYA, G.: Effect of metal ions on the utilization of glucose and on the influence of insulin on it by the isolated rat diaphragm. Biochem. J. **79**, 369 (1961)

BHATTACHARYA, G.: Influence of Li^+ on glucose metabolism in rats and rabbits. Biochim. biophys. Acta (Amst.) **93**, 644 (1964)

BIHLER, I., CAVERT, H.M., FISHER, R.B.: A differential effect of inhibitors of sugar penetration into the isolated rabbit heart. J. Physiol. (Lond.) **180**, 168 (1965)

BIHLER, I.: The action of cardiotonic steroids on sugar transport in muscle, *in vitro*. Biochim. biophys. Acta (Amst.) **163**, 401 (1968)

BIHLER, I., HOLLANDS, M., DRESEL, P.E.: Stimulation of sugar transport by a factor released from gas-perfused hearts. Canad. J. Physiol. Pharmacol. **48**, 327 (1970)

BIHLER, I., SAWH, P.C.: The effect of alkali metal ions on sugar transport in muscle: Interaction with the sugar carrier or indirect effect. Biochim. biophys. Acta (Amst.) **225**, 56 (1971a)

BIHLER, I., SAWH, P.C.: Regulation of sugar transport in muscle: Effect of increased external potassium *in vitro*. Biochim. biophys. Acta (Amst.) **241**, 302 (1971b)

BIHLER, I., SAWH, P.C.: Effects of diphenylhydantoin on the transport of Na^+ and K^+ and the regulation of sugar transport in muscle in vitro. Biochim. biophys. Acta (Amst.) **249**, 240 (1971c)

BIHLER, I., SAWH, P.C., ELBRINK, J.: A specific sugar transport mechanism in smooth muscle and its regulation. Fed. Proc. **30**, Abstr. 256 (1971)
BITTAR, E.E.: Insulin and the sodium pump of the Maia muscle fiber. Nature (Lond.) **214**, 726 (1967)
BLAUSTEIN, M.P., HODGKIN, A.L.: The effect of cyanide on the efflux of calcium from squid axons. J. Physiol. (Lond.) **200**, 497 (1969)
BLEEHEN, N.M., FISHER, R.B.: The action of insulin in the isolated rat heart. J. Physiol. (Lond.) **123**, 260 (1954)
BOCEK, R.M., BASINGER, G.M., BEATTY, C.H.: Comparison of glucose uptake and carbohydrate utilization in red and white muscle. Amer. J. Physiol. **210**, 1108 (1966)
BOCEK, R.M., BEATTY, C.H.: Effect of insulin on the carbohydrate metabolism of fetal rhesus monkey muscle. Endocrinology **85**, 615 (1969)
BODEL, P.T., RUBINSTEIN, D., MCGARRY, E.E., BECK, J.C.: Utilization of free fatty acids by diaphragm in vitro. Amer. J. Physiol. **203**, 311 (1962)
BODO, R., MARKS, H.P.: The action of insulin on the aseptically perfused heart. J. Physiol. (Lond.) **63**, 242 (1927)
BOLTE, H.D., LÜDERITZ, B.: Membranpotentiale bei experimentellem Kaliummangel. Pflügers Arch. ges. Physiol. **301**, 254 (1968)
BOWER, B.F., GRODSKY, G.M.: Uptake of glucose dependent on insulin in the isolated bladder of the toad. Nature (Lond.) **198**, 391 (1963)
BROUGHER, J.C.: Blood calcium as affected by insulin. Amer. J. Physiol. **80**, 411 (1927)
BRUSH, J.S.: Purification and characterization of a protease with specificity for insulin from rat muscle. Diabetes **20**, 140 (1971)
BYGRAVE, F.L.: The ionic environment and metabolic control. Nature (Lond.) **214**, 667 (1967)
CAMPBELL, G.D.: Oral hypoglycemic agents. London and New York: Academic Press 1969
CARLIN, H., HECHTER, O.: Effects of insulin on the permeability of D- and L-xylose and D- and L-arabinose in rat diaphragm muscle. J. gen. Physiol. **45**, 309 (1961)
CHAIN, E.B., MANSFORD, K.R.L., OPIE, L.H.: Effects of insulin on the pattern of glucose metabolism in the perfused working and Langendorff heart of normal and insulin-deficient rats. Biochem. J. **115**, 537 (1969)
CHAPLER, C.K., STAINSBY, W.N.: Carbohydrate metabolism in contracting dog skeletal muscle in situ. Amer. J. Physiol. **215**, 995 (1968)
CHAUDRY, I.H., GOULD, M.K.: Kinetics of glucose uptake in isolated soleus muscle. Biochim. biophys. Acta (Amst.) **177**, 527 (1969)
CHAUDRY, I.H., GOULD, M.K.: Effect of externally added ATP on glucose uptake by isolated rat soleus muscle. Biochim. biophys. Acta (Amst.) **196**, 327 (1970)
CHRISTENSEN, N.J., ØRSKOV, H.: The relationship between endogenous serum insulin concentration and glucose uptake in the forearm muscles of nondiabetics. J. clin. Invest. **47**, 1262 (1968)
CLARK, C.M.: Carbohydrate metabolism in the isolated fetal rat heart. Amer. J. Physiol. **220**, 583 (1971)
CLAUSEN, T.: The effect of intraperitoneally injected insulin, glucagon, growth hormone and cortisol on the *in vivo* glycogen synthesis in the mouse diaphragm. Acta endocr. (Kbh.) **50**, 115 (1965a)
CLAUSEN, T.: The relationship between the transport of glucose and cations across cell membranes in isolated tissues. I. Stimulation of glycogen deposition and inhibition of lactic acid production in diaphragm, induced by ouabain. Biochim. biophys. Acta (Amst.) **109**, 164 (1965b)
CLAUSEN, T.: The relationship between the transport of glucose and cations across cell membranes in isolated tissues. II. Effects of K^+-free medium, ouabain and insulin upon the fate of glucose in rat diaphragm. Biochim. biophys. Acta (Amst.) **120**, 361 (1966)
CLAUSEN, T.: The relationship between the transport of glucose and cations across cell membranes in isolated tissues. III. Effect of Na^+ and hyperosmolarity on glucose metabolism and insulin responsiveness in isolated rat hemidiaphragm. Biochim. biophys. Acta (Amst.) **150**, 56 (1968a)
CLAUSEN, T.: The relationship between the transport of glucose and cations across cell membranes in isolated tissues. IV. The "insulin-like" effect of Li^+. Biochim. biophys. Acta (Amst.) **150**, 66 (1968b)
CLAUSEN, T.: Electrolytes and hormonal control of fat-cell metabolism. In: Adipose tissue, regulation and metabolic functions, p. 66 (B. JEANRENAUD and D. HEPP, eds.). Stuttgart: Thieme Verlag and New York: Academic Press 1970
CLAUSEN, T.: Role of insulin in ion transport in muscle and adipose tissue. Jugoslav. Physiol. Pharmacol. Acta **5**, 363 (1969)

Clausen, T., Gliemann, J., Vinten, J., Kohn, P.G.: Stimulating effect of hyperosmolarity on glucose transport in adipocytes and muscle cells. Biochim. biophys. Acta (Amst.) **211**, 233 (1970)

Clausen, T., Kohn, P.G.: K^+-ions, swelling, and sugar transport in muscle, in Na^+-linked transport of organic solutes, p. 177 (E. Heinz, ed.). Berlin-Heidelberg-New York: Springer 1972

Clausen, T.: Cations, glucose metabolism, and insulin action. Thesis, Århus University, 1972

Clausen, T., Harving, H., Dahl-Hansen, A.B.: The relationship between the transport of glucose and cations across cell membranes in isolated tissues. VIII. The effect of membrane stabilizors on the transport of K^+, Na^+ and glucose in muscle, adipocytes and erythrocytes. Biochim. biophys. Acta (Amst.) **298**, 393 (1973)

Clauser, H., Volfin, P., Eboué-Bonis, D.: Effect of insulin on the ^{32}P-mononucleotide and phosphocreatine labelling in the isolated diaphragm of the normal, the hypophysectomized, and the hypophysectomized growth-hormone treated rat. Gen. comp. Endocr. **2**, 369 (1962)

Coimbra, A.: Radioautographic studies of glycogen synthesis in the striated muscle of rat tongue. Amer. J. Anat. **124**, 361 (1968)

Coore, H.G., Denton, R.M., Martin, B.R., Randle, P.J.: Regulation of adipose tissue pyruvate dehydrogenase by insulin and other hormones. Biochem. J. **125**, 115 (1971)

Cori, C.F., Cori, G.T.: The influence of epinephrine and insulin injections on hexosephosphate content of muscle. J. biol. Chem. **94**, 581 (1931)

Cori, G.T., Closs, J.O., Cori, C.F.: Fermentable sugar in heart and skeletal muscle. J. biol. Chem. **103**, 13 (1933)

Cosmos, E., Harris, E.J.: In vitro studies of the gain and exchange of calcium in frog striated muscle. J. gen. Physiol. **44**, 1121 (1960)

Cowan, D.W., Wright, H.N.: The interrelationship between blood sugar, blood calcium, and blood coagulability. Amer. J. Physiol. **100**, 40 (1932)

Craig, J.W., Larner, J.: Influence of epinephrine and insulin on UDPG-alfa-glucan transferase and phosphorylase in muscle. Nature (Lond.) **202**, 971 (1964)

Craig, J.W., Rall, T.W., Larner, J.: The influence of insulin and epinephrine on adenosine 3′,5′-phosphate and glycogen transferase in muscle. Biochim. biophys. Acta (Amst.) **177**, 213 (1969)

Crane, R.K.: Intestinal absorption of sugars. Physiol. Rev. **40**, 789 (1960)

Crane, R.K.: Uphill outflow of sugar from intestinal epithelial cells induced by reversal of the Na^+ gradient: its significance for the mechanism of Na^+-dependent active transport. Biochem. biophys. Res. Commun. **17**, 481 (1964)

Creese, R., Northover, J.: Maintenance of isolated diaphragm with normal sodium content. J. Physiol. (Lond.) **155**, 343 (1961)

Creese, R.: Sodium fluxes in diaphragn muscle and the effects of insulin and serum proteins. J. Physiol. (Lond.) **197**, 255 (1968)

Csaky, T.Z., Wilson, J.E.: The fate of 3-O-methylglucose in the rat. Biochim. biophys. Acta (Amst.) **22**, 185 (1956)

Csaky, T.Z.: Effect of cardioactive steroids on the active transport of nonelectrolytes. Biochim. biophys. Acta (Amst.) **74**, 160 (1963)

Cuatrecasas, P.: Interaction of insulin with the cell membrane: The primary action of insulin. Proc. nat. Acad. Sci (Wash.) **63**, 450 (1969)

Curran, P.F.: Ion transport in intestine and its coupling to other transport processes. Fed. Proc. **24**, 993 (1965)

Danforth, W.H., Helmreich, E.: Regulation of glycolysis in muscle. I. The conversion of phosphorylase b to phosphorylase a infrog sartorius muscle. J. biol. Chem. **239**, 3133 (1964)

Danforth, W.H.: Glycogen synthetase activity in skeletal muscle. Interconversion of two forms and control of glycogen synthesis. J. biol. Chem. **240**, 588 (1965)

Davidson, M.B.: Studies on the mechanism of pentobarbital-induced glucose intolerance. Horm. Metab. Res. **3**, 243 (1971)

Davies, D.T., Dickens, F., Dodds, E.C.: Observations on the preparation, properties and source of the parathyroid hormone. Part I. Biochem. J. **20**, 694 (1926)

Daw, J.C., Berne, R.M.: Effect of sympathectomy on cardiac UDPG-glycogen transferase activity in the cat. Amer. J. Physiol. **213**, 1480 (1967)

Delcher, H.K., Shipp, J.C.: Effect of pH, pCO_2 and bicarbonate on metabolism of glucose by perfused rat heart. Biochim. biophys. Acta (Amst.) **121**, 250 (1966)

DeMello, W.C.: Effect of insulin on the membrane resistance of frog skeletal muscle. Life Sci. **6**, 959 (1967)

Dickens, F., Randle, P.J., Whelan, W.J.: Carbohydrate metabolism and its disorders. London and New York: Academic Press 1968

Dieterle, P., Gmeiner, K.H., Henner, J.: Evidence for peripheral release of insulin during muscular work in man. Horm. Metab. Res. **4**, 54 (1972)

DRUMMOND, G.I., SEVERSON, D.L., SULAKHE, P.V.: Nature of hormone and fluoride stimulation of adenyl cyclase in muscle. In: Insulin action, p. 277 (I.B. FRITZ, ed.). New York and London: Academic Press 1972

DULLY, C.C., BOCEK, R.M., BEATTY, C.H.: Presence of two or more glucose-6-phosphate pools in voluntary skeletal muscle and their sensitivity to insulin. Endocrinology **84**, 855 (1969)

DUNAND, P., BLONDEL, B., GIRARDIER, L., JEANRENAUD, B.: Alfa-aminoisobutyric acid uptake by cultured beating heart cells. Biochim. biophys. Acta (Amst.) **255**, 462 (1972)

DUNDEE, J.W.: Effect of thiopentone on blood sugar and glucose tolerance. Brit. J. Pharmacol. **11**, 458 (1956)

DURLACH, J.: Les relations entre magnésium et glucides. Diabetes **19**, 99 (1971)

EBOUÉ-BONIS, D., CHAMBAUT, A.M., VOLFIN, P., CLAUSER, H.: Action sélective de la N-éthylmaléimide sur la stimulation par l'insulin du métabolisme du diaphragme en survie. Bull. Soc. Chim. biol. (Paris) **49**, 415 (1967)

ELBRINK, J., BIHLER, I.: The effect of stimulation frequency and of ouabain on the intracellular penetration of L-arabinose in rabbit ventricular muscle. Life Sci. in press (1973)

ELLISON, R.J., WILSON, W.P., WEISS, E.B.: Changes in cerebral potassium during insulin hypoglycemia. Proc. Soc. exp. Biol. (N.Y.) **98**, 128 (1958)

EVANS, G.: The glycogen content of the rat heart. J. Physiol. (Lond.) **82**, 468 (1934)

FAHIMI, H.D., KARNOVSKY, M.J.: Cytochemical localization of two glycolytic dehydrogenases in white skeletal muscle. J. Cell Biol. **29**, 113 (1966)

FARISS, B.L., LUTCHER, C.L.: Diphenylhydantoin-induced hyperglycemia and impaired insulin release. Effect of dosage. Diabetes **20**, 177 (1971)

FELIX, J.M., SUTTER, M.T., SUTTER, B.C.J.: Circulating insulin and tissular reactivity to insulin in the rat during the perinatal period. Horm. Metab. Res. **3**, 71 (1971)

FENICHEL, R.L., BECHMANN, W.H., ALBURN, H.E.: Pituitary and adrenal influence on reduced insulin B-chain induced hyperglycemia. Diabetes **17**, 67 (1968)

FISHER, R.B., LINDSAY, D.B.: The action of insulin on the penetration of sugars into the perfused heart. J. Physiol. (Lond.) **131**, 526 (1956)

FISHER, R.B., ZACHARIAH, P.: The mechanism of the uptake of sugars by the rat heart and the action of insulin on this mechanism. J. Physiol. (Lond.) **158**, 73 (1961)

FISHER, R.B., WILLIAMSON, J.R.: The effects of insulin adrenaline and nutrients on the oxygen uptake of the perfused rat heart. J. Physiol. (Lond.) **158**, 102 (1961)

FISHER, R.B., GILBERT, J.C.: The effect of insulin on the kinetics of pentose permeation of the rat heart. J. Physiol. (Lond.) **210**, 297 (1970)

FREYGANG, W.H., JR., GOLDSTEIN, D.A., HELLAM, D.C., PEACHEY, L.D.: The relation between the late after potential and the size of the transverse tubular system of frog muscle. J. gen. Physiol. **48**, 235 (1964)

FRITZ, I.B.: Effects of insulin on glucose and palmitate metabolism by resting and stimulated rat diaphragms. Amer. J. Physiol. **198**, 807 (1960)

FRITZ, I.B., KAPLAN, E.: Effects of glucose on fatty acid oxidation by diaphragms from normal and alloxan-diabetic fed and starved rats. Amer. J. Physiol. **198**, 39 (1960)

FRITZ, G.R., KNOBIL, E.: The effect of insulin on extracellular space and tissue-water content of the isolated rat diaphragm. Biochim. biophys. Acta (Amst.) **78**, 773 (1963)

FUHRMAN, F.A.: Glycogen, glucose tolerance and tissue metabolism in potassium-deficient rats. Amer. J. Physiol. **167**, 314 (1951)

GARDNER, L.I., TALBOT, N.B., COOK, C.D., BERMAN, H., URIBE, C.: The effect of potassium deficiency on carbohydrate metabolism. J. Lab. clin. Med. **35**, 592 (1950)

GARLAND, P.B., NEWSHOLME, E.A., RANDLE, P.J.: Effect of fatty acids, ketone bodies, diabetes and starvation on pyruvate metabolism in rat heart and diaphragm muscle. Nature (Lond.) **195**, 381 (1962)

GARLAND, P.B., RANDLE, P.J., NEWSHOLME, E.A.: Citrate as an intermediate in the inhibition of phosphofructokinase in rat heart muscle by fatty acids. Nature (Lond.) **200**, 169 (1963)

GARLAND, P.B., NEWSHOLME, E.A., RANDLE, P.J.: Regulation of glucose uptake by muscle. 9. Effects of fatty acids and ketone bodies, and of alloxan-diabetes and starvation, on pyruvate metabolism and on lactate/pyruvate and L-glycerol 3-phosphate/dihydroxyacetone phosphate concentration ratios in rat heart and rat diaphragm muscles. Biochem. J. 93, 665 (1964)

GARLAND, P.B., RANDLE, P.J.: Regulation of glucose uptake by muscle. 10. Effects of alloxan-diabetes, starvation, hypophysectomy and adrenalactomy, and of fatty acids, ketone bodies and pyruvate, on the glycerol output and concentrations of free fatty acids, longchain fatty acylcoenzyme A, glycerol phosphate and citrate-cycle intermediates in rat heart and diaphragm muscles. Biochem. J. **93**, 678 (1964)

GARRATT, C.J., CAMERON, J.S., MENZINGER, G.: The association of ^{131}I-iodo-insulin with rat diaphragm muscle and its effect on glucose uptake. Biochim. biophys. Acta (Amst.) **115**, 179 (1966)

GARRATT, C.J., BUTTERFIELD, W.J.H., ABRAMS, M.E., STERKY, G., WHICHELOW, M.J.: Effect of exercise on peripheral uptake of ^{131}I-iodo-insulin and glucose in nondiabetics. Metabolism **21**, 36 (1972)

GEMMILL, C.L.: The effect of insulin on the glycogen content of isolated muscles. Bull. Johns Hopk. Hosp. **66**, 232 (1940)

GEMMILL, C.L.: The effects of glucose and of insulin on the metabolism of the isolated diaphragm of the rat. Bull. Johns Hopk. Hosp. **68**, 329 (1941)

GEVERS, W., DOWDLE, E.: The effect of pH on glycolysis in vitro. Clin. Sci. **25**, 343 (1963)

GILBOE, D.P., NUTTALL, F.Q.: The role of ATP and glucose-6-phosphate in the regulation of glycogen synthetase D phosphatase. Biochem. biophys. Res. Commun. **48**, 898 (1972)

GOLD, A.H.: The effect of diabetes and insulin on liver glycogen synthetase activation. J. biol. Chem. **245**, 903 (1970)

GOLDBERG, N.D., VILLAR-PALASI, C., SASKO, H., LARNER, J.: Effects of insulin treatment on muscle 3′,5′-cyclic adenylate levels *in vivo* and *in vitro*. Biochim. biophys. Acta (Amst.) **148**, 665 (1967)

GOLDSTEIN, M.S., MULLICK, V., HUDDLESTON, B., LEVINE, R.: Action of muscular work on transfer of sugars across cell barriers: comparison with action of insulin. Amer. J. Physiol. **173**, 212 (1953)

GOLDSTEIN, M.S.: Humoral nature of hypoglycemia in muscular exercise. Amer. J. Physiol. **200**, 67 (1961)

GORDEN, P., SHERMAN, B.M., SIMOPOULOS, A.P.: Glucose intolerance with hypokaliemia: an increased proportion of circulating proinsulin-like component. J. clin. Endocr. **34**, 235 (1972)

GOULD, M.K., RAWLINSON, W.A.: Effect of electrical stimulation and training on muscle pentose transport. Amer. J. Physiol. **211**, 141 (1966a)

GOULD, M.K., RAWLINSON, W.A.: Effect of natural exercise on pentose transport in rat skeletal muscle. Amer. J. Physiol. **211**, 147 (1966b)

GOULD, M.K., CHAUDRY, I.H.: The action of insulin on glucose uptake by isolated rat soleus muscle. I. Effects of cations. Biochim. biophys. Acta (Amst.) **215**, 249 (1970)

GOURLEY, D.R.H., FISHER, K.C.: Role of citrate in stimulation of oxygen consumption by insulin in frog muscle. Amer. J. Physiol. **179**, 378 (1954)

GOURLEY, D.R.H.: Separation of insulin effects on K^+ content and O_2 consumption of frog muscle with cardiac glycosides. Amer. J. Physiol. **200**, 1320 (1961)

GOURLEY, D.R.H., BETHEA, M.D.: Insulin effects on adipose tissue sodium and potassium. Proc. Soc. exp. Biol. (N.Y.) **115**, 821 (1964)

GOURLEY, D.R.H.: Effect of insulin on potassium exchange in normal and ouabain-treated skeletal muscle. J. Pharmacol. exp. Ther. **148**, 339 (1965)

GOURLEY, D.R.H., KYU SUH, T.: An apparent increase in water content of frog sartorius muscle exposed to insulin and carbohydrate intermediates. Canad. J. Physiol. Pharmacol. **44**, 871 (1966)

GOURLEY, D.R.H., BRUNTON, L.L.: Insulin-like effects of puromycin on lactate metabolism in frog skeletal muscle. Biochim. biophys. Acta (Amst.) **184**, 43 (1969)

GROSSMAN, S.H., MANCHESTER, K.L.: Response to insulin by guinea-pig taenia coli. Nature (Lond.) **211**, 1300 (1966)

GUIDOTTI, G.G., KANAMEISHI, D., FOA, P.P.: Chick embryo heart as a tool for studying cell permeability and insulin action. Amer. J. Physiol. **201**, 863 (1961)

GUIDOTTI, G.G., LORETI, L., GAJA, G., FOA, P.P.: Glucose uptake in the developing chick embryo heart. Amer. J. Physiol. **211**, 981 (1966)

HACKEL, D.B.: Effect of insulin on cardiac metabolism of intact normal dogs. Amer. J. Physiol. **199**, 1135 (1960)

HALDANE, J.B.S., WIGGLESWORTH, V.B., WOODROW, C.E.: The effect of reaction changes on human carbohydrate and oxygen metabolism. Proc. roy. Soc. B **96**, 15 (1924)

HALES, C.N., PERRY, M.C.: The role of ions in the hormonal control of adipose tissue. In: Adipose tissue, regulation and metabolic functions, p. 63 (B. JEANRENAUD and D. HEPP, eds.). Stuttgart: Thieme Verlag and London-New York: Academic Press 1970

HALL, J.C.: The effect of insulin on intact muscle from normal and alloxan-diabetic rats. J. biol. Chem. **235**, 6 (1960)

HAMMARSTEN, J.F., SMITH, W.O.: Serum magnesium and other electrolytes in insulin-induced hypoglycemia. Amer. J. Psychiat. **112**, 1956

HARROP, G.A., BENEDICT, E.M.: The participation of inorganic substances in carbohydrate metabolism. J. biol. Chem. **59**, 683 (1924)

HAUGAARD, E.S., SMITH, M.J., HAUGAARD, N.: Effects of thiols and disulfides on glucose utilization and insulin action in the isolated rat diaphragm. Biochem. Pharmacol. **21**, 517 (1972)

HAVIVI, E., WERTHEIMER, H.E.: A muscle activity factor increasing sugar uptake by rat diaphragms in vitro. J. Physiol. (Lond.) **172**, 342 (1964)

HECHTER, O., LESTER, G.: Cell permeability and hormone action. Recent Progr. Hormone Res. **16**, 139 (1960)

HEINZ, E. (ed.): Na-linked transport of organic solutes. Berlin-Heidelberg-New York: Springer 1972

HELMREICH, E., CORI, C.F.: Studies on tissue permeability. II. The distribution of pentoses between plasma and muscle. J. biol. Chem. **224**, 663 (1957)

HENDERSON, M.J., MORGAN, H.E., PARK, C.R.: Regulation of glucose uptake in muscle. IV. The effect of hypophysectomy on glucose transport, phosphorylation, and insulin sensitivity in the isolated perfused heart. J. biol. Chem. **236**, 273 (1961)

HEPBURN, J., LATCHFORD, J.K.: Effect of insulin (pancreatic extract) on the sugar consumption of the isolated surviving rabbit heart. Amer. J. Physiol. **52**, 177 (1922)

HIATT, N., YAMAKAWA, T., DAVIDSON, M.B.: Necessity for insulin in transfer of infused K to intracellular fluid. Metabolism **23**, 43 (1974)

HIDER, R.C., FERN, E.B., LONDON, D.R.: The effect of insulin on free amino acid pools and protein synthesis in rat skeletal muscle *in vitro*. Biochem. J. **125**, 751 (1971)

HODGKIN, A.L., NAKAJIMA, S.: The effect of diameter on the electrical constants of frog skeletal muscle fibres. J. Physiol. (Lond.) **221**, 105 (1972)

HOESCHEN, R.J.: The effect of ouabain on substrate metabolism in the isolated perfused rat heart. Canad. J. Physiol. Pharmacol. **49**, 412 (1971)

HOLLOSZY, J.O., NARAHARA, H.T.: Studies in tissue permeability. X. Changes in permeability to 3-O-methylglucose associated with contraction of isolated frog muscle. J. biol. Chem. **240**, 3493 (1965)

HOLLOSZY, J.O., NARAHARA, H.T.: Enhanced permeability to sugar associated with muscle contraction. J. gen. Physiol. **50**, 551 (1967a)

HOLLOSZY, J.O., NARAHARA, H.T.: Nitrate ions: potentiation of increased permeability to sugar associated with muscle contraction. Science **155**, 573 (1967b)

HOLM, J., SCHERSTÉN, T.: In vitro metabolism of glucose by human skeletal muscle. Method and normal values. Scand. J. clin. Lab. Invest. **29**, 99 (1972)

HUIJING, F., NUTTALL, F.Q., VILLAR-PALASI, C., LARNER, J.: UDPG-alfa-1,4-glucan alfa-4-glycosyltransferase in heart. Regulation of the activity of the transferase *in vivo* and *in vitro* in rat. A dissociation in the action of insulin on transport and on transferase conversion. Biochim. biophys. Acta (Amst.) **177**, 204 (1969)

ILSE, D., ONG, S.: Studies on the sugar carrier in skeletal muscle. Biochim. biophys. Acta (Amst.) **211**, 602 (1970)

INGLE, J., NEZAMIS, J.E., RICE, K.L.: Work output and blood glucose values in normal and in diabetic rats subjected the stimulation of muscle. Endocrinology **46**, 505 (1950)

IRWIN, R.L., OLIVER, K.L.: Prevention of relaxation in slow skeletal muscle by inhibition of active transport of sodium. Amer. J. Physiol. **218**, 1216 (1970)

ISAACSON, A.: Caffeine-induced contractures and related calcium movements of muscle in hypertonic media. Experientia (Basel) **25**, 1263 (1969)

JEFFERSON, J.S., KOEHLER, J.O., MORGAN, H.E.: Effect of insulin on protein synthesis in skeletal muscle of an isolated perfused preparation of rat hemicorpus. Proc. nat. Acad. Sci. (Wash.) **69**, 816 (1972)

JERVELL, J.: The antagonistic effect of human plasma albumin on the insulin stimulated glucose uptake of the isolated rat diaphragm. Acta physiol. scand. **65**, 33 (1965)

JESSUP, D.C., WIBERG, G.S.: Insulin bioassay using glycogen deposition in a single rat diaphragm. Diabetes **10**, 201 (1961)

JORI, A., BERNARDI, D., FARATTINI, S.: Chlorpromazine and glucose metabolism. Int. J. Neuropharmacol. **3**, 553 (1964)

KAESS, H., SENFT, G., LOSERT, W., SITT, R., SCHULTZ, G.: Mechanismus der gesteigerten glykogenolytischen Wirkung des Diazoxids im Kaliummangel. Naunyn-Schmiedebergs Arch. exp. Path. Pharmak. **253**, 395 (1966)

KAFKA, M.S., PAK, C.Y.C.: Effects of polypeptide and protein hormones on lipid monolayers. I. Effect of insulin and parathyroid hormone on monomolecular films of monooctadecyl phosphate and stearic acid. J. gen. Physiol. **54**, 134 (1969)

KAJI, H., PARK, C.R.: Stimulation of phosphate uptake by insulin and its relation to sugar transport in the perfused rat heart. Fed. Proc. **20**, 190 (1961)

KALANT, N., BEITNER, R.: Intracellular compartmentation of glycolytic phosphate esters. J. biol. Chem. **246**, 504 (1971)

KAMMINGA, C.E., WILLEBRANDS, A.F., GROEN, J., BLICKMAN, J.R.: Effect of insulin on the potassium and inorganic phosphate content of the medium in experiments with isolated rat diaphragms. Science **111**, 30 (1950)

KARPATKIN, S., HELMREICH, E., CORI, C.F.: Regulation of glycolysis in muscle. In: Current aspects of biochemical energetics, p. 127 (N.O. KAPLAN and E. KENNEDY, eds.). New York-London: Academic Press 1966

KARPATKIN, S., BRAUN, J.: Solubilization and partial purification of sarcoplasmic reticulum-bound hexokinase of frog skeletal muscle. Biochim. biophys. Acta (Amst.) **242**, 89 (1971)

KATZEN, H.M., SCHIMKE, R.T.: Multiple forms of hexokinase in the rat: tissue distribution, age dependency, and properties. Proc. nat. Acad. Sci. (Wash.) **54**, 1218 (1965)

KATZEN, H.M.: Hexokinase. In: Protein and polypeptide hormones, part 3, p. 822 (M. MARGOULIES, ed.). Amsterdam: Excerpta Medica 1969

KATZEN, H.M., SODERMAN, D.D. WILEY, C.E.: Multiple forms of hexokinase. Activities associated with subcellular particulare and soluble fractions of normal and streptozotocin diabetic rat tissues. J. biol. Chem. **245**, 4081 (1970)

KELLER, D.M., LOTSPEICH, W.D.: Phlorizin inhibition of the insulin expansion of the galactose space in the eviscerate rat. J. biol. Chem. **234**, 995 (1959)

KERLY, M., OTTAWAY, J.H.: The effect of diet on the metabolism of glucose and acetate by rat diaphragm muscle. J. Physiol. (Lond.) **123**, 534 (1954)

KERNAN, R.P.: The role of lactate in the active excretion of sodium by frog muscle. J. Physiol. (Lond.) **162**, 129 (1962)

KERR, S.E.: The effect of insulin and of pancreatectomy on the distribution of phosphorus in the blood. J. biol. Chem. **78**, 35 (1928)

KIEN, G.A., GOMOLL, A.W., SHERROD, T.R.: Action of digoxin and insulin on transport of glucose through myocardial cell membrane. Proc. Soc. exp. Biol. (N.Y.) **103**, 682 (1960)

KIEN, G.A., SHERROD, T.R.: The effect of digoxin on the intermediary metabolism of the heart as measured by glucose-C^{14} utilization in the intact dog. Circulat. Res. **8**, 188 (1960)

KIPNIS, D.M., CORI, C.F.: Studies on tissue permeability. III. The effect of insulin on pentose uptake by the diaphragm. J. biol. Chem. **224**, 681 (1957)

KIPNIS, D.M.: Regulation of glucose uptake by muscle: functional significance of permeability and phosphorylating activity. Ann. N.Y. Acad. Sci. **82**, 354 (1959)

KIPNIS, D.M., HELMREICH, E., CORI, C.F.: Studies of tissue permeability. IV. The distribution of glucose between plasma and muscle. J. biol. Chem. **234**, 165 (1959)

KIPNIS, D.M., CORI, C.F.: Studies of tissue permeability. VI. The penetration and phosphorylation of 2-deoxyglucose in the diaphragm of diabetic rats. J. biol. Chem. **235**, 3070 (1960)

KIPNIS, D.M., PARRISH, J.E.: Role of Na^+ and K^+ on sugar (2-deoxy-glucose) and amino acid (alfa-aminoisobutyric acid) transport in striated muscle. Fed. Proc. **24**, 1051 (1965)

KLEINZELLER, A., KOTYK, A.: Cations and transport of galactose in kidney-cortex slices. Biochim. biophys. Acta (Amst.) **54**, 367 (1961)

KOHN, P.G., CLAUSEN, T.: The relationship between the transport of glucose and cations across cell membranes in isolated tissues. VI. The effect of insulin, ouabain, and metabolic inhibitors on the transport of 3-O-methylglucose and glucose in rat soleus muscles. Biochim. biophys. Acta (Amst.) **225**, 277 (1971)

KOHN, P.G., CLAUSEN, T.: The relationship between the transport of glucose and cations across cell membranes in isolated tissues. VII. The effects of extracellular Na^+ and K^+ on the transport of 3-O-methylglucose in rat soleus muscle. Biochim. biophys. Acta (Amst.) **255**, 798 (1972)

KONO, T., COLOWICK, S.P.: Stereospecific sugar transport caused by uncouplers and SH-inhibitors in rat diaphragm. Arch. Biochem. **93**, 514 (1961)

KRAHL, M.E.: The action of insulin on cells. New York-London: Academic Press 1961

KREBS, H.A., EGGLESTON, L.V.: The effect of insulin on oxidations in isolated muscle tissue. J. Physiol. (Lond.) **32**, 913 (1938)

KREISBERG, R.A., WILLIAMSON, J.R.: Metabolic effects of ouabain in the perfused rat heart. Amer. J. Physiol. **207**, 347 (1964)

KUZUYA, T., SAMOLS, E., WILLIAMS, R.H.: Stimulation by hyperosmolarity of glucose metabolism in rat adipose tissue and diaphragm in vitro. J. biol. Chem. **240**, 2277 (1965)

KYPSON, J., TRINER, L., NAHAS, G.G.: Effects of ouabain and K^+-free medium on activated lipolysis and epinephrine-stimulated glycogenolysis. J. Pharmacol. exp. Ther. **159**, 8 (1968a)

KYPSON, J., TRINER, L., NAHAS, G.G.: The effects of cardiac glycosides and their interaction with catecholamines on glycolysis and glycogenolysis in skeletal muscle. J. Pharmacol. exp. Ther. **164**, 22 (1968b)

LANDAU, B.R., SIMS, E.A.H.: On the existence of two separate pools of glucose-6-phosphate in rat diaphragm. J. biol. Chem. **242**, 163 (1967)

Larner, J., Villar-Palasi, C., Richman, D.J.: Insulin stimulated glycogen formation in rat diaphragm. Ann. N. Y. Acad. Sci. **82**, 345 (1959)
Larner, J., Villar-Palasi, C., Brown, N.B.: UDPG-alfa-1,4-glucan alfa-4-glycosyltransferase in heart. Two forms of the enzyme, interconversion reactions and properties. Biochim. biophys. Acta (Amst.) **178**, 470 (1969)
Law, R.O.: The distribution of ^{14}C-sucrose within the skeletal muscle of the rat *in vitro*. J. Physiol. (Lond.) **190**, 71 (1967)
Lazarus, N.R., Penhos, J.C., Tanase, T., Michaels, L., Gutman, R., Racant, L.: Studies on the biological activity of porcine proinsulin. J. clin. Invest. **49**, 487 (1970)
LeFevre, P.G., Marshall, J.K.: Conformational specificity of a biological sugar transport system. Amer. J. Physiol. **194**, 333 (1958)
Leloir, L.F., Cardini, C.E.: Biosynthesis of glycogen from uridine diphosphate glucose. J. Amer. chem. Soc. **79**, 6340 (1957)
Levine, R., Goldstein, M., Klein, S., Huddlestun, B.: The action of insulin on the distribution of galactose in eviscerated, nephrectomized dogs. J. biol. Chem. **179**, 985 (1949)
Levine, R., Goldstein, M.S.: On the mechanism of action of insulin. Recent Progr. Hormone Res. **11**, 343 (1955)
Levine, R.: Cell membrane as a primary site of insulin action. Fed. Proc. **24**, 1071 (1965)
Liébecq, C.: Effet stimulant de l'insuline sur la consommation du glucose par le diaphragme et integrité cellulaire. Arch. int. Physiol. Biochim. **64**, 503 (1956)
Lipman, R.L., Raskin, P., Love, T., Triebwasser, J., Lecocq, F.R., Schnure, J.J.: Glucose intolerance during decreased physical activity in man. Diabetes **21**, 101 (1972)
Litwack, G. (ed.): Biochemical actions of hormones I. New York-London: Academic Press 1970
Lotspeich, W.D., Wheeler, A.H.: Insulin, anaerobiosis and phlorizin in entry of D-galactose into skeletal muscle. Amer. J. Physiol. **202**, 1065 (1962)
Lundholm, L., Mohme-Lundholm, E.: Effect of insulin on the carbohydrate metabolism of smooth muscle. Acta physiol. scand. **57**, 130 (1963)
Lundholm, L., Rall, T., Vamos, N.: Influence of K^+-ions and adrenaline on the adenosine-3',5'-monophosphate content in rat diaphragm. Acta physiol. scand. **70**, 127 (1967)
Lundsgaard, E.: The phosphate exchange between blood and tissue in experiments with artificially perfused livers and hind limb preparations. Skand. Arch. Physiol. **80**, 291 (1938)
Lundsgaard, E.: On the mode of action of insulin. Upsala Läk.- Fören. Förh. **45**, 143 (1939)
Mackler, B., Lichtenstein, H., Guest, G.M.: Effects of ammonium chloride acidosis on the action of insulin in dogs. Amer. J. Physiol. **166**, 191 (1951)
Mahler, R.J., Szabo, O., Penhos, J.C.: Antagonism to insulin action on the perfused hind limb of the rat by a reduced insulin B chain-albumin complex. Diabetes **17**, 1 (1968)
Manchester, K.L.: Stimulation by insulin of incorporation of ^{32}P-phosphate and ^{14}C from acetate into lipid and protein of isolated rat diaphragm. Biochim. biophys. Acta (Amst.) **70**, 208 (1963)
Manery, J.F., Gourley, D.R.H., Fisher, K.C.: The potassium uptake and rat of oxygen consumption of isolated frog skeletal muscle in the presence of insulin and lactate. Canad. J. Biochem. **34**, 893 (1956)
Marinetti, G.V., Shlatz, L., Reilly, K.: Hormone — membrane interactions, in Insulin action (I.B. Fritz, ed.). New York-London: Academic Press 1972
Martin, B.R., Denton, R.M., Pask, H.T., Randle, P.J.: Mechanisms regulating adipose tissue pyruvate dehydrogenase. Biochem. J. **129**, 763 (1972)
Martin, H.E., Wertman, M.: Serum potassium, magnesium, and calcium levels in diabetic acidosis. J. clin. Invest. **26**, 217 (1947)
Mennear, J.H., Miya, T.S.: Chlorpromazine-induced glucose intolerance in the mouse. Proc. Soc. exp. Biol. (N.Y.) **133**, 770 (1970)
Menozzi, P.G., Polleri, A.: Rapporti tra potassoi ed effetto insulinico nel muscolo isolato. Arch. E. Maragliano Pat. Clin. **17**, 677 (1961)
Meyer, F., Heilmeyer, L.M.G., Jr., Haschke, R.H., Fischer, E.H.: Control of phosphorylase activity in a muscle glycogen particle. I. Isolation and characterization of the protein-glycogen complex. J. biol. Chem. **245**, 6642 (1970)
Meyerhof, O., Himwich, H.E.: Beiträge zum Kohlenhydratstoffwechsel des Warmblütermuskels, insbesondere nach einseitiger Fetternährung. Arch. ges. Physiol. **205**, 415 (1924)
Milner, R.D.G., Hales, C.N.: The sodium pump and insulin secretion. Biochim. biophys. Acta (Amst.) **135**, 375 (1967)
Mondon, C.E., Burton, S.D., Grodsky, G.M., Ishida, T.: Glucose tolerance and insulin response of potassium-deficient rat and isolated liver. Amer. J. Physiol. **215**, 779 (1968)
Moore, R.D.: The ionic effects of insulin. Abstr. Biophys. Soc. Ann. Meeting, San Francisco, febr. 24—26, 1965, p. 122

MOORTHY, K.A., GOULD, M.K.: Synthesis of glycogen from glucose and lactate in isolated rat soleus muscle. Arch. Biochem. **130**, 399 (1969)

MORGAN, H.E., RANDLE, P.J., REGEN, D.M.: Regulation of glucose uptake by muscle: 3. The effects of insulin, anoxia, salicylate and 2:4-dinitrophenol on membrane transport and intracellular phosphorylation of glucose in the isolated rat heart. Biochem. J. **73**, 573 (1959)

MORGAN, H.E., HENDERSON, M.J., REGEN, D.M., PARK, C.R.: Regulation of glucose uptake in muscle. I. The effects of insulin and anoxia on glucose transport and phosphorylation in the isolated, perfused heart of normal rats. J. biol. Chem. **236**, 253 (1961a)

MORGAN, H.E., CADENAS, E., REGEN, D.M., PARK, C.R.: Regulation of glucose uptake in muscle. II. Rate-limiting steps and effects of insulin and anoxia in heart muscle from diabetic rats. J. biol. Chem. **236**, 262 (1961b)

MORGAN, H.E., REGEN, D.M., PARK, C.R.: Identification of a mobile carrier-mediated sugar transport system in muscle. J. biol. Chem. **239**, 369 (1964)

MORGAN, H.E., NEELY, J.R., WOOD, R.E., LIÉBECQ, C., LIEBERMEISTER, H., PARK, C.R.: Factors affecting glucose transport in heart muscle and erythrocytes. Fed. Proc. **24**, 1040 (1965)

MORGAN, H.E., NEELY, J.R.: Insulin and membrane transport. In: Handbook of Physiology, section 7: Endocrinology, p. 323. Baltimore: Williams and Wilkins 1972

MORIWAKI, T., LANDAU, B.R.: Fructose and glucose metabolism in the normal and diabetic rat diaphragm *in vitro*. Arch. Biochem. **97**, 544 (1962)

MORTIMORE, G.E.: Effect of insulin on potassium transfer in isolated rat liver. Amer. J. Physiol. **200**, 1315 (1961)

MULCAHY, P.D., WINEGRAD, A.I.: Effects of insulin and alloxan diabetes on glucose metabolism in rabbit aortic tissue. Amer. J. Physiol. **203**, 1038 (1962)

NAKADA, H.I., MORITA, T.N., WICK, A.N.: Studies on the relationships between insulin, glucosamine, and glucose in rat diaphragms. J. biol. Chem. **215**, 803 (1955)

NAKADA, H.I.: The metabolism of fructose by isolated rat diaphragms. J. biol. Chem. **219**, 319 (1956)

NARAHARA, H.T., ÖZAND, P., CORI, C.F.: Studies of tissue permeability. VII. The effect of insulin on glucose penetration and phosphorylation in frog muscle. J. biol. Chem. **235**, 3370 (1960)

NARAHARA, H.T., ÖZAND, P.: Studies on tissue permeability. IX. The effect of insulin on the penetration of 3-O-methylglucose-^{3}H in frog muscle. J. biol. Chem. **238**, 40 (1963)

NARAHARA, H.T.: Biological activity of proinsulin. In: Insulin action, p. 63 (I.B. FRITZ, ed.). New York-London: Academic Press 1972

NEEDHAM, D.M.: Machina Carnis. Cambridge University Press, p. 451, 1971

NEELY, J.R., LIEBERMEISTER, H., MORGAN, H.E.: Effect of pressure development on membrane transport of glucose in isolated rat heart. Amer. J. Physiol. **212**, 815 (1967)

NEPTUNE, E.M., SUDDUTH, H.C., FASH, F.J., FOREMAN, D.R.: Quantitative participation of fatty acid and glucose substrates in oxidative metabolism of excised rat diaphragm. Amer. J. Physiol. **196**, 269 (1959)

NEWSHOLME, E.A., RANDLE, P.J.: Regulation of glucose uptake in muscle. V. The effects of anoxia, insulin, adrenaline and prolonged starvation on concentrations of hexose phosphate in isolated rat diaphragm and perfused isolated rat heart. Biochem. J. **80**, 655 (1961)

NEWSHOLME, A.E., RANDLE, P.J.: Regulation of glucose uptake by muscle. VII. Effects of fatty acids, ketone bodies and pyruvate, and of alloxan-diabetes, starvation, hypophysectomy and adrenalectomy, on the concentrations of hexose phosphates, nucleotides and inorganic phosphate in perfused rat heart. Biochem. J. **93**, 641 (1964)

NORMAN, D., MENOZZI, P., REID, D., LESTER, G., HECHTER, O.: Action of insulin on sugar permeability in rat diaphragm muscle. J. gen. Physiol. **42**, 1277 (1959)

NUTTALL, F.Q.: Mechanism of insulin action on glycogen synthesis. In: Handbook of Physiology, section 7: Endocrinology, p. 395. Baltimore: Williams and Wilkins 1972

ÖZAND, P., NARAHARA, H.T., CORI, C.F.: Studies of tissue permeability. VIII. The effect of anaerobiosis on glucose uptake in frog sartorius muscle. J. biol. Chem. **237**, 3037 (1962)

ÖZAND, P., NARAHARA, H.T.: Regulation of glycolysis in muscle. III. Influence of insulin, epinephrine, and contraction on phosphofructokinase activity in frog skeletal muscle. J. biol. Chem. **239**, 3146 (1964)

OFFERIJNS, F.G.J., WESTERINK, D., WILLEBRANDS, A.F.: The relation of potassium deficiency to muscular paralysis by insulin. J. Physiol. (Lond.) **141**, 377 (1958)

OKA, T., TOPPER, Y.J.: Dynamics of insulin action on mammary epithelium. Nature (Lond.) **239**, 216 (1972)

OPIE, L.H., EVANS, J.R., SHIPP, J.C.: Effect of fasting on glucose and palmitate metabolism of perfused rat heart. Amer. J. Physiol. **205**, 1203 (1963)

Opie, L.H., Mansford, K.R.L., Owen, P.: Effects of increased heart work on glycolysis and adenine nucleotides in the perfused heart of normal and diabetic rats. Biochem. J. **124**, 475 (1971)

Otsuka, M., Ohtsuki, I.: Mechanisms of muscular paralysis by insulin with special reference to periodic paralysis. Amer. J. Physiol. **219**, 1178 (1970)

Oyama, J., Grant, R.L.: Effect of insulin on glucose uptake by mouse diaphragm tissue. Proc. Soc. exp. Biol. (N.Y.) **100**, 90 (1959)

Ozawa, E., Hosoi, K., Ebashi, S.: Reversible stimulation of muscle phosphorylase b kinase by low concentrations of calcium ions. J. Biochem. (Tokyo) **61**, 531 (1967)

Pain, V.M., Manchester, K.L.: The influence of electrical stimulation in vitro on protein synthesis and other metabolic parameters or rat extensor digitorum longus muscle. Biochem. J. **118**, 209 (1970)

Park, C.R., Bornstein, J., Post, R.L.: Effect of insulin on free glucose content of rat diaphragm in vitro. Amer. J. Physiol. **182**, 12 (1955)

Park, C.R., Johnson, L.H., Wright, J.H., Jr., Batsel, H.: Effect of insulin on transport of several hexoses and pentoses into cells of muscle and brain. Amer. J. Physiol. **191**, 13 (1957)

Park, C.R., Reinwein, D., Henderson, M.J., Cadenas, E., Morgan, H.E.: The action of insulin on the transport of glucose through the cell membrane. Amer. J. Med. **26**, 674 (1959)

Park, C.R., Morgan, H.E., Henderson, M.J., Regen, D.M., Cadenas, E., Post, R.L.: The regulation of glucose uptake in muscle as studied in the perfused rat heart. Recent Progr. Hormone Res. **17**, 493 (1961)

Park, C.R., Crofford, O.B., Kono, T.: Mediated (nonactive) transport of glucose in mammalian cells and its regulation. J. gen. Physiol. **52**, 296s (1968)

Parrish, J.E., Kipnis, D.M.: Effects of Na^+ on sugar and amino acid transport in striated muscle. J. clin. Invest. **43**, 1994 (1964)

Paul, D.H.: The effects of anoxia on the isolated rat phrenic-nerve-diaphragm preparation. J. Physiol. (Lond.) **155**, 358 (1961)

Pearson, O.H., Hastings, A.B., Bunting, H.: Metabolism of cardiac muscle: Utilization of ^{14}C labelled pyruvate and acetate by rat heart slices. Amer. J. Physiol. **158**, 261 (1949)

Perry, M.C., Hales, C.N.: Factors affecting the permeability of isolated fat cells from the rat to ^{42}K potassium and ^{36}Cl chloride ions. Biochem. J. **117**, 615 (1970)

Piras, R., Rothman, L.B., Cabib, E.: Regulation of muscle glycogen synthetase by metabolites. Differential effects on the I and D forms. Biochemistry **7**, 56 (1968)

Plenge, P., Mellerup, E.T., Rafaelsen, O.J.: Lithium action on glycogen synthesis in rat brain, liver and diaphragm. J. psychiat. Res. **8**, 29 (1970)

Pollack, H., Millet, R.F., Essex, H.E., Mann, F.C., Bollman, J.L.: Serum phosphate changes induced by injections of glucose into dogs under various conditions. Amer. J. Physiol. **110**, 117 (1934)

Post, R.L., Morgan, H.E., Park, C.R.: Regulation of glucose uptake in muscle. III. The interaction of membrane transport and phosphorylation in the control of glucose uptake. J. biol. Chem. **236**, 269 (1961)

Rabinowitz, D., Zierler, K.L.: Role of free fatty acids in forearm metabolism in man, quantitated by use of insulin. J. clin. Invest. **41**, 2191 (1962)

Rafaelsen, O.J.: Action of phenothiazine derivatives on carbohydrate uptake of isolated rat diaphragm and isolated rat spinal cord. Psychopharmacologia (Berl.) **2**, 185 (1961)

Rafaelsen, O.J., Clausen, T.: Fate of glucose in isolated rat spinal cord and diaphragm incubated in the absence and presence of insulin. J. Neurochem. **7**, 52 (1961)

Rafaelsen, O.J.: Glycogen content of rat diaphragm after intraperitoneal injection of insulin and other hormones. Acta physiol. scand. **61**, 314 (1964)

Rafaelsen, O.J., Lauris, V., Renold, A.E.: Localized intraperitoneal action of insulin on rat diaphragm and epididymal adipose tissue *in vivo*. Diabetes **14**, 19 (1965)

Randle, P.J., Smith, H.: Regulation of glucose uptake by muscle. II. The effects of insulin, anaerobiosis and cell poisons on the penetration of isolated rat diaphragm by sugars. Biochem. J. **70**, 501 (1958)

Randle, P.J., Garland, P.B., Hales, C.N., Newsholme, E.A., Denton, R.M., Pogson, C.I.: Interaction of metabolism and the physiological role of insulin. Recent Progr. Hormone Res. **17**, 1 (1966)

Randle, P.J.: Blood glucose homeostasis, glucose utilization. In: Nobel symposium, No. 13, p. 173 (E. Cerasi and R. Luft, eds.). Stockholm: Almquist and Wiksel 1970

Rasmussen, H.: Cell communication, calcium ion, and cyclic adenosine monophosphate. Science **170**, 404 (1970)

REGEN, D.M. DAVIS W.W., MORGAN, H.E., PARK, C.R.: The regulation of hexokinase and phosphofructokinase activity in heart muscle. Effects of alloxan diabetes, growth hormone, cortisol, and anoxia. J. biol. Chem. **239**, 43 (1964)

RESNICK, O., HECHTER, O.: Studies on the permeability of galactose in muscle cells of the isolated rat diaphragm. J. biol. Chem. **224**, 941 (1957)

REUTER, H., SEITZ, N.: The dependence of calcium efflux from cardiac muscle on temperature and external ion composition. J. Physiol. (Lond.) **195**, 451 (1968)

REUTER, H., BLAUSTEIN, M.P., HAEUSLER, G.: Na-Ca exchange and tension development in arterial smooth muscle. Phil. Proc. roy. Soc. B (Lond.) B **265**, 87 (1973)

RIESER, P., RIESER, C.H.: Anabolic response of diaphragm muscle to insulin and to other pancreatic proteins. Proc. Soc. exp. Biol. (N.Y.) **116**, 669 (1964)

RIESER, P.: Enzymatic hypoglycemia in alloxan diabetic rats. Proc. Soc. exp. Biol. (N.Y.) **119**, 532 (1965)

RIESER, P.: Insulin, membranes, and metabolism. Baltimore: Williams and Wilkins 1967

RIKLIS, E., QUASTEL, J.H.: Effects of cations on sugar absorption by isolated surviving guinea pig intestine. Canad. J. Biochem. **36**, 347 (1958)

ROCH-NORLUND, A.E., BERGSTRÖM, J., CASTENFORS, H., HULTMAN, E.: Muscle glycogen in patients with diabetes mellitus. Glycogen content before treatment and the effect of insulin. Acta med. scand. **187**, 445 (1970)

ROCH-NORLUND, A.E., BERGSTRÖM, J., HULTMAN, E.: Muscle glycogen and glycogen synthetase in normal subjects and in patients with diabetes mellitus. Scand. J. clin. Lab. Invest. **30**, 77 (1972)

RODBELL, M.: Metabolism of isolated fat cells. I. Effects of hormones on glucose metabolism and lipolysis. J. biol. Chem. **239**, 375 (1964)

RODBELL, M.: Metabolism of isolated fat cells. II. The similar effects of phospholipase C (clostridium perfringens alfa toxin) and of insulin on glucose and amino acid metabolism. J. biol. Chem. **241**, 130 (1966)

ROGUS, E., PRICE, T., ZIERLER, K.L.: Sodium plus potassium-activated, ouabain-inhibited adenosine triphosphatase from a fraction of rat skeletal muscle, and lack of insulin effect on it. J. gen. Physiol. **54**, 188 (1969)

ROJAS, E., HIDALGO, C.: Effect of temperature and metabolic inhibitors on ^{45}Ca outflow from squid giant axon. Biochim. biophys. Acta (Amst.) **163**, 550 (1968)

RUBENSTEIN, A.H., MELANI, F., STEINER, D.F.: Circulating proinsulin: immunology, measurement, and biological activity. In: Handbook of Physiology, section 7: Endocrinology, p. 515. Baltimore: Williams and Wilkins 1972

RUDERMAN, N.B., TOEWS, C.J., SHAFRIR, E.: Role of free fatty acids in glucose homeostasis. Arch. intern. Med. **123**, 299 (1969)

RUDERMAN, N.B., HOUGHTON, C.R.S., HEMS, R.: Evaluation of the isolated perfused rat hindquarter for the study of muscle metabolism. Biochem. J. **124**, 639 (1971)

RUDOLPH, W., HAUER, G.: Der Stoffwechsel des menschlichen Herzens unter dem Einfluß von Insulin. I. Untersuchungen über Koronardurchblutung, Sauerstoffaufnahme und Kohlendioxidabgabe des Myokards. Klin. Wschr. **47**, 486 (1969)

RUDOLPH, W., HAUER, G., DIETZE, G.: Der Stoffwechsel des menschlichen Herzens unter dem Einfluß von Insulin. II. Untersuchungen über die myokardiale Aufnahme von Glucose, Lactat und Pyruvat. Klin. Wschr. **47**, 814 (1969)

SAGILD, U., ANDREASEN, P.B.: Glucose tolerance and insulin responsiveness in experimental potassium depletion. Acta med. scand. **169**, 243 (1961)

SARKAR, A.K., OTTAWAY, J.H.: Inorganic phosphate metabolism by the perfused rat heart. Biochem. J. **84**, 57p (1962)

SCHLENDER, K., WEI, S.H., VILLAR-PALASI, C.: UDP-glucose: glycogen alfa-4-glucosyltransferase I kinase activity of purified muscle protein kinase. Cyclic nucleotide specificity. Biochim. biophys. Acta (Amst.) **191**, 272 (1969)

SCHONFELD, G., KIPNIS, D.M.: Effects of fatty acids on carbohydrate and fatty acid metabolism of rat diaphragm. Amer. J. Physiol. **215**, 513 (1968)

SCHULTZ, S.G., CURRAN, P.F.: Coupled transport of sodium and organic solutes. Physiol. Rev. **50**, 637 (1970)

SEEMAN, P., ROTH, S.: All lipid-soluble anaesthetics protect red cells. Nature (Lond.) **231**, 284 (1971)

SHANES, A.M.: Electrochemical Aspects of physiological and pharmacological action in excitable cells. Part I. The resting cell and its alterations by extrinsic factors. Pharmacol. Rev. **10**, 61 (1958)

SHAW, W.N., STADIE, W.C.: Coexistence of insulin-responsive and insulin-non-responsive glycolytic systems in rat diaphragm. J. biol. Chem. **227**, 115 (1957)

Shaw, W.N., Chance, R.E.: Effect of porcine proinsulin in vitro on adipose tissue and diaphragm of the normal rat. Diabetes **17**, 737 (1968)

Shaw, W.N., Stadie, W.C.: Two identical Embden-Meyerhof enzyme systems in normal rat diaphragm differing in cytological location and response to insulin. J. biol. Chem. **234**, 2491 (1959)

Shen, L.C., Villar-Palasi, C., Larner, J.: Hormonal alteration of protein kinase sensitivity to 3′,5′-cyclic AMP. Physiol. Chem. **2**, 536 (1970)

Shigel, T., Imai, S., Murase, H.: Contracture of slow muscle fibre induced by cardiac active steroids. Naunyn-Schmiedebergs Arch. exp. Path. Pharmak. **244**, 510 (1963)

Shorr, E., Barker, S.B.: *In vitro* action of insulin on minced avian and mammalian muscle. Biochem. J. **33**, 1798 (1939)

Sims, E.A., Landau, B.R.: Insulin responsive and nonresponsive pools of glucose-6-phosphate in diaphragmatic muscle. Fed. Proc. **25**, 835 (1966)

Smith, C.H., Brown, N.E., Larner, J.: Molecular characteristics of the totally dependent and independent forms of glycogen synthase of rabbit skeletal muscle. II. Some chemical characteristics of the enzyme protein and of its change on interconversion. Biochim. biophys. Acta (Amst.) **242**, 81 (1971)

Smith, G.H., Randle, P.J., Battaglia, F.C.: The mechanism of action of insulin in muscle. Mem. Soc. Endocrin. **11**, 124 (1961)

Soderling, T.R., Kickenbottom, J.P., Reimann, E.M., Hunkeler, F.L., Walsh, D.A., Krebs, E.G.: Inactivation of glycogen synthetase and activation of phosphorylase kinase by muscle adenosine 3′,5′-monophosphate-dependent protein kinases. J. biol. Chem. **245**, 6317 (1970)

Søvik, O.: Effect of insulin on the isolated rat diaphragm in the presence and in the absence of puromycin and actinomycin D. Acta physiol. scand. **63**, 325 (1965)

Søvik, O.: The action of insulin on glycogen synthesis in rat diaphragm. Acta physiol. scand. **68**, 246 (1966)

Søvik, O.: The effect of puromycin on glycogen synthetase. Biochim. biophys. Acta (Amst.) **141**, 190 (1967)

Spergel, G., Schmidt, P., Stern, A., Bleicher, S.J.: Effects of hypokaliemia on carbohydrate and lipid metabolism in the rat. Diabetes **16**, 312 (1967)

Stadie, W.C., Zapp, J.A., Jr., Lukens, F.D.W.: The effect of insulin upon oxidations of isolated minced muscle tissue. J. biol. Chem. **132**, 411 (1940)

Stadie, W.C., Zapp, J.A., Jr.: The effect of insulin upon the synthesis of glycogen by rat diaphragm in vitro. J. biol. Chem. **170**, 55 (1947)

Stadie, W.C., Haugaard, N., Perlmutter, M.: Effect of insulin upon pyruvate utilization by pigeon muscle. J. biol. Chem. **172**, 567 (1948)

Stadie, W.C., Haugaard, N., Marsch, J.B., Hills, A.G.: The chemical combination of insulin with muscle (diaphragm) of normal rat. Amer. J. med. Sci. **218**, 265 (1949)

Stauffacher, W., Renold, A.E.: Effect of insulin in vivo on diaphragm and adipose tissue of obese mice. Amer. J. Physiol. **216**, 98 (1969)

Steiner, D.F., Freinkel, N. (ed.): Handbook of physiology, section 7: Endocrinology. Baltimore: Williams and Wilkins 1972

Steiner, D.F., Kemmler, W., Clark, J.L., Oyer, P.E., Rubenstein, A.H.: The biosynthesis of insulin. In: Handbook of physiology, section 7: Endocrinology, p. 175. Baltimore: Williams and Wilkins 1972

Stout, R.W.: The effect of insulin on the incorporation of sodium (1-^{14}C)-acetate into the lipids of the rat aorta. Diabetologia **7**, 367 (1971)

Strändell, B.: On the influence of exercise on the blood sugar, especially in connection with glucose ingestion. Acta med. scand. Suppl. to vol. 55 (1934)

Surmaczynska, B., Metz, R.: Hormonal and immunological properties of insulin fragments. I. The individual peptide chains. Endocrinology **85**, 368 (1969)

Torres, H.N., Birnbaumer, L., Del Carmen Garcia Fernandez, M., Bernard, E., Belocopitow, E.: Glycogen metabolism in muscle homogenates. Arch. Biochem. **116**, 59 (1966)

Treasure, T., Toseland, P.A.: Hyperglycemia due to phenytoin toxicity. Arch. Dis. Childh. **46**, 563 (1971)

Triner, L., Killian, P., Nahas, G.G.: Ouabain hypoglycemia: Insulin mediation. Science **162**, 560 (1968)

Valencia, R.: Études des cations mineraux (K, Na, Ca, Mg) sous l'influence de l'insuline et dans e diabete. These Medical, Paris (1954)

Vasyanin, S.I., Serebryakov, V.S.: The effect of electrical stimulation on the distribution of sugars in the frog sartorius muscles. Biofizika **13**, 368 (1968)

Villar-Palasi, C., Larner, J.: Insulin-mediated effect on the activity of UDPG-glycogen transglycosylase of muscle. Biochim. biophys. Acta (Amst.) **39**, 171 (1960)

VILLAR-PALASI, C., LARNER, J.: Insulin treatment and increased UDPG-glycogen transglycosylase activity in muscle. Arch. Biochem. **94**, 436 (1961)

VILLAR-PALASI, C.: The hormonal regulation of glycogen metabolism in muscle. Vitam. and Horm. **26**, 65 (1969)

VILLAR-PALASI, C., LARNER, J.: Glycogen metabolism and glycolytic enzymes. Ann. Rev. Biochem. **39**, 639 (1970)

VILLEE, C.A., HASTINGS, A.B.: The utilization in vitro of ^{14}C-labelled acetate and pyruvate by diaphragm muscle of rat. J. biol. Chem. **181**, 131 (1949)

VINOGRADOVA, N.A.: Distribution of non-penetrating sugars in the frog's sartorius muscle under hypo- and hypertonic conditions. Tsitologia **10**, 831 (1968)

VINOGRADOVA, N.A., DOROSHENKO, N.V., NIKOLSKII, N.N., TROSHIN, A.S.: Regulation of transport of sugars in muscle fibers. Biofizika **13**, 365 (1968)

VOLFIN, P., CHAMBAUT, A.M., EBOUÉ-BONIS, D., CLAUSER, H., BRINKHOFF, O., BREMER, H., MEIENHOFER, J., ZAHN, H.: Biological activity of natural and synthetic insulin A-chain preparations on the isolated rat diaphragm. Nature (Lond.) **203**, 408 (1964)

WAHREN, J.: Human forearm muscle metabolism during exercise. IV. Glucose uptake at different work intensities. Scand. J. clin. Lab. Invest. **25**, 129 (1970)

WAHREN, J., FELIG, P., AHLBORG, G., JORFELDT, L.: Glucose metabolism during leg exercise in man. J. clin. Invest. **50**, 2715 (1971)

WALAAS, O., WALAAS, E., WICK, A.N.: The stimulatory effect by insulin on the incorporation of ^{32}P radioactive inorganic phosphate into intracellular inorganic phosphate, adenine nucleotides and guanine nucleotides of the intact isolated rat diaphragm. Diabetologia **5**, 79 (1969)

WALKER, B.G., PHEAR, D.N., MARTIN, F.I.R., BAIRD, C.W.: Inhibition of insulin by acidosis. Lancet ii, 964 (1963)

WANSON, J.-C., DROCHMANS, P.: Rabbit skeletal muscle glycogen. A morphological and biochemical study of glycogen beta-particles isolated by the precipitation-centrifugation method. J. Cell Biol. **38**, 130 (1968)

WEIS, L.S., NARAHARA, H.T.: Regulation of cell membrane permeability in skeletal muscle. J. biol. Chem. **244**, 3084 (1969)

WEITZEL, G., RENNER, R., GUGLIELMI, H.: Insulinähnliche Activität von Arginylverbindungen in vitro. Hoppe-Seylers Z. physiol. Chem. **352**, 1617 (1971)

WERMERS, G.W., CAVERT, H.M., HARRIS, J.O., QUELLO, C.F.: Glycogen metabolism in perfused contracting whole rat diaphragm muscle. Amer. J. Physiol. **219**, 1434 (1970)

WHANG, R., REYES, R., RODGERS, D.: Response of serum Mg and K to glucose and insulin infusion in uremic dogs. Metabolism **18**, 439 (1969)

WHELAN, W.J. (ed.): Control of glycogen metabolism. London-New York: Academic Press 1968

WIELAND, O., SIESS, E., SCHULZE-WEITMAR, H., v. FUNCKE, H.G., WINTON, B.: Active and inactive forms of pyruvate dehydrogenase in rat heart and kidney: Effect of diabetes, fasting, and refeeding on pyruvate dehydrogenase interconversion. Arch. Biochem. **143**, 593 (1971)

WIGGLESWORTH, V.B., WODROW, C.E., SMITH, W., WINTER, L.B.: On the effect of insulin on blood phosphate. J. Physiol. (Lond.) **57**, 447 (1922)

WILBRANDT, W., ROSENBERG, T.: The concept of carrier transport and its corollaries in pharmacology. Pharmacol. Rev. **13**, 109 (1961)

WILLIAMS, B.J., MAYER, S.E.: Hormonal effects on glycogen metabolism in the rat heart in situ. Molec. Pharmacol. **2**, 454 (1966)

WILLIAMS, G.R.: A continuous flow method for the determination of glucose uptake by excised rat diaphragm. J. gen. Physiol. **42**, 1139 (1959)

WILLIAMS, T.F., EXTON, J.H., FRIEDMANN, N., PARK, C.R.: Effects of insulin and adenosine 3',5'-monophosphate on K^+ flux and glucose output in perfused rat liver. Amer. J. Physiol. **221**, 1645 (1971)

WILLIAMSON, J.R., KREBS, H.A.: Acetoacetate as fuel of respiration in the perfused rat heart. Biochem. J. **80**, 540 (1961)

WOHLTMANN, H.J., NARAHARA, H.T.: Binding of insulin-^{131}I by frog sartorius muscle. J. biol. Chem. **241**, 4931 (1966)

WOLLENBERGER, A.: Metabolic action of the cardiac glycosides. I. Influence on respiration of heart muscle and brain cortex. J. Pharmacol. exp. Ther. **91**, 39 (1947)

YOUNG, D.A.B.: Hypothalamic (photoperiodic) control of a seasonal antagonism to insulin in the rat heart. J. Physiol. (Lond.) **178**, 530 (1965)

YOUNG, D.A.B., BALANT, L.: Intraperitoneal test of insulin activity on the rat diaphragm in vivo: factors controlling the variability of response. Acta endocr. (Kbh.) **71**, 103 (1972)

ZIERLER, K.L.: Increase in resting membrane potential of skeletal muscle produced by insulin. Science **126**, 1067 (1957)

Zierler, K.L.: Effect of insulin on membrane potential and potassium content of rat muscle. Amer. J. Physiol. **197**, 515 (1959a)
Zierler, K.L.: Hyperpolarization of muscle by insulin in a glucose-free environment. Amer. J. Physiol. **197**, 524 (1959b)
Zierler, K.L.: Effect of insulin on potassium efflux from rat muscle in the presence and absence of glucose. Amer. J. Physiol. **198**, 1066 (1960)
Zierler, K.L., Rabinowitz, D.: Effect of very small concentrations of insulin on forearm metabolism. Persistence of its action on potassium and free fatty acids without its effect on glucose. J. clin. Invest. **43**, 950 (1964)
Zierler, K.L., Rogus, E., Hazlewood, C.F.: Effect of insulin on potassium flux and electrolyte content of muscles from normal and from hypophysectomized rats. J. gen. Physiol. **49**, 433 (1966)
Zierler, K.L.: Possible mechanisms of insulin action on membrane potential and ion fluxes. Amer. J. Med. **40**, 735 (1966)
Zierler, K.L.: Insulin, ions, and membrane potentials. In: Handbook of Physiology, section 7: Endocrinology, p. 347. Baltimore: Williams and Wilkins 1972

E. Metabolic Effects on Adipose Tissue in vitro

Robert L. Jungas

"**Das Fettgewebe . . . steht . . . im Zentrum der Stoffwechselvorgänge**" — Schur and Löw, 1928.

I. Introduction and Early Studies

It is now widely recognized that adipose tissue represents one of the major targets for insulin's action in many species. The principal metabolic functions of adipose tissue which are regulated by insulin are lipogenesis and lipolysis. In some species lipogenesis in adipose tissue is rather sluggish, e.g., humans, and in these cases the major function of insulin in adipose tissue appears to be the regulation of triglyceride uptake and of its subsequent release in the form of free fatty acids (FFA) and glycerol (Gries, 1970). In other species such as most birds, insulin appears to have very little effect on either lipogenesis or lipolysis in adipose tissue (Goodridge, 1964; Goodridge and Ball, 1966). Because of these species differences this review will be restricted to the rat and mouse whose adipose tissues are extremely active metabolically and also particularly sensitive to the action of insulin. These species have been therefore the most thoroughly studied. In most cases little distinction will be made between studies utilizing segments of adipose tissue and those employing isolated adipocytes, since as shown by Rodbell (1965) the stromal cells of adipose tissue contribute very little to the tissue's overall glucose metabolism despite their large number. The action of insulin on brown adipose tissue, an organ which differs rather fundamentally both in function and metabolism from the more abundant white or unilocular adipose tissue, will not be considered.

Wide recognition of adipose tissue as an important site of action of insulin was surprisingly slow to develop. Reports appearing in the German literature shortly after insulin became available clearly suggested that adipose tissue was a target of insulin action.

Indeed three groups of investigators working independently had arrived at this conclusion by the late twenties. Thus both ARNDT (1926, 1928) and HOFFMAN and WERTHEIMER (1927) observed that the administration of insulin to dogs induced a deposition of glycogen in the fat depots. Failing to find glycogen in the serum these workers concluded that the glycogen was synthesized within the adipocytes and subsequently converted to fat in this tissue. Both reports stress the view that adipose tissue is not merely an inert storage depot for fat but is metabolically very active. Indeed SCHUR and LÖW (1928) drawing on similar experimental data arrived at the startling conclusion that adipose tissue was to be regarded as perhaps the major site of action of insulin. However it was to be another 30 years before the work of WINEGRAD and RENOLD (1958a) and their reiteration of this same conclusion brought to adipose tissue the wide attention it deserved.

Why, one might ask, were the earlier reports so widely ignored by contemporary biochemists and physiologists who continued to regard the liver as the major site of fat synthesis and looked with lethargic eyes on that dull and inert storage depot, adipose tissue? The reader is referred to WERTHEIMER (1965) for an authoritative account, but it may be helpful to point out that among the peculiar features of rat adipose tissue was its apparent failure to respond to insulin administered *in vivo*. Thus although ARNDT (1926) and HOFFMAN and WERTHEIMER (1927) were able to demonstrate glycogen deposition in dog adipose tissue following insulin administration, similar experiments were commonly negative on the favorite laboratory species, the rat (WERTHEIMER, 1928; LÖW and KRCMA, 1929; RICHTER, 1931; TUERKISCHER and WERTHEIMER, 1942). Since during this period the major criteria available for detecting metabolic changes within distinct tissues were the appearance and composition of the tissue in question, these negative results strongly encouraged the prevailing attitude of disinterest in adipose tissue. It was not until the middle forties that WERTHEIMER succeeded in inducing glycogen deposition in rat adipose tissue by the administration of insulin (WERTHEIMER, 1943, 1945). TUERKISCHER and WERTHEIMER (1946) investigated the requirements for this action of insulin in some detail, noting especially that the glycogen deposition response was favored by adrenalectomy of the rats and was prevented by the simultaneous administration of epinephrine. FAWCETT (1948) confirmed the basic findings using histochemical techniques.

Evidence for a direct local action of insulin on rat adipose tissue was provided in 1950 by RENOLD *et al.* who noted hypertrophy of adipose tissue immediately surrounding the site of insulin injections. It thus appeared likely that insulin promoted de novo synthesis of fat within adipose tissue, that it enhanced the deposition of fat synthesized elsewhere, or that it restrained fat mobilization. We now recognize that all three processes are subject to regulation by insulin.

Interest centered first on the process of de novo fatty acid synthesis. The occurrence of this process in isolated adipose tissue *in vitro* was demonstrated by SHAPIRO and WERTHEIMER (1948) using deuterated water and by FELLER (1954) using [^{14}C]acetate. HAUSBERGER *et al.* (1954) were the first to show that [^{14}C] glucose could be converted to fatty acids by segments of adipose tissue and that the rate of this process was enhanced by administration of insulin to the donor rats. Lipogenesis from carbohydrate by adipose tissue *in vitro* had been established far earlier however by the manometric studies of QUAGLIARIELLO and SCOZ (1930), RUSKA and QUAST (1935), HENLE and SZPINGIER (1936), and FELIX and EGER (1939). The studies of HAUSBERGER *et al.* were of great significance for they emphasized the quantitative importance of lipogenesis in adipose tissue. On a nitrogen basis rat adipose tissue was found to convert glucose to fatty acids some 500 times more rapidly than liver. These findings coupled with the studies of lipogenesis in mouse liver and adipose tissue *in vivo* by FAVARGER and GERLACH (1955, 1958) forced the abandonment of the earlier belief that liver was the major site of lipogenesis in these species.

KRAHL (1951) and ITZHAKI and WERTHEIMER (1957) appear to have been the first to demonstrate an effect of insulin added *in vitro* on white adipose tissue. They observed that high concentrations of insulin (1 unit/ml or 7 μM) increased the glucose uptake by 15—100% depending on the anatomical source of the tissues and the dietary status of the donor rats. HAUGAARD and MARSH (1952) had reported a 20% increase in oxygen consumption upon the addition of insulin to adipose tissue incubated in a phosphate buffer containing glucose but devoid of bicarbonate, though subsequent workers could not confirm this finding (BREIBART and ENGEL, 1954; ITZHAKI and WERTHEIMER, 1957; JUNGAS and BALL, 1961).

It was the appearance of the now classic papers of WINEGRAD and RENOLD (1958a, 1958b), however, which brought to the attention of endocrinologists the extraordinary responsiveness of adipose tissue metabolism to the action of insulin. For the first time massive increases amounting to an order of magnitude were demonstrated in lipogenesis from glucose in response to what was at that time regarded as a minute concentration of insulin (0.1 unit/ml, 0.7 μM). At about the same time a report appeared (GORDON and CHERKES, 1958) indicating that insulin also exerted a major inhibitory influence on the release of FFA from adipose tissue incubated in the presence of serum albumin and glucose. With the realization just emerging that FFA represented the principal form in which stored fat was mobilized from the depot stores (DOLE, 1956; GORDON and CHERKES, 1956; GORDON *et al.*, 1957; RESHEF *et al.*, 1958) these findings indicated that the major physiological processes occurring in adipose tissue, namely, lipogenesis from glucose and the storage and mobilization fat, were subject to regulation by insulin. Insulin thus came to be regarded as one of the hormones most vital to the proper functioning of this tissue, and intense interest was aroused in the possible role which abnormalities of adipose tissue function might play in the pathological disturbances of diabetes mellitus.

The immediate result of these remarkable discoveries was an explosive growth of interest in adipose tissue metabolism which in turn generated an avalanche of papers documenting the manifold actions of insulin and other hormones on this tissue. These studies culminated in the exhaustive review of the subject edited by RENOLD and CAHILL in 1965. The present review will deal only lightly with topics thoroughly covered in that volume and will concentrate on the refinements in our knowledge of the action of insulin on adipose tissue developed since that time.

Numerous reviews relating to this subject have appeared since 1965. Of particular note is the review of JEANRENAUD (1968), the volume edited in 1970 by JEANRENAUD and HEPP, and the recent review by AVRUCH *et al.* (1972). Other reviews deserving mention include RANDLE *et al.* (1966), GRIES and STEINKE (1967), GLIEMANN (1969), BJORNTORP and OSTMAN (1971), and FAIN (1973).

II. Description of the Effects of Insulin

1. Membrane Transport of D-glucose and Related Sugars

a) Recognition of Sugar Transport as a Major Locus of Insulin Action

It is currently well established that the transport of glucose across the plasma membrane of fat cells is normally the major rate-limiting step in the utilization of glucose by adipose tissue and that insulin's major action on carbohydrate metabolism in this tissue is to accelerate this translocation process. It is now also widely recognized that insulin exerts a variety of additional effects on adipose tissue metabolism which appear to be quite independent of the action of insulin on sugar transport. This current viewpoint represents a considerable modification of the status of thinking in the field from that which prevailed a dozen years ago.

At that time it was possible to maintain a far simpler notion of the action of insulin on adipose tissue which ascribed the entirety of its effects to an acceleration of sugar transport, presumably through an action on the glucose carrier mechanism. This interpretation was a natural one for early workers on adipose tissue metabolism since the action of insulin on glucose transport in muscle had already been established by the time detailed study of adipose tissue began. Indeed in their key papers in 1958, WINEGRAD and RENOLD emphasized that all of the effects of insulin which they had observed were consistent with this simple unifocal view of the action of insulin.

This interpretation of the action of insulin dominated thinking on this subject for several years after the appearance of these papers, drawing support primarily from the following observations:

i) Insulin accelerated the metabolism of glucose through all of the metabolic pathways available to it. There did not appear to be any pronounced channeling of the glucose carbon through a particular metabolic route. Insulin seemed simply to drive more glucose carbon in all directions through the available metabolic machinery of the adipocyte (WINEGRAD and RENOLD, 1958b).

ii) Insulin failed to accelerate the utilization of substances which entered the metabolic machinery at points other than via the glucose carrier, e.g., pyruvate and acetate (WINEGRAD and RENOLD, 1958a).

iii) No effects of insulin could be demonstrated on any enzymatic process in a cell-free system.

iv) The pattern of glucose conversion to various endproducts was similar whether glucose utilization was increased by the addition of insulin at low glucose concentrations or simply by increasing the medium glucose concentration (JEANRENAUD and RENOLD, 1959).

v) Certain processes were accelerated by insulin only if glucose was present in the incubation medium, e.g., fatty acid synthesis from pyruvate or acetate (WINEGRAD and RENOLD, 1958a) and protein synthesis from glycine (HERRERA and RENOLD, 1960) or other amino acids (CARRUTHERS and WINEGRAD, 1962). In each such instance the sole addition of glucose also accelerated the process and it seemed reasonable to propose that insulin acted solely by providing additional glucose to the metabolic mill.

vi) The only hormonal ation whose mechanism was at all understood at that time concerned the activation of glycogen phosphorylase by hormones such as epinephrine and glucagon acting via cyclic-AMP (RALL and SUTHERLAND, 1958; SUTHERLAND and RALL, 1958). Insulin was reported not to affect adipose tissue phosphorylase activity even in the presence of glucose (VAUGHAN, 1960) and thus was assumed not to be included in that group of hormones acting on intracellular processes by way of cyclic-AMP.

vii) The report of an action of insulin on adipose tissue hexokinase activity (MACLEOD *et al.*, 1960) was discounted because of the acknowledged difficulty of measuring accurately the intracellular glucose concentration in a tissue where the aqueous cytoplasmic volume is so minute. Direct assays of hexokinase in cell extracts revealed no effect of insulin (HERNANDEZ and SOLS, 1963).

There were however several observations which though difficult to reconcile with the simple unifocal view of insulin action, were not given emphasis by most workers. They were regarded simply as observations which could not yet be fully explained. The most troubling were the following:

i) KRAHL (1959) found that the incorporation of radioactivity from [3-^{14}C] pyruvate into protein was increased 30% by insulin even when no glucose was present. This finding was confirmed by CARRUTHERS and WINEGRAD (1962) using [2-^{14}C]pyruvate. The effect could be demonstrated even when tissue from fasted rats was employed. Moreover the addition of glucose did not increase the conversion of pyruvate carbon to protein in the presence or absence of insulin. Thus an effect of insulin either on protein synthesis or degradation and apparently independent of either glucose or amino acid transport was indicated. However because the conversion of labeled glycine, proline, or histidine to protein was not affected by insulin in the absence of glucose, no clear interpretation of this result could be given.

ii) LEONARDS and LANDAU (1960) conducted a thorough study of the patterns of glucose carbon disposition in various endproducts when glucose uptake was increased either by elevating the medium concentration or by the addition of insulin. They concluded that "insulin has an action other than on cell-wall permeability or the phosphorylation of glucose", primarily for two reasons:

a) Whereas conversion of glucose carbon to fatty acids was increased either by insulin or by elevating the glucose concentration, conversion to glyceride-glycerol was increased only by increasing the glucose concentration. Insulin lowered the fraction of glucose carbon appearing in glyceride-glycerol.

b) Conversely, conversion of glucose carbon to glycogen was greatly increased by insulin but was increased only slightly by elevating the concentration of glucose. Insulin preferentially channeled glucose carbon into glycogen.

In their similar earlier study JEANRENAUD and RENOLD (1959) had reached a different conclusion (see above) but they had considered primarily the conversion of glucose to fatty acids and CO_2 and had only limited data on glyceride-glycerol and glycogen. Insufficient attention was given by many workers to this important study of LEONARDS and LANDAU. Additional evidence suggesting a more direct action of insulin upon glycogen synthesis was provided by PITTMAN and BOSHELL (1963) who noted that while oxytocin stimulated glucose oxidation to an extent similar to that seen with insulin, it had no effect on the conversion of glucose carbon to glycogen, whereas insulin increased glycogen synthesis from medium glucose 5-fold.

With the realization in 1962 (JUNGAS and BALL) that insulin had an important antilipolytic effect in addition to its effect on glucose uptake, the way was opened for explaining the observations of LEONARDS and LANDAU on glucose metabolism (see below). Subsequent studies however have not yet fully clarified the effects of insulin on protein metabolism. They have also shed very little light indeed on the manner by which insulin accelerates glucose transport. The available information on this most vital problem will now be summarized.

b) Evidence that the Transport of D-glucose is Accelerated by Insulin

Although measurements of the action of insulin on glucose uptake, one of the most outstanding of which was the study by LIBERMAN (1961), were clearly consistent with an action of the hormone on glucose transport they obviously could not distinguish effects on translocation from those on glucose phosphorylation. To do so it was necessary to make measurements of the intracellular concentration of glucose in adipocytes. Such measurements are extremely difficult both because of the small amount of intracellular water (only some 5% of the tissue fresh weight represents intracellular water) and because of the unfavorable ratio of intra- to extra-cellular water (about 15% of the tissue wet weight is extracellular water).

It was not until 1965 that the first successful measurements of intracellular glucose were reported (CROFFORD and RENOLD, 1965a). Prior to that time several observations had been made which indirectly suggested that membrane translocation was the major rate-limiting step in the utilization of glucose and that insulin activated this process:

i) DIPIETRO (1963) and HERNANDEZ and SOLS (1963) presented evidence indicating that extracts of adipose tissue contained a single hexokinase (later recognized to be a group of isozymes) which acted on both glucose and fructose. It displayed a far lower affinity for fructose ($K_m = 3$ mM) than for glucose ($K_m = 0.05$ mM). Nevertheless when glucose and fructose were presented simultaneously to adipose tissue in the absence of insulin, the presence of glucose did not interfere with the utilization of fructose (FROESCH and GINSBERG, 1962; FAIN, 1964a). If transport were not the process limiting glucose entry, intracellular glucose should accumulate when glucose is presented and competitively inhibit the phosphorylation of fructose by hexokinase. When both glucose and fructose were present in high concentration and insulin was added glucose utilization was enhanced while fructose consumption was severely diminished, indicating that insulin increased glucose transport sufficiently to permit intracellular glucose to accumulate and interfere with fructose metabolism.

ii) The concentration of glucose required for half-maximal rates of glucose utilization (K_u) in the absence of insulin in 100—1000 times higher than the K_m of hexokinase (FROESCH and GINSBERG, 1962; HERNANDEZ and SOLS, 1963; BAKER and RUTTER, 1964). Barring an active process extruding glucose, this result suggests that either a diffusion or a transport process prior to hexokinase action limits glucose utilization.

iii) A limited permeability of the adipose tissue membranes to sugars was indicated by the slow entry of poorly utilized sugars such as N-acetylglucosamine (HERNANDEZ and SOLS, 1963) and D-xylose (MENOZZI *et al.*, 1961). The entry of D-xylose appeared to be increased by insulin.

Despite these suggestive results no firm conclusions regarding the action of insulin on glucose transport could be drawn until the work of CROFFORD and RENOLD (1965a, b). Using segments of rat adipose tissue and tritiated water or 3-O-methylglucose (3-OMG) to measure the intracellular water and sorbitol or sucrose to measure extracellular water, they found the tissue had an extracellular space of about 13 μL/100 mg fresh weight and an intracellular water space of 4.1 ± 0.3 μL/100 mg. When tissue from normally-fed rats was incubated at 25° with glucose but no insulin the tissue content of glucose was observed to be less than that which the extracellular water would contain were the concentration of glucose in this water the same as in the incubation medium. Thus a negative value was calculated for the intracellular glucose space. The addition of insulin caused the calculated intracellular glucose space to become even more negative at low medium glucose concentrations (5 mM) but less negative when the medium glucose was high (80 mM). The result at low medium glucose concentration indicated that insulin acted either on the membrane transport or the phosphorylation step rather than on the process, presumably simple diffusion, whereby glucose traverses the extracellular spaces. The result at high medium glucose concentration, where this diffusion process is less likely to limit glucose utilization, indicated that the effect of insulin on glucose phosphorylation, if any, must be of lesser magnitude than the effect on membrane translocation.

In an effort to obtain a more straightforward demonstration of the action of insulin on glucose transport CROFFORD and RENOLD turned to the use of adipose tissue from fasted-refed rats which presents itself in thinner lamellae and is very responsive to insulin. However, even with this special tissue and at low temperatures (17°) it was not possible to demonstrate an effect of insulin uniquely on the membrane transport step at normal levels of glucose (5 mM). Insulin clearly did cause an accumulation of intracellular glucose when the medium glucose concentration was raised to 20 mM (360 mg %) provided the tissue was kept cold. It was also evident from the data of CROFFORD and RENOLD that more intracellular glucose tended to be present when glucose utilization was enhanced by the addition of insulin than when similar rates of uptake were achieved by increasing the medium glucose concentration. Thus insulin was more effective in increasing glucose transport relative to glucose phosphorylation than was mere elevation of the external glucose concentration.

DENTON *et al.* (1966) and SAGGERSON and GREENBAUM (1970a) also could not detect any free intracellular glucose in adipose tissue incubated with insulin under physiological conditions.

Subsequent studies either on isolated fat cells or on tissue segments have not yet produced a completely satisfactory demonstration of an action of insulin on glucose transport at 37° with concentrations of glucose normally seen *in vivo*. It might be imagined that such a demonstration could be more easily achieved by utilizing isolated fat cells rather than intact segments of adipose tissue. This however has not proven to be the case. CROFFORD *et al.* (1966) found that the ratio of intracellular water to extracellular water in fat cells collected by filtration was about 1 to 8 rather than the more favorable ratio of 1 to 3 observed with tissue segments. Moreover the membranes of the isolated cells were apparently more permeable to small molecules since in cell preparations the sorbitol space was equal to the 3-OMG space rather than to the inulin space as in tissue segments. It is hardly surprising to find that membrane functions are altered in cells whose membranes have been exposed for prolonged periods to the mixture of lytic enzymes termed "collagenase" (KONO, 1969).

It may therefore be useful to mention the following additional indirect experiments in support of the view that under physiological conditions insulin does accelerate the rate of glucose transport into adipocytes:

i) The addition of glucose to tissue previously equilibrated with 3-OMG leads to a fall in the steady-state intracellular 3-OMG concentration (CROFFORD and RENOLD, 1965b). This is strong evidence for the existence of a mobile carrier able to transport both glucose and 3-OMG. Presumably the added glucose competes with 3-OMG for entry, but since the glucose cannot accumulate intracellularly, the exit of 3-OMG is less markedly reduced. This asymmetry results in the "countertransport" of 3-OMG upon the addition of glucose. When insulin is present this effect of glucose is much reduced, apparently because insulin allows the accumulation of additional intracellular glucose by promoting the transport step (CROFFORD *et al.*, 1966; CROFFORD, 1967).

ii) CLAUSEN (1969) reported that the rate of efflux of 3-OMG from tissue segments was enhanced up to 6-fold by insulin. This apparently reflects the action of insulin on the glucose carrier mechanism.

c) Transport Studies in Ghosts

Subcellular preparations have also been employed for assessing the effect of insulin on glucose transport. RODBELL (1967a) obtained a preparation of closed membranous sacs of about one-tenth or less the volume of fat cells by rupturing cells osmotically. These sacs, termed "ghosts", had within them many of the cellular enzymes but very little fat. When cells were ruptured in the presence of ATP, NAD^+, and $NADP^+$, the ghosts obtained would metabolize glucose at very slow rates — roughly 5% of that of cells containing the same amount of protein. Furthermore, the ghosts responded to insulin in that glucose consumption was increased about 50% — again about 5% of the percentage increase seen with intact cells. The glucose transport mechanism, though functioning, is apparently severely crippled since the transport step still seemed to limit the rate of glucose utilization (RODBELL, 1967b) despite the major losses of intracellular enzymes which are incurred during the preparation of the ghosts and their much higher surface to volume ratio. Obviously great caution must be exercised in extrapolating the findings obtained on such preparations to more physiological situations.

By omitting the cofactors ATP, NAD^+, and $NADP^+$, ILLIANO and CUATRECASAS (1971a) obtained ghosts in which glucose transport could be studied with little interference from glucose metabolism. D-Glucose entered such ghosts at rates roughly 10-fold greater than L-glucose, and with a K_t of 3.3 mM. Insulin increased the rate of entry and exit of D-glucose, but not L-glucose, by 2-fold or less, though about 40% of the preparations failed to respond. Significantly, the rate of efflux of D-glucose was accelerated by the addition of 3-OMG to the bathing medium. Such "accelerated exchange diffusion" is very strong evidence for the existence of a mobile glucose carrier. One explanation of the phenomenon is based on the assumption that the carrier is less mobile when empty. Thus supplying external 3-OMG hastens the return of the carrier to the inner membrane surface and accelerates the exit of glucose.

d) Characteristics of the Effect of Insulin on D-glucose Uptake

The concentration of insulin required to accelerate glucose entry into adipocytes is much lower when isolated fat cells are examined than when tissue segments are employed. With cells half-maximal responses are seen with about 5 μUnits/ml (0.04 nM) (HEPP *et al.*, 1967; CROFFORD, 1968; GLIEMANN, 1968, 1970) whereas 50—150 μUnits/ml (0.4—1.2 nM) are required with tissue segments (BALL and MERRILL, 1961; DOISY, 1963; BAKER and RUTTER, 1964; GLIEMANN, 1968). This difference in sensitivity to insulin is probably due primarily to two factors — more ready access of the hormone to the cells in the isolated cell preparation, and less proteolytic degradation by the cells provided the "collagenase" used in their preparation is scrupulously removed (GLIEMANN, 1968). In an heroic experiment GLIEMANN (1970) demonstrated that partial responses to insulin resulted from each cell responding in a graded manner to insulin rather than from all-or-none responses by individual cells differing in their sensitivity to insulin.

The extreme sensitivity of isolated adipocytes to insulin poses something of a dilemma. If the sensitivity of the cells is as great *in vivo* where serum insulin levels rarely fall as low as 5 μUnits/ml even in the lymph (RASIO *et al.*, 1965) it would seem the cells must always be experiencing nearly the full action of insulin. This problem is especially acute with regard to the antilipolytic action of insulin which

Table 1. *Representative Data Illustrating the Kinetic Characteristics of Glucose Utilization in Adipose Tissue Segments and Isolated Adipocytes. The term Ku is used to represent the concentration of medium glucose required for half-maximal rates of glucose uptake. Generally the utilization rate has been measured over a period of an hour or longer, though most authors have found the rate to be linear during this period. Assessment of glucose uptake has been either by measurement of disappearance from the medium or by summing the amount of glucose carbon converted to the major endproducts, CO_2 and lipid*

Author	Preparation	Ku (mM) Basal	Insulin	V_{max} Insulin/Basal	Comments
Froesch and Ginsberg (1962)	Tissue	3—4	—	—	Based on 3 points in range 2—44 mM. Fructose present at same concentration as glucose
Hernandez and Sols (1963)	Tissue	(1)	—	—	Based on net gas exchange. Rate at 200 mM was 3-times that at 3 mM
Baker and Rutter (1964)	Tissue	60	7	1—2	Based on 6 points in range 2—36 mM
Crofford and Renold (1965)	Tissue	90—140	7—12	1	Based on 3 points in range 10—86 mM (Basal) or 3—22 mM (insulin). Refed rats
Denton *et al.* (1966)	Tissue	1.6—2.4	1.6—2.4	2.5	Based on 6 points in range 1.5—11 mM. Fasted rats, 16 h
Rodbell (1966)	Cells	0.8	0.3	2.5	Range studied, 0.5—3 mM
Kuo *et al.* (1967)	Cells	0.5	—	—	Range studied, 0.3—3 mM
Caygill and Stein (1967)	Cells	0.4—2.9	0.4—2.9	1—1.5	Used rats of 300—450 g
Gliemann (1970)	Cells	5	1.7	3—4	Range studied, 0.4—20 mM, Non-linear 2 mM with insulin

is seen at even lower levels of insulin (see below). As it is extremely unlikely that this is in fact the case, some factor(s) must lower the sensitivity of the cells *in vivo* to about the range observed *in vitro* with tissue segments.

The fact that the biological response to insulin changes in a sigmoidal manner as the insulin concentration is changed (CROFFORD, 1968; GLIEMANN, 1968; LAVIS and WILLIAMS, 1970) probably does not reflect the kinetic characteristics of the insulin-receptor combination. It is more likely an artifact resulting either from the presence of excess insulin receptors or from the presence of processes competing for insulin when its concentration is very low, such as proteolytic degradation or adsorption to glassware.

It is experimentally extremely difficult to evaluate accurately the kinetic parameters K_u and V_{max} associated with glucose uptake and thus to assess the influence of insulin on these parameters. Representative data bearing on this question are displayed in Table 1. The estimates for K_u using tissue segments are spread over an extraordinarily large range. More careful inspection suggests that two processes might be involved, one displaying a K_u in the range of 2 mM and a second with a K_u in the region of 100 mM. Insulin appears to lower the K_u only of the latter process and to raise the V_{max} only of the former. One interpretation is that the higher affinity process represents the operation of the insulin-sensitive glucose carrier mechanism while the low affinity process is a less specific insulin-insensitive entry process. Insulin would appear to lower the K_u of this latter process only because it increases the relative contribution of the concomitantly occurring high affinity mechanism. Isolated cells do not display the low affinity mechanism though glucose concentrations sufficiently high to reveal it may not have been studied.

e) Effect of Insulin on the Transport of Other Sugars

The entry or metabolism of a variety of sugars is affected by insulin. D-Mannose utilization is increased by insulin in a manner very similar to that of D-glucose, differing only in that mannose utilization is about two-thirds as great as glucose (BALL and COOPER, 1960; WOOD *et al.*, 1961; HERNANDEZ and SOLS, 1963). As mannose and glucose share a common hexokinase (DIPIETRO, 1963; HERNANDEZ and SOLS, 1963) the lesser utilization of mannose probably reflects the stereospecificity of this enzyme. Transport of mannose has not been studied, though CROFFORD and RENOLD (1965b) reported that the addition of mannose did not decrease the intracellular glucose space and under certain conditions actually increased it. Competition between glucose and mannose utilization (WOOD *et al.*, 1961; CROFFORD and RENOLD, 1965b) is thus likely to occur primarily at the level of phosphorylation, though additional competition at the transport step is not excluded.

The metabolism of D-fructose by adipose tissue is also enhanced by insulin though less dramatically than that of D-glucose. BALL and COOPER (1960) found the insulin effect on fructose utilization only about one-third of that seen with glucose and subsequent workers have reported similar findings (FROESCH and GINSBERG, 1962; POZZA and GHIDONI, 1962; FAIN, 1964a; LEONARDS and LANDAU, 1964; FROESCH *et al.*, 1967; COORE *et al.*, 1971). In the absence of insulin, fructose entry can be accelerated more effectively than glucose by increases in the concentration of sugar in the medium (FROESCH and GINSBERG, 1962). These authors as well as FAIN (1964a) concluded that an insulin-insensitive pathway for fructose entry was present with a K_u of about 30 mM. Whether this is the same entry process as the one suggested above for glucose with a K_u of 100 mM is unknown. The affinity of fructose for the insulin-sensitive glucose carrier has not been determined because of interference from the insulin-independent process, but it is probably considerably lower than that of glucose since the utilization of glucose and fructose is additive at low sugar concentrations (FROESCH and GINSBERG, 1962). Thus glucose fails to impair fructose utilization under these conditions apparently because fructose utilization is limited by the phosphorylation step and intracellular glucose is low, while fructose fails to impair glucose utilization because transport is limiting and fructose has a low affinity for the glucose carrier.

No sugars besides the three already mentioned are rapidly utilized by adipose tissue (HERNANDEZ and SOLS, 1963). Evidence for a sluggish utilization of D-galactose especially at high concentrations has been presented (BALL and COOPER, 1960; BALLY *et al.*, 1960; BUCKLE *et al.*, 1961; POZZA and GHIDONI, 1962; MERTZ and ROGINSKI, 1963) but the results may merely reflect small glucose impurities in the galactose preparations (HERNANDEZ and SOLS, 1963). Sorbitol is slowly metabolized (FROESCH and GINSBERG, 1962; CROFFORD *et al.*, 1965) and insulin accelerates this process several-fold. Neither glucose nor fructose inhibited the oxidation of [U-^{14}C] sorbitol even in the presence of insulin and when isolated fat cells were employed (CROFFORD *et al.*, 1965). Phloretin and 3-OMG were effective inhibitors. Thus a distinct insulin-sensitive carrier mechanism responsible for sorbitol entry may exist whose physiological function is unknown. Neither L-glucose, L-arabinose, or D-xylose is metabolized by adipose tissue, though insulin appears to favor the entry of these sugars (MENOZZI *et al.*, 1961; CROFFORD and RENOLD, 1965b; BRAY and GOODMAN, 1968).

f) Role of Monovalent Cations in Sugar Uptake

Possible influences of the ionic composition of the medium on the metabolism of adipose tissue and its response to insulin were of concern to early investigators. HAGEN *et al.* (1959) noted that omitting Na^+ from the medium seriously disturbed the pattern of net gas exchange exhibited by the tissue. It appeared that basal glucose uptake was greater in the absence of Na^+ while the response to insulin was seriously impaired. Similar though less striking effects were seen when K^+ was omitted. CAHILL *et al.* (1959a) also found that the omission of K^+ led to an increase in glucose oxidation and conversion to fatty acids and glycogen. They also noted that the response to insulin was diminished in the absence of K^+. ZAHND *et al.* (1960) reported similar findings as did LEONARDS *et al.* (1962).

The above studies were performed primarily with the view of discovering the optimal conditions under which to incubate adipose tissue *in vitro*. Little attention was paid to the detailed mechanisms by which the cations might exert their influences on tissue metabolism. Interest in this latter aspect was kindled about 5 years later with the growing awareness of the importance of inorganic ions in the membrane transport of organic molecules. Perhaps of greatest impact was the discovery of the role of Na^+ in the active transport of sugars (CRANE, 1965) and of amino acids (PARRISH and KIPNIS, 1964). The observation by CLAUSEN (1966) that ouabain, known as an inhibitor of the Na^+-K^+-activated ATPase, stimulated the conversion of glucose to glycogen in diaphragm *in vitro* suggested that ion involvement might not be limited to translocation mechanisms capable of uphill transport. Interest was thereby renewed in the earlier work of BEIGELMAN and HOLLANDER (1962, 1963, 1964) who had shown that insulin increased the resting electrical potential across adipocyte membranes even in the absence of glucose.

Consequently a reinvestigation of the role of cations in the action of insulin on adipose tissue was initiated. The results confirmed the earlier findings concerning the major role of Na^+ both in restraining glucose entry in the absence of insulin and in permitting greatly increased entry in the presence of insulin (LETARTE and

RENOLD, 1967). Whether these results should be interpreted as evidence for a direct role for Na^+ in the operation of the glucose carrier (LETARTE and RENOLD, 1969) is not yet clear. CLAUSEN (1970) found that the effect of insulin on 3-OMG efflux from adipocytes was not affected by the replacement of Na^+ by Li^+, K^+, or choline, while confirming the fact that insulin fails to augment glucose oxidation or conversion to lipid in the absence of Na^+. Thus the requirement for Na^+ may be largely at steps subsequent to the transport function. Since so drastic a maneuver as omitting Na^+ may have a multitude of consequences to cellular function causing, for example, alterations in membrane potentials, in gradients for other ions especially Ca^{++} and K^+, in levels of ATP, etc., it is not at all clear what role, if any, Na^+ per se might play in glucose transport or in the action of insulin on this process.

The role of K^+ in the transport of glucose has also been given additional study. This ion behaves as though it were a simple non-competitive inhibitor of basal glucose uptake, being capable of lowering the V_{max} about 2.5-fold (LETARTE *et al.*, 1969). Ouabain prevents the inhibition by even high levels of K^+ and thus in its presence appears to have an insulin-like action on glucose uptake. In the absence of K^+ ouabain is ineffective. The inhibitory action of K^+ is remarkable in that it is prevented not only by ouabain but also by insulin. This observation prompted a test of the action of insulin on the Na^+-K^+-activated ATPase of adipocyte plasma membranes (MODOLELL and MOORE, 1967) but no effect could be demonstrated (LETARTE *et al.*, 1969). Data presently available are insufficient to define the K_i for the inhibitory action of K^+, and it is not clear whether insulin merely raises the K_i for K^+ or whether the inhibition is overcome in a non-competitive manner. While K^+ may be more directly involved in the glucose uptake process than Na^+, it is not known whether the effects of K^+ lack are due to the absence of the ion itself, or are due to secondary changes in the functioning of the Na^+-K^+ pump or in the cytoplasmic level of K^+.

A second remarkable feature of the action of K^+ is that even as it impairs glucose uptake it activates adenylate cyclase (HO *et al.*, 1967) and promotes lipolysis (MOSINGER and KUJALOVA, 1966; BLEICHER *et al.*, 1966a, b; HO *et al.*, 1966). This unusual coupling between effects on lipolysis and on glucose utilization whether induced by insulin or by a variety of agents which mimic some of the actions of insulin (RODBELL and JONES, 1966; KUO *et al.*, 1966; KUO, 1970) has played a major role in theoretical conceptions of the mechanism of action of insulin. The meaning of the association noted between changes in adenylate cyclase, glucose uptake and lipolysis remains, however, to be established.

2. Glycogen Metabolism

The earliest action of insulin on adipose tissue to be discovered was its ability to promote the accumulation of glycogen (ARNDT, 1926; HOFFMAN and WERTHEIMER, 1927; SCHUR and LÖW, 1928). This effect of insulin can now be understood in terms of its action on the enzymes responsible for glycogen synthesis and degradation, glycogen synthetase and glycogen phosphorylase. The discovery of the vital role of cyclic-AMP in the regulation of both of these enzymes (SUTHERLAND and RALL, 1960; ROSELL-PEREZ and LARNER, 1964), and of the role of insulin in regulating another cyclic-AMP-dependent process, lipolysis (JUNGAS and BALL, 1963), suggested that insulin might also be capable of affecting these enzymes. This was confirmed by JUNGAS (1966) who showed that homogenates prepared from tissue previously exposed to insulin had elevated glycogen synthetase activity and diminished phosphorylase activity. Although it appeared that the effect of insulin was to increase the fraction of synthetase in the "I" or independent form and to diminish the fraction of phosphorylase in the "a" or phospho form, no firm conclusions can be reached until these enzymes have been obtained in purified form from adipose tissue and their kinetic properties have been defined. The action of insulin on glycogen synthetase activity has been confirmed by SHAFRIR *et al.* (1970) and that on phosphorylase by JUNGAS and SCHWARTZ (1970).

These effects of insulin on the activities of glycogen synthetase and phosphorylase fit well with what is known of the role played by glycogen in adipose tissue metabolism. Significant glycogen accumulation in this tissue is seen normally only during the first days of refeeding starved animals, particularly when the diet contains substantial amounts of carbohydrate (GIERKE, 1906; TUERKISCHER and WERTHEIMER, 1942). The capacity of adipose tissue to convert glucose to fatty acids is drastically reduced by fasting (HAUSBERGER and MILSTEIN, 1955) and this deficiency cannot be rapidly overcome (HERRERA *et al.*, 1965). Presumably the diminished lipogenesis results from a drop in the level of certain key enzymes involved more or less directly in the lipogenic process, but just which enzymes are most crucial in this regard is not yet known (FLATT, 1970). In any event when vigorous refeeding is initiated by a hungry animal hexose carbon must be stored as glycogen until the enzymatic machinery required for rapid lipogenesis is resynthesized. As a result glucose carbon often flows to triglyceride via glycogen, a fact which so impressed early investigators that many concluded that glycogen was actually a necessary intermediate on the lipogenic pathway. Since refeeding on carbohydrate is normally accompanied by large elevations in plasma insulin, the appropriateness of insulin's effects on glycogen synthetase and phosphorylase activity is apparent.

The action of insulin on these two enzymes accounts for most but not all of the effects of this hormone on glycogen metabolism. The preferential channeling of glucose or fructose carbon to glycogen frequently observed upon addition of insulin presumably results from the activation of glycogen synthetase (JEANRENAUD and RENOLD, 1959; LEONARDS and LANDAU, 1960, 1964; PITTMAN and BOSHELL, 1963; SHAFRIR and KERPEL, 1964). When glycogen-rich tissue obtained from fasted rats refed briefly a high carbohydrate diet is incubated *in vitro* in the absence of glucose, active glycogenolysis occurs with the carbon flowing primarily to glyceride-glycerol, lactate, and fatty acids. Insulin markedly reduces the rate of disappearance of the glycogen and of release of lactate (JUNGAS and BALL, 1964; FROESCH *et al.*, 1965, 1967) and pyruvate (HALPERIN, 1970), presumably primarily as a consequence of the reduction in phosphorylase activity. For reasons still unknown this effect of insulin cannot be demonstrated under anaerobic conditions (JUNGAS and BALL, 1964). Similarly if tissue is first incubated with ^{14}C-labeled glucose or fructose to generate [^{14}C]glycogen *in situ*, the disappearance of glycogen radioactivity during subsequent incubation is retarded by insulin (FROESCH *et al.*, 1967).

The flow of glycogen carbon to glyceride-glycerol in tissue from refed rats is also reduced by insulin, in large part because of the reduction in lipolysis and hence in the supply of fatty acids available for reesterification (JUNGAS and BALL, 1964; JUNGAS, 1970a; BALL, 1970). However the flow of glycogen carbon to fatty acids is not diminished but increased. Suggestive evidence that this occurred was obtained by manometric measurements which revealed a rise in the Respiratory Quotient when insulin was added to glycogen-rich tissue incubated in the absence of glucose (JUNGAS and BALL, 1964). This was subsequently confirmed by the use of tritiated water, which provides a means of accurately measuring the total rate of fatty acid synthesis in adipose tissue (JUNGAS, 1968). Lipogenesis from endogenous sources was found to increase about 50% upon the addition of insulin

(Jungas, 1969; Halperin, 1970). The change in the pattern of disposition of glycogen carbon caused by insulin, namely, less formation of lactate and increased formation of fatty acids, provided the first indication that insulin in some manner activated pyruvate dehydrogenase (see below).

3. Fatty Acid Synthesis

The major metabolic fates of glucose carbon in either adipose tissue or isolated adipocytes from normally-fed rats incubated *in vitro* without added hormones are CO_2 and glyceride-glycerol (Cahill *et al.*, 1959b; Rodbell, 1964). When glucose uptake is accelerated by a substance which also enhances lipolysis, such as epinephrine, ACTH, or glucagon, these remain the major end-products of glucose metabolism (Cahill *et al.*, 1960a; Vaughan, 1961; Leboeuf and Cahill, 1961; Rodbell, 1965). However when glucose uptake is enhanced by raising its concentration in the bathing medium or by a substance which simultaneously diminishes lipolysis, such as insulin, the major endproduct is fatty acid (Jeanrenaud and Renold, 1959; Leonards and Landau, 1960; Rodbell, 1964). This holds true until the concentrations of both glucose and insulin reach very high levels. Then glucose uptake becomes greater than the tissue's capacity for lipogenesis and the excess incoming carbon is converted to glycogen. Insulin thus appears to promote fatty acid synthesis from glucose primarily as a secondary consequence of its actions on glucose translocation and on lipolysis.

While this general conclusion regarding the role on insulin in lipogenesis is widely accepted, evidence for additional effects of insulin at specific steps in the metabolic pathway leading from intracellular glucose to fatty acids has appeared from time to time. In considering these observations it is important to bear in mind that our knowledge of the factors which regulate lipogenesis in adipose tissue is very incomplete. However, it now seems likely that the upper limit on the rate at which glucose can be converted into fatty acids is determined not by the maximal catalytic capacity of any enzyme directly involved in this conversion, but by the capacity of the tissue to dispose of the excess ATP (or NADH) generated as a byproduct of the lipogenic process (Flatt and Ball, 1966; Flatt, 1970; Halperin and Robinson, 1970; Saggerson, 1972a, b). The precise enzymatic steps at which excess ATP and NADH (or lack of ADP and NAD^+) act to restrain further increases in lipogenesis are not known, but probably include pyruvate dehydrogenase (Saggerson and Greenbaum, 1970b; Randle and Denton, 1972; Taylor *et al.*, 1973) and phosphofructokinase (Jungas, 1969).

In discussing the action of insulin on lipogenesis it is convenient to divide the process into three stages:

1. intracellular glucose to pyruvate, 2. pyruvate to intramitochondrial citrate, and 3. intramitochondrial citrate to cytoplasmic fatty acid.

a) Conversion of Intracellular Glucose to Pyruvate

There is little evidence to suggest that insulin augments the phosphorylation of glucose in any manner other than by increasing its intracellular concentration. The capacity of the tissue to phosphorylate glucose exceeds its capacity for lipogenesis (see above). It is likely that any effect which insulin might have on the tissue's hexokinase activity would assume importance primarily when the rate of glucose uptake is very high and approaches the phosphorylative capacity of the tissue. Under these conditions excess glucose-6-phosphate is generated and much of it simply spills over into glycogen. Regulation of hexokinase activity therefore is unlikely to be of major importance to lipogenesis.

It was established by HERNANDEZ and SOLS (1963) that homogenates prepared from tissue exposed to insulin had unaltered total hexokinase activity and BORREBAEK and SPYDEVOLD (1969) and BORREBAEK (1970) have confirmed this finding. The latter author noted that a larger proportion of the hexokinase activity in homogenates prepared from tissue of fasted rats could be recovered in the mitochondrial fraction if the tissue was exposed to insulin prior to homogenization. This was true even in the absence of medium glucose and is of special interest since KOSOW and ROSE (1968) reported that hexokinase bound to mitochondria is less subject to inhibition by its products. The true intracellular location of hexokinase may of course not be accurately reflected by its distribution in homogenates, especially in a tissue so rich in lipid.

No strong evidence is available in support of an action of insulin on any enzyme involved in the conversion of glucose-6-phosphate to pyruvate. Since under certain conditions insulin can lower the level of cyclic-AMP in adipose tissue (BUTCHER *et al.*, 1966) and in isolated fat cells (BUTCHER *et al.*, 1968), and since cyclic-AMP is a particularly potent deinhibitor of adipose tissue phosphofructokinase (DENTON and RANDLE, 1966), it is possible that insulin could indirectly influence the activity of this enzyme. Measurements of the intracellular concentrations of the adenine nucleotides, fructose-6-phosphate, and fructose-1,6-bisphosphate revealed that the reaction catalyzed by this enzyme is far from equilibrium but failed to provide any evidence for an effect of insulin on its activity (HALPERIN and DENTON, 1969; SAGGERSON and GREENBAUM, 1970a).

The observation by BRAY (1967a) that high concentrations (10 μM) of dibutyryl-cyclic-AMP competitively inhibit 6-phosphogluconate dehydrogenase in extracts of fat cells cannot be considered compelling evidence for a role of physiological levels of cyclic-AMP in the regulation of this enzyme. In this regard it should be pointed out that the proportion of glucose-6-phosphate which enters the pentose cycle relative to that traversing the Embden-Meyerhof pathway is usually somewhat increased by insulin (FLATT and BALL, 1964; LANDAU and KATZ, 1964; KATHER *et al.*, 1972a). This proportion, however, should not be regarded as an independent variable. Rather, it seems to be determined by the supply of $NADP^+$ (KATZ and WALS, 1971; KATHER *et al.*, 1972b) and hence is dependent upon the rates of other metabolic processes which produce or consume this cofactor and not upon the activities of the enzymes which comprise the pentose cycle. The influence of insulin or other hormones on the proportion of glucose-6-phosphate which enters the pentose cycle is therefore likely to be very indirect.

b) Conversion of Pyruvate to Intramitochondrial Citrate

The reactions involved in this segment of the lipogenic pathway occur within the mitochondria of the adipocyte (MARTIN and DENTON, 1970) and include those catalyzed by the pyruvate dehydrogenase complex, pyruvate carboxylase, and citrate synthetase. It has recently been found that insulin activates pyruvate dehydrogenase and the available evidence suggests that this activation is a significant factor in the acceleration of lipogenesis by insulin.

The effect of insulin on pyruvate dehydrogenase activity (PDH) was discovered nearly simultaneously by two groups working independently. JUNGAS (1969), noting that insulin increased fatty acid synthesis from endogenous sources, probably mostly glycogen, while it diminished lactate production, concluded that the hormone must increase the activity of PDH. He suggested (incorrectly) that this might be a reflection of changes in the concentrations of acetyl CoA or NADH which were known to be inhibitors of the dehydrogenase (GARLAND and RANDLE, 1964; WIELAND *et al.*, 1969). It was not until the discovery by LINN *et al.* (1969a, b) of the existence of phospho- and dephospho-forms of the enzyme differing in their catalytic activity that the way was opened for the demonstration of an hormonal involvement in the regulation of PDH. JUNGAS (1970a) proceeded to show that fatty acid synthesis from medium pyruvate or lactate was increased by insulin and that extracts prepared from tissue previously exposed to insulin in the absence of substrate had slightly increased pyruvate dehydrogenase activity. DENTON *et al.* (1971) and COORE *et al.* (1971) incubated tissue with [U-^{14}C] fructose and found that insulin increased fatty acid synthesis from this precursor while decreasing the release of both lactate and pyruvate. Struck by the increase in lipogenesis at a time when tissue levels of pyruvate appeared to be lowered, they were also led to assay homogenates for PDH and found 2-fold increases in extracts prepared from tissue previously exposed to insulin. No changes were found in pyruvate carboxylase, citrate synthase, or glutamate dehydrogenase.

Earlier, FAIN (1964b) had noted in passing that insulin could increase the incorporation of radioactivity from [2-^{14}C]pyruvate into fatty acids. In a more thorough study HALPERIN (1970, 1971; HALPERIN and ROBINSON, 1971) found that insulin would increase fatty acid synthesis from low (0.25 mM) but not from high concentrations (25 mM) of medium pyruvate. This result probably explains why earlier investigators working with high levels of pyruvate failed to observe the effect of insulin on lipogenesis from pyruvate (WINEGRAD and RENOLD, 1958a; KRAHL, 1959).

Evidence has been presented by COORE *et al.* (1971) that insulin activates PDH by increasing the fraction of the enzyme protein present in the active (dephospho-) form. Just how insulin achieves this result is not yet known. There is no evidence for any involvement of cyclic-nucleotides in the regulation of either pyruvate dehydrogenase kinase or phosphatase (COORE *et al.*, 1971; JUNGAS and TAYLOR, 1972; SIESS and WIELAND, 1972; HUCHO *et al.*, 1972). It has recently been found that pyruvate dehydrogenase phosphatase requires low levels of Ca^{++} (DENTON *et al.*, 1972; PETTIT *et al.*, 1972) and changes in the intramitochondrial level of this ion may therefore play an important role in the response to insulin (RANDLE and DENTON, 1972). Alternatively, the effect of insulin might be mediated via changes in the mitochondrial ratio of ATP/ADP (TAYLOR *et al.*, 1973). It is also possible that a unique second messenger is generated when insulin combines with its receptor on the adipocyte plasma membrane and that this substance penetrates into the mitochondrial matrix to influence pyruvate dehydrogenase activity.

The importance of the activation of pyruvate dehydrogenase by insulin is emphasized by two facts. The first is that the activity of PDH in tissue extracts is lower than that of any other enzyme known to be involved in the conversion of glucose to fatty acids, i.e., PDH appears to be a strong candidate for a pacemaker enzyme (SAGGERSON and GREENBAUM, 1970b; COORE *et al.*, 1971). The second is that the product of PDH, acetyl CoA, is required for the functioning of pyruvate carboxylase (UTTER and KEECH, 1963). Thus by facilitating the conversion of pyruvate to acetyl CoA, insulin may indirectly augment pyruvate carboxylation to oxalacetate, thereby greatly favoring the generation of mitochondrial citrate.

It should also be mentioned that high levels of cellular pyruvate lead to activation of PDH (JUNGAS and TAYLOR, 1972; MARTIN *et al.*, 1972) probably by interfering with the action of PDH kinase (LINN *et al.*, 1969b). The unusual dependence of the rate of fatty acid synthesis from pyruvate on the medium concentration of pyruvate (HALPERIN, 1971) and the failure of insulin to accelerate this process at high levels of pyruvate (HALPERIN, 1970) may derive from this fact. No explanation can yet be given for the apparent rise in the affinity of PDH for pyruvate in tissue exposed to insulin (HALPERIN, 1971), as the K_m of PDH in extracts of adipose tissue is not affected by insulin (Coore *et al.*, 1971; Jungas and Taylor, 1972).

c) Conversion of Intramitochondrial Citrate to Fatty Acids

Lipogenesis is completed by the exit of citrate from the mitochondria via the tricarboxylate exchange carrier, its cleavage into acetyl CoA and oxalacetate, and the conversion of cytoplasmic acetyl CoA into long chain fatty acids by acetyl CoA carboxylase and fatty acid synthetase. During active lipogenesis in adipose tissue some 90% or more of the citrate formed intramitochondrially exits to the cytoplasm to be converted to fatty acids leaving only a small fraction to enter the tricarboxylic acid cycle (Winegrad and Renold, 1958b; Flatt and Ball, 1964; Landau and Katz, 1964). The factors which control the partitioning of citrate between these alternate metabolic routes are not well understood, but evidence has recently been obtained suggesting that insulin may exert an indirect controlling influence at this crucial metabolic branchpoint.

The exit of citrate through the mitochondrial inner membrane is facilitated by an anion exchange carrier which couples the exit of citrate with the entrance of another anion such as malate (Halperin *et al.*, 1969; Martin and Denton, 1970). In liver this citrate transport process has recently been shown to be competitively inhibited by low concentrations of fatty acyl CoA (Halperin *et al.*, 1972). Since insulin lowers the concentration of fatty acyl CoA in adipose tissue (Denton and Halperin, 1968; Saggerson and Greenbaum, 1970a) it may well promote the escape of mitochondrial citrate. This important observation by Halperin *et al.* (1972) offers direct support for the often expressed view that the regulation of the rate of transport of substances into or out of mitochondria will prove to be important features of metabolic control.

Little is known of the factors which regulate the rate at which cytoplasmic citrate is converted to fatty acids. The vast increase in lipogenesis from glucose caused by the addition of insulin is not associated with a rise in tissue citrate concentration (Denton *et al.*, 1966; Halperin and Denton, 1969; Saggerson and Greenbaum, 1970a). Thus citrate itself is unlikely to be an important regulatory substance under these conditions. Moreover this observation implies that some reaction lying between citrate and fatty acids is facilitated by insulin. This speculation is supported by the finding that insulin increases the incorporation of radioactivity from leucine into fatty acids even in the absence of glucose (Goodman, 1964; Smith and Beigelman, 1968; Meikle and Klain, 1972; but see also Christophe and Wodon, 1964). Three factors deserve mention in this regard. The first is the decrease in fatty acyl CoA caused by insulin. This may alleviate inhibitory influences of this substance on this portion of the pathway, for example on acetyl CoA carboxylase (Bortz and Lynen, 1963; Goodridge, 1972). The second is based on the recent finding that cyclic-AMP somehow inhibits the conversion of acetyl CoA to fatty acids in liver (Berthet, 1960; Tepperman and Tepperman, 1972; Bricker and Levey, 1972). If this proves to be true in adipose tissue as well, the ability of insulin to lower cyclic-AMP may contribute to its ability to accelerate this segment of the lipogenic pathway. (See also Murthy and Steiner, 1970; Steiner and Murthy, 1971.) Thirdly, Carlson and Kim (1973) have recently confirmed the finding of Inoue and Lowenstein (1972) that acetyl CoA carboxylase is subject to phosphorylation. The activity of acetyl CoA carboxylase appears to be regulated by phosphorylation in a manner precisely analagous to pyruvate dehydrogenase, and may therefore also be influenced by insulin.

It should be emphasized that once cytoplasmic citrate is "irreversibly" cleaved to acetyl CoA and oxalacetate, the acetate fragment is virtually committed to lipogenesis. Moreover, the capacity of the tissue to convert acetyl CoA to fatty acids is considerably greater than the highest rates of lipogenesis normally achieved from glucose (FLATT and BALL, 1966). Rate control between acetyl CoA and fatty acids is therefore unlikely to be of primary importance in the regulation of fatty acid synthesis from glucose. Additional attention to the possible regulatory role of the citrate cleavage enzyme in adipose tissue seems warranted.

The intriguing observation by BENJAMIN and GELLHORN (1964) that adipose tissue removed from diabetic rats fails to introduce the normal number of double bonds into newly synthesized fatty acids deserves mention. This defect cannot however be remedied by the addition of insulin to tissue incubated *in vitro*. Diabetic rats must be treated with insulin for 6—12 h to restore olefinic fatty acid synthesis and the synthesis of new enzymes is apparently required (GELLHORN and BENJAMIN, 1966).

4. Triglyceride Metabolism

a) Esterification of Fatty Acids

The hydrolysis of tryglycerides and subsequent reesterification of a portion of the fatty acids so liberated is a constantly occurring process of major quantitative significance in adipose tissue (CAHILL *et al.*, 1959b; BALL and JUNGAS, 1961). Indeed under nearly all conditions examined to date the quantity of free fatty acids (FFA) generated by the hydrolysis of glycerides far exceeds the amount of fatty acids produced by *de novo* synthesis. For example, even in tissue incubated in the presence of excess glucose and insulin, when lipolysis is near its slowest and fatty acid synthesis near its most rapid rate, the quantity of fatty acids liberated by lipolysis is 2—8 times the amount synthesized *de novo* (CAHILL *et al.*, 1959b; FLATT and BALL, 1966; LANDAU and KATZ, 1965; DENTON and HALPERIN, 1968; SAGGERSON and GREENBAUM, 1970a). This ratio may be increased to 30 in isolated fat cells (RODBELL, 1965). Thus to the extent that the rate of triglyceride synthesis is dependent upon the supply of fatty acids it is much more closely linked to the rate of lipolysis than it is to the rate of fatty acid synthesis.

These considerations probably explain why insulin is relatively ineffective in promoting the conversion of medium glucose (CAHILL *et al.*, 1959b; LEONARDS and LANDAU, 1960) or fructose (LEONARDS and LANDAU, 1964; FROESCH, 1965) to glyceride-glycerol. By restraining lipolysis, insulin limits the supply of fatty acids; hence triglyceride synthesis cannot be greatly increased despite the abundance of glycerol-3-phosphate available. In fact in tissue from fasted-refed animals the total rate of triglyceride synthesis as measured by the incorporation of tritiated water into glyceride-glycerol, is reduced nearly 50% by insulin even in the presence of glucose (JUNGAS, 1970a). Only under rather unusual conditions, as when both insulin and large amounts of a potent lipolytic agent are present (JUNGAS and BALL, 1963; SAGGERSON and GREENBAUM, 1970a) or when high levels of fatty acid are added to the bathing medium (BALLY *et al.*, 1960; SAGGERSON and GREENBAUM, 1970a), is the total rate of fatty acid esterification greatly increased by insulin. Insulin does, however, considerably increase the percentage of fatty acids liberated by lipolysis which are reesterified, provided glucose is present. It is commonly assumed that this effect of insulin results from an increased supply of glycerol-3-phosphate for the reesterification process, though attempts to verify this assumption have met with limited success (DENTON and HALPERIN, 1968; HALPERIN and DENTON, 1969; SAGGERSON and GREENBAUM, 1970a, b).

The assembly of triglycerides from FFA and glycerol-3-phosphate in adipose tissue follows the same route as in liver (STEINBERG *et al.*, 1961) only the enzymes involved may be more closely associated with mitochondria than with microsomes

(ANGEL and FARKAS, 1970). A small but metabolically very active pool of diglycerides is present in adipocytes and when lipogenesis is very rapid, as in the presence of insulin, up to a quarter of the newly synthesized lipid may be recovered from this fraction (ANGEL and FARKAS, 1970; WINAND *et al.*, 1971). No evidence has been obtained that any enzyme involved in the assembly of triglycerides is influenced by insulin.

b) Hydrolysis of Triglycerides

One of the most important properties of insulin both in terms of its effects on adipose tissue metabolism and on the energy metabolism of the whole animal is its ability to inhibit the hydrolysis of triglycerides in adipose tissue and hence to inhibit the mobilization of depot fat. The discovery of this effect of insulin was greatly facilitated by the observation that glycerol is very poorly utilized in adipose tissue (SHAPIRO *et al.*, 1957; WIELAND and SUYTER, 1957; CAHILL *et al.*, 1960b; STEINBERG *et al.*, 1961; MARGOLIS and VAUGHAN, 1962). Taken together with the fact that the process of lipolysis appears to be largely irreversible, this means that the flux through the lipase reactions *in situ* can be approximately determined simply by measuring the rate of glycerol release from the tissue. This rare opportunity to conveniently monitor the activity of an intracellular enzyme led to the rapid accumulation of information concerning the regulation of the triglyceride lipase by a variety of hormones (VAUGHAN and STEINBERG, 1963; JUNGAS and BALL, 1963). Homogenates of adipose tissue hydrolyze diglycerides and monoglycerides much more rapidly than triglycerides (STRAND *et al.*, 1964; VAUGHAN *et al.*, 1964) and major quantities of mono and diglycerides do not accumulate in adipose tissue even when lipolysis is quite rapid (VAUGHAN and STEINBERG, 1963; SCOW *et al.*, 1965; WINAND *et al.*, 1971). Thus the hydrolysis of stored triglycerides appears to be limited by the enzyme removing the first fatty acid moiety. This enzyme is referred to as the "hormone-sensitive" lipase (RIZACK, 1961; VAUGHAN *et al.*, 1964).

The first indication that the activity of this lipase could be reduced by insulin was the observation by PERRY and BOWEN (1962) that the release of fatty acids from adipose tissue was lowered by the addition of insulin even when no glucose was present. These authors however did not measure glycerol release and assumed that insulin lowered the release of fatty acids by promoting their esterification using glycerol-3-phosphate from endogenous sources. It was not until the demonstration that insulin lowered the release of glycerol (JUNGAS and BALL, 1963; MAHLER *et al.*, 1964) that the antilipolytic action of insulin was established. Since this effect of insulin could be readily observed in the absence of glucose, it became apparent that insulin had important effects on lipid metabolism which were independent of glucose transport. With the realization of the enormous influence which the supply of fatty acids from adipose tissue exerts on the metabolism of liver, heart, skeletal muscle and other organs, the inhibition of lipolysis has come to be regarded as one of the most significant metabolic actions of insulin.

Insulin is effective in lowering lipolysis in tissue incubated without any added lipolytic agent in the presence or absence of glucose, especially if the tissue is obtained from fasted-refed animals (BALL and JUNGAS, 1963; FROESCH *et al.*, 1965). The antilipolytic action of insulin is most dramatically revealed, however, when it is added together with low concentrations of a hormone which normally activates lipolysis, such as epinephrine, norepinephrine, ACTH or glucagon (JUNGAS and BALL, 1963; MAHLER *et al.*, 1964; RODBELL and JONES, 1966; FAIN *et al.*, 1966; HEPP *et al.*, 1969; MINEMURA and CROFFORD, 1969; LEFEBVRE and LUYCKX, 1969). The increased lipolysis induced in fat cells by low levels of theophylline or a prolonged incubation with growth hormone and a glucocorticoid is also blocked by insulin (FAIN *et al.*, 1965, 1966; RODBELL and JONES, 1966). However, if caffeine or theophylline is added along with a lipolytic hormone or if very high levels of the lipolytic hormone are employed, the inhibitory effect of insulin is overcome. Thus a large surge of norepinephrine released perhaps in response to a sudden stress would initiate the release of FFA from the depot fat stores even if it should occur at a moment, for example after a meal, when insulin levels were high.

For reasons that are currently not understood the quantity of insulin required to block lipolysis is lower than that needed to accelerate glucose uptake. For example, HEPP *et al.* (1967) using isolated fat cells found that 8 μUnits of insulin per ml (0.05 nM) were required to achieve a half-maximal effect on glucose oxidation whereas only 1.3 μUnits per ml (0.01 nM) produced a half-maximal inhibition of glycerol release in the presence of 0.5 μg ACTH per ml. Similar results have been reported by others (FAIN *et al.*, 1966; SOLOMON *et al.*, 1970; MINEMURA *et al.*, 1970; KONO, 1972) but not by CUATRECASAS (1972a). The higher sensitivity of lipolysis to insulin may be important in preventing a wasteful cyclic process of lipolysis and reesterification from occurring when glucose uptake is increased by insulin. This circumstance may also help to explain why a partial deficiency of insulin, as in maturity-onset diabetes, may lead to elevated levels of blood glucose and glucosuria without a concomitant ketosis (FAIN and ROSENBERG, 1972). If a single class of insulin receptors exists in the fat cell plasma membrane, this finding suggests that a lesser fraction of them need be occupied by insulin to restrain lipolysis than to promote glucose uptake (KONO, 1972). The physiological dilemma presented by the extraordinary sensitivity of lipolysis to insulin has been alluded to previously.

It is currently believed by most investigators that the ability of insulin to inhibit lipolysis derives from its ability to lower cellular levels of cyclic-AMP (but see FAIN and ROSENBERG, 1972, for another view). The fact that a variety of hormones share the property of activating both lipolysis and glycogen phosphorylase first suggested that cyclic-AMP might be involved in the regulation of the hormone-sensitive lipase (VAUGHAN, 1960; HAGEN, 1961; FRERICHS and BALL, 1962). This suspicion was reinforced with the demonstration that homogenates prepared from tissue exposed to a lipolytic hormone such as ACTH or epinephrine exhibited increased triglyceride lipase activity (HOLLENBERG *et al.*, 1961; RIZACK, 1961; VAUGHAN *et al.*, 1964) and that under certain conditions the addition of cyclic-AMP to tissue homogenates enhanced its lipolytic activity (RIZACK, 1964). It was not until 1970 however that a truly convincing demonstration of the role of cyclic-AMP in activating the hormone-sensitive lipase was provided by CORBIN *et al.* (1970) and by HUTTUNEN *et al.* (1970a, b). In no case could insulin be shown to affect lipase activity when added directly to cell-free homogenates, though homogenates prepared from tissue previously exposed to insulin did exhibit a reduced lipolytic activity (BALL and JUNGAS, 1964; LÖFFLER and WEISS, 1970; SCHWARTZ and JUNGAS, 1971). The mechanism by which insulin lowers cyclic-AMP in adipose tissue will be discussed below.

Several aspects of the antilipolytic action of insulin remain poorly understood. Among these the following deserve mention:

i) Adipose tissue or isolated fat cells removed from fasting animals exhibit accelerated lipolysis (GORDON and CHERKES, 1958; RESHEF *et al.*, 1958). There is disagreement in the literature as to whether or not insulin is effective *in vitro* in blocking this increased lipolysis. PERRY and BOWEN (1962), BUCKLE (1963), JUNGAS and BALL (1964), and JUNGAS and SCHWARTZ (1970) have presented data suggesting that insulin is ineffective in reducing lipolysis induced by fasting while MAHLER *et al.* (1964) and FAIN *et al.* (1966) found insulin to be effective.

ii) Concentrations of insulin greater than about 100 μUnits per ml (0.7 nM) are less effective in blocking lipolysis than smaller amounts (JUNGAS and BALL, 1963; LAVIS *et al.*, 1970; ALLEN and CLARK, 1971). The effect of insulin on adenylate cyclase also diminishes at high concentrations of insulin (HEPP, 1972; ILLIANO and CUATRECASAS, 1972). This is reminiscent of the inhibition of an enzyme be excess substrate and may derive from similar causes, e.g., two molecules of insulin may bind to a single receptor with mutual interference preventing activation of the receptor. Excess insulin however has not been found to have diminished effectiveness in stimulating glucose uptake.

iii) The antilipolytic effect of insulin can not be observed in all species. Outstanding exceptions are rabbits (HAGEN, 1963; RUDMAN *et al.*, 1968a, b), cows (METZ and VAN DEN BERGH, 1972), and birds. Bird adipose tissue releases abundant glycerol and FFA in response to glucagon, but insulin not only fails to inhibit the lipolytic action of glucagon, it actually enhances it (GOODRIDGE and BALL, 1965; GOODRIDGE, 1968; LANGSLOW and HALES, 1969). Insulin also fails to stimulate lipogenesis from glucose in avian adipose tissue (GOODRIDGE, 1964; GOODRIDGE and BALL, 1966).

iv) Under certain conditions the antilipolytic effect of insulin on rat adipose tissue can be reduced or eliminated by the addition of rapidly utilized substrates such as glucose, fructose, or pyruvate (JUNGAS and BALL, 1963; BALLY *et al.*, 1965; HALL and BALL, 1970). The effect is readily seen when tissue is incubated with both epinephrine and glucose, but no albumin. The addition of insulin now may cause a striking increase in lipolysis rather than an inhibition. This unusual response is not seen in tissue from fasted-refed animals nor from certain batches of normally-fed rats (JUNGAS, unpublished results). The reasons for the erratic nature of this response are not known.

In attempting to understand this bizarre "lipolytic" action of insulin it is important to recall that cellular levels of ATP must be maintained if lipolysis is to proceed (RIZACK, 1961; BALL and JUNGAS, 1963). Epinephrine depresses cellular ATP levels (HEPP *et al.*, 1968b; HALPERIN and DENTON, 1969; BIHLER and JEANRENAUD, 1970) and the further addition of glucose or pyruvate restores ATP and considerably enhances the release of FFA and glycerol (HO, 1970; ANGEL *et al.*, 1971). The "lipolytic" effect of insulin may therefore simply reflect its ability to promote the oxidation of carbohydrate substrates, thus enabling the cells to maintain their ATP levels sufficiently high to permit lipolysis to proceed.

v) Some suggestive evidence has recently been obtained indicating that in addition to its effects on lipolysis insulin may hinder the release of newly formed FFA from the adipocyte (SCHIMMEL and GOODMAN, 1972). The transport of FFA out of the fat cell is poorly understood but may occur in part by pinocytosis (CUSHMAN, 1970). Further study particularly of the possible role of cations in FFA transport is needed.

Which, one might ask, contributes more importantly to the ability of insulin to lower FFA release from adipose tissue *in vivo*, increased reesterification or decreased lipolysis? No precise answer can be given, though BOTTERMANN *et al.* (1966) have presented evidence that increased esterification plays an important role. It should be emphasized, however, that merely increasing FFA esterification is an inefficient means of decreasing FFA release. There are two reasons for this. First, large quantities of ATP are consumed in the esterification process. Second, FFA themselves inhibit lipolysis (JUNGAS, 1970b) and removing them by esterification may permit a compensatory rise in lipolysis to occur. The obvious efficiencies realized by blocking FFA production at its source argues strongly for its biological importance.

It might be useful to summarize briefly the hierarchy of restraints which can be brought to bear upon FFA release from adipose tissue. The first and most exquisitely sensitive mechanism is that brought into play by insulin, as just discussed. When this mechanism fails or is reduced in effectiveness, as in diabetes or fasting, FFA release can be curtailed by the process of glycerogenesis (Reshef and Shapiro, 1970). Glycerol-3-phosphate can be generated in adipose tissue from pyruvate (Ballard *et al.*, 1970) and this process is facilitated in diabetes or fasting by a rise in phosphoenolpyruvate carboxykinase activity (Reshef *et al.*, 1969; Shafrir *et al.*, 1970; Saggerson and Tomassi, 1971). However it cannot proceed rapidly at physiological pyruvate concentrations unless short chain fatty acids or possibly ketone bodies are present (Reshef and Shapiro, 1970). Thus the glycerogenic restraint may be important in limiting ketosis during fasting. For unknown reasons short-chain fatty acids fail to augment glycerogenesis in diabetic animals, a fact which may contribute to the excessive ketosis in this condition. Thirdly, if these mechanisms are insufficient, a build-up of FFA and ketones in plasma and hence in adipose tissue cytoplasm will occur and both of these substances are able to directly block the lipolytic process (Hellman *et al.*, 1969; Bjorntorp, 1966; Nakano and Ishii, 1970; Hotta *et al.*, 1971; Jungas, 1970b). Finally, if even this should prove insufficient, FFA levels become excessive, adipocyte ATP levels fall, and lipolysis is halted (Ho, 1970; Angel *et al.*, 1971). The regulatory effects of insulin on FFA release thus are seen to be superimposed upon a variety of less sensitive, less efficient, and possibly more primitive control mechanisms.

c) Uptake of Triglycerides

Triglycerides presented in the form of chylomicrons or very low density lipoproteins can be taken up from circulating plasma by adipose tissue. For this to occur rapidly the triglycerides associated with these massive lipoprotein molecules must be hydrolyzed to FFA and glycerol. Apparently this hydrolysis occurs at the inner surfaces of the endothelial cells lining the capillary walls, and the FFA so liberated make their way through the capillary walls and extracellular spaces to reach the adipocytes. The details of this uptake process are not yet fully understood, but the rate-limiting step is probably the initial hydrolytic cleavage catalyzed by the enzyme known as the "clearing-factor lipase" or "lipoprotein lipase". This enzyme is apparently synthesized within adipocytes and secreted into the extracellular spaces from which it migrates to its binding sites on the inner surfaces of the capillaries. The enzyme can be released from these binding sites by heparin. A brief recent review has been given by Robinson and Wing (1970).

Factors regulating the activity of the clearing-factor lipase can be conveniently studied in adipose tissue removed from rats which have been fasted overnight. Such tissue contains only about 10% of the normal levels of clearing-factor lipase activity. When this tissue is incubated *in vitro* in a suitable medium the activity of the lipase rises over a period of hours to values approaching those seen in tissue of fed animals. When this incubation is performed at 25° the only components which must be added to the medium to achieve a maximal increase in activity are amino acids, glucose, insulin, bicarbonate and inorganic ions (Robinson and Wing, 1970). The rise is inhibited by substances able to elevate tissue cyclic-AMP levels such as catecholamines, ACTH, glucagon, TSH, theophylline or puromycin (Wing and Robinson, 1968; Nestel and Austin, 1969) and by dibutyryl-cyclic-AMP (Wing and Robinson, 1968). The rise in activity is enhanced by agents capable of lowering cyclic-AMP including insulin (Salaman and Robinson, 1966; Wing *et al.*, 1966; Austin and Nestel, 1968) and nicotinic acid (Nikkilä and Pykälistö, 1968). The pattern of regulation of the clearing-factor lipase is thus seen to be the exact opposite of the "hormone-sensitive" lipase involved in fat mobilization. Many features of the regulation of the clearing-factor lipase remain to be clarified but it now appears likely that insulin will be found to play a highly significant role.

5. Tissue Respiration and ATP Production

The synthesis of palmitic acid from glucose in adipose tissue may be described formally by an expression of the following type:

$$4\ C_6H_{12}O_6 + O_2 \rightarrow C_{16}H_{32}O_2 + 8\ CO_2 + 8\ H_2O$$

The exact amount of oxygen consumed in the process depends on the fraction of glucose-6-phosphate which enters the pentose cycle but it cannot be less than that given above. Two important conclusions are immediately obvious:

i) The ratio of CO_2 produced to O_2 consumed (Respiratory Quotient) during lipogenesis is far greater than one. Therefore any substance such as insulin which accelerates lipogenesis will tend to raise the R.Q.

ii) The conversion of glucose to fatty acids requires oxygen or its equivalent. Substances increasing lipogenesis will therefore raise the tissue's oxygen consumption.

Ample experimental confirmation of these predictions has been obtained. BALL *et al.* (1959) were the first to demonstrate the striking effect of insulin on the net gas exchange of adipose tissue. Tissue incubated with glucose but no insulin produces CO_2 more slowly than it consumes O_2 (R.Q. less than 1). The addition of insulin causes an abrupt rise in CO_2 evolution and the R.Q. becomes much greater than one. Indeed measurements of the excess CO_2 produced in response to insulin provide one of the most sensitive and accurate bioassays for insulin-like activity (BALL and MERRILL, 1961; DOISY, 1963; FRERICHS *et al.*, 1965). FLATT and BALL (1964) and JUNGAS (1968) have noted a direct correlation between the rates of fatty acid synthesis and of excess CO_2 production. No additional actions of insulin besides its effects on lipogenesis need therefore be postulated to account for its effect on tissue net gas exchange.

The above considerations also explain why insulin is able to increase the O_2 consumption of adipose tissue only when the tissue is incubated in a bicarbonate-containing medium (JUNGAS and BALL, 1961; FLATT and BALL, 1963; HEPP *et al.*, 1968a). Without bicarbonate lipogenesis cannot be accelerated (GIBSON *et al.*, 1958) and insulin has very little effect on O_2 uptake (HAUGARD and MARSH, 1952; BREIBART and ENGEL, 1954; ITZHAKI and WERTHEIMER, 1957; ORTH *et al.*, 1960; LYNN *et al.*, 1960; WINEGRAD and SHAW, 1963).

Insulin has a much more dramatic effect on O_2 uptake when added in the presence of glucose and high levels of a lipolytic agent such as epinephrine (JUNGAS and BALL, 1963). In this case the increased O_2 uptake can be fully accounted for by the increased esterification of fatty acids caused by insulin (BALL and JUNGAS, 1961) as discussed previously. Under other conditions, for example in tissue from fasted-refed animals, insulin diminishes O_2 uptake (JUNGAS and BALL, 1964). Again the effect is readily explained by the decrease in fatty acid esterification resulting from the powerful antilipolytic action of insulin in this tissue. By relating the decrease in ATP consumption associated with the change in the rate of fatty acid esterification to the change in O_2 consumption an estimate of 3.0 was obtained for the P/O ratio, indicating that mitochondria within intact white adipose tissue are efficiently coupled.

More recently it has been reported that insulin increases the rate of incorporation of radioactivity from medium $^{32}P_i$ into the ATP of adipose tissue or isolated fat cells even when no glucose is present (HEPP *et al.*, 1968b). The explanation for this observation is not yet apparent. No rise in oxygen uptake occurs under these conditions so that if ATP synthesis is increased a rise in the P/O ratio would be implied. As noted above there is reason to believe that adipose tissue mitochondria *in situ* are normally efficiently coupled. The possibility that the effect is secondary to an enhancement of phosphate transport by insulin was discredited though perhaps not completely ruled out.

6. Amino Acid Metabolism and Protein Synthesis

Adipose tissue is capable of incorporating amino acids into protein at a rate ten-times greater than that of diaphragm on a nitrogen basis (Herrera and Renold, 1960). Nevertheless the action of insulin on protein synthesis in adipose tissue has not been extensively investigated. The available information suggests, but does not prove, that insulin may be capable of accelerating protein synthesis in this tissue.

The processes of protein synthesis and protein degradation are normally maintained in a delicate balance in most cells of an adult animal. When adipose tissue or isolated adipocytes are incubated *in vitro* this balance is destroyed and proteolysis proceeds far more rapidly than protein synthesis. For example in the outstanding study of protein metabolism in isolated fat cells by Minemura *et al.* (1970) it was found that in the basal state amino acids were generated by proteolysis some 6-times more rapidly than they were utilized by the protein synthetic machinery. While this circumstance of negative nitrogen balance is not unusual for a tissue incubated *in vitro* it is important to bear it in mind when considering the possible action of an anabolic hormone such as insulin on these processes. It may be very difficult to find experimental conditions under which the full anabolic influence of a hormone can be exhibited in a tissue whose metabolic balance has been so strongly distorted by unknown factors.

One factor which almost certainly plays an important role in permitting the fullest expression of anabolic functions such as protein synthesis is the cellular supply of ATP. Circumstances which favor the maintenance of high ATP stores may therefore indirectly promote protein synthesis. This is especially true under *in vitro* conditions where cellular ATP often falls well below the levels seen in fresh tissue. Several perplexing observations concerning the effects of insulin on protein synthesis can, I believe, be given plausible explanations on this basis.

Krahl in 1959 reported that insulin increased the incorporation of radioactivity from [3-^{14}C]pyruvate into protein about 30% without altering the conversion of medium pyruvate to lipids and in the absence of glucose. This observation has been repeatedly confirmed (Carruthers and Winegrad, 1962; Fain, 1964b; Herrera and Renold, 1965) and was originally regarded as evidence for an effect of insulin on protein synthesis independent of glucose or amino acid transport. However it was soon found that under the conditions of these experiments insulin failed to increase the conversion of either labeled amino acids (Herrera and Renold, 1960; Carruthers and Winegrad, 1962; Christophe and Wodon, 1964; Krahl, 1964; Herrera and Renold, 1965; Miller and Beigelman, 1966) or acetate (Krahl, 1959; Herrera and Renold, 1965) into protein unless either pyruvate or glucose was also present, in which cases increases of 20—60% were seen. As previously discussed, it is now recognized that insulin can augment the oxidation of either glucose or pyruvate and thus favor the generation of ATP from either source. These effects of insulin on label incorporation into protein may therefore be secondary to its effects on carbohydrate oxidation. This interpretation is supported by the observation that under the conditions of these experiments the simple addition of glucose or pyruvate is sufficient to increase amino acid incorporation (Carruthers and Winegrad, 1962; Christophe and Wodon, 1964; Krahl, 1964; Herrera and Renold, 1965) suggesting that energy availability may be limiting in the absence of these substrates. The powerful inhibition of the incorporation of amino acids into protein caused by large amounts of epinephrine or ACTH (Herrera and Renold, 1960; Christophe and Wodon, 1964) may also be a reflection of the fall in cellular ATP levels caused by these agents.

Attempts to demonstrate an effect of insulin on amino acid transport in adipose tissue or isolated adipocytes have been uniformly without success. Goodman (1966) demonstrated that the non-utilizable amino acid analog, amino isobutyric acid (AIB), was actively accumulated by adipose tissue but neither the rate of accumulation nor the concentration ratio achieved in the steady state were affected by insulin whether or not glucose was present. Others have reported similar findings using intact tissue (Bruchhausen, 1968), isolated cells (Touabi and Jeanrenaud, 1969; Minemura *et al.*, 1970) or adipocyte ghosts (Clausen and Rodbell, 1969). Under conditions where ATP is limiting insulin may exert a small favorable effect on the steady state concentration ratio of AIB either by increasing glucose oxidation or by limiting lipolysis (Touabi and Jeanrenaud, 1969; Vassalli and Jeanrenaud, 1970).

The picture which thus emerged from a dozen or so reports spread over nearly a decade was that insulin played at best a minor and perhaps secondary role in the regulation of protein synthesis in adipose tissue. Recently, however, evidence has been presented suggesting that insulin may have a more direct role in the regulation of protein synthesis or degradation. Smith and Beigelman (1968) and Bruchhausen (1968) found that insulin increased the incorporation of radioactive leucine into protein in the absence of oxidizable carbohydrate. These observations were confirmed and extended in the more complete study of Minemura *et al.* (1970). Working with isolated fat cells provided with a balanced mixture of amino acids, these workers demonstrated that insulin increased the incorporation of labeled leucine into protein by nearly 100%, of alanine and glycine by about 50%, and of serine by about one-third. Importantly, under their conditions the addition of glucose or pyruvate did not appreciably enhance this effect of insulin. Minemura *et al.* (1970) also found that insulin caused a decrease of 25—35% in the release of amino acids from cells incubated without glucose and in the presence of puromycin. This "antiproteolytic" effect of insulin had been noted earlier by Christophe and Wodon (1964). Jarett *et al.* (1972) have also reported an increased incorporation of labeled amino acids into protein by insulin in the absence of carbohydrate.

At present it is difficult to give a clear interpretation of these results. If one accepts the fairly straightforward demonstration of the antiproteolytic action of insulin, the effects on labeled amino acid incorporation into protein may be regarded at least in part as secondary consequences of this action. Quantitative assessment requires a knowledge of how rapidly intra- and extracellular amino acid pools exchange and of the half-life of the newly synthesized proteins. While it is likely that insulin affects the rate of protein synthesis as well as degradation, currently available data fall short of providing a clear demonstration of this point.

III. Analysis of the Mechanism of Action of Insulin

1. The Insulin Receptor

There can be little doubt that the effects of insulin on adipocytes are initiated by the combination of the hormone with receptor proteins located primarily or exclusively on the outer surface of the cell's plasma membrane. As this topic is discussed in detail elsewhere in this volume only a few comments will be added here.

At present very little information concerning the insulin receptor can be regarded as established fact. Indeed the receptor's very existence is largely an assumption. The major experimental difficulty is to identify the receptor molecules in a cell-free system. It is a relatively simple task to isolate and purify a substance from plasma membranes with a high binding affinity for insulin, and substantial progress toward this goal has already been achieved (see Chapter 3.1). However to establish that the substance so isolated is the physiologically relevant insulin receptor will require the demonstration that the combination of insulin with the binding substance has significance for some biological function. Even then an extrapolation of questionable validity from an *in vitro* model system to the intact cell will probably be necessary.

It is important to stress that we cannot identify the receptor on the basis of its physical or chemical properties. We do not know how many receptor molecules to expect to find per unit of cell surface nor can we anticipate what affinity an isolated receptor will show for insulin. Reasonable arguments can be advanced to suggest that the concentration of insulin required to yield half-maximal binding with the isolated receptor should be either much lower or much higher than the hormone concentration which yields half-maximal biological response. It follows that the binding affinity of a substance for insulin has limited value as a criterion on which to base the identification of the receptor to say nothing of attempting to judge whether the isolated substance has retained its natural state. Thus an experimental approach in which the exposed receptors of the intact cells are chemically modified by a selective procedure such as affinity-labeling may prove useful in identifying the receptor after cell rupture. Speculations concerning the insulin receptor or receptors are likely to continue relatively uninhibited by experimental findings for some time to come.

2. Correlation with Tissue cyclic-AMP Concentration

Since the discovery of the antilipolytic action of insulin in 1962 it has been suspected that cyclic-AMP might play a role in mediating some of the biological effects of insulin. This suspicion has been greatly strengthened with the realization that the activity of at least four enzymes is influenced by insulin in the manner to be expected were insulin to decrease the availability of cyclic-AMP. These enzymes are the hormone-sensitive lipase, glycogen phosphorylase, glycogen synthetase and the clearing-factor lipase. In each case insulin is capable of altering the activity of these enzymes when added to tissue apparently in the "basal state", that is, tissue incubated in the absence of any other hormone added *in vitro*. This may simply indicate that such tissue remains under the influence of lipolytic hormones to which it was exposed *in vivo*. These observations constitute strong but inconclusive evidence that one of the important functions of insulin in adipose tissue is to decrease the availability of cyclic-AMP thereby countering the influences of a variety of other hormones which act by elevating the concentration of this nucleotide (JUNGAS, 1966). Nevertheless, the possibility that insulin might alter the activity of these enzymes by additional mechanisms remains attractive, particularly in the cases of glycogen synthetase (LARNER, 1972) and the clearing-factor lipase (ROBINSON and WING, 1970). Additional mechanisms also appear to be involved in the action of insulin on pyruvate dehydrogenase (RANDLE and DENTON, 1972) and on glucose transport (RODBELL *et al.*, 1968; BRAY and GOOD-

MAN, 1968; PARK *et al.*, 1969). The possible involvement of cyclic-GMP in the action of insulin deserves serious consideration.

Direct experimental tests of the hypothesis that insulin lowers the availability of cyclic-AMP in adipocytes have met with limited success. It has not been possible to detect any change in the basal level of tissue or adipocyte cyclic-AMP (or cyclic-GMP) upon the addition of insulin (BUTCHER *et al.*, 1966; KUO and DE RENZO, 1969; JARETT *et al.*, 1972; FAIN and ROSENBERG, 1972). Only when the level of cyclic-AMP is first inflated by a lipolytic hormone, or by caffeine, or by both together, is it possible to demonstrate a fall in cyclic-AMP in response to insulin (BUTCHER *et al.*, 1966; BUTCHER *et al.*, 1968; KUO and DE RENZO, 1969). These data provide strong support for the view that cyclic-AMP is involved in the action of insulin though some authors have drawn from them the unwarranted conclusion that cyclic-AMP is not important in mediating the effects of insulin on tissue in the basal state. The difficulty of interpretation resides in the astonishingly high level of cyclic-AMP found in basal tissue. As pointed out by PARK *et al.* (1969) and many other authors the amount of cyclic-AMP in either basal tissue or adipocytes would produce a concentration of approximately 5 micromolar if evenly distributed throughout the intracellular water. The concentration required for half-maximal activation of adipose tissue cyclic-AMP dependent protein kinase is about 100 times lower (CORBIN and KREBS, 1969). Thus if the kinase is to remain in the non-activated state only a minute fraction of the total cyclic-AMP in the basal tissue could have free access to the enzyme. It is not known whether this tiny "active pool" of cellular cyclic-AMP is always a constant proportion of the total tissue cyclic-AMP, or whether its size is independently variable. Thus the influence of insulin on this functionally active portion of the tissue cyclic-AMP pool cannot be determined by current techniques. Indeed even a several-fold expansion of the active pool of cyclic-AMP might pass unnoticed. In this regard the rather good correlations between total cyclic-AMP levels and the activities of the hormone-sensitive lipase, glycogen phosphorylase, and glycogen synthetase recently observed by MAYER *et al.* (1972) are of great interest. However, firm conclusions regarding the role of cyclic-AMP in the action of insulin may have to await the development of more definitive methods for evaluating the intracellular distribution of cyclic-AMP. Thus just as in the studies of the insulin receptor, our attempts to pry into the secrets of a promising candidate for the role of intracellular mediator of insulin action are currently being stymied by experimental insufficiencies.

3. Role of Adenylate Cyclase

Insulin could diminish the availability of cyclic-AMP in at least 3 ways: it could lower adenylate cyclase activity, it could raise phosphodiesterase activity, or it could alter the intracellular distribution of the massive cyclic-AMP pool in favor of increased sequestration. Only the first two of these possibilities are currently amenable to investigation and in each case promising results have been obtained.

It was suggested by JUNGAS (1966) on the basis of some rather crude experiments that insulin reduced the activity of adenylate cyclase in adipose tissue. Since that time several workers using more sophisticated techniques have provided ample confirmation of this action of insulin. These latter positive findings followed an interim period characterized by negative reports. Thus RODBELL *et al.* (1968), CRYER *et al.* (1969), FAIN and ROSENBERG (1972), and COMBRET and LAUDAT (1972) could not detect any effect of insulin on the adenylate cyclase of fat cell ghosts whether or not an activator such as ACTH, epinephrine, or NaF was also present.

Williams *et al.* (1968) measured adenylate cyclase activity in intact adipocytes and again insulin was without effect on basal activity, though it appeared to block the stimulation of adenylate cyclase by epinephrine or isoproterenol under some conditions. Vaughan and Murad (1969) found no effect of insulin on the adenylate cyclase of particles isolated from fat cells, and Allen and Clark (1971) obtained negative results in fat cell homogenates. In 1971 however Hepp reported that low concentrations of insulin (100 μUnits/ml; 0.7 nM) were effective in blocking the rise in adenylate cyclase activity caused by glucagon in a plasma membrane preparation from rat or mouse liver. This result was confirmed and extended by Hepp and Renner (1972) and by Illiano and Cuatrecasas (1972) who found that the activation of adenylate cyclase by catecholamines or ACTH could also be inhibited, that only 5 μUnits of insulin per ml were required, and that plasma membrane preparations from fat cells yielded similar results. Illiano and Cuatrecasas mentioned that the basal adenylate cyclase of fat cell membranes could be lowered by insulin whereas Hepp (1972) found this to be true with liver membranes but not with fat cell ghosts.

These reports represent the first successes in that long-sought goal, the demonstration of effects of physiological concentrations of insulin in a cell-free system. They constitute therefore strong evidence that the enzymic processes being measured lie near to the core of at least some of the biological actions of insulin (Hepp, 1972; Illiano and Cuatrecasas, 1972). It will be of interest to determine whether other substances capable of depressing adenylate cyclase activity will exhibit insulin-like effects on adipose tissue metabolism. Substances already fulfilling this prediction include niacin (Butcher *et al.*, 1968; Allen and Clark, 1971) and the small serum polypeptide termed "non-suppressible insulin-like activity" or NSILA (Hepp, 1972).

4. Role of Phosphodiesterase

Further evidence that insulin lowers the availability of cyclic-AMP in adipocytes has come from measurements of the phosphodiesterase (PDE) which degrades cyclic-AMP to 5′-AMP (Butcher and Sutherland, 1962). Considerable confusion arose concerning the role of insulin in regulating PDE until it was realized that several diesterases with widely different kinetic properties were present in adipocytes (Murad *et al.*, 1970; Loten and Sneyd, 1970; Thompson and Appleman, 1971). An enzyme with high affinity for cyclic-AMP ($K_m = 1$ μM or less) is present along with much greater amounts of an enzyme with low affinity ($K_m = 40$ μM or higher). It is assumed though not yet proven that these are distinct and separable enzymes.

Loten and Sneyd (1970) reported that the activity of the low K_m enzyme was influenced by insulin. They found that homogenates prepared from either intact tissue or adipocytes which had been exposed to insulin as briefly as 3 min showed an increase of about 50% in the V_{max} of the low K_m diesterase. There was no change in the K_m and insulin had no effect if added directly to the homogenates. These findings have been confirmed by Vaughan (1972), by Zinman and Hollenberg (1972) and in my laboratory (unpublished data). It is necessary to conduct the assay for the low K_m PDE at very low concentrations of cyclic-AMP, preferably 0.1 μM or below, in order to reduce interference by the far more abundant hormone-insensitive PDE. The failure to observe this precaution probably accounts for the negative reports of other workers concerning this action of insulin (Blecher *et al.*, 1968; Hepp *et al.*, 1969; Allen and Clark, 1971; Fain and Rosenberg, 1972).

To date it has not been possible to influence the activity of the PDE by the addition of insulin to a cell-free system. In particular the PDE of a fat cell membrane preparation whose adenylate cyclase was sensitive to insulin failed to respond to insulin (ILLIANO and CUATRECASAS, 1972). The action of insulin on PDE may therefore be no more direct than its influence on, for example, the hormone-sensitive lipase. However in the case of the PDE no effect of epinephrine could be detected (CLARK and JUNGAS, unpublished experiments). CHEUNG (1970) described a heat stable protein which served as an activator of PDE in several tissues and we have noticed a similar substance in adipose tissue (WACHOLTZ and JUNGAS, unpublished experiments). Its role in the regulation of PDE activity remains to be determined. The physiological function of the very abundant PDE of high K_m is obscure.

It is difficult to estimate the contribution which changes in PDE make to the lowering of cyclic-AMP availability in the presence of insulin. There is disagreement concerning the effectiveness of insulin in blocking the actions of added cyclic-AMP. GOODMAN (1969) found insulin did block the effects of cyclic-AMP on lipolysis while HEPP *et al.* (1969) reported insulin to be ineffective. There is wide agreement that insulin is ineffective in blocking the actions of dibutyryl cyclic-AMP on adipocytes (BLECHER *et al.*, 1968; GOODMAN, 1969; HEPP *et al.*, 1969; HALL and BALL, 1970; SOLOMON *et al.*, 1970; JARETT *et al.*, 1972; FAIN and ROSENBERG, 1972; but see BROWN *et al.*, 1969). The mode of action of this analog is, however, not entirely clear. For example, despite the fact that dibutyryl cyclic-AMP is not a substrate for adipose tissue PDE (BLECHER, 1971), FAIN (1968) and GOODMAN (1969) reported that theophylline potentiated the effects of this analog. Dibutyryl cyclic-AMP can be hydrolyzed to cyclic-AMP by tissue extracts (BLECHER, 1971) and in some tissues acts as an inhibitor of PDE (HEERSCHE *et al.*, 1971). Thus dibutyryl cyclic-AMP may act in part by causing an elevation of intracellular cyclic-AMP, which could explain the potentiation of its effects by theophylline. In this case however it is not clear why insulin should be ineffective against dibutyryl cyclic-AMP if the activation of PDE plays an important role in insulin action.

5. Reflections

A few brief personal remarks may be appropriate in concluding this review. The sobering fact is that we understand the mechanism of action of insulin on adipose tissue little better today than we did a decade ago. The major difference is that we now have experimental facts to justify what were only suspicions and hypotheses 10 years ago. However very little really new in the way of concepts has appeared. For many years it has been assumed that insulin initiates its metabolic actions by combining with a substance in the cell's plasma membrane, and that this substance must be at least partly protein in order to account for the high affinity and specificity of the response. It has been further assumed that upon combination with insulin this receptor substance undergoes a change in conformation which is transmitted to neighboring molecules in the membrane, some of which are enzymes or transport carriers. More recently it has even been imagined that the conformational repercussions of the insulin-receptor combination might extend to the lipid moieties of the membrane with the result that major changes in the physical properties of the proteolipid lamellae of the membrane might result (BLECHER, 1965; RODBELL, 1966; RODBELL *et al.*, 1968). In any event it is supposed that the rather direct consequence of the insulin-receptor combination is a change in the conformation and hence of the biological activity of a variety of enzymes and/or carrier molecules located in the plasma membrane, and that these conformational perturbations are transmitted largely within the membrane itself. According to this view the membrane is where the action is and cytoplasmic components play at best a secondary or subsidiary role in mediating the effects of insulin. The implication is that the action of insulin on glucose transport is a more direct or immediate effect of the hormone than for example its effect on glycogen synthetase or pyruvate dehydrogenase. The practical consequence of this conception of insulin action is seen in recent efforts to isolate a purified plasma membrane fraction of the cell which might then be used to investigate the mode of action of insulin.

I wish to register certain reservations concerning these assumptions as to the mechanism of action of insulin and to offer a slightly modified viewpoint as the basis for further experimentation. To begin at a rather basic level, the "conventional model" for insulin action just described envisions a series of membranal events initiated by insulin with the sole energy source drawn upon to cause these events to occur being the energy released by the combination of the insulin molecule with its receptor. It is therefore of interest to attempt to estimate the order of magnitude of the energy made available in this way. There is not space here to go into this matter in detail, but if one takes the data currently available concerning the putative insulin receptor the value obtained is astonishingly small — only some 2000 calories per mole, i.e., about that of a single hydrogen bond. This value is of course no more dependable than the assumption that the properties of the isolated insulin binding substance (CUATRECASAS, 1972b) reflect those of the physiological receptor. I mention it only to draw serious attention to the difficulties which arise in a model for hormone action which requires the hormone not only to act as the signal, but also to provide the energy for initiating the response.

From this point of view one of the interesting features of the concept that cyclic-AMP serves as a second-messenger in mediating hormone action (SUTHERLAND *et al.*, 1965) is that cellular ATP is implicated as an energy source used ultimately to operate the control mechanisms. Indeed it is not obvious that this feature is merely incidental. I believe serious attention should be given to the possibility that a cytoplasmic second messenger is involved in mediating the action of insulin on glucose transport. At present reasonably strong arguments can be advanced to rule out cyclic-AMP as this messenger (BRAY, 1967; RODBELL *et al.*, 1968; BRAY and GOODMAN, 1968; BLECHER *et al.*, 1969). However cyclic-AMP has also been discredited as a possible messenger in mediating the effect of insulin on pyruvate dehydrogenase, only in this case it is obvious that some sort of cytoplasmic messenger must be involved since the enzyme is confined within the mitochondria.

Several intriguing experimental findings may be cited which hint at the possibility of a cytoplasmic involvement in the action of insulin on glucose transport. Fat cell ghosts though grossly depleted in cytoplasmic enzymes, nevertheless are capable of utilizing glucose at slow rates and they do give a sluggish response to insulin (RODBELL, 1967b). However when small membranous vesicles were prepared from fat cells under conditions which caused the virtually complete loss of cytoplasmic enzymes and of the ability to metabolize glucose, it was found that although a stereospecific transport system for glucose was still operative in the vesicles, they were no longer capable of responding to insulin (MARTIN and CARTER, 1970; CARTER and MARTIN, 1972; CARTER *et al.*, 1972). Such vesicles will bind insulin and apparently retain an intact receptor (HAMMOND *et al.*, 1972). In muscle the effect of insulin on sugar transport is characterized by a substantial time lag between the moment of insulin binding and the moment when transport begins to increase (WOHLTMANN and NARAHARA, 1967). Electrical stimulation on the other hand initiates an immediate rise in sugar transport. If the sugar carrier system of the membrane is capable of rapid activation what causes the delay in the response to insulin ? Conformational changes of a protein in response to binding ligands are normally very rapid and may even precede the binding. Diffusional processes within the membrane might be involved or cytoplasmic intermediates may have to accumulate. In liver insulin appears to have no effect on sugar transport, whereas a variety of cytoplasmic effects are well documented. One might have imagined that the most direct effects of insulin would be of widest occurence with secondary or indirect effects varying more widely from tissue to tissue. I would urge therefore that careful consideration be given to the possible role of cytoplasmic factors in mediating what appears on the surface to be intra-membranous effects of insulin.

References

Allen, D.O., Clark, J.G.: Effect of various antilipolytic compounds on adenylate cyclase and phosphodiesterase activity in isolated fat cells. Advanc. Enzymol. Reg. **9**, 99—112 (1971)

Angel, A., Farkas, J.: Structural and chemical compartments in adipose cells. Horm. Metab. Res. Suppl. **2**, 152—161 (1970)

Angel, A., de Sai, K., Halperin, M.L.: Free fatty acids and ATP levels in adipocytes during lipolysis. Metabolism **20**, 87—99 (1971)

Arndt, H.J.: Experimentell-morphologische Untersuchungen über den Glykogen- und Fettstoffwechsel in ihren gegenseitigen Beziehungen. Verh. dtsch. path. Ges. **21**, 297—303 (1926)

Arndt, H.J.: Vergleichend-morphologische und experimentelle Untersuchungen über den Kohlehydrat- und Fettstoffwechsel der Gewebe. Beitr. path. Anat. **79**, 523—591 (1928)

Austin, W., Nestel, P.J.: The effect of glucose and insulin in vitro on the uptake of triglycerides and on lipoprotein lipase in fat pads from normal, fed rats. Biochim. biophys. Acta (Amst.) **164**, 59—63 (1968)

Avruch, J., Carter, J.R., Martin, D.B.: The effect of insulin on the metabolism of adipose tissue. In: Handbook of Physiology. Section 7: Endocrinology, Vol. I, pp. 545—562. Washington: Amer. Physiol. Soc. 1972

Baker, W.K., Rutter, W.J.: Influence of insulin and environmental factors on glucose uptake in epididymal adipose tissue. Arch. Biochem. **105**, 68—79 (1964)

Ball, E.G.: Some considerations of the multiplicity of insulin action on adipose tissue. Horm. Metab. Res. Suppl. **2**, 102—107 (1970)

Ball, E.G., Cooper, O.: Studies on the metabolism of adipose tissue. III. The response to insulin by different types of adipose tissue in the presence of various metabolites. J. biol. Chem. **235**, 584—588 (1960)

Ball, E.G., Jungas, R.L.: On the action of hormones which accelerate the rate of oxygen consumption and fatty acid release in rat adipose tissue in vitro. Proc. nat. Acad. Sci. (Wash.) **47**, 932—941 (1961)

Ball, E.G., Jungas, R.L.: Studies on the metabolism of adipose tissue. XIII. The effect of anaerobic conditions and dietary regime on the response to insulin and epinephrine. Biochemistry **2**, 586—592 (1963)

Ball, E.G., Jungas, R.L.: Some effects of hormones on the metabolism of adipose tissue. Recent Progr. Hormone Res. **20**, 183—214 (1964)

Ball, E.G., Merrill, M.A.: A manometric assay of insulin and some results of the application of the method to sera and islet-containing tissues. Endocrinology **69**, 596—607 (1961)

Ball, E.G., Martin, D.B., Cooper, O.: Studies on the metabolism of adipose tissue. I. The effect of insulin on glucose utilization as measured by the manometric determination of carbon dioxide output. J. biol. Chem. **234**, 774—780 (1959)

Ballard, F.J., Hanson, R.W., Leveille, G.A.: Phosphoenol-pyruvate carboxykinase and the synthesis of glyceride-glycerol from pyruvate in adipose tissue. J. biol. Chem. **242**, 2746—2750 (1967)

Bally, P.R., Cahill, G.F., Jr., Leboeuf, B., Renold, A.E.: Studies on rat adipose tissue in vitro. V. Effects of glucose and insulin on metabolism of palmitate-1-^{14}C. J. biol. Chem. **235**, 333—336 (1960)

Bally, P.R., Kappeler, H., Froesch, E.R., Labhart, A.: Effects of glucose on spontaneous limitation of lipolysis in isolated adipose tissue: A potential regulatory mechanism. Ann. N.Y. Acad. Sci. **131**, 143—156 (1965)

Beigelman, P.M., Hollander, P.B.: Effect of insulin upon resting electrical potential of adipose tissue. Proc. Soc. exp. Biol. (N.Y.) **110**, 590—595 (1962)

Beigelman, P.M., Hollander, P.B.: Effect of insulin and rat weight upon rat adipose tissue membrane resting electrical potential (REP). Diabetes **12**, 262—267 (1963)

Beigelman, P.M., Hollander, P.B.: Effects of hormones upon adipose tissue membrane electrical potentials. Proc. Soc. exp. Biol. (N.Y.) **116**, 31—35 (1964)

Benjamin, W., Gellhorn, A.: Effect of diabetes and insulin on the biosynthesis of individual fatty acids in adipose tissue. J. biol. Chem. **239**, 64—69 (1964)

Berthet, J.: Action du glucagon et de l'adrenaline sur le metabolisme des lipides dans le tissu hepatique. Proc. 4th Int. Congr. Biochem. **17**, 107 (1960)

Bihler, I., Jeanrenaud, B.: ATP content of isolated fat cells. Effects of insulin, oubain, and lipolytic agents. Biochim. biophys. Acta (Amst.) **202**, 496—506 (1970)

Bjorntorp, P.: Effect of ketone bodies on lipolysis in adipose tissue in vitro. J. Lipid Res. **7**, 621—626 (1966)

Bjorntorp, P., Ostman, J.: Human adipose tissue dynamics and regulation. Advanc. Metab. Disord. **5**, 277—327 (1971)

Blecher, M.: Phospholipase C and mechanisms of action of insulin and cortisol on glucose entry into free adipose cells. Biochem. biophys. Res. Commun. **21**, 202—209 (1965)

Blecher, M.: Biological effects and catabolic metabolism of 3',5'-cyclic nucleotides and derivatives in rat adipose tissue and liver. Metabolism **20**, 63—77 (1971)

Blecher, M., Merlino, N.S., Ro'Ane, J.T.: Control of the metabolism and lipolytic effects of cyclic 3',5'-adenosine monophosphate in adipose tissue by insulin, methyl xanthines, and nicotinic acid. J. biol. Chem. **243**, 3973—3977 (1968)

Blecher, M., Merlino, N.S., Ro'Ane, J.T., Flynn, P.D.: Independence of the effects of epinephrine, glucagon, and ACTH on glucose utilization from those on lipolysis in isolated rat adipose cells. J. biol. Chem. **244**, 3423—3429 (1969)

Bleicher, S.J., Lewis, A., Farber, L., Goldner, M.G.: Effect of mono- and divalent cations on in vitro lipolysis. Proc. Soc. exp. Biol. (N.Y.) **121**, 980—982 (1966a)

Bleicher, S.J., Farber, L., Lewis, A., Goldner, M.G.: Electrolyte-activated lipolysis in vitro: Modifying effect of calcium. Metabolism **15**, 742—748 (1966b)

Borrebaek, B.: Mitochondria-bound hexokinase of the rat epididymal adipose tissue and its possible relation to the action of insulin. Biochem. Med. **3**, 485—497 (1970)

Borrebaek, B., Spydevold, O.: The effects of insulin and glucose on mitochondrial-bound hexokinase activity of rat epididymal adipose tissue. Diabetologia **5**, 42—43 (1969)

Bortz, W.M., Lynen, F.: Elevation of long chain acyl CoA derivatives in livers of fasted rats. Biochem. Z. **339**, 77—82 (1963)

Bottermann, P., Schwarz, K., Schulze-Solde, R., Dambacher, M.: Untersuchungen über den Fettstoffwechsel bei der Fettsucht. Diabetologia **1**, 180—186 (1966)

Bray, G.A.: Inhibition of glucose oxidation in adipose tissue by dibutyryladenosine-3',5'-phosphate. Biochem. biophys. Res. Commun. **28**, 621—627 (1967a)

Bray, G.A.: Effects of epinephrine corticotropin, and thyrotropin on lipolysis and glucose oxidation in rat adipose tissue. J. Lipid Res. **8**, 300—307 (1967b)

Bray, G.A., Goodman, H.M.: Effects of epinephrine on glucose transport and metabolism in adipose tissue of normal and hypothyroid rats. J. Lipid Res. **9**, 714—719 (1968)

Breibart, S., Engel, F.: Influence of cortisone and insulin on the respiratory activity of rat adipose tissue in vitro. Endocrinology **55**, 70—76 (1954)

Bricker, L.A., Levey, G.S.: Evidence for regulation of cholesterol and fatty acid synthesis in liver by cyclic adenosine 3'-5'-monophosphate. J. biol. Chem. **247**, 4914—4915 (1972)

Brown, J.D., Stone, D.B., Steele, A.A.: Mechanism of action of antilipolytic agents: Comparison of the effects of insulin, tolbutamide, and phenformin on lipolysis induced by dibutyryl cyclic-AMP plus theophylline. Metabolism **18**, 926—929 (1969)

Bruchhausen, F. von: Hemmung des alpha-amino-isobuttersäure-Transportes in das isolierte Fettgewebe durch N-6-O-2'-dibutyryl-adenosin-3',5'-phosphat. Z. Physiol. Chem. **349**, 1437—1439 (1968)

Buckle, R.M.: Mobilization of free fatty acids from adipose tissue from normal and diabetic subjects. Influence of glucose and insulin. Diabetes **12**, 133—140 (1963)

Buckle, R.M., Rubinstein, D., McGarry, E.E., Beck, J.C.: Factors influencing the release of free fatty acids from rat adipose tissue. Endocrinology **69**, 1009—1015 (1961)

Butcher, R.W., Sutherland, E.W.: Adenosine 3',5'-phosphate in biological materials. I. Purification and properties of cyclic 3',5'-nucleotide phosphodiesterase and use of this enzyme to characterize adenosine 3',5'-phosphate in human urine. J. biol. Chem. **237**, 1244—1250 (1962)

Butcher, R.W., Sneyd, J.G.T., Park, C.R., Sutherland, E.W., Jr.: Effect of insulin on adenosine 3',5'-monophosphate in the rat epididymal fat pad. J. biol. Chem. **241**, 1651—1653 (1966)

BUTCHER, R.W., BAIRD, C.E., SUTHERLAND, E.W.: Effects of lipolytic and antilipolytic substances on adenosine 3′,5′-monophosphate levels in isolated cells. J. biol. Chem. **243**, 1705—1712 (1968)

CAHILL, G.F., JR., JEANRENAUD, B., LEBOEUF, B., RENOLD, A.E.: Effects of insulin on adipose tissue. Ann. N.Y. Acad. Sci. **82**, 403—411 (1959a)

CAHILL, G.F., JR., LEBOEUF, B., RENOLD, A.E.: Studies on rat adipose tissue in vitro. III. Synthesis of glycogen and glyceride-glycerol. J. biol. Chem. **234**, 2540—2543 (1959b)

CAHILL, G.F., JR., LEBOEUF, B., FLINN, R.B.: Studies on rat adipose tissue in vitro. IV. Effect of epinephrine on glucose metabolism. J. biol. Chem. **235**, 1246—1250 (1960a)

CAHILL, G.F., JR., LEBOEUF, B., RENOLD, A.E.: Factors concerned with regulation of fatty acids metabolism by adipose tissue. Amer. J. clin. Nutr. **8**, 733—742 (1960b)

CARLSON, C.A., KIM, K.-H.: Regulation of hepatic acetyl CoA carboxylase by phosphorylation and dephosphorylation. J. biol. Chem. **248**, 378—380 (1973)

CARRUTHERS, B.M., WINEGRAD, A.I.: Effects of insulin on amino acid and RNA metabolism in rat adipose tissue. Amer. J. Physiol. **202**, 605—610 (1962)

CARTER, J.R., JR., MARTIN, D.B.: Glucose-uptake by isolated particles from rat epididymal adipose tissue cells. Proc. nat. Acad. Sci. (Wash.) **64**, 1343—1348 (1972)

CARTER, J.R., JR., AVRUCH, J., MARTIN, D.B.: Glucose transport in plasma membrane vesicles from rat adipose tissue. J. biol. Chem. **247**, 2682—2687 (1972)

CAYGILL, C.P.J., STEIN, W.O.: Glucose uptake by isolated fat cells and the influence of insulin. Biochem. J. **105**, 17P (1967)

CHEUNG, W.Y.: Cyclic 3′,5′-nucleotide phosphodiesterase. Demonstration of an activator. Biochem. biophys. Res. Commun. **38**, 533—538 (1970)

CHRISTOPHE, J., WODON, C.: Metabolisme *in vitro* du tissu adipeux. I. Controles hormonaux du metabolisme *in vitro* de la L-leucine dans le tissu adipeux epididymaire du rat normal. Arch. int. Physiol. Biochim. **72**, 100—115 (1964)

CLAUSEN, T.: Relationship between transport of glucose and cations across cell membranes in isolated tissues. I. Stimulation of glycogen deposition and inhibition of lactic acid production in diaphragm induced by ouabain. Biochim. biophys. Acta (Amst.) **109**, 164 (1966)

CLAUSEN, T.: The relationship between the transport of glucose and cations across cell membranes in isolated tissues. V. Stimulating effect of ouabain, potassium-free medium and insulin on efflux of 3-O-methylglucose from epididymal adipose tissue. Biochim. biophys. Acta (Amst.) **183**, 625—634 (1969)

CLAUSEN, T.: Electrolytes and the hormonal control of organic metabolism in adipocytes. Horm. Metab. Res. Suppl. **2**, 66—70 (1970)

CLAUSEN, T., RODBELL, M.: The metabolism of isolated fat cells. 8. Amino acid transport in ghosts. J. biol. Chem. **244**, 1258—1262 (1969)

COMBRET, Y., LAUDAT, P.: Adenyl cyclase activity in a plasma membrane fraction purified from "ghosts" of rat fat cells. FEBS Letters **21**, 45—48 (1972)

COORE, H.G., DENTON, R.M., MARTIN, B.R., RANDLE, P.J.: Regulation of adipose tissue pyruvate dehydrogenase by insulin and other hormones. Biochem. J. **125**, 115—127 (1971)

CORBIN, J.D., KREBS, E.G.: A cyclic AMP-stimulated protein kinase in adipose tissue. Biochem. biophys. Res. Commun. **36**, 328—336 (1969)

CORBIN, J.D., REIMANN, E.M., WALSH, D.A., KREBS, E.G.: Activation of adipose tissue lipase by skeletal muscle cyclic-AMP stimulated protein kinase. J. biol. Chem. **245**, 4849—4851 (1970)

CRANE, R.K.: Na^+-dependent transport in the intestine and other animal tissues. Fed. Proc. **24**, 1000—1006 (1965)

CROFFORD, O.B.: Countertransport of 3-O-methyl glucose in incubated rat epididymal adipose tissue. Amer. J. Physiol. **212**, 217—220 (1967)

CROFFORD, O.B.: The uptake and inactivation of native insulin by isolated fat cells. J. biol. Chem. **243**, 362—369 (1968)

CROFFORD, O.B., RENOLD, A.E.: Glucose uptake by incubated rat epididymal adipose tissue. J. biol. Chem. **240**, 14—21 (1965a)

CROFFORD, O.B., RENOLD, A.E.: Glucose uptake by incubated rat epididymal adipose tissue: Characteristics of the glucose transport system and action of insulin. J. biol. Chem. **240**, 3237—3244 (1965b)

CROFFORD, O.B., JEANRENAUD, B., RENOLD, A.E.: Effect of insulin on the transport and metabolism of sorbitol by incubated rat epididymal adipose tissue. Biochim. biophys. Acta (Amst.) **111**, 429—439 (1965)

CROFFORD, O.B., STAUFFACHER, W., JEANRENAUD, B., RENOLD, A.E.: Glucose transport in isolated fat cells. Helv. Physiol. Acta **24**, 45—57 (1966)

CRYER, P.E., JARETT, L., KIPNIS, D.M.: Nucleotide inhibition of adenyl cyclase activity in fat cell membranes. Biochim. biophys. Acta (Amst.) **177**, 586—590 (1969)

CUATRECASAS, P.: Discussion. In: "Insulin Action", p. 190—191. New York-London: Academic Press 1972a
CUATRECASAS, P.: Properties of the insulin receptor isolated from liver and fat cell membranes. J. biol. Chem. **247**, 1980—1991 (1972b)
CUSHMAN, S.W.: Pinocytic activity in the isolated adipose cell. Horm. Metab. Res. Suppl. **2**, 162—166 (1970)
DENTON, R.M., HALPERIN, M.L.: Control of fatty acid and triglyceride synthesis in rat epididymal adipose tissue. Biochem. J. **110**, 27—38 (1968)
DENTON, R.M., RANDLE, P.J.: Citrate and regulation of adipose tissue phosphofructokinase. Biochem. J. **100**, 420—423 (1966)
DENTON, R.M., RANDLE, P.J.: Stimulation by calcium ions of pyruvate dehydrogenase phosphate phosphatase. Biochem. J. **128**, 161—163 (1972)
DENTON, R.M., COORE, H.G., MARTIN, B.R., RANDLE, P.J.: Insulin activates pyruvate dehydrogenase in rat epididymal adipose tissue. Nature (Lond.) **231**, 115—116 (1971)
DENTON, R.M., YORKE, R.E., RANDLE, P.J.: Measurement of concentrations of metabolites in adipose tissue and effects of insulin, alloxan-diabetes and adrenaline. Biochem. J. **100**, 407—419 (1966)
DIPIETRO, D.L.: Hexokinase of white adipose tissue. Biochim. biophys. Acta (Amst.) **67**, 305—312 (1963)
DOISY, R.J.: Plasma insulin assay and adipose tissue metabolism. Endocrinology **72**, 273—278 (1963)
DOLE, V.P.: Relation between non-esterified fatty acids of plasma and metabolism of glucose. J. clin. Invest. **35**, 150—154 (1956)
FAIN, J.N.: Effect of dexamethasone and 2-deoxy-D-glucose on fructose and glucose metabolism by incubated adipose tissue. J. biol. Chem. **239**, 958—962 (1964a)
FAIN, J.N.: Effect of puromycin on incubated adipose tissue and its response to dexamethasone, insulin, and epinephrine. Biochim. biophys. Acta (Amst.) **84**, 636—642 (1964b)
FAIN, J.N.: Effect of dibutyryl-3',5'-AMP, theophylline, and norepinephrine on lipolytic action of growth hormone and glucocorticoid in white fat cells. Endocrinology **82**, 825—830 (1968)
FAIN, J.N.: Mode of action of insulin. In: The Biochemistry of the Hormones, Vol. 8, MTP Intl. Rev. of Science, Biochemistry Series, 1973, In press
FAIN, J.N., ROSENBERG, L.: Antilipolytic action of insulin on fat cells. Diabetes **21**, 414—425 (1972)
FAIN, J.N., KOVACEV, V.P., SCOW, R.O.: Effect of growth hormone and dexamethasone on lipolysis and metabolism in isolated fat cells of the rat. J. biol. Chem. **240**, 3522—3529 (1965)
FAIN, J.N., KOVACEV, V.P., SCOW, R.O.: Antilipolytic effect of insulin in isolated fat cells of the rat. Endocrinology **78**, 773—778 (1966)
FAVARGER, P., GERLACH, J.: Recherches sur la synthese des graisses. II. Les roles respectivement du foie, adipeux, et certain autres tissues. Helv. Physiol. Acta **13**, 96—105 (1955)
FAVARGER, P., GERLACH, J.: Recherches sur la synthese des graisses. IV. Importance de la lipogenese hepatique; etude experimentale critique. Helv. physiol. pharmacol. Acta **66**, 188—200 (1958)
FAWCETT, D.W.: Histological observations on the relation of insulin to the deposition of glycogen in adipose tissue. Endocrinology **42**, 454—462 (1948)
FELIX, K., EGER, W.: Die Bildung von Fett aus Kohlehydrat in den Fettorganen. II. Mitteilung. Dtsch. Arch. klin. Med. **184**, 446—457 (1939)
FELLER, D.D.: Metabolism of adipose tissue. I. Incorporation of acetate carbon into lipids by slices of adipose tissue. J. biol. Chem. **206**, 171—180 (1954)
FLATT, J.P.: Conversion of carbohydrate to fat in adipose tissue: an energy-yielding and, therefore, self-limiting process. J. Lipid Res. **11**, 131—143 (1970)
FLATT, J.P., BALL, E.G.: Studies on the metabolism of adipose tissue. XIV. The manometric determination of total CO_2 production and oxygen consumption in bicarbonate buffer. Biochem. Z. **338**, 73—83 (1963)
FLATT, J.P., BALL, E.G.: Studies on the metabolism of adipose tissue. XV. An evaluation of the major pathways of glucose catabolism as influenced by insulin and epinephrine. J. biol. Chem. **239**, 675—685 (1964)
FLATT, J.P., BALL, E.G.: Studies on the metabolism of adipose tissue. XIX. An evaluation of the major pathways of glucose catabolism as influenced by acetate in the presence of insulin. J. biol. Chem. **241**, 2862—2869 (1966)
FRERICHS, H., BALL, E.G.: Studies on the metabolism of adipose tissue. XI. Activation of phosphorylase by agents which stimulate lipolysis. Biochemistry **1**, 501—509 (1962)
FRERICHS, H., REICH, U., CREUTZFELDT, W.: Insulinsekretion in vitro. I. Hemmung der glucoseinduzierten Insulinabgabe durch Insulin. Klin. Wschr. **43**, 136—140 (1965)

FROESCH, E.R.: Fructose metabolism in adipose tissue from normal and diabetic rats. In: Handbook of Physiology, Section 5: Adipose Tissue, p. 281—293. Washington: Amer. Physiol. Soc. 1965

FROESCH, E.R., GINSBERG, J.L.: Fructose metabolism of adipose tissue. I. Comparison of fructose and glucose metabolism in epididymal adipose tissue of normal rats. J. biol. Chem. **237**, 3317—3324 (1962)

FROESCH, E.R., BURGI, H., BALLY, P., LABHART, A.: Insulin inhibition of spontaneous adipose tissue lipolysis and effects upon fructose and glucose metabolism. Molec. Pharmacol. **1**, 280—296 (1965)

FROESCH, E.R., WALDVOGEL, M., MEYER, V.A., JAKOB, A., LABHART, A.: Effects of 5-methyl-pyrazole-3-carboxylic acid on adipose tissue. I. Inhibition of lipolysis, effects on glucose, fructose, and glycogen metabolism in vitro and comparison with insulin. Molec. Pharmacol. **3**, 429—441 (1967)

GARLAND, P.B., RANDLE, P.J.: Control of pyruvate dehydrogenase in the perfused rat heart by the intracellular concentration of acetyl-coenzyme A. Biochem. J. **91**, 6c—7c (1964)

GELLHORN, A., BENJAMIN, W.: Fatty acid biosynthesis and RNA function in fasting, aging and diabetes. Advanc. Enzymol. Reg. **4**, 19—41 (1966)

GIBSON, D.M., TITCHENER, E.B., WAKIL, S.J.: Studies on the mechanism of fatty acid synthesis. V. Bicarbonate requirement for the synthesis of long-chain fatty acids. Biochim. biophys. Acta (Amst.) **30**, 376—383 (1958)

GIERKE, E. VON: Zum Stoffwechsel des Fettgewebes. Verh. dtsch. path. Ges. **10**, 182—185 (1906)

GLIEMANN, J.: Glucose metabolism and response to insulin of isolated fat cells and epididymal fat pads. Acta physiol. scand. **72**, 481—491 (1968)

GLIEMANN, J.: Action of insulin on isolated fat cells. Dan. med. Bull. **16**, Suppl. **4**, 1—42 (1969)

GLIEMANN, J.: Studies on the action of insulin on isolated fat cells. Horm. Metab. Res. Suppl. **2**, 116—119 (1970)

GOODMAN, H.M.: Stimulatory action of insulin on leucine uptake and metabolism in adipose tissue. Amer. J. Physiol. **206**, 129—132 (1964)

GOODMAN, H.M.: Alpha amino isobutyric acid transport in adipose tissue. Amer. J. Physiol. **211**, 815—820 (1966)

GOODMAN, H.M.: The effects of insulin on lipolysis evoked by cyclic AMP and its dibutyryl analog. Proc. Soc. exp. Biol. (N.Y.) **130**, 97—100 (1969)

GOODRIDGE, A.G.: The effect of insulin, glucagon and prolactin on lipid synthesis and related metabolic activity in migrating and non-migrating finches. Comp. Biochem. Physiol. **13**, 1—26 (1964)

GOODRIDGE, A.G.: Lipolysis in vitro in adipose tissue from embryonic and growing chicks. Amer. J. Physiol. **214**, 902—907 (1968)

GOODRIDGE, A.G.: Regulation of the activity of acetyl coenzyme A carboxylase by palmitoyl coenzyme A and citrate. J. biol. Chem. **247**, 6946—6952 (1972)

GOODRIDGE, A.G., BALL, E.G.: Studies on the metabolism of adipose tissue. XVII. In vitro effects of insulin, epinephrine and glucagon on lipolysis and glycolysis in pigeon adipose tissue. Comp. Biochem. Physiol. **16**, 367—381 (1965)

GOODRIDGE, A.G., BALL, E.G.: Lipogenesis in the pigeon: in vitro studies. Amer. J. Physiol. **211**, 803—808 (1966)

GORDON, R.S., JR., CHERKES, A.: Unesterified fatty acids in human blood plasma. J. clin. Invest. **35**, 206—212 (1956)

GORDON, R.S., JR., CHERKES, A.: Production of unesterified fatty acids from isolated rat adipose tissue incubated in vitro. Proc. Soc. exp. Biol. (N.Y.) **97**, 150—151 (1958)

GRIES, F.A.: Hormonal control of human adipose tissue metabolism in vitro. Horm. Metab. Res. Suppl. **2**, 167—171 (1970)

GRIES, F.A., STEINKE, J.: Insulin and human adipose tissue in vitro: a brief review. Metabolism **16**, 693—696 (1967)

HAGEN, J.H.: Effects of glucagon on the metabolism of adipose tissue. J. biol. Chem. **236**, 1023—1027 (1961)

HAGEN, J.H.: Effect of insulin on concentration of plasma glycerol. J. Lipid Res. **4**, 46—51 (1963)

HAGEN, J.H., BALL, E.G., COOPER, O.: Studies on the metabolism of adipose tissue. II. The effect of changes in the ionic composition of the medium upon the response to insulin. J. biol. Chem. **234**, 781—786 (1959)

HALL, C.L., BALL, E.G.: Factors affecting lipolysis rates in rat adipose tissue. Biochim. biophys. Acta (Amst.) **210**, 209—220 (1970)

HALPERIN, M.L.: An additional role for insulin in the control of fatty acid synthesis independent of glucose transport. Canad. J. Biochem. **48**, 1228—1233 (1970)

HALPERIN, M.L.: Studies on the conversion of pyruvate into fatty acids in white adipose tissue. Biochem. J. **124**, 615—621 (1971)
HALPERIN, M.L., DENTON, R.M.: Regulation of glycolysis and L-glycerol 3-phosphate concentration in rat epididymal adipose tissue in vitro. Role of phosphofructokinase. Biochem. J. **113**, 207—214 (1969)
HALPERIN, M.L., ROBINSON, B.H.: The role of cytoplasmic redox potential in control of fatty acid synthesis from glucose, pyruvate and lactate in white adipose tissue. Biochem. J. **116**, 235—240 (1970)
HALPERIN, M.L., ROBINSON, B.H.: Mechanism of insulin action on control of fatty acid synthesis independent of glucose transport. Metabolism **20**, 78—86 (1971)
HALPERIN, M.L., ROBINSON, B.H., MARTIN, B.R., DENTON, R.M.: Permeability of rat white adipose tissue mitochondria to citrate, isocitrate and 2-oxoglutarate. Nature (Lond.) **223**, 1369—1371 (1969)
HALPERIN, M.L., ROBINSON, B.H., FRITZ, I.B.: Effects of palmityl CoA on citrate and malate transport by rat liver mitochondria. Proc. nat. Acad. Sci. (Wash.) **69**, 1003—1007 (1972)
HAMMOND, J.M., JARETT, L., MARIZ, I.K., DAUGHADAY, W.H.: Heterogeneity of insulin receptors on fat cell membranes. Biochem. biophys. Res. Commun. **49**, 1122—1128 (1972)
HAUGAARD, N., MARSH, J.B.: Effect of insulin on the metabolism of adipose tissue from normal rats. J. biol. Chem. **194**, 33—40 (1952)
HAUSBERGER, F.X., MILSTEIN, S.W.: Dietary effects on lipolysis in adipose tissue. J. biol. Chem. **214**, 483—488 (1955)
HAUSBERGER, F.X., MILSTEIN, S.W., RUTMAN, R.J.: Influence of insulin on glucose utilization in adipose and hepatic tissue *in vitro*. J. biol. Chem. **208**, 431—438 (1954)
HEERSCHE, J.N.M., FEDAK, S.A., AURBACH, G.D.: The mode of action of dibutyryl adenosine 3′,5′-monophosphate on bone tissue *in vitro*. J. biol. Chem. **246**, 6770—6775 (1971)
HELLMAN, D.E., SENIOR, B., GOODMAN, H.M.: Anti-lipolytic effects of beta-hydroxybutyrate. Metabolism **18**, 906—915 (1969)
HENLE, W., SZPINGIER, G.: Der Stoffwechsel des isolierten Fettgewebes. III. Über den echten R. Q. und seine Beeinflussung durch Nährstoffe *in vitro* und *in vivo*. Arch. exp. Path. Pharmakol. **180**, 672—689 (1936)
HEPP, K.D.: Inhibition of glucagon-stimulated adenyl cyclase by insulin. FEBS Letters **12**, 263—266 (1971)
HEPP, K.D.: Adenylate cyclase and insulin action. Europ. J. Biochem. **31**, 266—276 (1972)
HEPP, K.D., RENNER, R.: Insulin action on the adenyl cyclase system: Antagonism to activation by lipolytic hormones. FEBS Letters **20**, 191—194 (1972)
HEPP, D., POFFENBARGER, P.L., ENSINCK, J.W., WILLIAMS, R.H.: Effects of nonsuppressible insulin-like activity and insulin on glucose oxidation and lipolysis in the isolated adipose cell. Metabolism **16**, 393—401 (1967)
HEPP, D., CHALLONER, D.R., WILLIAMS, R.H.: Respiration in isolated fat cells and the effects of epinephrine. J. biol. Chem. **243**, 2321—2327 (1968a)
HEPP, D., CHALLONER, D.R., WILLIAMS, R.H.: Studies on the action of insulin in isolated adipose tissue cells. I. Stimulation of incorporation of ^{32}P-labeled inorganic phosphate into mononucleotides in the absence of glucose. J. biol. Chem. **243**, 4020—4026 (1968b)
HEPP, K.D., MENAHAN, L.A., WIELAND, O., WILLIAMS, R.H.: Studies on the action of insulin in isolated adipose tissue cells. II. 3′,5′-nucleotide phosphodiesterase and antilipolysis. Biochim. biophys. Acta (Amst.) **184**, 554—565 (1969)
HERNANDEZ, A., SOLS, A.: Transport and phosphorylation of sugars in adipose tissue. Biochem. J. **86**, 166—172 (1963)
HERRERA, M.G., RENOLD, A.E.: Hormonal effects on glycine metabolism in rat epididymal adipose tissue. Biochim. biophys. Acta (Amst.) **44**, 165—167 (1960)
HERRERA, M.G., RENOLD, A.E.: Amino acid and protein metabolism. In: Handbook of Physiology, Section 5: Adipose Tissue, p. 375—383. Washington: Amer. Physiol. Soc. 1965
HERRERA, M.G., PHILIPPS, G.R., RENOLD, A.E.: Stimulation of metabolic activity of adipose tissue from fasted rats by prolonged incubation *in vitro*. I. Requirement for glucose and insulin. Biochim. biophys. Acta (Amst.) **106**, 221—233 (1965)
HO, R.J.: Dependence of hormone-stimulated lipolysis on ATP and cyclic AMP levels in fat cells. Horm. Metab. Res. Suppl. **2**, 83—87 (1970)
HO, R.J., JEANRENAUD, B., RENOLD, A.E.: Oubain-sensitive fatty acid release from isolated fat cells. Experientia (Basel) **22**, 86—87 (1966)
HO, R.J., JEANRENAUD, B., POSTERNAK, T., RENOLD, A.E.: Insulin-like action of ouabain. II. Primary antilipolytic effect through inhibition of adenyl cyclase. Biochim. biophys. Acta (Amst.) **144**, 74—82 (1967)
HOFFMAN, A., WERTHEIMER, E.: Stoffwechselregulationen. VIII. Zur Physiologie des Fettgewebes und der Fettablagerung. Pflügers Arch. ges. Physiol. **217**, 728—746 (1927)

HOLLENBERG, C.H., RABEN, M.S., ASTWOOD, E.B.: Lipolytic response to corticotropin. Endocrinology **68**, 589—598 (1961)

HOTTA, N., SIREK, A., SIREK, O.V.: Inhibitory effect of beta-hydroxybutyrate on lipolysis stimulated by dihydroergotamine and growth hormone *in vitro*. Canad. J. Physiol. Pharmacol. **49**, 87—91 (1971)

HUCHO, F., RANDALL, D.D., ROCHE, T.E., BURGETT, M.W., PELLEY, J.W., REED, L.J.: α-keto acid dehydrogenase complexes. XVII. Kinetic and regulatory properties of pyruvate dehydrogenase kinase and pyruvate dehydrogenase phosphatase from bovine kidney and heart. Arch. Biochem. **151**, 328—340 (1972)

HUTTUNEN, J.K., STEINBERG, D., MAYER, S.E.: Protein kinase activation and phosphorylation of a purified hormone-sensitive lipase. Biochem. biophys. Res. Commun. **41**, 1350—1356 (1970a)

HUTTUNEN, J.K., STEINBERG, D., MAYER, S.E.: ATP-dependent and cyclic-AMP-dependent activation of rat adipose tissue lipase by protein kinase from rabbit skeletal muscle. Proc. nat. Acad. Sci. (Wash.) **67**, 290—295 (1970b)

ILLIANO, G., CUATRECASAS, P.: Glucose transport in fat cell membranes. J. biol. Chem. **246**, 2472—2479 (1971)

ILLIANO, G., CUATRECASAS, P.: Modulation of adenylate cyclase activity in liver and fat cell membranes by insulin. Science **175**, 906—908 (1972)

INOUE, H., LOWENSTEIN, J.M.: Acetyl coenzyme A carboxylase from rat liver. Purification and demonstration of different subunits. J. biol. Chem. **247**, 4825—4832 (1972)

ITZHAKI, S., WERTHEIMER, E.: Metabolism of adipose tissue *in vitro*: nutritional factors and effects of insulin. Endocrinology **6**, 72—78 (1957)

JARETT, L., STEINER, A.L., SMITH, R.M., KIPNIS, D.M.: The involvement of cyclic-AMP in the hormonal regulation of protein synthesis in rat adipocytes. Endocrinology **90**, 1277—1284 (1972)

JEANRENAUD, B.: Adipose tissue dynamics and regulation, revisited. Ergebn. Physiol. **60**, 57—140 (1968)

JEANRENAUD, B., HEPP, D.: Adipose tissue: regulation and metabolic functions. Horm. Metab. Res. Suppl. **2**, (1970)

JEANRENAUD, B., RENOLD, A.E.: Studies on rat adipose tissue *in vitro*. IV. Metabolic patterns produced in rat adipose tissue by varying insulin and glucose concentrations independent from each other. J. biol. Chem. **234**, 3082—3087 (1959)

JEANRENAUD, B., HEPP, D., RENOLD, A.E.: The influence of lipolysis on energy metabolism of isolated cells. Horm. Metab. Res. Suppl. **2**, 76—79 (1970)

JUNGAS, R.L.: Role of cyclic-3′,5′-AMP in the response of adipose tissue to insulin. Proc. nat. Acad. Sci. (Wsh.) **56**, 757—763 (1966)

JUNGAS, R.L.: Fatty acid synthesis in adipose tissue incubated in tritiated water. Biochemistry **7**, 3708—3717 (1968)

JUNGAS, R.L.: Factors regulating the rate of fatty acid synthesis in adipose tissue. In: Proc. VIth Cong. p. 334—342, Int. Diabetes Fed., Amsterdam: Excerpta Medica 1969

JUNGAS, R.L.: Effect of insulin on fatty acid synthesis from pyruvate, lactate, or endogenous sources in adipose tissue: Evidence for the hormonal regulation of pyruvate dehydrogenase. Endocrinology **86**, 1368—1375 (1970a)

JUNGAS, R.L.: Effects of biogenic amines on adipose tissue metabolism. In: Biogenic amines as physiological regulators, p. 181—206. Englewood Cliffs, New Jersey: Prentice-Hall 1970b

JUNGAS, R.L., BALL, E.G.: Studies on the metabolism of adipose tissue. VII. A comparison of the effects of insulin and a growth-hormone preparation on oxygen consumption in bicarbonate and phosphate buffers. Biochim. biophys. Acta (Amst.) **54**, 304—314 (1961)

JUNGAS, R.L., BALL, E.G.: An anti-lipolytic action of insulin on adipose tissue. Fed. Proc. **21**, 202 (1962)

JUNGAS, R.L., BALL, E.G.: Studies on the metabolism of adipose tissue. XII. The effects of insulin and epinephrine on free fatty acid and glycerol production in the presence and absence of glucose. Biochemistry **2**, 383—388 (1963)

JUNGAS, R.L., BALL, E.G.: Studies on the metabolism of adipose tissue. XVII. *In vitro* effects of insulin upon the metabolism of the carbohydrate and triglyceride stores of adipose tissue from fasted-refed rats. Biochemistry **3**, 1696—1702 (1964)

JUNGAS, R., SCHWARTZ, J.P.: Studies on the lipases of adipose tissue. Horm. Metab. Res. Suppl. **2**, 37—40 (1970)

JUNGAS, R.L., TAYLOR, S.I.: Influence of insulin, epinephrine and substrates on pyruvate dehydrogenase activity of adipose tissue. In: Insulin Action, p. 369—413. New York-London: Academic Press 1972

KATHER, H., RIVERA, M., BRAND, K.: Interrelationship and control of glucose metabolism and lipogenesis in isolated fat cells. Biochem. J. **128**, 1089—1096 (1972a)

KATHER, H., RIVERA, M., BRAND, K.: Interrelationship and control of glucose metabolism and lipogenesis in isolated fat cells. Biochem. J. **128**, 1097—1102 (1972b)

KATZ, J., WALS, P.A.: Effects of phenazine methosulfate on glucose metabolism in rat adipose tissue. Arch. Biochem. **147**, 405—418 (1971)

KONO, T.: Destruction of insulin effector system of adipose tissue cells by proteolytic enzymes J. biol. Chem. **244**, 1772—1778 (1969)

KONO, T.: The insulin receptor of fat cells: The relationship between the binding and physiological effects of insulin. In: Insulin Action, p. 171—203. New York-London: Academic Press 1972

KOSOW, D.P., ROSE, I.A.: Ascites tumor mitochondrial hexokinase. II. Effect of binding on kinetic properties. J. biol. Chem. **243**, 3623—3630 (1968)

KRAHL, M.E.: The effect of insulin and pituitary hormones on glucose uptake in muscle. Ann. N.Y. Acad. Sci. **54**, 649—670 (1951)

KRAHL, M.E.: Incorporation of [^{14}C]amino acid precursors into adipose tissue protein: An insulin stimulation not involving glucose or amino acid transport. Biochim. biophys. Acta (Amst.) **35**, 556 (1959)

KRAHL, M.E.: Stimulation of peptide synthesis in adipose tissue by insulin without glucose. Amer. J. Physiol. **206**, 618—620 (1964)

KUO, J.F.: Effects of insulin and substances having insulin-like activity on adipose cells: Sugar utilization, lipolysis, adenyl cyclase-cyclic AMP system and cyclic AMP-dependent protein kinase. Horm. Metab. Res. Suppl. **2**, 112—115 (1970)

KUO, J.F., DE RENZO, E.C.: A comparison of the effects of lipolytic and antilipolytic agents on adenosine-3′,5′-monophosphate levels in adipose cells as determined by prior labeling with adenine-8-^{14}C. J. biol. Chem. **244**, 2252—2260 (1969)

KUO, J.F., HOLMLUND, C.E., DILL, I.K., BOHONOS, N.: Insulin-like activity of a microbial protease on isolated fat cells. Arch. Biochem. **117**, 269—274 (1966)

LANDAU, B.R., KATZ, J.: A quantitative estimation of the pathways of glucose metabolism in rat adipose tissue *in vitro*. J. biol. Chem. **239**, 697—704 (1964)

LANDAU, B.R., KATZ, J.: Pathways of glucose metabolism. In: Handbook of Physiology. Section 5: Adipose Tissue, p. 253—271. Washington: Amer. Physiol. Soc. 1965

LANGSLOW, D.R., HALES, C.N.: Lipolysis in chicken adipose *in vitro*. J. Endocr. **43**, 285—294 (1969)

LARNER, J.: Insulin and glycogen synthetase. Diabetes **21**, Suppl. **2**, 428—438 (1972)

LAVIS, V.R., WILLIAMS, R.H.: Studies of the insulin-like actions of thiols upon isolated fat cells. J. biol. Chem. **245**, 23—31 (1970)

LAVIS, V.R., HEPP, D., WILLIAMS, R.H.: Paradoxical failure of a high concentration of insulin to suppress hormone-stimulated lipolysis by isolated fat cells. Diabetes **19**, 371 (1970)

LEBOEUF, B., CAHILL, G.F., JR.: Studies on rat adipose tissue *in vitro*. VIII. Effect of a preparation of pituitary ACTH and growth hormone on glucose metabolism. J. biol. Chem. Chem. **236**, 41—46 (1961)

LEFEBVRE, P.J., LUYCKX, A.S.: Effect of insulin on glucagon enhanced lipolysis *in vitro*. Diabetologia **5**, 195—197 (1969)

LEONARDS, J.R., LANDAU, B.R.: A study of the equivalence of metabolic proteins in rat adipose tissue: Insulin versus glucose concentration. Arch. Biochem. **91**, 194—200 (1960)

LEONARDS, J.R., LANDAU, B.R.: Metabolism of fructose by adipose tissue, and the effect of insulin. Endocrinology **74**, 142—144 (1964)

LEONARDS, J.R., LANDAU, B.R., BARTSCH, G.: Assay of insulin and insulin-like activity with rat epididymal fat pad. J. Lab. clin. Med. **60**, 552—570 (1962)

LETARTE, J., RENOLD, A.E.: Glucose metabolism in fat cells stimulated by insulin and dependent on sodium. Nature (Lond.) **215**, 961—962 (1967)

LETARTE, J., RENOLD, A.E.: Ionic effects on glucose transport and metabolism by isolated mouse fat cells incubated with or without insulin. III. Effects of replacement of Na^+. Biochim. biophys. Acta (Amst.) **183**, 366—374 (1969)

LETARTE, J., JEANRENAUD, B., RENOLD, A.E.: Ionic effects on glucose transport and metabolism by isolated mouse fat cells incubated with or without insulin. II. Effect of replacement of K^+ and of ouabain. Biochim. biophys. Acta (Amst.) **183**, 357—365 (1969)

LIBERMAN, L.L.: Testing small insulin concentrations by means of isolated epididymal rat fat. Bull. exp. Biol. Med. **52**, 121—124 (1961)

LINN, T.C., PETTIT, F.H., REED, L.J.: Alpha-keto acid dehydrogenase complexes. X. Regulation of the activity of the pyruvate dehydrogenase complex from beef kidney mitochondria by phosphorylation and dephosphorylation. Proc. nat. Acad. Sci. (Wash.) **62**, 234—241 (1969a)

LINN, T.C., PETTIT, F.H., HUCHO, F., REED, L.J.: Alpha-keto acid dehydrogenase complexes. XI. Comparative studies of regulatory properties of the pyruvate dehydrogenase complexes from kidney, heart and liver mitochondria. Proc. nat. Acad. Sci. (Wash.) **64**, 227—234 (1969b)

Löffler, G., Weiss, L.: Lipase activities in adipose tissue. Horm. Metab. Res. Suppl. **2**, 32—36 (1970)

Loten, E.G., Sneyd, J.G.T.: An effect of insulin on adipose tissue adenosine 3′,5′-cyclic monophosphate phosphodiesterase. Biochem. J. **120**, 187—193 (1970)

Löw, A., Krcma, A.: Insulin und Nahrungsdepots. Biochem. Z. **206**, 360—368 (1929)

Lynn, W.S., Macleod, R.M., Brown, R.H.: Effects of epinephrine, insulin, and corticotrophin on metabolism of rat adipose tissue. J. biol. Chem. **235**, 1904—1911 (1960)

Macleod, R.M., Brown, R., Lynn, W.S.: *In vitro* stimulation of hexokinase by insulin. J. clin. Invest. **39**, 1008 (1960)

Mahler, R., Stafford, W.S., Tarrant, M.E., Ashmore, J.: The effect of insulin on lipolysis. Diabetes **13**, 297—302 (1964)

Margolis, S., Vaughan, M.: α-Glycerol-PO_4 synthesis and breakdown in homogenates of adipose tissue. J. biol. Chem. **237**, 44—48 (1962)

Martin, B.R., Denton, R.M.: Intracellular localization of enzymes in white adipose tissue fat cells and permeability properties of fat-cell mitochondria. Biochem. J. **117**, 861—877 (1970)

Martin, B.R., Denton, R.M., Pask, H.T., Randle, P.J.: Mechanisms regulating adipose tissue pyruvate dehydrogenase. Biochem. J. **129**, 763—773 (1972)

Martin, D.B., Carter, J.R., Jr.: Insulin-stimulated glucose uptake by subcellular particles from adipose tissue cells. Science **167**, 873—874 (1970)

Mayer, S., Khoo, J., Steinberg, D., Jarett, L.: Comparison of phosphorylase and lipase activation in adipocytes by epinephrine. Fed. Proc. **31**, 555abs. (1972)

Meikle, A.W., Klain, G.J.: Effect of fasting and fasting-refeeding on conversion of leucine into CO_2 and lipids in rats. Amer. J. Physiol. **222**, 1246—1250 (1972)

Menozzi, P.G., Bognanni, I., Balestreri, R.: Meccanismo di azione dell'insulina sul tessuto adiposo. Arch. E. Maragliano **17**, Pat Clin. 829—833 (1961)

Mertz, W., Roginski, E.E.: Effect of Cr^{+++} on galactose entry in rat epididymal fat tissue. J. biol. Chem. **238**, 868—872 (1963)

Metz, S.H.M., van den Bergh, S.G.: Effects of volatile fatty acids, ketone bodies, glucose and insulin on lipolysis in bovine adipose tissue. FEBS Letters **21**, 203—206 (1972)

Miller, L.V., Beigelman, P.M.: Stimulation by insulin of protein synthesis in isolated fat cells. Proc. Soc. exp. Biol. (N.Y.) **122**, 73—75 (1966)

Minemura, T., Crofford, O.B.: Insulin-receptor interaction in isolated fat cells. I. The insulin-like properties of p-chloromercuribenzene sulfonic acid. J. biol. Chem. **244**, 5181—5188 (1969)

Minemura, T., Lacy, W.W., Crofford, O.B.: Regulation of the transport and metabolism of amino acids in isolated fat cells. J. biol. Chem. **245**, 3872—3881 (1970)

Modolell, J.B., Moore, R.O.: ATPase activities of rat epididymal adipose tissue. Biochim. biophys. Acta (Amst.) **135**, 319—332 (1967)

Mosinger, B., Kujalova, V.: K^+-dependent lipomobilizing effect of adrenaline on incubated adipose tissue. Biochim. biophys. Acta (Amst.) **116**, 174—177 (1966)

Murad, F., Manganiello, V., Vaughan, M.: Effects of guanosine 3′,5′-monophosphate on glycerol production and accumulation of adenosine 3′,5′-monophosphate by fat cells. J. biol. Chem. **245**, 3352—3360 (1970)

Murthy, V.K., Steiner, G.: Stimulation of lipogenesis by insulin, a direct *in vitro* effect independent of glucose. Clin. Res. **18**, 461 (1970)

Nakano, J., Ishii, T.: Effect of ketone bodies on hormone-, theophylline-, and dibutyryl cyclic AMP-induced lipolysis and on cyclic AMP-phosphodiesterase. Res. Commun. Chem. Path. Pharm. **1**, 485—496 (1970)

Nestel, P.J., Austin, W.: Relationship between adipose lipoprotein lipase activity and compounds which affect intracellular lipolysis. Life Sci. **8**, 157—164 (1969)

Nikkilä, E.A., Pykälistö, O.: Induction of adipose tissue lipoprotein lipase by nicotinic acid. Biochim. biophys. Acta (Amst.) **152**, 421—423 (1968)

Orth, R.D., O'Dell, W.D., Williams, R.H.: Some hormonal effects on the metabolism of acetate-1-C^{14} by rat adipose tissue. Amer. J. Physiol. **198**, 640—644 (1960)

Park, C.R., Sneyd, J.G.T., Corbin, J.D., Jefferson, L., Exton, J.: Role of cyclic adenylate in the actions of insulin. In: Proc. 6th Cong. Intl. Diabetes Fed., p. 5—15. Amsterdam: Excerpta Medica 1969

Parrish, J.E., Kipnis, D.M.: Effects of Na^{++} on sugar and amino acid transport in striated muscle. J. clin. Invest. **43**, 1994—2002 (1964)

Perry, W.F., Bowen, H.F.: Factors affecting the *in vitro* production of non-esterified fatty acid from adipose tissue. Canad. J. Biochem. **40**, 749—755 (1962)

Pettit, F.H., Roche, T.E., Reed, L.J.: Function of calcium ions in pyruvate dehydrogenase phosphatase activity. Biochem. biophys. Res. Commun. **49**, 563—571 (1972)

Pittman, J.A., Jr., Boshell, B.R.: Stimulation of glucose oxidation without glycogen deposition by oxytocin and vasopressin. Biochim. biophys. Acta (Amst.) **74**, 151—153 (1963)

Pozza, G., Ghidoni, A.: Action of insulin upon glucose, fructose, and galactose utilization by rat epididymal fat pad. Clin. chim. Acta **7**, 55—57 (1962)

Quagliariello, G., Scoz, G.: Ricerche sul metabolismo dei Grassi VIII. Boll. Soc. ital. Biol. sper. **5**, 117—119 (1930)

Rall, T.W., Sutherland, E.W.: Formation of a cyclic adenine ribonucleotide by tissue particles. J. biol. Chem. **232**, 1065—1076 (1958)

Randle, P.J., Denton, R.M.: Rate control by insulin and its mechanism. In press (1972)

Randle, P.J., Garland, P.B., Hales, C.N., Newsholme, E.A., Denton, R.M., Pogson, C.I.: Interactions of metabolism and the physiological role of insulin. Recent Progr. Hormone Res. **22**, 1—48 (1966)

Rasio, E.A., Soeldner, J.S., Cahill, G.F., Jr.: Insulin and insulin-like activity in serum and lymph. Diabetologia **1**, 125—127 (1965)

Renold, A.E., Cahill, G.F.: Handbook of Physiology. Section V: Adipose Tissue. Washington: Amer. Physiol. Soc. 1965

Renold, A.E., Marble, A., Fawcett, D.W.: Action of insulin on deposition of glycogen and storage of fat in adipose tissue. Endocrinology **46**, 55—66 (1950)

Reshef, L., Shapiro, B.: The physiological function and regulation of glycerogenesis in adipose tissue. Horm. Metab. Res. Suppl. **2**, 136—142 (1970)

Reshef, L., Shafrir, E., Shapiro, B.: *In vitro* release of unesterified fatty acids by adipose tissue. Metabolism **7**, 723—730 (1958)

Reshef, L., Hanson, R.W., Ballard, F.J.: Glyceride-glycerol synthesis from pyruvate. Adaptive changes in phosphoenolpyruvate carboxykinase and pyruvate carboxylase in adipose tissue and liver. J. biol. Chem. **244**, 1994—2001 (1969)

Richter, F.: Experimentelle Untersuchungen über das Vorkommen von Glykogen im Fettgewebe. Beitr. path. Anat. **86**, 65—82 (1931)

Rizack, M.A.: An epinephrine-sensitive lipolytic activity in adipose tissue. J. biol. Chem. **236**, 657—662 (1961)

Rizack, M.A.: Activation of an epinephrine-sensitive lipolytic activity from adipose tissue by adenosine 3′,5′-monophosphate. J. biol. Chem. **239**, 392—395 (1964)

Robinson, D.S., Wing, D.R.: Regulation of adipose tissue clearing factor lipase activity. Horm. Metab. Res. Suppl. **2**, 41—46 (1970)

Rodbell, M.: Metabolism of isolated fat cells. I. J. biol. Chem. **234**, 375—380 (1964)

Rodbell, M.: The metabolism of isolated fat cells. In: Handbook of Physiology, Section 5: Adipose Tissue, p. 471—482. Washington: Amer. Physiol. Soc. 1965

Rodbell, M.: Metab. of isolated fat cells. II. The similar effects of phospholipase C (Clostridium perfringens α toxin) and of insulin on glucose and amino acid metabolism. J. biol. Chem. **241**, 130—139 (1966)

Rodbell, M.: Metabolism of isolated fat cells. V. Preparation of "ghosts" and their properties; adenylate cyclase and other enzymes. J. biol. Chem. **242**, 5744—5750 (1967a)

Rodbell, M.: Metabolism of isolated fat cells. VI. The effects of insulin, lipolytic hormones, and theophylline on glucose transport and metabolism in "ghosts". J. biol. Chem. **242** 5751—5756 (1967b)

Rodbell, M., Jones, A.B.: Metabolism of isolated fat cells. III. The similar inhibitory action of phospholipase C (Clostridium perfringens α toxin) and of insulin on lipolysis stimulated by lipolytic hormones and theophylline. J. biol. Chem. **241**, 140—142 (1966)

Rodbell, M., Jones, A.B., Chiappe de Cingolani, G.E., Birnbaumer, L.: The actions of insulin and catabolic hormones on the plasma membrane of the fat cells. Recent Progr. Hormone Res. **24**, 215—254 (1968)

Rosell-Perez, M., Larner, J.: Studies on UDPG-α-glucan transglucosylase. IV. Purification and characterization of two forms from rabbit skeletal muscle. Biochemistry **3**, 75—81 (1964)

Rudman, D., Garcia, L.A., Del Rio, H., Akgun, S.: Further observations on cleavage of bovine insulin by rat adipose tissue. Biochemistry **7**, 1864—1874 (1968a)

Rudman, D., Garcia, L.A., Del Rio, A.: Effect on mammalian adipose tissue of fragments of bovine insulin and of certain synthetic peptides. Biochemistry **7**, 1875—1881 (1968b)

Ruska, H., Quast, A.: Der Stoffwechsel des isolierten Fettgewebes. II. Abhängigkeit von Tiergewicht, Wachstum und Ernährungsform. Arch. exp. Path. Pharmakol. **179**, 217—225 (1935)

Saggerson, E.D.: The regulation of glyceride synthesis in isolated white-fat cells. The effects of palmitate and lipolytic agents. Biochem. J. **128**, 1057—1068 (1972a)

SAGGERSON, E.D.: The regulation of glyceride synthesis in isolated white fat cells. The effects of acetate, pyruvate, lactate, palmitate, electron-acceptors, uncoupling agents and oligomycin. Biochem. J. **128**, 1069—1078 (1972b)

SAGGERSON, E.D., GREENBAUM, A.L.: Regulation of triglyceride synthesis and fatty acid synthesis in rat epididymal adipose tissue. Biochem. J. **119**, 193—220 (1970a)

SAGGERSON, E.D., GREENBAUM, A.L.: Regulation of triglyceride synthesis and fatty acid synthesis in rat epididymal adipose tissue: Effect of altered diet and hormonal conditions. Biochem. J. **119**, 221—242 (1970b)

SAGGERSON, E.D., TOMASSI, G.: The regulation of glyceride synthesis from pyruvate in isolated fat cells. The effects of palmitate and alteration of dietary status. Europ. J. Biochem. **23**, 109—117 (1971)

SALAMAN, M.R., ROBINSON, D.S.: Clearing factor lipase in adipose tissue. A medium in which the enzyme activity of tissue from starved rats increases *in vitro*. Biochem. J. **99**, 640—647 (1966)

SCHIMMEL, R.J., GOODMAN, H.M.: Release of pre-formed free fatty acids from adipose tissue: Acceleration by cyclic adenosine 3′-5′-phosphate. Endocrinology **90**, 1391—1395 (1972)

SCHUR, H., LÖW, A.: Studien über den Kohlehydrat-Stoffwechsel. Wien. klin. Wschr. **41**, 225—229; 261—266 (1928)

SCHWARTZ, J.P., JUNGAS, R.L.: Studies on the hormone-sensitive lipase of adipose tissue. J. Lipid Res. **12**, 553—562 (1971)

SCOW, R.O., STRICKER, F.A., PICK, T.Y., CLARY, T.R.: Effect of ACTH on free fatty acid release and diglyceride content in perfused rat adipose tissue. Ann. N.Y. Acad. Sci. **131**, 288—301 (1965)

SHAFRIR, E., KERPEL, S.: Fatty acid esterification and release as related to carbohydrate metabolism of adipose tissue. Arch. Biochem. **105**, 237—246 (1964)

SHAFRIR, E., GUTMAN, A., GORIN, E., OREVI, M.: Regulatory aspects in carbohydrate metabolism of adipose tissue: Glycolysis, glycogen synthesis, and glyceroneogenesis. Horm. Metab. Res. Suppl. **2**, 130—135 (1970)

SHAPIRO, B., WERTHEIMER, E.: Synthesis of fatty acids in adipose tissue *in vitro*. J. biol. Chem. **173**, 725—728 (1948)

SHAPIRO, B., CHOWERS, I., ROSE, G.: Fatty acid uptake and esterification in adipose tissue. Biochim. biophys. Acta (Amst.) **23**, 115—120 (1957)

SIESS, E.A., WIELAND, O.H.: Purification and characterization of pyruvate dehydrogenase phosphatase from pig-heart muscle. Europ. J. Biochem. **26**, 96—105 (1972)

SMITH, M.J., BEIGELMAN, P.M.: L-leucine-U-C^{14} metabolism in isolated fat cells. Proc. Soc. exp. Biol. (N.Y.) **129**, 621—623 (1968)

SOLOMON, S.S., BRUSH, J.S., KITABCHI, A.E.: Antilipolytic activity of insulin and proinsulin on ACTH and cyclic nucleotide-induced lipolysis in the isolated adipose cell of rat. Biochim. biophys. Acta (Amst.) **218**, 167—169 (1970)

STEINBERG, D., VAUGHAN, M., MARGOLIS, S.: Studies of tryglyceride biosynthesis in homogenates of adipose tissue. J. biol. Chem. **236**, 1631—1637 (1961)

STEINER, G., MURTHY, V.K.: Increased lipogenesis by insulin independent of its action on glucose transport. Diabetes **20**, Suppl. 1, 379 (1971)

STRAND, O., VAUGHAN, M., STEINBERG, D.: Rat adipose tissue lipases: activity against triglycerides compared with activity against lower glycerides. J. Lipid Res. **5**, 554—562 (1964)

SUTHERLAND, E.W., RALL, T.W.: Fractionation and characterization of a cyclic adenine ribonucleotide formed by tissue particles. J. biol. Chem. **232**, 1077—1091 (1958)

SUTHERLAND, E.W., RALL, T.W.: The relation of adenosine-3′,5′-phosphate and phosphorylase to the actions of catecholamines and other hormones. Pharmacol. Rev. **12**, 265—299 (1960)

SUTHERLAND, E.W., ØYE, I., BUTCHER, R.W.: The action of epinephrine and the role of the adenyl cyclase system in hormone action. Recent Progr. Hormone Res. **21**, 623—646 (1965)

TAYLOR, S.I., MUKHERJEE, C., JUNGAS, R.L.: Studies on the mechanism of activation of adipose tissue pyruvate dehydrogenase by insulin. J. biol. Chem. **248**, 73—81 (1973)

TEPPERMAN, H.M., TEPPERMAN, J.: Mechanism of inhibition of lipogenesis by 3′,5′-cyclic AMP. In: Insulin Action, p. 543—569. New York-London: Academic Press 1972

THOMPSON, W.J., APPLEMAN, M.M.: Characterization of cyclic nucleotide phosphodiesterase of rat tissues. J. biol. Chem. **246**, 3145—3150 (1970)

TOUABI, M., JEANRENAUD, B.: α-Aminoisobutyric acid uptake in isolated mouse fat cells. Biochim. biophys. Acta (Amst.) **173**, 128—140 (1969)

TUERKISCHER, E., WERTHEIMER, E.: Glycogen and adipose tissue. J. Physiol. (Lond.) **100**, 385—409 (1942)

TUERKISCHER, E., WERTHEIMER, E.: Factors influencing deposition of glycogen in adipose tissue of the rat. J. Physiol. (Lond.) **104**, 361—365 (1946)

UTTER, M.F., KEECH, D.B.: Pyruvate carboxylase. I. Nature of the reaction. J. biol. Chem. **238**, 2603—2608 (1963)

VASSALLI, J.D., JEANRENAUD, B.: Lipolysis and α-aminoisobutyric acid uptake in isolated fat cells. Effects of insulin and lipolytic agents. Biochim. biophys. Acta (Amst.) **202**, 477—485 (1970)

VAUGHAN, M.: Effects of hormones on phosphorylase in adipose tissue. J. biol. Chem. **235**, 3049—3053 (1960)

VAUGHAN, M.: Effects of hormones on glucose metabolism in adipose tissue. J. biol. Chem. **236**, 2196—2199 (1961)

VAUGHAN, M.: The role of insulin in regulation of cyclic AMP metabolism. In: Insulin Action, p. 297—318. New York-London: Academic Press 1972

VAUGHAN, M., MURAD, F.: Adenyl cyclase activity in particles from fat cells. Biochemistry **8**, 3092—3099 (1969)

VAUGHAN, M., STEINBERG, D.: Effect of hormones on lipolysis and esterification of free fatty acids during incubation of adipose tissue *in vitro*. J. Lipid Res. **4**, 193—199 (1963)

VAUGHAN, M., BERGER, J.E., STEINBERG, D.: Hormone-sensitive lipase and monoglyceride lipase activities in adipose tissue. J. biol. Chem. **239**, 401—409 (1964)

WERTHEIMER, E.: Stoffwechselregulationen. X. Über Glykogen in Fettgewebe und über die Möglichkeit der Umwandlung von Fett in Kohlehydrat. Pflügers Arch. ges. Physiol. **219**, 190—201 (1928)

WERTHEIMER, E.: Glycogen in adipose tissue after insulin injection. Nature (Lond.) **152**, 565—566 (1943)

WERTHEIMER, E.: Glycogen in adipose tissue. J. Physiol. (Lond.) **103**, 359—366 (1945)

WERTHEIMER, H.E.: Introduction — a perspective. In: Handbook of Physiology, Section 5: Adipose Tissue, p. 5—11. Washington: Amer. Physiol. Soc. 1965

WIELAND, O., SUYTER, M.: Glycerokinase: Isolierung und Eigenschaften des Enzyms. Biochem. Z. **329**, 320—331 (1957)

WIELAND, O., VON JAGOW-WESTERMANN, B., STUKOWSKI, B.: Kinetic and regulatory properties of heart muscle pyruvate dehydrogenase. Z. Physiol. Chem. **350**, 329—334 (1969)

WILLIAMS, R.H., WALSH, S.A., HEPP, D.K., ENSINCK, J.W.: Method for measuring hormonal effects on conversion of adenosine triphosphate to adenosine 3′,5′-monophosphate by isolated lipocytes. Metabolism **17**, 653—668 (1968)

WINAND, J., FURNELLE, J., WODON, C., CHRISTOPHE, J.: Spectrum of fatty acids synthesized in situ and metabolic heterogeneity of free fatty acids and glycerides within isolated rat adipocytes. Biochim. biophys. Acta (Amst.) **239**, 142—153 (1971)

WINEGRAD, A.I., RENOLD, A.E.: Studies on rat adipose tissue *in vitro*. I. J. biol. Chem. **233**, 267—272 (1958a)

WINEGRAD, A.I., RENOLD, A.E.: Studies on rat adipose tissue *in vitro*. II. J. biol. Chem. **233**, 273—276 (1958b)

WINEGRAD, A.I., SHAW, W.N.: Effects of alloxan diabetes and insulin on the oxidative metabolism of adipose tissue. J. biol. Chem. **238**, 524—527 (1963)

WING, D.R., ROBINSON, D.S.: Clearing-factor lipase in adipose tissue. Studies with puromycin and actinomycin. Biochem. J. **106**, 667—676 (1968)

WING, D.R., SALAMAN, M.R., ROBINSON, D.S.: Clearing-factor lipase in adipose tissue. Factors influencing the increase in enzyme activity produced on incubation of tissue from starved rats *in vitro*. Biochem. J. **99**, 648—656 (1966)

WOHLTMANN, H.J., NARAHARA, H.T.: Binding of insulin-I^{131} by isolated frog sartorious muscles. J. biol. Chem. **241**, 4931—4939 (1967)

WOOD, F.C., JR., LEBOEUF, B., RENOLD, A.E., CAHILL, G.F., JR.: Metabolism of mannose and glucose by adipose tissue and liver slices from normal and alloxan-diabetic rats. J. biol. Chem. **236**, 18—21 (1961)

ZAHND, G.R., DAGENAIS, Y.M., THORN, G.W.: Ionic effects upon glucose metabolism of rat adipose tissue with and without hormonal stimulation *in vitro*. Acta endocr. (Kbh.) Suppl. **51**, 947 (1960)

ZINMAN, B., HOLLENBERG, C.H.: Abstracts 4th Intl. Cong. Endocrinology, p. 157. Amsterdam: Excerpta Medica 1972

F. Direct In Vitro Effects of Insulin on Liver Metabolism

HANS-DIETER SÖLING and CLAUS-DIETER SEUFERT

With 3 Figures

In vivo studies of direct effects of insulin on liver metabolism are complicated by counterregulatory processes. The isolated perfused liver and the recently developed isolated liver cell preparation permit the study of these insulin effects under well-defined conditions.

I. Effects of Insulin on the Net Glucose Balance and on Glycogen Metabolism

HAFT and MILLER (1958) and MORTIMORE (1963) were the first to describe a net uptake of glucose by isolated perfused livers from fed rats in the presence of insulin. Similar observations were made by SÖLING *et al.* (1966a) who reported a net uptake of glucose (glucose concentration 11.1 mM) when insulin (0.9 U/h) was infused intraportally. No effect of insulin was seen in livers from starved or diabetic rats (SÖLING *et al.*, 1966b). In contrast to these results BODEN and WILLMS (1966) observed an increased uptake of ^{14}C-labeled glucose by livers from diabetic but not from normal rats when insulin was infused intraportally at a rate of 8 U/3 h. Since the ability of glucose to penetrate the liver cell seems to be relatively independent of the presence of insulin (CAHILL *et al.*, 1958), the effect of insulin on the net balance of glucose must proceed via an action on the metabolism of intracellular glucose. The increased net uptake of glucose by livers from fed rats was not accompanied by an increased net production of L-lactate or pyruvate (SÖLING *et al.*, 1966a). Thus it is likely that the increased net uptake of glucose resulted mainly from an enhanced synthesis or a decreased breakdown of liver glycogen. This observation is supported by recent experiments of WAGLE *et al.* (1973), who observed a significant increase in the glycogen content of isolated rat liver cells in the presence of insulin.

How does insulin affect glycogen metabolism *in vitro*? HERS *et al.* (1970) recently reviewed the present knowledge on the regulation of hepatic glycogen metabolism. A rough schema of the regulation is presented in Fig. 1.

There are 2 basic regulatory mechanisms:

1. Direct regulation by glucose itself,
2. Regulation via 3′,5′-cAMP.

Since there is no evidence that insulin affects the availability of glucose for the first regulatory mechanism, insulin must act via the second mechanism, namely by affecting the availability of 3′,5′-cAMP. This hypothesis is supported by the finding that the effects of insulin on the net glucose balance of isolated perfused livers or isolated liver cells are much more clear-cut under conditions in which the synthesis or release of 3′,5′-cAMP is stimulated (e.g. by glucagon) than in the non-stimulated state.

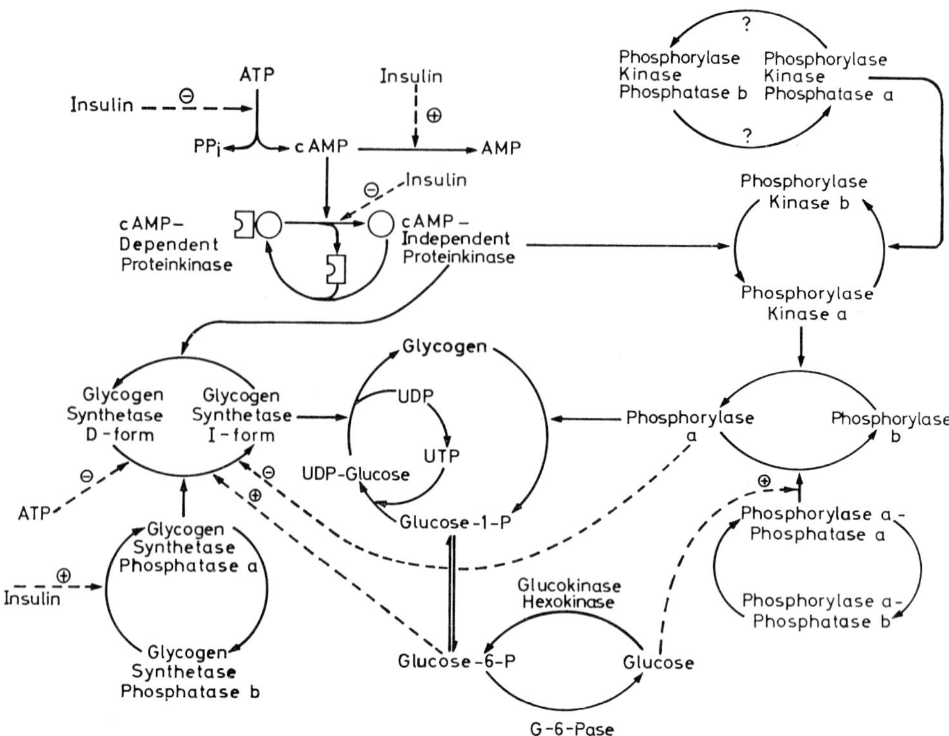

Fig. 1. Control of glycogen metabolism by insulin and some metabolic factors. Stimulation of a reaction is indicated by a (+) symbol, inhibition by a (—) symbol. The schema represents possible control points as far as they are discussed in the present literature. Whether insulin really affects glycogen metabolism under physiological conditions at all steps indicated in the schema remains an open question. The control by glucose is shown in the lower part of the figure. The schema does not include control by glucagon and catecholamines and leaves out most of the allosteric control mechanisms

Several groups have found inhibition of glucagon-stimulated glycogenolysis in isolated perfused rat livers (EXTON *et al.*, 1971a, 1972; GLINSMAN and MORTIMORE, 1968; JEFFERSON *et al.*, 1968; LEWIS *et al.*, 1971; MACKRELL and SOKAL, 1969; WILLIAMS *et al.*, 1971) or isolated rat liver cells (JOHNSON *et al.*, 1972). EXTON *et al.* (1972) brilliantly worked out the insulin-glucagon dose relationship in isolated perfused rat liver. Insulin can completely inhibit the effects of $1\cdot10^{-10}$ M glucagon, partially inhibit the effects of $5\cdot10^{-10}$ to $5\cdot10^{-8}$ M glucagon, but has no effect on glucagon concentrations of 10^{-8} M and higher. The glucagon-stimulated release of 3',5'-cAMP into the medium was likewise inhibited by insulin, and the glucagon/insulin dose relationship was similar to that observed for the effect on glucose output (Fig. 2).

The addition of 3',5'-cAMP to the perfusion medium also enhanced glycogenolysis in isolated perfused livers from rats (EXTON *et al.*, 1971a, 1972; GLINSMAN and MORTIMORE, 1968; JEFFERSON *et al.*, 1968; WILLIAMS *et al.*, 1971), guinea pigs (SÖLING *et al.*, 1970) or mice (ASSIMACOPOULOS-JEANNET *et al.*, 1973), as well as in isolated rat liver cells (JOHNSON *et al.*, 1972; GARRISON and HAYNES, 1973). Insulin inhibited the glycogenolytic action of low but not of high concentrations of 3',5'-cAMP (WILLIAMS *et al.*, 1971). The effects of $2.4\cdot10^{-5}$ M 3',5'-cAMP were strong-

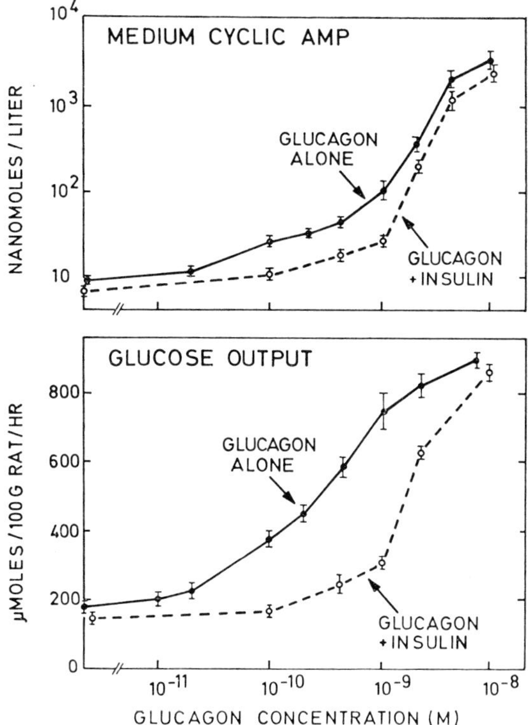

Fig. 2. Insulin-inhibition of glucagon-stimulated glucose production and cyclic AMP release in rat livers perfused with recirculating medium. Livers from fed rats were perfused for 1 h with recirculating medium. Glucagon was infused at a constant rate to produce the final concentrations shown on the abscissa of the lower panel. The concentration of glucagon given is that which would have been produced in the medium after 1 h assuming no degradation (certainly an overestimate). Insulin when present was infused at 2.5 mU/min. Glucose production (lower panel) was measured over the hour of perfusion. Medium cyclic AMP (upper panel) was measured at the end of the perfusion. (From EXTON *et al.*, 1972)

ly inhibited by insulin during liver perfusion, but insulin was ineffective at 3′,5′-cAMP concentrations of $9.6 \cdot 10^{-5}$ M or higher (WILLIAMS *et al.*, 1971). Similarly EXTON *et al.* (1971a) could, with insulin, completely inhibit the effect of 3′,5′-cAMP infused at a rate of 0.3 µmole/min during perfusion of isolated rat livers, whereas they could only partially inhibit the effect of 0.6—1.2 µmoles/min of 3′,5′-cAMP.

The *in vitro* stimulation of glycogenolysis by the 3′,5′-cAMP analogue N^6-2′-O-dibutyryl-3′,5′-cAMP was not inhibited by insulin (WILLIAMS *et al.*, 1971). Since 3′,5′-cAMP stimulates (among other effects) a protein kinase which catalyzes the phosphorylation of phosphorylase kinase (activation) and of glycogen synthetase (inactivation), it seems likely that glucagon, catecholamines and cyclic nucleotides (3′,5′-cAMP, 3′,5′-cGMP) stimulate glycogenolysis not only by activating the phosphorylase reaction but also by inhibiting the glycogen synthetase reaction. MACKRELL and SOKAL (1969) did not find a clear relationship between the effects of insulin on glycogenolysis on one hand and on the activity of phosphorylase on the other hand: The inhibitory effect of insulin on glycogenolysis induced in isolated perfused rat livers by 8.6 pmoles of glucagon was much greater than that on phosphorylase. When 28.7 pmoles of glucagon were used, 0.3 units of insulin still inhibited glycogenolysis but had no effect on phosphorylase. When the concentrations of glucagon were raised to levels between 86 and 287 pmoles, insulin was still able to inhibit ureogenesis, but had no effect on glycogenolysis or phosphorylase activity. These observations fit well with the earlier findings of Glinsman and Mortimore (1968), who likewise found in isolated perfused rat livers an inhibition by insulin of glucagon-induced glycogenolysis but not of glucagon-induced activation of phosphorylase.

There remains, however, the problem of how insulin could affect glycogen turnover in the isolated perfused liver without prior stimulation by glucagon, catecholamines or 3′,5′-cAMP (see page 420). One could speculate that adenylate cyclase was already in a slightly stimulated state due to the surgical operation procedure and that insulin added to the perfusion medium counteracted this process, thus enhancing glycogen synthesis relative to glycogenolysis.

An increased uptake of glucose due to an insulin-mediated stimulation of glycogen synthesis can of course only occur when the phosphorylation of glucose is not rate limiting. This condition is fulfilled in livers from fed rats, as is illustrated by the finding that an increase of the glucose concentration in the medium above 10—11 mM leads to a net uptake of glucose by isolated rat liver even in the absence of insulin (Soskin *et al.*, 1938; Cahill *et al.*, 1959; McCraw *et al.*, 1968). The same holds also for isolated rat liver cells (Wagle *et al.*, 1973). Most of the glucose taken up under these conditions is incorporated into glycogen as a consequence of the glucose-mediated insulin independent stimulation of glycogen synthetase (for review see Hers *et al.*, 1970). Hue and Hers (1974) pointed out that due to the stimulation of glycogen synthetase, glucose-6-phosphate is pulled in the direction of glycogen synthesis leading to a decreased concentration of glucose-6-phosphate. The consequence is a decrease in the rate of the glucose-6-phosphatase reaction. Thus, an increased supply of external glucose could itself inhibit glucose release. However, as Miller *et al.* (1973) recently showed, the "insulin-independent" activation of glycogen synthetase and of glycogen synthesis by glucose no longer works

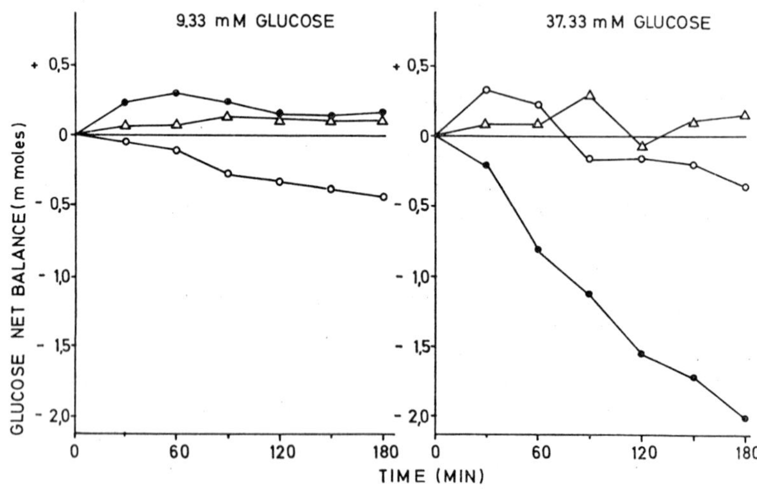

Fig. 3. Changes of the net glucose balance in experiments with isolated perfused livers from fed rats (●), guinea pig (○) and chickens (△) after increasing the glucose concentration in the medium from 9.33—33.33 mM. Only rat livers respond with a net uptake of glucose

in isolated perfused livers from alloxan diabetic rats. Apparently, insulin plays a permissive role in the occurrence of the glucose effect.

Similarly, in species which have only low or nearly no glucokinase activity (guinea pig, man, birds) (and in this respect resemble the diabetic rat), an increase in the concentration of glucose in the medium does not lead to a significant uptake of glucose (Fig. 3). In these species no *in vitro* effect of insulin on the net uptake of glucose can be expected. This situation does not, of course, exclude the possibility that, in these species, insulin affects the glucose net balance across the liver under the condition of glucagon- or epinephrine-induced glycogenolysis. At present, studies of the *in vitro* effect of insulin on glucagon- or epinephrine-stimulated glycogenolysis in isolated livers or liver cells from species with low or absent glucokinase activity are lacking.

II. In Vitro Effects of Insulin on Gluconeogenesis in Liver

Very often the expressions "gluconeogenesis" and "glucose release" are used synonymously. This usage has led to the widespread idea that insulin per se is able to inhibit gluconeogenesis. However, if one restricts the term gluconeogenesis to the formation of free glucose (and glycogen) from all sources except glycogen, one has considerable difficulties in proving an effect of insulin on gluconeogenesis, if the liver is in a "basic" state, i.e. if gluconeogenesis is not stimulated by glucagon, catecholamines or 3′,5′-cAMP.

Mortimore (1963) observed inhibition of urea formation from endogenous sources in isolated perfused livers from non-diabetic rats, but this finding could not be confirmed by Söling *et al.* (1966a) or by Haft and Miller (1958) under similar conditions. In isolated liver cells from 48-hour-fasted rats, gluconeogenesis from a saturating concentration of L-lactate, pyruvate or L-alanine was stimulated rather than inhibited by insulin without a significant effect on the production of urea (Table 1) (Söling, Kehl, and Heinz, unpublished results).

In contrast to these results, Rudorff *et al.* (1970a and b) reported that insulin (20 mU/ml + 1 U insulin/h intraportally) significantly inhibited gluconeogenesis from 10 mM L-alanine in isolated perfused livers from rats (Rudorff *et al.*, 1970b) and normal but not New Zealand obese mice (Rudorff *et al.*, 1970a).

The picture is quite different if one studies the *in vitro* effects of insulin in the presence of low concentrations of either glucagon, epinephrine or 3′,5′-cAMP.

In 1966, Sokal demonstrated that glucagon stimulated gluconeogenesis from endogenous sources in isolated perfused livers from rats starved for 24 h concomitantly with an increase in the release of urea. The latter had already been shown by Miller in 1960 with isolated perfused livers from fed rats.

Later, numerous groups demonstrated also stimulation of gluconeogenesis from exogenous sources by glucagon in experiments with isolated perfused rat livers. When fructose or dihydroxyacetone was used as a glycogenic substrate, gluconeogenesis was not stimulated by glucagon in isolated perfused rat livers (Exton and Park, 1968). This finding could not be confirmed by Blair *et al.* (1973a, b), who described stimulation of gluconeogenesis not only from L-lactate, but also from propionate, fructose, dihydroxyacetone and xylitol in isolated perfused rat livers. These findings of Blair *et al.* (1973a, b) were confirmed by Zahlten *et al.* (1973) for dihydroxyacetone and xylitol and by us (Söling, Kehl and Heinz, unpublished results) for propionate in isolated rat liver cells (Tab. 1).

Lewis *et al.* (1970) and Exton *et al.* (1972) found that the action of glucagon or of epinephrine on gluconeogenesis in isolated perfused rat livers was accompanied by an intracellular increase of 3′,5′-cAMP and by an increased release of

Table 1. *Effects of glucagon, insulin and glucagon + insulin on glucose formation by isolated liver cells from 48-hour-starved rats in the presence of various precursors. The initial precursor concentration was always 10 mM. The initial concentration of glucagon was 2.7 · 10^{-7}M and that of insulin 1 mU/ml. The incubation was performed for 60 min at 37° C*

Condition	No precursor	L-Lactate	Propionate	Glycerol	L-Alanine
		Net formation of glucose (nmoles · g liver cells^{-1} · min^{-1})			
Control	63 ± 5	649 ± 51	399 ± 23	629 ± 52	354 ± 13
Glucagon	—	866 ± 56	481 ± 44	660 ± 34	380 ± 9
Insulin	—	700 ± 62	482 ± 18	773 ± 50	336 ± 31
Glucagon + Insulin .	—	838 ± 60	662 ± 35	816 ± 49	424 ± 21

3′,5′-cAMP from unknown intracellular compartments into the perfusion medium. 3′,5′-cAMP or its N^6,2′-O-dibutyryl derivative likewise stimulated gluconeogenesis from endogenous sources (Menahan and Wieland, 1967, 1969) as well as from exogenous substrates (L-lactate, pyruvate, L-alanine) in isolated perfused rat livers (Conn and Kipnis, 1969; Exton and Park, 1968, 1969) and in isolated rat liver cells (Johnson *et al.*, 1972). In accordance with the central role of 3′,5′-cAMP is the finding that in isolated rat liver cells from alloxan diabetic rats the level of 3′,5′-cAMP as well as the rate of gluconeogenesis from exogenous substrates (L-lactate, pyruvate, L-alanine) is higher than that in liver cells from non-diabetic rats (Ingebretsen *et al.*, 1972). A similar observation has been made with livers from starved rats (Selawry *et al.*, 1973). Because there is a considerable increase in the activities of the gluconeogenic key enzymes, especially phosphoenolpyruvate carboxykinase, in the livers of diabetic or starved rats, it is, of course, impossible to decide whether the increased level of 3′,5′-cAMP is really responsible for the increased rate of gluconeogenesis under these circumstances.

Insulin added to the perfusion or incubation medium inhibits the effect of glucagon on gluconeogenesis. Glinsman and Mortimore (1968) describe, among other effects (see below), inhibiton of glucagon-stimulated glucose production in isolated perfused rat liver. Mackrell and Sokal (1969) and Menahan and Wieland (1969) have confirmed this finding. The latter authors found in addition a significant inhibition of glucagon-stimulated endogenous gluconeogenesis by insulin. Johnson *et al.* (1972) recently reported that insulin significantly suppressed glucagon-stimulated gluconeogenesis in isolated liver cells from starved rats.

Exton *et al.* (1973) reported on the effects of an intraportal infusion of 10 mU/h of insulin on the net release of glucose, the formation of glycogen and the incorporation of ^{14}C-radioactivity from (U-^{14}C) labeled L-lactate into glucose and glycogen by livers from alloxan diabetic rats. There was a small decrease in glucose output and in incorporation of radioactivity into glucose, and no change in urea production. On the other hand, in diabetic rats given insulin *in vivo* prior to liver perfusion, a highly significant reduction in glucose production and in incorporation of ^{14}C-radioactivity into glucose could already be observed when the liver was excised 30 min after the *in vivo* application of insulin. These results show clearly the complex nature of the *in vivo* effects of insulin on liver metabolism as compared to its *in vitro* effects. When glucagon was infused intraportally (0.2 pmole/h) during perfusion of livers from diabetic rats, a simultaneous infusion of 600 mU/h of insulin did not significantly inhibit the glucagon-induced stimulation of glucose output, ^{14}C- incorporation from (U-^{14}C)-L-lactate into glucose and ureogenesis during the first hour, but the effect of glucagon on all 3 parameters was significantly inhibited by insulin during the second hour (Exton *et al.*, 1973).

Examination of the effect of insulin on gluconeogenesis stimulated by 3′,5′-cAMP or N^6-2′O-dibutyryl-3′,5′-cAMP gave contradictory results: GLINSMAN and MORTIMORE (1968) observed a significant inhibition of the 3′,5′-cAMP-stimulated release of glucose and of the net uptake of L-lactate when insulin (0.2 mU/h) was simultaneously infused together with 0.84 mg/h of 3′,5′-cAMP. However, no effect was observed by the same authors when 2.4 mg/h of 3′,5′-cAMP was used. MENAHAN and WIELAND (1967) did not find an inhibition of N^6-2′O-dibutyryl-3′,5′-cAMP-stimulated ureogenesis and gluconeogenesis from exogenous sources in isolated perfused rat livers.

This discrepancy could result from the different methods of application, because MENAHAN and WIELAND (1967) administered the 3′,5′-cAMP-derivative as a large single dose (final concentration $1 \cdot 10^{-6}$ M). However, it is more probable that the difference results from the different chemical structure of the N^6-2′O-dibutyryl-3′,5′-cAMP (see below).

The way in which glucagon, epinephrine or 3′,5′-cAMP could stimulate, and insulin inhibit, gluconeogenesis *in vitro* is still open to discussion:

WILLIAMSON (1967) proposed that insulin inhibits gluconeogenesis by inhibiting glucagon- or 3′,5′-cAMP-stimulated lipolysis. This argument was based mainly on the finding that in isolated perfused rat liver, gluconeogenesis from pyruvate and from L-lactate was stimulated by fatty acids (SÖLING *et al.*, 1964; 1968b; STRUCK *et al.*, 1965, 1966; WILLIAMSON *et al.*, 1966, 1969a and b; WILLIAMSON, 1967; MENAHAN *et al.*, 1968; ROSS *et al.*, 1969). An inhibition of lipolysis would, therefore, decrease not only ketogenesis, but also gluconeogenesis.

FRÖHLICH and WIELAND (1971), however, found that glucagon is able to further enhance gluconeogenesis in isolated perfused rat livers even in the presence of large concentrations of long-chain fatty acids. This result would not fit with the concept that glucagon stimulates gluconeogenesis only via lipolysis and the resulting increased rate of fatty acid oxidation.

On the other hand, in isolated perfused livers from guinea pigs (SÖLING *et al.*, 1970; ARINZE and HANSON, 1973), mice (LOTEN *et al.*, 1974), cats (ARINZE and HANSON, 1973) and pigeons (SÖLING *et al.*, 1973), fatty acids did not stimulate but rather inhibit gluconeogenesis. The effects of glucagon and 3′,5′-cAMP were studied in two of these species: Glucagon as well as 3′,5′-cAMP or its N^6-2-O-dibutyryl-derivative failed to stimulate gluconeogenesis from L-lactate, pyruvate or L-alanine in isolated perfused guinea pig liver, but enhanced glycogenolysis, as well as ketogenesis and ureogenesis (SÖLING *et al.*, 1970). Similar findings were recently reported by ASSIMACOPOULOS-JEANNET *et al.* (1973) and by LOTEN *et al.* (1974). These authors found no significant stimulation of gluconeogenesis from L-lactate in isolated perfused mouse liver by glucagon or 3′,5′-cAMP, whereas glycogenolysis was clearly enhanced by both agents.

The finding that glucagon and 3′,5′-cAMP are ineffective in those species in which increased fatty acid oxidation also failed to stimulate gluconeogenesis would favor the concept of J.R. Williamson. Unfortunately, data on the effect of insulin on gluconeogenesis in isolated perfused livers or in liver cells from species other than rat are lacking.

EXTON *et al.* (1971c) concluded, mainly on the basis of crossover plots of intracellular substrate patterns, that in rat liver, glucagon or 3′,5′-cAMP acts by enhancing the phosphoenolpyruvate carboxykinase reaction. This conclusion is, however, not compatible with the recent findings of ZAHLTEN *et al.* (1973), BLAIR *et al.* (1973a, b) and our own data (SÖLING, KEHL and HEINZ, unpublished results), that glucagon can stimulate gluconeogenesis from substrates not involved in the phosphoenolpyruvate carboxykinase step (propionate, dihydroxyacetone, glycerol, fructose, xylitol).

A carbon-sparing effect of glucagon, e.g. by inhibition of pyruvate kinase or pyruvate oxidation (Zahlten *et al.*, 1973; Blair *et al.*, 1973a, b), would provide an explanation which best fits all data obtained. The other possibility is an effect of glucagon or of 3′,5′-cAMP on the phosphofructokinase/fructose-1,6-diphosphatase step. The stimulating effect of glucagon on pyruvate transport into the mitochondria as described by Adam and Haynes (1969) would not be contradictory to this view.

III. The Mode of Action of Insulin on 3′,5′-cAMP-Mediated Processes in Vitro

The data summarized in the foregoing sections justify a short synopsis of the *in vitro* effects of insulin on the cyclic nucleotide system in the liver.

There are several theoretical explanations of how insulin may affect 3′,5′-cAMP-mediated processes *in vitro*:

1. Insulin could decrease the synthesis of 3′,5′-cAMP by inhibiting adenylate cyclase;
2. Insulin could inhibit the release of 3′,5′-cAMP from endogenous compartments;
3. Insulin could enhance the breakdown of 3′,5′-cAMP by stimulating 3′,5′-cAMP phosphodiesterase;
4. Insulin could inhibit the effects of 3′,5′-cAMP at the site of its action.

Inhibition of adenylate cyclase activity by insulin has been found in mouse liver by Hepp (1971). Under the same conditions adenylate cyclase activity was also inhibited by insulin antibody-resistant insulin-like activity (non-suppressible insulin-like activity, NSILA; Hepp, 1972). In accordance with these findings, Illiano and Cuatrecasas (1972) described the inhibition of adenylate cyclase activity in isolated liver membranes by insulin at a concentration of $1 \cdot 10^{-11}$ M (1.38 μU/ml).

Pohl *et al.* (1971) could not find an effect of 10 mU/ml insulin on basal- or glucagon-stimulated adenylate cyclase from isolated liver plasma membranes. However, as shown by Hepp (1972), the inhibitory effect of insulin increases only up to concentrations of 100 μU/ml. Higher concentrations of insulin have less, and concentrations of 1 mU/ml and higher have no effect at all. But this argument would not hold for the findings of Leray *et al.* (1973), who failed to affect adenylate cyclase activity from rat liver plasma membranes by insulin concentrations from 48 μU/ml to 2.88 mU/ml.

On the other hand, Senft *et al.* (1968) described activation of 3′,5′-cAMP phosphodiesterase activity by insulin, which has been confirmed by Loten and Sneyd (1970) who also showed, that cAMP-phosphodiesterases with different K_M values for 3′,5′-cAMP exhibited different sensitivities towards the activating effect of insulin. House *et al.* (1972) isolated a 3′,5′-cAMP phosphodiesterase-containing subfraction from rat liver plasma membranes. In this preparation insulin at near physiological concentrations effectively stimulated 3′,5′-cAMP phosphodiesterase activity within 30 sec. When large amounts of insulin were added to the medium during perfusion of isolated rat livers, Menahan *et al.* (1969) were unable to detect an effect on 3′,5′-cAMP phosphodiesterase activity.

The fact that several authors found *in vitro* an inhibitory action of insulin on the effects of 3′,5′-cAMP but not on those of N^6-2′-O-dibutyryl-3′,5′-cAMP on glycogenolysis and gluconeogenesis favors the concept that insulin acts by enhancing 3′,5′-cAMP phosphodiesterase activity, as was pointed out by Exton *et al.* (1972).

Recently, TOLBERT *et al.* (1973) showed in experiments with isolated rat liver cells that the β-adrenergic catecholamine isoproterenol led to an increase in the level of 3',5'-cAMP which was at least as high as that observed with equimolar concentrations of epinephrine. However, only epinephrine enhanced gluconeogenesis under these conditions. The authors discuss the possibility that epinephrine stimulates gluconeogenesis independently of the rise in the level of 3',5'-cAMP, which would be in contrast to the mode of action of glucagon, which is believed to act on gluconeogenesis via 3',5'-cAMP. That there are basic differences between glucagon and catecholamines in this respect is supported by the finding that stimulation of gluconeogenesis by epinephrine is accompanied by a much smaller increase in the level of 3',5'-cAMP than is stimulation by equi-effective doses of glucagon (EXTON and PARK, 1968, 1969; EXTON *et al.*, 1971b).

The rise in the level of 3',5'-cAMP effected by glucagon is without effect on glycogenolysis and gluconeogenesis if the membrane potential is altered by perfusion with a medium free of sodium ions (FRIEDMANN, 1972).

EXTON *et al.* (1971a) recently reported that 3',5'-cGMP acts on glycogen metabolism, gluconeogenesis and potassium release in a manner similar to that of 3',5'-cAMP. However, the effects of 3',5'-cGMP could not be influenced by insulin. This fact would favor the concept that insulin acts mainly by affecting the synthesis, breakdown or the intracellular distribution of 3',5'-cAMP, and not so much by inhibiting the metabolic effects of 3',5'-cAMP itself.

IV. Effects of Insulin on Electrolyte Metabolism

The marked disturbance of the electrolyte balance during diabetic coma indicates that insulin may have a direct effect on hepatic electrolyte metabolism. Several clear-cut *in vivo* effects of insulin on electrolyte metabolism have been described, but the results obtained *in vitro* are contradictory, especially if one tries to correlate them with other effects of insulin and of other hormones.

MORTIMORE (1961) found that insulin inhibits almost completely the release of potassium by isolated perfused rat livers. This effect was accompanied by a decreased release of water from the organ. KESTENS *et al.* (1963) obtained similar results without affecting the net balance of glucose across the liver. In contrast to these reports, SÖLING *et al.* (1966a) were unable to detect a significant effect of insulin on the net balance of glucose or inorganic phosphate in experiments with livers from 20 h starved normal or alloxan diabetic rats, although insulin led to a net uptake of glucose in experiments with livers from non-diabetic fed rats. The release of potassium by isolated perfused livers from alloxan diabetic rats was significantly elevated in comparison with non-diabetic controls, but remained unaffected by the presence of insulin (0.9 U/h intraportally) (SÖLING *et al.*, 1966a). The reason for the inefficiency of insulin in the experiments of SÖLING *et al.* (1966a) remains unclear. In experiments with isolated perfused dog liver LAMBOTTE (1968) observed that insulin inhibited the release of potassium without affecting the glucose net balance. The effect of insulin on potassium metabolism could be abolished by the prior addition of ouabaine.

The effect of insulin apparently requires an intact active ion transport system. Since insulin exerts a similar effect on potassium metabolism in muscle it is likely that the mechanism of action is the same: ZIERLER (1959) showed that in muscle, after addition of insulin, a hyperpolarization of the cell membrane precedes the effect on the potassium balance. KERNAN (1961) explained the recovery of the membrane potential in muscle in the presence of insulin in terms of a decreased membrane permeability for sodium. LAMBOTTE (1968) arrived at the conclusion that this explanation is also valid for the liver.

PARK *et al.* (1972) as well as GLINSMAN and MORTIMORE (1968) assumed, on the other hand, that all direct effects of insulin on liver metabolism, including the effect on glucagon- or 3′,5′-cAMP-mediated potassium release, result from a decrease in the intracellular level of 3′,5′-cAMP. In experiments with isolated perfused dog livers LAMBOTTE (1968) could stimulate potassium release with epinephrine, but not with 3′,5′-cAMP. This result seems difficult to understand in terms of the concept of PARK *et al.* (1972). In LAMBOTTE's experiments 3′,5′-cAMP had a stimulatory effect on glycogenolysis. On the other hand, BURTON *et al.* (1967) were able to produce in isolated perfused rat livers an inhibitory effect of insulin on the efflux of potassium under conditions where insulin did not significantly affect release of glucose from glycogen. In contrast to the findings of Lambotte obtained with isolated perfused dog livers, not only glucagon but also 3′,5′-cAMP stimulated the efflux of potassium from isolated perfused rat liver (GLINSMAN and MORTIMORE, 1968). Stimulation by glucagon and by 3′,5′-cAMP could be inhibited by insulin.

Epinephrine inhibited the effect of insulin on the potassium balance in isolated perfused livers from dogs (LAMBOTTE, 1968) and rats (LULY *et al.*, 1972). This action of epinephrine could be inhibited in dog liver by phenoxybenzamine, an α-receptor blocking agent, whereas in rat liver the action of epinephrine on membrane bound Na^+-K^+-ATPase was antagonized by propranolol, a typical β-receptor blocking substance. Several effects on the potassium balance which had not been detected with the classical recirculating perfusion technique, were found when non-recirculating systems ("open systems") were used instead. WILLIAMS *et al.* (1971) observed that the addition of glucagon, epinephrine or 3′,5′-cAMP to such a non-recirculating perfusion system elicited an immediate net influx of potassium into isolated rat livers followed by a net efflux. The influx phase was particularly pronounced during perfusion at low temperature (27°C). Apparently, the influx phase which is accompanied by a Ca^{++} efflux represents a direct response to the increased availability of 3′,5′-cAMP. In these experiments, insulin inhibited the efflux of potassium during the second phase, but had no detectable effect on the early phase of potassium influx. The inhibitory effect of insulin could only be seen when submaximal doses of 3′,5′-cAMP were used, and it disappeared completely in the presence of saturating concentrations of 3′,5′-cAMP. Insulin did not diminish the stimulatory effect of N^6-2′O-dibutyryl-3′,5′-cAMP on the efflux of calcium and glucose (WILLIAMS *et al.*, 1971). These results are in accordance with the idea that insulin decreases the level of that fraction of 3′,5′-cAMP which gets into contact with the regulatory systems for intracellular potassium and glucose. Apparently, a clear-cut effect of insulin on the hepatic potassium balance can be seen only if the level of this fraction of 3′,5′-cAMP is sufficiently elevated. Ignoring intrinsic species differences, differences in the level of "free" 3′,5′-cAMP could be one reason for the contradictory results with respect to the effect of insulin on hepatic potassium metabolism.

The mechanism by which 3′,5′-cAMP acts on the hepatic potassium balance is still unknown. Also unknown is whether the effect of insulin involves 3′-5′-cAMP at all, or whether insulin affects the activity of membrane bound Na^+-K^+-ATPase directly by altering the physicochemical properties of the plasma membrane. The latter idea corresponds to the model proposed by KRAHL (1972), according to which the insulin receptor in the plasma membrane is directly coupled to the Mg^{++}-stimulated Na^+-K^+-ATPase.

LULY *et al.* (1972) showed, however, that not only epinephrine and glucagon but also 3′,5′-cAMP reduce *in vitro* the activity of the plasma membrane bound

Na^+-K^+-ATPase in rat liver. Insulin alone had no effect on the ATPase activity but partially abolished the inhibitory effect of the two hormones.

The finding that insulin is able to reduce the hormone (glucagon, epinephrine) stimulated loss of potassium would support the concept that the loss of potassium observed during liver perfusion involves Na^+-K^+-ATPase and does not result merely from an unspecific change of the plasma membrane cation permeability.

However, a recent report of FRIEDMANN (1972) makes it doubtful that the membrane bound Na^+-K^+-ATPase plays a central role in the effect of hormones on hepatic potassium movements: The addition of glucagon or of 3',5'-cAMP to the perfusion medium led to a parallel biphasic response of potassium and sodium from the isolated perfused rat liver. During a short initial phase potassium and sodium were taken up in exchange for protons leaving the liver cell. This phase was followed by a more pronounced uptake of protons and a release of potassium and sodium ions. It was mentioned previously that the metabolic action of glucagon, but not its ability to increase the level of 3',5'-cAMP, depends on an intact membrane potential. Therefore, the antiglucagon effects of insulin *in vitro* on hepatic metabolism must be confined to the cAMP-system itself but could include also a cAMP-independent effect on the liver cell membrane.

V. Effects of Insulin on Hepatic Lipid Metabolism

No effect of insulin on the uptake of long-chain non-esterified fatty acids was observed by SÖLING *et al.* (1966a) in experiments with isolated perfused livers from normal and alloxan diabetic rats, or by TOPPING and MAYES (1972) in isolated livers from fed rats perfused with diluted rat blood. Only PENHOS *et al.* (1968) described an enhanced uptake of long-chain fatty acids by isolated perfused rat livers when insulin was added to the perfusion medium. HAFT and MILLER (1958) were the first to report an inhibition by insulin of ketone body formation by isolated rat livers. However, PENHOS *et al.* (1968) were unable to confirm this finding. SÖLING *et al.* (1966a) likewise found no effect of insulin (0.9 U/h intraportally) on ketone body formation by isolated perfused livers form normal or alloxan diabetic rats, and TOPPING and MAYES (1972) did not observe an effect of insulin on the formation of ^{14}C-ketone bodies from (1-^{14}C) oleate.

On the other hand, POLEDNE and MAYES (1970) observed earlier an inhibitory effect of insulin *in vitro* on ketone body production from endogenous sources in livers from starved rats. For full understanding of the difficulties in assessing the *in vitro* effect of insulin on liver metabolism, one has to mention that all studies referred to were performed with the recirculating perfusion system. In this system no difference in the production of ketone bodies by livers from normal and from alloxan diabetic rats has been found (SÖLING *et al.*, 1966a). However, when livers from normal and from alloxan diabetic rats were compared in an open perfusion system, it became evident that the rate of production of ketone bodies from endogenous as well as from exogenous fatty acids is significantly higher with livers from diabetic animals (SÖLING *et al.*, 1974; SEUFERT *et al.*, 1974). Therefore it cannot be excluded that in this system, *in vitro* effects of insulin may become visible. Moreover, we have recently shown (SÖLING *et al.*, 1974; SEUFERT *et al.*, 1974) that the isolated perfused rat liver produces not only ketone bodies but also free acetate from fatty acids and that the formation of acetate is significantly increased in states of insulin deficiency. Therefore, effects of insulin must not be restricted necessarily to ketogenesis alone.

When isolated perfused rat livers were first perfused with insulin, the stimulating effect of glucagon on ketogenesis was significantly inhibited (MENAHAN and

WIELAND, 1969). This finding is in accordance with the view that glucagon stimulated ketogenesis by activation of a 3′,5′-cAMP sensitive triglyceride lipase. For a discussion of the *in vitro* effects of insulin on the hepatic adenylate cyclase — and 3′,5′-cAMP phosphodiesterase system, the reader is referred to page 420.

Fatty acid synthesis is significantly decreased in states of insulin deficiency. An *in vitro* effect of insulin on fatty acid synthesis, however, has been reported only by HAFT (1967) in experiments with isolated perfused livers from fasted, but not from fed rats. HAFT observed that insulin at an initial level of 1 mU/ml in the perfusion medium and during continuous infusion of 30 mU/h enhanced not only the incorporation of radioactivity from ^{3}H-acetate but also from (1-^{14}C) D-glucose into fatty acids and cholesterol.

How does insulin affect lipogenesis *in vitro*?

Several factors have been claimed to contribute to the low rate of lipogenesis in states of insulin deficiency:

1. a lack of generation of reducing equivalents due to low activities of the pentose phosphate cycle and of malic enzyme;
2. a decreased activity of acetyl-CoA carboxylase;
3. a decreased activity of citrate cleavage enzyme (for the case of fatty acid synthesis from glucose);
4. a decreased activity of pyruvate dehydrogenase due to a higher degree of interconversion of the enzyme into the phosphorylated inactive from.

None of the 4 parameters has ever been shown to be directly influenced by insulin *in vitro*. HAFT (1967) reported that the effect of insulin was less marked in the presence of high concentrations of glucose and that high concentrations of glucose alone stimulated fatty acid synthesis from both glucose and acetate provided that livers from fed rats were used. Thus it is likely that the *in vitro* effect of insulin is mediated by enhancement of glucose metabolism. Increased metabolism of glucose could affect fatty acid synthesis in several ways:

1. An increased rate of generation of α-glycerophosphate would favor esterification of fatty acids and as a result lower the concentration of long-chain acyl-CoA compounds which are supposed to inhibit acetyl-CoA carboxylase and (by their oxidation) to shift the equilibrium of the pyruvate dehydrogenase interconversion reaction in the direction of the inactive form.
2. An increased turnover of glucose through the pentose phosphate cycle would lead to enhanced formation of reducing equivalents for fatty acid synthesis. The increased rate of fatty acid synthesis would in turn decrease the intramitochondrial ATP/ADP ratio due to its energy demand and thus favor the interconversion of pyruvate dehydrogenase to the active form.

Both mechanisms would explain why in the experiments of HAFT insulin stimulated fatty acid synthesis from acetate as well as from glucose. The weak point in this argument is that is has never been shown that insulin *in vitro* really stimulates the flux of glucose through the glycolytic chain or the pentose phosphate cycle.

WIELAND *et al.* (1972) observed in rat liver a rapid conversion of pyruvate dehydrogenase to the active form shortly after an *in vivo* injection of insulin. However, this effect was completely abolished when the decrease in the plasma levels of long-chain free fatty acids was overcome by an infusion of oleate. This finding is in accordance with the idea that insulin does not affect the pyruvate dehydrogenase interconversion reaction in a direct manner.

TOPPING and MAYES (1972) have shown in an series of excellent experiments that insulin *in vitro* has a significant effect on the intracellular disposal of the long-chain fatty acids by isolated perfused rat livers. In these experiments the livers were perfused with whole diluted rat blood. The insulin level in the perfusion medium was elevated by injecting the blood donor rats with glucose prior to sacrifice.

Under these conditions insulin had the following effects:

It increased the release of triglycerides as very low density lipoprotein complexes and the incorporation of ^{14}C-radioactivity from (1-^{14}C) oleate into very low density lipoproteins as well as the total esterification rate. Insulin inhibited significantly the formation of $^{14}CO_2$ from (1-^{14}C) oleate. In these experiments fructose alone had effects on all these parameters which were similar to those of insulin. Insulin and fructose administered together were no more effective than either of the two agents alone. Insulin also had an effect on the incorporation of radioactivity from (Meth-^{3}H) acetate into total lipids and the lipid moiety of the very low density lipoproteins. But this effect was not significant in the experiments in which rat insulin (given together with the medium as mentioned above) was used and was completely abolished by the presence of fructose. Surprisingly, when fructose was given together with bovine insulin instead of rat insulin, the ^{3}H-incorporation into total lipids and into the very low density lipoprotein lipids was significantly stimulated. Unfortunately, TOPPING and MAYES (1972) did not include any data from a group receiving only bovine insulin. Since the concentration of bovine insulin used (about 1.34 mU/ml) was certainly much higher than the concentrations of rat insulin in the blood of the glucose-loaded donor rats, we feel that this phenomenon has nothing to do with an additive effect of bovine insulin and fructose, but with the much higher concentration of biologically active insulin.

The concentration of bovine insulin in the experiments of HAFT (1967, see page 424) was in the same range as that in the bovine insulin experiments of TOPPING and MAYES (1972). In the experiments of TOPPING and MAYES (1972) insulin as well as fructose stimulated the esterification of long-chain fatty acids and the secretion of esterified fatty acids as very low density lipoprotein complexes. The higher rate of esterification led to a decreased rate of fatty acid oxidation, which may explain the decreased rate of ketone body formation described by other authors (POLEDUE and MAYES, 1970; HAFT and MILLER, 1958). TOPPING and MAYES (1972) explain their findings mainly on the basis of an inhibition by insulin of the reactions leading to activation of hepatic triglyceride lipase(s), whereas the effect of fructose is explained mainly as the result of increased esterification following the enhanced formation of α-glycerophosphate. Both the insulin mediated and the fructose mediated mechanisms tend to lower the intracellular concentration of long-chain acyl-CoA compounds, which would explain the similarities of the metabolic effects of insulin and fructose. The main difference between the actions of these two factors in the experiments of TOPPING and MAYES (1972) was that insulin stimulated the incorporation of ^{3}H-radioactivity from (Meth-^{3}H) acetate into long-chain fatty acids whereas fructose inhibited this process.

High concentrations of fructose lead to a considerable drop in the hepatic concentrations of adenine nucleotides and in the ATP/ADP ratio *in vivo* (MÄENPÄÄ *et al.*, 1968; RAIVIO *et al.*, 1969; SÖLING and BERNHARD, 1971) and possibly also in the isolated perfused rat liver (PATZELT *et al.*, 1973). This phenomenon may have limited fatty acid synthesis in the experiments of TOPPING and MAYES (1972) in the presence of fructose. In accordance with this view is the observation by HAFT (1967) that glucose had the same stimulatory effect on the incorporation of ^{3}H-radioactivity from (Meth-^{3}H) acetate into liver lipids as insulin in experiments with isolated livers from fed rats.

So far, there is no evidence for a direct *in vitro* effect of insulin on acetyl-CoA carboxylase, and the insulin-mediated induction of the enzyme needs far too much time to affect lipogenesis from acetate during the relatively short time of perfusion, which lasted only 2 h.

Considering all facts, an inhibitory effect of insulin on the activation of hepatic triglyceride lipase(s) is the most likely mechanism by which insulin exerts its various *in vitro* effects on the hepatic metabolism of lipids. This concept is in accordance with the observation that the greater the concentration of glucose, the lesser is the *in vitro* effect of insulin on hepatic lipid metabolism, since large concentrations of glucose favor re-esterification of long-chain fatty acids, the net effect on lipolysis being similar to that of insulin.

VI. Effects of Insulin on the Metabolism of Amino Acids and Proteins

As early as 1937 Bach and Holmes observed inhibition of urea production by rat liver slices in the presence of insulin. In 1956 Miller *et al.* found that insulin as well as growth hormone led to a positive nitrogen balance in isolated perfused rat livers. In these experiments the medium contained a physiological mixture of amino acids and glucose. Later, Miller (1960) showed that the effects of these hormones were not dependent on the presence of exogenous amino acids in the medium. Söling *et al.* (1966a) described the effect of the *in vitro* addition of insulin (0.9 U/h intraportally) on the balance of α-amino acids in isolated perfused livers from normal and diabetic rats. In the absence of insulin, livers from normal and from diabetic animals exhibited a similar net release of free amino acids. In the presence of insulin, the net release of amino acids was converted into a net uptake of α-amino acids in livers from normal and from diabetic rats.

Three main factors are responsible for the over-all nitrogen balance in the liver:

1. Transport of α-amino acids into the liver cell and between the intracellular compartments;
2. Protein synthesis;
3. Protein breakdown.

The non-metabolizable α-amino acid α-aminoisobutyric acid (AIB) has been used as a tool in studying amino acid transport. Chambers *et al.* (1965) were the first to describe that insulin as well as hydrocortisone stimulated the uptake of AIB by isolated perfused rat livers. The effects of both hormones were additive. The effect of hydrocortisone, but not that of insulin, was abolished by the α-receptor blocking agent phenoxybenzamine. However, the effect of insulin could be partially inhibited by concentrations of actinomycin D which inhibited already the synthesis of DNA-like RNA.

Miller and Griffin (1972) confirmed the finding of Chambers *et al.* (1965) and found in addition that insulin enhanced also the net uptake of the naturally occurring α-amino acids. The pH dependency of the uptake of AIB by isolated perfused rat livers was significantly reduced by insulin.

The interpretation of the *in vitro* effects of hormones on hepatic amino acid and protein metabolism in liver is complicated by the finding that insulin and glucagon are known to antagonize each other with respect to glycogenolysis, gluconeogenesis, ketogenesis and ureogenesis, but share several effects with respect to protein metabolism. Malette *et al.* (1969), using the nonrecirculating rat liver perfusion technique, observed effects of glucagon similar to those already mentioned for insulin: Glucagon stimulated the hepatic uptake of AIB. Moreover, glucagon enhanced the intracellular utilization of L-glycine, L-alanine, L-glutamate and L-phenylalanine.

JOHN and MILLER (1969) determined in a very careful study the requirements for the synthesis of several secretory proteins by the isolated perfused rat liver. They perfused livers from fed rats for up to 12 h and examined the effects of the following factors:

1. A physiological mixture of L-amino acids
2. Hydrocortisone
3. Growth hormone
4. Insulin.

They measured the net synthesis of fibrinogen, a_1-acid glycoprotein, a_2-globulin and haptoglobin, and the incorporation of radioactivity from (1-^{14}C) lysine into total liver protein. Only two factors out of the four were essential, namely a-amino acids and insulin.

JOHN and MILLER (1969) interpreted their results in terms of a stimulation of protein synthesis by insulin since inhibition of protein breakdown, as had been determined earlier by the same authors (1966), would not have been sufficient to explain the increased net production of proteins. On the other hand, an inhibitory effect of insulin on proteolysis was established not only by the findings of JOHN and MILLER (1966), but also by the more recent studies of MORTIMORE and MONDON (1970). The latter authors prelabeled *in vivo* hepatic proteins in rats. When the livers of these rats were perfused, insulin significantly reduced the release of ^{14}C-valine by the liver.

How insulin affects proteolysis *in vitro* is still a matter of speculation. Glucagon promotes the liberation of lysosomal enzymes. Among these lysosomal enzymes are certainly proteases (GUDER *et al.*, 1970). However, it is all but certain that only lysosomal proteases are responsible for the degradation of proteins under physiological conditions. Moreover, whether insulin really inhibits the effects of glucagon on the release of lysosomal enzymes has never been studied. In addition, the inhibitory effect of insulin on proteolysis is observed also in the absence of glucagon.

This finding, of course, does not exclude the possibility that inhibition of the proteolytic effects of glucagon or of 3′,5′-cAMP contributes to the anticatabolic *in vitro* effects of insulin, as is indicated by the inhibitory effect of insulin on glucagon- or 3′,5′-cAMP-stimulated ureogenesis (see page 417 ff.).

The experiments of JOHN and MILLER (1969) seem to indicate that under *in vitro* conditions insulin leads to a general stimulation of protein synthesis. One has tried to explain this action of insulin by an effect on one or several very early steps of protein synthesis. On the basis of *in vivo* findings of LANGAN (1969), it was thought that insulin might affect the availability of translatable DNA by enhancing the phosphorylation of specific sites on the lysine-rich F_1 histones. This explanation was hampered by the fact that glucagon and 3′,5′-cAMP had the same effect *in vivo* as insulin. It was recently shown by MALLETTE *et al.* (1973) that in the isolated perfused rat liver glucagon and 3′,5′-cAMP but not insulin were able to enhance the phosphorylation of lysine-rich histones. The *in vivo* effect of insulin on histone phosphorylation was probably elicited by an enhanced secretion of glucagon and/or catecholamines following insulin-induced hypoglycemia. Unfortunately, MALLETTE *et al.* (1973) did not mention whether insulin inhibited *in vitro* the effects of glucagon on histone phosphorylation in the isolated perfused rat liver.

There are only a few examples in which insulin affected the turnover of specific proteins *in vitro:*

Tyrosine α-ketoglutarate aminotransferase (TAT) is by far the most extensively studied enzyme. HAGER and KENNEY (1968) demonstrated with isolated perfused rat livers that not only glucagon and hydrocortisone but also insulin increased the activity of TAT *in vitro*. The effects of insulin and glucagon did not correlate with changes in the levels of 3′5′-cAMP. The increase in TAT activity could be abolished by actinomycin D irrespective of whether hydrocortisone, glucagon or insulin was the stimulatory hormone. BARNETT and WICKS (1971) induced TAT in hepatoma cell cultures with N^6-2′O-dibutyryl-3′5′-cAMP. This effect was thought to take place at the post-transcriptional level. N^6-2′O-dibutyryl-3′5′-cAMP had no effect on the degradation of TAT under these conditions.

Stimulation of TAT synthesis in the perfused rat liver is in sharp contrast to the results of *in vivo* studies in which lack of insulin leads to an increased activity which can be lowered to normal values upon treatment with insulin (SÖLING *et al.*, 1968a). Moreover, hormonal effects on TAT are complex: LEVITAN and WEBB (1969) induced TAT in rats *in vivo* with cortisol for 4 h. Subsequently, the livers were perfused and the effect of various factors examined. Inhibitors of protein synthesis (cycloheximide or 8-azaguanine) but not pyridoxal, L-tyrosine, L-tryptophane, α-ketoglutarate, glucagon or insulin prevented the decrease in enzyme activity during perfusion. JERVELL and SEGLEN (1969) found that in isolated perfused rat livers cycloheximide inhibited the synthesis of TAT but had no effect on its degradation. However, when insulin was added to the perfusion medium 15 min prior to the addition of cycloheximide, the degradation of TAT was completely inhibited. The inefficiency of cycloheximide in blocking the degradation of TAT in the absence of insulin could be observed also under conditions in which TAT had been induced *in vitro* by glucocorticoids. SEGLEN (1971) suggests that insulin and cycloheximide exert only an indirect influence on the turnover of TAT which might be mediated by the intracellular supply of amino acids. This suggestion is supported by experiments with isolated perfused rat livers in which amino acids had indeed been shown to affect TAT turnover (LEVITAN and WEBB, 1969; KNOX and SHARMA, 1968).

Indirect hormonal effects also provide the best explanation of why hormones like insulin and glucagon, known to act as antagonists *in vivo*, had a similar action on TAT activity *in vitro*. Interestingly, glucagon as well as insulin affects *in vitro* (isolated perfused rat liver) the activity of TAT but not that of tryptophane pyrrolase.

Extensive studies concerning these problems have been performed, especially with hepatoma cell cultures. Hepatoma cells usually exhibit signs of dedifferentiation combined with a loss of sensitivity towards hormonal factors. But as long as responses to hormones are detectable in these cells, they can still be used as indicators for similar effects of the hormones in normal cells.

Insulin as well as dialyzed serum increases TAT activity in HTC cells, a special hepatoma line (GELEHRTER and TOMKINS, 1969), when the cells were previously stimulated by steroids. The steroid effect, but not the stimulation exerted by insulin or serum, was abolished by actinomycin D. Similar observations were made by REEL *et al.* (1970) in Reuber hepatoma cell cultures in which actinomycin D was also unable to abolish the *in vitro* effect of insulin.

Although insulin and serum seem to act on the post-transcriptional steps of TAT synthesis, insulin as well as serum was able to induce TAT without prior stimulation by steroids (GELEHRTER, 1973). If one assumes that steroids act by derepression, it is unclear how insulin and serum could stimulate synthesis of TAT *in vitro* in the non-derepressed state. The effect of serum, although similar to that of insulin, cannot be explained on the basis of insulin in the serum, since the effects of insulin and serum were additive even at saturating concentrations of insulin (GELEHRTER and TOMKINS, 1970). Induction by sepharose-bound insulin in cultured rat liver cells has recently been described by DAVIDSON *et al.* (1973).

PEP-carboxykinase, one of the gluconeogenic key enzymes, responds to insulin differently than does TAT: While insulin *in vitro* in Reuber H 35 hepatoma cell culture elicits an additive increase in the TAT activity in the presence of steroids or of N^6-2′O-dibutyryl-3′5′-cAMP, it abolishes completely the steroid- or N^6-2′O-dibutyryl-3′5′-cAMP-induced increase in PEP-carboxykinase activity. From these experiments it appears that the influence of insulin is enzyme specific and not merely an influence upon the 3′5′-cAMP system or upon the general action of glucocorticoids.

Another enzyme affected by insulin *in vitro* is pyruvate kinase. GERSCHENSON and ANDERSSON (1971) observed a significant increase in the activity of this enzyme in rat hepatoma cell culture in the presence of insulin. The induction could be blocked by cycloheximide or actinomycin D.

The activity of ornithine-decarboxylase increases significantly in isolated perfused rat liver in the presence of insulin or glucagon. This induction was inhibited by actinomycin D (MALLETTE and EXTON, 1973). There is some support for the idea that insulin may affect the turnover of ornithine-decarboxylase also under physiological conditions, since the activity of this enzyme disappeared during starvation, but reappeared within 1—2 h upon refeeding (DOMSCHKE and SÖLING, 1973). Whether some of the *in vitro* effects of insulin on protein synthesis in liver result indirectly from an effect of insulin on ornithine-decarboxylase activity remains an open question. But since ornithine-decarboxylase is a key enzyme for the synthesis of polyamines and since this group of biological substances has very general effects on protein synthesis (for a review see BACHRACH, 1973), it might well be that such a relation exists.

It is known from *in vivo* studies that in states of severe insulin deficiency, the size distribution of the hepatic polysomes is altered and indicates an increase in the relative amount of the lighter polysomes. EKREN *et al.* (1971) studied the effects of insulin on the size distribution of polysomes in isolated perfused rat livers. When the livers were perfused in the absence of amino acids in the medium, insulin enhanced rather than inhibited the breakdown of heavy polysomes. Amino acids alone inhibited this change in livers from normal but not in those from diabetic rats. Addition of insulin together with amino acids resulted in a significant increase in the relative amount of heavier polysomes in livers from normal as well as from diabetic rats. The way in which insulin exerts this effect is as yet unknown. The effect on the polysome distribution may be a secondary result of an effect of insulin on the metabolism of amino acids.

Microsomes from alloxan diabetic rats have a diminished capacity to incorporate ^{14}C-leucine into nascent proteins (ROBINSON, 1961; DOELL, 1960; KORNER, 1960). Attemps to compensate this effect by adding insulin *in vitro* failed. However, COHEN and GRINBLAT (1971) recently reported that in their experiments, insulin *in vitro* stimulated the incorporation of ^{3}H-phenylalanine by hepatic microsomes from pancreatectomized diabetic rats. An effect of insulin on processes residing in the soluble cell fraction appears unlikely, since in these experiments soluble fractions from non-diabetic rats were used together with the microsomes from livers of diabetic animals. The microsomes in these experiments were only washed with KCl, whereas WOOL and CAVICCHI (1967) used desoxycholate-treated microsomes. Since the ribosomes are normally attached to intracellular membranous structures, it may well be that this binding had been destroyed by the desoxycholate treatment, rendering them resistent to *in vitro* effects of insulin.

Nothing but pure speculation can be offered thus far as to how insulin acts *in vitro* on the translation process in the cell free system.

References

Adam, P.A.J., Haynes, R.C., Jr.: Control of hepatic mitochondrial CO_2 fixation by glucagon, epinephrine, and cortisol. J. biol. Chem. **244**, 6444—6450 (1969)

Arinze, I.J., Hanson, R.W.: Mitochondrial redox state and the regulation of gluconeogenesis in the isolated perfused cat liver. FEBS Letters **31**, 280—282 (1973)

Assimacopoulos-Jeannet, F., Exton, J.H., Jeanrenaud, B.: Control of gluconeogenesis and glycogenolysis in perfused livers of normal mice. Amer. J. Physiol. **225**, 25—32 (1973)

Bach, S.J., Holmes, E.G.: The effect of insulin on carbohydrate formation in the liver. Biochem. J. **31**, 89—100 (1937)

Bachrach, U.: Function of naturally occurring polyamines. New York-London: Academic Press 1973

Barnett, C.A., Wicks, W.D.: Regulation of phosphoenolpyruvate carboxykinase and tyrosine transaminase in hepatoma cell cultures. I. Effects of glucocorticoids, N^6,$O^{2'}$-dibutyryl-cyclic adenosine 3',5'-monophosphate and insulin in Reuber H35 cells. J. biol. Chem. **246**, 7201—7206 (1971)

Blair, J.B., Cook, D.E., Lardy, H.A.: Influence of glucagon on the metabolism of xylitol and dihydroxyacetone in the isolated perfused rat liver. J. biol. Chem. **248**, 3601—3607 (1973a)

Blair, J.B., Cook, D.E., Lardy, H.A.: Interaction of propionate and lactate in the perfused rat liver. J. biol. Chem. **248**, 3608—3614 (1973b)

Boden, G., Willms, B.: Einfluß von Insulin auf Kohlenhydrat- und Fettstoffwechsel der perfundierten Leber bei normalen und alloxandiabetischen Ratten. Klin. Wschr. **44**, 579—583 (1966)

Burton, S.D., Mondon, C.E., Ishida, T.: Dissociation of potassium and glucose efflux in isolated perfused rat liver. Amer. J. Physiol. **212**, 261—266 (1967)

Cahill, G.F., Jr., Ashmore, J., Earle, A.S., Zottu, S.: Glucose penetration into liver. Amer. J. Physiol. **192**, 491—496 (1958)

Cahill, G.F., Jr., Ashmore, J., Renold, A.E., Hastings, A.B.: Blood glucose and the liver. Amer. J. Med. **26**, 264—282 (1959)

Chambers, J.W., Georg, R.H., Bass, A.D.: Effect of hydrocortisone and insulin on uptake of α-amino-isobutyric acid by isolated perfused rat liver. Molec. Pharmacol. **1**, 66—76 (1965)

Cohen, M.P., Grinblat, L.: Stimulation with insulin in vitro of protein synthesis by diabetic hepatic microsomes. FEBS Letters **15**, 299—301 (1971)

Conn, H.O., Kipnis, D.M.: The effect of various 3',5'-cyclic nucleotides on gluconeogenesis and glycogenolysis in the perfused rat liver. Biochem. biophys. Res. Commun. **37**, 319—326 (1969)

Davidson, M.B., Van Herle, A.J., Gerschenson, L.E.: Insulin and sepharose-insulin effects on tyrosine transaminase levels in cultured rat liver cells. Endocrinology **92**, 1442—1446 (1973)

Doell, R.G.: The effect of injected insulin on the amino acid incorporating system of rat liver. Biochim. biophys. Acta (Amst) **39**, 237—241 (1960)

Domschke, S., Söling, H.D.: Polyamine metabolism in rat liver: Effect of starvation and refeeding. Horm. Metab. Res. **5**, 97—101 (1973)

Ekren, T., Jervell, K.F., Seglen, P.O.: Insulin and amino-acid regulation of polysomes in perfused, diabetic rat liver. Nature (Lond.) **229**, 244—245 (1971)

Exton, I.H., Hardman, I.G., Williams, T.F., Sutherland, E.W., Park, C.R.: Effects of guanosine 3',5'-monophosphate on the perfused rat liver. J. biol. Chem. **246**, 2658—2664 (1971a)

Exton, J.H., Harper, S.C., Tucker, A.L., Ho, R.I.: Effects of insulin on gluconeogenesis and cyclic AMP levels in perfused livers from diabetic rats. Biochim. biophys. Acta (Amst.) **329**, 23—40 (1973)

Exton, J.H., Lewis, S.B., Ho, R.I., Park, C.R.: The role of cyclic AMP in the control of hepatic glucose production by glucagon and insulin. Adv. Cycl. Nucleot. Res. **1**, 91—101 (1972)

Exton, J.H., Park, C.R.: Control of gluconeogenesis in liver. II. Effects of glucagon, catecholamines, and adenosine 3',5'-monophosphate on gluconeogenesis in the perfused rat liver. J. biol. Chem. **243**, 4189—4196 (1968)

Exton, J.H., Park, C.R.: Control of gluconeogenesis in liver. III. Effects of L-lactate, pyruvate, fructose, glucagon, epinephrine, and adenosine 3',5'-monophosphate on gluconeogenic intermediates in the perfused rat liver. J. biol. Chem. **244**, 1424—1433 (1969)

EXTON, J.H., ROBINSON, G.A., SUTHERLAND, E.A., PARK, C.R.: Studies on the role of adenosine 3′,5′-monophosphate in the hepatic actions of glucagon and catecholamines. J. biol. Chem. **246**, 6166—6177 (1971b)

EXTON, J.H., UI, M., PARK, C.R.: Mechanism of glucagon action on gluconeogenesis. In: Regulation of gluconeogenesis. New York-London: Academic Press 1971c

FRIEDMANN, N.: Effects of glucagon and cyclic AMP on ion fluxes in the perfused liver. Biochim. biophys. Acta (Amst.) **274**, 241—252 (1972)

FRÖHLICH, J., WIELAND, O.: Dissociation of gluconeogenic and ketogenic action of glucagon in the perfused rat liver. In: Regulation of gluconeogenesis. New York-London: Academic Press 1971

GARRISON, I.C., HAYNES, R.C., JR.: Hormonal control of glycogenolysis and gluconeogenesis in isolated rat liver cells. J. biol. Chem. **248**, 5333—5343 (1973)

GELEHRTER, T.D.: Mechanism of hormonal induction of enzymes. Metabolism **22**, 85—100 (1973)

GELEHRTER, T.D., TOMKINS, G.M.: Control of tyrosine aminotransferase synthesis in tissue culture by a factor in serum. Proc. nat. Acad. Sci. (Wash.) **64**, 723—730 (1969)

GELEHRTER, T.D., TOMKINS, G.M.: Posttranscriptional control of tyrosine aminotransferase synthesis by insulin. Proc. nat. Acad. Sci. (Wash.) **66**, 390—397 (1970)

GERSCHENSON, L.E., ANDERSSON, M.: Regulation of the pyruvate kinase of an established rat liver cell line (RLC) in culture by insulin, glucose and serum. Biochem. biophys. Res. Commun. **43**, 1211—1218 (1971)

GLINSMAN, W.H., MORTIMORE, G.E.: Influence of glucagon and 3′,5′-cAMP on insulin responsiveness of the perfused rat liver. Amer. J. Physiol. **215**, 553—559 (1968)

GUDER, W., HEPP, K.D., WIELAND, O.: The catabolic action of glucagon in rat liver. The influence of age, nutritional state and renal function on the effect of glucagon on lysosomal N-acetyl-β, D-glucosaminidase. Biochim. biophys. Acta (Amst.) **222**, 593—605 (1970)

HAFT, D.E.: Effects of insulin on glucose metabolism by the perfused normal rat liver. Amer. J. Physiol. **213**, 219—230 (1967)

HAFT, D.E., MILLER, L.L.: Alloxan diabetes and demonstrated direct action of insulin on metabolism of isolated perfused rat liver. Amer. J. Physiol. **192**, 33—42 (1958)

HAGER, C.B., KENNEY, F.T.: Regulation of tyrosine-α-ketoglutarate transaminase in rat liver. VII. Hormonal effects on synthesis in the isolated perfused rat liver. J. biol. Chem. **243**, 3296—3300 (1968)

HEPP, K.D.: Inhibition of glucagon-stimulated adenyl cyclase by insulin. FEBS Letters **12**, 263—266 (1971)

HEPP, K.D.: Adenylate cyclase and insulin action. Effect of insulin, non-suppressible insulin-like material and diabetes on adenylate-cyclase activity in mouse liver. Europ. J. Biochem. **31**, 266—276 (1972)

HERS, H.G., STALMANS, W., DE WULF, H., LALOUX, M., HUE, L.: Regulation of glycogen metabolism. In: Regulation of hepatic metabolism. Alfred Benzon Symposium VI. Copenhagen: Munksgaard p. 237—249 (1974)

HERS, H.G., DE WULF, H., STALMANS, W.: The control of glycogen metabolism in the liver. FEBS Letters **12**, 73—82 (1970)

HOUSE, P.D.R., POULIS, P., WEIDEMANN, M.J.: Isolation of a plasma-membrane subfraction from rat liver containing an insulin-sensitive cyclic AMP phosphodiesterase. Europ. J. Biochem. **24**, 429—437 (1972)

HUE, L., HERS, H.-G.: Utile and futile cycles in the liver. Biochem. biophys. Res. Commun. **58**, 540—548 (1974)

ILLIANO, G., CUATRECASAS, P.: Modulation of adenylate cyclase activity in liver and fat cell membranes by insulin. Science **175**, 906—908 (1972)

INGEBRETSEN, W.R., JR., MOXLEY, M.A., ALLEN, D.O., WAGLE, S.R.: Studies on gluconeogenesis, protein synthesis and cyclic AMP levels in isolated parenchymal cells following insulin withdrawal from alloxan diabetic rats. Biochem. biophys. Res. Commun. **49**, 601—607 (1972)

JEFFERSON, L.S., EXTON, J.H., SUTHERLAND, E.W., PARK, C.R.: Role of adenosine 3′,5′-monophosphate in the effects of insulin and anti-insulin serum on liver metabolism. J. biol. Chem. **243**, 1031—1038 (1968)

JERVELL, K.F., SEGLEN, P.O.: Tyrosine transaminase degradation in perfused liver after inhibition of protein synthesis by cycloheximide. Biochim. biophys. Acta (Amst.) **174**, 398—400 (1969)

JOHN, D.W., MILLER, L.L.: Influence of actinomycin D and puromycin on net synthesis of plasma albumin and fibrinogen by the isolated perfused rat liver. J. biol. Chem. **241**, 4817—4824 (1966)

John, D.W., Miller, L.L.: Regulation of net biosynthesis of serum albumin and acute phase plasma proteins. Induction of enhanced net synthesis of fibrinogen, α_2-acid glycoprotein, α_1(acute phase)-globulin, and haptoglobin by amino acids and hormones during perfusion of the isolated normal rat liver. J. biol. Chem. **244**, 6134—6142 (1969)

Johnson, M.E.M., Das, N.M., Butcher, F.R., Fain, J.N.: The regulation of gluconeogenesis in isolated rat liver cells by glucagon, insulin, dibutyryl cyclic adenosine monophosphate, and fatty acids. J. biol. Chem. **247**, 3229—3235 (1972)

Kernan, R.P.: Insulin and the membrane potential of frog sartorius muscle. Biochem. J. **80**, 23 (1961)

Kestens, P.J., Haxhe, J.J., Lambotte, L., Lambotte, C.: The effect of insulin on the uptake of potassium and phosphate by the isolated perfused canine liver. Metabolism **12**, 941—950 (1963)

Knox, W.E., Sharma, C.: Enzyme induction in perfused rat liver by glucagon and other agents. Enzym. biol. clin. **9**, 21—30 (1968)

Korner, A.: Alloxan diabetes and in vitro protein biosynthesis in rat liver microsomes and mitochondria. J. Endocr. **20**, 256—265 (1960a)

Krahl, M.E.: Insulin action at the molecular level, facts and speculations. Diabetes **21**, Suppl. 2, 695—702 (1972)

Lambotte, L.: La regulation du potassium hepatique. Collection "Medico-Monographes D'Agreges." Bruxelles: Editions Arscia S.A. 1968

Langan, T.A.: Phosphorylation of liver histone following the administration of glucagon and insulin. Proc. nat. Acad. Sci. (Wash.) **64**, 1276—1283 (1969)

Lardy, H.A., Zahlten, R., Stratman, F.W., Cook, D.E.: Regulation of gluconeogenesis by glucagon. In: Regulation of hepatic metabolism. Alfred Benzon Symposium VI, p. 19. Copenhagen: Munksgaard 1974

Leray, F., Chambaut, A.M., Perrenoud, M.L., Hanoune, I.: Adenylate-cyclase activity of rat liver plasma membranes. Hormonal stimulations and effect of adrenalectomy. Europ. J. Biochem. **38**, 185—192 (1973)

Levitan, I.B., Webb, T.E.: Regulation of tyrosine transaminase in the isolated perfused rat liver. J. biol. Chem. **244**, 4684—4688 (1969)

Lewis, S.B., Exton, J.H., Ho, R.I., Park, C.R.: Dose responses of glucagon (2×10^{-12} to 1×10^{-6} M) in the perfused rat liver. Fed. Proc. **29**, 379 Abs. (1970)

Lewis, S.B., Exton, I.H., Ho, R.I., Park, C.R.: Interactions of insulin, glucagon, epinephrine and cyclic AMP in the perfused rat liver. Fed. Proc. **30**, 1205 Abs. (1971)

Loten, E.G., Assimacopoulos-Jeannet, F., Le Marchand, Y., Singh, A., Jeanrenaud, B.: Regulation of carbohydrate and lipid metabolism in the liver and adipose tissue of normal and diabetic mice. Advanc. Enzyme Reg. **12**, 45—71 (1974)

Loten, E.G., Sneyd, I.G.T.: An effect of insulin on adipose tissue 3',5'-cyclic adenosine monophosphate phosphodiesterase. Biochem. J. **120**, 187—193 (1970)

Luly, P., Barnabei, O., Tria, E.: Hormonal control in vitro of plasma membrane-bound (Na^+-Na^+)-ATPase of rat liver. Biochim. biophys. Acta (Amst.) **282**, 447—452 (1972)

Mackrell, D.I., Sokal, J.E.: Antagonism between the effects of insulin and glucagon on the isolated liver. Diabetes **18**, 724—732 (1969)

Mallette, L.E., Exton, J.H.: Stimulation by insulin and glucagon of ornithine decarboxylase activity in perfused rat livers. Endocrinology **93**, 640—644 (1973)

Mallette, L.E., Exton, J.H., Park, C.R.: Effects of glucagon on amino acid transport and utilization in the isolated perfused rat liver. J. biol. Chem. **244**, 5724—5728 (1969)

Mallette, L.E., Neblett, M., Exton, J.H., Langan, T.A.: Phosphorylation of lysine-rich histone in the isolated perfused rat liver. Effects of glucagon, cyclic adenosine 3',5'-monophosphate, and insulin. J. biol. Chem. **248**, 6289—6291 (1973)

Mäenpää, P.H., Raivio, K.O., Kekomäki, M.P.: Liver adenine nucleotides: Fructose-induced depletion and its effect on protein synthesis. Science **161**, 1253—1254 (1968)

McCraw, E.F., Peterson, U.J., Yarnell, G., Ashmore, J.: Autoregulation of glucose in the isolated perfused rat liver. Advanc. Enzyme Reg. **6**, 57—65 (1968)

Menahan, L.A, Hepp, K.D., Wieland, O.: Liver 3':5'-nucleotide phosphodiesterase and its activity in rat liver perfused with insulin. Europ. J. Biochem. **8**, 435—443 (1969)

Menahan, L.A., Ross, B.D., Wieland, O.: Studies on the mechanism of fatty acid and glucagon stimulated gluconeogenesis in the perfused rat liver. In: Stoffwechsel der isoliert perfundierten Leber. Berlin-Heidelberg-New York: Springer 1968

Menahan, L.A., Wieland, O.: Glucagon-like action of N^6,2'-O-dibutyryl cyclic 3',5'-AMP on perfused rat liver. Biochem. biophys. Res. Commun. **29**, 880—885 (1967)

Menahan, L.A., Wieland, O.: Interactions of glucagon and insulin on the metabolism of perfused livers from fasted rats. Europ. J. Biochem. **9**, 55—62 (1969)

Miller, L.L.: Glucagon: A protein catabolic hormone in the isolated perfused rat liver. Nature (Lond.) **185**, 248 (1960)

MILLER, L.L., BURKE, W.T., HAFT, D.E.: In: Some Aspects of Amino Acid Supplementation. New Brunswick, New Jersey: Rutgers University Press 1956

MILLER, L.L., GRIFFIN, E.E.: Direct effects of insulin on amino acid and protein metabolism in the isolated perfused rat liver: Insulin, the hormone essential for positive nitrogen balance. In: Action of Insulin, Chapter 19. New York-London: Academic Press 1972

MILLER, T.B., JR., HAZEN, R., LARNER, J.: An absolute requirement for insulin in the control of hepatic gluconeogenesis by glucose. Biochem. biophys. Res. Commun. **53**, 466—474 (1973)

MORTIMORE, G.E.: Effect of insulin on potassium transfer in isolated rat liver. Amer. J. Physiol. **200**, 1315—1319 (1961)

MORTIMORE, G.E.: Effect of insulin on release of glucose and urea by isolated perfused rat liver. Amer. J. Physiol. **204**, 699—704 (1963)

MORTIMORE, G.E., MONDON, C.E.: Inhibition by insulin of valine turnover in liver. Evidence for a general control of proteolysis. J. biol. Chem. **245**, 2375—2383 (1970)

PARK, C.R., LEWIS, S.B., EXTON, J.H.: Relationship of some hepatic actions of insulin to the intracellular level of cyclic adenylate. Diabetes **21**, Suppl. 2, 439—446 (1972)

PATZELT, C., LÖFFLER, G., WIELAND, O.: Interconversion of pyruvate dehydrogenase in the isolated perfused rat liver. Europ. J. Biochem. **33**, 117—122 (1973)

PENHOS, J.C., WU, C.H., LEMBERG, A., DAUNAS, J., BRODOFF, B., SODERO, A., LEVINE, R.: The effect of insulin on the metabolism of lipids and on urea formation by the perfused rat liver. Metabolism **17**, 246—259 (1968)

POHL, S.L., BIRNBAUMER, L., RODBELL, M.: The glucagon-sensitive adenyl cyclase system in plasma membranes of rat liver. I. Properties. J. biol. Chem. **246**, 1849—1856 (1971)

POLEDNE, R., MAYES, P.A.: Lipolysis and the regulation of fatty acid metabolism in the liver. Biochem. J. **119**, 47P (1970)

RAIVIO, J., KEKOMÄKI, M.P., MÄENPÄÄ, P.H.: Depletion of liver adenine nucleotides induced by D-fructose. Biochem. Pharmacol. **18**, 2615—2624 (1969)

REEL, J.R., LEE, K.L., KENNEY, F.T.: Regulation of tyrosine-α-ketoglutarate transaminase in rat liver. VIII. Induction by hydrocortisone and insulin in cultured hepatoma cells. J. biol. Chem. **245**, 5800—5805 (1970)

ROBINSON, W.S.: Alloxan diabetes and insulin effects on the amino acid incorporation activity of rat liver microsomes. Proc. Soc. exp. Biol. (N.Y.) **106**, 115—118 (1961)

ROSS, B.D., HEMS, R., FREEDLAND, R.A., KREBS, H.A.: Carbohydrate metabolism of the perfused rat liver. Biochem. J. **105**, 869—875 (1969)

RUDORFF, K.H., HUCHTERMEYER, H., WINDECK, R., STAIB, W.: Über den Einfluß von Insulin auf die Alaningluconeogenese in der isoliert perfundierten Leber von New Zealand obese mice. Europ. J. Biochem. **16**, 481—486 (1970a)

RUDORFF, K.H., WINDECK, R., STAIB, W.: Effect of proinsulin on the metabolism of alanine in isolated perfused rat livers. In: Regulation of gluconeogenesis. New York: Academic Press 1970b

SEGLEN, P.O.: Regulation of tyrosine transaminase degradation in the isolated perfused rat liver by cycloheximide and insulin. Biochim. biophys. Acta (Amst.) **230**, 319—326 (1971)

SELAWRY, H., GUTMAN, R., FINK, G., RECANT, L.: The effect of starvation of tissue adenosine 3′-5′-monophosphate levels. Biochem. biophys. Res. Commun. **51**, 198—204 (1973)

SENFT, G., SCHULTZ, G., MUNSKE, K., HOFFMANN, M.: Influence of insulin on cyclic 3′,5′-AMP phosphodiesterase activity in liver, skeletal muscle, adipose tissue, and kidney. Diabetologia **4**, 322—329 (1968)

SEUFERT, C.D., GRAF, M., JANSON, G., KUHN, A., SÖLING, H.D.: Formation of free acetate by isolated perfused livers from normal, starved and diabetic rats. Biochem. biophys. Res. Commun. **57**, 901—909 (1974)

SÖLING, H.D., BERNHARD, G.: Interconversion of inactive to active pyruvate dehydrogenase in rat liver after fructose application in vivo. FEBS Letters **13**, 201—203 (1971)

SÖLING, H.D., GRAF, M., SEUFERT, C.D.: On the regulation of incomplete oxidation of fatty acids by livers from normal, starved and diabetic rats. Alfred Benzon Symp., VL, 1973. p. 695. Copenhagen: Munksgaard 1974

SÖLING, H.D., KAPLAN, J., ERBSTOESZER, M., PITOT, H.C.: The role of hormones in glucose repression in rat liver. Advanc. Enzyme Reg. **7**, 171—182 (1968a)

SÖLING, H.D., KATTERMANN, R., SCHMIDT, H.: The relationship between the cytoplasmic redox-state and ketogenesis in the liver cell, and the problem of triosephosphate block in diabetes mellitus. Excerpta med. (Amst.) (Intern. Congr. Ser.) **74**, 55 Abs. (1964)

SÖLING, H.D., KLEINEKE, J., WILLMS, B., JANSON, G., KUHN, A.: Relationship between intracellular distribution of phosphoenolpyruvate carboxykinase, regulation of gluconeogenesis and energy cost of glucose formation. Europ. J. Biochem. **37**, 233—243 (1973)

Söling, H.D., Kneer, P., Drägert, W., Creutzfeldt, W.: Die Wirkung von Insulin auf den Stoffwechsel der isolierten perfundierten Leber normaler und alloxandiabetischer Ratten. II. Stoffwechseländerungen unter dem Einfluß intraportaler Insulininfusionen. Diabetologia **2**, 32—44 (1966a)

Söling, H.D., Koschel, R., Drägert, W., Kneer, P., Creutzfeldt, W.: Die Wirkung von Insulin auf den Stoffwechsel der isolierten perfundierten Leber normaler und alloxandiabetischer Ratten. I. Stoffwechsel isoliert perfundierter Leber von normalen und alloxandiabetischen Ratten unter verschiedenen experimentellen Bedingungen. Diabetologia **2**, 20—31 (1966b)

Söling, H.D., Willms, B., Friedrichs, D., Kleineke, J.: Regulation of gluconeogenesis by fatty acid oxidation in isolated perfused livers of starved and non-starved rats. Europ. J. Biochem. **4**, 364—372 (1968b)

Söling, H.D., Willms, B., Kleineke, J., Gehlhoff, M.: Regulation of gluconeogenesis in guinea pig liver. Europ. J. Biochem. **16**, 289—302 (1970)

Sokal, J.E.: Effect of glucagon on gluconeogenesis by the isolated perfused rat liver. Endocrinology **78**, 538—548 (1966)

Sokal, J.E., Sarcione, E.J., Henderson, A.M.: Relative potency of glucagon and epinephrine as hepatic glycogenolytic agents. Studies with the isolated perfused rat liver. Endocrinology **74**, 930—938 (1964)

Soskin, S., Essex, H.E., Herrick, J.F., Mann, F.C.: The mechanism of regulation of the blood sugar by the liver. Amer. J. Physiol. **124**, 558—567 (1938)

Struck, E., Ashmore, J., Wieland, O.: Stimulierung der Gluconeogenese durch langkettige Fettsäuren und Glucagon. Biochem. Z. **343**, 107—110 (1965)

Struck, E., Ashmore, J., Wieland, O.: Effects of glucagon and long chain fatty acids on glucose production by isolated perfused rat liver. Advanc. Enzyme Reg. **4**, 219—224 (1966)

Tolbert, M.E.M., Butcher, F.R., Fain, J.N.: Lack of correlation between catecholamine effects on cyclic adenosine 3′:5′-monophosphate and gluconeogenesis in isolated rat liver cells. J. biol. Chem. **248**, 5686—5692 (1973)

Topping, D.L., Mayes, P.A.: The immediate effects of insulin and fructose on the metabolism of the perfused liver. Biochem. J. **126**, 296—311 (1972)

Wagle, S.R., Ingebretsen, W.R., Jr., Sampson, L.: Studies on the in vitro effects of insulin on glycogen synthesis and ultrastructure in isolated rat liver hepatocytes. Biochem. biophys. Res. Commun. **53**, 937—943 (1973)

Wieland, O., Patzelt, C., Löffler, G.: Active and inactive forms of pyruvate dehydrogenase in rat liver. Effect of starvation and refeeding and of insulin treatment on pyruvate-dehydrogenase interconversion. Europ. J. Biochem. **26**, 426—433 (1972)

Williams, T.F., Exton, J.H., Friedmann, N., Park, C.R.: Effects of insulin and adenosine 3′5′-monophosphate on K^+flux and glucose output in the perfused rat liver. Amer. J. Physiol. **221**, 1645—1651 (1971)

Williamson, J.R.: Effects of fatty acids, glucagon and anti-insulin serum on the control of gluconeogenesis and ketogenesis in rat liver. Advanc. Enzyme Reg. **5**, 229—255 (1967)

Williamson, J.R., Browning, E.T., Scholz, R.: Control mechanisms of gluconeogenesis and ketogenesis. I. Effects of oleate on gluconeogenesis in perfused rat liver. J. biol. Chem. **244**, 4607—4616 (1969a)

Williamson, J.R., Browning, E.T., Thurman, R.G., Scholz, R.: Inhibition of glucagon effects in perfused rat liver by (+)-decanoyl carnitine. J. biol. Chem. **244**, 5055—5064 (1969b)

Williamson, J.R., Kreisberg, R.A., Felts, W.P.: Mechanism for the stimulation of gluconeogenesis by fatty acids in perfused rat liver. Proc. nat. Acad. Sci. (Wash.) **56**, 247—254 (1966)

Wool, I.G., Cavicchi, P.: Protein synthesis by skeletal muscle ribosomes. Effects of diabetes and insulin. Biochemistry (Wash.) **6**, 1231—1242 (1967)

Zahlten, R., Stratman, F.W., Lardy, H.A.: Regulation of glucose synthesis in hormone-sensitive isolated rat hepatocytes. Proc. nat. Acad. Sci. (Wash.) **70**, 3213—3218 (1973)

Zierler, K.L.: Hyperpolarization of muscle by insulin in a glucose-free environment. Amer. J. Physiol. **197**, 524—526 (1959)

G. Action of Insulin on Some Other Organs and on Differentiation

Franz v. Bruchhausen

With 1 Figure

I. Action on Stomach Function and Exocrine Pancreas

1. Action on Stomach Function

The literature on this topic up to 1952 was comprehensively reviewed by Bachrach. A recent review has been presented by Groza (1972).

The first observations on the influence of insulin (at that time as noncrystalline preparations) on gastric secretion go back to Detre and Sivo (1925). In these early studies many contradictory findings were made concerning gastric secretion in respect of the hypoglycemia concomitantly induced by high doses of noncrystalline insulin preparations and the directly or indirectly altered vagal tonus (for literature, see Boldyreff and Stewart, 1932). Later it became necessary to differentiate between hypoglycemia-induced effects and other effects of insulin on gastric secretion, for example, direct effects on gastric mucosa and side-effects of concomitant hypokalemia.

a) Stimulation of Gastric Secretion by Insulin Hypoglycemia (Fig. 1)

The hypoglycemic basis of the increased gastric secretion stimulated by parenteral administration of insulin has long been suggested. Surprisingly, goats do not respond in this manner (Hill, 1952) and chickens show only inhibitory effects (Long, 1967; Ruoff and Sewing, 1972; Burhol, 1973). In man, the inverse

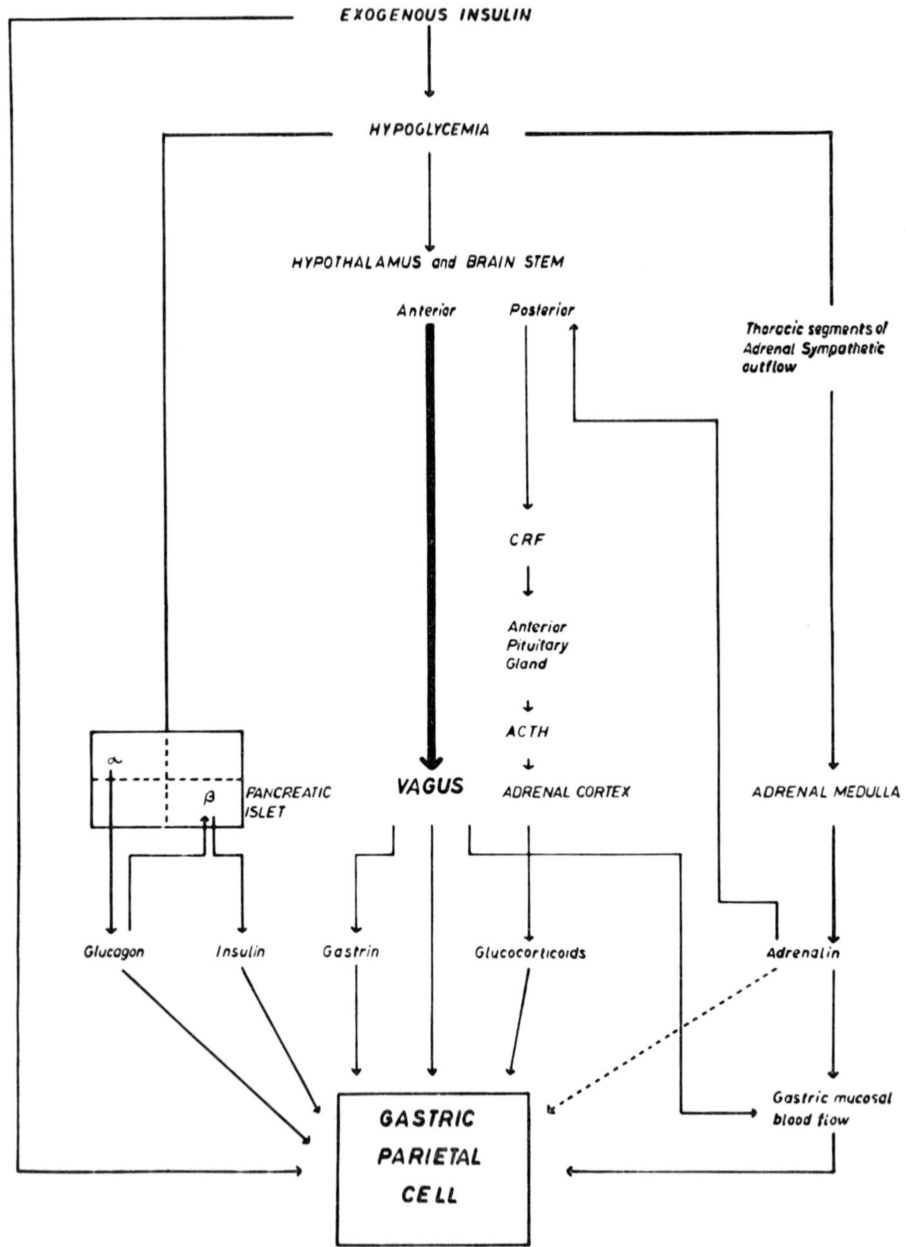

Fig. 1. Scheme showing possible influence of insulin and insulin hypoglycemia on the gastric parietal cell. (After Hodge, Masarei and Catchpole, 1972, with modifications)

relationship of the gastric secretion curve and the blood sugar curve was noted early (MEYER, 1930). Administration of glucose was found to suppress (LABARRE and CESPEDES, 1931) or delay (HELLER, 1931) gastric secretion in animals and man, but once gastric secretion is induced, glucose injection has little influence (HELLER, 1931). It is generally accepted that, for stimulation by insulin injection, the glucose concentration in blood must be below a critical value (KEMP *et al.*, 1968a) of about 50 mg% (ROHOLM, 1930; JEMERIN *et al.*, 1943; DAVIS *et al.*, 1965; DEMAND *et al.*, 1968), or 40 mg% if glucose oxidase methods are used (LANGER, 1972). An insulin dose of about 0.2 U/kg is therefore necessary. The same is true for alloxan-diabetic dogs, as carefully studied by SUGAWARA *et al.* (1971). The "all-or-none" nature of the effect is now being questioned. Optimal insulin doses have been found for the rat (LEE and THOMPSON, 1967) and dose-response relationships exist for the dog (HIRSCHOWITZ and O'LEARY, 1964; COOKE, 1969; SPENCER and GROSSMAN, 1971a), for cats (STENING and ISENBERG, 1969) and for man (BARON, 1970a). Thus peak acid output above a critical value correlates to some extent with the lowest concentrations of blood glucose reached by insulin; hypoglycemia below 15 mg% inhibits insulin-stimulated acid secretion in man. (For further data, see ISENBERG *et al.*, 1969a, b; JONES *et al.*, 1970; BARON *et al.*, 1972; COWLEY and BARON, 1972, 1973).

Two phases of gastric secretion after insulin have been observed. In the early phase (1—2 h) a fall in blood sugar is immediately followed by an increase in acid-rich juice (DAVIS and BROOKS, 1962). This reaction resembles stimulation of the anterior hypothalamus and is blocked by vagotomy (FRENCH *et al.*, 1953; PORTER *et al.*, 1953). Simultaneous recording of blood sugar and gastric secretion in beagles with gastric fistulas showed (DAVIS and BROOKS, 1963) that the gastric response follows the blood sugar with some delay and sometimes lasts longer. The late response resembling stimulation of the posterior hypothalamus (FRENCH *et al.*, 1953; PORTER *et al.*, 1953) has been described, but seems not to be a consistent finding (DAVIS and BROOKS, 1963). That corticosteroids or catecholamines somehow intervene in this case (SUN and SHAY, 1960; FRENCH *et al.*, 1953; MATUOKA *et al.*, 1966) has been questioned (DAVIS and BROOKS, 1963; DAVIS, BROOKS and ROBERT, 1965). In man these early and late responses to hypoglycemia are less clearcut, probably because the basal acid production is not as low as in the beagle (SUN and SHAY, 1960). A critical review on the problem of delayed-phase gastric secretion has appeared (BACHRACH, 1963). The inconstant occurrence of this phase could be attributed to the effect of special parasympathetic excitatory fibers.

Generally, one can assume that within limits the output of hydrochloric acid is paralleled by pepsin output. Thus, the stimulation of pepsin secretion by gastrin or pentagastrin in man is now well established (MAKHLOUF *et al.*, 1966; WORMSLEY *et al.*, 1966; DEMAND *et al.*, 1968; MAKHLOUF *et al.*, 1968; JEPSON *et al.*, 1968; AUBREY and FORREST, 1970; LIMBOSCH *et al.*, 1971). The same holds true for insulin-stimulated secretion (TEPPERMAN *et al.*, 1972). For an earlier review, see HIRSCHOWITZ (1967). The excess responsiveness of pepsin to stimulants like insulin, induced in normal subjects by gastrin (pentagastrin) infusion can, however, be greater than that of acid. This effect is absent in vagotomized patients (LIMBOSCH *et al.*, 1971). In the dog the same enhancement by insulin of pepsin secretion has been found in comparison to pentagastrin (CHARBION, 1972). In patients with gastric resections increased pepsin and mucoprotein secretion can persist even in the absence of acid secretion (GLASS and WOLF, 1950). In man (GLASS and BOYD, 1950) and dog (MENGUY and THOMPSON, 1967; WISE and BALLINGER, 1971) mucous secretion is increased by insulin hypoglycemia. Vagotomy prevents this effect. As with pentagastrin, the output and concentration of intrinsic factor (Castle factor) can be elicited by insulin hypoglycemia (ARDEMAN *et al.*, 1964; LANGER *et al.*, 1972).

As to other components of gastric juice during stimulation by insulin, the secretion is rich in sodium and chloride and poor in potassium (LEE and THOMPSON, 1967; DEMAND *et al.*, 1968) with a close correlation between sodium and H^+ concentrations (LEE and THOMPSON, 1968).

Acute administration of high doses of insulin at frequent intervals induced hemorrhagic erosions and ulcerations in the stomach of cats (HANKE, 1934) and rats (KIM and SHORE, 1963). As with reserpine, these lesions are correlated with a high gastric acid output and a 30% decrease in the histamine content of gastric tissue. In contrast to reserpine, insulin-induced secretion and lesions could be prevented by vagotomy. On the other hand only changes due to reserpine were impeded by monoamine oxidase inhibitors (KIM and SHORE, 1963). The insulin-induced lesions can therefore be interpreted as due to the combined action of gastric acid and neural effects on the stomach. Thus, epithelial alterations precede alterations in secretory cells and are necrotic in character. Sometimes a typical peptic ulceration is produced (HANKE, 1934).

The induction of secretory effects by hypoglycemia is generally ascribed to intracellular absence of metabolizable glucose in the brain (HIRSCHOWITZ and SACHS, 1965; COLIN-JONES and HIMSWORTH, 1969) or locally in the stomach (SPENCER and GROSSMAN, 1971b). The similarity of action of 2-desoxy-D-glucose (2-DG) (DUKE *et al.*, 1965; HIRSCHOWITZ and SACHS, 1965; MIGNON *et al.*, 1972) and 3-O-methylglucose (COLIN-JONES and HIMSWORTH, 1969) underscores this statement. For further literature on 2-DG in this respect, see ISENBERG (1972).

KERR and PRESHAW (1969) consider that direct stimulation of the dorsal nuclei of the vagus is elicited by hypoglycemia in the cat, and application of pressure near the vagus nuclei produces gastric secretion (NORTON *et al.*, 1972), yet a hypothalamic localization has generally been favored. KADEKARO *et al.* (1972), using the technique of surgical or coagulative lesions in cats, implicated the intrafascicular neurons of the medial forebrain bundle coming from the hypothalamus. This corresponds with findings in rats in which lateral hypothalamic regions are linked to secretory function (COLIN-JONES and HIMSWORTH, 1970). These authors used topical stimulation by 2-DG. The importance of the more ventrolateral nuclei of the hypothalamus for secretion has been stressed by RIDLEY and BROOKS (1965) as well as by MISHER and BROOKS (1966) for the rat. A more direct demonstration of hypothalamic participation in insulin hypoglycemia in the dog came from JÖGI *et al.* (1949) and DAVIS *et al.* (1968). Lesions of the lateral anterior hypothalamic nuclei presumably interrupt connections with feeding centers and with the vagal nuclei of the brainstem. Electrical stimulation of the posterior hypothalamic nucleus in rats elicits gastric secretion in cases in which pronounced hypoglycemia develops (MORRISEY and STEPHENS, 1972). With respect to increased food intake caused by insulin hypoglycemia, destruction of the same hypothalamic area prevents it (EPSTEIN and TEITELBAUM, 1967). For more on cerebral localization of gastric secretion regulation, see BROOKS (1967).

The participation of specific transmitters has to be elucidated. BUGAJSKI and HANO (1972) have found that in cats simultaneous doses of 5 mg/kg 5-hydroxytryptamine prevent the insulin-induced increase in gastric secretion, though hypoglycemia and hypokalemia are unaltered.

There is no doubt that the effects of gastric acid secretion in the peripheral nerves are propagated over the vagus nerve. The centrally induced effects of insulin and also of 2-DG (FEINBLATT and GELFAND, 1966) are abolished by vagotomy, xylocaine block of exteriorized vagi (BREMER and DUBOIS, 1963), or application of atropine sulfate. Consequently, pentobarbital depresses the gastric secretion produced by insulin more strongly than that caused by histamine (POWELL and HIRSCHOWITZ, 1967). A practical application of these findings has been to substitute for the formerly proposed (MEYER, 1930) histamine test an insulin test (Hollander test) in order to check the adequacy of vagotomy (HOLLANDER, 1948). There is much literature about this test and its success (for review, see BARON, 1970b; for criteria, see HOLLANDER, 1946; WADDELL, 1957; BACHRACH, 1962; STEMPIEN, 1962; ROSS and KAY, 1964; BANK *et al.*, 1967; SPENCER *et al.*, 1969; GILLESPIE *et al.*, 1972; GROSSMAN, 1972; for the influence of the diabetic state, see LANGER, 1972; for the influence of β-sympathetic blockade, see READ *et al.*, 1972). A less dangerous application by infusion has been proposed by CARTER *et al.* (1972) and DOZOIS *et al.* (1972). LIMBOSCH *et al.* (1971) considered the pepsin response more sensitive than that of hydrochloric acid for testing the completeness of vagotomy. Unilateral vagotomy seems to reduce the insulin response to acid secretion, at least in dogs and cats (STENING and ISENBERG, 1969). Because of the crossing of some vagal fibers, division of the thoracic rather than the cervical vagus provokes a more pronounced restraint (STENING and GROSSMAN, 1970). Basal acid secretion seems not to be under vagal control (MOORE, 1973).

Three major mechanisms are proposed by which vagal stimulation could influence gastric secretion (NYHUS *et al.*, 1960; EMÅS, 1973): (1) direct stimulation of oxyntic cells, especially in man, first assumed by GLASS *et al.* (1950), GLASS and WOLFF (1950), VARRO *et al.* (1954) and especially by PEVSNER and GROSSMAN (1955), PASSARO and GROSSMAN (1964) and their sensitization to gastrin; (2) antral (hormonal) stimulation; (3) extragastric (hormonal) influences.

The mediation of vagal stimulation by histamine was once assumed, but has now been questioned. Never data indicate that gastrin has an important role in vagal stimulation (for reviews, see BACHRACH, 1963; UVNÄS, 1969; KORMAN *et al.*, 1971). The indirect function of gastrin in vagal stimulation was formerly suggested by UVNÄS (1942), LIM and MOZER (1951), BURSTALL and SCHOFIELD (1953), VARRO *et al.* (1954), WOODWARD *et al.* (1957), OBERHELMAN *et al.* (1957), PE THEIN and SCHOFIELD (1960, 1962), NYHUS *et al.* (1960), and OLBE (1964). Parallel with insulin-induced gastric secretion, the biologically determined gastrin content of canine mucosa increases and then decreases (GROZA *et al.*, 1971). This humoral mediation of gastrin is often overshadowed by the strict inhibitory influences of hydrochloric acid (PE THEIN and SCHOFIELD, 1960; ANDERSSON, 1960).

Another finding that favors gastrin mediation is that under maximal stimulation of acid secretion by pentagastrin infusion in man, no further increases in acid response were seen (HALTER *et al.*, 1970; LIMBOSCH *et al.*, 1971), whereas with histamine a further response is sometimes seen (CHECKETTS *et al.*, 1968). In dogs, dose-response studies show that there is no potentiation or synergism between histamine and pentagastrin in secretion; this is in contrast to many earlier findings (HIRSCHOWITZ *et al.*, 1973).

Radioimmunoassay of gastrin under insulin-stimulated gastric secretion has shown an increase of gastrin in the plasma of dog (JAFFE *et al.*, 1970; TEPPERMAN *et al.*, 1972) and man (HANSKY and CAIN, 1969; GANGULI and ELDER, 1971; HANSKY *et al.*, 1971a, b; KORMAN *et al.*, 1971; STAGG *et al.*, 1971; STADIL, 1972). This corresponds well with the data on secretion and applies to several other stimulants, e.g. food (WYLLIE *et al.*, 1972; NILSSON *et al.*, 1972; TEPPERMAN *et al.*, 1972; BROUGH *et al.*, 1972) or electrical vagal stimulation (LANCIAULT *et al.*, 1971; LANCIAULT *et al.*, 1973a, 1973b). In some cases the values vary considerably (GANGULI and ELDER, 1971; STAGG *et al.*, 1971) with respect to insulin. After truncal vagotomy there is no increase in plasma gastrin levels (KORMAN *et al.*, 1972) or only slight elevation (JAFFE *et al.*, 1972). Resection of the antrum also prevents gastrin release in man (STADIL and REHFELD, 1972; MCGUIGAN and TRUDEAU, 1972). Furthermore antral acidification abolishes gastrin release in response to insulin in man (FEURLE *et al.*, 1973) and dogs (CSENDES *et al.*, 1972) though acid secretion is not reduced by more than 60% (CSENDES *et al.*, 1972). This vagal gastrin release does not mean that basal gastrin release is dependent on vagal influences alone (MOORE, 1973), since atropine leaves basal plasma gastrin levels unaltered (WALSH *et al.*, 1971; NILSSON *et al.*, 1972; TEPPERMAN *et al.*, 1972), but atropine itself prevents gastrin-induced gastric secretion in some animals (GREGORY and TRACY, 1961; BORG and EMÅS, 1970; JOHANSSON *et al.*, 1971). On the other hand, there is some evidence that the gastrin released in turn elicits contractions, for instance in intestine, by releasing acetylcholine (VIZI *et al.*, 1972, 1973).

The highest gastrin levels due to insulin hypoglycemia were obtained in patients with duodenal ulcer (HANSKY *et al.*, 1971a, b). Nevertheless, the maximal responses (about 30 min after administration) to pentagastrin and insulin differ in some way in man, particularly in ulcer patients (EMÅS and BORG, 1972). Thus, the gastrin mechanism does not explain the full secretion picture and a preoperative insulin test is hence of value (EMÅS and BORG, 1972).

Though gastrin (or pentagastrin) may be a trophic hormone of the upper gastrointestinal tract (WILLEMS *et al.*, 1972; MILLER *et al.*, 1973) the short-lasting gastrin release that can be induced by insulin does not seem to be sufficient. Insulin effects on histidine decarboxylase (KAHLSON *et al.*, 1967), ascribed to release of gastrin (JOHNSON *et al.*, 1969) are consequently lacking in antrectomized rats (AURES *et al.*, 1970; HAKANSON and LIEDBERG, 1970) or in acidified conditions where gastrin release is reduced (ROSENGREN and SVENSSON, 1969). The role of the enzyme is critically discussed by JOHNSON (1971).

Astonishingly enough, even after complete vagotomy (established by several criteria) a minor gastrin release persists after insulin injection (BYRNES and SCRATCHERD, 1972; STADIL, 1972). It therefore follows that hypoglycemia must be able to release gastrin other than by vagal stimulation alone. However, the lower response to insulin after vagotomy seems due primarily to reduction of the responsiveness of the oxyntic glands rather than to abolition of gastrin release. Observations of KEMP *et al.* (1968c) with a technique of combined antral denervation and fundic serosal incision revealed the importance of the vagally connected Meissner plexus for the function of the parietal cells. Moreover, the responsiveness towards pentagastrin infusion is greater in innervated than in denervated gastric pouch of the dog. This indicates that cholinergic factors play an important role in the response of the parietal cells to this agent (BROOKS *et al.*, 1971).

Today it is generally accepted that increasing the tone of the smooth muscle of the stomach is an integral part of the action of physiologic (ABBOTT and ROSSI, 1965) and other hormonal gastric stimulants. Known inhibitors of gastric secretion likewise relax gastric muscles. Only xanthines and related compounds combine increased secretory effects with decreased motor activity (see below). Thus an increase in gastric motor activity (rate, amplitude, tonus) due to insulin hypoglycemia was very early observed (BULATAO and CARLSON, 1924) and later confirmed (see BACHRACH, 1953; LORBER and SHAY, 1962). Interaction with the vagus was assumed because the excitomotoric effects of insulin were inhibited by atropine (QUIGLEY *et al.*, 1929) or bilateral vagotomy (QUIGLEY and TEMPLETON, 1930b). As expected, they were not seen in the (denervated) Heidenhain pouch of the dog (TEMPLETON and QUIGLEY, 1930). In the canine Heidenhain pouch, unlike the stomach, an inhibitory, hypoglycemia-related action of insulin was observed (LORBER, 1961; LORBER and SHAY, 1962; KEMP *et al.*, 1968c). Naturally, the actual motor activity depends on the algebraic summation of augmentative impulses over the vagi and inhibitory impulses over the sympathetic fibers. In the dog, stimulation of gastric motility by insulin differs considerably from that of feeding in that it has a lag phase (NELSON *et al.*, 1966). Maximal effects of insulin on blood glucose and stimulation of acid secretion and motility, however, develop at the same time, as shown by SUGAWARA *et al.* (1971). This parallel behavior is also seen in alloxan-diabetic dogs, in which maximal effects are reached later (SUGAWARA *et al.*, 1971). The reversal of insulin effects by infusion of glucose has been described (LORBER and SHAY, 1962).

A purely humoral interpretation, i.e. that gastrin release induces esophageal motility (or pressure), was proposed by CASTELL (1971). In favor of this hypothesis are the above-mentioned findings of STADIL (1972) that gastrin is released in completely vagotomized patients. Castell's hypothesis, however, is questioned by GROSSMAN (1971) and HANSKY *et al.* (1972). One explanation may be that, in contrast to normal and incompletely vagotomized patients, who respond to insulin hypoglycemia with release of gastrin into serum, completely vagotomized patients have a high basal level of serum gastrin and this is not altered by insulin hypoglycemia (HANSKY *et al.*, 1972), but is changed by local stimulation due to a protein meal (KORMAN *et al.*, 1972). Ten times higher concentrations of pentagastrin are needed for electrical activity and motor activity than for H^+ secretion in man (KWONG *et al.*, 1971). As regards gastric emptying, no parallelism to antral motility under pentagastrin infusion has been found in the dog (COOKE *et al.*, 1972).

b) Inhibitory Actions of Insulin

Inhibitory actions of insulin on gastric secretion and gastric motility have been observed in both dog (COLLAZO and DOBREFF, 1924; TEMPLETON and QUIGLEY, 1930; NECHELES *et al.*, 1941; DAVIS and BROOKS, 1962; EISENBERG *et al.*, 1963; JORDAN and QUINTANA, 1964; HIRSCHOWITZ, 1966; HIRSCHOWITZ and ROBBINS, 1966; TSUKAMOTO *et al.*, 1967) and man (MAHLER, 1930; ROBERTSON *et al.*, 1950a; OLSON and NECHELES, 1953, 1955; SCHAPIRO *et al.*, 1967; DEMAND *et al.*, 1968; LIMBOSCH *et al.*, 1971). In the cat no inhibitory action is found (SPENCER and GROSSMAN, 1971b). In man the effect is detected only under special conditions, especially after infusion of stimulants (pentagastrin) and/or vagotomy. In dogs, too, inhibitory effects of glucagon-free insulin are far more pronounced in denervated pouches (JORDAN and QUINTANA, 1964). The role of hypoglycemia is still controversial. Clearcut prevention of inhibition during (indirect) gastrin stimulation by glucose infusion was seen by JORDAN and QUINTANA (1964), as earlier suggested by KARVINEN and KARVONEN (1953) or NECHELES *et al.* (1940). BARON (1970a) noted the inhibitory action of very strong hypoglycemia. He assumed anoxia in the parietal cells to be the cause. The parallelism of inhibition to the fall in blood sugar is backed by the similar effects of tolbutamide (WEISS and SCIALES, 1961).

The inhibitory effect of insulin, at least in part, is independent of hypoglycemia (EISENBERG *et al.*, 1963; HIRSCHOWITZ and ROBBINS, 1966) because neither glucose nor glucagon completely reverses the inhibitory effect (HIRSCHOWITZ and SACHS, 1966); doses higher than those required to produce hypoglycemia are necessary (HIRSCHOWITZ, 1966a). It has nothing to do with the inhibitory effects of large doses of gastrin injected into dogs (MASTER *et al.*, 1969), because the corresponding concentrations are unlikely to be reached, and application of glucagon-free insulin during gastrin infusion reduces gastrin-induced acid secretion (JORDAN and QUIN-

TANA, 1964). It is also independent of sympathetic discharge, as revealed by FORREST and CODE (1954a, b) and GEZIRI *et al.* (1958), although catecholamines (especially epinephrine) often become elevated in blood (see BACHRACH, 1963); this type has been ascribed to glucagon impurities (see BACHRACH, 1963; GROZA, 1972). On the other hand, the inhibitory action of insulin was prevented by injection or infusion of potassium salts with respect to secretory function (HIRSCHOWITZ and SACHS, 1966; KEMP *et al.*, 1968) in the main stomach, but not in the Heidenhain pouch of the dog (SPENCER and GROSSMAN, 1971b) and not with respect to motor responses (KEMP *et al.*, 1968b). In this latter case reversal has been obtained by glucose infusion (KEMP *et al.*, 1968).

In chickens, which do not respond with gastric secretion to insulin hypoglycemia or 2-desoxy-D-glucose, the inhibitory action of insulin (LONG, 1967) is more pronounced than that of 2-DG (RUOFF and SEWING, 1972). This corresponds to the findings of SPENCER and GROSSMAN (1970) in dogs. Somewhat higher doses of 2-DG may stimulate gastric secretion in chickens (BURHOL, 1973).

Inhibitory effects of insulin on gastric motility have likewise been described (QUIGLEY and TEMPLETON, 1930a; NECHELES *et al.*, 1940; OBERHELMAN *et al.*, 1957; NELSON *et al.*, 1966; TSUKAMOTO *et al.*, 1967; SUGAWARA *et al.*, 1971) as preceding stimulatory effects. In the review by BACHRACH (1953) the inhibitory effect on gastric motility was interpreted as complex: direct action on gastric musculature, influence of epinephrin, and stimulation of vagal inhibitory fibers. Newer data in the past two decades have not resolved the problem. Since 2-DG depresses gastric motility (TSUKAMOTO *et al.*, 1967) and secretion (EISENBERG *et al.*, 1966) only slightly, vagal participation must be limited. As mentioned, the effects of insulin on motility are not blocked by infusion of potassium ions, in contrast to inhibition of secretion (HERRERA *et al.*, 1967) and it has been suggested "that insulin inhibits secretion and motility by a different mechanism, or that these two inhibitory effects of insulin have different sensitivities to the protective effect of potassium ions" (SINGLETON, 1969).

It is now well accepted that during insulin hypoglycemia there is a sustained decrease in serum potassium (QUIGLEY and TEMPLETON, 1930a; NECHELES *et al.*, 1941; OBERHELMAN *et al.*, 1957; NELSON *et al.*, 1966; TSUKAMOTO *et al.*, 1967; SUGAWARA *et al.*, 1971). This is generally correlated in the conscious dog with inhibitory effects on the water and acid content of gastric juice (HIRSCHOWITZ and SACHS, 1972). These studies were undertaken because it had been found that application of K^+ counteracted the inhibitory effects of insulin (HIRSCHOWITZ and SACHS, 1966). K^+ can be replaced by Rb^+ in reversing the inhibitory action of insulin on gastric secretion (HIRSCHOWITZ and SACHS, 1967). With frog mucosa, the removal of potassium ions almost completely stops H^+ secretion (DAVIS *et al.*, 1965).

c) Direct Mucosal Stimulation of Acid Secretion

That insulin has an inhibitory action on intestine and stomach *in vitro* has been questioned and attributed to impurities. Nevertheless, several lines of evidence make it probable that either insulin itself or insulin hypoglycemia acts directly on the stomach. As pointed out by PEVSNER and GROSSMAN (1955), the experimental infusion of acetylcholine into the regional gastric arteries evoked an effect on oxyntic cells. Under conditions of pouch denervation in the dog, some stimulation of acid and pepsin secretion by insulin hypoglycemia takes place without any increase in gastrin secretion (TEPPERMAN *et al.*, 1972). The same holds true for sham feeding (PRESHAW, 1970; TEPPERMAN *et al.*, 1972). When meat extract is compared with insulin as a stimulant of gastrin release in man, meat extract evokes the same peak as gastrin in serum, but its stimulatory response on gastric secretion is less. This means that insulin has a further direct component (WYLLIE *et al.*, 1972). A similar conclusion was reached by OLBE (1964) using resection techniques. The above-mentioned measurement of gastrin release by STADIL (1972) in the case of vagotomy allows the same interpretation of the direct influence of insulin hypoglycemia on the parietal glands. On the other hand, GROZA and DINA-CORNEANU (1971) suggested that insulin, by stimulating glucose utilization, could supply the substrate energy for the secretion of hydrogen ions into the gastric juice. No data are given, however, to support this hypothesis. For 2-DG the inhibition of gastric secretion in frog mucosa has been attributed to a direct mechanism (SACHS *et al.*, 1965). Special local cholinergic receptors were described by DOSS and VAN ZWIETEN (1972).

d) Participation of Intracellular Mediation in Oxyntic Cells

The direct or indirect (by vagus or gastrin release) action of insulin on gastric secretion should be discussed briefly in the light of humoral mediation within the oxyntic cell. At the present time many aspects seem to be controversial.

The view that gastric secretion might be mediated generally by endogenous cyclic adenosine 3′,5′-monophosphate (cAMP) (LEVINE, 1970; MERTZ, 1969; SCRATCHERD and CASE, 1969; MERTZ *et al.*, 1970; MERTZ, 1970; LEVINE and WILSON, 1971; BIECK, 1972) has been supported by several observations and interpretations. First, in amphibia stomach the correlation between cAMP concentrations and gastric secretion, assessed by several criteria and under various conditions, was very high (HARRIS *et al.*, 1969; ROSEN *et al.*, 1971). Furthermore, cAMP or its dibutyryl derivative (DBcAMP) added to amphibian mucosa preparations directly stimulated acid secretion (HARRIS and ALONSO, 1965; HARRIS *et al.*, 1969; WAY and DURBIN, 1969; NAKAJIMA *et al.*, 1970). In mammals it has been observed that methyl xanthines, known inhibitors of cAMP phosphodiesterase (PDE), potentiate stimulated gastric acid secretion in guinea pigs and cats (ROTH and IVY, 1944; MERENDINO *et al.*, 1945; WOOD, 1948), in dogs (MERENDINO *et al.*, 1945; ROBERTSON and IVY, 1949), in the monkey (SMITH *et al.*, 1960), and in man (ROTH and IVY, 1944; MERENDINO *et al.*, 1945; KRASNOW and GROSSMAN, 1949; MERTZ, 1969; COHEN *et al.*, 1971; DEBAS *et al.*, 1971; BITTNER *et al.*, 1972). Further evidence came from BIECK (1972) and BIECK *et al.* (1973): in dogs an increased release of cAMP into gastric juice in a dose-dependent manner, shortly before secretion, has been found after stimulation by food, pentagastrin, and histamine. The local action is presumed because Heidenhain pouches react in the same manner as the innervated stomach. The same good correlations exist between low levels of cAMP and hydrochloric acid in gastric juice in case of inhibition by prostaglandin E_2 or insulin given intravenously (BIECK, 1972). Direct perfusion of rat stomach by solutions containing DBcAMP and xanthine derivatives gave stimulatory results (SHAW and RAMWELL, 1968). Some measurements of the cAMP content in gastric mucosa furthermore support its having a role in secretion. This has been shown for histamine stimulation (DOMSCHKE *et al.*, 1972a, 1973; KARPPANEN and WESTERMANN, 1973; DOUSA and CODE, 1974) and for circadian secretion rhythm (DOMSCHKE *et al.*, 1971, 1972b). Mild stimulation of gastric secretion by infusion of exogenous cAMP in man has been reported (MERTZ *et al.*, 1971). In the dog, however, infusion of cAMP (LEVINE *et al.*, 1967) or DBcAMP (MAO *et al.*, 1972) decreases or leaves unaltered gastric secretion, possibly due to hemodynamic effects. A similar report for rats came from TAFT and SESSIONS (1972).

These observations should be interpreted with caution, however, because inhibitory actions on gastric function of cAMP (and other adenosine nucleotides) seem possible at higher concentrations (SANDERS *et al.*, 1966). Such high concentrations, however, decrease gastric mucosal blood flow in the case of cAMP (WILSON and LEVINE, 1969) and other nucleotides (LIVINE *et al.*, 1967). Some evidence shows that the involvement of cAMP differs depending on whether histamine or gastrin acts as stimulant (KARPPANEN *et al.*, 1974).

If stimulants like gastrin or histamine act via the cAMP mechanism, one would expect corresponding alterations in the committed enzyme activities. Several things, however, prevent strong alterations in the resulting cAMP levels: (1) the action of phosphodiesterase (PDE) as the destroying enzyme for cAMP depends on pre-existent (high) cAMP concentrations; (2) more than one pool of cAMP seems to exist in other tissues; (3) all measurements must take into account that mucosa contains a variety of cells that respond differently. So measurements of cAMP are not convincing in one direction or the other (BROOKS, 1970).

MAO *et al.* (1971, 1972), measuring adenylate cyclase and PDE in the dog, found *in vitro* inhibition of PDE by theophylline and papaverine only; under certain conditions *in vivo* no inhibition of gastric secretion was found. In both cases histamine elicits gastric secretion without alteration of adenylate cyclase activity. This means that, at least in the dog, the mediation of acid secretion by cAMP is limited (MAO *et al.*, 1973). A correlation between the stimulation of adenylate cyclase activity and gastric secretion caused by histamine and analogs was found only in the fundic part of the rabbit gastric mucosa (SUNG *et al.*, 1973).

Some discrepancies may derive from the fact that the somewhat higher cAMP concentrations found initially after stimulation by gastrin analogs (NARUMI and MAKI, 1973; RUOFF and SEWING, 1973) and other stimulants of gastric secretion may also act on other enzyme systems to elicit gastric secretion. Observations of this kind were made by SALGANIK *et al.* (1972), NARUMI and KANNO (1973), and NARUMI and MAKI (1973) for HCO_3^--stimulated, Mg^{++}-dependent ATPase and/or carbonic anhydrase in mitochondria of rat mucosa cells.

Some good evidence for a connection between gastric secretion and low cAMP concentrations has been found and extended (AMER, 1972), for instance, the biphasic nature from stimulation to inhibition of PDE by gastrin and cholecystokinin (CCK) on several tissues, which has been carefully analyzed in purified extracts by kinetically proved methods (AMER and MCKINNEY, 1972), and similar biphasic actions on gastric secretion (see MASTER *et al.*, 1969; JOHNSON and GROSSMAN, 1971; SVENSSON and EMÅS, 1971). The action of histamine may be similarly interpreted. Though histamine is claimed to stimulate adenylate cyclase of gastric mucosa in guinea pigs (PERRIER and LASTER, 1969), rats (BERSIMBAEV *et al.*, 1971), and rabbits (SUNG *et al.*, 1973), this action is unlikely to contribute to gastric secretion because it is blocked by antihistaminics (PERRIER and LASTER, 1969). It is more likely that histamine acts by stimulation of PDE, as found by AMER (1971) for rabbit fundic mucosa or by HONEYMAN and GOODMAN (1971) in enzyme preparations of heart and intestine. This stimulation is resistant to antihistaminics. The consequence of this interpretation would be that low concentrations of cAMP in oxyntic cells are associated with stimulated gastric secretion, as supported by several other pharmacological considerations (AMER, 1972).

One important exception from Amer's concept is that methylxanthines and imidazole, in contrast to all other stimulants of gastric secretion, lower gastric tone (ROBERTSON *et al.*, 1950b). Thus, a nonspecific effect, not related to cAMP, on gastric secretion has been claimed (AMER, 1972). Considerable changes in the regional blood flow to the stomach elicited such gastric secretion (JACOBSON, 1970). An alteration in membrane permeability, especially for calcium ions or other mechanisms, may likewise interfere. Further, metabolic reactions in connection with the second messenger have to be elucidated. Another candidate for mediation of gastric acid secretion seems to be cGMP (AMER, 1974). Several gastric acid stimulants all stimulated guanylyl cyclase of rabbit fundic mucosa before the secretion response (AMER and MCKINNEY, 1974). Some kind of regulation may derive from the differing sensitivity of PDE toward cAMP and cGMP, as revealed by its varying inhibition ratios against different inhibitors (AMER, 1974). In addition to these aspects, the direct actions of insulin must be considered. No actual measurements have yet been made of these.

References

ABBOTT, D.D., ROSSI, G.V.: The relationship of gastrin activity to antral motility: A review. Amer. J. Pharm. **137**, 15—23 (1965)

AMER, M.S.: Effects of aspirin, other analgesics, histamine and some antihistamines on 3′,5′-cyclic adenosine monophosphate (cAMP) phosphodiesterase (PDE) activity from rabbit liver. Abstr. Amer. Pharm. Ass., Acad. Pharm. Sci. **1**, 120 (1971)

AMER, M.S.: Cyclic AMP and gastric secretion. Amer. J. dig. Dis. **17**, 945—953 (1972)

AMER, M.S.: Cyclic AMP and gastric acid secretion. Amer. J. dig. Dis. **19**, 71—74 (1974)

AMER, M.S., MCKINNEY, G.R.: Studies with cholecystokinin *in vitro*. IV. Effects of cholecystokinin and related peptides on phosphodiesterase. J. Pharmacol. exp. Ther. **183**, 535—548 (1972)

AMER, M.S., MCKINNEY, G.R.: The possible role of cyclic GMP in gallbladder contraction and gastric acid secretion in rabbits. Pharmacologist **15**, 157 (1973)

ANDERSON, S.: Inhibitory effects of hydrochloric acid in antrum and duodenum on gastric secretory response to insulin hypoglycemia in Pavlov pouch dog. Acta physiol. scand. **50**, 23—31 (1960)

ARDEMAN, S., CHANARIN, I., DOYLE, J.C.: Studies on secretion of gastric intrinsic factor in man. Brit. med. J. **1964II**, 600—603

AUBREY, A.D., FORREST, P.M.: Effects of histamine acid phosphate and pentagastrin on gastric secretion in normal human subjects. Gut **11**, 395—404 (1970)

AURES, D., JOHNSON, L.R., WAY, L.W.: Gastrin: obligatory intermediate for activation of gastric histidine decarboxylase activity in the rat. Amer. J. Physiol. **219**, 214—216 (1970)

BACHRACH, W.H.: Action of insulin hypoglycemia on motor and secretory functions of the digestive tract. Physiol. Rev. **33**, 566—592 (1953)

BACHRACH, W.H.: Laboratory criteria for the completeness of vagotomy. Amer. J. dig. Dis. **7**, 1071—1084 (1962)

BACHRACH, W.H.: On the question of a pituitary-adrenal component in the gastric secretory response to insulin hypoglycemia. Gastroenterology **44**, 178—189 (1963)

BANK, S., MARKS, I.N., LOUW, J.H.: Histamine and insulin stimulated gastric acid secretion after selective and truncal vagotomy. Gut **8**, 36—41 (1967)

BARON, J.H.: Dose-response relationships of insulin hypoglycaemia and gastric acid in man. Gut **11**, 826—836 (1970a)

BARON, J.H.: Clinical use of gastric function tests. Scand. J. Gastroent. **5**, Suppl. 6, 9—46 (1970b)

BARON, J.H., COWLEY, D.J., GUTIERREZ, L.V., IWEZE, F.I., SPENCER, J., TINKER, J.: Dose-response of gastric acid to insulin in patients with duodenal ulcer. Gastroenterology **62**, 203—206 (1972)

BERSIMBAEV, R.I., ARGUTINSKAYA, S.V., SALGANIK, R.I.: The stimulating action of gastrin pentapeptide and histamine on adenyl cyclase activity in rat stomach. Experientia (Basel) **27**, 1389—1390 (1971)

BIECK, P.R.: Role of cyclic AMP in the regulation of gastric secretion in dogs and human. Adv. Cyclic Nucleotide Res. **1**, 149—161 (1972)

BIECK, P.R., OATES, A., ROBISON, G.A., ADKINS, R.B.: Cyclic AMP in the regulation of gastric secretion in dogs and humans. Amer. J. Physiol. **224**, 158—164 (1973)

BITTNER, R.R., KRAAS, E., BEGER, H.G., MEVES, M.: The action of theophylline on gastric secretion stimulated by means of gastrin. Z. Gastroent. **10**, 461—466 (1972)

BOLDYREFF, E.B., STEWART, J.F.: A study of gastric secretion caused by insulin. J. Pharmacol. exp. Ther. **46**, 419—429 (1932)

BORG, I., EMÅS, S.: Effect of atropine on the gastric acid response to histamine acid. Scand. J. Gastroent. **5**, 369—374 (1970)

BREMER, A., DUBOIS, A.: Effects du blocage instantané des nerfs vagus sur la sécrétion acide de l'estomac. J. Physiol. (Paris) **55**, 210—211 (1963)

Brooks, F.P.: Central neural control of acid secretion. In: Handbook of Physiology, Vol. 6, II: Alimentary canal (Code, Ed.), Verlag American Physiolog. Soc., p. 805—826 (1967)
Brooks, A.M., Stening, G.F., Grossman, M.I.: Effect of gastric vagal denervation on inhibition of acid secretion by secretin. Amer. J. dig. Dis. **16**, 193—202 (1971)
Brooks, F.P.: Report of a symposium on gastrointestinal hormones. Amer. J. dig. Dis. **15**, 1045—1046 (1970)
Brough, B.J., Korman, M.G., Hansky, J.: Gastrin and acid studies in the pouch dog. I. The response to food and insulin hypoglycaemia. Scand. J. Gastroent. **7**, 519—523 (1972)
Bugajski, J., Hano, J.: Action of serotonin on insulin-stimulated gastric secretion, blood glucose and serum electrolyte levels in the cat. Diss. pharm. pharmacol. **24**, 435—446 (1972)
Bulatao, E., Carlson, A.J.: Contributions to the physiology of the stomach. Influence of experimental changes in blood sugar level on gastric hunger contractions. Amer. J. Physiol. **69**, 107—115 (1924)
Burhol, P.G.: Stimulation by 2-deoxy-D-glucose and inhibition by insulin of gastric secretion in fistula chickens. Scand. J. Gastroent. **8**, 761—764 (1973)
Burstall, P.A., Schofield, B.: Secretory effects of psychic stimulation and insulin hypoglycemia on Heidenhain gastric pouches in dogs. J. Physiol. (Lond.) **120**, 383—408 (1953)
Byrnes, D., Scratcherd, T.: Vagotomy and gastrin secretion. Gut **13**, 848 (1972)
Carter, D.C., Dozois, R.R., Kirkpatrick, J.R.: Insulin infusion test of gastric secretion. Brit. med. J. **1972II**, 202—204
Castell, D.O.: Changes in lower esophageal sphincter pressure during insulin-induced hypoglycemia. Gastroenterology **61**, 10—15 (1971)
Charbion, G.A.: Pentagastrin-induced gastric secretion in dogs. Modulation by drugs acting on the tone of the autonomic nervous system. Digestion **5**, 275—283 (1972)
Checketts, R.G., Gillespie, I.D., Kay, A.W.: Insulin potentiation of the augmented histamine response. Gut **9**, 683—687 (1968)
Cohen, M.M., Debas, H.T., Holubitsky, I.B., Harrison, R.C.: Caffeine and pentagastrin stimulation of human gastric secretion. Gastroenterology **61**, 440—444 (1971)
Colin-Jones, D.G., Himsworth, R.L.: The secretion of gastric acid in response to a lack of metabolizable glucose. J. Physiol. (Lond.) **202**, 97—109 (1969)
Colin-Jones, D.G., Himsworth, R.L.: The location of the chemoreceptor controlling gastric acid secretion during hypoglycaemia. J. Physiol. (Lond.) **206**, 397—409 (1970)
Collazo, J.A., Dobreff, M.: Insulinwirkung auf die Absonderung der Verdauungssäfte. Klin. Wschr. **3**, 1226 (1924)
Cooke, A.R.: Acid and pepsin secretion in response to endogenous and exogenous cholinergic stimulation and pentapeptide. Aust. J. exp. Biol. med. Sci. **47**, 197—202 (1969)
Cooke, A.R., Chvasta, T.E., Weisbrodt, N.W.: Effect of pentagastrin on emptying and electrical and motor activity of the dog stomach. Amer. J. Physiol. **223**, 934—938 (1972)
Cowley, D.J., Baron, J.H.: Gastric acid secretion and changes in blood-glucose after insulin in another healthy man. Brit. J. Surg. **59**, 305 (1972)
Cowley, D.J., Baron, J.H.: Insulin-stimulated gastric acid secretion after vagotomy in man: A dose-response study. Amer. J. dig. Dis. **18**, 544—550 (1973)
Csendes, A., Walsh, J.H., Grossman, M.I.: Effects of atropine and antral acidification on gastrin release and acid secretion in response to insulin and feeding in dogs. Gastroenterology **63**, 257—263 (1972)
Davis, R.A., Brooks, F.P.: Variability of gastric secretory response to insulin hypoglycemia in fistulous beagle dogs. Amer. J. Physiol. **202**, 1070—1072 (1962)
Davis, R.A., Brooks, F.P.: Gastric secretion, continuously recorded blood sugar, and plasma steroids after insulin. Amer. J. Physiol. **204**, 143—146 (1963)
Davis, R.A., Brooks, F.P., Robert, C.M.N.: Gastric secretory response to graded insulin hypoglycemia. Amer. J. Physiol. **208**, 6—8 (1965)
Davis, R.A., Brooks, F.P., Steckel, D.: Gastric secretory changes after anterior hypothalamic lesions. Amer. J. Physiol. **215**, 600—604 (1968)
Davis, T.L., Rutledge, J.R., Keese, D.C., Bajondas, F.J., Rehm, W.S.: Acid secretion, potential, and resistance of frog stomach in K^+-free solutions. Amer. J. Physiol. **209**, 146—152 (1965)
Debas, H.T., Cohen, M.M., Holubitsky, I.B., Harrison, R.C.: Caffeine-stimulated acid and pepsin secretion: Dose-response studies. Scand. J. Gastroent. **6**, 453—457 (1971)
Demand, H.A., Gross, H.U., Berg, G.: Effects of continuous insulin infusions on unstimulated human gastric secretion. Part I. Interrelations between insulin dosage, blood sugar and gastric secretory changes. Part II. Quantitative changes of the gastric juice pattern. Gastroenterology **54**, 1038—1049 (1968)
Detre, L., Sivo, R.: Insulin und Magensekretion. Z. ges. exp. Med. **46**, 594—599 (1925)

DOMSCHKE, W., CLASSEN, M., DEMLING, L.: Circadian rhythmicity of gastric secretion and cyclic 3',5'-adenosine monophosphate contents of gastric mucosa in rats. Scand. J. Gastroent. **7**, 39—41 (1972b)

DOMSCHKE, W., DOMSCHKE, S., CLASSEN, M., DEMLING, L.: Cyclisches Adenosin-3',5'-monophosphat und die Magensekretion. Naturwissenschaften **58**, 628 (1971)

DOMSCHKE, W., DOMSCHKE, S., CLASSEN, M., DEMLING, L.: Histamin und die Magensekretion der Ratte: Adenosin-3'5'-monophosphat als "second messenger". Naturwissenschaften **59**, 521 (1972a)

DOMSCHKE, W., DOMSCHKE, S., CLASSEN, M., DEMLING, L.: Histamine and cyclic 3',5'-AMP in gastric acid secretion. Nature (Lond.) **241**, 454—455 (1973)

DOSS, J., VAN ZWIETEN, P.A.: Cholinergic receptors involved in the production of gastric acid. Arch. int. Pharmacodyn. **197**, 245—160 (1972)

DOUSA, T.P., CODE, CH.F.: Effect of histamine and its methyl derivatives on cyclic AMP metabolism in gastric mucosa and its blockade by an H_2 receptor antagonist. J. clin. Invest. **53**, 334—337 (1974)

DOZOIS, R.R., CARTER, D.C., KIRKPATRICK, J.R.: Patterns of gastric secretory response to an insulin infusion in vagotomized patients. Brit. J. Surg. **59**, 905 (1972)

DUKE, W.W., HIRSCHOWITZ, B.I., SACHS, G.: Vagal stimulation of gastric secretion in man by deoxy-D-glucose. Lancet **1965II**, 871—876

EISENBERG, M.M., EMÅS, G.S., GROSSMAN, M.I.: Comparison of the effect of 2-DG and insulin on gastric acid secretion in dogs. Surgery **60**, 111—117 (1966)

EISENBERG, M.M., WOODWARD, E.R., QUINTANA, R., DRAGSTEDT, L.R.: Insulin inhibition of gastric secretion. J. surg. Res. **3**, 479—484 (1963)

EMÅS, S.: Review: Vagal influences on gastric acid secretion. Scand. J. Gastroent. **8**, 1—4 (1973)

EMÅS, S., BORG, I.: Comparison of the gastric acid responses to pentagastrin and insulin hypoglycemia in male and female ulcer patients. Digestion **5**, 140—152 (1972)

EPSTEIN, A.N., TEITELBAUM, P.: Specific loss of the hypoglycemic control of feeding in recovered lateral rats. Amer. J. Physiol. **213**, 1159—1167 (1967)

FEINBLATT, I., GELFAND, T., SMITH, G.P.: Gastric acid response to 2-deoxy-D-glucose in chronic fistula rats. Proc. Soc. exp. Biol. (N.Y.) **123**, 241—242 (1966)

FEURLE, G., ARNOLD, R., EYDT, M., FUCHS, K., KETTERER, H., CREUTZFELDT, W.: Unterschiedlicher Anstieg des Serum-Gastrins während Insulinhypoglykämie mit und ohne gleichzeitige Aspiration des Magensaftes. Dtsch. med. Wschr. **98**, 1879—1880 (1973)

FORREST, A.P.M., CODE, C.F.: Effect of postganglionic sympathectomy on canine gastric secretion. Amer. J. Physiol. **177**, 425—429 (1954a)

FORREST, A.P.M., CODE, C.F.: The effect of sympathectomy and vagotomy on the inhibition by insulin of histamine-induced secretion in separated (Heidenhain) canine pouches. Amer. J. Physiol. **177**, 430—432 (1954b)

FRENCH, J.D., LONGUIRE, R.L., PORTER, R.W., MOVIUS, H.J.: Extravagal influences on gastric hydrochloric acid secretion induced by stress stimuli. Surgery **34**, 621—632 (1953)

GANGULI, P.C., ELDER, J.B.: Effect of insulin hypoglycemia on plasma gastrin concentration and gastric acid secretion in normal subjects. Gut **12**, 861 (1971)

GEZIRI, M.F., ROBERTSON, C., PEZAK, L.F., WOODWARD, E.R.: The effect of sympathectomy and adrenalectomy on gastric inhibitory property of insulin. Surgery **43**, 606—609 (1958)

GILLESPIE, G., ELDER, J.B., SMITH, I.S., KENNEDY, F., GILLESPIE, I.E., KAY, A.W., CAMPBELL, E.H.G.: Analysis of basal acid secretion and its relation to the insulin response in normal and duodenal ulcer subjects. New criterion for the insulin test. Gastroenterology **62**, 903—911 (1972)

GLASS, G.B.J., BOYD, L.J.: Patterns of response of gastric mucoprotein and acid to insulin; correlation with the underlying disease in the non-operated stomach of man. Gastroenterology **15**, 438—453 (1950)

GLASS, G.B.J., PUGH, B.L., WOLF, S.: Correlation of acid, pepsin and mucoprotein secretion by human gastric glands. J. appl. Physiol. **2**, 571—579 (1950)

GLASS, G.B.J., WOLF, S.: Hormonal mechanisms in nervous mediation of gastric acid secretion in humans. Proc. Soc. exp. Biol. (N.Y.) **73**, 535—537 (1950)

GREGORY, R.A., TRACEY, H.J.: The preparation and properties of gastrin. J. Physiol. (Lond.) **156**, 523—543 (1961)

GROSSMAN, M.I.: How does insulin stimulate the lower esophageal sphincter ? Gastroenterology **61**, 119—120 (1971)

GROSSMAN, M.I.: Insulin test results should be expressed as a number, not as positive or negative. Gastroenterology **63**, 1089 (1972)

GROZA, P.: Consideratii privind mecanismul gastrostimulator al insulinei. Fiziol. norm. si pat. **18**, 97—110 (1972)

GROZA, P., DINA-CORNEANU, M.: Researches on the post-insulin secretion of the stomach. Rev. roum. Physiol. **8**, 485—495 (1971)

GROZA, P., DINA-CORNEANU, M., IONESCU, S.: Dynamics of gastrin under the secreto-stimulating effect of insulin. Rev. roum. Physiol. **8**, 497—502 (1971)

HÅKANSON, R., LIEDBERG, G.: The role of endogenous gastrin in the activation of histidine decarboxylase activity in the rat. Effect of antrectomy and vagal denervation. Europ. J. Pharmacol. **12**, 94—103 (1970)

HALTER, F., ESTERMAN, C., MULLER W.A.: Effects of combinations of pentagastrin and insulin on gastric acid secretion in man. In: Proc. 4th World Congr. Gastroenterol. Copenhagen, p. 203 (1970)

HANKE, H.: Experimentelle Untersuchungen über hormonelle Ulcuserzeugung. I. Die akute erosive Insulin-Gastritis und ihre Pathogenese. Z. ges. exp. Med. **93**, 447—464 (1934)

HANSKY, J., CAIN, M.D.: Radioimmunoassay of gastrin in human serum. Lancet **1969II**, 1388—1390

HANSKY, J., KORMAN, M.G., COWLEY, D.J., BARON, J.H.: Plasma-gastrin levels in patients with duodenal ulcer after insulin hypoglycemia. Brit. J. Surg. **58**, 863 (1971a)

HANSKY, J., KORMAN, M.G., COWLEY, D.J., BARON, J.H.: Serum gastrin in duodenal ulcer. II. Effects of insulin hypoglycemia. Gut **12**, 959—962 (1971b)

HANSKY, J., SOVENY, C., KORMAN, M.G.: Role of the vagus in insulin-mediated gastrin release. Gastroenterology **63**, 387—391 (1972)

HARRIS, J.B., ALONSO, D.: Stimulation of the gastric mucosa by adenosine-3′,5′-monophosphate. Fed. Proc. **24**, 1368—1376 (1965)

HARRIS, J.B., NIGON, K., ALONSO, D.: Adenosine-3′,5′-monophosphate: intracellular mediator for methyl xanthine stimulation of gastric secretion. Gastroenterology **57**, 377—384 (1969)

HELLER, H.: Der Einfluß des Insulins auf die Magentätigkeit. Z. ges. exp. Med. **79**, 607—629 (1931)

HERRERA, F., KEMP, D.R., TSUKAMOTO, M., EISENBERG, M.M.: Insulin inhibition of gastric secretion and motility: the potassium reversal effect. Surg. Forum **18**, 300—303 (1967)

HILL, K.J.: The effect of insulin on the secretion of gastric juice in the goat. Quart. J. exp. Physiol. **37**, 143 (1952)

HIRSCHOWITZ, B.I.: Quantitation of inhibition of gastric electrolyte secretion by insulin in the dog. Amer. J. dig. Dis. **11**, 173—182 (1966a)

HIRSCHOWITZ, B.I.: Characteristics of inhibition of gastric electrolyte secretion by insulin. Amer. J. dig. Dis. **11**, 183—198 (1966b)

HIRSCHOWITZ, B.I.: Secretion of pepsinogen. In: Handbook of Physiology, Vol. 6, II: Alimentary canal (CODE, Ed.), Verlag: American Physiol. Soc., p. 889—918, 1967

HIRSCHOWITZ, B.I., O'LEARY, D.K.: Dose dependence of insulin-stimulated gastric secretion. Amer. J. dig. Dis. **9**, 379—397 (1964)

HIRSCHOWITZ, B.I., ROBBINS, R.C.: Direct inhibition of gastric electrolyte secretion by insulin, independent of hypoglycaemia or the vagus. Amer. J. dig. Dis. **11**, 199—212 (1966)

HIRSCHOWITZ, B.I., SACHS, G.: Vagal gastric secretory stimulation by 2-deoxy-D-glucose. Amer. J. Physiol. **209**, 452—460 (1965)

HIRSCHOWITZ, B.I., SACHS, G.: Reversal of insulin inhibition of gastric secretion by intravenous injection of potassium. Amer. J. dig. Dis. **11**, 217—230 (1966)

HIRSCHOWITZ, B.I., SACHS, G.: Insulin inhibition of gastric secretion: reversal by rubidium. Amer. J. Physiol. **213**, 1401—1405 (1967)

HIRSCHOWITZ, B.I., SACHS, G.: KCl reversal of insulin inhibition and fade in pentagastrin-stimulated gastric secretion. Amer. J. Physiol. **223**, 305—309 (1972)

HIRSCHOWITZ, B.I., SACHS, G., HUTCHINSON, G.: Lack of potentiation or synergism between histamine and pentagastrin in the fistula dog. Amer. J. Physiol. **224**, 509—513 (1973)

HODGE, A.J., MASAREI, J.R., CATCHPOLE, B.N.: The role of the sympathetic nervous system in hypoglycaemia-stimulated gastric secretion. Gut **13**, 341—345 (1972)

HOLLANDER, F.: The insulin test for the presence of intact nerve fibers after vagal operations for peptic ulcer. Gastroenterology **7**, 607—614 (1946)

HOLLANDER, F.: Laboratory procedures in the study of vagotomy (with particular reference to the insulin test). Gastroenterology **11**, 419—425 (1948)

HONEYMAN, T., GOODMAN, H.M.: Histamine activities, cyclic nucleotide phosphodiesterase. Fed. Proc. **30**, 435 (1971)

ISENBERG, J.I.: Insulin versus 2-deoxy-D-glucose: or "2-DG or not 2-DG": an unanswered question. Gastroenterology **63**, 701—704 (1972)

ISENBERG, J.I., STENING, G.F., GROSSMAN, M.I.: Dose-response relation for stimulation of gastric secretion by insulin in man. Gastroenterology **56**, 1254 (1969a)

ISENBERG, J.I., STENING, G.F., WARD, S., GROSSMAN, M.I.: Relation of gastric secretory response in man to dose of insulin. Gastroenterology **57**, 395—398 (1969b)

JACOBSON, E.D.: Comparison of prostaglandin E_1 and norepinephrine on the gastric mucosal circulation. Proc. Soc. exp. Biol. (N.Y.) **133**, 516—519 (1970)

JAFFE, B.M., CLARK, R.J., WILLIAMS, J.A.: Gastrin response to selective and parietal cell vagotomies. Surg. Forum **23**, 324—325 (1972)

JAFFE, B.M., MCGUIGAN, W.T., NEWTON, W.H.: Immunochemical measurement of the vagal release of gastrin. Surgery **68**, 196—201 (1970)

JEMERIN, E.E., HOLLANDER, F., WEINSTEIN, V.A.: A comparison of insulin and food as stimuli for the differentiation of vagal and non-vagal gastric pouches. Gastroenterology **1**, 500—512 (1943)

JEPSON, K., DUTHIE, H.L., FAWCETT, A.N., GUMPERT, J.R., JOHNSTON, D., LARI, J., WORMSLEY, K.G.: Acid and pepsin response to gastrin I, pentagastrin, tetragastrin, histamine and pentagastrin snuff. Lancet **1968II**, 139—141

JÖGI, P., STRÖM, G., UVNÄS, B.: The origin in the CNS of gastric secretory impulses induced by hypoglycemia. Acta physiol. scand. **17**, 212—221 (1949)

JOHANSSON, I., LUNDELL, L., SVENSSON, S.E.: Inhibition of gastric secretion by atropine in conscious rats. J. Physiol. (Lond.) **217**, 723—735 (1971)

JOHNSON, L.R.: Control of gastric secretion: no room for histamine. Gastroenterology **61**, 106—118 (1971)

JOHNSON, L.R., GROSSMAN, M.I.: Intestinal hormones as inhibitors of gastric secretion. Gastroenterology **60**, 120—144 (1971)

JOHNSON, L.R., JONES, R.S., AURES, D., HÅKANSON, R.: Effect of antrectomy on gastric histidine decarboxylase activity in the rat. Amer. J. Physiol. **216**, 1051—1053 (1969)

JONES, R.S., GEIST, R.E., HALL, A.D.: Comparison of dose-response relations of insulin and 2-deoxy-D-glucose for biliary and gastric acid secretion in dogs. Gastroenterology **59**, 665—670 (1970)

JORDAN, P.H., QUINTANA, R.: Insulin inhibition of gastrin-stimulated gastric secretion. Gastroenterology **47**, 617—625 (1964)

KADEKARO, M., TIMO-IARIA, C., VALLE, L.E.R., VELHA, L.P.E.: Site of action of 2-deoxy-D-glucose mediating gastric secretion in the cat. J. Physiol. (Lond.) **221**, 1—13 (1972)

KAHLSON, G., ROSENGREN, E., THUNBERG, R.: Accelerated mobilization and formation of histamine in the gastric mucosa evoked by vagal excitation. J. Physiol. (Lond.) **190**, 455—463 (1967)

KARPPANEN, H.O., WESTERMANN, E.: Increased production of cyclic AMP in gastric tissue by stimulation of $histamine_2$ (H_2)-receptors. Naunyn-Schmiedebergs Arch. Pharmak. **279**, 83—87 (1973)

KARPPANEN, H.O., NEUVONEN, P.I., BIECK, P.R., WESTERMANN, E.: Effect of histamine, pentagastrin and theophylline on the production of cyclic AMP in isolated gastric tissue of the guinea pig. Naunyn-Schmiedebergs Arch. Pharmak. **284**, 15—23 (1974)

KARVINEN, E., KARVONEN, M.J.: Effect of insulin hypoglycaemia on histamine induced Heidenhain pouch secretion in the dog. Acta physiol. scand. **27**, 350—370 (1953)

KEMP, D.R., HERRERA, F., ISAZA, J., EISENBERG, M.M.: On the critical nature of blood sugar levels in the vagal stimulation of gastric acid secretion in normal and diabetic dogs. Surgery **64**, 958—966 (1968a)

KEMP, D.R., HERRERA, F., TSUKAMOTO, M., EISENBERG, M.M.: Insulin-potassium effect on gastric acid secretion and antral motility in dogs. Gastroenterology **54**, 190—196 (1968b)

KEMP, D.R., HERRERA-FERNANDEZ, F., WOODWARD, E.R., DRAGSTEDT, L.R.: Meissner's plexus and the mechanism of vagal stimulation of gastric secretion. Gastroenterology **55**, 76—80 (1968c)

KERR, F.W.L., PRESHAW, R.M.: Secretomotor function of the dorsal motor nucleus of the vagus. J. Physiol. (Lond.) **205**, 405—415 (1969)

KIM, K.S., SHORE, P.A.: Mechanism of action of reserpine and insulin on gastric amines and gastric acid secretion, and the effect of monoamine oxidase inhibition. J. Pharmacol. exp. Ther. **141**, 321—325 (1963)

KORMAN, M.G., BROUGH, B.J., HANSKY, J.: Gastrin and acid studies in the pouch dog. II. Effect of truncal vagotomy on response to food and insulin hypoglycaemia. Scand. J. Gastroent. **7**, 525—529 (1972)

KORMAN, M.G., HANSKY, J., SCOTT, P.R.: Serum gastrin in duodenal ulcer. III. Effect of vagotomy and pylorectomy. Gut **13**, 39—42 (1972)

KORMAN, M.G., SOVENY, C., HANSKY, J.: Radioimmunoassay of gastrin: the response of serum gastrin to insulin hypoglycaemia. Scand. J. Gastroent. **6**, 71—75 (1971)

KRASNOW, S., GROSSMAN, M.I.: Stimulation of gastric secretion in man by theophylline ethylene diamine. Proc. Soc. exp. Biol. (N.Y.) **71**, 335—336 (1949)

KWONG, N.K., BROWN, B.H., WHITTAKER, G.E., DUTHIE, H.L.: Response of the electrical activity, motor activity and acid secretion of the human stomach to pentagastrin and histamine stimulation. Scand. J. Gastroent. **6**, 145—158 (1971)

La Barre, J., de Cespedes, C.: Le relèvement brusque de la glycémie par injection de dextrose supprime-t-il l'exagération post-insulinique de la sécrétion gastrique? C. R. Soc. Biol. (Paris) **106**, 482—483 (1931)

Lanciault, G., Bonoma, C., Brooks, F.P.: Measurement of endogenous gastrin release in response to vagal stimulation. Fed. Proc. **30**, 478 Abs. (1971)

Lanciault, G., Bonoma, C., Brooks, F.P.: Vagal stimulation, gastrin release, and acid secretion in anesthetized dogs. Amer. J. Physiol. **225**, 546—552 (1973b)

Lanciault, G., Bonoma, C., Karreman, G., Brooks, F.P.: Kinetics of gastrin release and degradation in response to electrical vagal stimulation in the dog. Proc. Soc. exp. Biol. (N.Y.) **142**, 740—743 (1973a)

Langer, L.: Pentagastrin- and insulin-induced secretion in diabetes mellitus. Acta med. scand. **191**, 471—475 (1972)

Langer, L., Dotevall, G., Walan, A.: Intrinsic factor secretion following pentagastrin and insulin stimulation in diabetes mellitus. Acta med. scand. **192**, 433—437 (1972)

Lee, Y.H., Thompson, J.H.: Dose response of gastric secretion, and electrolyte output in pylorus-ligated rats to insulin hypoglycemia. Experientia (Basel) **23**, 300—302 (1967)

Lee, Y.H., Thompson, J.H.: The relationship between osmolality and electrolytes in rat gastric juice following histamine and insulin hypoglycaemia. Europ. J. Pharmacol. **3**, 212—216 (1968)

Levine, R.A.: The role of cyclic AMP in hepatic and gastrointestinal function. Gastroenterology **59**, 280—300 (1970)

Levine, R.A., Cafferta, E.P., McNally, E.F.: Inhibitory effect of adenosine 3′,5′-monophosphate on gastric secretion and gastrointestinal motility *in vivo*. Rec. Adv. Gastroent. **1**, 408—410 (1967)

Levine, R.A., Wilson, D.E.: The role of cyclic AMP in gastric secretion. Ann. N.Y. Acad. Sci. **185**, 363—375 (1971)

Lim, R.K.S., Mozer, P.: Does vagus excitation liberate pyloric gastrin? Fed. Proc. **10**, 84 (1951)

Limbosch, J.M., de Graef, J., Gerard, A.: Effect of insulin on acid and pepsin secretion in vagotomized and non-vagotomized patients already stimulated by pentagastrin. Scand. J. Gastroent. **6**, 183—188 (1971)

Long, J.F.: Gastric secretion in unanesthesized chickens. Amer. J. Physiol. **212**, 1303—1307 (1967)

Lorber, S.H.: Mechanisms concerned in the control of gastric motor function. Amer. J. med. Sci. **242**, 518 (1961)

Lorber, S.H., Shay, H.: Effect of insulin and glucose on gastric motor activity of dogs. Gastroenterology **43**, 564—574 (1962)

Mahler, P.: Beiträge zur Chemie des menschlichen Magensaftes. Wien. Arch. inn. Med. **19**, 413—450 (1930)

Makhlouf, G.M., McManus, I.P.A., Card, W.I.: Action of pentapeptide (ICI 50123) on gastric acid secretion in man. Gastroenterology **51**, 455—465 (1966)

Makhlouf, G.M., Moore, E.W., Blum, A.: Models for the secretion of pepsin and other proteins by the human stomach. Gastroenterology **55**, 457—464 (1968)

Mao, C.C., Jacobson, E.D., Shanbour, L.L.: Mucosal cyclic AMP and secretion in the dog stomach. Amer. J. Physiol. **225**, 893—896 (1973)

Mao, C.C., Shanbour, L.L., Hodgkins, D.S., Jacobson, E.D.: Cyclic AMP and gastric secretion. Lab. clin. Med. **78**, 830 (1971)

Mao, C.C., Shanbour, L.L., Hodgkins, D.S., Jacobson, E.D.: Adenosine 3′,5′-monophosphate (cyclic AMP) and secretion in the canine stomach. Gastroenterology **63**, 427—438 (1972)

Master, S.P., Bedi, B.S., de Sousa, A.P., Gillespie, I.E.: Sustained inhibition of gastric secretion by repeated rapid intravenous injections of gastrin. Gastroenterology **56**, 875—881 (1969)

Matuoka, Y., Yasumitu, T., Sibata, M., Konaka, K.: Insulin-induced gastric secretion in adrenalectomized dogs. Kumamoto med. J. **19**, 183—189 (1966)

McGuigan, J.E., Trudeau, W.L.: Serum gastrin levels before and after vagotomy and pyloroplasty or vagotomy and antrectomy. New Engl. J. Med. **286**, 184—188 (1972)

Menguy, R., Thompson, A.E.: Regulation of secretion of mucus from the gastric antrum. Ann. N.Y. Acad. Sci. **140**, 797—803 (1967)

Merendino, K.A., Judd, E.S., Baronofsky, I., Litow, S.S., Lannin, G., Wangensteen, O.H.: Influence of caffeine on ulcer genesis. Experimental production of gastric ulcer in guinea pigs and cats with caffeine, together with a study of its effect upon gastric secretions in dog and man. Surgery **17**, 650—666 (1945)

Mertz, D.P.: Effect of theophylline on acid secretion of stimulated human gastric mucosa. Experientia (Basel) **25**, 269—278 (1969)

Mertz, D.P.: Nucleotide metabolism and gastric acid secretion. Klin. Wschr. **48**, 831—838 (1970)

Mertz, D.P., Mann, K., Jahr, R.: Effect of adenosine-3′,5′-cyclic monophosphate on basal gastric acid secretion in human. Klin. Wschr. **49**, 936—939 (1971)

Mertz, D.P., Wick, T., Thongbhoubesra, T., Walloschek, C.: Über die akute Wirkung verschiedener pharmakologischer Substanzen auf die Säuresekretion am stimulierten menschlichen Magen. Klin. Wschr. **48**, 821—822 (1970)

Meyer, P.F.: Über die Wirkungen des Insulins auf die Magensekretion. Klin. Wschr. **34**, 1578—1581 (1930)

Mignon, M., Varro, V., Vatier, J., Bonfils, S.: 2-DDG stimulation of gastric acid and pepsin secretion in dogs. Acta hepato-Gastroenterol. **19**, 464—469 (1972)

Miller, L.R., Jacobson, E.D., Johnson, L.R.: Effect of pentagastrin on gastric mucosal cells grown in tissue culture. Gastroenterology **64**, 254—267 (1973)

Misher, A., Brooks, F.P.: Electrical stimulation of hypothalamus and gastric secretion in the albino rat. Amer. J. Physiol. **211**, 403—406 (1966)

Moore, J.G.: High gastric acid secretion after vagotomy and pyloroplasty in man. Evidence for nonvagal mediation. Amer. J. dig. Dis. **18**, 661—669 (1973)

Morrissey, S., Stephens, D.N.: The role of the posterior hypothalamus in gastric acid secretion. J. Physiol. (Lond.) **221**, 14P—15P (1972)

Nakajima, S., Shoemaker, R.L., Hirschowitz, B.I., Sachs, G.: Comparison of action of aminophylline and pentagastrin on *Necturus* gastric mucosa. Amer. J. Physiol. **219**, 1259—1262 (1970)

Narumi, S., Kanno, M.: Effects of gastric acid stimulants and inhibitors on the activities of HCO_3-stimulated, Mg^{2+}-dependent ATPase and carbonic anhydrase in rat gastric mucosa. Biochim. biophys. Acta (Amst.) **311**, 80—89 (1973)

Narumi, S., Maki, Y.: Possible role of cyclic AMP in gastric acid secretion in rat. Activation of carbonic anhydrase. Biochim. biophys. Acta (Amst.) **311**, 90—97 (1973)

Necheles, H., Olson, W.H., Morris, R.: Depression of gastric motility by insulin. Amer. J. dig. Dis. **8**, 270—273 (1941)

Necheles, H., Olson, W.H., Morris, R.: Effect of hypoglycemia on gastric motility. Amer. J. Physiol. **129**, 429 (1940)

Nelson, T.S., Eigenbrodt, E.H., Keoshian, L.A.: Motor response of the canine stomach to insulin and feeding. Arch. Surg. **92**, 379—385 (1966)

Nilsson, G., Simon, I., Yalow, R.S., Berson, S.A.: Plasma gastrin and gastric acid responses to sham feeding and feeding in dogs. Gastroenterology **63**, 51—59 (1972)

Norton, L., Fuchs, E., Eiseman, B.: Gastric secretory response to pressure on vagal nuclei. Amer. J. Surg. **123**, 13—18 (1972)

Nyhus, L.M., Chapman, N.D., de Vito, R.V., Harkins, H.N.: The control of gastrin release. An experimental study illustrating a new concept. Gastroenterology **39**, 582—589 (1960)

Oberhelman, H.A., Rigler, S.P., Dragstedt, L.R.: Significance of innervation in the function of the gastric antrum. Amer. J. Physiol. **190**, 391—395 (1957)

Olbe, L.: Effect of resection of gastrin-releasing regions on acid response to sham feeding and insulin hypoglycemia in Pavlov pouch dogs. Acta physiol. scand. **62**, 169—175 (1964)

Olson, W.H., Necheles, H.: Initial depression of human gastric secretion by insulin. Gastroenterology **24**, 362—368 (1953)

Olson, W.H., Necheles, H.: Primary depression of gastric secretion by insulin in normal men. J. Amer. med. Ass. **159**, 1013—1014 (1955)

Passaro, E.P., Grossman, M.I.: Effect of vagal innervation on acid and pepsin to histamine and gastrin. Amer. J. Physiol. **206**, 1068—1076 (1964)

Perrier, C.V., Laster, L.: Adenyl cyclase activity of guinea-pig gastric mucosa. Clin. Res. **17**, 596 (1969)

Pe Thein, M., Schofield, B.: Feeding responses in separated fundic pouches in dogs before and after isolation of the innervated antrum. J. Physiol. (Lond.) **154**, 53P—54P (1960)

Pe Thein, M., Schofield, B.: Biphasic feeding responses in separated fundic pouches in dogs and their relation to the pyloric antrum. Gastroenterology **43**, 436—447 (1962)

Pevsner, L., Grossman, M.I.: The mechanism of vagal stimulation of gastric acid secretion. Gastroenterology **28**, 493—499 (1955)

Porter, R.W., Movius, H.J., French, I.D.: Hypothalamic influences on hydrochloric acid secretion of the stomach. Surgery **33**, 875—880 (1953)

Powell, D.W., Hirschowitz, B.I.: Sodium pentobarbital depression of histamine or insulin-stimulated gastric secretion. Amer. J. Physiol. **212**, 1001—1006 (1967)

Preshaw, R.M.: Gastric acid output after sham feeding and during release or infusion of gastrin. Amer. J. Physiol. **219**, 1409—1416 (1970)

QUIGLEY, J.P., JOHNSON, V., SOLOMON, E.I.: Action of insulin on the motility of the gastrointestinal tract. I. Action on the stomach of normal fasting man. Amer. J. Physiol. **90**, 89—98 (1929)

QUIGLEY, J.P., TEMPLETON, R.D.: The action of insulin on the motility of the gastrointestinal tract. IIIa. Action on the pyloric pouch, b. Action on the stomach following double splanchnicotomy. Amer. J. Physiol. **91**, 475—481 (1930a)

QUIGLEY, J.P., TEMPLETON, R.D.: Action of insulin on the motility of the gastrointestinal tract. IV. Action on the stomach following double vagotomy. Amer. J. Physiol. **91**, 482—487 (1930b)

READ, R.C., THOMPSON, B.W., HALL, W.H.: Conversion of Hollander tests in man from positive to negative: beta-adrenergic blockade with propranolol hydrochloride. Arch. Surg. **104**, 573—578 (1972)

RIDLEY, P.T., BROOKS, F.P.: Alterations in gastric secretion following hypothalamic lesions producing hyperphagia. Amer. J. Physiol. **209**, 319—323 (1965)

ROBERTSON, C., IVY, A.C.: Effect of some xanthine derivatives on gastric secretion. Fed. Proc. **8**, 133 (1949)

ROBERTSON, C., LANGLOIS, C.I., MARTIN, G.G., SZLEZCK, G., GROSSMAN, M.I.: Release of gastrin in response to bathing the pyloric mucosa with acetylcholine. Amer. J. Physiol. **163**, 27—33 (1950a)

ROBERTSON, C., ROSIERE, C.E., BLICKENSTAFF, D., GROSSMAN, M.I.: The potentiating action of certain xanthine derivatives on gastric acid secretion responses in the dog. J. Pharmacol. exp. Ther. **99**, 323—365 (1950b)

ROHOLM, K.: Clinical investigations into effect of intravenous injections of insulin: Gastric secretion in normal individuals. Acta med. scand. **73**, 472—492 (1930)

ROSEN, H., CHANDLER, J.G., MULTER, F., ORLOFF, J.M.J.: The role of cyclic adenosine 3′,5′-monophosphate in gastric secretion. Surg. Forum **22**, 291—293 (1971)

ROSENGREN, E., SVENSSON, S.E.: The role of the antrum and the vagus nerve in the formation of gastric mucosal histamine. J. Physiol. (Lond.) **205**, 275—288 (1969)

ROSS, B., KAY, A.W.: The insulin test after vagotomy. Gastroenterology **46**, 379—386 (1964)

ROTH, I.A., IVY, A.C.: The effect of caffeine on gastric secretion in dog, cat and man. Amer. J. Physiol. **141**, 454—461 (1944)

RUOFF, H.-J., SEWING, K.-F.: Hemmung der Magensaftsekretion von Hühnern durch Atropin, Insulin und 2-Desoxy-D-Glucose. Naunyn-Schmiedebergs Arch. Pharmakol. **273**, 219—229 (1972)

RUOFF, H.-J., SEWING, K.-F.: Cyclic 3′,5′-adenosine monophosphate in the rat gastric mucosa after starvation, feeding, and pentagastrin. Scand. J. Gastroent. **8**, 241—243 (1973)

SACHS, G., SHOEMAKER, R., HIRSCHOWITZ, B.I.: Action of 2-deoxy-D-glucose on frog gastric mucosa. Amer. J. Physiol. **209**, 461—466 (1965)

SALGANIK, R.I., ARGUTINSKAYA, S.V., BERSIMBAEV, R.I.: The stimulating action of gastrin, pentapeptide, histamine and cyclic adenosine 3′,5′-monophosphate on carbonic anhydrate in rat stomach. Experientia (Basel) **28**, 1190—1191 (1972)

SANDERS, S.S., WHITE, A.S., REHM, W.S.: Effect of adenosine compounds on motility of frog gastric mucosa. Fed. Proc. **25**, 514 (1966)

SCHAPIRO, H., CUMMINS, A.J., WRUBLE, L.D.: Insulin depression of human gastric secretion. Arch. Surg. **94**, 881—883 (1967)

SCRATCHERD, T., CASE, R.M.: The role of cyclic adenosine 3′,5′-monophosphate (cAMP) in gastrointestinal secretion. Gut **10**, 957—961 (1969)

SHAW, J.E., RAMWELL, P.W.: Inhibition of gastric secretion in rats by prostaglandin E_1. In: Prostaglandin Symposium for Experimental Biology (P.W. RAMWELL, J.E. SHAW, Eds.), p. 55—66. New York: Interscience 1968

SINGLETON, J.W.: Humoral effects of the pancreas upon the gastrointestinal tract. Gastroenterology **56**, 942—962 (1969)

SMITH, G.P., BROOKS, F.P., DAVIS, R.A., ROTHMAN, S.S.: Fasting gastric contents in the spider monkey. Amer. J. Physiol. **199**, 889—892 (1960)

SPENCER, J., BURNS, G.P., CHENG, F.C.Y., COX, A.G., WILLBOURN, R.B.: Differences between males and females in the Hollander insulin test. Gut **10**, 307—310 (1969)

SPENCER, J., GROSSMAN, M.I.: Inhibition of gastric secretion by insulin and 2-deoxyglucose. Gastroenterology **58**, 1052 (1970)

SPENCER, J., GROSSMAN, M.I.: The gastric secretory response to insulin: an "all-or-none" phenomenon? Gut **12**, 891—896 (1971a)

SPENCER, J., GROSSMAN, M.I.: Inhibition of gastric acid secretion by insulin and 2-deoxy-D-glucose. Brit. J. Surg. **58**, 295—296 (1971b)

STADIL, F.: Effect of vagotomy on gastrin release during insulin hypoglycemia in ulcer patients. Scand. J. Gastroent. **7**, 225—251 (1972)

STADIL, F., REHFELD, J.F.: Hypoglycaemic release of gastrin in man. Scand. J. Gastroent. **7**, 509—514 (1972)

STAGG, B.H., LEWIN, M.R., BOULOS, P.B., CLARK, C.G.: The release of gastrin in response to insulin, food and meat extract (Oxo). Brit. J. Surg. **58**, 863 (1971)

STEMPIEN, S.J.: Insulin gastric analysis: technic and interpretation. Amer. J. dig. Dis. **7**, 138—152 (1962)

STENING, G.F., GROSSMAN, M.I.: Effect of partial vagotomy in the neck or lower thorax on insulin-stimulated acid secretion in dogs. Gastroenterology **59**, 376—379 (1970)

STENING, G.F., ISENBERG, J.I.: Insulin-induced acid secretion after partial vagotomy in dogs and cats. Amer. J. Physiol. **217**, 962—964 (1969)

SUGAWARA, K., CHAWLA, R.C., EISENBERG, M.M.: Simultaneous observation of gastric motor and secretory response to vagal stimulation in normal and diabetic dogs. Surgery **70**, 325—333 (1971)

SUN, D.C.H., SHAY, H.: Mechanism of action of insulin hypoglycemia on gastric secretion in man. J. appl. Physiol. **15**, 697—703 (1960)

SUNG, C.P., JENKINS, B.C., BURNS, L.R., HACKNEY, V., SPENNEY, J.G., SACHS, G., WIEBELHAUS, V.D.: Adenyl and guanyl cyclase in rabbit gastric mucosa. Amer. J. Physiol. **225**, 1359—1363 (1973)

SVENSSON, S.O., EMÅS, S.: Effect of cholecystokinin on histamine- and pentagastrin-stimulated acid secretion in conscious cats. Scand. J. Gastroent. **6**, 371—376 (1971)

TAFT, R.C., SESSIONS, J.T.: Inhibition of gastric acid secretion by dibutyryl cyclic adenosine 3′,5′-monophosphate (Db-cAMP). Clin. Res. **20**, 43 (1972)

TEMPLETON, R.D., QUIGLEY, J.P.: The action of insulin on the motility of the gastro-intestinal tract. II. Action on the Heidenhain pouch. Amer. J. Physiol. **91**, 467—474 (1930)

TEPPERMAN, B.L., WALSH, J.H., PRESHAW, R.M.: Effect of antral denervation on gastrin release by sham feeding and insulin hypoglycemia in dogs. Gastroenterology **63**, 973—980 (1972)

TSUKAMOTO, M., HERRERA, F., KEMP, D.R., EMÅS, G.S., WOODWARD, E.R., EISENBERG, M.M.: Effect of vagal stimulation by 2-deoxy-D-glucose and insulin on gastric motility in dogs. Ann. Surg. **165**, 605—608 (1967)

UVNÄS, B.: The part played by the pyloric region in the cephalic phase of gastric secretion. Acta physiol. scand. **4**, Suppl. 13, 1—86 (1942)

UVNÄS, B.: Gastrin and vagus. Gastroenterology **56**, 812—815 (1969)

VARRO, V., OLAH, F., FAREDIN, E., FARAGO, A.: Contribution to the neurohormonal mechanism of gastric secretion. Acta med. hung. **5**, 143—148 (1954)

VIZI, S.E., BERTACCINI, G., IMPICCIATORE, M., KNOLL, J.: Acetylcholine-releasing effect of gastrin and related polypeptides. Europ. J. Pharmacol. **17**, 175—178 (1972)

VIZI, S.E., BERTACCINI, G., IMPICCIATORE, M., KNOLL, J.: Evidence that acetylcholine released by gastrin and related polypeptides contributes to their effect on gastro-intestinal motility. Gastroenterology **64**, 268—277 (1973)

WADDELL, W.R.: The acid secretory response to histamine and insulin hypoglycaemia after various operations on the stomach. Surgery **42**, 652—658 (1957)

WALSH, I.H., YALOW, R.S., BERSON, S.A.: The effect of atropine on plasma gastrin response to feeding. Gastroenterology **60**, 16—21 (1971)

WAY, L., DURBIN, R.P.: Inhibition of acid secretion *in vitro* by prostaglandin E_1. Nature (Lond.) **221**, 874—875 (1969)

WEISS, A., SCIALES, W.J.: The effect of tolbutamide on human basal gastric secretion. Ann. intern. Med. **55**, 406—475 (1961)

WILLEMS, G., VANSTEENKISTE, Y., LIMBOS+H, J.M.: Stimulating effect of gastrin on cell proliferation kinetics in canine fundic mucosa. Gastroenterology **62**, 583—589 (1972)

WILSON, D.E., LEVINE, R.A.: Decreased canine gastric mucosal blood flow induced by prostaglandin E_1: a mechanism for its inhibitory effect on gastric secretion. Gastroenterology **56**, 1268 (1969)

WISE, L., BALLINGER, W.F.: Effect of vagal stimulation and inhibition on gastric mucus and sulfated amino polysaccharide secretion. Ann. Surg. **174**, 976—982 (1971)

WOOD, D.R.: Caffeine and gastric secretion. Brit. med. J. **1948II**, 283—285

WOODWARD, E.R., ROBERTSON, C., FRIED, W., SCHAPIRO, H.: Further studies on the isolated gastric antrum. Gastroenterology **32**, 868—877 (1957)

WORMSLEY, K.G., MAHONEY, M.P., NG, M.: Effects of a gastrin-like pentapeptide (ICI 50123) on stomach and pancreas. Lancet **1966I**, 993—996

WYLLIE, J.H., BOULOS, P.B., LEWIN, U.R., STAGG, B.H., CLARK, C.G.: Plasma gastrin and acid secretion in man following stimulation by food, meat extract, and insulin. Gut **13**, 887—893 (1972)

2. Action on the Exocrine Pancreas

The influence of insulin and nutrition on the function of the pancreas is of special interest because the exocrine secretion process itself allows very little variation in the enzyme and solute content of the excreted juice. Any variations that do occur are regulated at the level of synthesis of the several components of pancreatic juice and depend mainly on nutritional factors. At present we are far from completely informed about the extent to which hormonal, autonomic neural, reflex neural, and nutritional factors interfere in these adaptational processes (for reviews, see Dupre, 1970; Christophe *et al.*, 1972; Harper, 1972; Ribet, Pascal and Frexinos, 1972a, b, c; Youngs, 1972; Brooks, 1973; Jamieson, 1973; Jorpes and Mutt, 1973).

a) Influence of Insulin on Exocrine Pancreas Secretion

Clinical observations over the last decade indicate in 30% of all diabetics and in more than 70% of human juvenile diabetics a decrease in the amylase secretion rate (Chey *et al.*, 1963). This was confirmed by Vacca *et al.* (1964), Herfort *et al.* (1972), Tympner *et al.* (1973) and by scintigraphic means (Lähdevirta, 1967). Apparently, this does not apply to milder forms of human diabetes (Bartelheimer and Ritter, 1960; Günther, 1961; Peters *et al.*, 1966). Several tests of pancreatic function showed that nearly all patients with maturity-onset diabetes had some kind of functional alteration (Baron and Nabarro, 1973). In contrast to patients with pancreatic tumors, this kind of alteration was reported not to occur in normal diabetics (Dreiling, 1951). In the diabetic state caused by insulin deficiency, the concentration of amylase in blood falls while that of proteolytic enzymes rises (Grossman *et al.*, 1944; Ben Abdeljlil *et al.*, 1965; Snook, 1968).

Two different cell types apparently participate in the exocrine secretion process, as shown by functional observations that differentiate between the excretion of water and electrolytes on the one hand and enzymes on the other (Ridderstap and Bonting, 1969; Rutten *et al.*, 1972). Water and electrolyte release is stimulated mainly by secretin; enzymes are released rather by vagal stimulation and by acetylcholine and its congeners. Like gastric secretion, pancreatic secretion is also regulated (see Harper, 1967; Preshaw, 1967; Grossman, 1971; Harper, 1972).

The pancreatic acinar cells are under direct vagal control (Harper *et al.*, 1959; Hayama *et al.*, 1963; Dean and Matthews, 1968, 1972; Lenninger, 1971; Lenninger and Ohlin, 1971; Konturek *et al.*, 1972). It seems possible that insulin acts on pancreatic enzyme secretion by way of vagal mechanisms in three ways: (1) by direct extragastric vagal innervation of the pancreas; (2) by vagal release of gastrin from the stomach; (3) by release of pancreozymin (and secretin) as a result of duodenal acidification (see Grossman, 1971; Harper, 1972; Brooks, 1973). Histologically, vagal stimulation causes a diminution in the zymogen granula within the pancreatic acinar cells (Harper and McKay, 1948).

As discussed in section A, gastrin is released directly by insulin hypoglycemia and secretin, and other duodenal hormones are released indirectly by acidification. These two processes presumably exert secondary effects on pancreatic secretion and emphasize the well-known fact of gastric participation in the regulation of pancreatic secretion. One of the best arguments for the indirect character of the secretion-stimulating properties of insulin derives from experiments performed by Couture *et al.* (1972) with rat pancreatic tissue *in vitro*; this tissue performs well functionally, but does not respond to insulin. These authors, however, did not

Abbreviations: CCK = cholecystokinin-pancreozymin; cAMP = cyclic 3′,5′-adenosine monophosphate; DBcAMP = dibutyryl-cAMP.

prevent inactivation of insulin by the tissue. Moreover, in batch incubation and perfusion experiments DANIELSON (1974) found that (basal and CCK-stimulated) secretion of amylase was even reduced by a concentration of 100 μg/ml of insulin.

In hypoglycemia in several animal species, stimulation of protein secretion has been found (BAYLISS and STARLING, 1902; THOMAS and CRIDER, 1947; EISENBERG and GROSSMAN, 1966) in contrast to findings of BAXTER (1932). Equivalent findings were made in man by FRISK and WELIN (1937), LAGERLÖF and WELIN (1937), PFIFFER *et al.* (1952), DREILING *et al.* (1952). Otherwise, hypoglycemia in combination with vagotomy reduced amylase secretion in the dog (ROUTLEY *et al.*, 1952) and in the rat (LIN and ALPHIN, 1959) as well as the amylase response to secretion in man (DREILING *et al.*, 1952). After highly selective vagotomy, which leaves the innervation for the pancreas intact, high amylase values are found after hypoglycemic doses of insulin, similar to those of unoperated patients (SMITH *et al.*, 1973). This points to a modest direct vagal effect. More detailed measurements of the secretion response to insulin hypoglycemia were done by GUPTA *et al.* (1973). They used 0.2 U/kg of insulin in dogs and found a lowered pancreatic bicarbonate output in cases of open gastric fistula, i.e. when secretion release and action does not play a role. On the other hand, protein output (enzymes) was remarkably high and began earlier, suggesting vagal stimulation; the response was similar to that seen after a meat meal, but no gastrin measurements were made. Direct vagal influences play a minor role (BEESLEY *et al.*, 1972). Thus, by far the most important vagal factor effecting induced secretion is the release of gastrin. If this is the case, pancreatic stimulation by gastrin must have the same characteristics as insulin hypoglycemia. Qualitatively, gastrin, which contains the same C-terminal pentapeptide as cholecystokinin-pancreozymin (MUTT and JORPES, 1967), and its congeners stimulate both the rate of flow and to a more pronounced degree the rate of protein secretion of the pancreas (PRESHAW *et al.*, 1965a; BESWICK *et al.*, 1968; EMÅS *et al.*, 1968; MORRIS *et al.*, 1968; STENING and GROSSMAN, 1969; PETERSON and BERSTAD, 1971; DOCKRAY, 1973). The use of open gastric fistula in addition to pancreatic fistula excluded any indirect effect above secondary CCK-pancreozymin release (PRESHAW *et al.*, 1965a). Generally, antrally released gastrin plays a physiological role in the pancreatic secretory response, for instance, in feeding (PRESHAW *et al.*, 1965b). Species differences may exist (DOCKRAY, 1973). In contrast to the dog (VAGNE and GROSSMAN, 1969), in the rat and man (WORMSLEY *et al.*, 1966; PETERSON and BERSTAD, 1971) pancreatic secretion takes place with more than gastric secretion-stimulating doses.

The participation of cAMP in the stimulus — secretion coupling of exocrine pancreas has been suggested (see LEVINE, 1970; BROOKS, 1973; SCRATCHERD and CASE, 1973; CASE, 1973b), in which by analogy insulin could interact. There may be no strict correlation between stimulation, e.g. by secretin, CCK and acetylcholine, and alterations in endogenous cAMP content (JOHNSON *et al.*, 1970; BENZ *et al.*, 1972). More work must be done on this subject before this question can be settled. In view of the many observations made on different pancreas preparations concerning the mediation of cAMP in hydromineral and enzymatic secretion, it may be said that the effects of cAMP or its dibutyryl derivative are surprisingly weak and that the effects of theophylline become apparent only with high doses or concentrations. CASE *et al.* (1972) who saw after-rises of cAMP not followed by secretion responses, pointed out that the regulation system is more complex, namely that the gland consists not only of acinar but of other types as well, and that synthetic mechanisms exist to replenish the enzyme stores. This last argument, however, has been questioned by MORISSET and WEBSTER (1971).

A more likely reason seems that calcium ions take part in the secretion process (Hokin, 1966; Case and Clausen, 1971; Robberecht and Christophe, 1971; Argent *et al.*, 1972; Heisler *et al*, 1972; Kanno, 1972; Case, 1973a, b; Case *et al.*, 1973). Hypercalcemia stimulates pancreas secretion in man (Goebell *et al.*, 1973). Microtubuli may participate (see Christophe *et al.*, 1972) or not (Benz *et al.*, 1972).

b) Influence of Insulin on Synthesis of Pancreatic Juice Components

Two approaches have been used to reveal the influence of insulin on enzyme biosynthesis. First, the enzyme content within the pancreas has been followed during chronic application of insulin; secondly, and more convincingly, the radioactive label of the enzyme protein was determined after administration of radioactive amino acid(s) with and without insulin. In this case precursor problems arise. One must also ask whether the biosynthesis of exportable enzymes follows upon or is completely independent of the secretion process (for references in controversial findings, see Morisset and Webster, 1972; Bauduin *et al.*, 1973). Differences in dose, application time, observation time, manner of stimulation, and mode of preparation may account for the discrepancies. The finding that synthesis is inhibited after secretion (attributed to shortage of energy supply) in rat pancreas pieces has further complicated the debate (Bauduin *et al.*, 1973). In any case, the adaptation of biosynthesis to secretional needs takes place slowly (Webster *et al.*, 1972), possibly by polysomal adaptation or by alteration in the acinar cell (Black and Webster, 1973).

Several observations suggest that enzyme biosynthesis *in vivo* is stimulated by insulin. In hypophysectomized rats insulin (in addition to somatotropin, corticosterone and thyroxine) replenishes the reduced enzyme stores (Baker *et al.*, 1961). Yet chronic administration of insulin (2 U/day) to rats reduces the amylase content of the pancreas (Grossman *et al.*, 1944). Ben Abdeljlil *et al.* (1965) showed that the biosynthesis of amylase in alloxan-diabetic rats fell by several times and was promptly reversed by insulin *in vivo*. Paradoxically, this effect paralleled glucose concentration, though a diet rich in carbohydrate or glucose itself usually increases amylase synthesis. It was thought therefore that insulin alone, or insulin secreted by hyperglycemia, induced amylase synthesis. As measured by incorporation of valine from the intracellular pool, insulin restores the normal rate of amylase biosynthesis in alloxan-diabetic animals. Yet if insulin is given to rats on a protein-rich diet, it does not completely restore amylase synthesis, which is interpreted as an indirect influence of insulin (Palla *et al.*, 1968). The synthesis of chymotrypsinogen is slightly altered in the opposite way to amylase (Ben Abdeljlil *et al.*, 1965; Palla *et al.*, 1968). In a more detailed study with labeled leucine, Söling and Unger (1972) argue for the interaction of insulin at the transcriptional level and its permissive role in transcription. The following facts support this claim: in the very rapid diazoxide diabetes of rats (analyzed after 6 h) amylase in the pancreas is not decreased; the same is seen after actinomycin, which simultaneously inhibits leucine incorporation and enzyme secretion. When the effect of insulin in alloxan-diabetic rats is followed in dependence on time the delay observed is remarkable. The rate of incorporation of leucine into amylase by insulin is exceptionally high compared with that due to other pancreas proteins (including other enzymes), when determined 2 h after insulin administration. Further points are that it is counteracted by actinomycin and the lack of involvement of the adrenal gland. Therefore it has been postulated that insulin has an effect on amylase synthesis through its stimulation of amylase messenger RNA synthesis. Such an effect, however, could be exerted indirectly, i.e. by faster passage of glucose into the pancreatic cell (Söling and Unger, 1972). Some caution should be advised as to this suggestion. For several cases it is known that all hydrolases of the zymogen granules are synthesized at a proportional rate and with the same turnover time (CHRISTOPHE *et al.*, 1973; REGGIO, 1973). It may be questioned whether the direct action of insulin could be the messenger mediating dietary adaptation, for MORISSET and DUNNIGAN (1971) found that chronic administration of insulin to rats fed a protein-rich diet (with and without glucose supplement) decreased the pancreatic amylase content, so confirming the above-mentioned findings of GROSSMAN *et al.* (1944). Another argument against a direct action of insulin (COUTURE *et al.*, 1972) is that no action on biosynthesis is found in rat pancreatic tissue *in vitro* as mentioned above, and that a vagal-humoral action may be deduced from the findings *in vivo*. The time lag COUTURE *et al* found in the decrease of amylase content and amino acid incorporation in comparison to hypoglycemia after administration of high doses of insulin suggests a close relationship between these two processes, i.e. between vagally stimulated secretion and amylase synthesis.

c) Trophic Effects of Insulin on Exocrine Pancreas Tissue

A special role in the development of the acinar tissue cell has been attributed to insulin (HENDERSON, 1969). Thus, a trophic effect of insulin has been postulated because autoradiographs of mouse pancreas after intravenous injection of ^{35}S methionine showed a stronger enrichment in acinar cells around endocrine islets (HANSSON, 1959) and because zymogen granula are more abundant in the peri-insular acini and are decreased after islet destruction by alloxan (KRAMER and TAN, 1968). The improved uptake of amino acids into exocrine pancreas cells may be of primary importance, as suggested by the reduced amino acid uptake into the pancreas of diabetics (LÄHDEVIRTA, 1967; MELMED *et al.*, 1968). It is interesting to note that chronic administration of pentagastrin to normal and hypophysectomized rats induces hyperplasia of the pancreas (MAYSTON and BARROWMAN, 1971, 1973).

It seems possible that insulin deficiency may cause progressive damage to the acinar pancreas cells: fibrosis is described in man (CHEY *et al.*, 1963; VACCA *et al.*, 1964) and in experimental diabetes of dogs the same type of damage is seen (RICHARDSON and YOUNG, 1938; GROSSMAN and IVY, 1946). This damage may be accentuated by the inhibitory action of glucagon, which is secreted to a higher extent by diabetics (see YOUNGS, 1972). As mentioned, the amylase content is much reduced under such conditions (PALLA *et al.*, 1968). The alterations elicited in acinar cells by insulin deficiency are obviously highly complex.

References

ARGENT, B.E., CASE, R.M., FRASER, M.P., SCRATCHERD, T.: The effects of calcium on volume and amylase secretion from the perfused cat pancreas. J. Physiol. (Lond.) **224**, 29P—30P (1972)

BAKER, B.L., CLAPP, H.W., ANNABALL, C.R., DEWEY, M.M.: Elevation of proteolytic activity in the pancreas of hypophysectomized rats by hormonal therapy. Proc. Soc. exp. Biol. (N.Y.) **108**, 238—242 (1961)

BARON, J.H., NABARRO, J.D.: Pancreatic exocrine function in maturity onset diabetes mellitus. Brit. med. J. **4**, 25—27 (1973)

BARTELHEIMER, H., RITTER, U.: Das exkretorische Pankreas bei Diabetikern. Med. Klin. **55**, 700—703 (1960)

BAUDUIN, H., TONDEUR, T., v. SANDE, I., VINCENT, D.: Secretion and protein metabolism in the rat pancreas *in vitro*. Biochim. biophys. Acta (Amst.) **304**, 81—92 (1973)

BAXTER, S.G.: Blood-sugar concentration and pancreatic secretion in the rabbit. Quart. J. exp. Physiol. **21**, 355—363 (1932)

BAYLISS, W.M., STARLING, E.H.: The mechanism of pancreatic secretion. J. Physiol. (Lond.) **28**, 325—353 (1902)

BEESLEY, W.H., ORAHOOD, R., DUTTA, P., EISENBERG, M.M.: The role of vagal release of gastrin in pancreatic enzyme secretion. Brit. J. Surg. **59**, 912 (1972)

BEN ABDELJLIL, A., PALLA, J.C., DESNUELLE, P.: Effect of insulin on pancreatic amylase and chymotrypsinogen. Biochem. biophys. Res. Commun. **18**, 71—75 (1965)

BENZ, L., ECKSTEIN, B., MATTHEWS, E.K., WILLIAMS, J.A.: Control of pancreatic amylase release *in vitro*: effects of ions, cyclic AMP and colchicine. Brit. J. Pharmacol. **46**, 66—77 (1972)

BESWICK, I.B., HOWAT, H.T., MORRIS, A.I.: The effects of gastrin and peptide analogous releated to gastrin on cats. J. Physiol. (Lond.) **197**, 71P—72P (1968)

BLACK, O., WEBSTER, B.: Protein synthesis in pancreas of fasted pigeons. J. Cell Biol. **57**, 1—8 (1973)

BROOKS, F.P.: The neurohumoral control of pancreatic exocrine secretion. Amer. J. clin. Nutr. **26**, 291—310 (1973)

CASE, R.M.: Calcium and gastrointestinal secretion. Digestion **8**, 269—288 (1973a)

CASE, R.M.: Cellular mechanisms controlling pancreatic exocrine secretion. Acta hepato-Gastroenterol. **20**, 435—444 (1973b)

CASE, R.M., CLAUSEN, T.: Amylase secretion and calcium efflux from isolated rat pancreas. Gut **12**, 862 (1971)

CASE, R.M., CLAUSEN, T., SMITH, R.K.: Fluxes of (^{45}Ca) calcium ions in exocrine rat pancreas and their relation to protein secretion. Biochem. Soc. Transact. **1**, 857—858 (1973)

CASE, R.M., JOHNSON, M., SCRATCHERED, T., SHERRATT, H.S.A.: Cyclic adenosine 3′,5′-monophosphate concentration in the pancreas following stimulation by secretin, cholecystokinin-pancreozymin and acetylcholine. J. Physiol. (Lond.) **223**, 669—684 (1972)

CHEY, W.Y., SHAY, H., SHUMAN, C.R.: External pancreatic secretion in diabetes mellitus. Ann. intern. Med. **59**, 812—821 (1963)

CHRISTOPHE, J., ROBBERECHT, P., DESCHODT-LANCKMAN, M., VANDERMEERS, A., VANDERMEERS-PIRET, M.-C., CANNIS, J., RATHÉ, J.: Biologie cellulaire du pancréas exocrine. Bull. Acad. roy. Méd. Belg. **12**, 323—355 (1972)

CHRISTOPHE, J., VANDERMEERS, A., VANDERMEERS-PIRET, M.-C., RATHÉ, J., CAMUS, J.: The relative turnover time *in vivo* of the intracellular transport of five hydrolases in the pancreas of the rat. Biochim. biophys. Acta (Amst.) **308**, 285—295 (1973)

COUTURE, Y., DUNNIGAN, J., MORISSET, J.: Stimulation of pancreatic amylase secretion and protein synthesis by insulin. Scand. J. Gastroent. **7**, 257—263 (1972)

DANIELSON, Å.: Effects of glucose, insulin and glucagon on amylase secretion from incubated mouse pancreas. Pflügers Arch. **348**, 333—342 (1974)

DEAN, P.M., MATTHEWS, E.K.: Miniature depolarization potential in pancreatic acinar cells. J. Physiol. (Lond.) **198**, 90P—91P (1968)

DEAN, P.M., MATTHEWS, E.K.: Pancreatic acinar cells: measurement of membrane potential and miniature depolarization potentials. J. Physiol. (Lond.) **225**, 1—13 (1972)

DOCKRAY, G.J.: The action of gastrin and cholecystokinin-related peptides on pancreatic secretion in the rat. Quart. J. exp. Physiol. **58**, 163—169 (1973)

DREILING, A.D.: Studies in pancreatic function. IV. The use of the secretin test in the diagnosis of tumors in and about the pancreas. Gastroenterology **18**, 184—196 (1951)

DREILING, A.D., DRUCKERMAN, L.J., HOLLANDER, F.: The effect of complete vagisection and vagal stimulation on pancreatic secretion in man. Gastroenterology **20**, 578—586 (1952)

DUPRE, J.: Regulation of the secretions of the pancreas. Ann. Rev. Med. **21**, 299—316 (1970)

EISENBERG, M.M., GROSSMAN, M.I.: Pancreatic exocrine response to 2-deoxy-D-glucose, insulin and histamine. Surg. Forum **17**, 349 (1966)

EMÅS, S., BILLINGS, A., GROSSMAN, M.I.: Effects of gastrin and pentagastrin on gastric and pancreatic secretion in dogs. Scand. J. Gastroent. **3**, 234—240 (1968)

FRISK, A.R., WELIN, G.: The external pancreatic secretion and the discharge of bile during hypoglycemia following intravenous administration of insulin. Acta med. scand. **91**, 170—182 (1937)

GOEBELL, H., STEFFEN, CH., BALTZER, G., BODE, CH.: Stimulation of pancreatic secretion of enzymes by acute hypercalcaemia in man. Europ. J. clin. Invest. **3**, 98—104 (1973)

GROSSMAN, M.I.: Control of pancreatic secretion. In: The exocrine pancreas. Proc. Symp. Kingston 1969 (BECK, SINCLAIR, Eds.), p. 59 (1971)

GROSSMAN, M.I., GREENGARD, H., IVY, A.C.: On the mechanism of the adaptation of pancreatic enzymes to dietary composition. Amer. J. Physiol. **141**, 38—41 (1944)

GROSSMAN, M.I., IVY, A.C.: Effect of alloxan upon external secretion of the pancreas. Proc. Soc. exp. Biol. (N.Y.) **63**, 62—63 (1946)

GÜNTHER, O.: Zur Ätiologie des Diabetes mellitus. Akademievorl. Berl. 1961

GUPTA, S., ELDER, J.B., KAY, A.W.: Exocrine secretory responses of the pancreas to insulin and to a meat meal in dogs. Gut **14**, 54—58 (1973)

HANSSON, E.: The formation of pancreatic juice proteins studied with labelled amino acids. Acta physiol. scand. **46**, Suppl. 161, 1—99 (1959)
HARPER, A.A.: Hormonal control of pancreatic secretion. In: Handbook Physiol. Sect. 6, Alimentary canal, Vol. II (CODE, Ed.), p. 969—995 (1967)
HARPER, A.A.: The control of pancreatic secretion. Gut **13**, 308—317 (1972)
HARPER, A.A., KIDD, C., SCRATCHERD, T.: Vago-vagal reflex effects on gastric and pancreatic secretion and gastrointestinal motility. J. Physiol. (Lond.) **148**, 417—436 (1959)
HARPER, A.A., MCKAY, I.F.S.: The effects of pancreozymin and of vagal nerve stimulation upon the histological appearance of the pancreas. J. Physiol. (Lond.) **107**, 89—96 (1948)
HAYAMA, T., MAGEE, D.F., WHITE, T.T.: Influence of autonomic nerves on the daily secretion of pancreatic juice in dogs. Ann. Surg. **158**, 290—294 (1963)
HEISLER, S., FAST, D., TENENHOUSE, A.: Role of Ca^{++} and cyclic AMP in protein secretion from rat exocrine pancreas. Biochim. biophys. Acta (Amst.) **279**, 561—572 (1972)
HENDERSON, J.R.: Why are the islets of Langerhans? Lancet **1969II**, 469—470
HERFORT, K., ŠKRHA, F., ŠOBRA, J., HEYROVSKY, A.: The exocrine pancreas in metabolic diseases. Dtsch. Z. Verdau.- u. Stoffwechselkr. **32**, 3—10 (1972)
HOKIN, L.E.: Effects of calcium omission on acetylcholine-stimulated amylase secretion and phospholipid synthesis in pigeon pancreas slices. Biochim. biophys. Acta (Amst.) **115**, 219—221 (1966)
JAMIESON, J.D.: The secretory process in the pancreatic exocrine cell: Morphologic and biochemical aspects. In: Handb. exp. Pharmakol., Vol. XXXIV: Secretin, Cholesystokinin-Pancreozymin and Gastrin (Eds. J.E. JORPES, V. MUTT), p. 195—217. Berlin-Heidelberg-New York: Springer 1973
JOHNSON, M., SHERRATT, H.S.A., CASE, R.M., SCRATCHERD, T.: The effects of secretin, pancreozymin and acetylcholine on the concentration of adenosine 3′,5′-cyclic monophosphate in cat pancreas. Biochem. J. **120**, 8P—9P (1970)
JORPES, J.E., MUTT, V.: Secretin and Cholecystokinin (CCK). In: Handb. exp. Pharmakol., Vol. XXXIV: Secretin, Cholecystokinin, Pancreozymin and Gastrin (Eds. J.E. JORPES, V. MUTT), p. 1—179. Berlin-Heidelberg-New York: Springer 1973
KANNO, T.: Calcium-dependent amylase release and electrophysiological measurements in cells of the pancreas. J. Physiol. (Lond.) **226**, 353—371 (1972)
KONTUREK, S.J., RADECKI, T., BIERNAT, J., THOR, P.: Effect of vagotomy on pancreatic secretion evoked by endogenous and exogenous cholecystokinin and caerulein. Gastroenterology **63**, 273—278 (1972)
KRAMER, M.F., TAN, H.T.: The peri-insular acini of the pancreas of the rat. Z. Zellforsch. **86**, 163—170 (1968)
LAGERLÖF, H., WELIN, G.: Pancreatic secretion after secretin during insulin hypoglycemia and after graded amounts of secretin. Acta med. scand. **91**, 397—408 (1937)
LÄHDEVIRTA, J.: Testing of exocrine function of pancreas in diabetes mellitus by use of ^{75}Se-methionine and of secretion. Acta med. scand. **182**, 345—351 (1967)
LENNINGER, S.: Effects of parasympathomimetic agents and vagal stimulation on the flow in the pancreatic duct of the cat. Acta physiol. scand. 82, 345—353 (1971)
LENNINGER, S., OHLIN, P.: The flow of juice from the pancreatic gland of the cat in response to vagal stimulation. J. Physiol. (Lond.) **216**, 303—318 (1971)
LEVINE, R.A.: The role of cyclic AMP in hepatic and gastrointestinal function. Gastroenterology **59**, 280—300 (1970)
LIN, T.M., ALPHIN, R.S.: Vagal secretory nerves for pancreatic secretion in the rat. Amer. J. Physiol. **197**, 555—557 (1959)
MAYSTON, P.D., BARROWMAN, J.A.: The influence of chronic administration of pentagastrin on the rat pancreas. Quart. J. exp. Physiol. **56**, 113—122 (1971)
MAYSTON, P.D., BARROWMAN, J.A.: Influence of chronic administration of pentagastrin on the pancreas in hypophysectomized rats. Gastroenterology **64**, 391—399 (1973)
MELMED, R.N., AGNEW, J.E., BOUCHIER, I.A.D.: The normal and abnormal pancreatic scan. Quart. J. Med. **37**, 607—624 (1968)
MORISSET, J.A., DUNNIGAN, J.: Effects of glucose, amino acids and insulin on adaptation of exocrine pancreas to diet. Proc. Soc. exp. Biol. (N.Y.) **136**, 231—234 (1971)
MORISSET, J.A., WEBSTER, P.D.: *In vitro* and *in vivo* effects of pancreozymin, urecholine, and cyclic AMP on rat pancreas. Amer. J. Physiol. **220**, 202—208 (1971)
MORISSET, J.A., WEBSTER, P.D.: Effects of fasting and feeding on protein synthesis by rat pancreas. J. clin. Invest. **51**, 1—8 (1972)
MORRIS, A.I., BESWICK, F.B., HOWAT, H.T., MORLEY, J.S.: Action of gastrin and gastrin analogues on cat stomach and pancreas. Proc. 3. Symp. Europ. Pancreatic Club, Prag, p. 42—49 (1968)
MUTT, V., JORPES, J.E.: Isolation of aspartyl-phenylalanine amide from cholecystokinin-pancreozymin. Biochem. biophys. Res. Commun. **26**, 392—397 (1967)

Palla, J.C., Ben Abdeljlil, A., Desnuelle, P.: Action de l'insuline sur la biosynthèse de l'amylase et de quelques autres enzymes du pancréas de rat. Biochim. biophys. Acta (Amst.) **158**, 25—35 (1968)

Peters, N., Dicks, A.P., Hales, C.N., Sorner, M.: Exocrine and endocrine pancreatic function in diabetes mellitus and chronic pancreatitis. Gut **7**, 277 (1966)

Peterson, H., Berstad, A.: Effect of pentagastrin on pancreatic secretion in man. Proc. 5. Symp. Europ. Pancreatic Club, p. 39 bis (1971)

Pfiffer, R.B., Stephenson, H.E., Hinton, J.W.: The effect of thoracolumbar sympathectomy and vagus section on pancreatic function in man. Ann. Surg. **136**, 585—592 (1952)

Preshaw, R.M.: Integration of nervous and hormonal mechanisms for external pancreatic secretion. In: Handb. Physiol. Sect. 6, Alimentary canal, Vol. II (Code, ed.), p. 997—1005. Washington: Amer. Physiol. Soc. 1967

Preshaw, R.M., Cooke, A.R., Grossman, M.I.: Pancreatic secretion induced by stimulation of the pyloric gland area of the stomach. Science **148**, 1347—1348 (1965a)

Preshaw, R.M., Cooke, A.R., Grossman, M.I.: Stimulation of pancreatic secretion by a humoral agent from the pyloric gland area of the stomach. Gastroenterology **49**, 617—622 (1965b)

Reggio, H.: Influence de divers traitements in vivo sur la vitesse de sécrétion de l'amylase, de la lipase et du chymotrypsinogène par des coupes de pancréas de pigeon. Biochim. biophys. Acta (Amst.) **297**, 81—92 (1973)

Ribet, A., Pascal, J.-P., Frexinos, J.: Le pancréas exocrine. La nouv. Presse méd. **1**, 2633—2640 (1972a)

Ribet, A., Pascal, J.-P., Frexinos, J.: Le pancréas exocrine. La nouv. Presse méd. **1**, 2699—2706 (1972b)

Ribet, A., Pascal, J.-P., Frexinos, J.: Le pancréas exocrine. La nouv. Presse méd. **1**, 2759—2764 (1972c)

Richardson, K.C., Young, F.G.: Histology of diabetes induced by injection of anterior-pituitary extracts. Lancet **1938I**, 1098—1101

Ridderstap, A.S., Bonting, S.L.: Enzyme secretion by the isolated rabbit pancreas: Absence of a relation with the Na-K-activated ATPase. Studies on Na-K-activated ATPase, XXVII. Pflügers Arch. **313**, 53—61 (1969)

Robberecht, P., Christophe, J.: Secretion of hydrolases by perfused fragments of rat pancreas: Effect of calcium. Amer. J. Physiol. **220**, 911—917 (1971)

Routley, E.F., Mann, F.C., Bollman, J.L., Grindlay, J.H.: Effects of vagotomy on pancreatic secretion in dogs with chronic pancreatic fistula. Surg. Gynec. Obstet. **95**, 529—536 (1952)

Rutten, W.J., de Pont, J.J.H.H.M., Bonting, S.L.: Adenylate cyclase in the rat pancreas: properties and stimulation by hormones. Biochim. biophys. Acta (Amst.) **274**, 201—213 (1972)

Scratcherd, T., Case, R.M.: The secretion of electrolytes by the pancreas. Amer. J. clin. Nutr. **26**, 326—329 (1973)

Smith, R.B., Edwards, J.P., Johnston, J.D.: Does the vagal nerve-supply to the pancreas matter in man? Brit. J. Surg. **60**, 318 (1973)

Snook, J.T.: Effect of diet, adrenalectomy, diabetes, and actinomycin D on exocrine pancreas. Amer. J. Physiol. **215**, 1329—1333 (1968)

Söling, H.D., Unger, K.O.: The role of insulin in the regulation of α-amylase synthesis in the rat pancreas. Europ. J. clin. Invest. **2**, 199—212 (1972)

Stening, G.F., Grossman, M.I.: Gastrin-related peptides as stimulants of pancreatic and gastric secretion. Amer. J. Physiol. **217**, 262—266 (1969)

Thomas, J.E., Crider, J.O.: Changes in concentration of enzymes in pancreatic juice after giving insulin. Proc. Soc. exp. Biol. (N.Y.) **64**, 27—31 (1947)

Tympner, F., Domschke, S., Domschke, W., Classen, M., Demling, L.: Exokrine Pankreasfunktion beim juvenilen Diabetes mellitus. 28. Tagung der Deutschen Gesellschaft für Verdauungs- und Stoffwechselkrankheiten, Erlangen 1973

Vacca, J.B., Henke, W.J., Knight, W.A.: The exocrine pancreas in diabetes mellitus. Ann. intern. Med. **61**, 242—247 (1964)

Vagne, M., Grossman, M.I.: Gastric and pancreatic secretion in response to gastric distension in dogs. Gastroenterology **57**, 300—310 (1969)

Webster, P.D., Singh, M., Tucker, P.C., Black, O.: Effects of fasting and feeding on the pancreas. Gastroenterology **62**, 600—605 (1972)

Wormsley, K.G., Mahoney, M.P., Ng, M.: Effect of gastrin-like pentapeptide on stomach and pancreas. Lancet **1966I**, 993—996

Youngs, G.: Hormonal control of pancreatic endocrine and exocrine secretion. Gut **13**, 154—161 (1972)

II. Action on the Mammary Gland

In considering how insulin may modify or regulate metabolic reactions in the mammary gland, several aspects have to be taken into account. In addition to altered transport of metabolites into the tissue, this hormone has effects on the production and metabolism of proteins and sugars. These effects will now be reviewed in relation to the functional state of the gland.

1. General Metabolic Alterations

When the uptake and metabolism of glucose by lactating mammary gland slices was used as the criterion, insulin was found to lead to increased glucose utilization (Balmain *et al.*, 1950, 1954; Abraham *et al.*, 1957; McLean, 1960). Similar findings were made with prelacting explants (Moretti and de Ome, 1962; Moretti and Abraham, 1966). Direct evidence of acceleration of transport is lacking but, Abraham *et al.* (1957), by measuring the glucose remaining in the outside medium, were able to substantiate increased permeation. It has also been claimed that glucose phosphorylation can be modified by insulin. In contrast to the parallel changes observed in hexokinase type II activity and to the changes in insulin sensitivity of the tissue within the lactation cycle (Walters and McLean, 1967), the capacity of the mammary gland to phosphorylate glucose via soluble hexokinase was unchanged in alloxan diabetes (Walters and McLean, 1967). Most of the mitochondria-bound hexokinase (Bartley *et al.*, 1966) had vanished, however, in both alloxan diabetes and diabetes caused by anti-insulin serum (Walters and McLean, 1968b).

Because of the strong participation of the pentose phosphate pathway in the breakdown of glucose (Abraham *et al.*, 1954; McLean, 1960; Katz and Wals, 1972), 1-^{14}C-glucose yields more $^{14}CO_2$ than the uniformly labeled sugar (Abraham *et al.*, 1957). Maximum $^{14}CO_2$ could be produced by concentrations of insulin of 200 mU/ml (Abraham *et al.*, 1957) despite the fact that the coenzyme NADP is found almost completely in the reduced state (Glock and McLean, 1955; McLean, 1958). Under the influence of insulin the percentage increase in $^{14}CO_2$ production from 1-^{14}C-glucose doubled within 3 h, as did the percentage recovery of ^{14}C in fatty acids from either 1-^{14}C- or 6-^{14}C-labeled glucose. In the latter case $^{14}CO_2$-production fell slightly (Abraham *et al.*, 1957). This effect of insulin on fatty acids is not inhibited by effective concentrations of actinomycin (Mayne and Barry, 1965). In alloxan diabetes and diabetes provoked by anti-insulin serum, the expected decrease was seen in $^{14}CO_2$ production and fatty acid labeling from labeled glucose (Walters and McLean, 1968a). This effect cannot be attributed solely to the presence of a diffusion barrier for glucose in these forms of diabetes; it appears to be more complex since an electron acceptor (such as phenazinemethosulfate (PMS)) cancels out some of the metabolic decreases. On the other hand, the same proportion of the glucose entering the mammary gland cells was channeled through the glycolytic and nonglycolytic pathways, whether they were stimulated by insulin or not (Abraham *et al.*, 1957). Similar but less conclusive data were obtained from experiments in which insulin (10 U) was applied to lactating rats during anesthesia 1 h before the extirpation of the mammary gland on the second side and compared with the previously extirpated first side (McLean, 1960). Using the sensitive method of isolated mammary cells, Martin and Baldwin (1971) reported a somewhat higher contribution of the pentose phosphate pathway to glucose metabolism under insulin stimulation (50 μU/ml). High glucose concentrations did not reduce the insulin-induced threefold increase in $^{14}CO_2$-, ^{14}C-lipid-, and ^{14}C-lactose-production from (U-^{14}C) glucose.

In contrast to lactating mammary tissue of rats, tissues from pregnant rats showed a lower level of glucose utilization (BALMAIN and FOLLEY, 1951; FOLLEY, 1956; ABRAHAM and CHAIKOFF, 1959) and a nearly complete primary deficiency in insulin sensitivity in this (BALMAIN *et al.*, 1954; MCLEAN, 1960) and other respects (BALMAIN and FOLLEY, 1951). Insulin sensitivity increased with time of incubation (MAYNE and BARRY, 1970). On day 4 of lactation, however, insulin effects were found to be highly pronounced (MCLEAN, 1960). The fate of glucose in slices of lactating rats has been carefully studied by KATZ and WALS (1972). When interpreting experiments with slices, the contribution of adipose tissue cells in the control of milk fat production (LASFARGUES, 1957) must be taken into account. However, the apparently lower content of adipose tissue in lactating glands (WRENN, LAUDER and BITMAN, 1965) and the high insulin concentration needed to elicit an effect argues against any contribution by adipose tissue.

In this situation the use of mammary gland explants of mice, first introduced by ELIAS (1957), proved to be of value (MORETTI and ABRAHAM, 1966). With incubation for up to 96 h in culture, it was found that in the prelactating state insulin[1] sensitivity develops after some delay. The behavior stimulating glucose uptake and $^{14}CO_2$ production from ^{14}C-glucose and its conversion into ^{14}C-fatty acids then resembles that of the lactation period. Insulin induction causes glucose 6-phosphate dehydrogenase and 6-phosphogluconate dehydrogenase to be increased by some 60—80%, beginning 12 h after the addition of the hormone to midpregnant or latepregnant mammary explants (LEADER and BARRY, 1969). The inductive increases in these enzymes were confirmed and extended to phosphoglucose isomerase by RIVERA and CUMMINS (1971a, b). In mature virgin explants such induction appears 1—2 days later (FRIEDBERG *et al.*, 1970).

The importance of insulin to the successful culture of mammary gland tissue has been generally emphasized (ELIAS, 1959; ELIAS and RIVERA, 1959; TROWELL, 1959; RIVERA and BERN, 1961; PROP, 1961; LASFARGUES, 1962; KOZIOROWSKA, 1962; MORETTI and DE OME, 1962). The maintenance of explants, also dependent on cortisol, shows high variability with respect to the date of pregnancy (RIVERA and BERN, 1961). Without insulin (or insulin plus cortisol) necrosis would occur (ELIAS, 1959; RIVERA and BERN, 1961; RIVERA, 1964b). Insulin therefore has been claimed to be essential for the maintenance of RNA levels in mammary tissue cultures (MAYNE and BARRY, 1967). Insulin could improve the overall metabolic state of the cells and insure cell survival by simply augmenting the supply of glucose (MORETTI and ABRAHAM, 1966). It has also been claimed that access to the cells by other hormones is enhanced in the presence of insulin (RIVERA, 1964a). The exact process has yet to be clarified exactly (for further data, see below).

Under the stimulation of hormones, including insulin, the production of short-chain fatty acids (typical for milk fat) is increased in explants of rabbit mammary (pregnant or pseudopregnant) glands (STRONG *et al.*, 1972; for mouse explants, see WANG *et al.*, 1972; MAYNE and BARRY, 1970) in addition to the higher overall incorporation of U-^{14}C-acetate into fatty acids. This effect depends largely on the action of prolactin, but in combination with it insulin increases the overall rate and improves tissue viability (FORSYTH *et al.*, 1972). To some extent synthesis of DNA and RNA is a prerequisite for hormonally stimulated fatty acid synthesis (WANG *et al.*, 1972). Similar hormonal cooperation has been claimed to influence the production of lactose in rabbit mammary explants (DELOUIS and DENAMUR, 1972). As shown by WANG *et al.* (1972), these effects are species-dependent.

---

1 In this and the following experiments with explants *in vitro*, concentrations of 5 μg/ml were used for insulin, cortisol, or prolactin.

As regards amino acid transfer, insulin stimulates the uptake of ^{14}C α-amino-isobutyric acid (AIB) into pregnant but not into mature-virgin mouse mammary explants (FRIEDBERG *et al.*, 1970). In the latter, a certain insulin sensitivity develops between 24 and 48 h of culture, and in the last hours of this period the presence of insulin is necessary for an effect (FRIEDBERG *et al.*, 1970). This time lag is shortened by use of insulin adsorbed on Sepharose (OKA and TOPPER, 1971a), which is curious. In this case, a transient contact between the particle and the cell was suggested (OKA and TOPPER, 1972a; TOPPER and OKA, 1972; TOPPER *et al.*, 1972). Recently, however, a highly active soluble form of sepharose-bound insulin was found (OKA and TOPPER, 1974). According to WANG and AMOR (1971) there is no insulin dependence on AIB at midpregnancy.

2. Specific Functional Alterations

Mammogenesis and lactogenesis are controlled by several hormones (for older literature, see NANDI and BERN, 1961; COWIE, 1969; DENAMUR, 1969, 1971). Insulin plays a part in the hormonal control of protein synthesis in the lactating gland, which produces several milk proteins (for reviews, see TURKINGTON, 1968d; TOPPER, 1970; TURKINGTON, 1972). The cooperation of insulin, cortisol (hydrocortisone)[2] and prolactin (mammotropin), probably stemming from the alveolar secretory cell membrane (BIRKINSHAW and FALCONER, 1972), in minimal effective concentrations of 3×10^{-7}M, 10^{-8} and 10^{-8}M, respectively (STOCKDALE *et al.*, 1966; see also RIVERA, 1964b) has been studied by the mammary gland organ-culture technique. Their combined action elicits the appearance of alveolar secretion in midpregnant mouse tissue (ELIAS, 1959; RIVERA and BERN, 1961; JUERGENS *et al.*, 1965; MAYNE *et al.*, 1968). Maintenance of human explants in hormone-free media is described (CEREANI *et al.*, 1972). If explants of virgin-mouse tissue are given early exposure to prolactin *in vivo* or *in vitro*, the tissue is stimulable like midpregnant tissue (VONDERHAAR *et al.*, 1973). In this case a critical mitosis must be reached (OWENS *et al.*, 1973). It seems, that prolactin, though not itself mitogenic, renders the mammary epithelium sensitive to the mitogenic action of insulin or serum (OKA and TOPPER, 1972b). In comparison with the situation *in vivo*, the findings of MUKHERJEE *et al.* (1973) lend support to the proposed permissive role of insulin in maintaining the mitotic action of prolactin. Thus, in alloxan-diabetic rats, insulin deficiency lasting several days induced no detectable difference with respect to normal mammary labulo-alveolar development under the effect of prolactin and growth hormone (SUD, 1971) but interrupted the maintenance of lactation in the rat (SUD, 1972). The importance of prolactin was stressed by DILLEY (1971) for whole mammary glands in culture. In midpregnant animals receiving insulin alone, there were no alterations in epithelial cytology and no increase in casein synthesis (STOCKDALE *et al.*, 1966; JUERGENS *et al.*, 1965). The synthesis of milk proteins (JUERGENS *et al.*, 1965; LOCKWOOD *et al.*, 1966) and especially of casein-like phosphoproteins is stimulated by insulin together with cortisol and prolactin (TURKINGTON *et al.*, 1965), as shown by phosphate-32 incorporation, the last, rapid insulin-dependent step in casein synthesis (TURKINGTON and TOPPER, 1966; VOYTOVICH *et al.*, 1969). When ^{14}C-labeled amino acids are used as precursors, the unspecific *in vitro* stimulation by insulin of non-milk protein derived from epithelial cells (most likely a reflection of cell proliferation) contrasts with the far more pronounced stimulation of whey proteins (α-lactalbumin, β-lactoglobulin and casein) (LOCKWOOD *et al.*, 1966; LOCKWOOD *et al.*, 1967;

2 In this respect, cortisol can be replaced by corticosterone or aldosterone (RIVERA, 1964a, b; TURKINGTON *et al.*, 1967; OKA and TOPPER, 1971b).

Turkington *et al.*, 1967) found after the addition of cortisol and prolactin, which can reach 200—400% of the initial value. The special feature of the role of insulin, as pointed out by Stockdale and Topper (1966), is that by stimulating DNA synthesis it provides the basis for the initiation of casein synthesis, which follows 30 h later. The same holds true for specific enzyme-protein synthesis. As far as proteins A and B (= α-lactalbumin) of lactose synthetase (UDP-galactose: D-glucose 1-galactosyltransferase, EC2.4.1.22) are concerned, insulin is necessary before prolactin can elicit its special role as inducer (Turkington *et al.*, 1968). In midpregnant mouse explants the induction of A and B units is initiated fairly early in the presence of all three hormones (Palmiter, 1969a). Some modifications *in vivo* are attributed to interference by progesterone (Turkington and Hill, 1969).

To sum up briefly, insulin interferes in the overall changes in cell function (differentiation) by altering some environmental factors that are intimately associated with cell proliferation, as first proposed by Prop and Hendrix (1965) and Stockdale and Topper (1966). Numerically, the cells double (Mills and Topper, 1970) and are indistinguishable from other epithelial parent cells (Mills and Topper, 1969). This does not exclude the need for insulin at a later stage, e.g. for the phase after mitosis (G_1) (Lockwood *et al.*, 1967).

Several observations shed some light on how insulin stimulates DNA synthesis and cell proliferation in the "first conversion phase" in the mammary gland. A primary event seems to be accelerated protein synthesis (Marzluff *et al.*, 1969). Thus, suppression of protein synthesis has been reported to lead to reduced synthesis of DNA (Turkington, 1968a; Wang and Amor, 1971) and of DNA polymerase (Lockwood *et al.*, 1967). Then synthesis of DNA and histone follows coordinately about 12 h after insulin and lasts for at least 3 days (Marzluff *et al.*, 1969; for further data, see Stockdale and Topper, 1966; Lockwood *et al.*, 1967; Stockdale *et al.*, 1966; Turkington and Topper, 1967; Turkington, 1968a; Palmiter, 1969b; El Darwish and Rivera, 1970; Mayne and Barry, 1970; Koyama *et al.*, 1972). In this case, too, neither cortisol nor prolactin, nor both together, can induce changes to the same extent as insulin alone. Addition of prolactin, however, prolongs the duration of the period of DNA stimulation (Mayne and Barry, 1970) as one would expect from its own growth-promoting properties in this rat tissue (Dilley and Nandi, 1968). For several reasons the insulin effect on DNA synthesis is independent of glucose transport (Turkington *et al.*, 1967; Lockwood *et al.*, 1967). For time course and dependency on insulin, glucose and amino acids, see Skarda *et al.* (1971). Concomitantly with DNA synthesis, DNA polymerase is increased (Lockwood *et al.*, 1967). No preponderance of any particular histone fraction was found. On the other hand, nuclei of pre-incubated mammary gland explants of mice showed a 3-fold increase (maximal in 8 h) of DNA-dependent RNA polymerase activity by insulin; prolactin however stimulated RNA synthesis and polymerase activity only after previous incubation with insulin and cortisol (Turkington and Ward, 1969). This insulin-mediated effect was independent of glucose transport, since it persisted when fructose was substituted for glucose.

As expected, RNA synthesis in the mammary gland is stimulated by insulin (Mayne *et al.*, 1966, 1968; Stockdale *et al.*, 1966; Turkington and Ward, 1969; Palmiter, 1969a, b; Green and Topper, 1970; Mayne and Barry, 1970), as revealed by incorporation of ^{3}H- or ^{14}C-uridine or ^{14}C-adenine into RNA of mouse explants or rat slices. The effect on RNA starts immediately (Mayne *et al.*, 1966; Palmiter, 1969b), but some data are subject to correction because insulin appears to increase the precursor label in both cases, whether uridine (Rivera and Cum-

MINS, 1972) or adenine (MAYNE and BARRY, 1970) is used. Stimulation of RNA synthesis by insulin is more pronounced in pregnant than in lactating tissues (MAYNE *et al.*, 1966). Under these conditions, a similar time course and extent is provoked by the incorporation of leucine into tissue proteins. Studies with isolated mammary cells and Sepharose-bound insulin and/or prolactin show that these hormones elicit RNA synthesis from the cell membrane (TURKINGTON, 1970a).

Parallel with the increased incorporation of precursors into RNA, especially into preribosomal and ribosomal RNA (TURKINGTON, 1970b), found soon after the addition of insulin to mammary gland explants, there is also an increase in RNA polymerase (TURKINGTON and WARD, 1969; TURKINGTON and RIDDLE, 1969), RNA methylase (TURKINGTON, 1969), and in the phosphorylation of nuclear proteins (TURKINGTON and RIDDLE, 1969) and histone fractions (TURKINGTON and RIDDLE, 1969). Under the same conditions, increased labeling of histones by labeled amino acids follows about 4 h later (after increased phosphorylation (TURKINGTON and RIDDLE, 1969). With respect to the time course this coincides with increased DNA synthesis.

Both uridine incorporation into RNA and nuclear protein phosphorylation are markedly reduced by actinomycin D. Thus it appears that insulin interferes at the level of transcription (TURKINGTON and RIDDLE, 1969). On the other hand, the total number of ribosomes (monosomes and polysomes) increased under the influence of insulin on mammary gland explants (TURKINGTON and RIDDLE, 1970).

Morphologically, the increased DNA synthesis due to insulin, as revealed by thymidine incorporation, is paralleled by mitotic indices in the epithelium (STOCKDALE and TOPPER, 1966), autoradiography (STOCKDALE *et al.*, 1966; TURKINGTON, 1968a), and comparison of intact with de-epithelialized explants (LOCKWOOD *et al.*, 1967). As with other insulin-stimulated reactions, this effect, too, is retarded in mature-virgin mammary explants (TURKINGTON, 1968a; FRIEDBERG *et al.*, 1970) and is more pronounced than in midpregnant ones (TURKINGTON, 1968a). Colchicine renders the postmitotic G_1 phase susceptible to insulin-initiated DNA synthesis (TURKINGTON, 1968a). This role of insulin is understood to be permissive for several reasons (PALMITER, 1969b). Suppression of DNA synthesis by androgens (TURKINGTON and TOPPER, 1967) or suppression of mitosis by colchicine (STOCKDALE and TOPPER, 1966) therefore interrupts insulin-mediated proliferation.

Another aspect more closely related to the membrane interaction of insulin is the fact that two protein kinases (WADDY and MACKINLEY, 1971), designated as protein kinases I and II, and the cAMP-binding protein related to them were recovered from cultured mammary epithelial cells (MAJUMDER and TURKINGTON, 1971a, b). Addition of insulin to isolated mammary epithelial cells induced a stimulation of both protein kinase and cAMP-binding protein at 16 h of incubation (MAJUMDER and TURKINGTON, 1971b). The term induction seems justified here, because actinomycin D or cycloheximide inhibit this action of insulin. On the other hand, prolactin induces kinases and binding-protein rapidly, coordinately, and synergistically with insulin (MAJUMDER and TURKINGTON, 1971b). The action of cortisol is not necessary.

As a consequence within few hours insulin stimulates membrane and ribosomal phosphorylation by 120—160% with a maximum at 16 h (MAJUMDER and TURKINGTON, 1972). Similarly, prolactin stimulates this type of phosphorylation if explants are treated for 72 h with insulin and cortisol. The time course seems to be more rapid (maximal at 8 h) and is due to newly formed cells because colchicine inhibits this prolactin effect (MAJUMDER and TURKINGTON, 1972).

Once cell proliferation has been induced by insulin, cortisol is needed for building up the rough endoplasmic reticulum of mammary alveolar epithelial cells (Mills and Topper, 1969) and especially for the distribution of ribosomes into the membranes of rough endoplasmic reticulum (Oka and Topper, 1971b). Afterwards prolactin is necessary for the conversion of these cells into secretory cells (Lockwood *et al.*, 1967) and for the subsequent production of casein and α-lactalbumin and β-lactoglobulin (Turkington *et al.*, 1967).

In this postmitotic phase prolactin supported by insulin stimulates RNA synthesis (Turkington, 1968b, c; Turkington and Ward, 1969; Palmiter, 1969a; Turkington and Riddle, 1969; Green and Topper, 1970; Turkington, 1970b; Green *et al.*, 1971; Rillema, 1973) especially pre-ribosomal and ribosomal RNA (Turkington, 1970b), as reflected in the somewhat higher intracellular concentrations of ribosomes and polysomes (Turkington and Riddle, 1970), of tRNA and its aminoacyl acceptor activity (Turkington, 1969), and of total cellular RNA (Turkington, 1968b, c). In the presence of insulin, the phosphorylation of nuclear proteins and several histone fractions is also stimulated (Turkington and Riddle, 1969). According to Voytovich *et al.* (1969), the presence of insulin is necessary only for the very last hours of the postmitotic incubation period as measured by the ^{32}P-labeling of casein, which as the last step is presumably localized in the Golgi apparatus (Bingham *et al.*, 1972).

Independently of insulin, prolactin induces protein kinase and cAMP-binding protein in epithelial cells (Majumder and Turkington, 1971b). For the time course of events, see Oka and Topper (1971b).

Specific milk protein synthesis, as an expression of secretory responses, is attained as mentioned earlier; several other enzyme activities found to be increased (Jones and Forsyth, 1969; Leader and Barry, 1969) reflect general alterations toward normal lactation (Baldwin and Milligan, 1966; Gumaa *et al.*, 1973), most of which are prevented by addition of DBcAMP to the explants (Sapag-Hagar *et al.*, 1974). For earlier inductive effects of insulin alone, see above: (Leader and Barry, 1969).

A new method for the preparation of parenchymal cells of bovine mammary gland using collagenase and density-gradient centrifugation (Pitelka *et al.*, 1969) enabled favorable comparisons to be made between enzymatic and metabolic data (Abraham *et al.*, 1972). The hormonal aspects have been little studied until now. O'Keefe and Cuatrecasas (1974) also found insulin receptors irrespective of whether the cells derived from virgin or pregnant animals.

Because of the clearcut sequential hormonal influence on cell alteration toward its main (i.e. secretory) function, the mammary gland has been a valuable model for the study of cytodifferentiation and epithelial development.

As far as mammary carcinoma cells are concerned, hormonal control by insulin is limited. Glucose uptake, unlike that in normal mammary explants, is not stimulated by insulin in 5-day cultures of spontaneous mammary tumor (Moretti and De Ome, 1962), though a very early enhancement of glycolysis by insulin is reported (Woods and Vlahakis, 1974). Pre-neoplastic hyperplastic alveolar nodules (HAN) differ from these tumors in that they react to some extent to hormonal influences. Elias and Rivera (1959) have found data that support the stepwise decrease of hormone dependence in the development of mammary neoplasms. Cultures of mammary epithelial tumor likewise show increased cell attachment properties for serum and insulin (Hosick and Nandi, 1974).

References

ABRAHAM, S., CADY, P., CHAIKOFF, I.L.: Effect of insulin *in vitro* on pathways of glucose utilization, other than Embden-Meyerhof, in rat mammary gland. J. biol. Chem. **224**, 955—962 (1957)

ABRAHAM, S., CHAIKOFF, I.L.: Glycolytic pathways and lipogenesis in mammary glands of lactating and non-lactating normal rats. J. biol. Chem. **234**, 2246—2253 (1959)

ABRAHAM, S., HIRSCH, P.F., CHAIKOFF, I.L.: The quantitative significance of glycolysis and non-glycolysis in glucose utilization by rat mammary gland. J. biol. Chem. **211**, 31—38 (1954)

ABRAHAM, S., KERKOF, P.R., SMITH, S.: Characteristics of cells dissociated from mouse mammary gland. II. Metabolic and enzymatic activities of parenchymal cells from lactating glands. Biochim. biophys. Acta (Amst.) **261**, 205—218 (1972)

BALDWIN, R.L., MILLIGAN, L.P.: Enzymatic changes associated with the initiation and maintenance of lactation in the rat. J. biol. Chem. **241**, 2058—2066 (1966)

BALMAIN, J.H., FOLLEY, S.F.: Further observations on the *in vitro* stimulation by insulin of fat synthesis by lactating mammary gland slices. Biochem. J. **49**, 663—670 (1951)

BALMAIN, J.H., FOLLEY, S.F., GLASCOCK, R.F.: Relative utilization of glucose and acetate carbon for lipogenesis by mammary-gland slices, studied with tritium, ^{13}C and ^{14}C. Biochem. J. **56**, 234—239 (1954)

BALMAIN, J.H., FRENCH, T.H., FOLLEY, S.J.: Stimulation by insulin of *in vitro* fat synthesis by lactating mammary gland slices. Nature (Lond.) **165**, 807—808 (1950)

BARTLEY, J.C., ABRAHAM, S., CHAIKOFF, I.L.: Activity of several enzymes of liver, adipose tissue, and mammary gland of virgin pregnant and lactating mice. Proc. Soc. exp. Biol. (N.Y.) **123**, 670—675 (1966)

BINGHAM, E.W., FARRELL, H.M., BASCH, J.J.: Phosphorylation of casein. Role of the Golgi apparatus. J. biol. Chem. **247**, 8193—8194 (1972)

BIRKINSHAW, U., FALCONER, I.R.: The localization of prolactin labelled with radioactive iodine in rabbit mammary tissue. J. Endocr. **55**, 323—334 (1972)

CERIANI, R.L., CONTESSO, G.P., NATAF, B.M.: Hormone requirement for growth and differentiation of the human mammary gland in organ culture. Cancer Res. **32**, 2190—2196 (1972)

COWIE, A.T.: General hormonal factors involved in lactogenesis. In: Lactogenesis (REYNOLDS, FOLLEY, S.J., Eds.), p. 157—169. Philadelphia: University Press 1969

DELOUIS, C., DENAMUR, R.: Induction of lactose synthesis by prolactin in rabbit mammary gland explants. J. Endocr. **52**, 311—319 (1972)

DENAMUR, R.: Comparative aspects of hormonal control in lactogenesis. In: Progress in Endocrinology. Proc. III. Int. Congr. Endocrinol. Int. Congr. Series, No. 184, Excerpta Medica Found., p. 959—972 (1969)

DENAMUR, R.: Hormonal control of lactogenesis. J. Dairy Res. **38**, 237—264 (1971)

DILLEY, W.G.: Morphogenic and mitogenic effects of prolactin on rat mammary gland *in vitro*. Endocrinology **88**, 514—517 (1971)

DILLEY, W.G., NANDI, S.: Rat mammary gland differentiation *in vitro* in the absence of steroids. Science **161**, 59—60 (1968)

EL-DARWISH, I., RIVERA, E.M.: Temporal effects of hormones on DNA synthesis in mouse mammary gland *in vitro*. J. exp. Zool. **173**, 285—291 (1970)

ELIAS, J.J.: Cultivation of adult mouse mammary gland in hormone-enriched synthetic medium. Science **126**, 842—843 (1957)

ELIAS, J.J.: Effect of insulin and cortisol on organ cultures of adult mouse mammary glands. Proc. Soc. exp. Biol. (N.Y.) **101**, 500—502 (1959)

ELIAS, J.J., RIVERA, E.M.: Comparison of the responses to normal, precancerous and neoplastic mouse mammary tissues to hormones *in vitro*. Cancer Res. **19**, 505—511 (1959)

FOLLEY, S.J.: The physiology and biochemistry of lactation, p. 93—118. Springfield/Ill.: Ch. C. Thomas 1956

FORSYTH, I.A., STRONG, C.R., DILS, R.: Interactions of insulin, corticosterone and prolactin in promoting milk-fat synthesis by mammary explants from pregnant rabbits. Biochem. J. **129**, 929—935 (1972)

FRIEDBERG, S.H., OKA, T., TOPPER, I.J.: Development of insulin sensitivity by mouse mammary gland *in vitro*. Proc. nat. Acad. Sci. (Wash.) **67**, 1493—1500 (1970)

GLOCK, G., MCLEAN, P.: Levels of oxidized and reduced diphosphopyridine nucleotide and triphosphopyridine nucleotide in animal tissues. Biochem. J. **61**, 388—390 (1955)

GREEN, M.R., BUNTING, S.L., PEACOCK, A.C.: Changes in labeling pattern of ribonucleic acid from mammary tissue as a result of hormone treatment. Biochemistry **10**, 2366—2371 (1971)

Green, M.R., Topper, Y.J.: Some effects of prolactin, insulin and hydrocortisone on RNA synthesis by mouse mammary gland *in vitro*. Biochim. biophys. Acta (Amst.) **204**, 441—448 (1970)

Gumaa, K.A., Greenbaum, A.L., McLean, P.: Adaptive changes in satellite systems related to lipogenesis in rat and sheep mammary gland and in adipose tissue. Europ. J. Biochem. **34**, 188—198 (1973)

Hosick, H.L., Nandi, S.: Plating and Maintenance of Epithelial Tumor Cells in Primary Culture: Interacting Roles of Serum and Insulin. Exp. Cell Res. **84**, 419—425 (1974)

Jones, E.A., Forsyth, I.A.: Increases in the enzyme activity of mouse mammary explants induced by prolactin. J. Endocr. **43**, 41—43 (1969)

Juergens, W.G., Stockdale, F.E., Topper, Y.J., Elias, J.J.: Hormone-dependent differentiation of mammary gland *in vitro*. Proc. nat. Acad. Sci. (Wash.) **54**, 629—634 (1965)

Katz, J., Wals, P.A.: Pentose cycle and reducing equivalents in rat mammary-gland slices. Biochem. J. **128**, 879—899 (1972)

Koyama, H., Sinka, D., Dao, T.L.: Effects of hormones and 7,12-dimethyl benz(a)anthracene on rat mammary tissue grown in organ culture. Nat. Cancer Inst. Monogr. **48**, 1671—1680 (1972)

Koziorowska, J.: The influence of ovarian hormones and insulin on the mouse mammary glands cultivated *in vitro*. Acta med. pol. **3**, 237—245 (1962)

Lasfargues, E.Y.: Cultivation and behaviour *in vitro* of the normal mammary epithelium of the adult mouse. II. Observations on the secretory activity. Exp. Cell Res. **13**, 553—562 (1957)

Lasfargues, E.Y.: Concerning the role of insulin in the differentiation and functional activity of mouse mammary tissues. Exp. Cell Res. **28**, 531—542 (1962)

Leader, D.P., Barry, J.M.: Increase in activity of glucose 6-phosphate dehydrogenase in mouse mammary tissue cultured with insulin. Biochem. J. **113**, 175—182 (1969)

Lockwood, D.H., Stockdale, F.E., Topper, Y.J.: Hormone-dependent differentiation of mammary gland: Sequence of action of hormones in relation to cell cycle. Science **156**, 545—546 (1967)

Lockwood, D.H., Turkington, R.W., Topper, Y.J.: Hormone-dependent development of milk protein synthesis in mammary gland *in vitro*. Biochim. biophys. Acta (Amst.) **130**, 493—501 (1966)

Lockwood, D.H., Voytovich, A.E., Stockdale, F.E., Topper, Y.J.: Insulin-dependent DNA polymerase and DNA synthesis in mammary epithelial cells *in vitro*. Proc. nat. Acad. Sci. (Wash.) **58**, 658—664 (1967)

Majumder, G.C., Turkington, R.W.: Hormonal regulation of protein kinases and adenosine 3′,5′-monophosphate-binding protein in developing mammary gland. J. biol. Chem. **246**, 5546—5554 (1971a)

Majumder, G.C., Turkington, R.W.: Stimulation of mammary epithelial cell proliferation *in vitro* by protein factor(s) present in serum. Endocrinology **88**, 1506—1510 (1971b)

Majumder, G.C., Turkington, R.W.: Hormone-dependent phosphorylation of ribosomal and plasma membrane proteins in mouse mammary gland *in vitro*. J. biol. Chem. **247**, 7207—7217 (1972)

Martin, R.J., Baldwin, R.L.: Effects of insulin on isolated rat mammary cell metabolism. Glucose utilization and metabolite pattern. Endocrinology **89**, 1263—1269 (1971)

Marzluff, W.F., McCarty, K.S., Turkington, R.W.: Insulin-dependent synthesis of histones in relation to the mammary epithelial cell cycle. Biochim. biophys. Acta (Amst.) **190**, 517—526 (1969)

Mayne, R., Barry, J.M.: Actinomycin D does not inhibit the stimulation by insulin of fatty synthesis in mammary gland slices. Biochim. biophys. Acta (Amst.) **107**, 160—162 (1965)

Mayne, R., Barry, J.M.: Insulin maintains the level of RNA in mammary tissue cultures. Biochim. biophys. Acta (Amst.) **138**, 195—197 (1967)

Mayne, R., Barry, J.M.: Biochemical changes during development of mouse mammary tissue in organ culture. J. Endocr. **46**, 61—70 (1970)

Mayne, R., Barry, J.M., Rivera, E.M.: Stimulation by insulin of the formation of ribonucleic acid and protein by mammary tissues *in vitro*. Biochem. J. **99**, 688—693 (1966)

Mayne, R., Forsyth, I.A., Barry, J.M.: Stimulation by hormones of RNA and protein formation in organ cultures of the mammary glands of pregnant mice. J. Endocr. **41**, 247—253 (1968)

McLean, P.: Carbohydrate metabolism of mammary tissue. II. Levels of oxidised and reduced diphosphopyridine nucleotide and triphosphopyridine nucleotide in the rat mammrary gland. Biochim. biophys. Acta (Amst.) **30**, 316—324 (1958)

McLean, P.: Carbohydrate metabolism of mammary tissue. III. Factors in the regulation of pathways of glucose catabolism in the mammary gland of the rat. Biochim. biophys. Acta (Amst.) **37**, 296—309 (1960)

Mills, E.S., Topper, Y.J.: Mammary alveolar epithelial cells: Effect of hydrocortisone on ultrastructure. Science **165**, 1127—1128 (1969)

Mills, E.S., Topper, Y.J.: Some ultrastructural effects of insulin hydrocortisone and prolactin on mammary gland explants. J. Cell Biol. **44**, 310—328 (1970)

Moretti, R.L., Abraham, S.: Effects of insulin on glucose metabolism by explants of mouse mammary gland maintained in organ culture. Biochim. biophys. Acta (Amst.) **124**, 280—288 (1966)

Moretti, R.L., de Ome, K.B.: Effect of insulin on glucose uptake by normal and neoplastic mouse mammary tissues in organ cultures. J. nat. Cancer Inst. **29**, 321—329 (1962)

Mukherjee, A.S., Washburn, L.L., Banerjee, M.R.: Role of insulin as a "permissive" hormone in mammary gland development. Nature (Lond.) **246**, 159—160 (1973)

Nandi, S., Bern, H.A.: The hormones responsible for lactogenesis in BALB/cCrGl mice. Gen. comp. Endocr. **1**, 195—210 (1961)

Oka, T., Topper, Y.J.: Insulin-Sepharose and the dynamics of insulin action. Proc. nat. Acad. Sci. (Wash.) **68**, 2066—2068 (1971a)

Oka, T., Topper, Y.J.: Hormone-dependent accumulation of rough endoplasmic reticulum in mouse mammary epithelial cells *in vitro*. J. biol. Chem. **246**, 7701—7707 (1971b)

Oka, T., Topper, Y.J.: Dynamics of insulin action on mammary epithelium. Nature New Biology **239**, 216—217 (1972a)

Oka, T., Topper, Y.J.: Is prolactin mitogenic for mammary epithelium ? Proc. nat. Acad. Sci. (Wash.) **69**, 1693—1696 (1972b)

Oka, T., Topper, J.I.: A soluble super-active form of insulin. Proc. nat. Acad. Sci. (Wash.) **71**, 1630—1633 (1974)

O'Keefe, E., Cuatrecasas, P.: Insulin receptors in murine mammary cells: Comparison in pregnant and nonpregnant animals. Biochim. biophys. Acta (Amst.) **343**, 64—77 (1974)

Owens, I.S., Vonderhaar, B.K., Topper, Y.J.: Concerning the necessary coupling of development to proliferation of mouse mammary epithelial cells. J. biol. Chem. **248**, 472—477 (1973)

Palmiter, R.D.: Hormonal induction and regulation of lactose synthetase in mouse mammary gland. Biochem. J. **113**, 409—417 (1966a)

Palmiter, R.D.: Early macromolecular syntheses in cultured mammary tissue from mid-pregnant mice. Endocrinology **85**, 747—751 (1969b)

Pitelka, D.R., Kerkof, P.R., Garné, H.T., Smith, S., Abraham, S.: Characteristics of cells dissociated from mouse mammary glands. I. Methods of separation and morphology of parenchymal cells from lactating glands. Exp. Cell Res. **57**, 43—62 (1969)

Prop, F.J.: Sensitivity to prolactin of mouse mammary glands *in vitro*. Exp. Cell Res. **24**, 629—631 (1961)

Prop, F.J.A., Hendrix, S.E.A.M.: Effect of insulin on mitotic rate in organ cultures of total mammary glands of the mouse. Exp. Cell Res. **40**, 277—281 (1965)

Rillema, J.A.: Early actions of prolactin on uridine metabolism in mammary gland explants. Endocrinology **92**, 1673—1679 (1973)

Rivera, E.M.: Interchangeability of adrenocortical hormones in initiating mammary secretion *in vitro*. Proc. Soc. exp. Biol. (N.Y.) **116**, 568—572 (1964a)

Rivera, E.M.: Differential responsiveness to hormones of C3H and A mouse mammary tissues in organ culture. Endocrinology **74**, 853—864 (1964b)

Rivera, E.M., Bern, H.A.: Influence of insulin on maintenance and secretory stimulation of mouse mammary tissues by hormones in organ culture. Endocrinology **69**, 340—353 (1961)

Rivera, E.M., Cummins, E.P.: Differential actions of insulin on enzyme activities in mammary organ culture. J. cell. Physiol. **77**, 175—178 (1971a)

Rivera, E.M., Cummins, E.P.: Hormonal induction of dehydrogenase enzymes in mammary gland *in vitro*. Gen. comp. Endocr. **17**, 319—326 (1971b)

Rivera, E.M., Cummins, E.P.: Insulin stimulation of uridine incorporation into acid-soluble and acid-insoluble ribonucleotides of mammary gland explants. J. Endocr. **52**, 205—206 (1972)

Sapag-Hagar, M., Greenbaum, A.L., Lewis, D.J., Hallowes, R.C.: The effects of Dibutyryl cAMP on enzymatic and metabolic changes in explants of rat mammary tissue. Biochem. biophys. Res. Commun. **59**, 261—268 (1974)

Skarda, J., Green, C.D., Barry, J.M.: Initiation of deoxyribonucleic acid replication in mammary-gland organ cultures. Biochem. J. **124**, 65P (1971)

Stockdale, F.E., Juergens, W.G., Topper, Y.J.: A histological and biochemical study of hormone-dependent differentiation of mammary gland tissue *in vitro*. Develop. Biol. **13**, 266—281 (1966)

Stockdale, F.E., Topper, Y.J.: The role of DNA synthesis and mitosis in hormone-dependent differentiation. Proc. nat. Acad. Sci. (Wash.) **56**, 1283—1289 (1966)

Strong, C.R., Forsyth, I.A., Dils, R.: The effects of hormones on milk-fat synthesis in mammary explants from pseudopregnant rabbits. Biochem. J. **128**, 509—519 (1972)

Sud, S.C.: Importance of insulin for mammary growth. Indian J. exp. Biol. **9**, 307—311 (1971)

Sud, S.C.: Effect of alloxan diabetes on the lactational performance in rats. Indian J. exp. Biol. **10** 389—390 (1972)

Topper, Y.J.: Multiple hormone interactions in the development of mammary gland *in vitro*. Recent Progr. Hormone Res. **26**, 287—308 (1970)

Topper, Y.J., Oka, T.: Insulin and the mammary epithelium cell membrane. In: The Role of Membranes in Metabolic Regulation (M.A. Mehlmann, R.W. Hanson, Eds.), p. 341—347. New York: Academic Press 1972

Topper, Y.J., Oka, T., Owens, I.S., Vonderhaar, B.K.: Some aspects of mouse mammary gland development from maturity to early pregnancy. In vitro **8**, 228—234 (1972)

Trowell, O.A.: The culture of mature organs in a synthetic medium. Exp. Cell Res. **16**, 118—147 (1959)

Turkington, R.W.: Hormone-induced synthesis of DNA by mammary gland *in vitro*. Endocrinology **82**, 540—546 (1968a)

Turkington, R.W.: Induction of milk protein synthesis by placental lactogen and prolactin *in vitro*. Endocrinology **82**, 575—583 (1968b)

Turkington, R.W.: Inhibition of casein turnover by hydrocortisone during mammary gland differentiation *in vitro*. Biochim. biophys. Acta (Amst.) **158**, 274—280 (1968c)

Turkington, R.W.: Hormone-dependent differentiation of mammary gland *in vitro*. In: Curr. Top. Dev. Biol. (Moscona, Monroy, Eds.), Vol. **3**, p. 199—218 (1968 d)

Turkington, R.W.: Multiple hormonal interactions. The mammary gland. In: Biochemical Actions of Hormones, Vol. 2 (Ed. Litwack), p. 55—80. New York, London: Academic Press 1972

Turkington, R.W.: Hormonal regulation of transfer ribonucleic acid and transfer ribonucleic acid-methylating enzymes during development of the mouse mammary gland. J. biol. Chem. **244**, 5140—5148 (1969)

Turkington, R.W.: Hormonal regulation of rapidly labeled ribonucleic acid in mammary cells *in vitro*. J. biol. Chem. **245**, 6690—6697 (1970a)

Turkington, R.W.: Stimulation of RNA synthesis in isolated mammary cells by insulin and prolactin bound to Sepharose. Biochem. biophys. Res. Commun. **41**, 1362—1367 (1970b)

Turkington, R.W., Brew, K., Vanaman, T.C., Hill, R.L.: The hormonal control of lactose synthetase in the developing mouse mammary gland. J. biol. Chem. **243**, 3382—3387 (1968)

Turkington, R.W., Hill, R.L.: Lactose synthetase: progesterone inhibition of the induction of α-lactalbumin. Science **163**, 1458—1460 (1969)

Turkington, R.W., Juergens, W.G., Topper, Y.J.: Hormone-dependent synthesis of casein *in vitro*. Biochim. biophys. Acta (Amst.) **111**, 573—576 (1965)

Turkington, R.W., Juergens, W.G., Topper, Y.J.: Steroid structural requirements for mammary gland differentiation *in vitro*. Endocrinology **80**, 1139—1142 (1967)

Turkington, R.W., Lockwood, D.H., Topper, Y.J.: The induction of milk protein synthesis in post-mitotic mammary epithelial cells exposed to prolactin. Biochim. biophys. Acta (Amst.) **148**, 475—480 (1967)

Turkington, R.W., Riddle, M.: Hormone-dependent phosphorylation of nuclear proteins during mammary gland differentiation *in vitro*. J. biol. Chem. **244**, 6040—6046 (1969)

Turkington, R.W., Riddle, M.: Hormone-dependent formation of polysomes in mammary cells *in vitro*. J. biol. Chem. **245**, 5145—5152 (1970)

Turkington, R.W., Topper, Y.J.: Casein biosynthesis: evidence for phosphorylation of precursor proteins. Biochim. biophys. Acta (Amst.) **127**, 366—372 (1966)

Turkington, R.W., Topper, Y.J.: Androgen inhibition of mammary gland differentiation *in vitro*. Endocrinology **80**, 329—336 (1967)

Turkington, R.W., Ward, O.T.: Hormonal stimulation of RNA polymerase in mammary gland *in vitro*. Biochim. biophys. Acta (Amst.) **174**, 291—301 (1969)

Vonderhaar, B.K., Owens, I.S., Topper, Y.J.: An early effect of prolactin on the formation of α-lactalbumin by mouse mammary epithelial cells. J. biol. Chem. **248**, 467—471 (1973)

Voytovich, A.E., Owens, I.S., Topper, Y.J.: A novel action of insulin on phosphoprotein formation by mammary gland explants. Proc. nat. Acad. Sci. (Wash.) **63**, 213—217 (1969)

Waddy, C.T., Mackinlay, A.G.: Protein kinase activity from lactating bovine mammary gland. Biochim. biophys. Acta (Amst.) **250**, 491—500 (1971)

Walters, E., McLean, P.: Multiple forms of glucose adenosine triphosphate phosphotransferase in rat mammary gland. Biochem. J. **104**, 778—783 (1967)

Walters, E., McLean, P.: Effect of alloxan-diabetes and treatment with anti-insulin serum on pathways of glucose metabolism in lactating rat mammary gland. Biochem. J. **109**, 407—417 (1968a)

Walters, E., McLean, P.: The effect of anti-insulin serum and alloxan diabetes on the distribution and multiple forms of hexokinase in lactating rat mammary gland. Biochem. J. **109**, 737—741 (1968b)

Wang, D. Y., Amor, V.: A study on the effect of insulin on DNA, RNA and protein synthesis in mouse mammary gland tissue in organ culture. J. Endocr. **50**, 241—249 (1971)

Wang, D. Y., Halloweg, R. C., Bealing, J., Strong, C. R., Dils, R.: The effect of prolactin and growth hormone on fatty acid synthesis by pregnant mouse mammary gland in organ culture. J. Endocr. **53**, 311—321 (1972)

Woods, M. W., Vlahakis, G.: Immediate Effects on Insulin and Anti-Insulins on Glycolysis in Spontaneous Mammary Tumors in Mice. J. nat. Cancer Inst. **52**, 579—582 (1974)

Wrenn, T. R., Lauder, W. R., Bitman, J.: Rat mammary gland composition during pregnancy and lactation. J. Dairy Sci. **48**, 1517—1521 (1965)

III. Action on the Crystalline Lens

1. Diabetic and Sugar Cataract

Interest leading to studies of the influence of insulin on the crystalline lens arose from the fact that in diabetes mellitus, i.e. in long-lasting hyperglycemia, there is a high incidence of cataract (Caird *et al.*, 1964). Similar findings were made in experimental alloxan diabetes (Naidoff *et al.*, 1955). At the present time the common mechanism for all sugar cataracts is thought to be the high concentration of glucose, galactose, or xylose (found initially in the aqueous humor) and of these sugars and their metabolites (van Heyningen, 1959) in the lens (see Gabbay and Kinoshita, 1972). The cataract develops by an osmotic mechanism. Other mechanisms may contribute too, because diets rich in fat and protein delay or prevent the cataract development (Patterson *et al.*, 1965). This type of cataract possibly has only increased membrane permeability in common with other non-sugar types (see Barber, 1973).

In hyperglycemia, aldose reductase (alditol : NADP oxidoreductase, EC 1.1.1.21) leads to the formation of high concentrations of sorbitol from glucose, because the K_M for glucose for this enzyme is higher than for hexokinase and therefore more sorbitol is made than glucose 6-phosphate (Kinoshita *et al.*, 1963; Pottinger, 1967). This polyol, in turn, cannot leave the lens (Wick and Drury, 1951). To a lesser extent more fructose is formed by action of sorbitol dehydrogenase (L-iditol : NAD oxidoreductase, EC 1.1.1.14). Thus in the case of human diabetic cataracts high concentrations of sorbitol have been found (Pirie and van Heyningen, 1964), though it must be assumed that polyols are lost from the lens as the cataract matures (Patterson and Bunting, 1964). The same holds true for the alloxan-diabetic rat and rabbit lenses (van Heyningen, 1959; Kinoshita *et al.*, 1962b; Patterson and Bunting, 1965; Kuck, 1966) or after the incubation of rabbit lenses with high glucose concentrations (Chylack and Kinoshita, 1969).

More pronounced opacities of the lens are found in hypergalactosemia or produced *in vitro* by addition of galactose (Kinoshita, 1965; Kinoshita *et al.*, 1968), where galactitol (dulcitol) is formed. This is consequently prevented by addition of a suitable inhibitor of aldose reductase (Kinoshita *et al.*, 1968; Dvornik *et al.*, 1973). Galactokinase deficiency may contribute to the development of cataracts (Beutler *et al.*, 1973).

Secondary to osmotic effects several alterations have been observed: a decreased amino acid uptake (Reddy and Kinsey, 1963; Kinoshita *et al.*, 1965, 1969); an accumulation of Na^+ (Andrée, 1970); a decreased uptake of K^+ (^{86}Rb) (Kinoshita and Merola, 1964; Cotlier and Becker, 1965); a decreased content of reduced glutathione (Sippel, 1966a); a decreased inositol uptake (Broekhuyse, 1968; Stewart *et al.*, 1968); an increased pentose phosphate pathway (Kinoshita *et al.*, 1963, in contrast to Lerman and Zigman, 1965) and decreased glycolysis (Sippel, 1966b); and decreased protein synthesis (Dische *et al.*, 1956; Lerman and Zigman, 1965) and protein content of the lens (Sippel, 1966a). Within a few days of incubation in galactose, calf lens demonstrates decreased transparency (Kinoshita *et al.*, 1962a). Most of these alterations can be prevented if the lenses are incubated simultaneously in media of higher tonicity (Kinoshita, 1965; Kinoshita *et al.*, 1965). For reviews of galactose cataract, see Kinoshita (1965), Caird *et al.* (1969), Kuck (1970), and van Heyningen (1971).

Fewer data are available on experimental diabetic cataracts, but in general they support the above findings, e.g. for decreased amino acid transport in alloxan-treated (Reddy, 1965) and streptozotocin-treated animals (Laurent *et al.*, 1973), and also for increased passive permeability. For reviews of transport of organic molecules into lens, see REDDY (1973) and KEM and HO (1973). VARMA and KINOSHITA (1974), comparing streptozotocin-diabetic and galactosemic rat lenses, found higher aldose reductase activities (accompanied by lower polyol dehydrogenase activity) only in diabetic lenses.

Both galactose and diabetes (alloxan-induced) cataracts are similar in that fiber size is found to be greater (FRIEDENWALD and RYTEL, 1955) and small vacuoles in the cortical cells lead to opacities (KUWABARA *et al.*, 1969). In this cortical area an altered phosphatide turnover has been found (BROEKHUYSE, 1971) in comparison to normal lenses. In the course of diabetes mellitus, changes in the chemical composition of the basement membrane (lens capsule) have been reported (LAZAROW and SPEIDEL, 1964; PATERSON and HEATH, 1967; SRINIVASAN *et al.*, 1970; v. SALLMANN and GRIMES, 1971). This collagen- and glycoprotein-containing membrane tends to thicken, even though in alloxan-diabetic rat lenses the glycosidase activity is higher (CARLIN and COTLIER, 1971).

2. Hexose Transport in Lens

If polyol accumulation is the main, but surely not the only cause (CAIRD *et al.*, 1969) of diabetic lens opacities and cataracts, the question arises as to whether insulin has something to do with the transport of hexoses in lenses. This transport (see PATTERSON, 1965), however, has some peculiarities. Within the lens a free glucose pool is present. As with mature erythrocytes, no stimulation of glucose penetration is seen by altering the sodium and potassium gradients or by inhibiting oxidative phosphorylation (ELBRINK and BIHLER, 1972a). As already mentioned, aerobic glycolysis, the hexose monophosphate shunt, and the sorbitol pathway are especially active in lenses (CHYLACK, 1971). Furthermore, insulin normally does not readily enter the aqueous humor (GILES and HARRIS, 1958). Under *in vitro* conditions, insulin stimulation of sugar transport into the lens was observed by ROSS (1953) and confirmed by LEVARI, KORNBLUETH and WERTHEIMER (1961). There are, however, other reports which question these findings or limit the effects to insulin administration *in vivo* (HARRIS *et al.*, 1955; FARKAS and PATTERSON, 1957; GILES and HARRIS, 1959). In the case of *in-vivo* effects of insulin on glucose transport, a dependency on hepatic functions has been revealed by FARKAS and PATTERSON (1957). Furthermore, several minor effects were observed when glucose concentrations lower than 1 mg/ml were used (LEVARI *et al.*, 1961; FARKAS and ROBERSON, 1965; FARKAS and WEESE, 1970). On the other hand a careful study using 3-O-methylglucose, a nonmetabolizable glucose model, failed to show transport stimulation *in vivo* or *in vitro* by insulin or many other stimulants, although the sugar penetration is of facilitated-diffusion character (ELBRINK and BIHLER, 1972b). In this respect lens cells resemble mature erythrocytes rather than muscle or adipose cells.

3. Lens Differentiation

Insulin in higher concentrations influences lens cell differentiation. Much the same as with mammary gland explants (see Section B) insulin initiates the differentiation of lens epithelia in explants of chick embryo lens. In general, typical signs of differentiation are the elongation of epithelial cells, the appearance of longitudinally oriented microtubuli and synthesis of lens-specific proteins (δ-crystallin). Like serum (HARDING *et al.*, 1962; PHILPOTT and COULOMBRE, 1965; PIATIGORSKY *et al.*, 1972; ZWAAN and IKEDA, 1968) insulin promotes cell elongation (PIATIGORSKY, 1973) and microtubule assembly. Generally the involvement of the microtubular system can be demonstrated both histologically and by the inhibitory action of colchicin (Piatigorsky *et al.*, 1972). With insulin, the final stimulation of protein synthesis is lacking (Piatigorsky *et al.*, 1973). It seems unclear whether insulin like serum promotes the biosynthesis of RNA, especially of rRNA, which in lens epithelium in culture initiates fiber formation (Piatigorsky and Rothschild, 1971). Increases in RNA and DNA biosynthetic activity, however, are a prerequisite of proliferation of lens epithelium (Rothstein *et al.*, 1966; Piatigorsky *et al.*, 1973).

Some kind of mitotic inhibition by catecholamines has been found either on addition to rabbit lens in culture (Voaden, 1968; Leeson and Voaden, 1970) or when given systemically to rats (Miki, 1961; v. Sallmann and Grimes, 1971). This inhibition is potentiated by theophylline and therefore attributed to the mediation of cAMP (Grimes and v. Sallmann, 1972). No interference by insulin has been reported.

References

Andrée, G.: Natriumakkumulation in Kataraktlinsen. Ber. dtsch. ophthal. Ges. **70**, 352—358 (1970)

Barber, G.W.: Human cataractogenesis: A review. Exp. Eye Res. **16**, 85—94 (1973)

Beutler, E., Matsumoto, F., Kuhl, W., Krill, A., Levy, N., Sparkes, R., Degnan, M.: Galactokinase deficiency as a cause of cataracts. New Engl. J. Med. **288**, 1203—1206 (1973)

Broekhuyse, R.M.: Changes in myo-inositol permeability in the lens due to cataractous conditions. Biochim. biophys. Acta (Amst.) **163**, 269—272 (1968)

Broekhuyse, R.M.: Lipids in tissues of the eye. V. Phospholipid metabolism in normal and cataractous lens. Biochim. biophys. Acta (Amst.) **231**, 360—369 (1971)

Caird, F.I., Hutchinson, M., Pirie, A.: Cataract and diabetes. Brit. med. J. **1964II**, 665—668

Caird, F.I., Pirie, A., Ramsell, T.G.: Diabetes and the Eye. Oxford: Blackwell 1969

Carlin, R., Cotlier, E.: Glycosidases of the crystalline lens. II. Alterations in diabetic cataracts. Invest. Ophthal. **10**, 898—903 (1971)

Chylack, L.T., Jr.: Control of glycolysis in the lens. Exp. Eye Res. **11**, 280—293 (1971)

Chylack, L.T., Jr., Kinoshita, J.H.: A biochemical evaluation of a cataract induced in a high-glucose medium. Invest. Ophthal. **8**, 401—412 (1969)

Cotlier, E., Becker, B.: Rubidium-86 accumulation and dulcitol distributions in lenses of galactose-fed rats. Exp. Eye Res. **4**, 340—345 (1965)

Dische, Z., Borenfreund, E., Zelmenis, G.: Proteins and protein synthesis in rat lenses with galactose cataract. Arch. Ophthal. **55**, 633 (1956)

Dvornik, D., Sunard-Duquesne, N., Krami, M., Sestanj, K., Gabbay, K.H., Kinoshita, J.H., Varma, S.D., Merola, L.O.: Polyol accumulation in galactosemic and diabetic rats: Control by an aldose reductase inhibitor. Science **182**, 1146—1148 (1973)

Elbrink, J., Bihler, I.: Membrane transport of sugars in the rat lens. Canad. J. Ophthal. **7**, 96—101 (1972a)

Elbrink, J., Bihler, I.: Characteristics of the membrane transport of sugars in the lens of the eye. Biochim. biophys. Acta (Amst.) **282**, 337—351 (1972b)

Farkas, T.G., Patterson, J.W.: Insulin and the lens. Amer. J. Ophthal. **44**, 341—344 (1957)

Farkas, T.G., Roberson, S.L.: The effect of Cr^{3+} on the glucose utilization of isolated lenses. Exp. Eye Res. **4**, 124—126 (1965)

Farkas, T.G., Weese, W.C.: The role of aqueous humor, insulin and trivalent chromium in glucose utilization of rat lenses. Exp. Eye Res. **9**, 132—136 (1970)

Friedenwald, J.S., Rytel, D.: Contribution to the histopathology of cataract. Arch. Ophthal. **53**, 825—831 (1955)

Gabbay, K.H., Kinoshita, J.H.: Mechanism of development and possible prevention of sugar cataracts. Israel J. med. Sci. **8**, 1557—1561 (1972)

Giles, K.M., Harris, J.E.: Radioelectrophoretic patterns of aqueous and plasma after intravenous injection of J^{131}-labeled insulin into rabbits. Amer. J. Ophthal. **46**, 196—203 (1958)

Giles, K.M., Harris, J.E.: The accumulation of C^{14} from uniformly labeled glucose by the normal and diabetic rabbit lens. Amer. J. Ophthal. **48**, 508—516 (1959)

Grimes, P., v. Sallmann, L.: Possible cyclic adenosine monophosphate mediation in isoproterenol-induced suppression of cell division in rat lens epithelium. Invest. Ophthal. **11**, 231—235 (1972)

Harding, C.V., Rothstein, H., Newman, M.B.: The activation of DNA synthesis and cell division in rabbit lens *in vitro*. Exp. Eye Res. **1**, 457—465 (1962)

HARRIS, J.E., HAUSCHILDT, J.D., NORDQUIST, L.T.: Transport of glucose across the lens surfaces. Amer. J. Ophthal. **39**, 161—169 (1955)
VAN HEYNINGEN, R.: Formation of polyols by the lens of the rat with "sugar" cataract. Nature (Lond.) **184**, 194—195 (1959)
VAN HEYNINGEN, R.: Galactose cataract: a review. Exp. Eye Res. **11**, 415—428 (1971)
KERN, M.L., HO, C.K.: Localization and specificity of the transport system for sugars in the calf lens. Exp. Eye Res. **15**, 751—765 (1973)
KINOSHITA, J.H.: Cataracts in galactosemia. Invest. Ophthal. **4**, 786—799 (1965)
KINOSHITA, J.H., BARBER, G.W., MEROLA, L.O., TUNG, B.: Changes in the levels of free amino acids and myo-inositol in the galactose-exposed lens. Invest. Ophthal. **8**, 625—632 (1969)
KINOSHITA, J.H., DVORNIK, D., KRAME, M., GABBAY, K.H.: The effect of an aldose reductase inhibitor on the galactose-exposed rabbit lens. Biochim. biophys. Acta (Amst.) **158**, 472—475 (1968)
KINOSHITA, J.H., FUTTERMAN, S., SATOH, K., MEROLA, L.O.: Factors affecting the formation of sugar alcohols in ocular lens. Biochim. biophys. Acta (Amst.) **74**, 340—350 (1963)
KINOSHITA, J.H., MEROLA, L.O.: Hydration of the lens during the development of galactose cataract. Invest. Ophthal. **3**, 577—584 (1964)
KINOSHITA, J.H., MEROLA, L.O., DIKMAK, E.: The accumulation of dulcitol and water in rabbit lens incubated with galactose. Biochim. biophys. Acta (Amst.) **62**, 176—178 (1962a)
KINOSHITA, J.H., MEROLA, L.O., DIKMAK, E.: Osmotic changes in experimental galactose cataracts. Exp. Eye Res. **1**, 405—410 (1962b)
KINOSHITA, J.H., MEROLA, L.O., HAYMAN, S.: Osmotic effects on the amino acid-concentrating mechanism in the rabbit lens. J. biol. Chem. **240**, 310—315 (1965)
KUCK, J.F.R.: Sorbitol pathway metabolites in the diabetic rabbit lens. Invest. Ophthal. **5**, 65—74 (1966)
KUCK, J.F.R.: Cataract formation. In: Biochemistry of the Eye (C.N. GRAYMAN, Ed.), p. 319—371. London, New York: Academic Press 1970
KUWABARA, T., KINOSHITA, J.H., COGAN, D.G.: Electron microscopic study of galactose-induced cataract. Invest. Ophthal. **8**, 133—149 (1969)
LAURENT, CH., KERN, P., REGNAULT, F.: Transport of amino acids into the lens in the course of experimental diabetic cataract. Ophthal. Res. **4**, 114—121 (1973)
LAZAROW, A., SPEIDEL, E.: The chemical composition of the glomerular basement membrane and its relationship to the production of diabetic complication. In: Small blood vessels involvement in diabetes mellitus (SIPERSTEIN, COLWELL, MEYER, Eds.), p. 127—150. Washington: 1964
LEESON, S.J., VOADEN, M.: A chalone in the mammalian lens. II. Relative effects of adrenaline and noradrenaline on cell division in the rabbit lens. Exp. Eye Res. **9**, 67—72 (1970)
LERMAN, S., ZIGMAN, S.: The metabolism of the lens as related to aging and experimental cataractogenesis. Invest. Ophthal. **4**, 643—660 (1965)
LEVARI, R., KORNBLUETH, W., WERTHEIMER, E.: The effect of insulin on the uptake of monosaccharides by the rat lens. J. Endocr. **22**, 361—369 (1961)
LEVARI, R., WERTHEIMER, E., BERMAN, E.R., KORNBLUETH, W.: Effect of insulin on pathways of glucose oxidation in the rat lens. Nature (Lond.) **192**, 1075—1076 (1961)
MIKI, T.: Fluctuation in mitosis count of lens epithelium. Influence of age, season and adrenal hormones. Acta Soc. opthal. Jap. **65**, 2207—2224 (1961)
NAIDOFF, D., PINCUS, I.J., TOWN, A.E., SCOTT, M.E.: Cataracts in alloxan-diabetic rabbits. Amer. J. Ophthal. **39**, 510—517 (1955)
PATERSON, R.A., HEATH, H.: Chemical changes in human diabetes, cataractous and β,β-iminodipropionitrile-treated rat lens capsules. Exp. Eye Res. **6**, 233—238 (1967)
PATTERSON, J.W.: A review of glucose transport in the lens. Ophthalmology **4**, 667—679 (1965)
PATTERSON, J.W., BUNTING, K.W.: Lens cell membrane permeability and cataract formation. Proc. Soc. exp. Biol. (N.Y.) **115**, 1156—1158 (1964)
PATTERSON, J.W., BUNTING, K.W.: Changes associated with the appearance of mature sugar cataracts. Invest. Ophthal. **4**, 167—173 (1965)
PATTERSON, J.W., PATTERSON, M.E., KINSEY, V.E., REDDY, D.V.N.: Lens assays on diabetic and galactosemic rats receiving diets that modify cataract development. Invest. Ophthal. **4**, 98—103 (1965)
PHILPOTT, G.W., COULOMBRE, A.J.: Lens development. II. Differentiation of embryonic chick lens epithelial cells *in vitro* and *in vivo*. Exp. Cell Res. **38**, 635—644 (1965)
PIATIGORSKY, J.: Insulin initiation of lens fiber differentiation in culture: Elongation of embryonic lens epithelial cells. Develop. Biol. **30**, 214—216 (1973)
PIATIGORSKY, J., ROTHSCHILD, S.S.: Effect of serum on the synthesis of RNA and of DNA in the cultured lens epithelium of the chick embryo: initiation of lens fiber formation *in vitro*. Biochim. biophys. Acta (Amst.) **238**, 86—98 (1971)

Piatigorsky, J., Rothschild, S.S., Milstone, S.M.: Differentiation of lens fibers in explanted embryonic chick lens epithelia. Develop. Biol. **34**, 334—345 (1973)

Piatigorsky, J., Rothschild, S.S., Wollberg, M.: Stimulation by insulin of cell elongation and microtubule assembly in embryonic chick-lens epithelia. Proc. nat. Acad. Sci. (Wash.) **70**, 1195—1198 (1973)

Piatigorsky, J., Webster, H.F., Craig, S.P.: Protein synthesis and ultrastructure during the formation of embryonic chick lens fiber *in vivo* and *in vitro*. Develop. Biol. **27**, 176—189 (1972)

Piatigorsky, J., Webster, H.F., Wollberg, M.: Cell elongation in the cultured embryonic chick lens epithelium with and without protein synthesis. Involvement of microtubules. J. Cell Biol. **55**, 82—92 (1972)

Pirie, A., van Heyningen, R.: The effect of diabetes on the content of sorbitol, glucose, fructose and inositol in the human lens. Exp. Eye Res. **3**, 124—131 (1964)

Pottinger, P.K.: A study of three enzymes acting on glucose in the lens of different species. Biochem. J. **104**, 663—668 (1967)

Reddy, D.V.N.: Amino acid transport in the lens in relation to sugar cataracts. Invest. Ophthal. **4**, 700—708 (1965)

Reddy, D.V.N.: Transport of organic molecules in the lens. Exp. Eye Res. **15**, 731—750 (1973)

Reddy, D.V.N., Kinsey, V.E.: Transport of amino acids into intraocular fluids and lens in diabetic rabbits. Invest. Ophthal. **2**, 237—242 (1963)

Ross, E.J.: Insulin and the permeability of cell membranes to glucose. Nature (Lond.) **171**, 125 (1953)

Rothstein, H., Fortin, J., Youngerman, M.L.: Synthesis of macromolecules in epithelial cells of the cultured amphibian lens. I. DNA and RNA. Exp. Cell Res. **44**, 303—311 (1966)

v. Sallmann, L., Grimes, P.: Eye changes in streptozotocin diabetes in rats. Amer. J. Ophthal. **71**, 312—319 (1971)

v. Sallmann, L., Grimes, P.: Isoproterenol-induced changes of cell proliferation in rat lens epithelium. Invest. Ophthal. **10**, 943—947 (1971)

Sippel, T.O.: Changes in the water, protein, and glutathione contents of the lens in the course of galactose cataract development in rats. Invest. Ophthal. **5**, 568—575 (1966a)

Sippel, T.O.: Energy metabolism in the lens during development of galactose cataract in rats. Invest. Ophthal. **5**, 576—582 (1966b)

Srinivasan, S.R., Berenson, G.S., Radhakrishnamurthy, B.: Glycoprotein changes in diabetic kidneys. Diabetes **19**, 171—175 (1970)

Stewart, M.A., Kurien, M.M., Sherman, W.R., Cotlier, E.V.: Inositol changes in nerve and lens of galactose fed rats. J. Neurochem. **15**, 941—946 (1968)

Varma, S.D., Kinoshita, J.H.: Sorbitol pathway in diabetic and galactosemic rat lens. Biochim. biophys. Acta (Amst.) **338**, 632—640 (1974)

Voaden, M.: A chalone in the rabbit lens. Exp. Eye Res. **7**, 326—331 (1968)

Wick, A.N., Drury, D.R.: Action of insulin on the permeability of cells to sorbitol. Amer. J. Physiol. **166**, 421—423 (1951)

Zwaan, J., Ikeda, A.: Macromolecular events during differentiation of the chicken lens. Exp. Eye Res. **7**, 301—311 (1968)

IV. Action on Some Mesenchymal Tissues and Single Cells

1. Action on Fibrocytes and Mesenchymal Tissues

a) Action of Insulin on Fibroblasts in Culture

Human skin fibroblasts in culture bind ^{125}I-insulin (GAVIN *et al.*, 1972). There are assumed to be specific receptor sites on the surface of the cell because the biologic effects parallel binding strength in the case of insulin derivatives and because unlabeled insulin competes with the labeled hormone for binding sites (see also the chapter by TELL, KRUG and CUATRECASAS). In contrast to normal or leukemic lymphocytes and granulocytes, which react like liver cells and adipocytes in their affinity, specificity, kinetics, and temperature sensitivity for insulin, fibroblasts and erythrocytes require higher insulin concentrations and higher displacement concentrations for 50% displacement by unlabeled insulin. There may be certain other peptides competing for insulin binding sites as well (HINTZ *et al.*, 1972). Furthermore, some similarities exist between insulin receptor sites and binding sites of plant lectins or concanavalin A (CUATRECASAS and TELL, 1973). Concanavalin A receptor sites on plasma membranes of fibroblasts and lymphocytes appear to be concentrated as caps (COMOGLIO and GUGLIELMONE, 1972).

The presence of insulin receptor sites is not necessarily associated with insulin sensitivity towards glucose transport. Stimulation of transport, denied hitherto by most authors, has recently been found under starvation conditions in human fibroblasts (FUJIMOTO and WILLIAMS, 1974), in chick embryo fibroblasts and in HeLa cells in culture. Like insulin, pyruvate stimulates the entry of D-glucose into the cells by a factor of 3 to 5 (SHAW and AMOS, 1973). Both types of stimulation can be prevented by actinomycin D or cycloheximide, which indicates a typical mechanism for transport stimulation, different from that found in adipocytes or muscle cells. Another interesting finding is that insulin sensitivity of glucose transport begins when the cells have entered the S phase (MORELL and FROESCH, 1973). Furthermore a delayed insulin sensitivity after trypsinization of cultured cells has previously been described by GOLDSTEIN and LITTLEFIELD (1969) and confirmed by MORELL and FROESCH (1973), who found no difference whether the cells of origin were of normal or diabetic skin biopsy. The delay was ascribed to the recovery from trypsinization.

The role of insulin as a stimulator of the growth of fibroblasts is well documented. HERSHKO *et al.* (1971) referred to it as the positive pleiotypic effect of insulin, i.e. reversal of inhibition of the transport of diverse substrates combined with slowing of macromolecular synthesis and stimulation of protein degradation (KRAM *et al.*, 1973). Insulin exerts this pleiotypic response in more than physiological concentrations (i.e. 1—100 mU/ml). One explanation of the need for higher concentrations is that insulin decomposes with time (GERSHENSON *et al.*, 1972). It is clear that insulin acts on the growth of different tissues like serum (GEY and THALHIMER, 1924; v. HAAM and CAPPEL, 1940; LESLIE and DAVIDSON, 1951; LESLIE and PAUL, 1954; LIEBERMAN and OVE, 1959; PAUL and PEARSON, 1960; WAYMOUTH and REED, 1965; TEMIN, 1967, 1968; SCHWARTZ and AMOS, 1968; BLAKER *et al.*, 1971; HARDING *et al.*, 1971; GERSHENSON *et al.*, 1972). To this pleiotypic effect of insulin belongs the increased transport of diverse substrates. HARE (1972) showed this for uridine transport into mouse embryo cells in culture. Transport of phosphate and uridine increases very early, with a fall in intracellular cAMP content (ROZENGURT and DE ASUA, 1973). Kinetically similar results were obtained for polyoma-transformed cells (LEMKIN and HARE, 1973). Some enzyme activities may change (e.g. EDMINSON *et al.*, 1973).

The primary effect of serum or insulin may be to stimulate phospholipid turnover in the target membrane (KNOX and PASTERNAK, 1973). Like serum, and with a similar time course, insulin stimulates glucose consumption, lactate production, and DNA synthesis (MORELL and FROESCH, 1973). Under certain experimental conditions insulin appears to have a lower growth-promoting activity than serum. This difference is due to insulin inactivation by fibroblasts and can be cancelled by more frequent changes of medium (MORELL and FROESCH, 1973). On the other hand, all growth-promoting properties of insulin vanish in the presence of serum and therefore are not additive to those of serum (MORELL and FROESCH, 1973). SCHER *et al.* (1974) recently showed that a particular serum fraction lost insulin-like activity on heating, but retained the growth-promoting property. Similar pleiotypic effects are found to be associated with non-suppressible insulin-like activity (NSILA) (TEMIN, 1969; MORELL and FROESCH, 1973). Further data see RECHLER *et al.* (1974). The pleiotypic effect of NSILA is 20 times stronger than its other actions, e.g. in fat pads.

The time-dependent sequence of changes following insulin exposure has been elucidated most clearly in a careful study by VAHERI *et al.* (1973). Chick embryo cells in a density-inhibited culture state (G_1 phase) respond to 20—500 ng/ml (0.5—13 mU/ml) of insulin with an early increased sugar uptake (2-desoxyglucose) and a depressed leucine uptake, followed by stimulation of protein synthesis (incorporation of ^{3}H-labeled amino acids), RNA synthesis (incorporation of ^{3}H-uridine), and DNA synthesis (incorporation of ^{3}H-thymidine) 5—10 h after the addition of insulin. Thus the mitotic index and the total cell number increase at a steady rate in the first 40 h. Relatively large cells are seen within 3 h after the addition of insulin. Thus insulin initiates some degree of synchronization. The changes are most clearly demonstrable in the presence of serum, indicating that insulin in this case does not replace only the growth-promoting properties of serum. Effects of insulin on mitosis and growth (as of serum or proteases) can be prevented by exogenous DBcAMP (BOMBIK and BURGER, 1973). Though insulin bound to agarose is effective only to the extent that insulin is set free from the particles, there is no doubt that the modulation of the cell surface by insulin stimulates cell proliferation because insulin uptake into the cell is minimal. A pronounced promotion of specific surface membrane conformation and the regulation of polysome formation by insulin have been observed (EVANS *et al.*, 1974).

In normal fibroblasts, at least, the pleiotypic control seems to be associated with cAMP (KRAM *et al.*, 1973). Data concerning insulin stimulation of growth also lend support to the concept of mediation by cAMP. Generally insulin is assumed to lower cAMP levels in most cells by inhibition of adenylate cyclase (see chapter by VOLFIN and HANOUNE). Furthermore, in normal fibroblasts insulin stimulates cell growth, especially under conditions in which cAMP levels are high or are elevated by means of other agents, e.g. by addition of prostaglandin E_1 (OTTEN *et al.*, 1972). As revealed by direct measurement, cAMP concentration fell by some 30—40% within 10—30 min after addition of 125 mU/ml insulin to some fibroblast cells (OTTEN *et al.*, 1972). When stimulated by prostaglandin E_1, other unresponsive cells react to insulin by a reduction of up to 50% in the cAMP content (OTTEN *et al.*, 1972). This fall takes place well before stimulation of DNA synthesis can be detected. FRANK (1972) and ZIMMERMAN and RASKA (1972) point out that this stimulation of DNA synthesis depends on low cAMP levels because it is prevented by the addition of DBcAMP. Also cAMP, added exogenously, inhibits the DNA synthesis of fibroblasts (FROEHLICH and RACHMELER, 1972; TEEL and HALL, 1973; BOMBIK and BURGER, 1973).

Treatment of BHK fibroblasts with 0.1 nM (approx. 100 μU/ml) insulin leads to an inhibition of adenylate cyclase (DE ASÚA *et al.*, 1973), thus explaining why the decrease in intracellular cAMP levels can be prevented by DBcAMP and theophylline. The adenylate cyclase inhibition, furthermore, may explain some characteristics of transformation shown morphologically. The relation of adenylate cyclase to β-receptors and cell motility is best demonstrated by the decreased motility of L 929 fibroblasts due to catecholamines and its prevention by β-blocking agents (MADERSPACH and FARKAS, 1973).

Direct correlation between the doubling time of several species of fibroblast cells and the content of cAMP was found by OTTEN *et al.* (1971). Especially in the mitotic phase, the cAMP content is low (BURGER *et al.*, 1972).

A growth-regulation system with cAMP as mediator has been proposed (OTTEN *et al.*, 1971; SHEPPARD, 1971, 1972). According to the main concept of WILLINGHAM *et al.* (1972), cAMP plays a decisive role in blocking cell growth in the early G_1 and G_2 phases. Transport phenomena may contribute, for DBcAMP is known to depress amino acid transport (ROZENGURT and PARDEE, 1972) and nucleoside transport (HAUSCHKA *et al.*, 1972). This hypothesis explains the well-known contact inhibition by stimulation of the membrane-bound adenylate cyclase (BÜRK, 1968; HSIE and PUCK, 1971). Other factors could, however, interfere (SEIFERT and PAUL, 1972) and changes in pH may play a role (D'ARMIENTO *et al.*, 1973). Recent reports point to the cAMP-antagonistic effect of cGMP in fibroblasts (KRAM and TOMKINS, 1973); this nucleotide is increased by insulin to a considerable extent in adipose-tissue cells (ILLIANO *et al.*, 1973). Some fibroblast lines (chick-embryo fibroblasts) in slightly restrictive growth conditions respond with proliferation to many cyclic and noncyclic nucleotides in 10^{-4}M concentrations. It seems that in this case restoration of the purine nucleotide pool favors growth; only cGMP (10^{-6}M) released this type of fibroblast from density-dependent inhibition (HOVI and VAHERI, 1973). Alterations in cyclic purine nucleotides are, however, not found in any case of fibroblast stimulation (HOVI *et al.*, 1974).

Some type of self-regulation seems possible because, on treatment of fibroblasts with DBcAMP and theophylline, an increase in cAMP phosphodiesterase (PDE) activity occurs by enzyme induction, which contributes to lower cAMP levels (D'ARMIENTO *et al.*, 1972). In view of the close connections between the cAMP system and calcium, observations of the proliferative properties of Ca^{++} gain in importance. Without reasonable calcium concentrations in the medium, proliferation stops (GAIL *et al.*, 1973). BALK *et al.* (1973) have seen such dependence, which is much more pronounced in the presence of serum; insulin has not been examined. The role of calcium does not apply to transformed cells.

b) Action of Insulin on Skin and Wound Tissue

A wide range of observations has been made to assess how diabetes influences wound healing. Several types of experimental wounds have recently been studied in some detail: hard-tissue wounds (HERBSMAN *et al.*, 1966, 1968), dental-extraction wounds (ITOI, 1966; CHIBA, 1968), skin wounds (ROSENTHAL *et al.*, 1962; PRAKASH *et al.*, 1973), and oral wounds (GLICKMAN *et al.*, 1967; KRONMAN *et al.*, 1970; ABBEY *et al.*, 1972). In most cases a delay in the healing process has been reported.

This retardation is supported by the fact that the incorporation of 1-^{14}C-acetate into mucopolysaccharides is reduced in diabetic rats and restored by the application of insulin (SCHILLER and DORFMAN, 1957). It had been thought that in diabetes mellitus glucose utilization may be diverted to pathways insensitive to insulin (WINEGRAD and BURDEN, 1966). This view was supported by studies on adipose tissue of starved and diabetic rats, where insulin abolishes the diluting effect of glucuronolactone upon $^{14}CO_2$ production from U^{14}C-glucose (Winegrad and Shaw, 1964). However, Sanwald and Ritz (1969) and Ritz and Sanwald (1970) did not find that an improved function of glucuronic pathway in diabetic arterial tissue (homogenate) determined the rate of single steps of glucuronic pathways. The reduced tensile strength of abdominal sutured wounds of alloxan-diabetic rats tends also to normalize with insulin (Rosenthal *et al.*, 1962). The same holds true for enzyme decreases in skin due to starvation or in the diabetic state (Ziboh *et al.*, 1971).

On the other hand *in vitro* diabetic skin biopsies and granulation tissue do not differ from normal tissues in several respects. For instance, proline incorporation, hydroxyproline turnover, and the solubility and cross-linking of collagen do not differ significantly (Yep *et al.*, 1972). *In vivo* there may be decreased vascularization in the diabetic state, which leads to retarded wound healing. Generally in alloxan diabetes, some stimulation of collagenolysis by elevated collagenase activity has to be taken into account (Ramamurthy *et al.*, 1973).

As far as nondiabetic granulation tissue is concerned, such tissue depends on glucose more than does normal tissue. After application of insulin *in vivo*, the ATP content in carrageenin granuloma fell sharply and recovered with glucose application (Murakami and Ishibashi, 1972a). Insulin *in vitro* may alter hexokinase isoenzymes in this type of granuloma (Murakami and Ishibashi, 1972b). *In vitro* additions of 0.3 U/ml insulin to cotton-pellet granuloma tissue resulted in increased proline incorporation into protein when adrenalectomized or insulin-deficient rats were used (Eichhorn and Sniffen, 1964). Similar findings were presented by Mikkonen *et al.* (1966).

Insulin has been used to influence wound healing in the nondiabetic state as well (Stuck, 1932). An increase in tensile strength, measured as bursting strength, has been found in rats (Rosenthal, 1968; Udupa and Chansouria, 1971; Grewal *et al.*, 1972), providing the treatment with 3—8 U per day and per rat of insulin leads to a weight gain. If it does not, no such increase is seen (Gregory, 1965). Therefore it seems probable that the favorable effects of insulin on wound healing depend on its ability to stimulate protein synthesis. In embryonic chick skin stimulation of collagen biosynthesis (Bashey *et al.*, 1972) has been reported besides increased glucosamine incorporation into hyaluronic acid (Bashey and Fleischmajer, 1974). Topically applied insulin likewise increased tensile strength (Shankswalker, 1958) or weight of granulation tissue (Nagy *et al.*, 1960, quoting earlier literature).

In normal human (Kahlenberg and Kalant, 1966) and rat skin (Ziboh *et al.*, 1971) insulin in higher concentrations (1 U/ml) stimulated glucose uptake. The flow of glucose carbon uses glycolytic and shunt pathways to the same extent and leads to higher lipid synthesis (Ziboh *et al.*, 1971).

c) Action of Insulin on Cartilage and Bone

When *in-vitro* preparations of bone are used, insulin stimulates amino acid uptake or incorporation into proteins (Vaes and Nichols, 1962; Westenhall *et al.*, 1969; Hahn *et al.*, 1969, 1971) without stimulation of 3-O-methylglucose uptake (Hahn *et al.*, 1971). For these effects prolonged administration of reasonably low insulin concentrations (0.2 μU/ml) and uninhibited protein synthesis (Hahn *et al.*, 1971) are needed. Furthermore, insulin did not result in higher proline incorporation into newborn rat tibia (Schwartz *et al.*, 1970). With isolated bone cells in primary culture an increase of uridine phosphorylation was seen with concentrations as low as 4.6 ng/ml (120 μU/ml) (PECK and MESSINGER, 1970), which was not related solely to sulfhydryl effects (PECK *et al.*, 1971).

PRASAD and RAJAN (1970) found increased proliferation of cartilage cells due to insulin in embryonic chick tibia *in-vitro* preparations. In incubations of cartilage, insulin stimulates (in addition to amino acid incorporation) mucopolysaccharide biosynthesis (SALMON and DAUGHADAY, 1957) as well as incorporation of uridine into RNA and of thymidine into DNA (SALMON *et al.*, 1968). Minimal effective concentrations were 1—10 mU/ml (SALMON, 1960). In somewhat higher concentrations insulin stimulates bone resorption, as revealed by calcium and metabolite measurements in the medium (PUCHE *et al.*, 1973). With very high insulin concentrations applied to *in-vitro* bone preparations of the early embryonic phase, adverse effects have been demonstrated (CHEN, 1954; HAY, 1958; ZWILLING, 1959). Thus in certain phases of development, several abnormalities, e.g. in bone growth, have been observed due to this hormone *in vivo* (DURAISWAMI, 1950; LANDAUER, 1953). Rather high doses were used.

References

ABBEY, L.M., COHEN, M., SHKLAR, G.: The effect of streptozotocin-induced diabetes on the healing of artificially produced tongue wounds in rats. Oral Surg. **33**, 672—683 (1972)

D'ARMIENTO, M., JOHNSON, G.S., PASTAN, I.: Regulation of adenosine 3′,5′-cyclic monophosphate phosphodiesterase activity in fibroblasts by intracellular concentrations of cyclic adenosine monophosphate. Proc. nat. Acad. Sci. (Wash.) **69**, 459—462 (1972)

D'ARMIENTO, M., JOHNSON, G.S., PASTAN, I.: Fibroblasts and cAMP: Cyclic AMP measured in fibroblasts cultured at different pH values. Nature New Biology **242**, 78—80 (1973)

ASÚA, L.J. DE, SURIAN, E.S., FLAWIA, M.M., TORRES, H.N.: Effect of insulin and adenylate cyclase activity of BHK fibroblasts. Proc. nat. Acad. Sci. (Wash.) **70**, 1388—1392 (1973)

BALK, S.D., WHITFIELD, J.F., YOUDALE, T., BRAUN, A.C.: Roles of calcium, serum, plasma, and folic acid in the control of proliferation of normal and Rous sarcoma virus-infected chicken fibroblasts. Proc. nat. Acad. Sci. (Wash.) **70**, 675—679 (1973)

BASHEY, R.I., FLEISCHMAJER, R.: Increased synthesis of hyaluronic acid by insulin in embryonic chick skin. Proc. Soc. exp. Biol. (N.Y.) **145**, 18 (1974)

BASHEY, R.I., PERLISH, J.S., FLEISCHMAJER, R.: Stimulation of collagen synthesis in embryonic chick skin by insulin. Connect. Tiss. Res. **1**, 189—193 (1972)

BLAKER, G.I., BIRCH, I.R., PIRTS, S.J.: The glucose, insulin and glutamine requirements of suspension cultures of HeLa cells in a defined culture medium. J. Cell Sci. **9**, 529—537 (1971)

BOMBIK, B.M., BURGER, M.M.: cAMP and the cell cycle: Inhibition of growth stimulation. Exp. Cell Res. **80**, 88—94 (1973)

BURGER, M.M., BOMBIK, B.M., BRECKENRIDGE, B.M., SHEPPARD, J.R.: Growth control and cyclic alterations of cyclic AMP in the cell cycle. Nature New Biology **239**, 161—163 (1972)

BÜRK, R.R.: Reduced adenyl cyclase activity in a polyoma virus transformed cell line. Nature (Lond.) **219**, 1272—1273 (1968)

CHEN, J.M.: The effect of insulin on embryonic limb bones cultivated *in vitro*. J. Physiol. (Lond.) **125**, 148—162 (1954)

CHIBA, E.: Experimental studies of the recovery process of the tooth extraction wounds in alloxan-diabetic rats classified by blood sugar levels. Shikwa Gakuho **68**, 1471—1491 (1968)

COMOGLIO, P.M., GUGLIELMONE, R.: Two-dimensional distribution of concanavalin-A receptor molecules on fibroblast and lymphocyte plasma membranes. FEBS Letters **27**, 256—258 (1972)

CUATRECASAS, P., TELL, G.P.E.: Insulin-like activity of concanavalin A and wheat germ agglutinin — direct interactions with insulin receptors. Proc. nat. Acad. Sci. (Wash.) **70**, 485—489 (1973)

DURAISWAMI, P.K.: Insulin-induced skeletal abnormalities in developing chickens. Brit. med. J. **1950II**, 384—390

EDMINSON, P.D., SIEBKE, J.-C., TJÖTTA, E.: The effects of insulin, serum and glucose on total assayable activity and on soluble debris bound and latent activity of the hexokinases of normal and polyoma virus-transformed BHK 21 cells. Biochim. biophys. Acta (Amst.) **320**, 33—43 (1973)

EICHHORN, J.H., SNIFFEN, R.C.: Influence of cortisol and insulin on *in vitro* incorporation of amino acids into protein of granuloma tissue. Endocrinology **75**, 341—351 (1964)

Evans, R.B., Morhenn, V., Jones, A.L., Tomkins, G.M.: Concomitant Effects of Insulin on Surface Membrane Conformation and Polysome Profiles of Serum-starved Balb/C 3T3 Fibroblasts. J. Cell Biol. **61**, 95—106 (1974)

Frank, W.: Cyclic 3′:5′ AMP and cell proliferation in cultures of embryonic rat cells. Exp. Cell Res. **71**, 238—241 (1972)

Froehlich, J.E., Rachmeler, M.: Effect of adenosine 3′-5′-cyclic monophosphate on cell proliferation. J. Cell Biol. **55**, 19—31 (1972)

Fujimoto, W.Y., Williams, R.H.: Insulin Action on the Cultured Human Fibroblast. Glucose Uptake, Protein Synthesis, RNA Synthesis. Diabetes **23**, 443—448 (1974)

Gail, M.H., Boone, C.W., Thompson, C.S.: A calcium requirement for fibroblast motility and proliferation. Exp. Cell Res. **79**, 386—390 (1973)

Gavin, J.R., Roth, J., Jen, P., Freychet, P.: Insulin receptors in human circulating cells and fibroblasts. Proc. nat. Acad. Sci. (Wash.) **69**, 747—751 (1972)

Gershenson, L.E., Okigaki, T., Andersson, M., Molson, J., Davidson, M.B.: Fine structural and growth characteristics of cultured rat-liver cells. Exp. Cell Res. **71**, 49—58 (1972)

Gey, G.O., Thalhimer, W.: Observations on the effects of insulin introduced into the medium of tissue cultures. J. Amer. med. Ass. **82**, 1609 (1924)

Glickman, I., Smulow, J.B., Moreau, J.: Postsurgical periodontal healing in alloxan diabetes. J. Periodont. **38**, 93—99 (1967)

Goldstein, S., Littlefield, J.W.: Effect of insulin on the conversion of glucose-C-14 to C-14-O_2 by normal and diabetic fibroblasts in cultures. Diabetes **18**, 545—549 (1969)

Gregory, W.: Effect of insulin on the healing of bone wounds in albino rats. J. dent. Res. **44**, 487—492 (1965)

Grewal, R.S., Gupta, S.C., Singhal, G.M., Gupta, S.N.: Wound healing in relation to insulin. Int. J. Surg. **57**, 229—232 (1972)

Haam, E. v., Cappel, L.: Effect of hormones upon cells grown *in vitro*. II. The effects of the hormones from the thyroid, pancreas, and adrenal gland. Amer. J. Cancer **39**, 354—359 (1940)

Hahn, T.J., Downing, S.J., Phang, J.M.: Insulin effect on amino acid transport in bone. Biochim. biophys. Acta (Amst.) **184**, 675—677 (1969)

Hahn, T.J., Downing, S.J., Phang, J.M.: Insulin effect on amino acid transport in bone: dependence on protein synthesis and Na^+. Amer. J. Physiol. **220**, 1717—1723 (1971)

Harding, C.V., Reddan, J.R., Unakar, N.J., Bagchi, M.: The control of cell division in the ocular lens. Int. Rev. Cytol. **31**, 215—300 (1971)

Hare, J.D.: A labile, serum-dependent uridine uptake function in mouse embryo cells. Biochim. biophys. Acta (Amst.) **282**, 401—408 (1972)

Hauschka, P.V., Everhart, L.P., Rubin, R.W.: Alteration of nucleoside transport of Chinese hamster cells by dibutyryl adenosine 3′,5′-cyclic monophosphate. Proc. nat. Acad. Sci. (Wash.) **69**, 2542—2546 (1972)

Hay, M.F.: The effect of growth hormone and insulin on limb-bone rudiments of the embryonic-chick cultivated *in vitro*. J. Physiol. (Lond.) **144**, 490—504 (1958)

Herbsman, H., Kwon, K., Shaftan, G.W., Gordon, B., Foy, L.M., Enquist, I.: The influence of systemic factors on fracture healing. J. Trauma **6**, 75—85 (1966)

Herbsman, H., Powers, J.C., Hirschman, A., Shaften, G.W.: Retardation of fracture healing in experimental diabetes. J. surg. Res. **8**, 424—431 (1968)

Hershko, A., Mamont, P., Shields, R., Tomkins, G.M.: "Pleiotypic response". Nature (Lond.) **232**, 206—211 (1971)

Hintz, R.L., Clemmons, D.R., Underwood, L.E., van Dyk, J.J.: Competitive binding of somatomedin to the insulin receptors of adipocytes, chondrocytes, and liver membranes. Proc. nat. Acad. Sci. (Wash.) **69**, 2351—2353 (1972)

Hovi, T., Vaheri, A.: Cyclic AMP and cyclic GMP enhance growth of chick embryo fibroblasts. Nature New Biology **245**, 175—177 (1973)

Hovi, T., Keski-Oja, J., Vaheri, A.: Growth Control in Chick Embryo Fibroblasts; No Evidence for a Specific Role for Cyclic Purine Nucleotides. Cell **2**, 235—240 (1974)

Hsie, A.W., Puck, T.T.: Morphological transformation of Chinese hamster cells by dibutyryl adenosine cyclic 3′:5′-monophosphate and testosterone. Proc. nat. Acad. Sci. (Wash.) **68**, 358—361 (1971)

Illiano, G., Tell, G., Siegel, M., Cuatrecasas, P.: Guanosine 3′,5′-cyclic monophosphate and the action of insulin and acetylcholine. Proc. nat. Acad. Sci. (Wash.) **70**, 2443—2447 (1973)

Itoi, S.: Experimental studies of alveolar bone metabolism after dental extraction. II. A quantitative study of alveolar socket healing in alloxan-diabetic dogs. Bull. Stomat. Kyoto Univ. **6**, 230—253 (1966)

Kahlenberg, A., Kalant, N.: The effect of insulin and diabetes on glucose metabolism in humans. Canad. J. Biochem. **44**, 801 (1966)

KNOX, P., PASTERNAK, C.A.: Serum-mediated membrane changes. Biochem. Soc. Transact. **1**, 430—431 (1973)

KRAM, R., MAMONT, P., TOMKINS, G.M.: Pleiotypic control by adenosine 3′,5′-cyclic monophosphate: A model for growth control in animal cells. Proc. nat. Acad. Sci. (Wash.) **70**, 1432—1436 (1973)

KRAM, R., TOMKINS, G.M.: Pleiotypic control by cyclic AMP: Interaction with cyclic GMP and possible role of microtubules. Proc. nat. Acad. Sci. (Wash.) **70**, 1659—1663 (1973)

KRONMAN, J.H., COHEN, M.M., COTE, D., WAITZKEN, L.: Histologic and histochemical study of human diabetic gingiva. J. dent. Res. **49**, 177 (1970)

LANDAUER, W.: The effect of time of injection and of dosage on absolute and relative length of femur, tibiotarsus and tarsometarsus in chicken embryos treated with insulin or pilocarpine. Growth **17**, 87—109 (1953)

LEMKIN, J.A., HARE, J.D.: Nucleoside transport in normal and polyoma-transformed cells: Kinetic differences following adenosine and serum or insulin stimulation. Biochim. biophys. Acta (Amst.) **318**, 113—122 (1973)

LESLIE, I., DAVIDSON, J.N.: The effect of insulin on cellular composition and growth of chick-heart explants. Biochem. J. **49**, XLI—XLII (1951)

LESLIE, I., PAUL, J.: The action of insulin on the composition of cells and medium during culture of chick-heart explants. J. Endocr. **11**, 110—124 (1954)

LIEBERMAN, I., OVE, P.: Growth factors for mammalian cells in culture. J. biol. Chem. **234**, 2754—2758 (1959)

MADERSPACH, K., FARKAS, T.: The effect of catecholamines on cell motility in mouse fibroblasts. Life Sci. **12**, 413—418 (1973)

MIKKONEN, L., LAMPIAHO, K., KULONEN, E.: Effect of thyroid hormones, somatotrophin, insulin and corticosteroids on synthesis of collagen in granulation tissue both *in vivo* and *in vitro*. Acta endocr. (Kbh.) **51**, 23—31 (1966)

MORELL, B., FROESCH, E.R.: Fibroblasts as an experimental tool in metabolic and hormone studies. II. Effects of insulin and nonsuppressible insulin-like activity (NSILA-S) on fibroblasts in culture. Europ. J. clin. Invest. **3**, 119—123 (1973)

MURAKAMI, K., IHIBASHI, S.: Change in energy metabolism of proliferating granuloma tissue in response to insulin and 2-deoxyglucose. Horm. Metab. Res. **4**, 77—82 (1972a)

MURAKAMI, K., IHIBASHI, S.: Insulin-like effect of sulfhydryl inhibitor on hexokinase isoenzyme of rat granuloma tissue *in vitro* and the opposite effect of sulfhydryl compound. Endocr. jap. **19**, 115—119 (1972b)

NAGY, S., RÉDEI, A., KARÁDY, S.: The effect of insulin on production of granulation tissue in rats. Experientia (Basel) **16**, 121—123 (1960)

OTTEN, J., JOHNSON, G.S., PASTAN, I.: Cyclic AMP levels in fibroblasts: relationship to growth rate and contact inhibition of growth. Biochem. biophys. Res. Commun. **44**, 1192—1198 (1971)

OTTEN, J., JOHNSON, G.S., PASTAN, I.: Regulation of cell growth by cyclic adenosine 3′,5′-monophosphate. Effect of cell density and agents which alter cell growth on cyclic adenosine 3′,5′-monophosphate levels in fibroblasts. J. biol. Chem. **247**, 7082 (1972)

PAUL, J., PEARSON, E.S.: The action of insulin on the metabolism of cell cultures. J. Endocr. **21**, 287—294 (1960)

PECK, W.A., MESSINGER, K.: Nucleoside and ribonucleic acid metabolism in isolated bone cells. Effects of insulin and cortisol *in vitro*. J. biol. Chem. **245**, 2722—2729 (1970)

PECK, W.A., MESSINGER, K., CARPENTER, J.: Regulation of pyrimidine ribonucleoside incorporation in isolated bone cells. Stimulation by insulin and by 2,3-dihydroxy 1,4-dithiobutane (dithiotreitol). J. biol. Chem. **246**, 4439—4446 (1971)

PRAKASH, A., KAPUR, M., MAINI, B.S.: Wound healing in experimental diabetes: Histological, histochemical and biochemical studies. Indian J. med. Res. **61**, 1200—1206 (1973)

PRASAD, G.C., RAJAN, K.T.: Effect of insulin on bone in tissue culture. Acta orthop. scand. **41**, 44—56 (1970)

PUCHE, R.C., ROMANO, M.C., LOCATTO, M.E., FERRETTI, J.L.: The effect of insulin on bone resorption. Calcif. Tiss. Res. **12**, 8—15 (1973)

RAMAMURTHY, N.S., ZEBROWSKI, E.J., GOLUB, L.M.: Collagenolytic activity of gingivae from alloxan-diabetic rats. Diabetes **22**, 272—274 (1973)

RECHLER, M.M., PODSKALNY, J.M., GOLDFINE, I.D., WELLS, C.A.: DNA Synthesis in Human Fibroblasts: Stimulation by Insulin and by Nonsuppressible Insulin-like Activity (NSILA-S). J. clin. Endocr. **39**, 512—521 (1974)

RITZ, E., SANWALD, R.: Glucuronic acid cycle in arterial tissue. Z. ges. exp. Med. **153**, 237—245 (1970)

ROSENTHAL, S.P.: Acceleration of primary wound healing by insulin. Arch. Surg. **96**, 53—55 (1968)

Rosenthal, S. P., Lerner, B., Di Biase, F., Inquist, I. F.: Relation of strength to composition in diabetic wounds. Surg. Gynec. Obstet. **115**, 437—442 (1962)

Rozengurt, E., de Asua, L. J.: Role of cyclic 3′,5′-adenosine monophosphate in the early transport changes induced by serum and insulin in quiescent fibroblasts. Proc. nat. Acad. Sci. (Wash.) **70**, 3609—3612 (1973)

Rozengurt, E., Pardee, A. B.: Opposite effects of dibutyryl adenosine 3′,5′-cyclic monophosphate and serum on growth of Chinese hamster cells. J. cell. Physiol. **80**, 273—280 (1972)

Salmon, W. D.: Importance of amino acids in the actions of insulin and serum sulfation factor to stimulate sulfate uptake by cartilage from hypophysectomized rats. J. Lab. clin. Med. **56**, 673—681 (1960)

Salmon, W. D., Daughaday, W. H.: A hormonally controlled serum factor which stimulates sulfate incorporation by cartilage *in vitro*. J. Lab. clin. Med. **49**, 825—836 (1957)

Salmon, W. D., Du Vall, M. R., Thompson, E. Y.: Stimulation by insulin *in vitro* of incorporation of (^{35}S) sulfate and (^{14}C) leucine into protein-polysaccharide complexes, (^{3}H) uridine into RNA, and (^{3}H) thymidine into DNA of costal cartilage from hypophysectomized rats. Endocrinology **82**, 493—499 (1968)

Sanwald, R., Ritz, E.: Der Glucuronsäureabbauweg der Glucose in Aorten alloxandiabetischer Tiere. Verh. dtsch. Ges. inn. Med. **75**, 873—875 (1969)

Scher, C. D., Stathakos, D., Antoniades, H. N.: Dissociation of cell division stimulating capacity for BALB/C-3T3 from the insulin-like activity in human serum. Nature (Lond.) **247**, 279—281 (1974)

Schiller, S., Dorfman, A.: The metabolism of mucopolysaccharides in animals. IV. The influence of insulin. J. biol. Chem. **227**, 625—632 (1957)

Schwartz, A. G., Amos, H.: Insulin dependence of cells in primary culture: Influence on ribosome integrity. Nature (Lond.) **219**, 1366—1367 (1968)

Schwartz, P. L., Wettenhall, R. E. H., Tovedel, M. A., Bornstein, J.: A long-term effect of insulin on collagen synthesis by newborn rat bone *in vitro*. Diabetes **19**, 465—466 (1970)

Seifert, W., Paul, D.: Levels of cyclic AMP in sparse and dense cultures of growing and quiescent 3T3 cells. Nature New Biology **240**, 281—283 (1972)

Shankswalker, G. B.: The local effect of insulin on wound healing in rats. J. dent. Res. **37**, 84 (1958)

Shaw, S. N., Amos, H.: Insulin stimulation of glucose entry in chick fibroblasts and HeLa cells. Biochem. biophys. Res. Commun. **53**, 357—365 (1973)

Sheppard, J. R.: Restoration of contact-inhibited growth to transformed cells by dibutyryl adenosine 3′,5′ cyclic monophosphate. Proc. nat. Acad. Sci. (Wash.) **68**, 1316—1320 (1971)

Sheppard, J. R.: Difference in the cyclic adenosine 3′,5′-monophosphate levels in normal and transformed cells. Nature New Biology **236**, 14—16 (1972)

Stuck, W. G.: The effect of insulin on the healing of experimental fractures in the rabbit. J. Bone Jt. Surg. **14**, 109—115 (1932)

Teel, R. W., Hall, R. G.: Effect of dibutyryl cyclic AMP on the restoration of contact inhibition in tumor cells and its relationship to cell density and the cell cycle. Exp. Cell Res. **76**, 390—394 (1973)

Temin, H. M.: Studies on carcinogenesis by avian sarcoma viruses. VI. Differential multiplication of uninfected and of converted cells in response to insulin. J. cell. Physiol. **69**, 377—384 (1967)

Temin, H. M.: Carcinogenesis by avian sarcoma viruses. X. The decreased requirement for insulin-replaceable activity in serum for cell multiplication. Int. J. Cancer **3**, 771—787 (1968)

Temin, H. M.: Control of cell multiplication in uninfected chicken cells and chicken cells converted by avian sarcoma viruses. J. cell. Physiol. **74**, 9 (1969)

Udupa, K. N., Chansouria, J. P. N.: The role of protamine zinc insulin in accelerating wound healing in the rat. Brit. J. Surg. **58**, 673—675 (1971)

Vaes, G. M., Nichols, G.: Metabolism of glycine-1-C^{14} by bone *in vitro*: effects of hormones and other factors. Endocrinology **70**, 890—901 (1962)

Vaheri, A., Ruoslahti, E., Hovi, T., Nordling, S.: Stimulation of density-inhibited cell cultures by insulin. J. cell Physiol. **81**, 355—363 (1973)

Waymouth, C., Reed, D. E.: A reversible morphological change in mouse cells (strain L, clone NCTC 929) under the influence of insulin. Tex. Rep. Biol. Med. **23**, Suppl. 1, 413—419 (1965)

Westenhall, R. E. H., Schwartz, P. L., Bornstein, J.: Actions of insulin and growth hormone on collagen and chondroitin sulfate synthesis in bone organ cultures. Diabetes **18**, 280—284 (1969)

Willingham, M. C., Johnson, G. S., Pastan, I.: Control of DNA synthesis and mitosis in 3T3 cells by cyclic AMP. Biochem. biophys. Res. Commun. **48**, 743—748 (1972)

WINEGRAD, A.J., BURDEN, C.L.: L-Xylulose metabolism in diabetes mellitus. New Engl. J. Med. **274**, 298—305 (1966)
WINEGRAD, A.J., SHAW, W.N.: Glucoronic pathway activity in adipose tissue. Amer. J. Physiol. (Lond.) **206**, 165—168 (1964)
YEP, P., GULLANDER, S., RUCKER, R.B.: The effect of alloxan diabetes on skin collagen metabolism. Experientia (Basel) **28**, 508—509 (1972)
ZIBOH, V.A., RAULS, T.J., HSIA, S.L.: Adaptive changes of glycerol 3-phosphate dehydrogenase level in rat skin: effects of starvation, alloxan diabetes and insulin. Endocrinology **89**, 240—245 (1971)
ZIBOH, V.A., WRIGHT, R., HSIA, S.L.: Effects of insulin on the uptake and metabolism of glucose by rat skin *in vitro*. Arch. Biochem. **146**, 93—99 (1971)
ZIMMERMANN, J.E., RASKA, K.: Inhibition of adenovirus type 12-induced DNA synthesis in G^1-arrested BHK 21 cells by dibutyryl adenosine cyclic 3′,5′-monophosphate. Nature New Biology **239**, 145—147 (1972)
ZWILLING, E.: Micromelia as a direct effect of insulin. Evidence from *in vitro* and *in vivo* experiments. J. Morph. **104**, 159—179 (1959)

2. Action on Tumor Cells

At the present time we do not know what are the essential properties that distinguish malignant from normal cells. Research in the last few years has attempted to describe the properties exhibited by tumor cells that make them phenotypically different from normal cells. The most prominent recent contributions refer to decreased intercellular recognition (Dorsey and Roth, 1973), alterations of surface properties (Wallach, 1968; Inbar *et al.*, 1972), decreased hormonal regulation (Weber, 1973), and shifts in key enzymes or isoenzymes, followed by shifts from anabolic to more catabolic metabolism (Weber, 1973).

Several reports stated that tumor growth was found to be reduced in experimental diabetes (Salzberg and Griffin, 1952; Vangerow and McKee, 1955; Goranson and Tilser, 1955; Ingle, 1958, 1965; Garvie, 1968; Heuson and Legros, 1972; Puckett and Shingleton, 1972; Criss and Morris, 1973). Experiments in which insulin dependence is shown for mammary carcinomas (and also in organ culture) leave no doubt that insulin itself interferes in tumor growth and that insulin deprivation results in tumour regression (Heuson and Legros, 1972). Moreover, in non diabetic rats receiving insulin together with glucose (in drinking water), tumor weight increases several-fold (Heuson *et al.*, 1972). For leukemia cells in culture, insulin promotes growth in a serum-free medium (Moore *et al.*, 1966). Especially with hepatomas, growth was related in diabetic rats to a low-carbohydrate diet, or to fasting alone in normal rats. Alternatively, a high-glucose diet or insulin normalized tumor growth, a situation which repressed adenylate kinase and induced pyruvate kinase (Criss and Morris, 1973). In human male diabetics, observations of lower tumor incidence have been reported (Kessler, 1970). See also the thorough statistics of Rostlapil and Zrustová (1974).

Other tumors may react in the opposite manner in the diabetic state, as found by Wieser *et al.* (1967) with Zajdela H and Walker carcinoma 256. A direct anti-tumor effect of insulin in combination with glucagon has been suggested by Salter *et al.* (1958) and Johnson and Wright (1959).

Some tumor cell lines respond to insulin with increased glycogen content (Hilz and Tarnowski, 1970). In HeLa cells, however, due to a special regulation of glycogen synthetase, a decreased glycogen content was found with insulin (Alpers, 1966). High glycogen contents attributable to low intracellular cAMP levels can be reversed by addition of DBcAMP, but not by exogenous cAMP (Hilz and Tarnowski, 1970). In the latter case a nonspecific effect is seen and ascribed to adenosine set free from cAMP outside the cell (Hilz *et al.*, 1973). Such observations, which point to a stimulatory effect of cAMP on RNA biosynthesis in normal fibroblasts (Koblet, Kohler and Wyler, 1973), have to be interpreted with caution.

Tumor cells and transformed cells (whether transformed by oncogenic viruses, chemically, or spontaneously) show some similarity to their parent cells or their untransformed fibroblasts. Transformed fibroblasts respond to a smaller extent to density-induced inhibition of sugar transport (Bose and Zlotnik, 1973). Malignant cells generally have a defect of pleiotypic control (Holley and Kiernan, 1968; Temin, 1968; Hershko *et al.*, 1971), in which insulin plays a well-known role (see above). In this respect tumor cells resemble embryonic rat cells (Lieberman and Ove, 1959; Frank *et al.*, 1970). This does not exclude that some tumor cells (e.g. 3T3 fibroblasts) may react to insulin or serum by overgrowth (Temin, 1967; Yarnell and Schnebli, 1974).

Higher concentrations of insulin, which like serum or proteases stimulates confluent normal cells to growth (TEMIN, 1967; VAHERI *et al.*, 1973), decrease the cAMP content of normal 3T3 cells to the levels normally seen with transformed cells, e.g. 3T6 or py 3T3 cells (SHEPPARD, 1972). Similar observations were made by OTTEN *et al.* (1972). Since serum or proteases are also known to lower cAMP levels in normal cells (PASTAN and PERLMAN, 1971; SHEPPARD, 1972), there is ample evidence to support the more general role of cAMP in controlling growth. In a strain of murine plasma cell tumor insulin (0.5 U/ml) reversed growth inhibition by prostaglandins and cAMP (NASEEM and HOLLANDER, 1973).

The mechanism by which cAMP could interfere in cellular growth remains to be elucidated. WICKS *et al.* (1973) suggest by their studies on Reuber H 35 hepatoma cells that cAMP extends (retards) the DNA synthesis phase by interfering with the synthesis of desoxyribopyrimidine nucleosides. It is interesting to note that serum effects in previously serum-starved neuroblastoma cells are inhibited by DBcAMP; these effects include DNA synthesis, thymidine and desoxycytidine incorporation and their intracellular transport (FURMANSKI and LUBIN, 1973). In transformed 3T3 cells leucine transport is under the same influence (PAUL, 1973). HAMAZAKI (1973) found an additional thymidine kinase in Yoshida sarcoma cells which was inhibited by the addition of cAMP.

Generally lower cAMP contents have been found in transformed or rapidly growing cells (GRANNER *et al.*, 1968; HEIDRICK and RYAN, 1971; OTTEN *et al.*, 1971; SHEPPARD, 1971, 1972; WEISS *et al.*, 1971; OTTEN *et al.*, 1972; YOSHIKAWA-FUKADA and NOJIMA, 1972; GRIMES and SCHROEDER, 1973). Caution is advised in interpreting these results because in stationary-phase conditions somewhat higher adenylate cyclase activity and sensitivity towards glucagon, catecholamine and prostaglandin have been found. This, in turn, is more pronounced in normal than in malignant cell strains (MAKMAN, 1971).

A direct parallelism between the fall in cAMP content and the beginning of transformation has been neatly demonstrated by OTTEN *et al.* (1972) using temperature-dependent mutants of an oncogenic virus. The transformation could be prevented by means of agents that increase intracellular cAMP. Adenylate cyclase activity falls to the same extent (ANDERSON *et al.*, 1973). The immediate (within 3 h) fall in cAMP content after infection of contact-inhibited Balb/3T3 cells with SV 40 virus (REIN *et al.*, 1973) shows that viral gene expression leads to cAMP alteration before the onset of DNA synthesis stimulation some 15 h later. Serum, trypsin, and insulin more rapidly induce a fall in cAMP (REIN *et al.*, 1973).

Nevertheless, an imbalance in the cAMP-generating and -degrading system does not necessarily imply that actual alterations of cAMP content will be found (SHEPPARD *et al.*, 1973; WEBER, 1973), nor need cAMP-dependent protein kinase activities differ in virus-transformed cells from those in their normal counterparts (TROY *et al.*, 1973).

Soon after transformation with temperature-sensitive Rous sarcoma virus, adenylate cyclase activity decreases with a change in the K_M values for Mg-ATP (ANDERSON *et al.*, 1973). This finding confirms similar observations by BÜRK (1968), PEERY *et al.* (1971), YOSHIKAWA *et al.* (1972), and ANDERSON *et al.* (1973) for transformed cells, and by GRANNER *et al.* (1968) and MAKMAN (1970) for malignant cells. In any event, alterations in adenylate cyclase point to early plasma-membrane modification during transformation. On the other hand, there are reports of normal cyclase activity but altered glucagon sensitivity (ALLEN *et al.*, 1971). In hepatomas, especially high enzyme activities were reported. BROWN *et al.* (1970) comparing several lines of hepatomas, found the highest enzyme activities in the faster-growing ones. Similar observations came from BROWN *et al.*

(1969), PENNINGTON *et al.* (1970), THOMAS *et al.* (1973), and CHAYOTH *et al.* (1973). Careful measurements by EMMELOT and BOS (1971), however, indicated reduced enzyme activity in hepatoma lines. Similar data were reported by VAN WIJK *et al.* (1972) and TOMASI *et al.* (1973). Perhaps there is a very wide variation in the cell characteristics of different hepatoma lines (VAN WIJK *et al.*, 1972).

In transformed cells and in some tumor cells a low level of cAMP phosphodiesterase (PDE) was found (D'ARMIENTO *et al.*, 1972; SHARMA, 1972). It seems that generally in fibroblasts, whether untransformed or transformed, the concentrations of cAMP are regulated by the induction of PDE activities of the low-K_M type (D'ARMIENTO *et al.*, 1972). Induction of PDE was also found in a chemically transformed line of L929 fibroblasts (MANGANIELLO and VAUGHAN, 1972). In parallel with the increase in growth behavior from normal liver to hepatoma, an isoenzyme shift from high K_M to low K_M PDE activities was observed (CLARK *et al.*, 1973). This shift seems to be specific because it is not shared by newborn and regenerating livers (WEBER, 1973). Similar shift results were obtained by SCHRÖDER and PLAGEMANN (1972) in Novikoff hepatoma.

Further insight into the role of cAMP in growth control and thus in carcinogenesis was gained from studies with exogenous cAMP or its dibutyryl derivative (DBcAMP) with or without concomitant addition of theophylline, a PDE inhibitor. A peculiar property of tumor lines of fibroblasts is their decreased ability to transport exogenous cAMP or DBcAMP into the cell (RYAN and DURICK, 1972). It seems that this fact contributes to the loss of important mechanisms controlling the rate of cell division found in tumor cells (RYAN and CURTIS, 1973). Administration of (DB)cAMP to transformed cell lines decreases cell growth rate (BÜRK, 1968; RYAN and HEIDRICK, 1968; GERICKE and CHANDRA, 1969; HEIDRICK and RYAN, 1970; HSIE *et al.*, 1971; JOHNSON *et al.*, 1971; JOHNSON *et al.*, 1971a, b; PRASAD and HSIE, 1971; SHEPPARD, 1971; JOHNSON *et al.*, 1972; JOHNSON and PASTAN, 1972a, b; GRIMES and SCHROEDER, 1973); causes synchronization of cells in the G_2 phase (SMETS, 1972; WILLINGHAM *et al.*, 1972); increases cell adhesion (GAZDAR *et al.*, 1972; JOHNSON and PASTAN, 1972b); alters cell morphology (HSIE *et al.*, 1971; HSIE and PUCK, 1971; JOHNSON *et al.*, 1971b; SHEPPARD, 1971; GAZDAR *et al.*, 1972; JOHNSON and PASTAN, 1972a; PUCK, 1973) and favors organization of the microtubuli into parallel arrays (PUCK, 1973); diminishes cell mobility (JOHNSON *et al.*, 1972); restores some kind of contact inhibition (HEIDRICK and RYAN, 1971; HSIE *et al.*, 1971; JOHNSON *et al.*, 1971a; SHEPPARD, 1971, 1972; SMETS, 1972; ZACCHELLO *et al.*, 1972; GRIMES and SCHROEDER, 1973); alters agglutinability by plant lectins (SHEPPARD, 1971) and changes surface antigenic expression (KURTH and BAUER, 1973); increases collagen synthesis (HSIE *et al.*, 1971) and reduces the higher transport ability, e.g. for 2-desoxyglucose of py3T3 cells to normal levels (GRIMES and SCHROEDER, 1973). Glucose transport was not, however, normalized in every case (GAZDAR *et al.*, 1972). As a consequence of all these effects cAMP and DBcAMP have been called "reverse transformation agents" (PUCK, 1973). Many alterations were not seen with tumors of epithelial origin (JOHNSON *et al.*, 1971b). It is uncertain whether cAMP treatment has any influence on tumor cells *in vivo*. Favorable responses (GERICKE and CHANDRA, 1969; SELLER and BENSON, 1973; CHO-CHUNG and GULLINO, 1974) may be limited to certain conditions or kinds of tumor (PASTAN, 1973).

Whatever the modulating effect of cAMP may be, its influence cannot be fixed genotypically. In this connection it is of interest to know whether cAMP itself influences oncogenic transformation. SMITH *et al.* (1973) report that in the presence of DBcAMP the frequency of transformation increases 10-fold in the case of transformation of baby hamster kidney cells by simian virus 40 (SV40), a DNA virus.

Moreover, EBBESEN and HESSE (1972) found an inhibition of *in vitro* infection of fibroblasts by murine leukemia virus under high concentrations of insulin (8 U/ml). This penetration of virus seems to a certain extent to depend on the preexisting cAMP content of the cells (EBBESEN and ARNUNG, 1973).

In summary, the effects of insulin on the growth of tumor cells fit in well with present ideas on the role of the second messenger in growth regulation. Other substances and biochemical systems may interfere with the effects of insulin on cell growth.

References

ALLEN, D.O., MUNSHOWER, J., MORRIS, H.P., WEBER, G.: Regulation of adenyl cyclase in hepatomas of different growth rates. Cancer Res. **31**, 557—560 (1971)

ALPERS, J.B.: The influence of hexose and insulin on glycogen synthetase in HeLa cells. J. biol. Chem. **241**, 217—222 (1966)

ANDERSON, W.B., JOHNSON, G.S., PASTAN, I.: Transformation of chick-embryo fibroblasts by wild-type and temperature-sensitive Rous sarcoma virus alters adenylate cyclase activity. Proc. nat. Acad. Sci. (Wash.) **70**, 1055—1059 (1973)

ANDERSON, W.B., LOVELACE, E., PASTAN, I.: Adenylate cyclase activity is decreased in chick embryo fibroblasts transformed by wild-type and temperature sensitive Schmidt-Ruppin Rous sarcoma virus. Biochem. biophys. Res. Commun. **52**, 1293—1299 (1973)

D'ARMIENTO, M., JOHNSON, G.S., PASTAN, I.: Regulation of adenosine 3',5' cyclic monophosphate phosphodiesterase activity in fibroblasts by intracellular concentrations of cyclic adenosine monophosphate. Proc. nat. Acad. Sci. (Wash.) **69**, 459—462 (1972)

BOSE, S.K., ZLOTNICK, B.: Growth- and density-dependent inhibition of deoxyglucose transport in Balb 3T3 cells and its absence in cells transformed by murine sarcoma virus. Proc. nat. Acad. Sci. (Wash.) **70**, 2374—2378 (1973)

BROWN, H.D., CHATTOPADHYAY, MORRIS, H.P., PENNINGTON, S.N.: Adenyl cyclase activity in Morris hepatomas 7777, 7794 A and 9618 A. Cancer Res. **30**, 123—126 (1970)

BROWN, H.D., CHATTOPADHYAY, MORRIS, H.P., SPJUT, H.J., SPRATT, J.S., PENNINGTON, S.N.: Adenylcyclase activity in dimethylamino biphenyl-induced breast carcinoma. Biochim. biophys. Acta (Amst.) **192**, 372—375 (1969)

BÜRK, R.R.: Reduced adenyl cyclase activity in a polyoma virus transformed cell line. Nature (Lond.) **219**, 1272—1273 (1968)

CHAYOTH, R., EPSTEIN, S.M., FIELD, J.B.: Glucagon and prostaglandin E_1 stimulation of cyclic adenosine 3',5'-monophosphate levels and adenylate cyclase activity in benign hyperplastic nodules and malignant hepatomas of ethionine-treated rats. Cancer Res. **33**, 1970—1974 (1973)

CHO-CHUNG, Y.S., GULLINO, P.M.: *In vivo* inhibition of growth of two hormone-dependent mammary tumors by dibutyryl cyclic AMP. Science **183**, 87—88 (1974)

CLARK, I.F., MORRIS, H.P., WEBER, G.: Cyclic adenosine 3',5'-monophosphate phosphodiesterase activity in normal, differentiating, regenerating, and neoplastic liver. Cancer Res. **33**, 356—361 (1973)

CRISS, W.E., MORRIS, H.P.: Influence of hormones on the growth of hepatomes and induction of adenylate and pyruvate kinases. Cancer Res. **33**, 1023—1027 (1973)

DORSEY, I.K., ROTH, S.: Adhesive specificity in normal and transformed mouse fibroblasts. Develop. Biol. **33**, 249—256 (1973)

EBBESEN, P., ARNUNG, K.M.: Enhancement of the dye-exclusion cytotoxic test by insulin and inhibition by cyclic adenosine 3',5'-monophosphate and theophylline. Transplant. **16**, 476—478 (1973)

EBBESEN, P., HESSE, J.: Influence of hormones, poly I: C, polyvinylpyrrolidon and β-stimulators on *in vitro* infection with murine leukemia virus. Europ. J. Cancer **8**, 623—627 (1972)

EMMELOT, P., BOS, C.J.: Studies on plasma membranes. XIV. Adenyl cyclase in plasma membranes isolated from rat and mouse livers and hepatomas and its hormone sensitivity. Biochim. biophys. Acta (Amst.) **249**, 285—292 (1971)

FRANK, W., RISTOW, H.J., ZABEL, S.: Zur Regulation des Zellcyclus von embryonalen Rattenzellen in Kultur. Europ. J. Biochem. **14**, 392—398 (1970)

FURMANSKI, P., LUBIN, M.: Cyclic AMP and the expression of differentiated properties *in vitro*. In: The Role of Cyclic Nucleotides in Carcinogenesis (SCHULTZ, GRATZNER, Eds.). Miami Winter Symp. **6**, 239—261 (1973)

GARVIE, W.H.H.: The influence of alloxan diabetes on experimental cancer. Brit. J. Cancer **22**, 128—132 (1968)

Gazdar, A., Hatanaka, M., Herberman, R., Russell, E.: Effects of dibutyryl cyclic adenosine phosphate plus theophylline on murine sarcoma virus transformed non-producer cells. Proc. Soc. exp. Biol. (N.Y.) **141**, 1044—1050 (1972)

Gericke, D., Chandra, P.: Inhibition of tumor growth by nucleoside cyclic 3′,5′-monophosphates. Hoppe-Seylers Z. physiol. Chem. **350**, 1469—1471 (1969)

Goranson, E.S., Tilser, G.J.: Studies on the relationship of alloxan diabetes and tumor growth. Cancer Res. **15**, 626—631 (1955)

Granner, D., Chase, L.R., Aurbach, G.D., Tomkins, G.M.: Tyroxine amino-transferase: enzyme induction independent of adenosine 3′,5′-monophosphate. Science **162**, 1018—1020 (1968)

Grimes, W.J., Schroeder, J.L.: Dibutyryl cyclic adenosine 3′,5′-monophosphate sugar transport and regulatory control of cell division in normal and transformed cells. J. Cell Biol. **56**, 487—491 (1973)

Hamazaki, T.: Effect of adenosine 3′,5′-monophosphate on thymidine kinase in tumor cells. Gann **64**, 219—226 (1973)

Heidrick, M.L., Ryan, W.L.: Cyclic nucleotides on cell growth *in vitro*. Cancer Res. **30**, 376—378 (1970)

Heidrick, M.L., Ryan, W.L.: Adenosine 3′,5′-cyclic monophosphate and contact inhibition. Cancer Res. **31**, 1313—1315 (1971)

Hershko, A., Mamont, P., Shields, R., Tomkins, G.M.: "Pleiotypic response". Nature (Lond.) **232**, 206—211 (1971)

Heuson, J.-C., Legros, N.: Influence of insulin deprivation on growth of the 7,12-dimethylbenz(a)anthracene-induced mammary carcinoma in rats subjected to alloxan diabetes and food restriction. Cancer Res. **32**, 226—232 (1972)

Heuson, J.-C., Legros, N., Heimann, R.: Influence of insulin administration on growth of the 7,12-dimethylbenz(a)anthracene-induced mammary carcinoma in intact, oophorectomized, and hypophysectomized rats. Cancer Res. **32**, 233—238 (1972)

Hilz, H., Kaukel, E., Fuhrmann, U., Wagenhals, B.: Divergent action mechanism of cAMP and dibutyryl cAMP on cell proliferation and macromolecular synthesis in Hela S 3 cultures. Molecular cellular Biochem. **1**, 229—239 (1973)

Hilz, H., Tarnowski, W.: Opposite effects of cyclic AMP and its dibutyryl derivative on glycogen levels in Hela cells. Biochem. biophys. Res. Commun. **40**, 973—981 (1970)

Holley, R.W., Kiernan, J.A.: "Contact inhibition" of cell division in 3T3 cells. Proc. nat. Acad. Sci. (Wash.) **60**, 300—304 (1968)

Hsie, A.W., Jones, C., Puck, T.T.: Further changes in differentiation state accompanying the conversion of Chinese hamster cells to fibroblastic form by dibutyryl adenosine cyclic 3′,5′-monophosphate and hormones. Proc. nat. Acad. Sci. (Wash.) **68**, 1648—1652 (1971)

Hsie, A.W., Puck, T.T.: Morphological transformation of Chinese hamster cells by dibutyryl adenosine cyclic 3′:5′-monophosphate and testosterone. Proc. nat. Acad. Sci. (Wash.) **68**, 358—361 (1971)

Inbar, M., Ben-Bassat, H., Sachs, L.: Membrane changes associated with malignancy. Nature New Biology **236**, 3—4, 16 (1972)

Ingle, D.J.: Urinary glucose and tumor growth in partially depancreatized forcefed rats. Endocrinology **62**, 78—83 (1958)

Ingle, D.J.: Comparison of pancreatic and steroid diabetes in respect to tumor growth and glycosuria. Diabetes **14**, 93—95 (1965)

Johnson, A.M., Alper, C.A., Rosen, F.S., Craig, J.M.: Immunofluorescent hepatic localization of complement proteins: Evidence for a biosynthetic defect in hereditary angioneurotic edema (HANE). J. clin. Invest. **50**, 50a (1971)

Johnson, G.S., Friedman, R.M., Pastan, I.: Cyclic AMP-treated sarcoma cells acquire several morphological characteristics of normal fibroblasts. Ann. N.Y. Acad. Sci. **185**, 413—416 (1971a)

Johnson, G.S., Friedman, R.M., Pastan, I.: Restoration of several morphological characteristics of normal fibroblasts in sarcoma cells treated with adenosine 3′-5′ cyclic monophosphate and its derivatives. Proc. nat. Acad. Sci. (Wash.) **68**, 425—429 (1971b)

Johnson, G.S., Morgan, W.D., Pastan, I.: Regulation of cell motility by cyclic AMP. Nature (Lond.) **235**, 54—56 (1972)

Johnson, G.S., Pastan, I.: Role of 3′,5′-adenosine monophosphate in regulation of morphology and growth of transformed and normal fibroblasts. J. nat. Cancer Inst. **48**, 1377—1387 (1972a)

Johnson, G.S., Pastan, I.: Cyclic AMP increases the adhesion of fibroblasts to substratum. Nature New Biology **236**, 247—249 (1972b)

Johnson, I.S., Wright, H.F.: Anti-tumor activity of glucagon. Cancer Res. **19**, 557—560 (1959)

Kessler, I.: Cancer mortality among diabetics. J. nat. Cancer Inst. **44**, 673—686 (1970)

KOBLET, H., KOHLER, U., WYLER, R.: Stimulation of ribonucleic-acid synthesis in chick-embryo fibroblasts by exogenous adenosine 3′:5′-monophosphate. Europ. J. Biochem. **37**, 134—142 (1973)

KURTH, R., BAUER, H.: Influence of dibutyryl cyclic-AMP and theophylline on cell surface antigens on oncorna-virus transformed cells. Nature New Biology **243**, 243—245 (1973)

LIEBERMAN, I., OVE, P.: Growth factors for mammalian cells in culture. J. biol. Chem. **234**, 2754—2758 (1959)

MAKMAN, M.H.: Adenyl cyclase of cultured mammalian cells: activation by catecholamines. Science **170**, 1421—1423 (1970)

MAKMAN, M.H.: Conditions leading to enhanced response to glucagon, epinephrine, or prostaglandins by adenylate cyclase of normal and malignant cultured cells. Proc. nat. Acad. Sci. (Wash.) **68**, 2127—2130 (1971)

MANGANIELLO, V., VAUGHAN, M.: Prostaglandin E_1 effects on adenosine 3′:5′-cyclic monophosphate concentration and phosphodiesterase activity in fibroblasts. Proc. nat. Acad. Sci. (Wash.) **69**, 269—273 (1972)

MOORE, G.E., ITO, E., ULRICH, K., SANDBERG, A.A.: Culture of human leukemia cells. Cancer (Philad.) **19**, 713—723 (1966)

NASEEM, S.M., HOLLANDER, V.P.: Insulin reversal of growth inhibition of plasma cell tumor by prostaglandin or adenosine 3′,5′-monophosphate. Cancer Res. **33**, 1209—1212 (1973)

OTTEN, J., BADER, J., JOHNSON, G.S., PASTAN, I.: A mutation in a Rous sarcoma virus gene that controls adenosine 3′,5′-monophosphate levels and transformation. J. biol. Chem. **247**, 1632—1633 (1972)

OTTEN, J., JOHNSON, G.S., PASTAN, I.: Cyclic AMP levels in fibroblasts: relationship to growth rate and contact inhibition of growth. Biochem. biophys. Res. Commun. **44**, 1192—1198 (1971)

OTTEN, J., JOHNSON, G.S., PASTAN, I.: Regulation of cell growth by cyclic adenosine 3′,5′-monophosphate. Effect of cell density and agents which alter cell growth on cyclic adenosine 3′,5′-monophosphate levels in fibroblasts. J. biol. Chem. **247**, 7082 (1972)

PASTAN, I.: Discussion-remark. In: Role of Cyclic Nucleotides in Carcinogenesis (SCHULZ, GRATZNER, Eds.). Miami Winter Symp. **6**, 259 (1973)

PASTAN, I., PERLMAN, R.L.: Cyclic AMP in metabolism. Nature New Biology **229**, 5—7 (1971)

PAUL, D.: Quiescent SV 40 virus transformed 3T3 cells in culture. Biochem. biophys. Res. Commun. **53**, 745—753 (1973)

PEERY, C.V., JOHNSON, G.S., PASTAN, I.: Adenylcyclase in normal and transformed fibroblasts in tissue culture. Activation by prostaglandins. J. biol. Chem. **246**, 5785—5790 (1971)

PENNINGTON, S.N., BROWN, H.D., CHATTOPHADHYAY, S.K., CONAWAY, C., MORRIS, H.P.: Effect of sodium fluoride on the epinephrine responses of liver and hepatoma adenyl cyclase. Experientia (Basel) **26**, 139—140 (1970)

PRASAD, K.N., HSIE, A.W.: Morphologic differentiation of mouse neuroblastoma cells induced *in vitro* by dibutyryl adenosine 3′:5′-cyclic monophosphate. Nature New Biology **233**, 141—142 (1971)

PUCK, T.T.: Genetic-biochemical studies on the mammalian cell surface. In: The Role of Cyclic Nucleotides in Carcinogenesis (SCHULTZ, GRATZNER, Eds.). Miami Winter Symp. **6**, 283—302 (1973)

PUCKETT, C.L., SHINGLETON, W.W.: The effect of induced diabetes on experimental tumour growth in mice. Cancer Res. **32**, 789—790 (1972)

REIN, A., CARCHMAN, R.A., JOHNSON, G.S., PASTAN, I.: Simian virus 40 rapidly lowers cAMP levels in mouse cells. Biochem. biophys. Res. Commun. **52**, 899—904 (1973)

ROSTLAPIL, J., ZRUSTOVÁ, M.: Frequency of Malignant Tumours in Diabetes mellitus. Acta diabet. lat. **11**, 43—45 (1974)

RYAN, W.L., HEIDRICK, M.L.: Inhibition of cell growth *in vitro* by adenosine 3′5′-monophosphate. Science **162**, 1484—1485 (1968)

RYAN, W.L., CURTIS, G.L.: Chemical carcinogens and cyclic AMP. In: The Role of Cyclic Nucleotides in Carcinogenesis (SCHULTZ, GRATZNER, Eds.). Miami Winter Symp. **6**, 1—18 (1973)

RYAN, W.L., DURICK, M.A.: Adenosine 3′,5′-monophosphate and N^6-2-0-dibutyryl-adenosine 3′,5′-monophosphate transport in cells. Science **177**, 1002—1003 (1972)

SALTER, J.M., MEYER, R. DE, BEST, C.H.: Effect of insulin and glucagon on tumor growth. Brit. med. J. **1958II**, 5—7

SALZBERG, D.A., GRIFFIN, A.C.: Inhibition of azo dye carcinogenesis in the alloxan-diabetic rat. Cancer Res. **12**, 294 (1952)

SCHRÖDER, J., PLAGEMANN, P.G.W.: Cyclic 3′,5′-nucleotide phosphodiesterases of Novikoff rat hepatoma, mouse L, and HeLa cells growing in suspension culture. Cancer Res. **32**, 1082—1087 (1972)

Seller, M.J., Benson, P.F.: *In vivo* effect of adenosine 3',5'-monophosphate on Ehrlich ascites tumour cells. Europ. J. Cancer **9**, 525—526 (1973)

Sharma, R.K.: Studies on adrenocortical carcinoma of rat cyclic nucleotide phosphodiesterase activities. Cancer Res. **32**, 1734—1736 (1972)

Sheppard, J.R.: Restoration of contact-inhibited growth to transformed cells by dibutyryl adenosine 3':5' cyclic monophosphate. Proc. nat. Acad. Sci. (Wash.) **68**, 1316—1320 (1971)

Sheppard, J.R.: Difference in the cyclic adenosine 3',5'-monophosphate levels in normal and transformed cells. Nature New Biology **236**, 14—16 (1972)

Sheppard, J.R., Cromwell, R., Meyers, R., McLaughlin, W.J.: Metabolism of cyclic AMP in normal and transformed fibroblasts. In: The Role of Cyclic Nucleotides in Carcinogenesis (Schultz, Gratzner, Eds.). Miami Winter Symp. **6**, 19—37 (1973)

Smets, L.A.: Contact inhibition of transformed cells incompletely restored by dibutyryl cyclic AMP. Nature New Biology **239**, 123—124 (1972)

Smith, B.J., Defendi, Wigglesworth, N.U.: The effect of dibutyryl cyclic AMP on transformation by oncogenic viruses. Virology **51**, 230—232 (1973)

Temin, H.M.: Studies on carcinogenesis by avian sarcoma viruses. VI. Differential multiplication of uninfected and of converted cells in response to insulin. J. cell Physiol. **69**, 377—384 (1967)

Temin, H.M.: Carcinogenesis by avian sarcoma viruses. X. The decreased requirement for insulin-replaceable activity in serum for cell multiplication. Int. J. Cancer **3**, 771—787 (1968)

Thomas, E.W., Murad, F., Looney, W.B., Morris, H.P.: Adenosine 3',5'-monophosphate and guanosine 3',5'-monophosphate: Concentrations in Morris hepatomas of different growth rate. Biochim. biophys. Acta (Amst.) **297**, 564—567 (1973)

Tomasi, V., Rethy, A., Trevisani, A.: Soluble and membrane-bound adenylate cyclase of Yoshida hepatoma. In: The Role of Cyclic Nucleotides in Carcinogenesis (Schultz, Gratzner, Eds.). Miami Winter Symp. **6**, 127—152 (1973)

Troy, F.A., Vijay, I.K., Kawakami, T.G.: Cyclic 3',5'-AMP-dependent and independent protein kinase levels in normal and feline sarcoma virus transformed cells. Biochem. biophys. Res. Commun. **52**, 150—158 (1973)

Vaheri, A., Ruoslahti, E., Hovi, T., Nordling, S.: Stimulation of density-inhibited cell cultures by insulin. J. cell Physiol. **81**, 355—363 (1973)

Vangerow, M., McKee, R.W.: Metabolism of glucose, lactate, and alanine by Ehrlich ascites carcinoma cells from normal and alloxan-diabetic mice. Fed. Proc. **14**, 296 (1955)

Wallach, D.F.H.: Cellular membranes and tumor behavior: a new hypothesis. Proc. nat. Acad. Sci. (Wash.) **61**, 868—874 (1968)

Weber, G.: The molecular correlation concept of neoplasia and the cyclic AMP system. In: The Role of Cyclic Nucleotides in Carcinogenesis (Schultz, Gratzner, Eds.). Miami Winter Symp. **6**, 57—102 (1973)

Weiss, B., Shein, H.M., Snyder, R.: Adenylate cyclase and phosphodiesterase activity of normal and SV_{40} virus-transformed hamster astrocytes in cell culture. Life Sci. **10**, 1253 (1971)

Wicks, W.D., van Wijk, R., Clay, K., Bearg, C., Bevers, U.U., van Rijn, J.: Regulation of growth rate, DNA synthesis and specific protein synthesis by derivatives of cyclic AMP in cultured hepatoma. In: The Role of Cyclic Nucleotides in Carcinogenesis (Schultz, Gratzner, Eds.). Miami Winter Symp. **6**, 103—126 (1973)

Wieser, D., Pool, M., Mohr, U.: Wachstum von Transplantationstumoren auf Ratten mit Alloxandiabetes. Z. Naturwiss. **54**, 23 (1967)

van Wijk, R., Wicks, N.D., Clay, K.: Effects of derivatives of cyclic 3',5'-adenosine monophosphate on the growth, morphology and gene expression of hepatoma cells in culture. Cancer Res. **32**, 1905—1911 (1972)

Willingham, M.C., Johnson, G.S., Pastan, I.: Control of DNA synthesis and mitosis in 3T3 cells by cyclic AMP. Biochem. biophys. Res. Commun. **48**, 743—748 (1972)

Yarnell, M.M., Schnebli, H.P.: Release from density-dependent inhibition of growth in the absence of cell locomotion. J. Cell Sci. (in press)

Yoshikawa-Fukada, M., Nojima, T.: Biochemical characteristics of normal and virally transformed mouse cell lines. J. cell. Physiol. **80**, 421—430 (1972)

Zacchello, F., Benson, P.F., Gianelli, F., McGuire, M.: Induction of adenylate cyclase activity in cultured human fibroblasts during increasing cell population density. Biochem. J. **126**, 27P (1972)

3. Action on Blood Cells

a) Erythrocytes

It is generally assumed that insulin has no influence on glucose uptake into normal, nonnucleated erythrocytes (EADIE *et al.*, 1923; SOSKIN *et al.*, 1941; PLETSCHER *et al.*, 1955). In all these studies only net influxes of glucose were measured. Using a more detailed approach and measuring the maximal unidirectional net efflux of glucose and the exchange flux separately, ZIPPER and MAWE (1972) found a nearly 50% increase of glucose net influx due to insulin, whereas the more rapid exchange flux (3 times that of the net efflux) was unaltered. The insulin concentrations used were not particularly high (450 μU/ml), yet this insulin effect seems to be rather nonspecific because individual A and B chains and other agents (vasopressin, oxydized glutathione) had the same effect. In conclusion, a direct effect of insulin has been postulated on the free glucose carrier, which moves 4 times more slowly than the complexed carrier. An alteration in the transmembrane redox potential gradient in the presence of insulin has been found by DORMANDY (1966). Glucose transport can, however, be stimulated by noradrenalin *in vitro* and has been attributed to α-receptor stimulation (HADDEN *et al.*, 1971). To our knowledge no reports exist as to whether insulin actually interferes in this process. With high insulin concentrations (20 mU/ml), BURN (1962) demonstrated a somewhat slower increase in ATP content when erythrocytes previously low in ATP were incubated with adenosine, which increases the ATP content under such conditions. This curious effect was attributed to a decrease in the utilization of adenosine as substrate.

In erythrocytes previously treated with chymotrypsin, RIESER and RIESER (1964) found that high concentrations of insulin stimulate aldose-hexose transport into human erythrocytes. In view of the concept that erythrocytes have few (GAVIN *et al.*, 1972a) or no insulin receptor sites (ROBINSON *et al.*, 1972; KRUG *et al.*, 1972), some cryptic receptor sites may be moved to the outside by partial and nonspecific proteolysis.

It is interesting to note that the nonnucleated erythrocyte is the only cell type devoid of adenylate cyclase. Any activity found is probably restricted to reticulocytes in the preparation (GAUGER *et al.*, 1973). In patients with insulinoma, a higher activity of some glycolytic key enzymes was found, which fell after operation (KIMURA *et al.*, 1971). This points to an enzyme-inductive effect of variably high insulin concentrations in man. Formerly, an increase in lactate and pyruvate was found by ZURUKZOGLU (1966). When normal and prediabetic women were treated with hypoglycemic doses of insulin their erythrocytes showed a lower glucose consumption and lactate production, both attributable to growth hormone secretion (RAMASSO, 1970).

b) Granulocytes and Lymphocytes

In contrast to earlier assumptions (HELMREICH and EISEN, 1959) lymphocytes are not insensitive to insulin. Moreover, all white blood cells have surface sites which bind insulin specifically (GAVIN *et al.*, 1972a). The results are quantitatively similar with lymphocytes, cultured leukemic lymphocytes, and granulocytes. The 10-fold higher binding capacity of leukemic lymphocytes can be explained by their 10 times greater surface area. However, a highly variable number of receptor sites have been found by GAVIN *et al.* (1973) in several lines of lymphocytes. This partly explains the finding of KRUG *et al.* (1972), that erythrocytes, platelets, granulocytes, and normal lymphocytes have no binding sites. In the case of transformation by concanavalin A, however, lymphocytes gain receptor sites in parallel to the time course of transformation and of incorporation of ^{3}H-thymidine into nuclear DNA. Solubilized insulin receptor protein has been prepared from human lymphocytes by the use of nonionic detergent (Gavin *et al.*, 1972b). The release of receptors from cultured lymphocytes by incubation in serum-free neutral buffer alone for 70 min at 30° C has been demonstrated by Gavin *et al.* (1972) and used for preparation. For further details and for information on the similarity with insulin receptors of other tissues, see Gavin *et al.* (1973) and Tell *et al.* (Chapter A p 249). Some obese patients may have alterations in lymphocyte receptor sites (Archer *et al.*, 1973). Chronic exposure of lymphocytes to higher than normal insulin concentrations reduces the number of insulin receptor sites (Gavin *et al.*, 1974).

Several reports point to some stimulation by insulin of glucose transport in polymorphonuclear leukocytes, especially those of diabetic origin (Martin *et al.*, 1953; Dumm, 1957; Kalant and Schucker, 1962; Esmann, 1963; denied by Antonioli *et al.*, 1967) and in thymic lymphocytes of adrenalectomized rats (Boyett and Hofert, 1972). For this latter cell type, furthermore, an increased α-aminoisobutyric acid uptake by insulin was reported (Goldfine *et al.*, 1972). Both effects take place with reasonably low insulin concentrations; because they are inhibited by cycloheximide, it has been thought that protein synthesis participates in these transport effects of insulin. cAMP does not seem to be involved.

Within a few minutes after exposure of lymphocytes to mitogenic agents (phytohemagglutinin, concanavalin A) an increased Ca^{++} uptake was observed (Whitney and Sutherland, 1973) and after 20 min a rise in cGMP levels, followed at 72 h by increased DNA synthesis (Hadden *et al.*, 1972). In view of the findings of Illiano *et al.* (1973) of increased cGMP levels in adipocytes after insulin, one can speculate that insulin may induce similar alterations in lymphocytes.

Insulin as trophic hormone, e.g. in cases of deprived pituitary factors, given daily to rats over a period of several weeks, increased the weight of thymus and lymph nodes (Lundin and Angervall, 1970). Secondary hormonal reactions have, however, to be taken into account.

References

Antonioli, J., Felber, J.P., Vannotti, A.: Effet de l'insuline et de quelques autres facteurs sur la glycolyse des leucocytes humains mesures *in vitro*. Acta haemat. (Basel) **37**, 161—173 (1967)

Archer, J.A., Gorden, P., Gavin, J.R., Lesniak, M.A., Roth, J.: Insulin receptors in human circulating lymphocytes: application to the study of insulin resistance in man. J. clin. Endocr. **36**, 627—633 (1973)

Boyett, J.D., Hofert, J.F.: Stimulatory effect of insulin on glucose metabolism of thymus lymphocytes. Horm. Metab. Res. **4**, 163—167 (1972)

Burn, G.P.: Adenosine triphosphate content and glucose uptake of human erythrocytes and the influence of insulin. Biochim. biophys. Acta (Amst.) **59**, 347—354 (1962)

Dormandy, T.L.: The mechanism of insulin action. The effect of insulin on the allosteric properties of intracellular haemoglobin. J. Physiol. (Lond.) **183**, 378—406 (1966)

Dumm, M.E.: Glucose utilization and lactate production by leukocytes of patients with diabetes mellitus. Proc. Soc. exp. Biol. (N.Y.) **95**, 571—574 (1957)

Eadie, G.S., MacLeod, J.J.R., Noble, E.C.: Insulin and glycolysis. Amer. J. Physiol. **65**, 462—476 (1923)

Esmann, V.: Effect of insulin on human leukocytes. Diabetes **12**, 545—549 (1963)

Gauger, D., Palm, D., Kaiser, G., Quiring, K.: Adenyl cyclase activities in rat erythrocytes during stress erythopoiesis: localization of the enzyme in the reticulocytes. Life Sci. **13**, 31—40 (1973)

Gavin, J.R., Roth, J., Neville, D.M., de Meyts, P., Buell, D.N.: Insulin-dependent regulation of insulin-receptor concentrations: A direct demonstration in cell culture. Proc. nat. Acad. Sci. (Wash.) **71**, 84—88 (1974)

Gavin, J.R., Buell, D.N., Roth, J.: Water-suluble insulin receptors from human lymphocytes. Science **178**, 168—169 (1972)

Gavin, J.R., Gorden, P., Roth, J., Archer, J.A., Buell, D.N.: Characteristics of the human lymphocyte insulin receptor. J. biol. Chem. **248**, 2202—2207 (1973)

Gavin, J.R., Mann, D.L., Buell, D.N., Roth, J.: Preparation of solubilized insulin receptors from human lymphocytes. Biochem. biophys. Res. Commun. **49**, 870—876 (1972b)

Gavin, J.R., Roth, J., Jen, P., Freychet, P.: Insulin receptors in human circulating cells and fibroblasts. Proc. nat. Acad. Sci. (Wash.) **69**, 747—751 (1972a)

Goldfine, I.D., Gardner, J.D., Neville, D.M., Jr.: Insulin action in isolated rat thymocytes. I. Binding of ^{125}I-insulin and stimulation of α-aminoisobutyric acid transport. J. biol. Chem. **247**, 6919—6926 (1972)

Hadden, J.W., Hadden, E.M., Good, R.A.: Alpha-adrenergic stimulation of glucose uptake in human erythrocytes, lymphocytes, and lymphoblasts. Exp. Cell Res. **68**, 217—219 (1971)

Hadden, J.W., Hadden E.M., Haddox, M.K., Goldberg, N.D.: Guanosine 3′:5′-cyclic-monophosphate: a possible intracellular mediator of mitogenic influences in lymphocytes. Proc. nat. Acad. Sci. (Wash.) **69**, 3024—3027 (1972)

Helmreich, E., Eisen, H.: The distribution and utilization of glucose in isolated lymph-node cells. J. biol. Chem. **234**, 1958—1965 (1959)

Illiano, G., Tell, G., Siegel, M., Cuatrecasas, P.: Guanosine 3′:5′-cyclic monophosphate and the action of insulin and acetylcholine. Proc. nat. Acad. Sci. (Wash.) **70**, 2443—2447 (1973)

Kalant, N., Schucker, R.: Glucose utilization and insulin responsiveness of leucocytes in diabetes. Canad. J. Biochem. **40**, 899—903 (1962)

Kimura, H., Horiuchi, N., Kitamura, T., Morita, K.: Hormonal response of glycolytic key enzymes of erythrocytes in insulinoma. Metabolism **20**, 1119—1121 (1971)

Krug, M., Krug, F., Cuatrecasas, P.: Emergence of insulin receptors on human lymphocytes during *in vitro* transformation. Proc. nat. Acad. Sci. (Wash.) **69**, 2604—2608 (1972)

Lundin, P.M., Angervall, L.: Effect of insulin on rat lymphoid tissue. Path. europ. **5**, 273—278 (1970)

Martin, S.P., McKinney, G.R., Green, R., Becker, C.: The influence of glucose, fructose, and insulin on the metabolism of leukocytes of healthy and diabetic subjects. J. clin. Invest. **32**, 1171—1174 (1953)

Pletscher, A., v. Planta, P., Hunzinger, W.A.: Beeinflussung der Fructose- und Glukosepermeabilität von Erythrocyten durch Temperatur, Cortison und Insulin. Zum Kohlenhydratstoffwechsel VII. Helv. physiol. pharmacol. Acta **13**, 18—24 (1955)

Ramasso, J.C.: Metabolismo y fragilidad osmótica de eritrocitos humanos durante la hipoglucemia insulínica. Rev. Soc. argent. Biol. **46**, 72—77 (1970)

Rieser, P., Rieser, C.H.: Reversal of insulin resistance in red cell sugar transport. Arch. Biochem. **105**, 20—24 (1964)

Robinson, C.A., Boshell, B.R., Reddy, W.J.: Insulin binding to plasma membranes. Biochim. biophys. Acta (Amst.) **290**, 84—91 (1972)

Soskin, S., Levine, R., Hechter, O.: The relation between the phosphate changes in blood and muscle, following dextrose, insulin and epinephrine administration. Amer. J. Physiol. **134**, 40—46 (1941)

Whitney, R.B., Sutherland, R.M.: Characteristics of calcium accumulation by lymphocytes and alterations in the process induced by phytohemagglutinin. J. cell. Physiol. **82**, 9—20 (1973)

Zipper, H., Mawe, R.C.: The exchange and maximal net flux of glucose across the human erythrocyte. I. The effect of insulin, insulin derivatives and small proteins. Biochim. biophys. Acta (Amst.) **282**, 311—325 (1972)

Zurukzoglu, W.: The where and how of insulin. Lancet **1966II**, 746

H. Metabolic Alterations in the Body by Insulin

I. Effect of Insulin on the Fate of Glucose

ARNOLD HASSELBLATT

With 3 Figures

1. Introduction

Despite the abundance of available information on the effect of insulin on glucose metabolism in isolated tissues or organ systems, some questions can be answered only on the basis of data obtained from whole animals or man. Such questions concern the fate in the body, not of a single molecule of glucose, but rather of the entire mass of glucose present in the various tissue compartments. As to the effects of insulin, it may be anticipated at the very beginning of this discussion that this hormone reduces blood glucose levels by means other than opening up entirely new metabolic pathways for glucose molecules. Its action is rather to shift the existing balance between different metabolic pathways, thus altering the dynamic equilibrium. Insulin may therefore be expected to change the fate of glucose in a quantitative rather than in a qualitative manner.

We are aware today that insulin probably lowers the blood glucose concentration by means of two different mechanisms: by reducing hepatic glucose release, and by increasing peripheral glucose uptake. It thus hardly seems possible to give a simple answer to the most frequently asked question, which has inspired a variety of complicated experiments, i.e.:

Does insulin lower blood glucose by reducing glucose production or by stimulating glucose utilization?

This alternative is similarily expressed in the old controversy as to whether overproduction or underutilization of glucose is the primary cause of diabetic hyperglycemia. It is now realized that it is the quantitative aspect of this question that has to be discussed. The original question may therefore be reformulated as follows:

To what extent do the reduction of glucose production and the stimulation of glucose utilization contribute respectively to the hypoglycemic effect of insulin?

Other aspects may be introduced into the basic inquiry concerning how insulin affects the fate of glucose in the body. Thus, an additional question has been asked:

How does insulin change the volume of distribution of the glucose mass present in the body?

Any increase in this volume would lower the blood glucose concentration without necessarily affecting the rate of production or utilization of glucose. Experiments designed to answer such questions *in vivo* are of necessity more difficult to interpret than measurements performed on isolated tissues under well-defined conditions. Nevertheless, it is evident that data from *in vitro* systems can contribute only qualitative answers concerning the effect of insulin on the fate of glucose; they can never yield quantitative conclusions on rates of glucose flow in the body.

In vitro experiments are generally designed to allow no change to occur in the defined conditions except in the agent under investigation. However, the presence or absence of insulin never occurs as an isolated event in the living animal. The effects of insulin on the perfused liver, or on adipose or muscular tissue are discussed in the previous chapters; they illustrate the range of effects involved. Such *in vitro* experiments cannot, by their very nature, yield information concerning the extent to which these tissues participate in the overall effect of insulin in the whole body. One reason for this is that our information on glucose metabolism in various tissues of the body is incomplete. More important, in principle, is that the environment in the body is constantly changing and that different hormones selectively control the supply in various substrates. Insulin not only affects the tissue cells directly, it may also change their environment by lowering the level of free fatty acids or amino acids, to mention just a few examples. This is well illustrated by the isolated, perfused liver preparation. In perfusion experiments the liver is usually supplied with a single substrate (lactate, amino acids or glycerol) at a concentration high enough to saturate the enzymes responsible for gluconeogenesis and thus to induce glucose synthesis at the maximal rate. This is a reasonable approach when one desires to measure the capacity of the liver to synthesize glucose from various precursors. It is, however, a long way from anything that actually happens in the living animal or in man, as saturating levels of lactate or amino acids are never present in the blood perfusing the liver *in situ*. Thus any rise in the plasma level of lactate, whether due to exercise, catecholamines, or hypoxia, will supply additional precursor for hepatic gluconeogenesis and thus immediately increase the rate of glucose formation. By slight changes of lactate or amino acid levels in the blood, glucose production can be rapidly adjusted to changing demands (EXTON *et al.*, 1970). It has been shown that insulin hardly affects glucose production by the isolated perfused liver in the absence of glucagon or catecholamines, yet it can markedly affect hepatic gluconeogenesis by lowering plasma amino acid levels or inhibiting the uptake of glucogenic amino acids by the liver. Plasma levels of leucine, isoleucine, valine, tyrosine, threonine, and methionine have been found to decline in response to insulin (FELIG *et al.*, 1970), and insulin induces a steep decline in the release of these amino acids from the human forearm (POZEFSKY *et al.*, 1969). As the main glucogenic amino acids are less markedly affected by insulin, it may be a direct inhibitory effect on the hepatic utilization of alanine, glycine, and serine that is responsible for insulin reducing hepatic gluconeogenesis from amino acids (FELIG and WAHREN, 1971).

Once hypoglycemia has been allowed to develop in response to insulin, a sequence of counterregulatory reactions will ensue, including the release of catecholamines from the adrenal medulla and the sympathetic nerve endings (CANNON *et al.*, 1924), of steroids from the adrenal cortex (FROESCH, 1955), and of glucagon from the pancreatic islets (FOA *et al.*, 1952), all of which will grossly interfere with glucose metabolism.

Like hepatic glucose production, peripheral glucose utilization is greatly affected by the presence in the perfusing blood of substrates other than glucose. Thus, in muscle cells fatty acids (NEWSHOLME *et al.*, 1964; SHIPP *et al.*, 1964) or acetoacetate (WILLIAMSON and KREBS, 1961) are metabolized in preference to glucose. In diabetes plasma levels of both free fatty acids and ketone bodies are elevated, so they will compete with glucose for metabolization in the muscle. Insulin may stimulate glucose utilization in muscle in addition to its direct effect on the uptake of glucose (LEVINE *et al.*, 1950) by inhibiting lipolysis in adipose tissue (JUNGAS and BALL, 1963), thereby lowering plasma levels of free fatty acids and ketone bodies in blood. In addition to their direct interference with glucose metabolism, the free fatty acids may inhibit glucagon release (SEYFFERT and MADISON, 1967; EDWARDS *et al.*, 1969) and thus affect glucose homeostasis.

In adipose tissue, but not in muscle, high levels of free fatty acids may stimulate glucose uptake and glycolysis. Thus additional α-glycerophosphate is formed to esterify the free fatty acids present in excess and to store them as triglycerides (CAHILL *et al.*, 1960; LEBOEUF and CAHILL, 1961).

Insulin may thus affect the rate of glucose production and utilization by changing the levels of fatty acids, ketone bodies, or amino acids in addition to the changes it induces in various organ systems. If a new steady state is achieved in the presence of insulin and plasma glucose concentrations are maintained at a constant level, the amount of glucose entering the extracellular space will equal the amount being taken up by tissue cells. Then the rate of glucose production will equal the rate of glucose utilization. In the postabsorptive state, when no glucose is released from the gut, the liver is the main source of glucose. Net hepatic glucose output can be estimated by multiplying the arteriovenous difference in glucose concentration across the liver by the hepatic plasma flow. Such estimates are based on the unproven assumption that during the period of the experiment an equal fraction of the blood passing through the liver is being supplied by the hepatic artery and the portal vein, respectively. Any change in this ratio would affect the glucose concentration in the blood entering the liver and thus modify the basis for calculation of hepatic glucose release.

As the liver is not the only tissue capable of releasing glucose, hepatic glucose output will not equal total glucose production. In the postabsorptive state the kidney contributes 15—20% of the glucose inflow in man (CAHILL, 1967). However, our knowledge about possible changes in renal glucose release that might contribute to glucose homeostasis is very limited. Changes in the amount of glucose produced or utilized by the body will correlate best with hepatic glucose release if renal gluconeogenesis proceeds at a constant rate; this however, seems unlikely.

Finally, considerable difficulties are encountered because the method requires that catheters be inserted, not only into an artery and the hepatic vein, but also into the portal vein. Portal venous blood is unobtainable in intact man, so that true net hepatic glucose release has only been determined — in addition to animal data — in patients with cirrhosis of the liver in whom portal venous blood can be obtained from large and easily accessible portal vein collaterals (MYERS, 1950).

A different, and at first sight more promising approach to the exact measurement of body glucose turnover rates is based on isotope dilution. The dilution of a known amount of labeled glucose by unlabeled glucose molecules in the body should yield information on the total amount of glucose present. The rate of inflow of unlabeled endogenous glucose and the flow of the tagged glucose into the tissues may be estimated from the decay of plasma glucose specific activity.

Calculations based on data from such experiments yield information on the movements of the glucose pool, which intermixes rapidly with the label injected. As this rapidly intermixing glucose is not representative of the glucose present in any anatomically defined compartment, the physiological significance of such data may be limited. For this reason, experiments using isotope dilution techniques have sometimes been disappointing, especially when a single dose of tracer was injected and blood samples were drawn before equilibrium had been established.

2. Isotope Dilution Techniques

a) Definitions and Problems Arising from Incomplete Intermixing

The glucose molecules present in the body as such are molecules in solution. It seems reasonable, therefore, to assume that glucose molecules are homogeneously distributed within a space inside the body, which is bounded by membranes not freely permeable to glucose, and that glucose molecules intermix freely and rapidly within this space. Neither of these assumptions is, however, based on reality and the errors incurred by adhering to them will be discussed later. Nevertheless, a large body of experimental data has been obtained by assuming that body glucose is a rapidly intermixing entity, or at least that the errors induced by this assumption are of no practical significance.

The term "glucose pool" derives from similar lines of thought. A pool of material in steady-state turnover has been defined as "a collection of identical molecules from which deletions are made at a constant rate, along with simultaneous addition of new identical molecules at the same rate, the total pool size remaining unchanged" (STEELE, 1964). The term "pool" indicates that all the molecules should have an equal chance of exit and hence must be present in well-mixed solution. Thus defined, a pool comprises a given number of molecules that intermix freely and enter and leave, the pool by the same kinetic process. One could suppose the existence of different pools for the same species of molecules within the body, differing in their entry and removal rates, but in themselves offering homogeneous kinetic parameters. The simultaneous presence of such different pools would be expressed by adding different compartments, each characterized by the same kinetics for the molecules of glucose inside, but differing from each other in turnover rates and size.

The term "rapidly intermixing glucose pool" is not usually applied to denote a single well-defined and homogeneous pool. It is rather used to mean that kind of pool from which the measured data from isotope dilution experiments could have been derived, if intermixing of label were limited to a single pool. As this is not expected to be the case, however, the data will usually result from more or less complete intermixing of the injected labeled glucose within pools having different rates of exchange. Thus "pools" or "compartments" have in common that they are defined by kinetic parameters but not, it must be emphasized, by special anatomic correlates like blood plasma and extracellular fluid, or by organ systems like liver or kidney. One organ could well contain more than one compartment (GINSBERG and WILDE, 1954). Thus, even if it were possible to measure separately the size of a defined glucose pool, the space it occupies, and its turnover rate, these data as such would be of little physiological significance. It is rather the sum of all the movements of glucose between different compartments or pools, and of their entry and removal rates that could quantify the fate of glucose in the body.

Additional assumptions and facts have been introduced in order to facilitate calculation of flow rates from one compartment or pool to another, despite the limited number of individual tracers available and the fact that sampling is restricted to one compartment, usually plasma. It seems reasonable to assume that glucose from the liver or the kidney is released into the blood before being utilized by peripheral tissues. To meet this assumption one must envisage a more constrained system than one that allows free exchange of glucose molecules between all peripheral compartments. For this reason, the movements of glucose molecules within the body have been considered to conform to a system consisting of a central compartment plus a series of peripheral compartments, each of which communicates with any other only through the central one (WRENSHALL, 1955). The term "mammillary system" was coined by SHEPPARD and HOUSEHOLDER (1951) for a system defined in this way. If one wishes to calculate transfer rates in a mammillary system, intermixing of the injected tracer must be complete. As instantaneous intermixing of labeled and unlabeled molecules in the cell is unlikely to occur, methods have been developed for the calculation of transfer rates in biological systems containing compartments whose contents do not rapidly intermix. These methods are based on the extrapolation of all values to time zero, when all radioactivity is assumed to be present in a uniformly mixed state within the central, rapidly intermixing compartment. Under these conditions nonuniform mixing in peripheral compartments does not affect the calculated transfer rates (WRENSHALL, 1955). More recent developments indicate that practically all the glucose utilized stems from the rapidly mixing pool fraction (KATZ *et al.*, 1974b). If no glucose is leaving the slowly equilibrating fraction, the calculations to estimate flow rates of glucose in the nonsteady state may be improved (STEELE *et al.*, 1974). A noncompartmental approach to the estimation of glucose turnover rates has been proposed (KATZ *et al.*, 1974a): instead of compartmental units, the glucose system could be described by a model of tubes, communicating in labyrinthine manner with the rapidly intermixing pool.

The rapidly intermiscible fraction of the glucose pool is not necessarily the glucose present in the extracellular space. Equilibration of tracer is likely to occur more rapidly across the liver than with extracellular glucose molecules dissolved in the cerebrospinal fluid, the aqueous fluid of the eye, or the extracellular fluid of relatively avascular connective tissues. Again, it seems impossible to allocate glucose molecules to physiologically meaningful entities by measuring ease of mixing with injected tracer molecules. For the reasons mentioned, some early experiments, based on the assumption that injected ^{14}C-glucose equilibrates rapidly with total body glucose, gave variable and possibly misleading results.

When labeled glucose is given in a single injection and calculations of glucose production or utilization are based on the subsequent exponential decline of plasma specific activity, the results will be too high as long as mixing is incomplete. The label will be diluted not only by newly formed glucose but also by glucose molecules entering from less accessible compartments. On the other hand, ^{14}C-glucose will be lost not only as as result of glucose utilization but also by the exit of glucose into deeper compartments. The following example demonstrates how incomplete mixing can affect the actual experimental results. After a single intravenous injection of tracer both the slope and the extrapolated intercept of the specific activity decay curve at time zero of tracer injection changed by more than 50% when the time allowed for intermixing was increased from 15—140 min (WRENSHALL *et al.*, 1961).

Similarly, calculations of the glucose "space" of the body depend on complete intermixing of the tracer. This space is defined to "give total volume of fluid of the same glucose concentration as plasma that is required to contain the number of grams of glucose in the body pool" (Steele *et al.*, 1956). Correspondingly, experiments based on the assumption that injected ^{14}C-glucose equilibrates rapidly with the body glucose pool have yielded highly variable data for the glucose space. Thus, a single injection of labeled glucose was given to dogs and the exponential decline of plasma specific radioactivity with time was followed; extrapolation back to time zero gave a glucose space of 35—65% of body weight (Searle *et al.*, 1954), probably because metabolism of glucose took place before intermixing was complete. Following a single injection with subsequent constant infusion of labeled glucose, thus allowing for more complete intermixing, the same authors found a calculated glucose space of the order of 30% of the dog's weight, while the miscible glucose pool amounted to 2—3 g in dogs of 6—8 kg body weight.

The problems encountered when glucose mass, glucose space, or glucose turnover rates are calculated from isotope dilution data have been thoroughly analyzed by Steele (1964). It is evident that intermixing will be more complete when first a priming dose of labeled glucose is injected and subsequently an additional amount of label is infused, carefully balanced to compensate exactly for the dilution of label by endogenously produced glucose. The decay over time of plasma glucose specific activity was measured, and the resulting curve for one dog was analyzed by Steele (1964): it could only be defined as a function of two exponential terms, not one. The explanation favored by Steele (1964) for the presence of more than one exponential term is that a more slowly equilibrating glucose pool is present in the dog. In fact, previous experiments had revealed that about half of the intermiscible glucose mass is equilibrating slowly with the label, whether injected or infused. It is recommended, therefore, that samples of blood should not be taken earlier than 60 min after the priming dose of labeled glucose. Incomplete intermixing will most affect estimates of total-body free glucose and values derived from it, such as the glucose space. Isotope dilution techniques with access to the plasma compartment alone will measure total body free glucose in the dog with an uncertainty of $\pm 12\%$ (Steele, 1964). The data calculated by Steele (1964) for a 13.8-kg dog are: total glucose pool size between 3.75 and 4.75 g of glucose; glucose space between 27 and 34% of body weight.

The rates of glucose production and release may be estimated more precisely, even when intermixing is not complete. Following a single injection of tracer, the rate of appearance and disappearance of glucose has been calculated in diabetic animals by methods not assuming dynamic equilibrium (Henderson *et al.*, 1955). Because such measurements cover only movement out of the rapidly intermixing portion of body glucose, their physiological relevance has been questioned (Steele, 1964).

The capacity of a method based on repeated single injections of tracer to measure the same compartment as that characterized by constant infusion is limited by the time necessary to approximate uniform intermixing of tracer with traced substance (Wrenshall and Hetenyi, 1959). Intermixing times of 60—120 min were allowed following single injections of ^{14}C-glucose, and appearance rates of ^{12}C-glucose were calculated and compared to the known rates of glucose infusion into eviscerated dogs. Close agreement was established between calculated and measured rates (Wrenshall *et al.*, 1961). Despite additional evidence on the validity of the tracer-injection method (Cowan *et al.*, 1969), the authors subsequently applied a modified primed tracer-infusion technique (Cowan and Hetenyi, 1971), which allowed a constant specific activity of plasma glucose to be achieved within 40 min. The fraction of the glucose pool involved in any change in glucose flow rates is expected to depend on the slope of the change. The more rapid the change, the smaller the fraction of the total pool taking part. Thus, it is clear that body glucose responds as a single pool only to very slow changes. The physiological relevance of such a response may justly be questioned. Thus, movements of glucose through both the rapidly equilibrating and the slowly responding pool of body glucose are probably not representative of the glucose fluxes that ensure glucose homeostasis.

STEELE (1959) mentions an impressive example of how slow intermixing can interfere with the interpretation of results. ^{14}C-glucose has been used to measure changes in hepatic glucose release when exogenous glucose is supplied by injection. Following an injection of labeled glucose, plasma glucose specific radioactivity decays because of the release of unlabeled glucose from the liver. If no glucose were added to the blood, the specific activity would not decline further and the curve would level out into a plateau. Such a plateau has been observed to follow an intravenous glucose load (SEARLE and CHAIKOFF, 1952). This result may be interpreted as meaning that hepatic glucose release is suppressed in response to the glucose load, either by a rise of intracellular glucose concentration in the liver, or by stimulating the release of endogenous insulin from the pancreas gland. An identical response could equally well result from slow intermixing, as STEELE (1959) pointed out. The injected, unlabeled glucose load would mix initially only with the rapid pool, and subsequently the two opposing effects could act together. Continuing release of glucose from the liver would tend to reduce plasma glucose specific activity, while the entry of labeled glucose molecules from the more slowly equilibrating compartments would increase plasma glucose specific activity. With the two effects in balance, specific radioactivity would be maintained unchanged for some time, resulting in a plateau in the curve. In STEELE's experiments no plateau was seen when glucose of the same specific activity as that present in plasma was injected instead of unlabeled glucose. This finding favors the conclusion that failure to achieve homogeneous intermixing of injected label with body glucose is, in fact, responsible for the "plateau effect".

b) Recycling of Label

Recycling of labeled glucose may occur when ^{14}C-glucose molecules, after having been retained in the glycogen stores of the body, are released into the blood. It is well known since the experiments of STETTEN and STETTEN (1955) that turnover of the outer tiers of the liver glycogen molecule is far more rapid than that of the core. Labeled glucose may thus be concentrated in the outer tiers of liver glycogen and, when released by glycogenolysis, delay the fall in plasma specific activity. Insulin has been shown to induce a plateau effect in animals (DUNN *et al.*, 1957) and in man (REICHARD *et al.*, 1958). If hypoglycemia is allowed to develop in response to insulin, counterregulatory breakdown of liver glycogen should result in increased recycling of labeled glucose.

Recycling may also occur when labeled glucose is formed in the liver from the ^{14}C-lactate derived from the injected labeled glucose. ANDRES *et al.* (1956) calculated from their data, that some 20% of the total amount of glucose utilized is taken up by skeletal muscle in the resting basal state. About 60% of this can be accounted for by lactate production. From such data it can be estimated that approximately 12% of the ^{14}C-isotope injected as glucose may be released as lactate from skeletal muscles. The amount of glucose formed from labeled lactate has been roughly estimated in man by measuring the appearance of radioactivity in the carbon 6 of blood glucose after 1-^{14}C-glucose had been injected (REICHARD *et al.*, 1963). Replacement of blood glucose occurred at an average rate of 161 mg/kg/h, 12—20% of this glucose being derived by resynthesis from lactate.

Recycling of label is likely to occur when the experimental design favors glycogen breakdown in the liver or muscle. Thus, the release of labeled glucose from liver glycogen may be more prominent in insulin hypoglycemia (LANDAU and LEONARDS, 1960) than in the resting state under basal conditions (STEELE, 1964). It has been demonstrated by the use of tritiated glucose that recycling does indeed affect the data. The tritium in position 2 of the glucose molecule is much less involved in recycling than is the carbon isotope, as it is removed and rapidly incorporated into water in the hexose isomerase reaction. Any recycling delays the rate of disappearance of glucose from the blood, so that slower turnover rates may be expected to result from data based on u-^{14}C-glucose than from those based on 2-^{3}H-glucose. The turnover rate of tritiated glucose in rats was 3% of the glucose pool per min and 2% per min with ^{14}C-glucose (KATZ and DUNN, 1967). As the error caused by recycling amounted to one third in these experiments, the authors concluded that "^{14}C-glucose does not provide correct estimates of glucose turnover unless corrections are made for recycling".

When glucose labeled in position 2 and uniformly labeled ^{14}C-glucose were administered simultaneously, 25—35% of the glucose carbon was found to be recycled in rabbits and up to 30—40% in rats (KATZ *et al.*, 1974b). Some 3—4.5 mg/min per kg of glucose was synthesized by rabbits, with a mean of 4 mg/min per kg; in rats that had been fasted overnight the rate was 10 mg/min per kg body weight. The mean glucose pool size was 290 mg/kg in rabbits and was similar for rats when related to body weight.

These recent data may well be superior to those given in the following sections, as the degree to which recycling may occur has certainly been underestimated. Effects of insulin are not mentioned in this recent paper, so that the data given here have no immediate bearing on the present discussion.

Results indicating that a high degree of recycling may occur in dogs have been reported by ISSEKUTZ *et al.* (1972). In their experiments the turnover rates for glucose were 30—40% higher when calculated from measurements with 2-^{3}H-glucose than from those obtained with u-^{14}C-glucose. The rate of appearance of glucose was 99.99 mg/m^{2}/min for tritiated glucose as opposed to 74.35 mg/m^{2}/min when ^{14}C was employed as tracer.

The discrepancy between the two methods became even more marked when the dogs were pretreated with methylprednisolone. This glucocorticoid steroid increases the rate of gluconeogenesis and thus enhances recycling of glucose carbon.

c) Data from Studies Applying Isotope Dilution Techniques

α) Changes in the fate of body glucose induced by a deficient supply of insulin or by the diabetic state

Early experiments on the effect of alloxan diabetes on the fate of labeled glucose were done in rats, but most of the available information has been gained from dogs. Although the results obtained by different procedures are not strictly comparable, some of the data mentioned in this chapter have been included into Table 1.

Following an injection of labeled glucose, $^{14}CO_2$ is exhaled with a considerable time lag and yields rather indirect data on the amount of glucose utilized. For this reason, FELLER *et al.* (1950) stress the significance of isotope dilution techniques. The body glucose pool and its turnover rate were calculated from the plasma specific activity decay curve in rats injected with a single dose of labeled glucose. Intermixing was probably not complete in these experiments. Extrapolating the curve back to zero gave a body glucose pool of 130 mg/100 g body weight for normal rats; an amount equal to this was turned over about every 70 min, re-

Table 1. *Turnover-rates, pool size, and space of distribution of glucose in the normal and diabetic state. (R_a: Rate of appearance of glucose; R_d: Rate of disappearance of glucose; *transformed to fit into table)*

		Glucose pool g/kg b.wt.	Turnover-rate of glucose mg/kg b.wt./h	Glucose space % of body weight
FELLER *et al.* (1951)	normal dog	0.54	354	28—32%
	diabetic dog	2—3*	400—800*	
SEARLE *et al.* (1954)	normal dog	0.34—0.45	220—270	30%
	diabetic dog	increase about threefold	310—350	28%
STEELE *et al.* (1956b)	normal dog	0.284		27%
CHERRINGTON and VRANIC (1973)	normal dog		R_a: 171,6; R_d: 166.2	
VRANIC and WRENSHALL (1969)	normal dog		R_a: 154.2; R_d: 139.2	
	diabetic dog		R_a: 390.6; R_d: 392.4	
ISSEKUTZ *et al.* (1974)	diabetic dog		R_a: 402 ; R_d: 480	
BAKER *et al.* (1954)	normal man	0.15	62.1	17%
SHREEVE *et al.* (1956)	normal man	0.21	85	24%
	stable diabetes	0.87	100	26%
	labile diabetes	1.08	190	30%
REICHARD *et al.* (1961)	normal man	0.31	120	30%
	diabetics	0.51	109	29%
REICHARD *et al.* (1964)	normal man		161 (corrected for recycling)	
REICHARD *et al.* (1963)	diabetics	0.44	141	33%

sulting in a turnover rate of 100 mg/100 g/h. As was to be expected, almost twice this amount of glucose was calculated to be present in the alloxan-diabetic rat, and this large amount was also turned over within 70 min. Part of this glucose must be excreted in the urine, as slightly less glucose is converted to CO_2 by the alloxan-diabetic rat than by controls. Impaired glucose oxidation did not seem to be a major metabolic defect in the diabetic rats studied. Similarly, alloxan diabetes in rats did not appear to affect glucose oxidation very much in the experiments of WELT *et al.* (1952). These results are not really surprising because blood glucose levels were allowed to rise in these diabetic rats, and high glucose levels ensure glucose utilization, even in the absence of insulin.

It had been demonstrated previously (SOSKIN and LEVINE, 1937) that eviscerated dogs utilize less glucose at blood glucose levels of 100 mg/100 ml when deprived of the pancreas gland. At glucose levels of 400 mg/100 ml, the pancreatectomized preparation may utilize even more glucose than in the presence of endogenous insulin. A marked depression in glucose utilization was hardly to be expected when the diabetic rats were allowed to raise their blood glucose level and thus to compensate for the loss of insulin. The slight inhibition of glucose oxidation observed in these rats could stem from the fact that glucose was lost in the urine before optimal glucose levels could be built up in the blood. Free fatty acids and ketone bodies may be elevated in untreated diabetics, and both could have interfered with glucose oxidation in these experiments.

Glucose production was measured by WELT *et al.* (1952) in rats receiving a constant infusion of exogenous glucose at a rate sufficient to provoke glycosuria. A known amount of labeled glucose had been added to the infusion. From the difference in specific activity of the glucose injected and that excreted with the urine they calculated the amount of glucose formed from unlabeled sources. A constant level of specific activity of urinary glucose was attained between the

6th and 12th hours of infusion. For that period, intermixing of label may thus have been completed. Glucose formation was 17.5 mg/h in the normal rat, and 43.3 mg/h in the alloxan-diabetic rat. In comparison, normal rats utilized and thus produced 100 mg of glucose per 100 g body weight and hour according to the calculations of FELLER *et al.* (1950). There are two factors which may be responsible for the divergence of the data in the two sets of experiments: (a) incomplete intermixing of label will result in unduly high turnover rates, and (b) the glucose load infused to maintain glycosuria in normal rats may reduce hepatic glucose release. This effect is probably mediated in part by endogenous insulin and will be discussed in a subsequent chapter. It is of interest, however, that even diabetic rats produced less glucose than that calculated by FELLER *et al.* (1950) for utilization in normal rats.

Glucose pool size, glucose space, and turnover rates of body glucose have been calculated in normal and diabetic dogs. As estimated from a single injection of labeled glucose, the miscible glucose pool in normal dogs was about 0.54 g/kg body weight (FELLER *et al.*, 1951). Lower values (between 0.34 and 0.45 g/kg body weight) resulted from a priming injection plus infusion of label (SEARLE *et al.*, 1954). The size of the glucose pool was increased about threefold in diabetic dogs and restored to normal by insulin injection (FELLER *et al.*, 1951; SEARLE *et al.*, 1954).

If the miscible glucose pool is assumed to be present in a volume at a concentration equal to that in plasma, this volume may be calculated as a percentage of body weight. The glucose space has been estimated to constitute 28—32% of the weight of normal dogs (SEARLE *et al.*, 1954). STEELE *et al.* (1956) obtained a mean of 27% from 7 dogs. When the glucose of the erythrocytes is subtracted from the glucose pool, these authors arrive at a corrected space of 25% of body weight, which corresponds to the inulin space in dogs. The space occupied by diffusible glucose is of the same order of magnitude in the normal, diabetic, or the diabetic dog injected with insulin (SEARLE *et al.*, 1954). The increased glucose pool size in diabetics originates from a rise in glucose concentration rather than from an increased volume of distribution. It should be kept in mind, however, that the glucose space is not a real but a calculated volume, as uniform distribution of the body glucose pool is unlikely. For this reason, the fact that the glucose space is of similar size in the normal and the diabetic dog does not exclude different equilibration times. It is thus conceivable that the ratio of fast pool to slow pool is higher in diabetic than in normal dogs (COWAN and HETENYI, 1971) despite the fact that a similar overall glucose space can be calculated.

The rate of delivery of glucose from liver or kidneys has been measured in dogs by isotope dilution techniques. Again, data obtained from measurements following a single injection of labeled glucose are probably too high, because of incomplete intermixing. A turnover rate of 350 and 375 mg/kg/h has been calculated for two normal dogs (SEARLE and CHAIKOFF, 1952). The primed infusion technique resulted in a mean turnover rate of 220—270 mg/kg/h in normal dogs and 310—350 mg/kg/h in diabetic animals (SEARLE *et al.*, 1954). A rate of appearance of glucose of 154.2 mg/kg/h was calculated for normal dogs following successive injections of tracer (VRANIC and WRENSHALL, 1969) and this rate was elevated to 390.6 mg/kg/h in pancreatictomized dogs deprived of insulin for 2 days. A similar high rate of glucose appearance is given for the alloxan-streptozotocin-diabetic dog, namely 402 mg/kg/h (ISSEKUTZ *et al.*, 1974). Delivery of glucose has been measured by applying a primed infusion of tracer: the mean from 7 normal dogs that had been fasted for 18 h was 171.6 mg/kg/h (CHERRINGTON and VRANIC, 1973).

In diabetics, the body glucose pool is larger than normal, as glucose concentration is elevated throughout the extracellular space. The calculated glucose space is not affected by a deficiency of insulin whereas the rate of glucose turnover is markedly increased. Thus in diabetics, gluconeogenesis proceeds at an enhanced rate and supplies additional glucose to the glucose pool. At the same time more glucose is leaving the pool, perhaps mainly being excreted in the urine, as glucose oxidation is unchanged or even reduced in the diabetic state.

The results of animal experiments are confirmed by measurements done in man.

A glucose pool size of 0.15 g/kg body weight was calculated for 4 normal subjects (BAKER *et al.*, 1954); this value was later corrected to 0.21 g/kg and additional data were given from stable diabetics (0.87 g/kg) and labile diabetics (1.08 g/kg) (SHREEVE *et al.*, 1956). A mean of 0.31 g/kg calculated for 12 normal subjects by REICHARD *et al.* (1961) was found to be raised to 0.51 g/kg in 17 diabetic patients.

In the early paper of BAKER *et al.* (1952) the glucose space was calculated to comprise 17% (later corrected to 24%) of body weight in normal man. The slightly higher values for stable or labile diabetics (26 and 30%, respectively) did not differ significantly from the controls. REICHARD *et al.* (1961) gave almost identical figures for the mean glucose space in normal subjects (30%) and diabetic patients (29%).

The turnover of glucose in normal subjects was first estimated to proceed at a rate of 62.1 mg/kg/h (BAKER *et al.*, 1954), later raised to 85 mg/kg/h (SHREEVE *et al.*, 1956). A slightly higher rate was calculated for the 5 stable diabetics (100 mg/kg/h) while turnover was markedly elevated in 3 labile diabetics (190 mg/kg/h). REICHARD *et al.* (1961) found the rate of glucose turnover to be about 50% higher for normal subjects in the postabsorptive state (120 mg/kg/h). When the data were corrected for recycling of label by gluconeogenesis, a mean of 161 mg/kg/h was calculated (REICHARD *et al.*, 1964), while the individual data varied from 124—370 mg/kg/h. High and fluctuating blood glucose levels made estimation of replacement rates somewhat uncertain in diabetic patients, yielding data with a mean of 109 mg/kg/h (REICHARD *et al.*, 1961). Patients suffering from severe diabetes tended to have higher and those with mild diabetes lower replacement rates. Glucose turnover was not markedly changed in 4 diabetics from whom insulin had been withheld during the previous 24 h and whose blood glucose levels ranged from 155—368 mg/100 ml. The mean turnover rate was 141 mg/kg/h for these diabetics as compared to 161 mg/kg/h for 4 fasting normal subjects (REICHARD *et al.*, 1963).

In human subjects insulin deficiency does not affect the calculated glucose space; glucose pool size increases in diabetes while the rates of glucose turnover may be reduced, within the normal range, or elevated. This variability is to be expected as the severity of the metabolic disorder and its duration have some influence on the results. In addition, such individual factors as free fatty acids or ketone bodies in the blood affect both glucose utilization and production.

β) Changes in the fate of glucose induced by insulin

In stable diabetics glucose flow rates may approach a new steady state, with glucose appearing and disappearing at elevated rates and plasma glucose levels constant, although in the hyperglycemic range. This dynamic equilibrium is disturbed as soon as insulin is injected. The calculation of turnover rates has thus been based on methods that do not assume steady-state conditions (HENDERSON *et al.*, 1955).

When insulin is injected into normoglycemic animals and hypoglycemia is allowed to develop, counterregulatory effects are involved in the response. Thus, when sufficient insulin was injected into rats to lower blood glucose levels to about 30 mg/100 ml, labeled glucose was incorporated into muscle glycogen but no radioactivity was retained by the liver (LEVIN and WEINHOUSE, 1958). This result does not exclude the possibility that insulin may induce the liver to retain glucose. Hypoglycemia, however, causes breakdown of liver glycogen, thus reversing any effect insulin might have on hepatic glycogen formation. In addition, recycling is a source of error when labeled glucose is released from liver glycogen in response to hypoglycemia.

An error of this kind may be of relevance in experiments designed like those of DUNN *et al.* (1957). Labeled glucose was injected into normal dogs and the decay over time of plasma specific radioactivity was followed. It was calculated from the data for the first 30 min following the injection of label that, in a male dog of 11.7 kg, the glucose pool was 4.94 g, the glucose space 34% of body weight, and the glucose turnover rate 4.8 mg/kg/min. As the label was given by single injection, the intermixing of label was not likely to be complete at that time. On subsequent injection of 10 IU of insulin, the blood glucose fell within 20 min from 122 to 64 mg/100 ml. Immediately following insulin injection, plasma specific activity no longer declined but was maintained at an unchanged level throughout the initial hypoglycemic phase. It has been concluded from this result that no glucose was entering the blood and hence no dilution of label occurred. Insulin thus apparently suppresses hepatic glucose release and one quarter to one half of the total fall in blood sugar may be due to this reduced rate of entry of glucose. If release of labeled glucose, liberated from the outer tiers of liver glycogen in response to falling blood glucose levels, had occurred in these experiments, this would have contributed to the plateau observed in the plasma decay curve. Cessation of the decline in circulating glucose specific activity is not necessarily a result of cessation of hepatic glucose production. This has been demonstrated by the experiments of LANDAU and LEONARDS (1960), who injected 1-^{14}C-galactose into dogs together with unlabeled glucose. The glucose molecules formed from galactose were incorporated into the outer tiers of the liver glycogen. When insulin was subsequently injected, long periods of constant glucose specific activity, or even a rise above preinsulin levels occurred as labeled glucose was released from the liver into the blood.

It is clearly of great importance to prevent hypoglycemia in all experiments designed to demonstrate a hepatic effect of insulin, as has been well documented by ALTSZULER, DUNN, STEELE, WALL, and the other members of this group from 1957 to 1965. An early paper reported that insulin transiently lowered the rate of glucose inflow from about 4 to 2 g/m^2/h but that subsequently hepatic glucose release increased as hypoglycemia became more pronounced (WALL *et al.*, 1957). Thus insulin appeared to induce hypoglycemia by stimulating glucose uptake rather than by inhibiting glucose release. It was also noted that the "rate and amount of glucose inflow from the liver following insulin injection were related to the degree of hypoglycemia produced". When infusion of insulin was discontinued, a sudden increase was observed in the hepatic release of glucose, indicating that the presence of insulin did restrain glucose production in response to hypoglycemia (DUNN *et al.*, 1959).

A marked effect of insulin on heaptic glucose release was established in dogs with glycosuria caused by phlorizin. In these animals blood glucose levels were maintained by increased production of glucose. Insulin infusion reduced glucose release to prephlorizin levels (DUNN *et al.*, 1960).

A strong inhibitory effect of insulin on hepatic glucose production was observed in normal dogs, provided that enough glucose was also infused to limit hypoglycemia

(STEELE *et al.*, 1965). Giving insulin halved the release of newly formed glucose into the blood in dogs on a high carbohydrate or standard diet. Glucose release was reduced from a mean of 182 mg/kg/h to 102 mg/kg/h in the early phase and to 55 mg/kg/h in the late phase of insulin action. At the same time ^{14}C-glucose equivalents accumulated in liver glycogen while the rise in radioactivity in non-glycogen components was less pronounced (BISHOP *et al.*, 1965). Glucose uptake by all tissues rose from 182—382 during the early phase and to 694 mg/kg/h in the late phase. Thus, approximately four times as much glucose was utilized and less than one third was released from the liver in these experiments, while plasma glucose concentration was kept near its initial value by glucose infusion. The mean uptake of plasma glucose by the liver was increased to about 11 times the control rate and accounted for approximately 12% of the total glucose uptake.

Errors are not induced by hypoglycemia and counterregulatory factors in diabetic animals. Thus, HENDERSON *et al.* (1955), lowered plasma glucose levels from about 300 to 100 mg/100 ml within 3 h by injecting insulin into pancreatectomized, diabetic dogs. The findings compare well with those mentioned above: the rate of delivery of glucose was reduced from 4.53 to 1.27 mg/kg/min within 3 h following insulin injection. The rate of disappearance rose rapidly to 11.6 mg/kg/h but declined subsequently, reaching preinsulin levels at 90 min.

The effect of insulin has recently been studied in dogs made diabetic by injection of alloxan and streptozotocin (ISSEKUTZ *et al.*, 1974). Glucose kinetics were calculated by a primed constant-infusion isotope dilution technique, 2-^{3}H-glucose being used to minimize recycling. The blood glucose-lowering effect of a low dose of insulin was found to be due entirely to the decline in hepatic glucose output. In these dogs, which are still capable of releasing glucagon from the pancreatic α-cells, a small rise in plasma insulin will reduce the hepatic glucose release, which otherwise proceeds at an elevated rate. Higher doses of insulin resulted in an additional rise in the peripheral utilization of glucose.

Data from measurements in man are in agreement with these animal experiments. When insulin was injected subcutaneously to prevent a rapid hypoglycemic response, the drop in plasma glucose specific activity either "plateaued" or proceeded less rapidly, thus indicating that hepatic glucose release was suppressed (REICHARD *et al.*, 1960).

Although insulin affects both glucose production and glucose utilization, it did not increase the calculated glucose space in dogs (WRENSHALL and HETENYI, 1959). It is by reducing the amount of glucose in the body, i.e. the glucose pool (SEARLE *et al.*, 1954), that insulin restores normoglycemia in the diabetic dog.

γ) Effect of glucose loading on the fate of body glucose as measured by isotope dilution

Glucose, injected intravenously or taken orally, induces hyperglycemia and insulin release from the pancreas. Most hepatic effects of glucose loads in normal animals and man are thus considered to result from elevated levels of insulin in the portal venous blood that perfuses the liver. As discussed in a preceding chapter of this volume, high glucose levels can directly affect glucose release from the isolated perfused rat liver. This might explain why glucose inhibits endogenous glucose production to some extent, even in pancreatectomized dogs (HETENYI and WRENSHALL, 1968).

In dogs, labeled glucose was injected and the effects of a glucose load on the decay curves of plasma specific activity were measured (SEARLE and CHAIKOFF; 1952; REICHARD *et al.*, 1958). Both teams found that the decline in plasma specific activity was delayed or temporarily interrupted, producing a plateau in the curve. As mentioned previously, such a plateau may be interpreted as indicating that labeled glucose in the plasma is no longer diluted by glucose molecules released from the liver. This conclusion has, however, given rise to criticism. The results could not be reproduced in the experiments of Steele and Marks (1958). In two dogs anesthetized with pentobarbital, plasma glucose specific activity was maintained at a constant level by a continuous infusion of labeled glucose. When a load of glucose of the same specific activity as that in the infusion was injected, plasma specific activity failed to rise. This was taken to indicate either that glucose output from the liver continued or that recycling of label had been stimulated. Incomplete intermixing is likely to interfere in experiments where large quantities of unlabeled glucose are injected. Even if the specific activity of the glucose injected is not entirely identical to that present in the blood, stable tracer systems may be disturbed (Cowan and Hetenyi, 1971). When more concentrated labeled glucose is released into plasma from a slowly intermixing pool, any further decline in plasma specific radioactivity is prevented or delayed, even though glucose release from the liver may continue unchanged. It has been convincingly demonstrated that inhibition of hepatic glucose output is not the only possible reason for cessation of the exponential fall in plasma glucose specific activity (Steele, 1959). In eviscerated dogs, plasma glucose was maintained by constant intravenous infusion of glucose. When a single injection of labeled glucose was followed by a load of ^{12}C-glucose, a plateau in plasma specific activity resulted, despite the fact that hepatic glucose production was excluded in this preparation (Steele *et al.*, 1959). Thus the plateau effect may result in part from the slowness of mixing of about half of the total miscible glucose pool (Steele, 1959).

Although errors due to slow and incomplete intermixing do in fact occur, there is little reason to doubt that glucose will immediately reduce endogenous glucose release. Strong and convincing evidence for this belief has been furnished by the same authors who pointed out the possible pitfalls resulting from incomplete mixing of label (Bishop *et al.*, 1965). A glucose infusion raised plasma glucose levels by 29 mg/100 ml in the early phase and by 50 mg/100 ml in the late phase. Release of endogenous glucose was reduced from 182 to 96 or 35 mg/kg/h, respectively, while glucose uptake by all tissues rose from 182 to 436 or 706 mg/kg/h. Labeled glucose was retained by the liver and incorporated into glycogen.

As the effects of glucose are quite similar to those of insulin, there is little reason to doubt that they are mediated mainly by endogenous insulin. Some adjustment of glucose production to the rate of exogenous glucose infusion has also been observed in the pancreatectomized dog and must therefore occur independently of insulin (Hetenyi and Wrenshall, 1968). Infusions of unlabeled glucose at rates corresponding to 17—79% of the rate of hepatic glucose production correspondingly reduced endogenous glucose release in normal and diabetic dogs. In order to minimize incomplete intermixing, the authors later adopted a primed tracer infusion technique (Cowan and Hetenyi, 1971). In normal dogs the rate of appearance of endogenous glucose (2.3 ± 0.2 mg/kg/min) fell immediately in response to an intravenous injection of glucose. The same animals were subsequently pancreatectomized and the rate of appearance of glucose was found to be increased to 5.5 ± 0.9 mg/kg/min. Glucose then induced an initial drop in endogenous glucose production in 4 out of 5 animals. Thereafter the response in the rate of appearance was slight and could not easily be analyzed.

Such results in pancreatectomized dogs suggest that insulin release from the islet tissue is not the sole factor of relevance. In addition to insulin and the direct hepatic effects of glucose itself, a reduced supply in glucagon would favor the accumulation of glycogen in the liver of normal dogs.

3. Effect of Insulin on the Fate of Body Glucose as Measured by Catheterization Techniques

Despite their shortcomings, methods based on isotope dilution offer the only approach toward measuring the total amount of glucose, whether newly synthesized or originating from the body's glycogen stores. Estimates of glucose uptake or release that are based on direct measurements of arteriovenous gradients in glucose concentration will yield information on the net glucose balance across an organ such as the liver, or part of the body such as the human forearm. Blood is supplied to the liver by the hepatic artery and the portal vein; therefore glucose concentration within the portal vein, the hepatic artery, and the hepatic vein must be known in order to calculate net hepatic glucose release. In addition, information is required on the rate of plasma flow through the liver, usually measured by the clearance of dyes like rose bengal or bromsulphalein, which are removed by the liver from the perfusing blood. It is usually assumed that a constant proportion of the total hepatic blood flow is supplied by the portal vein or the hepatic artery. Madison *et al.* (1959a) have pointed out, however, that there is very little information available on possible changes in the ratio of blood supply from arterial or portal venous sources.

One main shortcoming of all direct measurements of glucose uptake and release is that data for dynamic flow rates are calculated from the concentrations that prevail at the moment of sampling. The assumption underlying such calculations is that rapid changes in glucose flow rates do not occur in steady-state conditions. The arterio-hepaticvenous glucose difference and the hepatic blood flow have been measured in man at intervals down to 30 sec (Bondy, 1952); spontaneous fluctuations were found to occur. Thus, although the data calculated from a single sample are reliable for the actual moment when the blood is withdrawn, they may not be very suitable for calculating overall metabolic balances.

a) Measurements of the Net Balance of Glucose across the Liver

Measurements of hepatic glucose release in diabetic dogs were carried out in an attempt to clarify whether diabetes mellitus originates from overproduction or underutilization of glucose. These two concepts were considered as mutually exclusive "rival theories". In the normal, nonanesthetized dog, hepatic glucose output was found to average 122 mg/kg/h (Lipscomb and Crandall, 1947), while a slightly higher figure was found for the pancreatectomized diabetic dog, namely 137 mg/kg/h, the difference being not statistically significant (Crandall and Lipscomb, 1947). Later, when the results from isotope dilution experiments were questioned, because slow intermixing of label with the miscible glucose pool was found to occur, Madison and his group set out to reestablish that insulin does in fact reduce hepatic glucose release. Their experiments were done on dogs bearing a shunt between portal vein and vena cava, so that only the hepatic artery delivered blood to the liver and the glucose gradient could be directly measured by the arteriovenous concentration difference. Although this procedure excludes sampling from the portal vein and eliminates any variation due to changes in the amount of blood contributed to the total hepatic blood flow by artery or portal vein, it may affect the physiological status of the liver. Hepatic blood flow is reduced by this procedure from 38.3 to 15 ml/kg/min (Madison *et al.*, 1959a). The fact that the liver is cut off from the direct supply of the pancreatic hormones, insulin and glucagon, via the portal vein may be of significance for the hepatic glucose metabolism. In diabetic dogs thus operated, heaptic glucose release was elevated from a control range of 25—45 mg/min to 77 mg/min and was reduced by insulin to 38 mg/min (MADISON *et al.*, 1959b). When glucose was given to mildly diabetic dogs with a blood glucose level of 148 mg/100 ml, the liver started to retain glucose at a concentration of 168—209 mg/100 ml. In severely diabetic dogs, blood glucose levels had to be raised to 350—490 mg/100 ml to induce a net uptake of glucose by the liver. Insulin promptly reduces the level at which the liver removes glucose from the perfusing blood down from the elevated diabetic range to a normal level of 140—168 mg/100 ml (MADISON *et al.*, 1959b; 1960b).

As opposed to these diabetic dogs, normal animals respond by hypoglycemia to the injection or infusion of insulin. As discussed above in connection with the tracer studies, a lowering of the glucose concentration normally maintained within the blood will evoke a series of counterregulatory reactions, which tends to increase glucose release from the liver. At least some of the controversy about the possible direct effects of insulin on hepatic glucose release could have been avoided if matched glucose infusions had been used to prevent hypoglycemic blood glucose levels. The central issue in the debate has usually been whether or not insulin reduces hepatic glucose release, and the published papers can be divided into those affirming and those denying such action.

It is useful, however, to consider the results in view of the factors that may interfere with the hepatic action of insulin. Thus, in one series of experiments, insulin failed to reduce hepatic glucose release in dogs threatened by hypoglycemia but did restrict the glucose output usually mobilized from the liver in response to low blood glucose levels (FINE and WILLIAMS, 1960). Insulin increased net uptake of glucose by the liver when given together with glucose to limit hypoglycemia (LEONARDS *et al.*, 1961).

Both the rate and the site of insulin administration are considered by MADISON *et al.* (1959a) to affect the quality of the response. A rapid intravenous injection primarily increased peripheral glucose uptake, while a slow infusion of insulin into the portal vein reduced hepatic glucose release from 42 to 24 mg/min.

A slow infusion of insulin, lowering arterial blood glucose level by 21 mg/100 ml within one hour, reduced hepatic glucose output in one dog from 25.5 to 13.2 mg/min and in a second dog from 47.8 to 17.0 mg/min (MADISON *et al.*, 1960a).

It is evident that, if it is desired to demonstrate a direct inhibitory effect of insulin on hepatic glucose release, it is important to prevent hypoglycemia so as to minimize interference by counterregulatory reactions. However, one can hardly write off all the results that fail to confirm the findings of MADISON and his group by claiming that the hepatic effects of insulin have been masked by counterregulation. Thus, insulin was infused into dogs at a dose that lowered blood glucose concentration from an initial 88 mg/100 ml to 75 mg/100 ml within one hour (SHOEMAKER *et al.*, 1960). The mean glucose output from the liver rose from 80—121 mg/min after insulin. Similarly, hepatic glucose output did not decrease in the period immediately following insulin but either remained unaltered or rose slightly in each of the animals studied (SHOEMAKER *et al.*, 1959). After 30 min, when insulin hypoglycemia became pronounced, there was a statistically significant rise in hepatic glucose release. In experiments on nonanesthetized dogs bearing indwelling catheters, a slow infusion into the portal vein of 0.2 IU of insulin per kg and h failed to significantly reduce the overall hepatic glucose output but greatly increased the peripheral utilization of glucose. It was concluded from these results that the hypoglycemia produced by insulin is not due to a reduction in the release of glucose from the liver (MARTIN *et al.*, 1959). Similarly, insulin failed to induce a marked reduction in hepatic glucose production in the experiments of FINE and WILLIAMS (1960) on normal, concious dogs. It did appear, however, to suppress the hepatic response to hypoglycemia, as there was a marked rise in glucose release following cessation of the infusion. Thus in these experiments insulin may have acted on the liver to maintain rather than to induce hypoglycemia.

One reason for the discrepancy in the results of measurements to determine the hepatic effects of insulin may lie in the diet fed to the dogs prior to the experiment. This point has been stressed by LEONARDS *et al.* (1961), as these authors, who belong to the same group that denied any hepatic effect of insulin two years earlier (MARTIN *et al.*, 1959), detected an immediate and perhaps direct effect of insulin on the liver of dogs fed a diet rich in carbohydrates. In dogs fed protein, insulin failed to reduce hepatic glucose output; it even failed to do so in one dog receiving glucose to prevent hypoglycemia.

The dog is a convenient animal for the insertion of indwelling catheters to study glucose gradients. However, the fact that the diet to which the animals had been adapted apparently had a decisive effect on the results raises the question whether the dog is indeed a suitable species for demonstrating the hepatic effects of insulin.

Catheters were inserted in rabbits into the femoral artery and vein and the portal vein. In order to prevent reflux of venous blood from the inferior vena cava, hepatic venous blood was withdrawn from a cannula pushed to a depth of 16 mm into the narrow vein irrigating the right superior lobe, which constitutes 7—8% of the total liver weight (Fig. 1). Experiments were done 6 h after the operation and anesthesia was maintained by an infusion of 7 mg/kg/h of pentobarbitone. The ganglionic blocking agent azamethonium bromide (1 mg/kg/h) had also been added to the infusion to minimize adrenergic reactions. Insulin infused at a rate of 0.2 IU/kg/h resulted in a hypoglycemic response. The glucose concentration in the femoral artery and vein is shown in Fig. 2; it can be seen that there

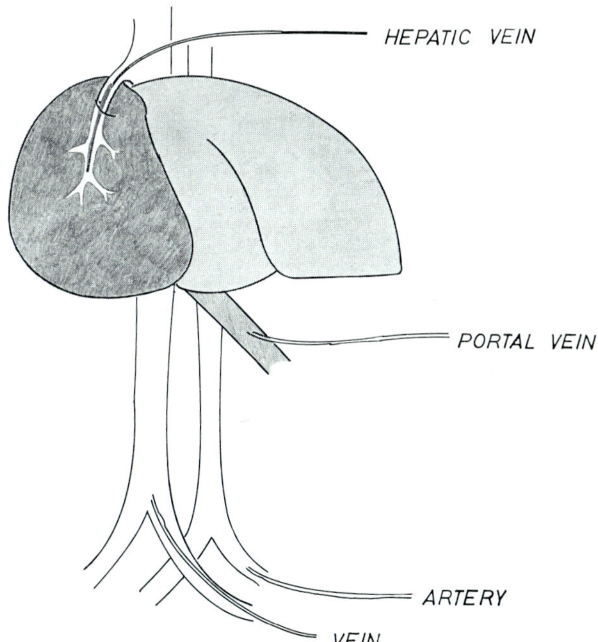

Fig. 1. Position of cannulae inserted in rabbits for sampling of blood from the femoral artery and vein, the portal vein, and the vein of the right superior lobe of the liver

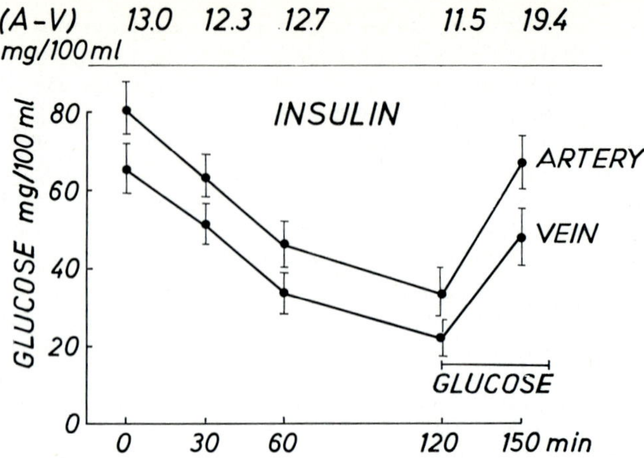

Fig. 2. Arterial and venous blood glucose concentration in rabbits receiving an infusion of 0.2 IU of insulin/kg/h. The arteriovenous gradient, given at the top, does not rise unless glucose (500 mg/kg/h) from 120—150 min is given by infusion in addition to insulin

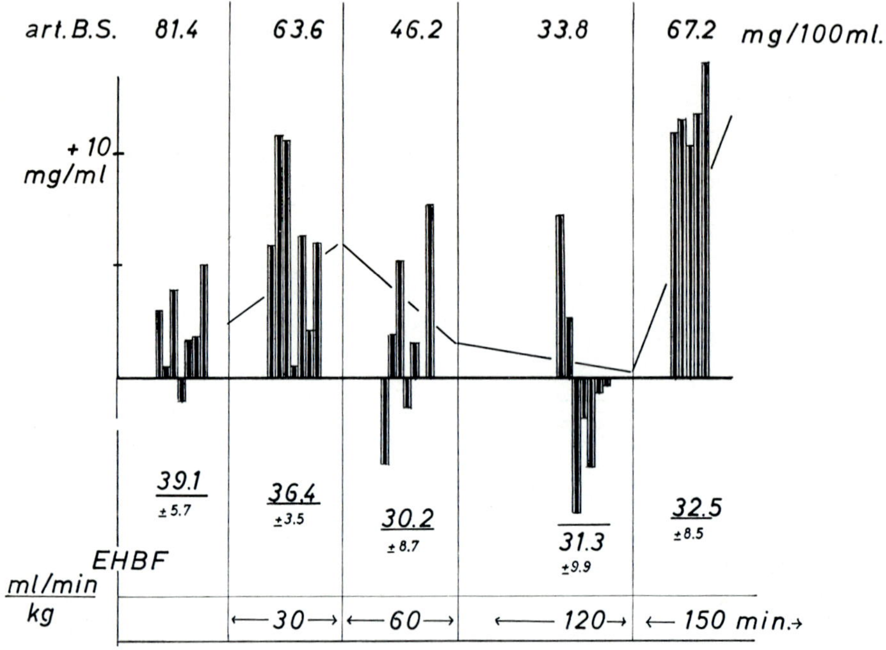

Fig. 3. Glucose gradient across the liver as calculated from the arterial, portal venous, and hepatic venous glucose concentration. The columns represent the data from individual animals. The estimated hepatic blood flow (EHBF) was measured by infusion of bromsulphalein. The net hepatic glucose uptake or release, calculated by multiplying the glucose gradient by the blood flow, is indicated by the smoothed line. Mean arterial blood sugar (art. B.S.) is given at the top

are no major changes in the glucose gradient across the hind leg; it did not decrease, although the arterial blood glucose fell to less than 40 mg/100 ml. The glucose gradient across the liver (Fig. 3) has been calculated by assuming that 8 parts of portal and 2 parts of arterial blood pass through the liver at any given time. The mean estimated hepatic blood flow is given underneath. After 30 min of insulin infusion, an increase in glucose uptake was observed in all the 7 experiments. When arterial blood glucose concentration had declined to less than 50 mg/100 ml, hepatic glucose uptake gave way to glucose release. For the last 30 min of the experiments glucose (500 mg/kg/h) was infused in addition to insulin. Although the initial blood glucose concentration was not reestablished by the glucose given, the hepatic glucose uptake was very markedly increased (Fig. 3), and the glucose gradient across the hind limb rose from 11.5—19.4 mg/100 ml (Fig. 2). It has been concluded from these experiments that glucose is initially retained by the liver in response to insulin (HASSELBLATT, 1961).

In these experiments in rabbits, as in those of MADISON *et al.* (1960a) and LANDAU *et al.* (1961) in dogs, the addition of glucose served to unmask an effect of insulin on hepatic glucose release.

In man, portal venous blood is not normally obtainable. The presence of large and easily accessible portal venous collaterals in 3 patients with cirrhosis of the liver enabled MYERS (1950) to sample portal venous blood. The difference in glucose concentration between portal vein and artery was insignificant and the authors thus felt justified in considering splanchnic glucose production as an approximation of hepatic glucose release. Net hepatic glucose output has been measured in 3 patients suffering from cirrhosis of the liver and bearing end-to-side portocaval anastomoses (CRAIG *et al.*, 1961). A single dose of 6—10 IU of glucagon-free insulin strikingly reduced hepatic glucose release and even induced a net glucose uptake in 2 subjects: 20 min before insulin the 3 livers released respectively 41.3, 127.8, and 42.5 mg of glucose per min; 50 min after insulin administration the corresponding data were —30.0, 51.0, and —5.9 mg/min. It is striking that here, as in the experiments of MADISON *et al.*, the most pronounced effects of insulin were measured when portal blood was not allowed to reach the liver directly. The positive results may thus be related to the fact that glucagon released into the portal vein is prevented from acting on the liver until it has been diluted by passing through the general circulation.

It may be concluded that in all probability insulin prevents hyperglycemia by reducing hepatic glucose release in addition to stimulating glucose utilization. This effect may be masked when hypoglycemia is allowed to develop and measures are taken to prevent a further drop in blood glucose levels. The hepatic effect of insulin is modified by factors such as diet or the manner of injection of insulin, and may differ between species. The finding that insulin reduces hepatic glucose release, or that it merely prevents the liver from responding to hypoglycemia by releasing additional glucose, may well reflect different states of the same effect of insulin. Even those experiments in which insulin induced hypoglycemia without lowering hepatic glucose release do not exclude the presence of a restraining effect of insulin, as described by FINE and WILLIAMS (1960). It is evident from this discussion that quantitative information on the effects of insulin on the release of glucose from the liver can only be obtained if blood glucose levels are not allowed to change during the period of measurement. Unfortunately, such standardized conditions have not been observed in most experiments. The effects of insulin on hepatic glucose release, as mentioned here, do not necessarily imply that insulin directly reduces hepatic glucose output. Experiments on the isolated perfused liver preparation, discussed by SÖLING and SEUFERT in a preceding chapter, offer little support for the hypothesis that insulin directly affects liver metabolism to a degree which might be of significance for the hypoglycemic response.

b) Effect of Insulin on Net Splanchnic Glucose Output

Portal venous blood can be obtained in man only under exceptional conditions, which is why the hepatic venous arterial glucose gradient has been used to estimate hepatic glucose release. The shortcomings of the method are evident, as the entire splanchnic area drained by the portal vein is included in such calculations. Measurements made on patients with cirrhosis and anastomoses have shown no measurable difference in glucose concentration as between samples taken simultaneously from the artery and portal vein under basal conditions (MYERS, 1950). This would not be expected to be the case, however, when insulin is injected, as glucose uptake into the spanchnic area, especially into adipose tissue, is likely to be stimulated by insulin.

That this occurs in dogs has been demonstrated by measuring simultaneously splanchnic net glucose output and true hepatic glucose release (SHOEMAKER *et al.*, 1959). In dogs, net splanchnic glucose release was significantly reduced by insulin from a mean of 3.9 to 2.1 mg/min. True hepatic glucose output did not decrease, however, but remained unchanged or rose slightly in each of the animals studied, the rise being more pronounced when hypoglycemia had developed. Measurements of net splanchnic glucose release and of the possible effects of insulin upon it thus seem to be of rather limited value for the discussion of direct effects of insulin on the glucose gradient across the liver. Nevertheless, the net splanchnic glucose production is of physiological significance, as it is in equilibrium with peripheral glucose utilization. MYERS (1950) calculated from his data that in man 162 g of glucose is released within 24 h; about 69% of this is used by the brain so that only 31% is available to other tissues. MYERS' calculation is based on a net splanchnic glucose release of 65 mg/min/m^2 body surface. This could equal 1.6 mg/min/kg, when this value would apply to a man of 70 kg body weight and 1.73 m^2 body surface. BONDY *et al.* (1949a) calculated that more than twice as much glucose is released from the splanchnic system in fasting man a mean of 3.5 mg/kg/min being given for net splanchnic glucose release in 9 normal subjects under fasting conditions. An injection of glucose resulted in immediate retention of glucose by the splanchnic region, and possibly also by the liver. In 5 patients with uncontrolled diabetes, glucose and urea were released from the splanchnic area at an increased rate (BONDY *et al.*, 1949b). Following insulin, the rate of splanchnic glucose production decreased and after latent periods of 45—75 min glucose was retained by the splanchnic system. Similarly, the rate of urea production was rapidly reduced by insulin. Rapid changes in the rate of hepatic gluconeogenesis are thus likely to occur in diabetic patients injected with insulin. The decline in urea production indicates that less amino acids are deaminated in the liver. Insulin has been shown to reduce plasma levels and efflux from forearm tissues of such amino acids, which do not serve as substrates for gluconeogenesis (POZEFSKY *et al.*, 1969). It is the uptake into the liver rather than the supply of the glucogenic precursors, alanine and lactate, that has been found to be reduced. In normal man amino acid reductions amounting to 30—60% have been observed in response to a glucose infusion (FELIG and WAHREN, 1971). The authors concluded that this effect was caused by endogenous insulin, released in response to hyperglycemia. On the other hand, insulin only slightly inhibited the utilization of exogenously supplied glucogenic substrates in recent experiments with healthy volunteers (DIETZE *et al.*, 1973), which employed a ^{133}Xe inhalation technique for the measurement of hepatic blood flow. Basal net splanchnic glucose production was calculated to amount to a mean of 8.43 ± 1.04 mg/100 g/min or to a total 180 g of glucose a day, assuming a liver weight of 1500 g. In order to compare this figure with the data given in the literature, we assume that the body weight of the volunteers was about 70 kg, and thus arrive at a glucose release of 1.8 mg/kg/min. This is nearer to the 1.6 mg/kg/min given by MYERS (1950) than to the 3.5 mg/kg/min calculated by BONDY *et al.* (1949a) or the 3.4 mg/kg/min found by FELIG and WAHREN (1971). DIETZE *et al.* (1973) infused lactate after a control period of 30 min. This caused splanchnic glucose release to rise to about twice the control level (16.33 ± 2.42 mg/100 g/min). Insulin reduced splanchnic glucose release in the presence of lactate although, contrary to the experiments of FELIG and WAHREN (1971), the liver continued to utilize glucogenic precursors.

Tissues other than the liver contribute to the splanchnic glucose balance and they may respond to insulin. Experiments showing that insulin may immediately reduce basal splanchnic glucose output in both normal and diabetic subjects (BEARN *et al.*, 1959) failed to furnish evidence for a hepatic effect of insulin. Nevertheless, results as those of FELIG and WAHREN (1971) indicate that such an effect must prevail in normal subjects receiving a low dose of glucose by infusion. An infusion of 2 mg of glucose kg/min raised arterial blood glucose concentration by 19 mg/100 ml and doubled the plasma immunoreactive insulin within 45 min. Despite this relatively small rise in insulin, hepatic glucose output fell by 85%. It is difficult to imagine that an effect of this magnitude could result solely from glucose uptake by extrahepatic tissues drained by the portal vein, and one is therefore tempted to agree with the authors, who state that the "liver is the primary target organ whereby glucose homeostasis is achieved with small increments in insulin".

4. Effect of Insulin on Glucose Utilization by the Extrahepatic Tissues

Glucose is almost immediately phosphorylated upon entering the cells of most tissues. Thus, all tissues except the liver were found to contain less glucose than plasma, and an especially low glucose level was found in testes and brain, amounting to one tenth of that present in the liver (GEY, 1956). The uptake of glucose by most cells is thus equivalent to phosphorylation and hence to glucose utilization. The uptake of glucose can be calculated from the arteriovenous difference in glucose concentration multiplied by the blood flow. Phosphorylation of glucose does not, however, imply immediate oxidation. Combustion of glucose, as measured by the production of $^{14}CO_2$ from ^{14}C-labeled glucose, although sometimes referred to as glucose "utilization", is a process differing from glucose uptake both in magnitude and in time course. The effect of insulin on the uptake and the oxidation of glucose will thus be discussed separately.

The stimulating effect of insulin on glucose uptake by the tissues that constitute the major part of the body mass, namely skeletal muscles and adipose tissue, is well recognized and has been dealt with in earlier chapters of this volume. Such direct effects of insulin on extrahepatic tissues are easily measured *in vitro*. It is not so easy to answer the basic question concerning the extent to which such peripheral effects of insulin actually contribute to the hypoglycemic response observed in the intact animal or in man. As previously discussed, the experimental design may affect the balance between hepatic and peripheral effects of insulin. Whenever hypoglycemia develops, the liver may respond with a release of glucose. Hypoglycemia would not persist if glucose were not taken up at a rapid rate by the tissues. A second, and probably equally extreme situation is produced when the fasting animals or human subjects are suddenly exposed to massive glucose loads. Experimental designs involving massive doses of both insulin and glucose may not be optimal for elucidating the peripheral and hepatic effects of endogenous insulin released from the islets of LANGERHANS to ensure the utilization of glucose slowly absorbed from the gut.

When a load of 100 g of glucose was given to healthy subjects, the resulting hyperglycemia was accompanied by a striking rise in the glucose gradient between capillary (arterial) and venous blood (SOMOGYI, 1948). Such data demonstrate the importance of the glucose uptake in the regulation of blood glucose levels, yet glucose tolerance depends not only on peripheral glucose uptake but is apparently affected by the liver as well. This conclusion was drawn by JACKSON *et al.* (1973), who studied dietary carbohydrate intolerance in normal subjects. Glucose tolerance was significantly impaired following a diet low in carbohydrates; at the same time the uptake of glucose by the forearm tissues was not delayed. These authors therefore considered, a reduced uptake of glucose by liver was to be the major cause of dietary carbohydrate intolerance.

Except in hyperglycemia, basal glucose uptake by the resting skeletal muscles is relatively small and may account for only 20% of total body glucose turnover as calculated from data obtained from the human forearm (ANDRES *et al.*, 1956). In the isolated perfused hindquarter of the rat, added glucose makes no more than a negligible contribution to the fuel of respiration, whereas glucose uptake increases sixfold when insulin is added (RUDERMAN *et al.*, 1971). The brain is probably the major site of glucose uptake, utilizing about 6.2 mg/min per 100 g of brain tissue in normal, resting young men (SCHEINBERG and STEAD, 1949). In lactating goats, however, 60—85% of the glucose used by the animal is taken up by the udder to form lactose and milk-fat glycerol (ANNISON and LINZELL, 1964). Glucose uptake is thus certainly dependent on the functional state of the tissues. There is some evidence that hormones may modify the insulin receptors of various tissues (GOLDFINE *et al.*, 1973), and it is tempting to suppose that tissue cells might thus be enabled to reduce their response to insulin. Moreover, some resistance to the stimulating effect of insulin on glucose uptake has been observed in persons exhibiting impaired glucose tolerance and in diabetic patients (OLEFSKY *et al.*, 1973).

When glucose utilization or combustion to CO_2 is compared in normal and diabetic animals, the effect of elevated glucose levels has to be considered. The classic experiments of SOSKIN and LEVINE (1937) demonstrated that the pancreatectomized dog can utilize glucose in the absence of insulin at "any rate of which the normal animal is capable". The lack of insulin is compensated for by elevating the blood glucose concentration. The authors stated that "the depancreatized dog at its usual hyperglycemic level utilizes as much or more sugar than the normal dog at its normal usual blood sugar level". It is thus conceivable that the rate of conversion of glucose to CO_2 may be only slightly reduced in alloxan-diabetic rats, as found in the experiments of FELLER *et al.* (1950). Following a single injection of labeled glucose, a turnover of 100 mg/100 g/h had been calculated for normal rats and twice that amount for diabetic rats. While 67 mg/100 g/h was oxidized to CO_2 by the controls, the diabetic rats oxidized 60 mg/100 g/h. When these studies were repeated in pancreatectomized dogs acutely deprived of insulin, the rate of glucose oxidation was found to be below normal (FELLER *et al.*, 1951). Insulin-controlled pancreatectomized dogs oxidized 1.5—2.0 g/h of glucose, yet only 0.5—0.8 g/h was transformed to CO_2 after insulin had been withdrawn for 72 h. Loss of glucose in the urine may have prevented plasma glucose levels from rising sufficiently to ensure adequate glucose utilization in these experiments. In addition, free fatty acids are likely to have been released from the adipose tissue of the acutely diabetic animals and may have inhibited glucose oxidation. This effect is less pronounced in alloxan-diabetic rats, which have already lost weight.

Experiments on eviscerated rabbits were designed to evaluate the effect of insulin on the calculated volume of distribution of labeled glucose (Drury and Wick, 1951). The tracer was given by single injection and 20 min was allowed for mixing. The glucose space made up between 23—30% of the body weight and was not changed by intravenous injection of 15—20 IU of insulin. Large amounts of glucose do, however, disappear from the blood and after a time lag the combustion of glucose to carbon dioxide by the extrahepatic tissues is increased (Wick *et al.*, 1951). Attempts to measure the oxidation of labeled glucose encounter the same problems as isotope dilution techniques due to incomplete intermixing. Intermixing of the labeled glucose with the body glucose mass is so slow that many hours or even days would be required in order to establish steady state conditions (Drury *et al.*, 1951). The problems arising from delayed intermixing can be reduced by employing a continuous infusion of the labeled substrate (Coxon and Robinson, 1959).

Stetten *et al.* (1951) were aware of these problems and in their experiments on rats infused glucose and the label at a rate that produced glycosuria. Measurements were made when the levels of the specific activity of urinary glucose reached constancy. In addition to the oxidation of labeled glucose to $^{14}CO_2$, the production of glucose from unlabeled sources has been measured in normal and alloxan-diabetic rats. While the amount of glucose oxidized was not greatly affected by the diabetic state, glucose production rose from 17.5—43.3 mg/rat/h.

5. Conclusions

The data discussed in the preceding sections give us little reason to assume that either insulin or the diabetic state affect the glucose space of the body. Insulin reduces blood glucose levels, not by diluting the glucose pool, but by reducing the amount of glucose present in the body.

The controversy as to whether or not insulin does reduce hepatic glucose release and if so, what is the possible physiological significance of this effect, is likely to continue. However, evidence has been presented here to show that insulin, when preventing hyperglycemia, does so in part by reducing the release of glucose into the blood.

When insulin has been employed to lower the blood glucose concentration from normoglycemic to hypoglycemic levels in fasting animals or in man, a hepatic effect has been less convincingly demonstrated. Whereas insulin did induce a net uptake of glucose or reduce hepatic glucose release in some experiments, in others it restrained the release of additional glucose from the liver in response to hypoglycemia or had no effect on hepatic glucose release. It is unlikely that the discrepancy in the results stems entirely from differences in the experimental procedures or in the diet the animals received prior to the fasting period preceding the actual measurements. Nevertheless, it is recognized that dietary factors, the animal species used, the rate of decline in blood glucose levels, and the route of administration of insulin can all affect the results.

Access to portal venous blood is usually impossible in man, so that it is difficult to obtain adequate data on the net hepatic glucose release from normal human subjects. Isotope dilution techniques have been applied to the study of glucose turnover in dogs (Steele *et al.*, 1974) and in sheep (Bergman *et al.*, 1974), but their applicability in man is limited.

Uptake of glucose will equal the rate of glucose production so long as the glucose pool and the glucose space do not change. Insulin reduces the glucose pool and thus interferes with estimations of glucose uptake based on the rate of appearance of glucose. The formation of labeled carbon dioxide from ^{14}C-glucose does not necessarily yield information pertinent to the amount of glucose utilized.

The stimulatory effect of insulin on the uptake of glucose by peripheral tissues has been amply studied on isolated tissues. Our knowledge about the way insulin affects glucose metabolism is derived from such experiments, but it should be remembered that they were not designed to yield quantitative information on how insulin affects the fate of glucose in the intact animal or in man.

References

Andres, R., Cadex, G., Zierler, K.L.: The quantitatively minor role of carbohydrate in oxidative metabolism by skeletal muscle in intact man in the basal state. Measurements of oxygen and glucose uptake and carbon dioxide and lactate production in the forearm. J. clin. Invest. **35**, 671—682 (1956)

Annison, E.F., Linzell, J.L.: The oxidation and utilization of glucose and acetate by the mammary gland of the goat in relation to their overall metabolism and to milk formation. J. Physiol. (Lond.) **175**, 372—385 (1964)

Baker, N., Shreeve, W.W., Shipley, R.A., Incefy, O.E., Miller, M.: C^{14} studies in carbohydrate metabolism. I. The oxidation of glucose in normal human subjects. J. biol. Chem. **211**, 575—592 (1954)

Bearn, A.G., Billing, B.H., Sherlock, S.: Response of the liver to insulin. Hepatic vein catheterization studies in man. In: Ciba Found. Sympos. on a scientific trends in medical research, p. 256. London: Churchill 1955

Bergman, E.N., Brockman, R.P., Kaufman, E.F.: Glucose metabolism in ruminants: comparison of whole body turnover with production by gut, liver, and kidneys. Fed. Proc. **33**, 1843—1854 (1974)

Bishop, J.S., Steele, R., Altszuler, N., Dunn, A., Bjerknes, C., de Bodo, R.C.: Effect of insulin on liver glycogen synthesis and breakdown in the dog. Amer. J. Physiol. **208**, 307—316 (1965)

Bondy, P.K.: Spontaneous fluctuations in glucose content of the hepatic venous blood in resting normal human beings. J. clin. Invest. **31**, 231—237 (1952)

Bondy, P.K., James, D.F., Farrar, B.W.: Studies of the role of the liver in human carbohydrate metabolism by the venous catheter technic. I. Normal subjects under fasting conditions and following the injection of glucose. J. clin. Invest. **28**, 238—244 (1949a)

Bondy, P.K., Bloom, W.L., Whitner, V.S., Farrar, B.W.: Studies on the role of the liver in human carbohydrate metabolism by the venous catheter technic. II. Patients with diabetic ketosis, before and after the administration of insulin. J. clin. Invest. **28**, 1126—1133 (1949b)

Cahill, G.F., Jr.: Some observations on hypoglycemia in man. Advanc. Enzyme Reg. 2, 137—148 (1967)

Cahill, G.F., Jr., Leboeuf, B., Flinn, R.B.: Studies on adipose tissue *in vitro*. IV. Effect of epinephrine on glucose metabolism. J. biol. Chem. **235**, 1246—1250 (1960)

Cannon, W.B., McIver, A.B., Bliss, S.W.: Studies on the conditions of activity of endocrine glands. XIII. A sympathetic and adrenal mechanism for mobilizing sugar in hypoglycemia. Amer. J. Physiol. **69**, 46—66 (1924)

Cherrington, A.D., Vranic, M.: Effect of arginine on glucose turnover and plasma free fatty acids in normal dogs. Diabetes **22**, 537—543 (1973)

Cowan, J.S., Hetenyi, G., Jr.: Glucoregulatory responses in normal and diabetic dogs recorded by a new tracer method. Metabolism **20**, 360—372 (1971)

Cowan, J.S., Schachter, D., Hetenyi, G., Jr.: Validity of a tracer injection method for studying glucose turnover in normal dogs. J. nucl. Med. **10**, 98—102 (1969)

Coxon, R.V., Robinson, R.J.: Movements of radioactive carbon dioxide within the animal body during oxidation of ^{14}C-labelled substrates. J. Physiol. (Lond.) **147**, 487—510 (1959)

Craig, J.W., Drucker, W.R., Miller, M., Woodward, H., Jr.: A prompt effect of exogenous insulin on net hepatic glucose output in man. Metabolism **10**, 212—220 (1961)

Crandall, L.A., Jr., Lipscomb, A.: A direct measurement of hepatic glucose production in experimental diabetes mellitus. Amer. J. Physiol. **148**, 312—318 (1947)

Dietze, G., Hepp, K.D., Wickmayr, M., Mehnert, H.: Application of a new method of measuring hepatic blood flow to metabolic balance studies in human liver. II. Regulation of glucose output by lactate and insulin. Diabetologia **9**, 65 (1973) (abstr.)

Drury, D.R., Wick, A.N.: Insulin and the volume of distribution of glucose. Amer. J. Physiol. **166**, 159—164 (1951)

Drury, D.R., Wick, A.N., Bancroft, R.W., MacKay, E.M.: Glucose utilization by the extrahepatic tissues. Amer. J. Physiol. **164**, 207—212 (1951)
Dunn, A., Altszuler, N., de Bodo, R.C.: Mechanism of action of insulin. Nature (Lond.) **183**, 1123—1124 (1959)
Dunn, D.F., Friedmann, B., Maass, A.R., Reichard, G.A., Weinhouse, S.: Effects of insulin on blood glucose entry and removal rates in normal dogs: J. biol. Chem. **225**, 225—237 (1957)
Dunn, A., Steele, R., Altszuler, N.: An effect of insulin on production of glucose during hepatic glycogenolysis. Nature (Lond.) **188**, 236—237 (1960)
Edwards, J.C., Howell, S.L., Taylor, K.W.: Fatty acids as regulator of glucagon secretion. Nature (Lond.) **224**, 808—809 (1969)
Exton, J.H., Mallette, L.E., Jefferson, L.S., Wong, E.H.A., Friedmann, N., Miller, T.B., Park, C.R.: The hormonal control of hepatic gluconeogenesis. Recent Progr. Hormone Res. **26**, 411—461 (1970)
Felig, P., Marliss, E., Ohman, J., Cahill, G.F., Jr.: Plasma amino acid levels in diabetic ketoacidosis. Diabetes **19**, 727—729 (1970)
Felig, P., Wahren, J.: Influence of endogenous insulin secretion on splanchnic glucose and amino acid metabolism in man. J. clin. Invest. **50**, 1702—1711 (1971)
Feller, D.D., Chaikoff, I.L., Strisower, E.H., Steele, G.L.: Glucose utilization in the diabetic dog, studied with C^{14} glucose. J. biol. Chem. **188**, 865—880 (1951)
Feller, D.D., Strisower, E.H., Chaikoff, I.L.: Turnover and oxidation of body glucose in normal and alloxan-diabetic rats. J. biol. Chem. **187**, 571—588 (1950)
Fine, M.B., Williams, R.H.: Effect of insulin infusion on hepatic output of glucose. Amer. J. Physiol. **198**, 645—648 (1960)
Foa, P.P., Santamaria, L., Weinstein, H.R., Berger, S., Smith, J.A.: Secretion of the hyperglycemic-glycogenolytic factor in normal dogs. Amer. J. Physiol. **171**, 32—36 (1952)
Froesch, R.: Die Funktion der Nebennierenrinde in der Insulingegenregulation. Schweiz. med. Wschr. **85**, 121—127 (1955)
Gey, K.F.: The concentration of glucose in rat tissue. Biochem. J. **64**, 145—150 (1956)
Ginsberg, J.M., Wilde, W.S.: Distribution kinetics of intravenous radiopotassium. Amer. J. Physiol. **179**, 63—75 (1954)
Goldfine, I.D., Kahn, C.R., Neville, D.M., Jr., Roth, J., Garrison, M.M., Bates, R.W.: Decreased binding of insulin to its receptors in rats with hormone induced insulin resistance. Biochem. biophys. Res. Commun. **53**, 852—857 (1973)
Hasselblatt, A.: Changes in the glucose concentration in the blood of the femoral artery and of the hepatic, portal and femoral vein during onset of tolbutamide- or insulin-hypoglycemia. Biochem. Pharmacol. **8**, 163 (1961) (abstr.)
Henderson, M.J., Wrenshall, G.A., Odense, P.: Effects of insulin on rates of glucose transfer in the depancreatized dog. Canad. J. Biochem. **33**, 926—939 (1955)
Hetenyi, G., Jr., Wrenshall, G.A.: Adaptive changes in rates of appearance and disappearance of glucose in dogs following step changes in the rate of glucose infusion. Canad. J. Physiol. Pharmacol. **46**, 391—398 (1968)
Issekutz, B., Jr., Allen, M., Borkow, I.: Estimation of glucose turnover in the dog with glucose-2-T and glucose-u-^{14}C. Amer. J. Physiol. **222**, 710—712 (1972)
Issekutz, B., Jr., Issekutz, T.B., Elalie, D., Borkow, I.: Effect of insulin infusions on the glucose kinetics in alloxan-streptozotocin diabetic dogs. Diabetologia **10**, 323—328 (1974)
Jackson, R.A., Advani, U., Perry, G., Rogers, J., Peters, N., Day, S., Pilkington, T.R.E.: Dietary diabetes. The influence of a low carbohydrate diet on forearm metabolism in man. Diabetes **22**, 145—159 (1973)
Jungas, R.L., Ball, E.G.: Studies on the metabolism of adipose tissue. XII. The effect of insulin and epinephrine on free fatty acid and glycerol production in the presence and absence of glucose. Biochemistry **2**, 383—388 (1963)
Katz, J., Dunn, A.: Glucose-2-t as a tracer for glucose metabolism. Biochemistry **6**, 1—5 (1967)
Katz, J., Rostami, H., Dunn, A.: Evaluation of glucose turnover, body mass and recycling with reversible and irreversible tracers. Biochem. J. **142**, 161—170 (1974a)
Katz, J., Dunn, A., Chenoweth, M.: Determination of synthesis, recycling and body mass of glucose in rats and rabbits *in vivo* with ^{3}H and ^{14}C-labelled glucose. Biochem. J. **142**, 171—183 (1974b)
Landau, B.R., Leonards, J.R.: Significance of changes in blood glucose specific activity following insulin administration. Amer. J. Physiol. **198**, 793—796 (1960)
Landau, B.R., Leonards, J.R., Barry, F.M.: Regulation of blood glucose concentration: response of liver to glucose administration. Amer. J. Physiol. **201**, 41—46 (1961)
Leboeuf, B., Cahill, G.F., Jr.: Studies on rat adipose tissue *in vitro*. VIII. Effect of preparations of pituitary adreno-corticotropic and growth hormones on glucose metabolism. J. biol. Chem. **236**, 41—46 (1961)

Leonards, J.R., Landau, B.R., Craig, J.W., Martin, F.I.R., Miller, M., Barry, F.M.: Regulation of blood glucose concentration: hepatic action of insulin. Amer. J. Physiol. **201**, 47—54 (1961)

Levin, H.W., Weinhouse, S.: Immediate effect of insulin on glucose utilisation in normal rats. J. biol. Chem. **232**, 749—760 (1958)

Levine, R., Goldstein, M.S., Huddleston, B., Klein, S.P.: Action of insulin on the permeability of cells to free hexoses as studied by its effect on the distribution of galactose. Amer. J. Physiol. **163**, 70—76 (1950)

Lipscomb, A., Crandall, L.A., Jr.: Hepatic blood flow and glucose output in normal unanesthetized dogs. Amer. J. Physiol. **148**, 302—311 (1947)

Madison, L.L., Combes, B., Strickland, W., Unger, R., Adams, R.: Evidence for a direct effect of insulin on hepatic glucose output. Metabolism **8**, 469—471 (1959a)

Madison, L.L., Combes, B., Adams, R., Strickland, W.: Evidence for a direct and immediate effect of insulin hepatic glucose output in diabetic and normal dogs. J. Lab. clin. Med. **54**, 920—921 (1959b) (abstr.)

Madison, L.L., Combes, B., Adams, R., Strickland, W.: The physiological significance of the secretion of endogenous insulin into the portal circulation. III. Evidence for a direct and immediate effect of insulin on the balance of glucose across the liver. J. clin. Invest. **39**, 507—522 (1960a)

Madison, L.L., Combes, B., Adams, R.: Insulin's control of the role of the liver in the disposition of a glucose load in diabetic and nondiabetic dogs. J. clin. Invest. **39**, 1009 (1960b) (abstr.)

Martin, F.I.R., Leonards, J.R., Craig, J.W., Barry, F.M., Miller, M., Ashmore, J., Shoemaker, W.: The effect of insulin on the hepatic output of glucose in the dog. J. Lab. clin. Med. **54**, 921—922 (1959) (abstr.)

Myers, J.D.: Net splanchnic glucose production in normal man and various disease states. J. clin. Invest. **29**, 1421—1429 (1950)

Newsholme, E.A., Randle, P.L., Manchester, K.L.: Regulation of glucose uptake by the muscle. 7. Effects of fatty acids, ketone bodies and pyruvate and diabetes and starvation, hypophysectomy and adrenalectomy on the concentration of hexose phosphates, nucleotides, and inorganic phosphate. Biochem. J. **93**, 641—651 (1964)

Olefsky, J., Farquar, J.W., Reaven, G.: Relationship between fasting plasma insulin level and resistance to insulin-mediated glucose uptake in normal and diabetic subjects. Diabetes **22**, 507—513 (1973)

Pozefsky, T., Felig, P., Tobin, J., Soeldner, J.S., Cahill, G.F., Jr.: Amino acid balance across the tissues of the forearm in postabsorptive man: effect of insulin at two dose levels. J. clin. Invest. **48**, 2273—2282 (1969)

Reichard, G.A., Friedmann, B., Maass, A.R., Weinhouse, S.: Turnover rates of blood glucose in normal dogs during hyperglycemia induced by glucose or glucagon. J. biol. Chem. **230**, 387—397 (1958)

Reichard, G.A., Jacobs, A.G., Kimbel, P., Hochella, N.J., Weinhouse, S.: Effects of insulin on blood glucose entry and removal rates in man. Diabetes **9**, 447—453 (1960)

Reichard, G.A., Jacobs, A.G., Kimbel, P., Hochella, N.J., Weinhouse, S.: Blood glucose replacement rates in normal and diabetic humans. J. appl. Physiol. **16**, 789—795 (1961)

Reichard, G.A., Moury, N.F., Hochella, N.J., Patterson, A.L., Weinhouse, S.: Quantitative estimation of the Cori cycle in the human. J. biol. Chem. **238**, 495—501 (1963)

Reichard, G.A., Moury, N.F., Hochella, N.J., Putnam, R.C., Weinhouse, S.: Metabolism of neoplastic tissue. XVII. Blood glucose replacement rates in human cancer patients. Cancer Res. **24**, 71—76 (1964)

Ruderman, N.B., Houghton, C.R.S., Hems, R.: Evaluation of the isolated perfused rat hindquarter for the study of muscle metabolism. Biochem. J. **124**, 639—651 (1971)

Scheinberg, P., Stead, E.A., Jr.: The cerebral blood flow in male subjects as measured by the nitrous oxide technique. Normal values for blood flow oxygen utilization, glucose utilization and peripheral resistance with observation of the effects of tilting and anxiety. J. clin. Invest. **28**, 1163—1171 (1949)

Searle, G.L., Chaikoff, I.L.: Inhibitory action of hypoglycemia on delivery of glucose to the blood stream by liver of normal dog. Amer. J. Physiol. **170**, 456—460 (1952)

Searle, G.L., Strisower, E.H., Chaikoff, I.L.: Glucose pool and glucose space in the normal and diabetic dog. Amer. J. Physiol. **176**, 190—194 (1954)

Seyffert, W.A., Madison, L.L.: Physiologic effects of metabolic fuels on carbohydrate metabolism. I. Acute effect of elevation of plasma free fatty acids on hepatic glucose output, peripheral glucose utilisation, serum insulin, and plasma glucagon levels. Diabetes **16**, 765—776 (1967)

Sheppard, C.W., Householder, A.S.: The mathematical basis of the interpretation of tracer experiments in closed steady-state systems. J. appl. Physics **22**, 510—520 (1951)

SHIPP, J.C., OPIE, L.H., CHALLONER, D.R.: Interaction between carbohydrate and fatty acid metabolism of isolated perfused rat heart. Metabolism **13**, 852—867 (1964)

SHREEVE, W.W., BAKER, N., MILLER, M., SHIPLEY, R.A., INCEFY, G.E., CRAIG, J.W.: C^{14} studies in carbohydrate metabolism. VI. The oxidation of glucose in diabetic human subjects. Metabolism **5**, 22—34 (1956)

SHOEMAKER, W.C., ASHMORE, J., CARRUTHERS, P.J., POWERS, I.C., SCHULMAN, M., FEINBERG, H.: Effect of insulin on hepatic carbohydrate and fat metabolism in normal and depancreatized dogs. Fed. Proc. **19**, 163 (1960) (abstr.)

SHOEMAKER, W.C., MAHLER, R., ASHMORE, J.: The effect of insulin on hepatic glucose metabolism in the unanesthetized dog. Metabolism **8**, 494—511 (1959)

SOMOGYI, M.: Studies of arteriovenous differences in blood sugar. I. Effect of alimentary hyperglycemia on the rate of extrapancreatic glucose assimilation. J. biol. Chem. **174**, 189—200 (1948)

SOSKIN, S., LEVINE, R.: Relationship between the blood sugar level and the rate of sugar utilization, affecting the theories of diabetes. Amer. J. Physiol. **120**, 761—770 (1937)

STEELE, R.: Use of C^{14}-glucose to measure hepatic glucose production following an intravenous glucose load or after injection of insulin. Metabolism **8**, 512—519 (1959)

STEELE, R.: Reflections on pools. Fed. Proc. **23**, 671—679 (1964)

STEELE, R., WALL, J.S., DE BODO, R.C., ALTSZULER, N.: Measurement of size and turnover rate of body glucose pool by the isotope dilution method. Amer. J. Physiol. **187**, 15—24 (1956)

STEELE, R., MARKS, P.A.: Production of glucose by the liver during hyperglycemia. Nature (Lond.) **182**, 1444—1445 (1958)

STEELE, R., BISHOP, J.S., LEVINE, R.: Does a glucose load inhibit hepatic sugar output? C^{14}-glucose studies in eviscerated dogs. Amer. J. Physiol. **197**, 60—62 (1959)

STEELE, R., BISHOP, J.S., DUNN, A., ALTSZULER, N., RATHGEB, J., DE BODO, R.C.: Inhibition by insulin of hepatic glucose production in the normal dog. Amer. J. Physiol. **208**, 301—306 (1965)

STEELE, R., ROSTAMI, H., ALTSZULER, N.: A two-compartment calculator for the dog glucose pool in the nonsteady state. Fed. Proc. **33**, 1869—1876 (1974)

STETTEN, DE WITT, JR., WELT, I.D., INGLE, D.J., MORLEY, E.H.: Rates of glucose production and oxidation in normal and diabetic rats. J. biol. Chem. **192**, 817—830 (1951)

STETTEN, M.R., STETTEN, DE WITT, JR.: Glycogen regeneration *in vivo*. J. biol. Chem. **213**, 723—732 (1955)

VRANIC, M., WRENSHALL, G.A.: Exercise, insulin and glucose turnover in dogs. Endocrinology **85**, 165—171 (1969)

WALL, J.S., STEELE, R., DE BODO, R.C., ALTSZULER, N.: Effect of insulin on utilization and production of circulating glucose. Amer. J. Physiol. **189**, 43—50 (1957)

WELT, I.D., STETTEN, DE WITT, JR., INGLE, D.J., MORLEY, E.H.: Effect of cortisone upon rates of glucose production and oxidation in the rat. J. biol. Chem. **197**, 57—66 (1952)

WICK, A.N., DRURY, D.R., BANCROFT, R.W., MACKAY, E.M.: Action of insulin on the extrahepatic tissues. J. biol. Chem. **188**, 241—249 (1951)

WILLIAMSON, J.R., KREBS, H.A.: Acetoacetate as fuel of respiration in the perfused rat heart. Biochem. J. **80**, 540—547 (1961)

WRENSHALL, G.A.: Working basis for the tracer measurement of transfer rates of a metabolic factor in biological systems containing compartments whose contents do not intermix rapidly. Canad. J. Biochem. **33**, 909—925 (1955)

WRENSHALL, G.A., HETENYI, G., JR.: Successive measured injections of tracer as a method for determining characteristics of accumulation and turnover in higher animals with access limited to blood. Metabolism **8**, 531—543 (1959)

WRENSHALL, G.A., HETENYI, G.,JR., BEST, C.H.: The validity of rates of glucose appearance in the dog calculated by the method of successive tracer injections. II. The influence of intermixing time following tracer injection. Canad. J. Biochem. **39**, 267—278 (1961)

II. Alterations in Fat Metabolism

Sigurd Sailer

1. Introduction

Carbohydrates and fat are the major metabolic fuels from which energy is obtained; with a few exceptions, the various tissues of the body are capable of burning either. Which of these fuels is used and to what extent depends on the nutritional state of the body, i.e. on the concentration of these fuels in the blood at the time of the demand for energy (Owen and Reichard, 1971). Of course, carbohydrates and fat are supplied and metabolized in a reciprocal fashion in various nutritional states in physiological as well as many pathological conditions. This interplay between carbohydrates and fatty acids is governed by many factors, one of the most important being insulin. The following section describes the role of insulin in regulating fat metabolism in the blood under normal circumstances and, as far as is known, the effects of hypo- and hyperinsulinemic states under different pathological conditions.

Cholesterol and phospholipids are not the main energy source and their metabolism is probably not regulated directly by insulin. Therefore, the following discussion is limited to the metabolism of free fatty acids (FFA) and triglycerides (TG). Detailed discussion of the action of insulin on lipid metabolism in various tissues is to be found elsewhere in this chapter.

2. Normal Metabolism of Lipids

a) Postprandial State

Dietary fat is absorbed after partial hydrolysis in the gut and is transported in the lymph mainly as TG in chylomicrons, in which the TG exist in the form of an oil droplet surrounded by an amphiphilic layer of phospholipids and proteins. The lymphatic route by passes the liver, and the bulk of the TG is hydrolyzed in the capillary beds of several extrahepatic tissues to liberate FFA and glycerol. Like glucose, the energy-rich FFA enter the tissues rapidly and serve as a readily available energy source. Alternatively, they can be esterified and stored in the form of TG, mainly in the adipose tissue.

During ingestion of an ordinary meal, insulin secreted from the pancreas is not necessary for the absorption of TG in the gut, but it facilitates the uptake and storage of TG in extrahepatic tissues. Storage of TG in adipose tissue is increased by insulin through

1) increased synthesis of lipoprotein lipase, the enzyme that splits the chylomicron TG and thus permits uptake of FFA into the cell;

2) increased formation of α-glycerophosphate from glucose; this is necessary for esterification of FFA before they can be stored as TG;

3) inhibition of an increased intracellular lipase activity (the so-called "hormone-sensitive lipase"); this prevents the formation of FFA from stored TG and their release into the blood stream. Thus, in the postprandial state, TG are stored in the adipose tissue, the concentration of FFA in the plasma is low, and carbohydrates provide the main energy source.

b) The Postabsorptive State (12—18 h after the Last Meal)

In the postabsorptive state, the body of an adult of normal weight contains about 12 kg of TG and about 0.5 kg of glycogen. In addition to supplying local energy needs, the liver glycogen is transported in the blood as glucose and most of the TG in adipose tissue are transported in the blood as FFA and glycerol. The increase in the rates of transport of FFA and glycerol can be attributed primarily to the increased activity of the hormone-sensitive lipase in adipose tissue due to the reduced availability of insulin, but may also be facilitated by enhanced secretion of lipolytic hormones. Glycogen stores are used up by 48 h after the last meal, so that the body then uses TG as the main fuel.

In the immediate postabsorptive state, about 7 g/h of FFA is released into the blood from adipose tissue, all of which is potentially available for energy needs. About 0.3 g of glycerol also enters the blood from this site; it is transported to the liver (and to a small extent to the kidney) and is there converted to glucose. Two days after the last meal the glycogen stores in the liver are depleted and the body becomes entirely dependent for the supply of glucose upon its synthesis from precursors, mainly glycerol and amino acids. Because insulin levels are reduced in this state, mobilization of glycerol from adipose tissue and of amino acids from muscle approximately doubles. The increased transport rates of these glucose precursors lead to a hepatic and renal glucose production of 2—3 g/h.

About 3 g/h of FFA is taken up by the liver. Hepatic FFA uptake is not under insulin regulation, but is rather a function of the plasma FFA concentration (FRIEDBERG *et al.*, 1961; HAVEL *et al.*, 1970; BASSO and HAVEL, 1970; VAN HARKEN *et al.*, 1969; FINE and WILLIAMS, 1960; SAILER *et al.*, 1967; SPITZER and MCELROY, 1960, 1962; SÖLING *et al.*, 1966a, b). One third of the uptake of FFA (1 g/h) is converted to ketone bodies (acetoacetate and β-hydroxybutyrate), one third (1 g/h) is oxidized completely to CO_2 and water, and the remaining third (1 g/h) is esterified with α-glycerophosphate to form TG. Some of these triglycerides are secreted by the liver in the form of lipoproteins (0.5 g/h). This is a complex energy-dependent process that requires the packaging of TG as lipoprotein and its transport through the endoplasmatic reticulum and Golgi apparatus to the extracellular space; from there it is exported to extrahepatic tissues for storage or oxidation.

Insulin may, however, be required to allow normal hepatic output of TG at any specific plasma concentration of FFA (WOODSIDE and HEIMBERG, 1972). About 0.5 g/h of esterified fatty acids is stored in the liver. In insulin deficiency, the secretion of TG does not keep pace with the increased rate of TG synthesis (2.0 g/h) as a result of the increased uptake of FFA by the liver (6.0 g/h), i.e. the increased concentration of FFA in the blood perfusing the liver. Fat accumulates in the liver (1.5 g/h) (Havel, 1972) and the output of TG in the form of TG-rich lipoproteins is low.

3. Effects of Severe Insulinopenia

The effects of severe insulin deficiency on fat metabolism resemble those of fasting; however, in some forms of diabetes mellitus the changes occur in a more exaggerated form.

a) Short-Term Insulin Deficiency (up to 6 h)

Short-term insulin deficiency can be observed when insulin-dependent diabetics are suddenly denied insulin; it can also be produced in animals by the administration of mannoheptulose or anti-insulin serum. Augmented fat mobilization is observed (Bierman *et al.*, 1957a) to occur when the effects of fat-mobilizing stimuli in adipose tissue are not counteracted by insulin (Jungas and Ball, 1963). Some of these stimuli also increase in intensity; for example, the secretion of glucagon rises. The early changes in hepatic metabolism are due to the increased influx of FFA as a result of the increased concentration of FFA in the blood perfusing the liver. TG synthesis increases as well as ketogenesis. This situation can also be reproduced by an intravenous infusion of norepinephrine. The mobilization of fat reaches a maximum 2—3 h after the onset of severe insulin deficiency in dog and man. At that time the utilization of ketones and TG-rich lipoproteins is still unimpaired. Glycogen stores in the liver diminish but TG accumulate in the liver cells. Hepatic glucose production increases, reflecting, besides increased glycogenolysis, increased gluconeogenesis from glycerol and amino acids.

b) Long-Term Insulin Deficiency (One Day or More)

The transition from short-term insulin deficiency to long-term deficiency is characterized by increasing hyperlipidemia and ketosis, with only a small change in the rate of fat mobilization. The fat content in the liver increases rapidly, especially when a fat-rich diet is given. Isotope studies in chronically depancreatized dogs (Basso and Havel, 1970) show that about 30% of FFA taken up by the liver is converted to ketone bodies, whereas an equal amount of ketones is derived from the abundant fat stores within the liver. A very small amount of the FFA taken up by the liver is converted to TG-rich liproproteins in this state (only about 2%).

In the perfused rat liver, the rate of TG output begins to fall as a function of time 6 h after administration of anti-insulin serum, reaching a minimum after 10 h (Woodside and Heimberg, 1972). Since a period of between 10 and 20 h was required to correct the biochemical lesion when insulin was given to the diabetic animal *in vivo*, one could conclude that severe insulin deficiency produces secondary changes in the liver which require a prolonged period of time to resolve. In summary, the rate of FFA uptake by the liver in normal and diabetic animals is a linear function of time and is constant over a wide range of concentrations. The hepatic output of TG in the form of TG-rich lipoproteins is also proportional to the mean FFA concentration and the liver FFA uptake, but in the diabetic both the relative and maximal rates of TG secretion are depressed; in other words, the diabetic liver secretes less TG than a normal liver at a given plasma FFA concentration. Thus, the hepatic production of ketone bodies and of glucose is elevated as compared with short-term deficiency of insulin, but that of TG is lowered. The rate of secretion of endogenous TG is also lower in patients with severe insulin deficiency (Sailer *et al.*, 1967). Therefore, hypertriglyceridemia must be due to defective utilization of TG in extrahepatic tissues.

Studies in laboratory animals indicate that after heparin injection there is a marked fall in lipoprotein lipase activity in adipose tissue and in the plasma (Meng and Goldfarb, 1959; Pav and Wenkeova, 1960; Schnatz and Williams, 1962, 1963; Kessler, 1963). The lowered postheparin lipoprotein lipase activity in the plasma and the delayed clearance of artificial chylomicrons from the plasma can be normalized by giving insulin injections (Kessler, 1962). In insulin-treated alloxan-diabetic rats after withdrawal of insulin the lipoprotein lipase showed decreased activity in adipose tissue (Schnatz and Williams, 1963). This is only to be expected since insulin plus glucose induces the formation of lipoprotein lipase in adipose tissue (Salaman, 1963). The effect can be blocked by puromycin (Eagle and Robinson, 1964).

Studies in man also suggest that the uptake of plasma TG in the tissues is impaired and that the activity of lipoprotein lipase is reduced (Bierman *et al.*, 1966; Bagdade *et al.*, 1967b, 1968; Brown, 1967). The enzyme deficiency is reversible with hormone repletion; insulin administration promptly restores postheparin lipoprotein lipase (Bagdade *et al.*, 1967b), improves TG removal (Bagdade *et al.*, 1968), and reduces plasma TG levels (Schlierf and Kinsell, 1965).

Therefore, various distinct mechanisms lead to hyperlipemia in different stages of severe insulinopenia: there is a gradual change from increased TG production by the liver in the early stages of insulin deficiency to a state of reduced production of lipoprotein by the liver, combined with lower utilization of TG-rich lipoproteins in the extrahepatic tissues.

One could speculate that the diminished protein synthesis in the diabetic liver is responsible for lowering lipoprotein production in the liver. In fact, in experimental diabetes mellitus, *in vitro* hepatic protein synthesis was markedly depressed in rats (Korner, 1960; Tragl and Reaven, 1971). Insulin deficiency is associated with a fall in the proportion of hepatic ribosomes that exist as polyribosomes (Tragl and Reaven, 1972; Wittman *et al.*, 1969). It has been suggested that the relative decrease in hepatic polysomes which results from the loss of rough endoplasmatic reticulum in diabetes is responsible for the decrease in hepatic protein synthesis (Reaven *et al.*, 1973). The decreased rate of apoprotein production could cause impaired secretion of TG-rich lipoproteins.

On the other hand, in the liver of rats treated with alloxan or anti-insulin serum, a low concentration of α-glycerophosphate was found (Kalkhoff *et al.*, 1966). A lowered concentration of α-glycerophosphate in the liver could be responsible for the markedly slower rate of esterification of FFA to plasma TG, although this pathomechanism does not seem very likely, because it does not explain the accumulation of fat (TG) in the diabetic liver.

The utilization of ketone bodies in chronically diabetic dogs withdrawn from insulin for 2 days is also impaired. Thus, the ketosis induced by in prolonged insulin deficiency is complex. It involves

1) increased supply of FFA to the liver;

2) increased ketogenesis from substrate stores within the liver;

3) defective utilization of ketone bodies in extrahepatic tissues. These abnormalities can be regarded as due respectively to increased lipolysis of TG in the adipose tissue, liver and skeletal muscle. It has been clearly shown that insulin rapidly inhibits lipolysis in adipose tissue, but this has not yet been demonstrated for liver and muscle.

The fact that changes in lipid metabolism during short-term insulin deficiency can be diminished by the administration of an inhibitor of fat mobilization suggests that the effects of insulin deficiency are mainly the result of increased TG mobilization. Similarly, the depletion of adipose stores by starvation diminishes the severity of ketosis during long-term insulin deficiency. For example, juvenile diabetes without ketosis is observed very frequently in undernourished populations. The depletion of adipose stores was also used to treat diabetes in the pre-insulin era.

4. Glycogenosis Type I

This form of Gierke's disease is due to a genetically determined deficiency of hepatic glucose-6-phosphatase. It is characterized by low insulin levels and hyperlipemia in addition to fasting hypoglycemia, increased fat mobilization, and ketosis. In contrast to short-term or prolonged insulin deficiency with augmented mobilization of TG, sufferers from this disease exhibit high *de novo* synthesis of fatty acids from citrate (Hülsmann *et al.*, 1970), a reduction of the fraction of plasma FFA converted to ketones in the postabsorptive state (from 35% to 20%), and enhanced conversion to lipoprotein TG (from 18% to 30%) (Havel *et al.*, 1969). Consequently, the rate of secretion of TG by the liver in form of very low density lipoproteins (VLDL-TG) is increased 3- to 4-fold, so that the hyperlipemia can be regarded as due to of overproduction of TG by the liver. Dihydroxyacetone, a precursor of the α-glycerophosphate required for TG synthesis, accumulates in the liver and hence could help to reduce oxidation of FFA by promoting TG synthesis.

It should be mentioned, however, that the lipoprotein lipase activity in the tissues, when measured as postheparin lipoprotein lipase in the plasma, is also lowered in such patients, due perhaps to their low plasma insulin concentration. This observation also suggests impaired utilization of the lipoproteins in G-6-P-deficient patients.

5. The Primary Lipodystrophies

Loss of fat, whether restricted to a limited area or involving all adipose tissue stores, is accompanied by characteristic changes in lipid metabolism. These changes are related to the fact that some of the actions of insulin are impeded (Piscatelli *et al.*, 1970). The usual fall in the level of FFA and glucose after intravenous injection of insulin is diminished. In spite of an almost total depletion of fat stores, the peripheral tissues continue to release into the blood appreciable quantities of FFA and glycerol in the usual proportions. The cause of the impaired antilipolytic action of insulin has not been ascertained, but the generalized loss of fat suggests that it may reflect the continuous activity of a potent lipolytic stimulus. The syndrome is further characterized by fatty liver and hyperlipemia. The hyperlipidemia probably results from stimulation of hepatic production of TG-rich lipoproteins due to the increased influx of FFA caused by ineffective storage of the fatty acids in adipose tissue, but it may also reflect retention of lipoprotein TG in the blood because of ineffective stimulation by insulin of lipoprotein lipase production in adipose tissue cells.

6. Excess Insulin and Endogenous Hypertriglyceridemia

At the other extreme, excess insulin, usually associated with obesity, could lead to hypertriglyceridemia. Although there is no direct evidence for this effect in man, many studies have shown a close relationship between elevated immunoreactive serum insulin levels, both in the basal state and after glucose stimulation, and plasma TG levels in normal and hypertriglyceridemic subjects (without chylomicronemia) (Farquhar *et al.*, 1966; Reaven, *et al.* 1967; Sailer *et al.*, 1968; Abrams *et al.*, 1969; Kuo and Feng, 1970; Eaton and Nye, 1973). However, correlation between TG concentration and insulin area after glucose loading was demonstrable only in hypertriglyceridemic patients without severe glucose intolerance, whereas in patients with glucosuria the insulin response after glucose was very poor, as is also the case in insulin-deficiency diabetes (Ford *et al.*, 1968; Sailer *et al.*, 1968; Glueck *et al.*, 1969; Bagdade *et al.*, 1971; Eaton and Nye, 1973). These findings do not support the hypothesis that hyperinsulinemia after glucose loading plays a major causal role in the development of endogenous hypertriglyceridemia. In addition, the following observations do not support the above-mentioned hypothesis:

1) patients with insulinoma have normal plasma TG concentration;
2) a very low concentration of plasma insulin is found in many patients with endogenous hypertriglyceridemia;
3) administration of insulin lowers the concentration of FFA in the plasma (the main precursor of endogenous plasma TG) (Dole, 1956; Bierman, 1957a) by inhibiting lipolysis in the adipose tissue (Bierman *et al.*, 1957b) and, probably as a result, decreases the overall rate of esterification of plasma FFA to plasma TG (Sailer *et al.*, 1967) and lowers the TG plasma concentration in both normal subjects and patients with diabetes mellitus (Schlierf and Kinsell, 1965; Bagdade *et al.*, 1967b);
4) the diurnal variations in plasma insulin and TG concentration also do not suggest that insulin plays a causative role in the development of endogenous hypertriglyceridemia (Schlierf and Dorow, 1973);
5) the formation of TG -fatty acids from plasma glucose-C does not seem to play a significant role (Sandhofer *et al.*, 1969).

It seems likely that obesity and glucose intolerance are associated with certain forms of endogenous hyperlipidemia in which hyperinsulinism is not the major determinant, though it is not excluded as influencing the lipemia. However, in nonobese subjects without glucose intolerance, TG concentration and insulin secretion seem closely related. Whether hypertriglyceridemia is the cause or the result of the hyperinsulinemia is still an open question, and both symptoms may yet be found to depend on a third metabolic disorder. The TG-lowering effect of diazoxide (Eaton and Nye, 1973) suggests that insulin concentration is at least one of the factors regulating plasma triglyceride concentration.

7. Endogenous Hyperlipemia and Insulin Resistance

Most cases of endogenous hyperlipemia (accumulation in the blood of TG-rich lipoproteins derived from the liver) are exacerbated by ingestion of carbohydrate-rich diets, and they are often accompanied by mildly impaired glucose tolerance with demonstrable insulin resistance (Sailer *et al.*, 1968). This phenomenon is not confined to a certain "lipoprotein pattern" of hyperlipoproteinemia (Glueck *et al.*, 1969; Sailer, 1973).

Some pathogenetic mechanisms have been put forward to explain the common association of insulin resistance with endogenous hyperlipemia; (1) it may simply reflect the common occurrence of obesity in hyperlipemic persons; (2) alterations in TG metabolism resulting from hyperlipemia per se may impede the action of insulin; (3) insensitivity to insulin may be an intrinsic component of at least some primary hyperlipemic states. Very recently, an alteration in the insulin receptors was found and was suggested to be in part responsible for insulin resistance, at least in obese patients (Archer *et al.*, 1973).

Obesity acquired in adult life is most prevalent in primary endogenous hyperlipemia. The characteristic elevation of both basal and glucose-stimulated insulin levels in obese subjects (Bagdade *et al.*, 1967a, 1971) associated with insulin resistance and elevated plasma TG concentrations and glucose intolerance is accompanied by obesity only in persons having a predisposition to hyperglycemia or hypertriglyceridemia. The "hypertrophic" obesity may simply be the phenotypic expression of these disorders. As in obese subjects without hyperlipemia, resistance is manifested to insulin in both its hypoglycemic and antilipolytic actions, and there is a similar increase in the level of insulin in the plasma. However, resistance to these actions of insulin is occasionally disproportionate to the extent of adiposity. Therefore, although hyperlipemia is favorably affected by weight reduction, insensitivity to insulin may be associated directly with at least some primary hyperlipemic states. The association of these two phenomena can also be observed in lipodystrophy, hyperadrenal corticism, chronic renal failure, liver cirrhosis, late pregnancy, and reactions to contraceptive steroids.

How hyperlipemia itself could induce a state of insulin resistance is not clear. Conceivably, the TG in plasma lipoproteins could compete with glucose as a fuel. Then we must ask how the altered action of insulin could promote hyperlipemia. The associated hyperinsulinism could lead to increased hepatic TG synthesis, as suggested by REAVEN *et al.* (1967). These authors observed a positive relationship between plasma insulin concentration and the increase in TG level produced by a high-carbohydrate diet. If this effect were due to hyperinsulinemia, the action of insulin on the liver might be impaired less than its effects in extrahepatic tissues. However, direct measurements show little difference between the metabolism of FFA in splanchnic tissues of normotriglyceridemic subjects and those of patients with primary endogenous hypertriglyceridemia (SAILER *et al.*, 1966; HAVEL *et al.*, 1970).

If in normal subjects insulin may either reduce TG synthesis in the liver (by reducing the influx of FFA from adipose tissue) or increase the uptake of TG in the extrahepatic tissues (by induction of lipoprotein lipase), a state of insulin resistance might then be accompanied by elevated levels of FFA in the postprandial state and/or by impairment of TG removal. Average rates of transport of endogenous TG in the blood are moderately elevated in subjects with primary endogenous hyperlipemia but usually remain within normal limits. Hence a lower rate of catabolism of TG-rich lipoproteins must be responsible for the developement of hypertriglyceridemia (SAILER *et al.*, 1966; HAVEL, 1968; HAVEL *et al.*, 1970; EATON *et al.*, 1969). Some studies in man have indicated that the activity of lipoprotein lipase is inversely related to plasma TG level, in which case impaired induction of lipoprotein lipase synthesis could be an additional manifestation of insulin resistance in hyperlipemic subjects.

It should be mentioned, however, that in some patients with primary endogenous hypertriglyceridemia, hyperinsulinemia, insulin resistance, decreased glucose tolerance, and obesity, the administration of insulin does not lead to a lowered plasma TG concentration, but, probably due to increased caloric intake after insulin administration, to an increase in body weight and in TG concentration (KALLIO and SAARIMAA, 1967; BRAUNSTEINER *et al.*, 1968).

8. Conclusions

The rate of insulin secretion and the concentration of insulin in the blood are perhaps the most important factors regulating the supply of energy to the body. After ingestion of a meal, lipids are stored in the form of TG, mainly in the adipose tissue, and carbohydrates are used principally as a fuel for energy. In the postabsorptive state and during early and late starvation, lipids can be used as fuel for energy, and glucose is burnt to CO_2 and water only by some tissues (brain, erythocytes, adrenals).

In order to perform this task of energy regulation, insulin promotes the uptake of TG into the fat cells and inhibits the liberation of FFA from the adipose tissue. Insulin is required in the liver to permit a normal rate of esterification of plasma FFA to endogenous TG as well as converting the FFA taken up by the liver to ketones.

In insulin deficiency, more FFA are converted to ketones and the rate of esterification of plasma FFA to plasma TG falls. We still do not know whether hyperinsulinemia combined with hyperglucosemia leads to hypertriglyceridemia, but many factors speak against such a hypothesis.

References

ABRAMS, M.E., JARRETT, R.J., KEEN, H., BOYNS, D.R., CROSSLEY, J.N.: Oral glucose tolerance and related factors in a normal population sample. II. Interrelationship of glycerides, cholesterol, and other factors with the glucose and insulin response. Brit. med. J. **1**, 599—602 (1969)

ARCHER, J.A., GORDEN, P., GAUIN, J.R., LESNIAK, M.A., ROTH, J.: Insulin receptors in human circulating lymphocytes: Application to the study of insulin resistance in man. J. clin. Endocr. **36**, 627—633 (1973)

BAGDADE, J.D., BIERMAN, E.L., PORTE, Jr. D.: The significance of basal insulin levels in the evaluation of the insulin response to glucose in diabetic and non-diabetic subjects. J. clin. Invest. **46**, 1549—1557 (1967a)

BAGDADE, J.D., PORTE, JR., D., BIERMAN, E.L.: Diabetic lipemia. A form of acquired fat-induced lipemia. New Engl. J. Med. **276**, 427—433 (1967b)

BAGDADE, J.D., PORTE, JR., D., BIERMAN, E.L.: Acute insulin withdrawal and the regulation of plasma triglyceride removal in diabetic subjects. Diabetes **17**, 127—132 (1968)

BAGDADE, J.D., BIERMAN, E.L., PORTE, JR., D.: The influence of obesity on the relationship between insulin and triglyceride levels in endogenous hypertriglyceridemia. Diabetes **20**, 664—673 (1971)

BASSO, L.V., HAVEL, R.J.: Hepatic metabolism of free fatty acids in normal and diabetic dogs. J. clin. Invest. **49**, 537—547 (1970)

BIERMAN, E.L., DOLE, V.P., ROBERTS, T.N.: An abnormality of nonesterified fatty acid metabolism in diabetes mellitus. Diabetes **6**, 475—479 (1957a)

BIERMAN, E.L., SCHWARTZ, I.L., DOLE, V.P.: Action of insulin on release of fatty acids from tissue stores. Amer. J. Physiol. **191**, 359—362 (1957b)

BIERMAN, E.L., AMARAL, J.A.P., BELKNAP, B.H.: Hyperlipemia and diabetes mellitus. Diabetes **15**, 675—679 (1966)

BRAUNSTEINER, H., HERBST, M., SAILER, S., SANDHOFER, F.: Diabetes mellitus bei primärer Hypertriglyceridämie mit Kontraindikation zur Insulinbehandlung. Wien. klin. Wschr. **80**, 415—417 (1968)

BROWN, D.F.: Triglyceride metabolism in the alloxandiabetic rat. Diabetes **16**, 90—95 (1967)

DOLE, V.P.: A relation between non-esterified fatty acids in plasma and the metabolism of glucose. J. clin. Invest. **35**, 150—154 (1956)

EAGLE, G.R., ROBINSON, D.S.: The ability of actinomycin D to increase clearing-factor lipase activity of rat adipose tissue. Biochem. J. **93**, 10C—11C (1964)

EATON, R.P., BERMAN, M., STEINBERG, D.: Kinetic studies of plasma free fatty acid and triglyceride metabolism in man. J. clin. Invest. **48**, 1560—1579 (1969)

EATON, R.P., NYE, W.H.R.: The relationship between insulin secretion and triglyceride concentration in endogenous lipemia. J. Lab. clin. Med. **81**, 682—695 (1973)

FARQUHAR, J.W., FRANK, A., GROSS, R.C., REAVEN, G.M.: Glucose, insulin, and triglyceride responses to high and low carbohydrate diets in man. J. clin. Invest. **45**, 1648—1656 (1966)

FINE, M.B., WILLIAMS, R.H.: Effect of fasting, epinephrine and glucose and insulin on hepatic uptake of nonesterified fatty acids. Amer. J. Physiol. **199**, 403—406 (1960)

FORD, S., JR., BOZIAN, R.C., KNOWLES, JR., H.C.: Interactions of obesity, and glucose and insulin levels in hypertriglyceridemia. Amer. J. clin. Nutr. **21**, 904—910 (1968)

FRIEDBERG, S.J., KLEIN, R.F., TROUT, D.L., BOGDONOFF, M.D., ESTES, Jr., E.H.: The incorporation of plasma free fatty acids into plasma triglycerides in man. J. clin. Invest. **40**, 1846—1855 (1961)

GLUECK, C.J., LEVY, R.L., FREDRICKSON, D.S.: Immunoreactive insulin, glucose tolerance, and carbohydrate inducibility in types II, III, IV and V hyperlipoproteinemia. Diabetes **18**, 739—748 (1969)

HAVEL, R.J.: Triglyceride and very low density lipoprotein turnover. Pıoc. 1968 Deuel Conf. on Lipids on the Turnover of Lipids and Lipoproteins, Carmel (Calif.), Feb. 21—24 (1968), p. 117—121

HAVEL, R.J., BALASSE, E.O., WILLIAMS, H.E., KANE, J.P., SEGEL, N.: Splanchnic metabolism in von Gierke's disease (glycogenosis type I). Trans. Ass. Amer. Phycns **82**, 305—323 (1969)

HAVEL, R.J., KANE, J.R., BALASSE, E.O., SEGEL, N., BASSO, L.V.: Splanchnic metabolism of free fatty acids and production of triglycerides of very low density lipoproteins in normotriglyceridemic and hypertriglyceridemic humans. J. clin. Invest. **49**, 2017—2035 (1970)

HAVEL, R.J.: Caloric homoestasis and disorders of fuel transport. New Engl. J. Med. **287**, 1186—1192 (1972)

HÜLSMANN, W.C., EIJKENBOOM, W.H.M., KOSTER, J.F., FERNANDES, J.: Glucose-6-Phosphatase deficiency and hyperlipaemia. Clin. chim. Acta **30**, 775—778 (1970)

JUNGAS, R.L., BALL, E.G.: Studies on the metabolism of adipose tissue. XII. The effects of insulin and epinephrine on free fatty acid and glycerol production in the presence and absence of glucose. Biochemistry **2**, 383—388 (1963)

KALKHOFF, R.K., HORNBROOK, K.R., BURCH, H.B., KIPNIS, D.M.: Studies of the metabolic effects of acute insulin deficiency. II. Changes in hepatic glycolytic and Krebs-cycle intermediates and pyridine nucleotides. Diabetes **15**, 451—456 (1966)

KALLIO, I.V.I., SAARIMAA, H.A.: Changes in blood lipids, postprandial lipemia and intravenous tolbutamide test response after insulin shock treatment. Amer. J. med. Sci. **254**, 619—622 (1967)

KESSLER, J.I.: Effect of insulin on release of plasma lipolytic activity and clearing of emulsified fat intravenously administered to pancreatictomized and alloxanized dogs. J. Lab. clin. Med. **60**, 747—755 (1962)

KESSLER, J.I.: Effect of diabetes and insulin on the activity of myocardial and adipose tissue lipoprotein lipase of rats. J. clin. Invest. **42**, 362—367 (1963)

KORNER, A.: Alloxan diabetes and in vitro protein biosynthesis in rat liver, microsomes and mitochondria. J. Endocr. **20**, 256—262 (1960)

KUO, P.T., FENG, L.Y.: Study of serum insulin in atherosclerotic patients with endogenous hypertriglyceridemia (types III and IV hyperlipoproteinemia). Metabolism **19**, 372—380 (1970)

MENG, H.C., GOLDFARB, J.L.: Heparin-induced lipemia clearing factor in rats. Role of the pancreas in its production. Diabetes 8, 211—217 (1959)

OWEN, O.E., REICHARD, JR., G.A.: Fuels consumed by man: the interplay between carbohydrates and fatty acids. Progr. biochem. Pharmacol. **6**, 177—213 (1971)

PAV, J., WENKEOVA, J.: Significance of adipose tissue lipoprotein lipase. Nature (Lond.) **185**, 926—927 (1960)

PISCATELLI, R.L., VIEWEG, W.V.R., HAVEL, R.J.: Partial lipodystrophy: metabolic studies in three patients. Ann. intern. Med. **73**, 963—970 (1970)

REAVEN, G.M., LERNER, R.L., STERN, M.P., FARQUHAR, J.W., NAKANISHI, R.: Role of insulin in endogenous hypertriglyceridemia. J. clin. Invest. **46**, 1756—1767 (1967)

REAVEN, E.P., PETERSON, D.T., REAVEN, G.M.: The effect of experimental diabetes mellitus and insulin replacement on hepatic ultrastructure and protein synthesis. J. clin. Invest. **52**, 248—262 (1973)

SAILER, S., SANDHOFER, F., BRAUNSTEINER, H.: Umsatzraten für freie Fettsäuren und Triglyceride im Plasma bei essentieller Hyperlipämie. Klin. Wschr. **44**, 1032—1036 (1966)

SAILER, S., SANDHOFER, F., BRAUNSTEINER, H.: Beziehungen zwischen Blutzuckerspiegel, Umsatzrate der freien Fettsäuren und Fettsäureneinbau in Plasmatriglyceride bei Diabetikern. Klin. Wschr. **45**, 86—91 (1967)

SAILER, S., BOLZANO, K., SANDHOFER, F., SPATH, P., BRAUNSTEINER, H.: Triglyceridspiegel und Insulinkonzentration im Plasma nach oraler Glukosegabe bei Patienten mit primärer kohlenhydratinduzierter Hypertriglyceridämie. Schweiz. med. Wschr. **98**, 1512—1518 (1968)

SAILER, S.: Indices of carbohydrate metabolism in patients with endogenous hypertriglyceridemia. Proceedings of the International Diabetes Federation, 8th Congress, Brussels July 15—20, 1973

SALAMAN, M.R., QUOTED BY ROBINSON, D.S.: Clearing factor lipase and fat transport. In: Advances in Lipid Research, **1**, 145 (eds. PAOLETTI R., and KRITCHEVSKY, D.). New York: Academic Press 1963

SANDHOFER, F., BOLZANO, K., SAILER, S., BRAUNSTEINER, H.: Quantitative Untersuchungen über den Einbau von Plasmaglucose-Kohlenstoff in Plasmatriglyceride und die Veresterungsrate von freien Fettsäuren des Plasmas zu Plasmatriglyceriden während oraler Zufuhr von Glucose bei primärer kohlenhydratinduzierter Hypertriglyceridämie. Klin. Wschr. **47**, 1086—1094 (1969)

Schlierf, G., Kinsell, L.W.: Effect of insulin in hypertriglyceridemia. Proc. Soc. exp. Biol. (N.Y.) **120**, 272—274 (1965)
Schlierf, G., Dorow, E.: Diurnal patterns of triglycerides, free fatty acids, blood sugar, and insulin during carbohydrateinduction in man and their modification by nocturnal suppression of lipolysis. J. clin. Invest. **52**, 732—740 (1973)
Schnatz, J.D., Williams, R.H.: Adipose tissue lipolytic activity during insulin lack. Clin. Res. **10**, 118 (1962)
Schnatz, J.D., Williams, R.H.: The effect of acute insulin deficiency in the rat on adipose tissue lipolytic activity and plasma lipids. Diabetes **12**, 174—178 (1963)
Söling, H.D., Koschel, R., Drägert, W., Kneer, P., Creutzfeldt, W.: Die Wirkung von Insulin auf den Stoffwechsel der isolierten perfundierten Leber normaler und alloxandiabetischer Ratten. I. Der Stoffwechsel isolierter perfundierter Lebern von normalen und alloxandiabetischen Ratten unter verschiedenen experimentellen Bedingungen. Diabetologia **2**, 20—31 (1966a); II. Stoffwechselveränderungen unter dem Einfluß intraportaler Insulininfusionen. Diabetologia **2**, 32—44 (1966b)
Spitzer, J.J., McElroy, Jr., W.T.: Some hormonal effects on uptake of free fatty acids by the liver. Amer. J. Physiol. **199**, 876—878 (1960)
Spitzer, J.J., McElroy, Jr., W.T.: Some hormonal influences on the hepatic uptake of free fatty acids in diabetic dogs. Diabetes **11**, 222—226 (1962)
Tragl, K.H., Reaven, G.M.: Effect of experimental diabetes mellitus on protein synthesis by liver ribosomes. Diabetes **20**, 27—32 (1971)
Tragl, K.H., Reaven, G.M.: Effect of insulin deficiency on hepatic ribosomal aggregation. Diabetes **21**, 84—88 (1972)
Van Harken, D.R., Dixon, C.W., Heimberg, M.: Hepatic lipid metabolism in experimental diabetes. V. The effect of concentration of oleate on metabolism of triglycerides and on ketogenesis. J. biol. Chem. **244**, 2278—2283 (1969)
Wittman, J.S., Lee, K.-L., Miller, O.N.: Dietary and hormonal influences on rat liver polysome profiles; fat, glucose and insulin. Biochim. biophys. Acta (Amst.) **174**, 536—542 (1969)
Woodside, W.F., Heimberg, M.: Hepatic metabolism of free fatty acids in experimental diabetes. Israel J. med. Sci. **8**, 309—316 (1972)

I. Modification of the Effects of Insulin by Hormonal Factors

NORMAN ALTSZULER

With 8 Figures

I. Introduction

Insulin exerts an influence on the metabolism of carbohydrate, fat, and protein. Its effects on carbohydrate metabolism have been studied most extensively and thorougly. This presentation will follow this emphasis. Various hormones may modify the effects of insulin on carbohydrate metabolism through actions on fat and protein metabolism. These effects will be considered briefly where applicable.

An appreciation of hormonal interactions on metabolism would be enhanced by some acquaintance with the techniques employed in these studies. The merits and limitations of the methods and parameters obtained in experiments using perfusion of organs, incubation of isolated tissues, tracer incorporation, and tracer dilution will not be pursued here, but more detailed discussion of some of these methods is available (STEELE, 1971; CSORBA, 1969; KRAHL, 1961; STADIE, 1954; ASHMORE and CAIN, 1969; ALTSZULER, 1974).

Much of this presentation will be based on studies performed *in vivo*. Such selection is appropriate, since the whole animal is the natural locale for evoked hormonal responses and hormonal interactions. The *in vitro* studies of limited and selective hormonal interactions have given some insight into the underlying biochemical events. Such data contribute significantly to our understanding of the events *in vivo*, and are discussed where applicable. Additional discussion of insulin action and antagonism to insulin may be found elsewhere (KATZEN and GLITZER, 1968; FRITZ, 1971; RANDLE *et al.*, 1964, 1966; WILLIAMS and ENSINCK, 1966).

II. Insulin

1. Effect on Blood Glucose Concentration

The ability of injected insulin to lower the blood glucose concentration is undoubtedly the best established effect of this hormone on carbohydrate metabolism. Injection of a very small dose of insulin (0.025 U/kg, i. v.) into a normal dog results, within a few minutes, in a fall in plasma glucose levels. The glucose concentration attains a nadir at 20—30 min followed by a prompt return to control levels at 45—60 min (DE BODO and SINKOFF, 1953). Since the plasma glucose concentration in the postabsorptive state is a resultant of glucose production and glucose utilization, knowledge of these rates allows evaluation of their role in the changes in glucose levels following insulin injection. Such measurements have been made under physiologic conditions with the use of radioisotopes. Studies in the dog reveal that the fall in plasma glucose following injection of insulin is due largely to an increased rate of glucose removal from the plasma (glucose uptake by the tissues) and to a lesser extent to a decrease in hepatic glucose output (glucose production). The restoration of the plasma glucose level to normal is due entirely to increased hepatic glucose output; indeed, glucose uptake remains above control values while plasma glucose concentrations are climbing back to normal (DE BODO *et al.*, 1963, 1963a).

2. Effect on Hepatic Glucose Output

The effect of insulin on hepatic glucose output has been debated by several groups of investigators. Insulin injection is claimed to increase, decrease or have no effect on hepatic glucose output. In experiments in intact dogs with chronically implanted transhepatic catheters, injection or infusion of insulin did not produce a decrease in hepatic glucose output (SHOEMAKER *et al.*, 1959; MAHLER *et al.*, 1959). In similar experiments, LEONARDS *et al.* (1961) reported that in dogs maintained on a high protein diet, insulin injection did not affect hepatic glucose output, but did lower it in dogs fed a high carbohydrate diet. In other experiments, using transhepatic catheterization, insulin administration was found to increase somewhat the hepatic glucose output (TARDING and SCHAMBYE, 1958).

On the other hand, ample evidence has been accumulated showing a decrease in hepatic glucose output with insulin administration. In the unanesthetized dog, with an Eck fistula, insulin administration produced a marked fall in hepatic glucose output. Since the Eck fistula involves translocation of the portal flow into the vena cava, which can alter liver metabolism, these findings were received with some reservations (see SHOEMAKER and ELWYN, 1969).

The decrease in hepatic glucose output following insulin injection was demonstrated more easily using isotope dilution techniques. Various degrees of inhibition were observed in the dog by WALL *et al.* (1957), DUNN *et al.* (1957), REICHARD *et al.* (1958), HETENYI *et al.* (1961); in the rabbit by BERSON *et al.* (1959); and in the human by JACOBS *et al.* (1958), REICHARD *et al.* (1960) and SEARLE *et al.* (1959).

In some experiments hepatic glucose output was measured simultaneously by transhepatic catherization and isotope dilution and qualitative and quantitative discrepancies were observed (TARDING and SCHAMBYE, 1958). More extensive discussion of the differences between these experiments can be found elsewhere (STEELE, 1966, SHOEMAKER and ELWYN, 1969).

One feature of many of the aforementioned experiments is that insulin was administered alone and hypoglycemia was allowed to develop, thereby evoking compensatory mechanisms which would increase hepatic glucose output. In experiments using ^{14}C-glucose, insulin infusion in normal dogs produced a transient decrease in hepatic glucose output in the first 5—10 min, and this was superseded by an increased glucose output with the hypoglycemia persisting (WALL *et al.*, 1957). The variable and often unimpressive magnitude of this initial decrease following insulin injection tended to minimize the significance of this effect. It was noted, however, that upon termination of the insulin infusion and without further fall in plasma glucose levels, there was a prompt increase in hepatic glucose output. Insulin infusion therefore prevented the normal response to hypoglycemia, and this was referred to as the "restraining" effect of insulin on hepatic glucose output (DUNN *et al.*, 1959). This phenomenon was later confirmed by the transhepatic catheterization technique (FINE and WILLIAMS, 1960). When hypoglycemia is prevented by the additional infusion of glucose, as shown in Fig. 1, the inhibitory effect of insulin on glucose output is clearly demonstrated. The necessity to avoid hypoglycemia in studying hepatic effects of insulin was emphasized earlier by BOUCKAERT and DE DUVE (1947), and this is convincingly reinforced in the aforementioned experiments.

3. Effect on Perfused Liver

The ability of insulin to decrease hepatic glucose output raises the question of whether insulin is producing this effect directly or indirectly. An answer to this question was sought in experiments with the isolated perfused liver. Initial attempts to demonstrate an inhibitory effect of insulin were unsuccessful (LUNDSGAARD *et al.*, 1936). With improved techniques of perfusion, a number of studies demonstrated distinct effects of insulin on the liver. HAFT and MILLER (1958) observed a decrease in hepatic glucose output in the 1- to 4-hour period following addition of insulin to perfused livers of alloxan-diabetic rats. This effect was less prominent or absent in livers from fed or fasted normal rats. MORTIMORE (1963), using further innovations which included the use of defibrinated red blood cells in the perfusion solution, observed that insulin decreased hepatic glucose output within 30 min after its addition to perfused livers from fed and fasted normal rats. JEFFERSON *et al.* (1968) reported similar findings, and in addition, with the aid of isotopes, showed that the decrease in net glucose production was due to suppression of glucose output rather than to enhanced glucose uptake by the perfused liver. The inhibitory effect of insulin appears to be directed at glucose derived from glycogenolysis (MORTIMORE *et al.*, 1967).

4. Effect of Endogenous Insulin on Hepatic Glucose Output

In view of the aforementioned inhibitory effects of administered insulin, it may be asked whether or not endogenous insulin has similar effects. Several lines of evidence suggest that it does. Administration of glucose alone into the whole animal decreases hepatic glucose output in a variety of species (ANNISON and WHITE, 1961; CHERRY and CRANDALL, 1937; COMBES *et al.*, 1961; LANDAU *et al.*, 1961; SOSKIN *et al.*, 1938; STEELE *et al.*, 1965). This inhibition has been attributed to the increased secretion of insulin which is evoked by the hyperglycemia.

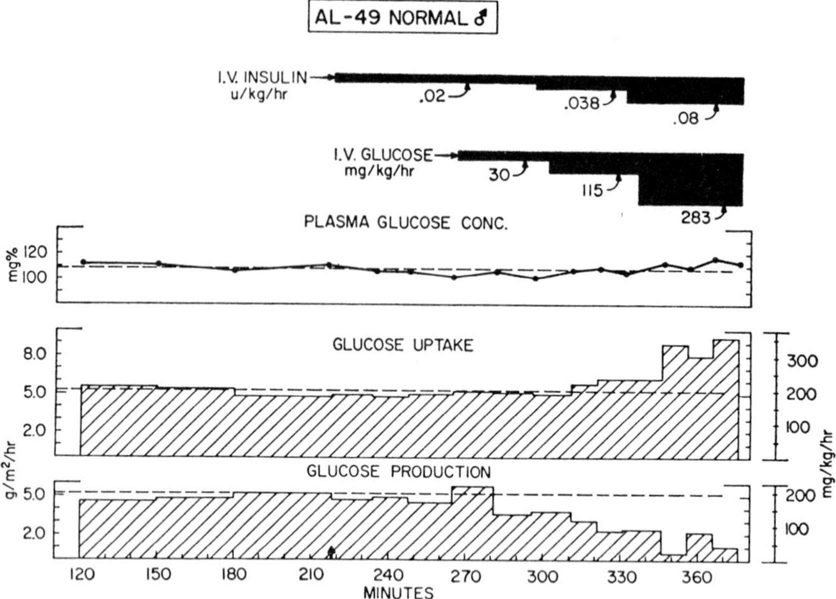

Fig. 1. Effects of continuous intravenous insulin infusion on plasma glucose concentration, glucose production, and glucose uptake, in a normal dog in the postabsorptive state, when hypoglycemia was prevented by intravenous glucose infusion in the amounts indicated. Zero time is the beginning of C^{14}-glucose infusion used to measure rates of overall glucose uptake and hepatic glucose production. Uptake and production are given relative to body surface area by reference to ordinate on left; relative to body weight be reference to ordinate on right. Dashed lines across graph represent the control value for uptake and production. (From DE BODO *et al.*, 1963 a)

More direct support for the participation of increased insulin secretion comes from the imaginative experiments of ISHIWATA *et al.* (1969) utilizing dogs in which the pancreas was exteriorized to allow its exclusion from the general circulation promptly and without further surgical procedures. Immediately upon separation of the pancreas from the circulation, a constant infusion of insulin is begun to just maintain normal blood glucose levels. Administration of glucose to these animals did not result in a decrease in hepatic glucose output, confirming the dependence of this effect no increased insulin secretion.

Another line of evidence indicates that endogenous insulin, even in the postabsorptive state, restrains hepatic glucose output. Injection of anti-insulin serum into normal dogs, in the postabsorptive state, as shown in Fig. 2, results in a prompt hyperglycemia which is due to a prompt increase in hepatic glucose output (ALTSZULER *et al.*, 1964). The adrenalectomized dog, maintained on cortisol and desoxycorticosterone, also shows a similar response to anti-insulin serum, indicating that epinephrine is not required in this response. Acute exclusion of the pancreas from the circulation, as described above, but without insulin replacement also results in a prompt increase in hepatic glucose output (WRENSHALL *et al.*, 1965), indicating that glucagon is not essential for this response. Livers removed from rats made acutely insulin-deficient by injection of anti-insulin serum also have a greater rate of glycogenolysis than livers from normal rats (JEFFERSON *et al.*, 1968).

Thus there is ample evidence from a variety of experimental approaches that insulin restrains or decreases hepatic glucose output. The two important mechanisms for making glucose available in the postabsorptive period are glycogenolysis and gluconeogenesis. The effect of insulin on these processes will now be considered.

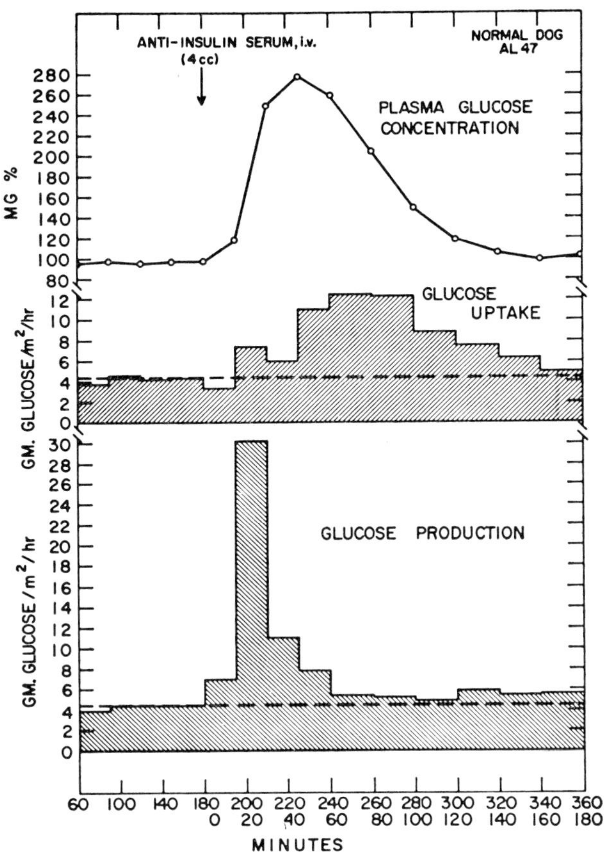

Fig. 2. Effect of guinea pig anti-insulin serum, injected intravenously in the normal dog, on plasma glucose concentration and rate of glucose uptake and glucose production. Zero time is the beginning of ^{14}C-glucose infusion which was used to measure hepatic glucose production and overall glucose uptake. (From ALTSZULER *et al.*, 1964)

5. Effect on Glycogen Concentration

The ability of insulin to increase glucose uptake and subsequently to increase glycogen deposition in skeletal muscle received early attention (see STADIE, 1954, this handbook, chapter p. 329). Similar effects were demonstrated in adipose tissue and liver (see STADIE, 1954). Glycogen deposition can occur without insulin, but, for a given rate of glucose uptake, more glycogen is deposited in the presence of insulin, suggesting a more specific insulin influence on glycogen synthesis. The comprehensive studies of Larner and associates (LARNER, 1972) documented that insulin stimulates the activity of glycogen synthetase (UDP-glucose-a-glucan transglucosylase), which catalyzes the conversion of UDP-glucose to glycoside chains of glycogen.

Infusion of insulin into the normal dog, along with sufficient glucose to prevent hypoglycemia, has been shown to decrease hepatic glycogenolysis and then to increase liver glycogen concentration (BISHOP *et al.*, 1965). In other studies, it was shown that such infusion of insulin and glucose resulted, within 7—13 min, in net conversion of liver glycogen synthetase D (dependent or active only in the presence of glucose-6-phosphate) to synthetase I (independent). The two forms of the enzyme are interconvertible, and insulin probably acts initially to enhance this conversion, thereby allowing glycogen formation to occur independently of the intracellular glucose-6-phosphate concentration (BISHOP and LARNER, 1967).

Insulin also has been shown to increase glycogen synthesis in isolated adipose tissue (LEONARDS and LANDAU, 1960). In this tissue, glycogen deposition may be a more specific effect of insulin than the enhancement of glucose uptake or oxidation of glucose to CO_2.

From the foregoing, it may be anticipated that interference with the effect of insulin on glucose uptake and glycogen synthesis, by various hormones, can affect hepatic glucose output.

6. Effect on Hepatic Gluconeogenesis

The key role that gluconeogenesis holds in supplying an adequate source of glucose to the organism is now well-recognized. The voluminous supporting data have been provided by studies using perfused tissues, labeled substrates, analyses of intermediary metabolites, and, more recently, analyses of adenosine 3′,5′-monophosphate (cyclic AMP). Excellent recent reviews of this subject are available (ASHMORE and WEBER, 1968; EXTON *et al.*, 1970). More detailed aspects of the effects of insulin on gluconeogenesis are discussed in other chapters. It is sufficient to point out that variations in such substrates as lactate, pyruvate, amino acids, and glycerol will have significant effects on gluconeogenesis. Insulin and various insulin "antagonists", such as growth hormone, glucocorticoids, glucagon, and epinephrine, have opposite effects on some of these substrates, and it appears likely that the antagonism between the hormones may be an indirect consequence of the changes in substrate.

The findings of JEFFERSON *et al.* (1968) suggest that insulin suppresses gluconeogenesis by diminishing the supply of amino acids to the liver, and also directly, by decreasing the activity of key enzymes involved in gluconeogenesis. Insulin also has been shown to lower the hepatic level of cyclic AMP when these were increased by glucagon and epinephrine.

7. Effect on Glucose Uptake

The effect of insulin to increase glucose uptake has been studied extensively in a variety of biological systems. These include eviscerated animals, perfused and excised tissues, and whole animals. More detailed discussion of these effects is given in other sections of this volume and in earlier reviews (KRAHL, 1961; RIGGS, 1970; ASHMORE and CARR, 1964; STADIE, 1954; RANDLE *et al.*, 1966; KIPNIS *et al.*, 1959).

The demonstration by LEVINE *et al.* (1949) that insulin increased the volume of distribution of galactose in the eviscerated dog suggested an action of insulin to increase permeability to glucose. Subsequent studies by many investigators redefined and characterized the process of glucose transport into the cell.

Studies using isolated tissues revealed that insulin enhanced glucose uptake by skeletal and heart muscle, adipose tissue, blood vessels, and lactating mammary glands. In a number of other tissues, e.g., nervous tissue, red blood cells, intestines, and kidneys, glucose transport is not dependent on insulin, although insulin might still affect it. It should be emphasized that adipose tissue is more sensitive than other tissues to the effect of insulin on glucose uptake. Also, glucose uptake by adipose tissue is increased by other hormones as well, e.g., epinephrine, ACTH, and growth hormone. These observations may be relevant to the interpretations and extrapolations from *in vitro* experiments to the whole animal.

In the whole animal, measurements of glucose production and uptake with the aid of radioisotopes revealed that infusion of insulin increases the amount of glucose disappearing from the plasma, i.e., glucose uptake by the tissues (see Fig. 1). This measurement represents the sum of glucose taken up by the various tissues, and it may be assumed that this represents uptake by tissues in which glucose transport is enhanced by insulin. Serial liver biopsy samples obtained during the insulin infusion revealed an increased uptake of glucose by the liver, indicating that this tissue is also responsive to insulin, although the liver cell is known to be permeable to glucose.

8. Comments

There is probably general agreement regarding the effects of insulin on carbohydrate metabolism. The underlying mechanisms still remain to be explored. The difficulty of doing this becomes evident when attempts are made to incorporate the known effects of insulin into a unitarian concept of insulin action. Thus, at present, it is difficult to relate the effects of insulin on glucose metabolism with its effect to increase uptake of amino acids and protein synthesis and to inhibit lipolysis, in the presence or absence of glucose.

It may be more fruitful to deal with a specific effect of insulin on a given tissue and to anticipate how other hormones alter this effect. There are many possible points of interaction. As shown by the exquisite experiments of CUATRECASAS (1969, 1972), insulin is initially bound to a receptor site on the cell membrane. The membrane has been shown to contain an insulin-degrading system also, which can quickly terminate the insulin stimulus (CROFFORD *et al.*, 1972). Furthermore, binding of the hormone is independent of its degradation (FREYCHET *et al.*, 1972). Insulin also affects the fate of glucose which enters the cell, by stimulating a variety of enzymes which lead to glycogen formation and glycolysis. Hormones antagonizing the various effects of insulin may act directly on the enzymes involved, or, indirectly, through an accumulation of intermediary metabolites which can inhibit other key enzymes. A further antagonism may occur at the level of substrates for gluconeogenesis.

The listing of potential sites of interaction between insulin and other hormones is intended mainly to focus attention on these key areas, in the hope of reaching a better understanding and of gaining more insight into the nature of these interactions.

III. Growth Hormone

1. Hypophysectomy — Effect on Glucose Production, Uptake, and Sensitivity to Insulin

Removal of the pituitary gland removes a number of hormones which directly or indirectly through their tropic actions, affect carbohydrate metabolism and responses to insulin. Despite the multiple hormone deficiency following hypophysectomy, it has been possible to assess the role of the individual hormones in the resulting abnormalities in carbohydrate metabolism. In this regard, the exaggerated hypoglycemic response to insulin which is characteristic of the hypophysectomized animal ("insulin hypersensitivity") has served as a useful tool (DE BODO and ALTSZULER, 1958). By comparing the insulin hypersensitivity following adrenalectomy and adrenalectomy-gonadectomy with that following hypophysectomy and the effects of various hormonal replacement therapies in these animals, DE BODO and SINKOFF (1953) and DE BODO *et al.* (1953) concluded that growth hormone, corticotropin (through its stimulation of cortisol secretion), and prolactin could significantly affect carbohydrate metabolism.

Table 1. *Effect of Growth Hormone Administration on Levels of Plasma Glucose and Insulin and Glucose Turnover in Normal and Hypophysectomized Dog*

Dog status	Plasma glucose conc. mg/100 ml	Plasma insulin conc. μU/ml	Glucose turnover[a] g/m^2/hour
Normal (30)[b]	101 ± 1[c]	18 ± 3	3.92 ± 0.13
Normal on GH R_x (7)	123 ± 3	138 ± 29	6.87 ± 0.32[e]
Hypophysectomized (7)	90 ± 2	7 ± 1	2.59 ± 0.27[e]
Hyphex on GH R_x (5)	111 ± 3	24 ± 5	3.93 ± 0.16[e]

[a] Measured in steady, postabsorptive state with ^{14}C-glucose (composite of data from DE BODO *et al.*, 1963a). Area based on formula: $m^2 = 0.2864 \times (\text{kg body wt})^{0.367} \times m$ (body length).

[b] Number of animals.

[c] Mean ± Standard Error of Mean.

[d] Bovine growth hormone 1 mg/kg per day for 4—7 days.

[e] Differences from respective control values are statistically significant, P = < 0.01.

In the postabsorptive state (18 h after meal), the hypophysectomized dog has a lower plasma glucose concentration than the normal dog. Using radioisotope techniques (WALL *et al.*, 1957), this was shown to be due to a depressed rate of hepatic glucose output. Overall glucose uptake by tissues is also depressed as is the plasma insulin concentration (Table 1). Studies on the mechanism of insulin hypersensitivity reveal that injection of a test dose of insulin (0.025 U/kg I.V.) results in a much greater increase in glucose uptake by the tissues than that produced in the normal animal, and this contributes to the more severe hypoglycemia in the operated animal. An additional important factor is that the hepatic glucose output in the operated animal does not increase sufficiently in response to low blood plasma glucose levels, thereby resulting in a more prolonged hypoglycemia.

These recent studies in dogs reinforce earlier observations obtained in various animals and in isolated tissues (see DE BODO and ALTSZULER, 1958; ALTSZULER, 1974). The fasted hypophysectomized dog was assumed to have a decreased glucose production on the basis of transhepatic catheterization measurements (CRANDALL and CHERRY, 1939) and the lower excretion of nitrogen than that in the normal fasted state (see DE BODO and ALTSZULER, 1958). Suggestive evidence that glucose uptake or utilization was inhibited came from reports that the eviscerated hypophysectomized dog required less glucose than the eviscerated normal one to maintain normal blood glucose levels (SOSKIN *et al.*, 1939). *In vitro* findings further confirmed this.

The comprehensive experiments of PARK *et al.* (1961), RANDLE *et al.* (1966), KIPNIS *et al.* (1959), HENDERSON *et al.* (1961), and RIDICK *et al.* (1962) characterized the regulation of glucose transport in rat muscle (heart and diaphragm). Uptake of

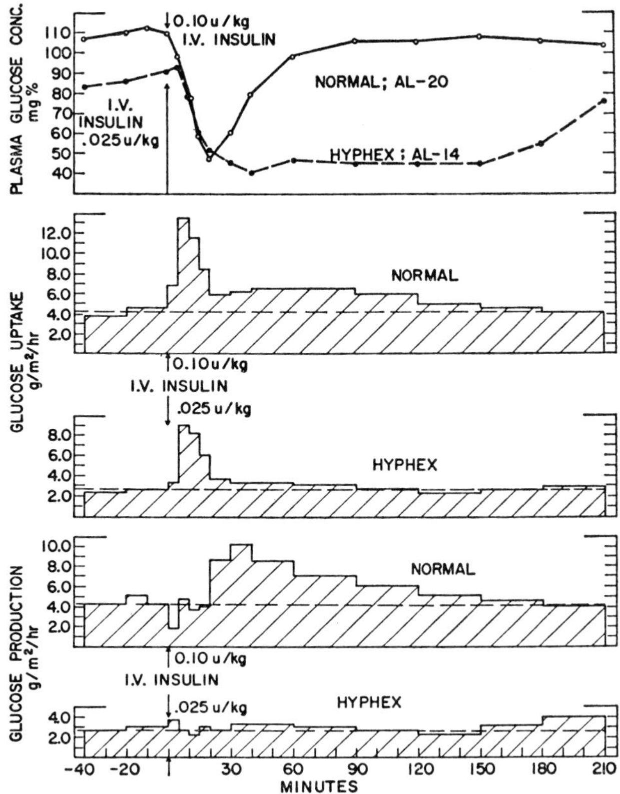

Fig. 3. Insulin hypersensitivity (plasma glucose concentration response) of a hypophysectomized dog to the injection, at zero time, of a small dose of insulin, shown by comparison with a normal dog given a larger dose of insulin. Glucose uptake, and the response of glucose production to insulin-induced hypoglycemia, are compared for the 2 dogs. For further description of the graph, see legend for Fig. 1. (From DE BODO *et al.*, 1963a)

glucose by these tissues excised from the hypophysectomized animal was diminished and, in the case of the heart, this was attributed to diminished plasma insulin levels which exist following hypophysectomy, rather than to a direct effect of the pituitary on glucose transport (HENDERSON *et al.*, 1961). This conclusion was based on the observation that removal of the pituitary gland in the diabetic rat did not alter glucose transport in the isolated heart, but it did sensitize glucose transport to administered insulin. Hypophysectomy may remove an inhibitory influence on phosphorylation of glucose, since this is depressed in the perfused heart of the alloxan-diabetic rat, but is restored to normal following hypophysectomy or adrenalectomy (RANDLE *et al.*, 1966). The epididymal fat tissue from hypophysectomized rats also show a diminished glucose uptake (MEZEY *et al.*, 1961). Other aspects of glucose uptake by adipose tissue of hypophysectomized animals have been investigated extensively (GOODMAN, 1968).

It can be anticipated that hormones which ameliorate the insulin hypersensitivity of the hypophysectomized or adrenalectomized animal would do this by reducing the excessive increase in glucose uptake following insulin injection and/or by enhancing the hepatic glucose output in response to the hypoglycemia (Fig. 3).

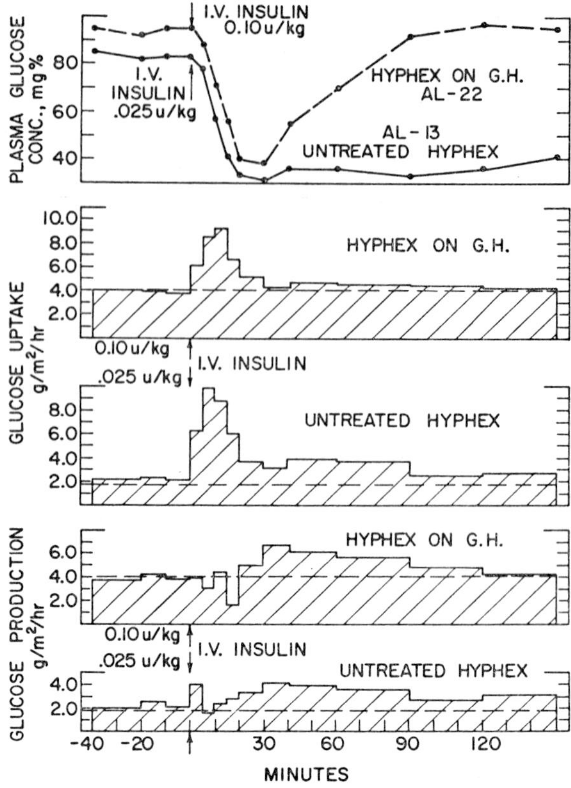

Fig. 4. Abolition of hypersensitivity to injection at zero time of a larger dose of insulin, brought about in a hypophysectomized dog by a growth hormone regimen (1 mg/kg/day for 4 days). Plasma glucose concentration, glucose uptake, and the response of glucose production to insulin-induced hypoglycemia are compared for an untreated hypophysectomized dog given a small dose of insulin and a growth hormone-treated hypophysectomized dog given a larger dose of insulin. For further description of the graph, see legend for Fig. 1. (From DE BODO *et al.*, 1963a)

2. Growth Hormone Administration in the Hypophysectomized Animal

Administration of very small doses of bovine growth hormone (0.02 mg/kg/day) to hypophysectomized dogs ameliorates their insulin hypersensitivity without significantly altering other parameters of carbohydrate metabolism (e.g., glucose tolerance test) (see DE BODO and ALTSZULER, 1957, 1958). Larger doses of growth hormone (1 mg/kg/day), which produce measurable body weight increments in the hypophysectomized rat, not only remove the insulin hypersensitivity of the hypophysectomized dog but also result in a less than normal hypoglycemic response to injected insulin ("insulin resistance"). Other changes in carbohydrate metabolism, e.g., impaired glucose tolerance, are also observed. It is noteworthy that concomitant administration of glucocorticoids with the growth hormone prevents the abnormal glucose tolerance and insulin resistance (DE BODO and SINKOFF, 1953).

Administration of the larger dose of growth hormone (1 mg/kg/day) to the hypophysectomized dog elevates to normal the fasting plasma concentration of glucose and insulin (Table 1). Hepatic glucose output and glucose uptake by the tissues are also restored to normal values (ALTSZULER *et al.*, 1959a). Injection of insulin into these animals no longer produces the exaggerated hypoglycemic response (Fig. 4). This is due largely to the attenuated increase in glucose uptake by the tissues. The additional contributing factor is the enhanced response of hepatic glucose output to the hypoglycemia (ALTSZULER *et al.*, 1959; DE BODO *et al.*, 1963a).

The increase in hepatic glucose output appears to be attuned to the degree of the induced hypoglycemia. With a small test dose of insulin (0.025 U/kg, i.v.), the induced hypoglycemia is minimal, and evokes only a small increase in hepatic glucose output. Larger doses of insulin (0.1—0.25 U/kg) result in a more severe hypoglycemia, and now the ability of the liver to increase glucose output significantly is clearly evident (ALTSZULER *et al.*, 1959). It is noteworthy that, although the growth hormone regimen enhances the hepatic glucose output in response to hypoglycemia, it does not improve the diminished hyperglycemic response to injected epinephrine or glucagon (see DE BODO and SINKOFF, 1953a; DE BODO and ALTSZULER, 1957).

In vitro studies, using the diaphragm, adipose tissue, or perfused heart of the rat, have sought to pinpoint the metabolic and enzymatic reactions which might be affected by growth hormone. Glucose transport and phosphorylation play key roles in regulating glucose uptake by these tissues. Glucose transport is the primary regulating step, but when this is accelerated and surmounted, phosphorylation may become rate-limiting. Thus, the action of growth hormone to impede the insulin-induced acceleration of glucose transport (HENDERSON *et al.*, 1961) may mask an effect on subsequent steps in the intermediary metabolism of glucose. Phosphorylation of glucose by the perfused heart of diabetic rat is diminished, but can be restored to normal by hypophysectomy, suggesting an inhibitory influence of some pituitary hormone. This is substantiated by the demonstrated inhibition of glucose phosphorylation by the perfused heart following growth hormone administration to the hypophysectomized diabetic rat (RANDLE *et al.*, 1966).

Additional sites in metabolism of glucose have been shown to be vulnerable to hormonal regulation (see RANDLE *et al.*, 1966; PARK *et al.*, 1961). Glucose utilization can be moderated by the activity of phosphofructokinase, and by pyruvate dehydrogenase, which regulates the conversion of pyruvate to acetyl coenzyme A. The activity of these enzymes is affected by similar factors. It is decreased when there is enhanced utilization of free fatty acids, as, for example, following growth hormone administration. Inhibition of these two enzymes observed in the diabetic rat can be removed by hypophysectomy, and inhibition is restored again by injection of growth hormone (RANDLE *et al.*, 1966).

Specific mechanisms, whereby administered growth hormone may affect the aforementioned enzymes, have been suggested, and these are discussed in detail elsewhere (RANDLE *et al.*, 1966). The findings implicate an indirect influence of growth hormone through its action to mobilize free fatty acids. Increased oxidation of free fatty acids alters intracellular concentration of key constituents (e.g., acetyl coenzyme A, citrate), which may affect the activity of pyruvate dehydrogenase and phosphofructokinase (RANDLE *et al.*, 1966).

Certain effects of growth hormone *in vitro* still remain to be understood. Addition of growth hormone to a glucose medium containing adipose tissue excised from the hypophysectomized rat results in a prompt increase in glucose uptake (GOODMAN, 1965). The stimulatory effect, which lasts several hours, is not converted into an inhibitory effect, but the stimulation can be prolonged by addition of inhibitors of protein synthesis. When growth hormone is injected into these animals, there is an inhibition of glucose uptake by the adipose tissue excised

$3^1/_2$ or 24 h later (GOODMAN, 1968). The initial stimulatory effect of growth hormone added *in vitro* is reminiscent of the insulin-like hypoglycemia seen following the first injection of growth hormone into normal rat or hypophysectomized dog (see DE BODO and ALTSZULER, 1957). The correlation of these early *in vivo* effects with those *in vitro* is still obscure.

3. Growth Hormone Administration in the Normal Animal

There is extensive documentation that growth hormone administration in the normal animal produces marked effects on carbohydrate metabolism. Various aspects of this are discussed in review articles and symposia (YOUNG, 1953; DE BODO and SINKOFF, 1953; DE BODO and ALTSZULER, 1955; ibid, 1957; CAMPBELL, 1955; SMITH *et al.*, 1955; PECILE and MULLER, 1968, 1972; KETTERER *et al.*, 1957; WEIL, 1965; MATSUZAKI and RABEN, 1965; LUFT and CERASI, 1968; KNOBIL and HOTCHKISS, 1964).

The effects of daily injection of bovine growth hormone (1 mg/kg/day) in the normal dog are shown in Table 1. This regimen usually causes only a moderate rise in plasma glucose concentration, but a very marked elevation in the plasma insulin levels in the postabsorptive state. Similar disappropriate elevations in plasma insulin levels have been reported in the dog by CAMPBELL and RASTOGI (1966) and in man by KIPNIS and STEIN (1964).

Hepatic glucose output is increased by the growth hormone regimen (Table 1). This effect may be due to the concomitant increase in liver glycogen concentration and the increased rate of liver glycogen breakdown observed at this time (BISHOP *et al.*, 1967). Overall glucose uptake is increased as shown in Table 1. However, in view of the hyperglycemia and marked hyperinsulinemia, the increase in glucose uptake is much less than expected. At a similar hyperglycemia obtained in the normal dog by glucose infusion, which caused only a moderate elevation in plasma insulin, there was a much greater increase (200—300%) in glucose uptake than that seen here. Thus, despite an increase in glucose uptake above basal values, the growth hormone regimen results in a "relative" inhibition of glucose uptake (DE BODO *et al.*, 1963).

The basis for the relative inhibition of glucose uptake remains to be explored. The increment in glucose uptake occurs in the presence of a resistance to endogenous and injected insulin. The resistance to endogenous insulin is evident from the small rise in glucose uptake, despite the presence of very high levels of insulin in the plasma (Table 1). The resistance to injected insulin is seen by the limited increase in glucose uptake following insulin injection (ALTSZULER *et al.*, 1968, 1968a). Injected insulin also is less effective in depressing hepatic glucose output, thus reflecting a resistance at this tissue (BISHOP *et al.*, 1967).

An impairment in removal of a glucose load has also been observed following administration of growth hormone in man (SCHALCH and KIPNIS, 1965) and in dog (CAMPBELL and RASTOGI, 1969). The magnitude of the impairment is even more impressive because the growth hormone regimen in the dog, by an unknown mechanism, causes excessive amounts of insulin to be secreted in response to a glucose load or ingestion of a meal (CAMPBELL and RASTOGI, 1966).

Further insight into the resistance to insulin may be obtained from studies in the fasted dog maintained on a growth hormone regimen. Fasting alone results in a decreased rate of glucose production and uptake. A growth hormone regimen with continued fasting failed to cause the usual increase in glucose production and uptake (RATHGEB *et al.*, 1970). Nevertheless, there still was a marked resistance to the hypoglycemic effect of injected and endogenous insulin. Thus, despite the absence of the usually observed effects of growth hormone on glucose metabolism, the response to insulin was attenuated.

4. Growth Hormone-Induced Diabetes

The term "diabetogenic" has been applied rather indiscriminately to describe the various effects of growth hormone on glucose metabolism. Frank diabetes, with hyperglycemia in excess of 180 mg%, and glucosuria, can be produced by an appropriate growth hormone regimen (Young, 1953; Campbell, 1955; de Bodo and Altszuler, 1955). In the normal dog, this usually can be produced by administration of bovine growth hormone, 3 mg/kg/day for 6—8 days. In the first 3—4 days, the rise in plasma glucose and insulin, and in glucose turnover, is similar to that seen with the smaller doses of growth hormone (1 mg/kg/day), which usually do not induce frank diabetes. At about day 4—6, the postabsorptive plasma glucose and insulin levels begin to rise further. Hepatic glucose output, however, shows only a slight further increase, indicating that the development of the marked hyperglycemia is due to a further inhibition of glucose uptake (Altszuler *et al.*, 1968, 1968a). Knowledge of the biochemical events which occur in the transition from the pre-diabetic state (4—6 days) to the diabetic state at 6—8 days should shed light on mechanisms contributing to the insulin resistance.

5. Comments

While most of our attention has been focused on the chronic influence of growth hormone, consideration should be given to the acute effects of growth hormone. This is appropriate, since plasma growth hormone levels have now been shown to fluctuate in response to a variety of stimuli (Glick *et al.*, 1965; Greenwood *et al.*, 1966).

Injection of growth hormone produces minimal, if any, acute changes in plasma glucose or insulin levels in man (Frohman *et al.*, 1967; Kipnis and Stein, 1964), dog (Campbell and Rastogi, 1966), or sheep (Bassett and Wallace, 1966). In the normal dog, infusion of growth hormone for a four-hour period did not produce changes in the basal rates of glucose production and uptake by the tissues (Altszuler *et al.*, 1968).

Nevertheless, other parameters of glucose metabolism have revealed that growth hormone may be exerting acute effects. A glucose load, administered at various times after intravenous injection of growth hormone in normal man, was found to be removed from the blood more rapidly than normal at 10 min after hormone injection, at a normal rate at 60 min, and at 50% of normal rate at 2 h (Schalch and Kipnis, 1965). Measurements of arterio-venous differences in blood glucose in forearm of normal man suggested an inhibitory effect of growth hormone on glucose uptake, within 12 min following its administration (Zierler, 1968; Zierler and Rabinowitz, 1964).

Although some aspects of the reported acute effects of growth hormone may be inconsistent, these will need to be reexamined in the light of new data. Recently, it was observed (Altszuler, unpublished data) that i.v. injection of growth hormone in the postabsorptive normal dog results, within 3 min, in a hyperglycemia which subsides by 15 min. The significance of this effect remains to be clarified, but it coincides with the period of increased glucose removal of a glucose load described above (Schalch and Kipnis, 1965). An additional factor, whose role in the growth hormone-mediated effects remains to be clarified, is the sulfation factro, or somatomedin (see Daughaday and Kipnis, 1966).

IV. Adrenal Glucocorticosteroids

1. Adrenalectomy — Effect on Glucose Production, Uptake, and Sensitivity to Insulin

Defects in carbohydrate metabolism due to adrenal deficiency in experimental animals were recognized in the early studies of LONG and LUKENS (1935) and BRITTON and SILVETTE (1932).

The adrenalectomized animal exhibits a number of abnormalities similar to those of the hypophysectomized animal, e.g., deficient hyperglycemic response to epinephrine and glucagon (DE BODO and ALTSZULER, 1958), and adrenal deficiency undoubtedly contributes to the metabolic alterations of the hypophysectomized animal. Nevertheless, certain differences can be demonstrated in the response of the two types of animals. The adrenalectomized animal is more sensitive than the normal animal to the hypoglycemic effect of insulin, but is less sensitive than the hypophysectomized animal. A small test dose of insulin (0.025 U/kg, i.v.) usually produces a normal hypoglycemic response in the adrenalectomized dog. Slightly larger doses of insulin (0.08 U/kg) clearly unmask the metabolic abnormality induced by adrenalectomy, which is reflected by a more severe and prolonged hypoglycemia than is seen in the normal animal. The insulin hypersensitivity is abolished by a regimen of cortisone or cortisol (0.8—1.2 mg/kg/day).

Despite the ample evidence that adrenalectomy alters metabolic responses to various provocative stimuli, e.g., injection of epinephrine or insulin, it is surprising that these abnormalities are not evident in the undisturbed, postabsorptive state. Rates of glucose production and overall glucose uptake by the tissues in the conscious adrenalectomized dog, measured by isotope dilution, were found to be normal (Table 2). Plasma glucose and insulin concentrations are only slightly lower than normal.

Table 2. *Effect of Cortisol Administration on Plasma Glucose and Insulin Levels and on Glucose Turnover in Normal, Adrenalectomized and Hypophysectomized Dog*

Dog status	Plasma glucose conc. mg/100 ml	Plasma insulin conc. μU/ml	Glucose turnover[a] g/m²/hour
Normal			
Control (30)[b]	101 ± 1[c]	18 ± 3	3.92 ± 0.13
Cortisol Rx[d] (15)	107 ± 6	21 ± 2	4.02 ± 0.26
Methylprednisolone Rx[e] (12)	97 ± 3	17 ± 2	5.30 ± 0.40[h]
Adrenalectomized[f]			
Control (9)	94 ± 6	11 ± 2	4.05 ± 0.41
Cortisol Rx[g] (9)	99 ± 2	15 ± 1	6.14 ± 0.60[h]
Hypophysectomized			
Control (9)	87 ± 2	7 ± 1	2.60 ± 0.24
Cortisol Rx[g] (6)	85 ± 2	21 ± 2	4.29 ± 0.08[h]

[a] Measured in steady, postabsorptive state with ^{14}C-glucose (composite of data from DE BODO *et al.*, 1963a; RATHGEB *et al.*, 1973). Area based on formula: $m^2 = 0.2864$ x (kg body wt)$^{0.367}$ x m (body length).

[b] Number of animals.

[c] Mean ± Standard Error of Mean.

[d] Cortisol acetate: 2 dogs (0.8—1.2 mg/kg/day, 5 days; 3 dogs: 5—5.5 mg/kg/day, 8 days).

[e] Methylprednisolone sodium succinate (Solu-Medrol®, Upjohn, 2—2.5 mg/kg/day for 3—4 days).

[f] Maintained on desoxycorticosterone acetate 2.5 mg/day.

[g] Cortisol acetate: 0.8—1.2 mg/kg/day for 5 days.

[h] Difference from respective control statistically significant, $p < 0.01$.

2. Glucocorticoid Administration in Hypophysectomized and Adrenalectomized Animals

Administration of glucocorticoids to adrenalectomized animals of many species raises blood glucose levels and increases liver and muscle glycogen. The glucocorticoids produce similar effects in the hypophysectomized animal which is also steroid deficient. In many respects, the hypophysectomized animal is a better model for demonstrating the effects of glucocorticoids, because it still can secrete epinephrine; the latter may modify the response to glucocorticoids (see below).

As shown in Table 2, the glucocorticoid regimen increases the rate of glucose turnover in the postabsorptive hypophysectomized dog. The increased hepatic glucose output is not surprising, since glucocorticoids increase gluconeogenesis. They may also increase liver glycogen content, but, since the untreated hypophysectomized dog has nearly normal amounts of liver glycogen (DE BODO and SINKOFF, 1953a), it is not clear that the steroids act to increase hepatic glucose output through this process. The glucose uptake by the tissues is also increased and this is accompanied by elevated plasma insulin levels. These findings may seem surprising in view of the substantial literature that steroids inhibit glucose utilization (see DE BODO and ALTSZULER, 1958; GLENN *et al.*, 1963; MUNCK, 1971; LANDAU, 1965; STEELE, 1974). Those conclusions, many based on indirect studies, will need to be reexamined in the light of these recent studies which utilize radioisotopes and are performed under more physiological conditions.

A glucocorticoid regimen in the hypophysectomized dog does ameliorate its insulin hypersensitivity (DE BODO and SINKOFF, 1953a). The excessive increase in glucose uptake following insulin injection is reduced to normal, and the hypoglycemia evokes a prompt and adequate increase in hepatic glucose output (ALTSZULER *et al.*, 1958). Large doses of insulin may still produce a more severe hypoglycemia in this animal than in the normal and steroid-treated adrenalectomized dog, suggesting that, in the hypophysectomized animal, a deficiency of other hormones, in addition to that of corticoids, is contributing to its insulin hypersensitivity. An insulin resistance, which occurs with growth hormone administration, has not been found to occur with steroid administration.

In view of the increase in glucose turnover produced by replacement doses of glucocorticoids in the hypophysectomized animal, it is surprising, as stated above, that the untreated adrenalectomized animal shows essentially normal rates of glucose turnover. As shown in Table 2, administration of glucocorticoids in replacement doses has little effect on plasma glucose and insulin levels, but hepatic glucose output and glucose uptake are markedly increased (ALTSZULER *et al.*, 1973). The insulin sensitivity in these animals is restored to normal. These findings support the view that glucocorticoids enhance, rather than impair, glucose uptake in the postabsorptive state.

3. Glucocorticoid Administration in the Normal Animal

The normal animal appears to be less responsive than the steroid-deficient one to the effects of glucocorticoids on glucose metabolism. Doses of cortisone which adequately maintain the adrenalectomized rat — 1—2 mg/kg (INGLE and BAKER, 1953)—or dog—0.8—1.5 mg/kg (DE BODO *et al.*, 1953)—have little effect in the normal animal. With large doses of glucocorticoids, a "steroid-diabetes", characterized by hyperglycemia and glucosuria, has been induced in the rat (INGLE *et al.*, 1951; INGLE, 1956), mouse (RASTOGI and CAMPBELL, 1970), guinea pig (KERN and LOGOTHETOPOULOS, 1970), hamster (CAMPBELL *et al.*, 1966), and rabbit (VOLK and LAZARUS, 1963). This type of diabetes is not demonstrated readily in the normal dog (CAMPBELL and RASTOGI, 1968; SIREK and BEST, 1952; DE BODO and ALTSZULER, 1955).

In normal man, responses have been varied (FAJANS, 1961), and the steroids have been reported to enhance, have no effect on, or impair the removal of a glucose load from the blood (see DE BODO and ALTSZULER, 1958). Nevertheless, a brief cortisone regimen has been used in conjunction with a glucose tolerance test to uncover latent diabetes (FAJANS and CONN, 1954). Since the abnormal glucose tolerance in the susceptible normal human occurs in the presence of substantial amounts of circulating insulin (PERLEY and KIPNIS, 1966), the impaired removal of glucose cannot be attributed to insulin deficiency. In this regard, the recent studies with large doses of glucocorticoids in another resistant species, the normal dog, are of great interest. Administration of methylprednisolone (4 mg/kg/day) to the normal dog was found to cause a $3^1/_2$-fold increase in the postabsorptive levels of plasma insulin on day 4, with only small elevations in plasma glucose levels (CAMPBELL and RASTOGI, 1968). The increases in plasma insulin levels were transient, the values returning to normal at about 7 days and remaining there for the duration of the steroid regimen. The fasting glucose values showed little further change throughout the regimen. Glucose tolerance tests and serum insulin responses, carried out at days 1, 4, 8, and 14 of the steroid regimen, revealed normal glucose removal at all times.

Serum insulin in response to the glucose load increased to a greater extent than in pre-steroid period only on days 1 and 4; on days 8 and 14, the insulin increase was even less than normal, and this did not impede glucose removal. Indeed, a comparison of the insulin increase with the amount of glucose removed would indicate that the steroid treatment enhanced glucose disposal. The enhanced glucose metabolism due to steroid administration is also seen in the postabsorptive state, using isotopes to measure glucose turnover. Thus, administration of methylprednisolone (2—4 mg/kg) to normal dogs for periods up to 17 days increased the rate of hepatic glucose output and glucose uptake by the tissues, without elevation of plasma glucose or insulin (ISSEKUTZ and ALLEN, 1972; ALTSZULER *et al.*, 1973).

In normal humans, administration of dexamethasone (8 mg/day) for only 3 days was found to increase fasting blood glucose levels by about 15 mg%, with no change in the plasma insulin level (PERLEY and KIPNIS, 1966). The increment in the insulin response to a glucose load was greater than in the non-treated individual, but the removal of glucose was slower. It is not certain that these findings in man are at variance with those in the normal dog (CAMPBELL and RASTOGI, 1968), since, in the latter, the steroid regimen was longer and the glucose loads were administered intravenously. The findings in the dog of an increased glucose turnover with normal insulin levels and an enhanced disposal of glucose loads, are inconsistent with an inhibitory effect of steroids on glucose uptake.

4. Comments

The ability of glucocorticoids to stimulate liver glycogen, gluconeogenesis, and hepatic glucose output is well-established. Some questions remain concerning the reports that infusion of adrenal steroids causes an initial decrease in hepatic glucose output, as observed by LECOCQ *et al.* (1964) in the anesthetized normal dog with an Eck fistula, and by NINOMIYA *et al.* (1965) in the normal and diabetic unanesthetized dog, using ^{14}C-glucose. These findings could not be confirmed in the unanesthetized normal dog, using ^{14}C-glucose (ALTSZULER *et al.*, 1973), nor in the adrenalectomized rat using ^{14}C-glucose (HAYNES and LU, 1969).

The effect of the glucocorticoids on glucose uptake by the tissues is less firmly established. The variable responses observed in a number of tissues and species and under differing experimental conditions have been discussed in great detail by LANDAU (1955), MUNCK (1971), and STEELE (1974). One difficulty in assessing these observations is the common tendency to expect that all tissues will be affected in a similar way by the steroids.

Inhibition of glucose uptake by glucocorticoids has been demonstrated in several tissues, e.g., skin, adipose tissue, and lymphoid tissue, and it has been suggested that such inhibition serves to trigger catabolic effects in these tissues, thereby supplying the metabolic fuel for the whole organism. The two reports (LECOCQ *et al.*, 1964; NINOMIYA *et al.*, 1965) that overall glucose uptake is inhibited acutely by steroid administration may be in harmony with the above. Nevertheless, there are numerous studies wherein glucocorticoid administration, in replacement doses, increases overall glucose uptake in the hypophysectomized (ALTSZULER *et al.*, 1958) and in the adrenalectomized (DE BODO *et al.*, 1963a) dog. Recent findings have revealed that, in dogs made epinephrine-deficient by adrenal demedullation, the overall glucose uptake was increased; following removal of the remaining adrenal cortex, the glucose uptake declined (RATHGEB *et al.*, 1973). These data were interpreted to indicate that endogenous glucocorticoids, unopposed by epinephrine, tended to increase overall glucose uptake. The role of epinephrine in moderating this effect of glucocorticoids remains obscure.

Further questions about the inhibitory effect of glucocorticoids can be raised, in view of the recent reports in several laboratories that a brief methylprednisolone regimen in normal dogs increases overall glucose uptake (NINOMIYA *et al.*, 1965; ISSEKUTZ and ALLEN, 1972; ALTSZULER *et al.*, 1973) and enhances removal of administered glucose load (CAMPBELL and RASTOGI, 1968). Insulin secretion in these studies was adequate, and its effectiveness to enhance glucose uptake was

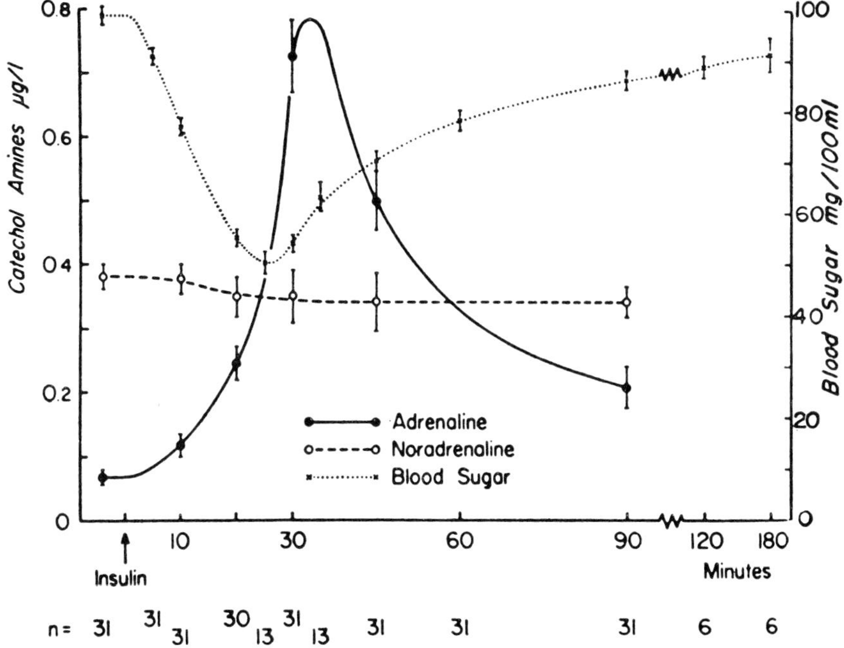

Fig. 5. Plasma catecholamine levels during insulin-induced hypoglycemia in man. n = number of determinations. (From VENDSALU, 1960). Similar findings were reported by GOLDFIEN *et al.* (1958)

unimpaired. Thus, on balance, the effect of glucocorticoids on overall glucose uptake in the normal dog, and perhaps in man, would appear to be one of stimulation rather than of inhibition. Additional discussion can be found elsewhere (ENSINCK and WILLIAMS, 1972).

V. Epinephrine

There is ample evidence of an interplay between insulin and epinephrine in their effects on carbohydrate metabolism. A release of epinephrine in response to insulin-induced hypoglycemia was demonstrated years ago by CANNON *et al.* (1924) and by ABE in 1924 (see DE BODO and ALTSZULER, 1958), who used the individual cat's own denervated heart and iris, respectively, to assay epinephrine discharge. More direct evidence is provided by measurements of the catecholamine in the plasma, as shown in Fig. 5. It may be noted that epinephrine levels do not rise in response to the mild decline of blood glucose, but do so when the hypoglycemia becomes more severe. This is in harmony with earlier observations (DE BODO and SINKOFF, 1953) that the adrenal denervated dog could still maintain a normal blood glucose level when subjected to mild exercise which resulted in extensive use of glucose. The adrenal demedullated animal, however, is more sensitive than the normal animal to the hypoglycemic effect of moderate doses of insulin (ZUCKER and BERG, see DE BODO and ALTSZULER, 1958), suggesting that epinephrine plays a counter-regulatory role against an excessive insulin effect.

1. Effect on Hepatic Glucose Output

The ability of injected epinephrine to increase blood glucose levels was first shown in 1901 by BLUM, and subsequently confirmed in many species (see DE BODO and ALTSZULER, 1958; ELLIS, 1956; HIMMS-HAGAN, 1967). The induced hyperglycemia is associated with a transient breakdown of liver glycogen and an increase in hepatic glucose output (HILDES *et al.*, 1949; BEARN *et al.*, 1952). The latter effect is in part a direct one on the liver, since epinephrine increases glucose output of the perfused liver of the dog (AMBRUS *et al.*, 1955) and of the cat (LUNDSGAARD, 1938). Concomitant with hepatic glycogenolysis, there is a breakdown of muscle glycogen resulting in elevated plasma levels of lactate (CORI and CORI, 1928; HILDES *et al.*, 1949), and subsequent conversion in the liver to glucose.

In the normal unanesthetized dog infusion of epinephrine, at 0.1 μg/kg/min causes a prompt rise of 12—15 mg% in plasma glucose by 15 min, a further slow rise to 30—35 mg% above control values at 60 min, with little further change for the remainder of a 3-hour infusion (ALTSZULER *et al.*, 1967). Hepatic glucose output, as measured with ^{14}C-glucose, is increased promptly, but returns to control values at about 60—90 min despite continued infusion. This transient effect is not due to exhaustion of liver glycogen, since the increase in hepatic glucose output is only moderate and not sufficient to deplete glycogen stores.

The stimulation of glycogenolysis by epinephrine is believed to be brought about by an activation of adenyl cyclase, which leads to increased formation of cyclic 3′-5′-adenosine monophosphate (cyclic AMP). This nucleotide in turn stimulates the conversion of inactive phosphorylase "b" to the active phosphorylase "a", thus allowing glycogenolysis to proceed. There is also much evidence, especially from the studies of EXTON and PARK (1972) and EXTON *et al.* (1970), that epinephrine also stimulates hepatic gluconeogenesis from lactate and alanine also via cyclic AMP.

Insulin has been shown to inhibit the epinephrine-induced glycogenolysis in the perfused cat liver (JEFFERSON *et al.*, 1968). The inhibitory effects may be mediated through cyclic AMP, since insulin lowers cyclic AMP levels in the perfused liver when these were previously elevated by epinephrine injection *in vivo* (EXTON *et al.*, 1970).

2. Effect on Glucose Uptake

An inhibitory effect of epinephrine on blood glucose utilization was proposed as early as 1906 by UNDERHILL and CLOSSON (1906). Similar conclusions were reached using the differences between the glucose concentration of arterial and venous blood (A-V difference). The A-V glucose difference during hyperglycemia produced by epinephrine was found to be less than that produced during glucose-induced hyperglycemia (see DE BODO and ALTSZULER, 1958).

The effects of epinephrine on glucose uptake by isolated tissues depend on the tissue employed. Addition of epinephrine increases glucose uptake by rat adipose tissue (HAGEN and BALL, 1960), whereas it decreases uptake by rat muscle (KIPNIS *et al.*, 1959; WALAAS and WALAAS, 1950). Studies in the whole animal suggest that the inhibitory effect of epinephrine is best demonstrated in the presence of insulin. In the eviscerated rat (INGLE and NEZAMIS, 1949) or dog (FRITZ *et al.*, 1957) infused with glucose only, the addition of epinephrine fails to raise blood glucose levels, whereas its addition to the combined infusion of glucose and insulin results in elevated blood glucose levels, presumably due to inhibition of glucose uptake.

In the experiments described above, using ^{14}C-glucose in the unanesthetized dog, infusion of epinephrine was found to produce a moderate hyperglycemia but glucose uptake did not increase (ALTSZULER *et al.*, 1967). Plasma insulin levels failed to increase despite the presence of hyperglycemia, reaffirming the well-established finding that epinephrine inhibits the usual insulin response to glucose, both *in vivo* (KOSAKA *et al.*, 1964; PORTE *et al.*, 1966; CERASI *et al.*, 1971; KRIS *et al.*, 1966) and *in vitro* (COORE and RANDLE, 1964; LERNMARK and HELLMAN, 1970).

Several mechanisms have been proposed to explain the inhibitory effect of epinephrine on glucose uptake. Epinephrine-induced glycogenolysis causes an increase in intracellular glucose-6-phosphate which inhibits hexokinase activity (KIPNIS *et al.*, 1959), and this consequently inhibits glucose transport into muscle. Another explanation relies on the concept developed by RANDLE *et al.* (1964) that free fatty acids released from triglycerides by the epinephrine-induced lipolysis may interfere with glucose uptake by various cells. The free fatty acids may exert this effect by inhibiting hexokinase and phosphofructokinase (PARK, 1964).

3. Comments

The physiologic significance of some of the described effects of epinephrine requires comment. In some studies, large doses of epinephrine have been used and notes of caution have been raised concerning the physiological extrapolations of these results. The basal secretion rate of epinephrine in man is reported to be about 0.008 μg/kg/min (VENDSALU, 1960). Infusion of epinephrine at rates of 0.07—0.14 μg/kg per min results in plasma levels of 0.5—0.8 μg/liter. It should be noted that similar plasma concentrations of endogenous epinephrine are observed during insulin-induced hypoglycemia (Fig. 5), indicating that administration of epinephrine within the above dosage ranges is still within physiologic bounds. As noted above, infusion of epinephrine at 0.1 μg/kg/min elevates plasma glucose and lactate levels, increases hepatic glucose output, and decreases liver glycogen in man (HILDES *et al.*, 1949) and in the dog (ALTSZULER *et al.*, 1967, 1971). Infusion of much smaller amounts of epinephrine, 3 mμg/kg/min, into normal subjects had no effect on the basal glucose levels; when a glucose load was superimposed, however, the plasma glucose levels were higher than those with glucose infusion alone, and there was also a 50% reduction in the usual increase in insulin secretion which occurs with hyperglycemia (CERASI *et al.*, 1971).

These experiments give credence to the physiologic significance of the studies discussed above. The conclusions are not at variance with the observations of SOKAL (1966) that in the rat stimulation of liver glycogenolysis required five to ten times larger doses of epinephrine than those needed to effect muscle glycogenolysis.

VI. Glucagon

Having survived an ignoble developmental period in which its status as a hormone was questioned, glucagon has now assumed an important role in the regulation of carbohydrate metabolism (see FOA, 1964; LAWRENCE, 1969; BLEICHER *et al.*, 1970). Its ability to produce hyperglycemia and to stimulate glycogenolysis is well-established. More recently, glucagon has been touted as an important stimulant of gluconeogenesis from substrates such as lactate, pyruvate, and alanine (EXTON *et al.*, 1970). Cyclic AMP appears to be the mediator of glycogenolysis (see SUTHERLAND and RALL, 1960) and of gluconeogenesis (EXTON *et al.*, 1970).

A potential physiologic role for glucagon was discerned from the skillful experiments of FOA (1972). In cross-circulation experiments in dogs, they found that, following insulin-induced hypoglycemia in the donor dog, its pancreatic vein blood, but not mesenteric blood, produced a rise in blood glucose in the recipient. With the development of a radioimmunoassay for glucagon (UNGER *et al.*, 1962), it was demonstrated directly that plasma glucagon levels increased in response to insulin hypoglycemia (Fig. 6). The rise is abated if hypoglycemia is terminated by glucose.

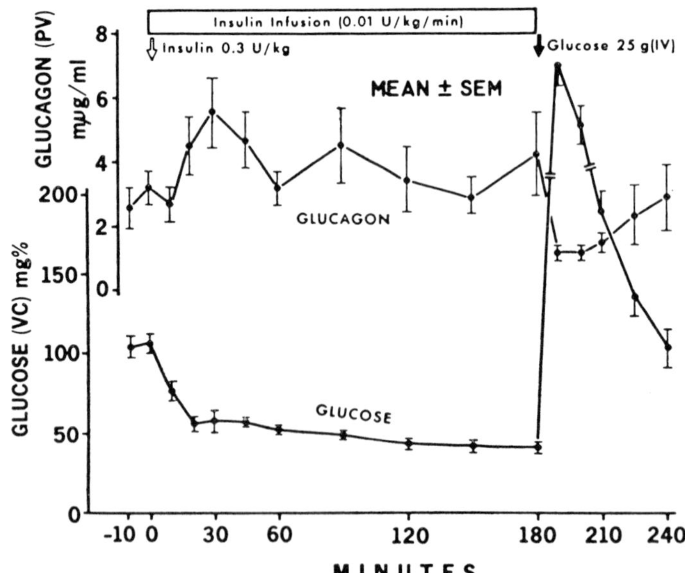

Fig. 6. Mean level ± SEM of plasma glucose in inferior vena cava (VC), and of glucagon in pancreaticoduodenal vein (PV) in seven conscious dogs during hypoglycemia indicated by insulin infusion and subsequent hyperglycemia. (From OHNEDA *et al.*, 1969)

1. Effect on Hepatic Glucose Output

From the early demonstration that glucagon activates liver phosphorylase, and consequently stimulates glycogenolysis, it could be anticipated that hepatic glucose output would be increased. This was subsequently demonstrated by various techniques using liver perfusion, transhepatic catheterization, and isotope dilution (see Foa, 1964; Exton *et al.*, 1972; Reichard *et al.*, 1958; Rathgeb *et al.*, 1966; Altszuler *et al.*, 1971; Williamson *et al.*, 1967). A rise in cyclic AMP levels in the liver is probably responsible for glycogenolysis, since doses of glucagon which are too low to activate adenyl cyclase also fail to produce glycogenolysis (Robison and Exton, quoted in Exton and Park, 1972).

Stimulation of gluconeogenesis by glucagon was first apparent in the experiments of Salter *et al.* (1957), who found that glucagon-treated rats, either fasted or force-fed, excreted greater amounts of nitrogen than the control animals. The difference was also observed in adrenalectomized animals, thus excluding the adrenal steroids as a mediating factor. The extensive studies of Park, Exton, and their associates (see Park *et al.*, 1972; Exton and Park, 1972) demonstrated in the perfused liver that glucagon causes a prompt (within a minute) stimulation of gluconeogenesis at doses only slightly higher than those needed to stimulate glycogenolysis.

2. Effect on Glucose Uptake

Since administration of glucagon produces a hyperglycemia, it might be anticipated that this would lead to an increase in glucose uptake by the tissues. With a few exceptions, an increase in glucose uptake was demonstrated in the eviscerated animal, and in the whole animal using A-V glucose differences (for references, see de Bodo and Altszuler, 1958) and radioisotopes (Reichard *et al.*, 1958; Rathgeb *et al.*, 1966; Altszuler *et al.*, 1971).

The hyperglycemia and enhanced glucose uptake during glucagon infusion are accompanied by elevated plasma insulin levels (Samols *et al.*, 1966; Rathgeb *et al.*, 1966; Altszuler *et al.*, 1971). The coexistence of elevated plasma levels of glucose and insulin would be expected to enhance glucose uptake markedly. However, a similar hyperglycemia and hyperinsulinemia produced in the normal dog by infusion of glucose resulted in a greater increase in glucose uptake than that observed during the glucagon-induced hyperglycemia (Altszuler *et al.*, 1971), suggesting a relative inhibition of glucose uptake by glucagon.

The site of interaction of insulin and glucagon on glucose uptake is not established. Glucagon does not appear to affect the key glycolytic enzymes (e.g., glycokinase, phosphofructokinase, pyruvate kinase), and there is no indication that its inhibitory effect is similar to that of epinephrine. The inhibitory effect may occur in the liver. During glucose-induced hyperglycemia, the liver participates in the removal of glucose from the plasma, whereas it is probable that glucagon prevents this during the glucagon-induced hyperglycemia. More direct experiments should resolve this problem.

The interaction of insulin and glucagon on hepatic glucose output is more clearly demonstrated. In the perfused rat liver, glucagon infusion increased glucose output and cyclic AMP release (the latter presumed to reflect elevated intracellular levels of cyclic AMP) (Park *et al.*, 1972). Addition of insulin to the glucagon perfusion first decreased cyclic AMP release, and this was followed promptly by a decrease in glucose output (Fig. 7). The ratio of insulin to glucagon in this interaction is critical (see Mackrell and Sokal, 1969; Park *et al.*, 1972).

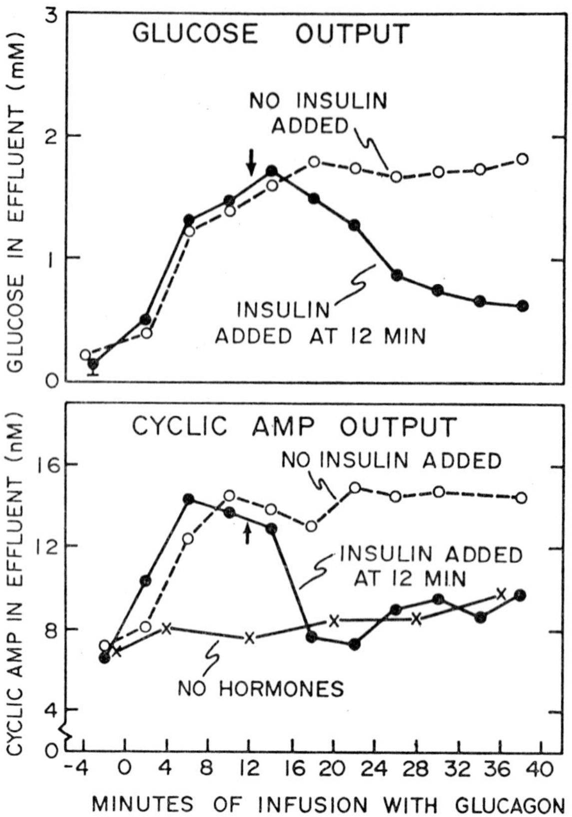

Fig. 7. Interaction of glucagon and insulin in the control of glucose output by the perfused rat liver. Livers of fed rats were perfused with recirculating media for a one-hour control period, and then perfusion without recirculation was begun at —4 min. Glucagon infusion was maintained from 0 time (except for the curve shown by x's) at a steady rate well below that giving a maximal effect. Insulin infusion was superimposed on the glucagon infusion where indicated. (From PARK *et al.*, 1972)

3. Comments

Stimulation by glucagon of hepatic glycogenolysis, gluconeogenesis, and hepatic glucose output appears to be closely linked to increased levels of cyclic AMP. Similar effects have been obtained by perfusion of liver with cyclic AMP (PARK *et al.*, 1972), and by infusion of dibutyryl cyclic AMP in the intact dog (ALTSZULER *et al.*, 1971a). The inhibitory effect of insulin on these processes has been attributed to a depression of hepatic cyclic AMP.

An interaction of insulin and glucagon on glucose uptake probably also occurs, although the metabolic sites of this occurrence are not defined. As indicated above, the hyperglycemia and hyperinsulinemia produced by glucagon results in a lesser increase in glucose uptake than is observed during glucose infusion. Infusion of dibutyryl cyclic AMP in the normal dog duplicates all the effects of glucagon (ALTSZULER *et al.*, 1971a). With both nucleotides, the inhibitory effect on glucose uptake was evident only when compared with uptake during glucose infusion, whereas epinephrine infusion prevented any significant increase in glucose uptake above the control values (ALTSZULER *et al.*, 1971).

Whether or not these interactions occur under physiologic conditions remains to be documented better. Increased plasma levels of glucagon are produced by fasting and by insulin-induced hypoglycemia (Fig. 6), but it is not established if they would occur at less severe hypoglycemia. Glucagon-secreting tumors have been reported, but defects in carbohydrate metabolism were not always present in these (for references, see FOA, 1972; UNGER, 1972). Acute glucagon deficiency has been produced by injection of glucagon anti-serum in laboratory animals, resulting in hypoglycemia (GREY *et al.*, 1970). Glucagon may be less essential as a provider of metabolic fuel in prolonged fasting, since, under such conditions, glucose-utilizing tissues, e.g., brain, adapt to the use of non-gluconeogenic substrates, e.g., ketones.

A more extensive discussion of the physiologic and pathologic status of glucagon can be found in recent reviews (FOA, 1972; UNGER, 1972).

VII. Prolactin and Human Placental Lactogen (HPL)

The influence of prolactin on mammary gland growth and lactation has been demonstrated in many species (see chapter p. 461). In the human, prolactin went undetected and its presence was doubted, until quite recently when the radioimmunoassay allowed detection of the small amounts present in the plasma. The effects of prolaction on overall metabolism have only recently begun to be explored, although the earlier observations (RIDDLE and BATES, 1939) in pigeons indicated that prolactin had calorigenic actions, it increased blood glucose levels, and it produced changes in lipid metabolism.

Studies in mammals have clearly demonstrated the effectiveness of prolactin to alter carbohydrate and lipid metabolism. In the hypophysectomized dog, daily administration of ovine prolactin at 1 mg/kg caused a small rise in the fasting blood glucose and attenuated the excessive hypoglycemic response to injected insulin (SINKOFF and DE BODO, 1953). The glucose tolerance was not affected, except that blood glucose levels no longer fell to severe hypoglycemic levels after the glucose load, which is characteristic of the hypophysectomized animal.

Under special circumstances, prolactin administration was shown to produce diabetes. This was observed in the partially-depancreatized dog and cat, and in the hypophysectomized adrenalectomized dog with only 15—18% of the pancreas remaining (for references, see DE BODO and ALTSZULER, 1958).

Daily administration of ovine prolactin in the normal dog (1 mg/kg) was shown to result in only a small rise in plasma glucose (about 6 mg/100 ml), but caused a significant increase in hepatic glucose output and overall glucose uptake (RATHGEB *et al.*, 1971). These effects occurred without changes in plasma insulin levels. Furthermore, infused insulin produced similar increases in glucose uptake in the prolactin-treated animal, as it did in the untreated animal. Thus, unlike the insulin resistance seen during growth hormone regimen, administration of prolactin in the normal dog does not antagonize endogenous or administered insulin. Prolactin and growth hormone have many similar metabolic effects, including those on free fatty acid turnover (WINKLER *et al.*, 1971), and the different effects with regard to insulin remain unexplained.

The human placental lactogen (HPL), or chorionic growth hormone-prolactin (CGP), is formed in the trophoblast tissue of the placenta. The duplicate nomenclature reflects the multiple effects of this polypeptide when determined by various bioassays. Although the impaired glucose tolerance and diminished sensitivity to insulin observed in pregnancy may be attributed to HPL, the evidence for this is not entirely convincing. HPL injection into normal volunteers had no significant effects on blood glucose, glucose tolerance, nor on insulin response to a glucose load (JOSIMOVICH and MINTZ, 1968). Other supporting and conflicting findings have been reported (see DAUGHADAY and KIPNIS, 1966; GRUMBACH *et al.*, 1968; HERRERA *et al.*, 1969), FRANTZ *et al.* (1972) and therefore conclusions concerning HPL must await more data.

VIII. Thyroid Hormones

The influence of thyroid hormones on carbohydrate metabolism can be discerned from the changes in hyper- and hypo-thyroidism. Hyperthyroid individuals may exhibit moderate elevation of blood glucose, increased rate of absorption of ingested sugars, and normal or impaired glucose tolerance (see DE BODO and ALTSZULER, 1958). There may be increased gluconeogenesis and glucose oxidation, glycogen depletion, ketogenesis, lipolysis, and a negative nitrogen balance (see TATA, 1964). Increased glucose utilization occurs in the hypothyroid rat and in adipose tissues excised from such an animal (HAGEN, 1960).

On the other hand, glucose uptake by the forearm muscle of hyperthyroid patients during intravenous glucose infusion was reported to be normal; it was postulated, however, that glucose uptake elsewhere, e.g., adipose tissue, might have increased, since blood glucose level during the infusion was lower than in the normal (BUTTERFIELD and WHICHELOW, 1964). Other recent studies in thyrotoxic individuals showed a normal glucose disappearance after intravenous glucose, and normal insulin secretion evoked by the hyperglycemia (ANDREANI *et al.*, 1970).

More striking changes from normal are seen in hypothyroidism. Such individuals may exhibit somewhat lower plasma glucose levels (ELRICK *et al.*, 1961) and reduced glucose removal from the plasma following glucose injection (ELRICK *et al.*, 1961; ANDREANI *et al.*, 1970). It is noteworthy that insulin levels in the postabsorptive state and during hyperglycemia were higher than in the normal or thyrotoxic individual, indicating that impaired glucose removal was not due to insulin deficiency (ANDREANI *et al.*, 1970).

Conclusion

Interpretations concerning the effect of thyroid hormones on insulin action, based on the above data, can be only tenuous. Administration of thyroid hormone to the hypothyroid individual would be expected to improve glucose ulilization and to reduce the excessive insulin secretion, i.e., to restore the normal status. It need not be inferred from this that thyroid hormone increases the sensitivity to insulin; it may well be that normalization of cell metabolism by thyroid allows a normal response to insulin.

The extensive data obtained in experimental animals have been reviewed (see DE BODO and ALTSZULER, 1958). As with the observations in humans, only mild changes in glucose metabolism have been observed following thyroidectomy or thyroid administration. It was concluded that the thyroid gland exerts a minor influence on the response to injected insulin (DE BODO and ALTSZULER, 1957).

IX. Concluding Remarks

It is evident from the foregoing presentation and from the extensive literature that a number of hormones can modify the effects of insulin on carbohydrate metabolism. Since these data have been obtained under a variety of experimental conditions, it may be pertinent to inquire whether or not such hormonal interactions have physiological significance. Several lines of evidence indicate that such interactions do moderate hormonal effects in physiologic situations.

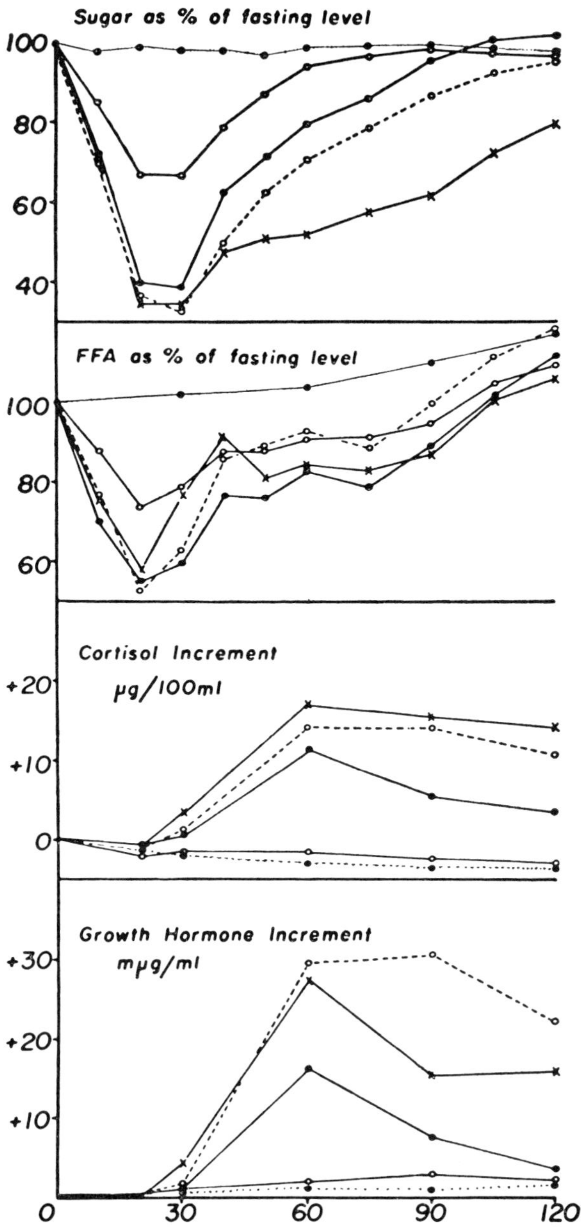

Fig. 8. The plasma sugar, FFA, cortisol, and growth hormone response to saline, ●.....●; to 0.025 units of insulin per kg, ○——○; to 0.05 units of insulin per kg, ●——●; to 0.10 units of insulin per kg, ○.........○; and to 0.15 units of insulin per kg, X——X, at 0, 30, 60, 90, and 120 min after insulin. (From GREENWOOD *et al.*, 1966). Similar responses of adrenal steroids were found by ARNER *et al.* (1962)

As discussed earlier, removal of various endocrine glands increases the sensitivity to the effect of insulin to increase glucose uptake and to induce hypoglycemia. This is observed following removal of the pituitary and the adrenal gland, and might occur following thyroidectomy, and possibly in isolated glucagon deficiency. Although injection of insulin with a consequent hypoglycemia is not a common physiologic phenomenon, it does serve to unmask this abnormality in metabolism, which may be unnoticed in the undisturbed steady state.

A demonstration of hormonal interactions involving endogenous insulin is evident from the glucose tolerance test. In the normal animal, following injection of a glucose load, the plasma glucose concentration declines from the peak value and stabilizes at the control values. In the hypophysectomized or hypophysectomized-adrenalectomized animal, a similar glucose load produces the initial hyperglycemia, but this is followed by a marked hypoglycemia, frequently terminating in convulsions which can be terminated by glucose administration (DE BODO and ALTSZULER, 1958). The hypoglycemia is attributed to secretion of insulin evoked by the hyperglycemia and to the excessive sensitivity of the hormone-deficient animal to even small amount of insulin. Administration of replacement doses of glucocorticoids or of growth hormone prevents the hypoglycemia.

A third line of evidence is derived from the observations that insulin hypoglycemia evokes the secretion of epinephrine (Fig. 5), glucagon (Fig. 6), and growth hormone and adrenal steroids (Fig. 8). Such responses viewed alone can offer only suggestive evidence, but taken together with the preceding data, reinforce the physiologic significance of the interaction between insulin and various other hormones.

Having given due emphasis to the interaction between insulin and other hormones, a note of caution should be added concerning making generalizations from the interactions discussed here. The various hormones have effects on fat and protein metabolism, as well as on carbohydrate metabolism, and the hormonal interactions may not apply to all substrates. This is exemplified by the fact that growth hormone and insulin have similar, rather than opposite, effects to increase amino acid uptake by cells and to increase protein synthesis, and are antagonistic only with regard to carbohydrate and fat metabolism. Similar reservations should be exercised in extrapolating the findings on one tissue to another. Thus, glucocorticoids are said to be catabolic in their overall effect on protein metabolism, yet they have very striking anabolic effects, in that they stimulate synthesis of various enzymes and markedly increase the protein content of liver and pancreas.

Finally, some thought might be given to future direction of investigation in this area. Clearly, the goal remains to determine the mechanism of action and of interaction of the hormones. The availability of radioimmunoassays for the various hormones has greatly enhanced our appreciation of the hormone fluxes in the blood. With regard to insulin, it has allowed KONO and BARHAM (1971) to observe that insulin-binding to tissues is not as firm as formerly believed (see STADIE, 1954), and that it could be readily removed from isolated adipose cells with a concomitant end of biological influence.

The recent reports on the insulin receptors have already enhanced our knowledge, and more information should be forthcoming. The reports to date (CUATRECASAS, 1969, 1972) indicate that conditions which diminish the biological effectiveness to insulin, e.g., diabetes, obesity, growth hormone administration, do not alter the number or affinity of binding sites for insulin on the adipose cell. This again puts the enphasis on the metabolic and enzymatic changes evoked by the hormones which eventually determine how the cell will respone to a given hormone.

References

ALTSZULER, N.: The actions of growth hormone on carbohydrate metabolism. In: Handbook of physiology, Section 7 (ed. by KNOBIL, E., SAWYER, W.H.). Washington, D.C.: Amer. Physiol. Soc. (in press, 1974)

ALTSZULER, N, MORRISON, A., GOTTLIEB, B., BJERKNES, C., RATHGEB, I., STEELE, R.: Effect of fasting and methyprednisolone on carbohydrate metabolism in the normal dog. Fed. Proc. **32**, 255 (1973)

ALTSZULER, N., MORRISON, A., STEELE, R., BJERKNES, C.: Metabolic effects of epinephrine, dibutyryl cyclic AMP, and glucagon infused intravenously into normal dogs. Ann. N. Y. Acad. Sci. **185**, 101—107 (1971)

ALTSZULER, N., RATHGEB, I., STEELE, R.: Mechanisms responsible for the hyperglycemia produced by the dibutyrul derivative of cyclic 3′,5′-adenosine monophosphate. Biochem. Pharmacol. **20**, 2813—2819 (1971a)

ALTSZULER, N., RATHGEB, I., WINKLER, B., BODO, DE, R.G., STEELE, R.: The effects of growth hormone on carbohydrate and lipid metabolism in the dog. Ann. N.Y. Acad. Sci. **148**, 441—458 (1968)

ALTSZULER, N., STEELE, R., DUNN, A., WALL, J.S., BODO, DE, R.C.: Diminution of insulin effect by growth hormone in hypophysectomized dogs; studies with C^{14} glucose. Amer. J. Physiol. **196**, 231—234 (1959)

ALTSZULER, N., STEELE, R., RATHGEB, I., BODO, DE, R.C.: Glucose metabolism and plasma insulin level during epinephrine infusion in the dog. Amer. J. Physiol. **212**, 677—682 (1967)

ALTSZULER, N., STEELE, R., RATHGEB, I., BODO, DE, R.C.: Influence of growth hormone on glucose metabolism and plasma insulin levels in the dog. In: Growth hormone (ed. by PECILE, A., MULLER, E.E.). Excerpta Medica Found., Int'l Comp. Series **158**, 309—318 (1968a)

ALTSZULER, N., STEELE, R., TOBIN, J., RATHGEB, I., BODO, DE, R.C.: Effect of anti-insulin serum on glucose production and uptake in dogs. Excerpta Medica Intern. Congr. Ser. **74**, 168 (1964)

ALTSZULER, N., STEELE, R., WALL, J.S., BODO, DE, R.C.: Mechanism of the "anti-insulin" action of 11,17-oxycorticosteriods in hypophysectomized dogs. Amer. J. Physiol. **192**, 219—226 (1958)

ALTSZULER, N., STEELE, R., WALL, J.S., DUNN, A., BODO, DE, R.C.: Effect of growth hormone on carbohydrate metabolism in normal and hypophysectomized dogs; studies with C^{14} glucose. Amer. J. Physiol. **196**, 121—124 (1959a)

AMBRUS, J.L., JOHNSON, G.C., CHERNICK, W.S., HARRISON, J.W.E.: Effect of epinephrine, insulin and glucagon on the regulation of blood sugar level by the isolated, transfused and the in situ liver. J. Pharmacol. **113**, 2 (1955)

ANDREANI, D., MENZINGER, G., FALLUCCA, F., ALIBERTI, G., TAMBURRANI, G., CASSANO, C.: Insulin levels in thyrotoxicosis and primary myxedema: response to intravenous glucose and glucagon. Diabetologia **6**, 1—7 (1970)

ANNISON, E.F., WHITE, R.R.: Glucose utilization in sheep. Biochem. J. **80**, 162—169 (1961)

ARNER, B., HEDNER, P., KARLEFORS, T.: Adrenocortical activity during induced hypoglycemia. Acta endocr. (Kbh.) **40**, 421—429 (1962)

ASHMORE, J., CARR, L.: Action of insulin on carbohydrate metabolism. In: Actions of Hormones on Molecular Processes (ed. by LITWACK, G., KRITCHEVSKY, D.). New York: John Wiley & Sons, Inc. 1964

ASHMORE, J., WEBER, G.: Hormonal control of carbohydrate metabolism in liver. In: Carbohydrate metabolism and its disorders. vol. 1 (ed. by DICKENS, F., RANDLE, P.J., WHELAN, W.J.). London: Academic Press 1968

BASSETT, J.M., WALLACE, A.L.C.: Short-term effects of ovine growth hormone on plasma glucose, free fatty acids and ketones in sheep. Metabolism **15**, 933—944 (1966)

BEARN, A.G., BILLING, B.H., SHERLOCK, S.: The response of the liver to insulin in normal subjects and in diabetes mellitus: Hepatic vein catheterization studies. Clin. Sci. **11**, 151—165 (1952)

BERSON, S.A., WEISENFELD, S., PASCULLO, M.: Utilization of glucose in normal and diabetic rabbits. Diabetes **8**, 116—127 (1959)

BISHOP, J.B., LARNER, J.: Rapid activation-inactivation of liver uridine diphosphate glucose-glycagon in vivo. J. biol. Chem. **242**, 1355—1356 (1967)

BISHOP, J.S., STEELE, R., ALTSZULER, N., DUNN, A., BJERKNES, C., BODO, DE, R.C.: Effects of insulin on liver glycogen synthesis and breakdown in the dog. Amer. J. Physiol. **208**, 307—316 (1965)

BISHOP, J.S., STEELE, R., ALTSZULER, N., RATHGEB, I., BJERKNES, C., BODO, DE, R.C.: Diminished responsiveness to insulin in the growth hormone treated normal dog. Amer. J. Physiol. **212**, 272—278 (1967)

Bleicher, S.J., Levy, L.J., Zarowitz, H., Spergel, G.: Glucagondeficiency hypoglycemia: a new syndrome. Clin. Res. **18**, 355 (1970)

Bodo, de, R.C., Altszuler, N.: Relationship of the adrenal cortex to the diabetogenic action of growth hormone. In: Hypophyseal growth hormone, nature and actions (ed. by Smith, R.W., Jr., Gaebler, O.H., Long, C.N.H.). New York: The Blakiston Division, McGraw-Hill Book Co. 1955

Bodo, de, R.C., Altszuler, N.: Metabolic effects of growth hormone and their physiologic significance. Vitam. and Horm. **15**, 205—258 (1957)

Bodo, de, R.C., Altszuler, N.: Insulin hypersensitivity and physiological insulin antagonists. Physiol. Rev. **38**, 389—445 (1958)

Bodo, de, R.C., Sinkoff, M.W.: The role of growth hormone in carbohydrate metabolism. Ann. N.Y. Acad. Sci. **57**, 23—60 (1953)

Bodo, de, R.C., Sinkoff, M.W.: Anterior pituitary and adrenal hormones in the regulation of carbohydrate metabolism. Recent Progr. Hormone Res. **3**, 511—563 (1953a)

Bodo, de, R.C., Sinkoff, M.W., Kurtz, M., Lane, N., Kiang, S.P.: Significance of adrenocortical atrophy in the carbohydrate metabolism of hypophysectomized dogs. Amer. J. Physiol. **173**, 11—21 (1953)

Bodo, de, R.C., Steele, R., Altszuler, N., Dunn, A., Bishop, J.S.: Effects of insulin on hepatic glucose metabolism and glucose utilization by tissues. Diabetes **12**, 16—28 (1963)

Bodo, de, R.C., Steele, R., Altszuler, N., Dunn, A., Bishop, J.S.: On the hormonal regulation of carbohydrate metabolism; studies with C^{14} glucose. Recent Progr. Hormone Res. **19**, 445—482 (1963a)

Bouckaert, J.P., de Duve, C.: The action of insulin. Physiol. Rev. **27**, 39—71 (1947)

Britton, S.W., Silvette, H.: Effects of cortico-adrenal extract on carbohydrate metabolism in normal animals. Amer. J. Physiol. **100**, 693—700 (1932)

Butterfield, W.J.H., Whichelow, M.J.: Are thyroid hormones diabetogenic? A study of peripheral glucose metabolism during infusions in normal subjects and hyperthyroid patients before and after treatment. Metabolism **13**, 620—628 (1964)

Campbell, J.: Diabetogenic actions of growth hormone. In: The hypophyseal growth hormone, nature and actions (ed. by Smith, R.W., Jr., Gaebler, O.H., Long, C.N.H.). New York: The Blakiston Division, McGraw-Hill Book Co., Inc. 1955

Campbell, J., Rastogi, K.S.: Growth hormone-induced diabetes and high levels of serum insulin in dogs. Diabetes **15**, 30—43 (1966)

Campbell, J., Rastogi, K.S.: Elevation in serum insulin, albumin and FFA, with gains in liver lipid and protein, induced by glucocorticoid treatment in dogs. Canad. J. Physiol. Pharmacol. **46**, 421—429 (1968)

Campbell, J., Rastogi, K.S.: Actions of growth hormone: Enhancement of insulin utilization with inhibition of insulin effect on blood glucose in dogs. Metabolism **18**, 930—944 (1969)

Campbell, J., Rastogi, K.S., Hausler, H.R.: Hyperinsulinemia with diabetes induced by cortisone, and the influence of growth hormone in the Chinese hamster. Endocrinology **79**, 749—756 (1966)

Cannon, W.B., McIver, M.A., Bliss, S.W.: Studies on the conditions of activity in endocrine glands. Amer. J. Physiol. **69**, 46—66 (1924)

Cerasi, E., Luft, R., Efendic, S.: Antagonism between glucose and epinephrine regarding insulin secretion. Acta med. scand. **190**, 411—417 (1971)

Cherry, I.S., Crandall, L.A.: The response of the liver to the oral administration of glucose. Amer. J. Physiol. **120**, 52—58 (1937)

Combes, B., Adams, R.H., Strickland, W., Madison, L.L.: The physiological significance of endogenous insulin into the portal circulation. IV. Hepatic uptake of glucose during glucose infusion in nondiabetic dogs. J. clin. Invest. **40**, 1706—1718 (1961)

Coore, H.G., Randle, P.J.: Regulation of insulin secretion studied with pieces of rabbit pancreas incubated in vitro. Biochem. J. **93**, 66—78 (1964)

Cori, C.F., Cori, G.T.: The mechanism of epinephrine action. I. The influence of epinephrine on the carbohydrate metabolism of fasting rats with a note on new formation of carbohydrates. J. biol. Chem. **79**, 309—319 (1928)

Crandall, L.A., Jr., Cherry, I.S.: The effects of insulin and glycine on hepatic glucose output in normal, hypophysectomized, adrenal denervated, and adrenalectomized dog. Amer. J. Physiol. **125**, 658—673 (1939)

Crofford, O.B., Rogers, N.L., Russell, W.G.: The effect of insulin on fat cells. An insulin degrading system extracted from plasma membranes of insulin responsive cells. Diabetes **21**, Suppl. 2, 403—413 (1972)

Csorba, T.R.: Isotope dilution studies of the effect of insulin and diabetes on glucose transfer rates. Horm. Metals Res. **1**, 97—107 (1969)

Cuatrecasas, P.: Interaction of insulin with cell membrane: the primary action of insulin. Proc. nat. Acad. Sci. (Wash.) **63**, 450—457 (1969)

CUATRECASAS, P.: The insulin receptor. Diabetes **21**, Suppl. 2, 396—402 (1972)
DAUGHADAY, W.H., KIPNIS, D.M.: The growth-promoting and anti-insulin actions of somatotropin. Recent Progr. Hormone Res. **22**, 49—93 (1966)
DUNN, A., ALTSZULER, N., BODO, DE, R.C., STEELE, R., ARMSTRONG, D.T., BISHOP, J.S.: Mechanism of action of insulin. Nature (Lond.) **183**, 1123—1124 (1959)
DUNN, D.F., FRIEDMAN, B., MAASS, A.R., REICHARD, G.A.,WEINHOUSE, S.: Effects of insulin on blood glucose entry and removal rates in dogs. J. biol. Chem. **225**, 225—237 (1957)
ELLIS, S.: The metabolic effects of epinephrine and related amines. Pharmacol. Rev. **8**, 485—562 (1956)
ENSINCK, J.W., WILLIAMS, R.H.: Hormonal and nonhormonal factors modifying man's response to insulin. In: Handbook of physiology, Section, 7 vol. 1 (ed. by STEINER, D.F., FREINKEL, N.). Washington, D.C.: Amer. Physiol. Soc. 1972
ELRICK, H., HEAD, C.J., JR., ARAI, Y.: Influence of thyroid function on carbohydrate metabolism and a new method for assessing response to insulin. J. clin. Endocr. **21**, 387—400 (1961)
EXTON, J.H., MALLETTE, L.E., JEFFERSON, L.S., WONG, E.H.A., FRIEDMANN, N., MILLER, T.B., JR., PARK, C.R.: The hormonal control of hepatic gluconeogenesis. Recent Progr. Hormone Res. **26**, 411—461 (1970)
EXTON, J.H., PARK, C.R.: Interaction of insulin and glucagon in the control of liver metabolism. In: Handbook of physiology, Section 7, vol. 1 (ed. by STEINER, D.F., FREINKEL, N.). Washington, D.C.: Amer. Physiol. Soc. 1972
FAJANS, S.S.: Some metabolic actions of corticosteroids. Metabolism **10**, 951—965 (1961)
FAJANS, S.S., CONN, J.W.: An approach to the prediction of diabetes mellitus by modification of the glucose tolerance test with cortisone. Diabetes **3**, 296—304 (1954)
FINE, M.B., WILLIAMS, R.H.: Effect of insulin infusion on hepatic output of glucose. Amer. J. Physiol. **198**, 645—648 (1960)
FOA, P.P.: Glucagon. Ergebn. Physiol. **60**, 141—219 (1964)
FOA, P.P.: The secretion of glucagon. In: Handbook of physiology, Section 7, vol. 1 (ed. by STEINER, D.F., FREINKEL, N.). Washington, D.C.: Amer. Physiol. Soc., p. 261—267 (1972)
FRANTZ, A.G., KLEINBERG, D.L., NOEL, G.L.: Studies on prolactin in man. Recent Progr. Hormone Res. **28**, 527—573 (1972)
FREYCHET, P., KAHN, R., ROTH, J., NEVILLE, D.M., JR.: Insulin interactions with liver plasma membranes. Independence of binding of the hormone and its degradation. J. biol. Chem. **247**, 3953—3961 (1972)
FRITZ, I.B.: Insulin actions on carbohydrate and lipid metabolism. In: Biochemical actions of hormones, vol. II (ed. by LITWICK, G.). New York: Academic Press 1971
FRITZ, I.B., SHATTON, J., MORTON, J.V., LEVINE, R.: Effects of epinephrine and insulin on glucose disappearance in eviscerated dogs. Amer. J. Physiol. **189**, 57—62 (1957)
FROHMAN, L.A., MACGILLIVRAY, M.H., ACETO, T., JR.: Acute effects of human growth hormone on insulin secretion and glucose utilization in normal and growth hormone deficient subjects. J. clin. Invest. **27**, 561—567 (1967)
GLENN, E.M., MILLER, W.L., SCHLAGEL, C.A.: Metabolic effects of adrenocortical steroids *in vivo* and *in vitro*: relationship to anti-inflammatory effects. Recent Progr. Hormone Res. **19**, 107—191 (1963)
GLICK, S.M., ROTH, J., YALOW, R.S., BERSON, S.A.: The regulation of growth hormone secretion. Recent Progr. Hormone Res. **21**, 241—270 (1965)
GOLDFIEN, A., ZILELI, M.S., DESPOINTES, R.H., BETHUNE, J.E.: The effect of hypoglycemia on the adrenal secretion of epinephrine and norepinephrine in the dog. Endocrinology **62**, 749—757 (1958)
GOODMAN, H.M.: In vitro actions of growth hormone on glucose metabolism in adipose tissue. Endocrinology **76**, 216—225 (1965)
GOODMAN, H.M.: Growth hormone and the metabolism of carbohydrate and lipid in adipose tissue. Ann. N.Y. Acad. Sci. **148**, 419—440 (1968)
GREENWOOD, F.C., LANDON, I., STAMP, T.C.B.: The plasma sugar, free fatty acid, cortisol and growth hormone response to insulin. J. clin. Invest. **45**, 429—436 (1966)
GREY, N., MCGUIGAN, J.E., KIPNIS, D.M.: Neutralization of endogenous glucagon by high titer glucagon antiserum. Endocrinology **86**, 1383—1388 (1970)
GRUMBACH, M.M., KAPLAN, S.L., SCIARRA, J.J., BURR, I.M.: Chorionic growth hormone — prolactin (CGP): Secretion, disposition, biological activity in man, and postulated function as the "growth hormone" of the second half of pregnancy. Ann. N. Y. Acad. Sci. **148**, 501—531 (1968)
HAFT, D.E., MILLER, L.L.: Alloxan diabetes and demonstrated direct action of insulin on metabolism of isolated perfused rat liver. Amer. J. Physiol. **192**, 33—42 (1958)
HAGEN, G.H.: Effect of insulin on the metabolism of adipose tissue from hyperthyroid rats. J. biol. Chem. **235**, 2600—2602 (1960)

Hagen, J.H., Ball, E.G.: Studies on the metabolism of adipose tissue. IV. The effect of insulin and adrenaline on glucose utilization, lactate production, and net gas exchange. J. biol. Chem. **235**, 1545—1549 (1960)

Haynes, R.C., Jr., Lu, Y.S.: Measurement of cortisol-stimulated gluconeogenesis in the rat. Endocrinology **85**, 811—814 (1969)

Henderson, M.J., Morgan, H.E., Park, C.R.: Regulation of glucose uptake in muscle. IV. The effect of hypophysectomy on glucose transport, phosphorylation, and insulin sensitivity in isolated, perfused heart. J. biol. Chem. **236**, 273—277 (1961)

Herrera, E., Knopp, R.H., Freinkel, N.: Carbohydrate metabolism in pregnancy. IV. Plasma fuels, insulin, liver composition, gluconeogenesis, and nitrogen metabolism during late gestation in the fed and fasted rat. J. clin. Invest. **48**, 2260—2272 (1969)

Hetenyi, G., Jr., Wrenshall, G.A., Best, C.H.: Rates of production, utilization, accumulation and apparent distribution space of glucose. Diabetes **10**, 304—311 (1961)

Hildes, J.A., Sherlock, S., Walshe, V.: Liver and muscle glycogen in normal subjects, in diabetes mellitus and in acute hepatitis. II. The effects of intravenous adrenaline. Clin. Sci. **7**, 297—314 (1949)

Himms-Hagen, J.: Sympathetic regulation of metabolism. Pharmacol. Rev. **19**, 367—461 (1967)

Houssay, B.A.: An argentine trail of hypophysial research. J. Endocr. **21**, 1—14 (1960)

Ingle, D.J., Nezamis, J.E.: Effect of epinephrine upon the tolerance of the eviscerated rat for glucose. Amer. J. Physiol. **156**, 361—364 (1949)

Ingle, D.J.: Experimental steroid diabetes. Diabetes **5**, 187—192 (1956)

Ingle, D.J., Baker, B.C.: Physiological and therapeutic effects of articotropin (ACTH) and cortisone. Springfield, Ill.: Charles C. Thomas 1953

Ingle, D.J., Prestrud, M.C., Li, C.H.: Effects of administering adrenocorticotropic hormone by continuous injection to normal rats. Amer. J. Physiol. **166**, 165—170 (1951)

Ishiwata, K., Hetenyi, G., Jr., Vranic, M.: Effect of D-glucose or D-ribose on the turnover of glucose in pancreatectomized dogs maintained on a matched intraportal infusion of insulin. Diabetes **18**, 820—827 (1969)

Issekutz, B., Jr., Allen, M.: Effect of catecholamines and methylprednisolone on carbohydrate metabolism of dogs. Metabolism **21**, 48—59 (1972)

Jacobs, G., Reichard, G., Goodman, E.H., Jr., Friedman, B., Weinhouse, S.: Action of insulin and tolbutamide on blood glucose entry and removal. Diabetes **7**, 358—364 (1958)

Jefferson, L.S., Exton, J.H., Butcher, R.W., Sutherland, E.W., Park, C.R.: Role of adenosinol 3′,5′-monophosphate in the effects of insulin and anti-insulin serum on liver metabolism. J. biol. Chem. **243**, 1031—1038 (1968)

Josimovich, J.B., Mintz, D.H.: Biological and immunochemical studies on human placental lactogen. Ann. N. Y. Acad. Sci. **148**, 488—500 (1968)

Katzen, H.M., Glitzer, M.S.: Insulin antagonists and disturbances in carbohydrate metabolism. In: Carbohydrate metabolism and its disorders (ed. by Dickens, F., Randle, P.J., Whelan, W.J.). London: Academic Press 1968

Kern, H., Logothetopoulos, J.: Steroid diabetes in the guinea pig. Studies on islet-cell ultrastructure and regeneration. Diabetes **19**, 145—154 (1970)

Ketterer, B., Randle, P.J., Young, F.G.: The pituitary growth hormone and metabolic processes. Ergebn. Physiol. **49**, 127—211 (1957)

Kipnis, D.M., Helmreich, E., Cori, C.F.: Studies of tissue permeability. IV. The distribution of glucose between plasma and muscle. J. biol. Chem. **234**, 165—170 (1959)

Kipnis, D.M., Stein, M.F.: Insulin antagonism: fundamental considerations. CIBA Found. Colloq. Endocrin. **15**, 156—191 (1964)

Knobil, E., Hotchkiss, J.: Growth hormone. Ann. Rev. Physiol. **26**, 47—74 (1964)

Kono, T., Barham, F.W.: The relationship between the insulin-binding capacity of fat cells and the cellular response to insulin: Studies with intact and trypsin-treated fat cells. J. biol. Chem. **246**, 6210—6216 (1971)

Kosaka, K., Ide, T., Kuzuya, T., Miki, E., Kuzuya, N., Okinaka, S.: Insulin-like activity in pancreatic vein blood after glucose loading and epinephrine hyperglycemia. Endocrinology **75**, 9—14 (1964)

Krahl, M.E.: The actions of insulin on cells. New York: Academic Press 1961

Kris, A.O., Miller, R.E., Wherry, F.E., Mason, J.W.: Inhibition of insulin secretion by infused epinephrine in rhesus monkeys. Endocrinology **78**, 87—97 (1966)

Landau, B.R.: Adrenal steroids and carbohydrate metabolism. Vitam. and Horm. **23**, 1—59 (1965)

Landau, B.B., Leonards, J.R., Barry, F.M.: Regulation of blood glucose concentration; response of liver to glucose administration. Amer. J. Physiol. **201**, 41—46 (1961)

Larner, J.: Insulin and glycogen synthetase. Diabetes **21**, Suppl. 2, 429—438 (1972)

LAWRENCE, A.M.: Glucagon. Ann. Rev. Med. **20**, 207—222 (1969)

LECOCQ, F.D., MEBANE, D., MADISON, L.L.: The acute effect of hydrocortisone on hepatic glucose output and peripheral glucose utilization. J. clin. Invest. **43**, 237—246 (1964)

LEONARDS, J.R., LANDAU, B.R.: A study of the equivalence of metabolic patterns in rat adipose tissue: insulin versus glucose concentration. Arch. Biochem. **91**, 194—200 (1960)

LEONARDS, J.R., LANDAU, B.R., CRAIG, J.W., MARTIN, F.I.R., MILLER, M., BARRY, F.M.: Regulation of blood glucose concentration; hepatic action of insulin. Amer. J. Physiol. **201**, 47—54 (1961)

LERNMARK, A., HELLMAN, B.: Effect of epinephrine and mannoheptulose on early and late phases of glucose-stimulated insulin release. Metabolism **19**, 614—618 (1970)

LEVINE, R., GOLDSTEIN, M., KLEIN, S., HUDDLESTUN, R.: The action of insulin on the distribution of galactose in eviscerated nephrectomized dogs. J. biol. Chem. **179**, 985—986 (1949)

LONG, C.N.H., LUKENS, F.D.W.: Effect of adrenalectomy and hypophysectomy upon experimental diabetes in the cat. Proc. Soc. exp. Biol. (N.Y.) **32**, 743—745 (1935)

LUFT, R., CERASI, E.: Human growth hormone in blood glucose homeostasis. In: Growth hormone (ed. by PECILE, A., MULLER, E.E.). Excerpta Medical Found., Int'l Congress Series 159, 1968

LUNDSGAARD, E.: The metabolism of the isolated liver. Bull. Johns Hopk. Hosp. **63**, 90—103 (1938)

LUNDSGAARD, E., NIELSEN, N.A., ORSKOV, S.L.: The carbohydrate metabolism of the isolated cat liver. Skand. Arch. Physiol. **73**, 296—313 (1936)

MACKRELL, D.J., SOKAL, J.E.: Antagonism between the effects of insulin and glucagon on the isolated liver. Diabetes **18**, 724—732 (1969)

MAHLER, R., SHOEMAKER, W.C., ASHMORE, J.: Hepatic action of insulin. Ann. N.Y. Acad. Sci. **82**, 452—459 (1959)

MATSUZAKI, F., RABEN, M.S.: Growth hormone. Ann. Rev. Pharmacol. **5**, 137—150 (1965)

MEZEY, A.P., FOLEY, H.T., ALTSZULER, N.: Effect of hypophysectomy and growth hormone on glucose uptake by rat epididymal fat tissue. Proc. Soc. exp. Biol. (N.Y.) **107**, 689—692 (1961)

MORTIMORE, G.E.: Effect of insulin on release of glucose and urea by isolated rat liver. Amer. J. Physiol. **204**, 699—704 (1963)

MORTIMORE, G.E., KING, E., JR., MONDON, C.E., GLINSMANN, W.H.: Effects of insulin on net carbohydrate alterations in perfused rat liver. Amer. J. Physiol. **212**, 179—183 (1967)

MUNCK, A.: Glucocorticoid inhibition of glucose uptake by peripheral tissues: old and new evidence, molecular mechanisms, and physiological significance. Perspect. Biol. Med. **14**, 265—289 (1971)

NINOMIYA, R., FORBATH, N.F., HETENYI, G.: Effect of adrenal steroids on glucose kinetics in normal and diabetic dogs. Diabetes **14**, 729—739 (1965)

OHNEDA, A., AGUILAR-PARADA, E., EISENTRAUT, A.M., UNGER, R.H.: Control of pancreatic glucagon secretion by glucose. Diabetes **18**, 1—10 (1969)

PARK, C.R.: Some factors regulating the utilization of carbohydrate. Int. Union. Biochem. Ser. **32**, 711—712 (1964)

PARK, C.R., LEWIS, S.B., EXTON, J.H.: Relationship of some hepatic actions of insulin to the intracellular level of cyclic adenylate. Diabetes **21**, Suppl. 2, 439—446 (1972)

PARK, C.R., MORGAN, H.E., HENDERSON, M.J., REGEN, D.M., CADENAS, E., POST, R.L.: The regulation of glucose uptake in muscle as studied in the perfused rat heart. Recent Progr. Hormone Res. **17**, 493—529 (1961)

PECILE, A., MULLER, E.E., Eds.: Growth hormone. Amsterdam: Excerpta Medical Found., Int'l Cong. Series 158, 1968

PECILE, A., MULLER, E.E., Eds.: Growth and growth hormone. Amsterdam: Excerpta Medical Found., Int'l Cong. Series 244, 1972

PERLEY, M., KIPNIS, D.M.: Effects of glucocorticoids on plasma insulin. New Engl. J. Med. **274**, 1237—1241 (1966)

PORTE, D., JR., GRABER, A.L., KUZUYA, T., WILLIAMS, R.H.: The effect of epinephrine on immunoreactive insulin levels in man. J. clin. Invest. **45**, 228—236 (1966)

RANDLE, P.J., GARLAND, P.B., HALES, C.N., NEWSHOLME, E.A.: The glucose fatty acid cycle and diabetes mellitus. CIBA Found. Colloq. Endocrin. **15**, 192—216 (1964)

RANDLE, P.J., GARLAND, P.B., HALES, C.N., NEWSHOLME, E.A., DENTON, R.M., POGSON, C.I.: Interactions of metabolism and the physiological role of insulin. Recent Progr. Hormone Res. **21**, 1—48 (1966)

RASTOGI, K.S., CAMPBELL, J.: Effect of growth hormone on cortisone-induced hyperinsulinemia and reduction in pancreatic insulin in the mouse. Endocrinology **87**, 226—232 (1970)

RATHGEB, I., ALTSZULER, N., STEELE, R., BODO, DE, R.C.: Glucagon infusion on glucose metabolism and insulin secretion in normal dogs. Fed. Proc. **25**, 378 (1966)

Rathgeb, I., Houssay, B.A., Ashkar, E., del Castillo, E.I., Steele, R., Altszuler, N.: Epinephrine deficiency potentiates cortisol elevation of glucose turnover in the dog. Endocrinology **93**, 1336—1341 (1973)

Rathgeb, I., Steele, R., Winkler, B., Altszuler, N.: Influence of fasting on changes in glucose metabolism induced by growth hormone injection in the normal dog. Diabetes **7**, 487—491 (1970)

Rathgeb, I., Winkler, B., Steele, R., Altszuler, N.: Effect of ovine prolactin administration on glucose metabolism and plasma insulin levels in the dog. Endocrinology **88**, 718—722 (1971)

Reichard, G.A., Friedmann, B., Maass, R., Weinhouse, S.: Turnover rates of blood glucose in normal dogs during hyperglycemia induced by glucose or glucagon. J. biol. Chem. **230**, 387—397 (1958)

Reichard, G.A., Jacobs, A.G., Kimbel, P., Hochella, N.J., Weinhouse, S.: Effects of insulin on blood glucose entry and removal rates in man. Diabetes **9**, 447—453 (1960)

Riddle, O., Bates, R.W.: The preparation, assay and actions of lactogenic hormone. In: Sex and Internal Secretions (ed. by Young, W.C.). Baltimore: Williams & Wilkins 1939

Ridick, F.A., Jr., Reisler, D.M., Kipnis, D.M.: The sugar transport system in striated muscle. Effect of growth hormone, hydrocortisone and alloxan-diabetes. Diabetes **11**, 171—178 (1962)

Riggs, T.R.: Hormones and transport across cell membranes. In: Biochemical actions of hormones (ed. by Litwack, G.). New York: Academic Press 1970

Salter, J.M., Davidson, I.W.F., Best, C.H.: The pathologic effects of large amounts of glucagon. Diabetes **6**, 248—252 (1957)

Samols, E., Marri, G., Marks, V.: Interrelationship of glucagon, insulin and glucose. The insulinogenic effect of glucagon. Diabetes **15**, 855—856 (1966)

Schalch, D.S., Kipnis, D.M.: Abnormalities in carbohydrate tolerance associated with elevated plasma non-esterified fatty acids. J. clin. Invest. **44**, 2010—2020 (1965)

Searle, G.L., Mortimore, G.E., Buckley, R.E., Reilly, W.A.: Plasma glucose turnover in humans as studied with C^{14} glucose. Diabetes **8**, 167—173 (1959)

Shoemaker, W.C., Elwyn, D.H.: Liver: functional interactions within the intact animal. Ann. Rev. Physiol. **31**, 227—268 (1969)

Shoemaker, W.C., Mahler, R., Ashmore, J.: The effect of insulin on hepatic glucose metabolism in the unanesthetized dog. Metabolism **8**, 494—511 (1959)

Sinkoff, M.W., Bodo, de, R.C.: Prolactin as an insulin antagonist. Arch. exp. Path. Pharmakol. **219**, 100—110 (1953)

Sirek, O., Best, C.H.: Intramuscular cortisone administration to dogs. Proc. Soc. exp. Biol. N.Y.) **80**, 594—598 (1952)

Sirek, O.V., Sirek, A.: The physiology of growth hormone. Ergebn. inn. Med. Kinderheilk. **21**, 217—263 (1964)

Smith, R.W., Gaebler, O.H., Long, C.N.H., eds.: The hypophyseal growth hormone, nature and actions. New York: The Blakiston Division, McGraw-Hill Book Co., Inc. 1955

Sokal, J.E.: Glucagon — an essential hormone. Amer. J. Med. **41**, 331—341 (1966)

Soskin, S., Essex, H.E., Herrick, J.F., Mann, F.C.: The mechanism of regulation of the blood sugar by the liver. Amer. J. Physiol. **124**, 558 (1938)

Soskin, S., Levine, R., Lehmann, W.: Influence of the hypophysis on carbohydrate metabolism. Amer. J. Physiol. **127**, 463—469 (1939)

Stadie, W.C.: Current concepts of the action of insulin. Physiol. Rev. **34**, 52—100 (1954)

Steele, R.: Influences of insulin on hepatic metabolism of glucose. Ergebn. Physiol. **57**, 91—189 (1966)

Steele, R.: Tracer probes in steady state systems. Springfield, Ill.: Charles C. Thomas 1971a

Steele, R.: The influence of corticosteroids on protein and carbohydrate metabolism. In: Handbook of physiology, Section 7 (ed. by Sayers, G.). Washington, D.C.: Amer. Physiol. Soc. (in press 1974)

Steele, R., Bishop, J.S., Dunn, A., Altszuler, N., Rathgeb, I., Bodo, de, R.C.: Inhibition by insulin of hepatic glucose production in the normal dog. Amer. J. Physiol. **208**, 301—306 (1965)

Sutherland, E.W., Rall, T.W.: The relation of adenosine-3′,5′-phosphate and phosphorylase to the actions of catecholamines and other hormones. Pharmacol. Rev. **12**, 265—299 (1960)

Tarding, F., Schambye, P.: The action of sulfonylureas and insulin on the glucose output from the liver of normal dogs. Endokrinologie **26**, 222—228 (1958)

Tata, J.R.: Biological action of thyroid hormones at the cellular and molecular levels. In: Actions of hormones on molecular processes (ed. by Litwak, G., Kritchevsky, D.). New York: Wiley 1964

UNDERHILL, F.P., CLOSSON, O.E.: Adrenalin glycosuria, and the influence of adrenal upon nitrogenous metabolism. Amer. J. Physiol. **17**, 42—54 (1906)

UNGER, R.H.: Circulating pancreatic glucagon and extrapancreatic glucagon-like materials. In: Handbook of physiology, Section 7, vol. 1 (ed. by STEINER, D.F., FREINKEL, N.). Washington, D.C.: Amer. Physiol. Soc. 1972

UNGER, R.H., EISENTRAUT, A.M., MCCALL, M.S., MADISON, L.L.: Measurements of endogenous glucagon in plasma and the influence of blood glucose concentration upon its secretion. J. clin. Invest. **41**, 682—689 (1962)

VENDSALU, A.: Studies on adrenaline and noradrenaline in human plasma. Acta physiol. scand., Suppl. 173, 1—123 (1960)

VOLK, B.W., LAZARUS, S.S.: Ultramicroscopic studies of rabbit pancreas during cortisone treatment. Diabetes **12**, 162—172 (1963)

WALAAS, O., WALAAS, E.: Effect of epinephrine on rat diaphragm. J. biol. Chem. **187**, 769—776 (1950)

WALL, J.S., STEELE, R., BODO, DE, R.C., ALTSZULER, N.: Effect of insulin on utilization and production of circulating glucose. Amer. J. Physiol. **189**, 43—50 (1957)

WALL, J.S., STEELF, R., BODO, DE, R.C., ALTSZULER, N.: Mechanism of insulin hypersensitivity in the hypophysectomized dog. Amer. J. Physiol. **189**, 51—56 (1957a)

WEIL, R.: Pituitary growth hormone and intermediary metabolism. I. The hormonal effect on the metabolism of fat and carbohydrate. Acta endocr. (Kbh.) Suppl. **98**, 1—92 (1965)

WILLIAMS, R.H., ENSINCK, J.W.: Secretion, fates and action of insulin and related products. Diabetes **15**, 623—654 (1966)

WILLIAMSON, J.R., GARCIA, A., RENOLD, A.E., CAHILL, G.F., JR.: Studies on the perfused rat liver. I. Effects of glucagon and insulin on glucose metabolism. Diabetes **15**, 183—187 (1967)

WINKLER, B., RATHGEB, I., STEELE, R., ALTSZULER, N.: Effect of ovine prolactin administration on free fatty acid metabolism in the normal dog. Endocrinology **88**, 1349—1352 (1971)

WRENSHALL, G.A., VRANIC, M., COWAN, J.S., RAPPAPORT, A.M.: Effects of sudden deprivation and restoration of insulin secretion on glucose metabolism in dogs. Diabetes **14**, 689—695 (1965)

YOUNG, F.G.: The growth hormone and diabetes. Recent Progr. Hormone Res. **8**, 471—510 (1953)

ZIERLER, K.L.: Effects of growth hormone on metabolism of muscle and adipose tissue of the forearm of man. In: Clinical Endocrinology II (ed. by ASTWOOD, E.B., CASSIDY, C.E.). New York: Grune and Stratton 1968

ZIERLER, K.C., RABINOWITZ, D.: Effect of very small concentration of insulin on forearm metabolism. Persistence of its action on potassium and free fatty acids without its effect on glucose. J. clin. Invest. **43**, 950—962 (1964)

Addendum

More recent studies concerned with insulin receptors in cells obtained from normal and insulin resistant animals have been reviewed by P. CUATRECASAS [Membrane receptors. Ann. Rev. Biochem. **43**, 169—214 (1974)], and by J. ROTH [Peptide hormone binding to receptors: A review of direct studies in vitro. Metabolism **22**, 1059—1073 (1973)]. The studies of Roth and associates indicate a decrease in insulin binding to liver and fat cell membranes of mice exhibiting insulin resistance. This would appear to be at variance with the conclusions of Cuatrecasas cited above. The isolation and synthesis of the hypothalamic hormone somatostatin or SRIF (somatotropin-release inhibiting factor) by GUILLEMIN and associates (P. BRAZEAU, W. VALE, R. BURGUS, N. LING, M. BUTCHER, J. RIVIER, R. GUILLEMIN: Hypothalamic polypeptide that inhibits the secretion of immunoreactive pituitary growth hormone). Science, **179**, 77—79 (1973), has added an important regulatory agent and a very useful tool for study of hormone secretion. This hormone decreases secretion of several hormones, such as growth hormone and glucagon, and is currently being used by a number of investigators to study the interrelationship between insulin and the various hormones which oppose some of the effects of insulin.

Acknowledgements

Original research quoted here was supported by grants from the United States Public Health Service (AM-1088) and the American Cancer Society (P-207).

Immunopathology of Insulin

A. Insulin Allergy, "Cellular" Antibodies and Insulitis

KONRAD FEDERLIN

With 9 Figures

I. Insulin Allergy

1. Introduction

Allergic reactions to insulin were observed even in the first year of insulin therapy. Four of the first 83 insulin-treated diabetics developed urticarial skin lesions (JOSLIN *et al.*, 1922). Although at that time it was a question of preparation, i.e., the insulin was very likely to be contaminated with numerous other animal proteins, similar side effects are still observed with the purified insulins now in use.

Allergic symptoms after parenteral administration of insulin are observed most often in the skin. In rare cases, however, the reaction of the organism may occur in other target organs or systemically. There are a few observations of thrombocytopenic purpura (CONSTAM, 1956; CAWLEY and BROWNE, 1970) and of non-thrombocytopenic purpura (KERN and LANGER, 1939), or of anemia due to immune-complexes at the surface of red cells (FAULK *et al.*, 1970) which can be considered allergic or "allergy-related" consequences of insulin therapy.

According to GOLDSTEIN (1971) also angioneurotic edema, serum sickness, and even gastrointestinal symptoms were observed. Whether the case described by BOULIN *et al.* (1955) of the development of polyarteritis nodosa following insulin administration can in fact be regarded as a consequence of insulin, remains doubtful. Secondary participation of different organs during anaphylaxis is discussed in the section on immediate type hypersensitivity to insulin.

2. Clinical Symptoms

a) Local Delayed Reaction

This type is expressed by a firm, painful local redness sometimes accompanied by itching and burning sensations at the point of injection and spreading to an area of 1—4 cm in diameter, although even larger areas have been observed (Fig. 1a, b). The reaction reaches its maximum of intensity within 24—36 h and recedes

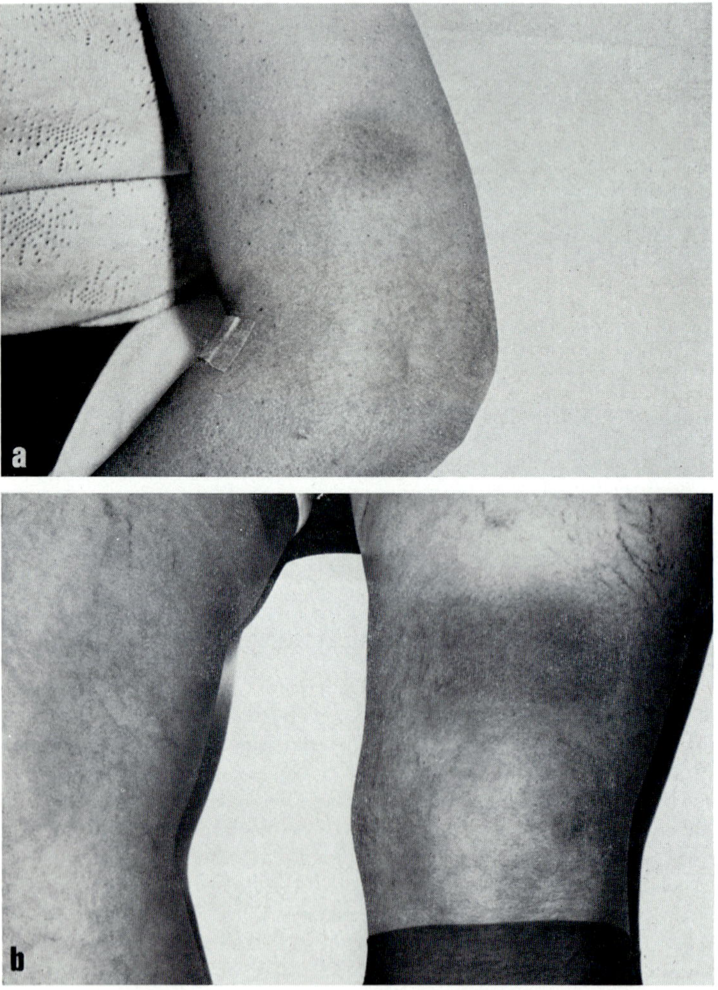

Fig. 1. a: Delayed allergic reaction to insulin, of a size which is most commonly observed. b: Marked local delayed allergic reaction of a size of 10 mm ∅

after 2—3 days. Sometimes residues can be seen for nearly a week. The symptoms vary widely in regard to time of initial onset and intensity and duration. The onset is usually observed during the first 8—10 days of insulin treatment but may appear as early as day 2 or 3. The latter occurs especially in patients in which

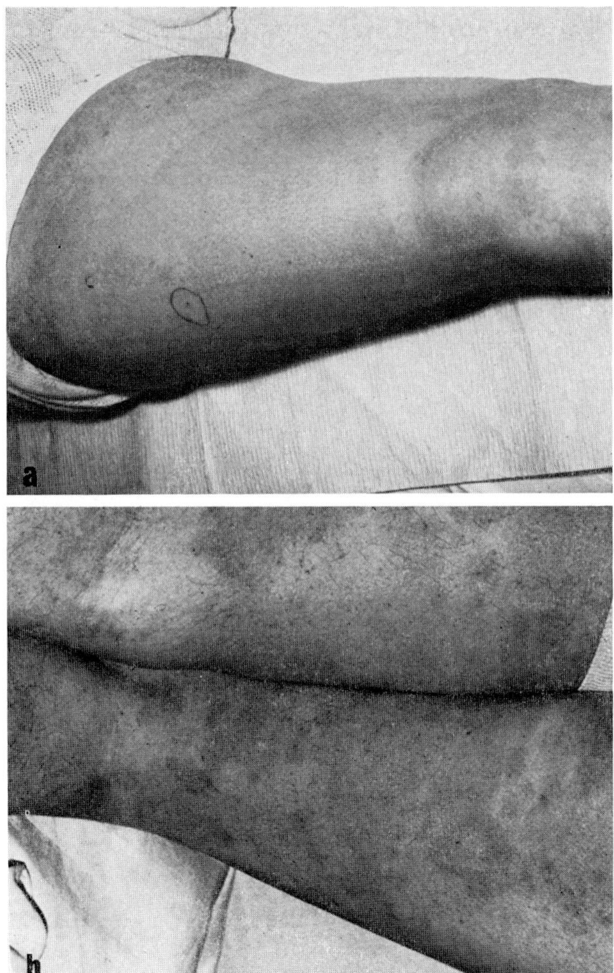

Fig. 2. a: Extensive local allergic reaction to insulin of the immediate type. b: Generalization of the reaction in the same patient after the following injection of insulin

insulin therapy was interrupted because of the introduction of therapy with sulfonylureas. The intensity of the allergic reaction is stronger when insulin is injected into the thigh than when it is injected into points of the upper arm or of the abdominal wall. On the other hand allergic reactions are not tolerated as well in the latter areas. In most cases the symptoms of delayed allergic reactions —

especially the mild forms — subside within a few days or within at least 2—3 weeks. However, longer periods of up to several months or 1 year have also been observed (ARKINS *et al.*, 1962; FEDERLIN, 1971).

The metabolic effect of insulin is little if at all affected by local allergies of the delayed type. Only if the size of the inflamed area reaches a diameter of 5—10 cm, elevated blood glucose levels may occur, probably as a result of local binding of insulin to lymphocytes and/or antibodies.

b) Immediate Local or Generalized Reactions

Immediate type reactions are expressed by local urticaria with itching and swelling, pale redness and occasional vesicles of the epidermis. In contrast to the delayed type allergy, this type occurs not only during the beginning of insulin treatment but also after years of treatment without complications. A very early onset is reported by WALKER (1926), who observed a generalized reaction 3 days after the initial injection.

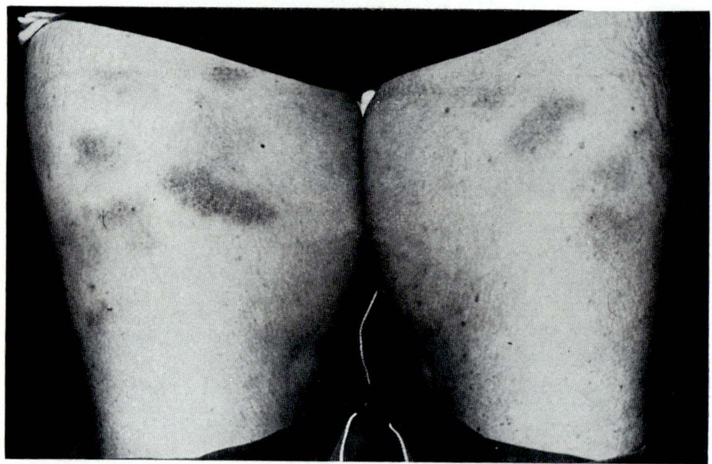

Fig. 3. "Delayed immediate" allergic reaction, difficult to classify, appearance after 6 h, combined with bleeding (mild Arthus reactions ?)

The area affected may reach a few cm in diameter but may also cover 20 cm or almost the whole thigh (Fig. 2a). The onset of the reactions usually starts about 20—30 min after the insulin injection. Continuation of insulin injections may lead to generalized reactions with erythema covering the whole body (Fig. 2b), generalized urticaria, pruritus, Quincke's edema, glottis edema, joint swelling, fever, bronchospasm and serious anaphylactic shock. In cases with marked sensitization such as that which occurs in allergies to other drugs, symptoms of hypersensitivity which require rapid therapeutic measures may also occur within a few minutes. According to our own experiences and pertinent literature, however, such situations — observed for example in allergies to penicillin — are extremely rare in patients allergic to insulin. Considering the large number of patients injecting insulin daily, fatal outcome is extremely rare. A few cases are reported by HANSEN (1957) and by MILLER (1962).

c) Other Types

Clinical experience shows that besides these two main types of allergic reactions there are skin manifestations due to insulin administration which cannot be classified clearly as either delayed or immediate type reactions. Some are characterized by local redness similar to that observed in the true delayed type but mostly less firm and occasionally followed by local bleeding (Fig. 3). In such cases the onset is earlier (4—6 h after injection) and the duration is shorter (12—24 h). DEVLIN (1968) described this type as "delayed immediate reaction". Whether such cases represent mild Arthus phenomena remains open.

True Arthus reactions are described by TUFT (1928), BARTELHEIMER (1952), SCHIRREN (1953), PORTER and HARTMANN (1970), in the latter, combined with lupus erythematosus cell phenomena. — Pigmentation (iron+melanin) of the skin in connection with allergic reactions to insulin was described by SCHEFFLER (1955). —

3. Frequency

Reports on the frequency of allergic reactions reflect a great variability. Furthermore accurate statistics of the true incidence of insulin allergy are difficult to secure because so many factors must be taken into account e.g., different commercial preparations, different species, types of insulin (regular insulin, insulins with retarded absorption of different degrees), clear-cut distinction among the types of reactions and so forth.

According to the survey by GOLDSTEIN (1971), the percentage of insulin allergy reported by different authors ranged from 1.05—55.8%.

ALLAN and SCHERER (1932) reported from a study of 18000 diabetics that 14% of the patients reacted allergically. In contrast PALEY and TUNBRIDGE (1952), on the basis of a survey of 147 patients, gave the figure of 55.8%. MARBLE (1959), from his experience with patients at the Joslin Clinic, stated that perhaps 25—33% of insulin-treated patients observe an allergic reaction once at some time during their treatment. According to MARBLE the number of patients exhibiting allergic symptoms depends mainly on the accuracy of observation, which is in agreement with our own observations. The files of the outpatient service in 1965 indicated that only 3 out of 77 patients evidenced allergic reactions to insulin, while regular personal control of each newly insulin-treated diabetic in 1966 led to a much higher incidence, namely 21 out of 54 (FEDERLIN, 1971).

Among the total number of cases of insulin allergy reported, the majority (81.7%) manifested mild symptoms while the remaining 18.3% showed severe local reactions (PALEY and TUNBRIDGE, 1952).

The authors encountered no generalized symptoms, but it is not known how many local reactions of the immediate type are included. Similarly, ALLAN and SCHERER (1932) reported a percentage of 82 for mild local reactions, 14 for severe local reactions and 4 for generalized reactions. Females seem to be more prone to allergy than males (MARBLE, 1959; DAWEKE, 1968) (65% to 35% according to PALEY and TUNBRIDGE, 1952).

The incidence of generalized reactions is much less frequent. ANDREANI and CORTI (1955) described 3 cases among 1522 insulin-treated diabetics, i.e. 0.2%. HANSEN (1957) estimated that generalized reactions constituted 1% of all the allergic reactions associated with insulin. On the basis of a rough calculation (20—30% allergic reactions in insulin-treated diabetics), this figure would lie approximately in the same range (0.2—0.3% of all insulin-treated diabetics). DEVLIN (1968) suggested a percentage of 0.1, while ALLAN and SCHERER (1932) found that 0.56% of their large number of patients (18,000) suffered from generalized allergic reactions. Interestingly, serious generalized allergic reactions were also observed in a group of non-diabetic psychiatric patients during shock therapy with insulin (DAHL, 1950). Anaphylactic reactions were found in 7 out of 1108 patients (0.6%), all 7 patients were women during menses. According to our own experience, generalized reactions to insulin occur in 0.3—0.4%.

4. Diagnostic Procedures

a) Skin Tests

Many studies have been performed using skin tests as a measure for reactiveness of the organism to insulin itself and to the different additives. The findings are controversial. They can be divided into two categories:

i) comparison of skin reactions between diabetics and healthy controls,

ii) comparison of different insulin preparations in regard to species (beef or pork) of purification and to additives, pH, or substances used for retarded absorption of the hormone (e.g. surfen, protamine, globin).

ad i)

GELFAND *et al.* (1954), using 1—2 units of insulin, and HAGEN *et al.* (1958), using 4 units as the test dose, found positive skin reactions of the immediate type to the same extent in insulin-treated diabetics, untreated diabetics, and healthy controls. Only regular insulin elicited a stronger response in diabetics than in normals (HAGEN *et al.*). WENIG and CALAP (1971), studying 20 nonallergic insulin treated diabetics and 70 healthy controls, had completely negative results using an intradermal skin test with a 10% insulin concentration (no details described).

ARKINS *et al.* (1962) found positive skin tests of the same type in 40 out of 76 insulin-treated patients, in 8 of 43 diabetics who had received no insulin for over 1 year and in 3 of 29 diabetics without any insulin therapy. Of 20 nondiabetic controls only 1 person had a positive skin reaction which was not repeatable. These authors used a dose of 0.16 units for the intradermal skin test, i.e. a concentration 10 times lower than that mentioned by the preceding authors. An even lower concentration was used in our own studies (0.04 units), the results of which are as follows:

Out of 18 nonallergic insulin-treated diabetics, 3 showed wheal and flare reactivity to the test dose, while out of 30 nonallergic healthy persons, none showed skin reactivity to insulin or additives (FEDERLIN *et al.*, unpublished).

ad ii)

Other studies concerned the influence of recrystallization, of the animal species used as the source of insulin and of the pH of the preparation used. In a study of 56 healthy controls and 84 nonallergic diabetics, HAGEN *et al.* (1958) found a more intense skin response to insulins from HOECHST Ltd. than to those from the NOVO Company, but they did not include information concerning what species-type of insulin was used for therapy in the cases studied. In order to clarify the role of the different possible factors, HAGEN and HAGEN (1959) examined healthy control persons and found that the size of testurtica and erythema was influenced only by the number of recrystallizations of the different insulins. Insulins recrystallized many times caused a weaker skin response than insulins recrystallized only once. The authors excluded any influence of the pH (2.8 versus 7.4) or of the buffer and the additives. On the other hand BERMONT (1967), using a test dose of 4 units, stated on the basis of a study in 150 nonallergic diabetics that skin reactivity of a nonallergic nature (so-called orthergy) was independent of the source of species but that solutions with acid or alkaline pH elicited enlarged skin reactions. However there was no information regarding the type of insulin used for pretreatment.

Recently LIEBERMAN *et al.* (1971) reported detailed examinations of 5 patients with immediate type allergy to insulin. Using 4 units of insulin or less as test doses, all 5 patients exhibited positive skin reactions to beef, pork, desalanated pork, sheep, human, chromatographically purified beef and synthetic insulin. All were most reactive to beef insulin and least reactive to human, sheep and synthetic. Pretreatment was done with beef-pork insulin (4 cases) or beef insulin (1 case). Of 50 nonallergic diabetics, 20 showed positive skin reactions (wheal and erythema). In 19 out of 20 patients the insulin being used for therapy produced positive results. Beef insulin purified by chromatography caused reactions in only 4 out of 20 subjects. This insulin and human insulin elicited the least reaction of the different varieties used (see above). Similar results were obtained in our own studies (FEDERLIN *et al.*, in press, 1974). Among 14 diabetics who developed allergy during treatment with bovine insulin (4 with delayed type, 10 with immediate type), there was no significant difference in skin reactivity using solutions of neutral or acid insulins. Furthermore all patients with immediate type allergy showed equal reactions to bovine and to porcine insulin. Chromatographically purified beef insulin led to positive results in 3 patients (3/10), indicating that one third of the patients had developed allergy against material which was removed by chromatography. All patients were pretreated with bovine insulin.

In conclusion it can be said that the value of skin tests in insulin immunology is limited and restricted to certain situations. There is no doubt that in patients with pronounced allergic reactions after injection of insulin, intradermal tests with the different components of the insulin preparations will help to clarify the role of species or of other factors in the induction of the immune response (KERP *et al.*, 1965; FEDERLIN *et al.*, 1966; DAWEKE, 1968; WENIG and CALAP, 1971; LIEBERMAN *et al.*, 1971). They may also help to distinguish clearly immediate type reactions from delayed reactions (Fig. 4) and indicate cross reactivity between the antibodies present and insulin from different species.

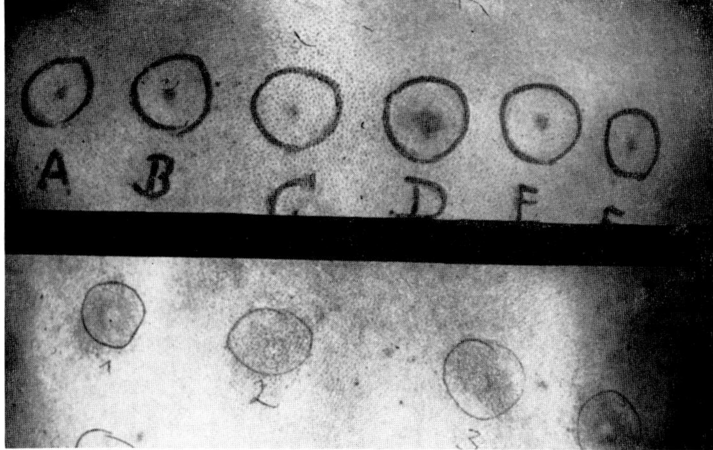

Fig. 4. Skin tests in insulin allergy: above: 24 h reactions in a patient with delayed allergy to insulin, below: 30 reactions in a patient with immediate type allergy to insulin

On the other hand, skin tests have also been found to be positive in a number of nonallergic insulin-treated diabetics and in patients with insulin resistance. There is only a weak correlation between the outcome of the skin test and the definite degree of hypersensitivity to insulin insofar as pronounced hypersensitivity of the immediate type causes regularly marked test reactions while mild reactions cannot be taken as an expression of clinical intolerance of the insulin used. In such cases it might be suggested that very low concentrations of skin-sensitizing antibodies are present which are not even clinically relevant.

For the test dose different amounts of insulin were used (from 4 to 0.04 units). To avoid the risk of anaphylactic shock, low doses are recommended in all cases suspected of immediate type allergy. Thus according to KERP *et al.* (1965) and to our experiences, a concentration of 0.04 units in 0.02 ml was found to be suitable for patients with either a low or a high degree of hypersensitivity.

b) Laboratory Findings (Cytological and Serological Studies)

α) Delayed allergic reaction

Using the skin test as a tool for measuring delayed hypersensitivity, McDEVITT (1964) demonstrated for the first time that sensitization of guinea pigs with insulin in incomplete Freuud's adjuvant resulted in typical reactions. CLARK and MUNOZ (1970) performed skin tests in guinea pigs with delayed hypersensitivity to insulin in order to compare the antigen-reactivity of sensitized lymphocytes with that of humoral antibodies in the search for antigen determinants.

In humans several attempts have been made to apply *in vitro* methods for the demonstration of delayed hypersensitivity. Antigen induced lymphocyte transformation was found in 6 patients with delayed allergic reactions to insulin and in 2 patients with the immediate form (FEDERLIN, KRIEGBAUM and FLAD, 1968). In 1967 already HALPERN, KY and AMACHE reported of two cases with generalized urticaria after insulin injections which showed lymphocyte transformation *in vitro* after adding of insulin Other investigations are based on the assumption that antigen-binding of sensitized lymphocytes indicates the state of cell-mediated immunity, i.e. delayed hypersensitivity (type IV reaction of COOMBS and GELL, 1968). Thus KERP *et al.* 1965) demonstrated binding of radioactive insulin to white blood cells in a case of severe local delayed allergy to insulin. FREI *et al.* (1965) found rosette formation between insulin-coated red cells and blood lymphocytes in a similar case. FEDERLIN *et al.* (1966) used immunofluorescence and immune adherence for the demonstration of antigen-binding to circulating white blood cells. In light of the new concepts of T- and B-lymphocytes, these findings probably were an expression of beginning antibody production, because B-cells (bone marrow-derived lymphocytes) which are capable of antigen-binding as mentioned previously are the precursors of plasma cells.

Nevertheless there is some evidence from experimental work for the assumption that the delayed allergic reactions to insulin in diabetics during the beginning of treatment may represent a state of delayed hypersensitivity. The occurrence of delayed allergic reactions of the skin after daily injections of small amounts of proteins in experimental animals — the so-called Jones-Mote-phenomenon (JONES and MOTE, 1934) — can be taken as a reliable parallel to delayed allergy in diabetics. —

Furthermore delayed hypersensitivity to insulin can be demonstrated *in vitro* with migration inhibition tests of peritoneal macrophages in guinea pigs (FEDERLIN *et al.*, 1969).

β) Immediate type allergy

Until recently the demonstration of reaginic antibodies as the underlying mechanism was possible only by *in vivo* methods. Therefore in the past the Prausnitz-Küstner technique (PRAUSNITZ and KÜSTNER, 1921) was used also in cases of insulin allergy. But because the use of human skin (i.e. the skin of another person) for this test was ethically dubious (risk of infection), later on the skin of other primates such as rhesus monkeys was used in the so-called allergic serum transfer test (LAYTON *et al.*, 1962). This technique could be employed also in cases with insulin allergy (FEDERLIN and GIGLI, 1968; FEDERLIN, 1971). Antibody was injected intracutaneously, and 48 h later antigen was given intravenously together with a dye. At the site of reaction the skin was colored within minutes. To avoid hypoglycemic shock which could interfere with the immunological reaction, insulin was made biologically inactive before use[1]. Recently also *in vitro* methods have been developed which permit demonstration of IgE-anti-insulin antibodies. PATTERSON *et al.* (1969) found localization of the anti-insulin reaginic antibody to an immunoglobulin other than G, A, M or D, presumably E. The antibody reacted only against extracted insulin including autologous insulin and not against endogenous circulating insulin. Shortly thereafter DOLOVICH *et al.* (1970) were able to demonstrate by the radioimmunodiffusion test the presence of IgE antibodies to bovine insulin in a patient with generalized allergic reactions. PATTERSON *et al.* (1973) in a detailed study described the use of radioimmunodiffusion and polystyrene tube immunoabsorbent assay in patients with immediate type allergy to insulin and in one case with combined IgE and IgG insulin resistance. Insulin binding by IgE correlated with the clinical state and declined with the Prausnitz-

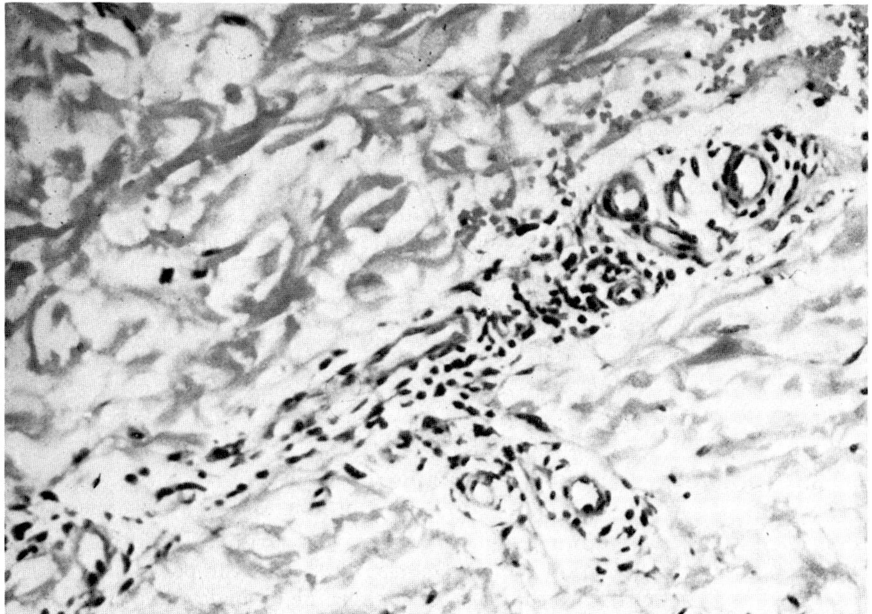

Fig. 5. Skin biopsy of a patient with local delayed allergy to insulin taken 24 h after insulin injection: perivascular lymphocytic infiltrates, HE-staining

1 Gift from Dr. Mager (Farbwerke Hoechst Ltd.).

Küstner titer of patients' sera. IgE-antibodies cross reacted with different insulins to a greater extent than did the IgG antibodies of patients with immunologic insulin resistance. The bovine "single component" insulin almost completely inhibited IgE or IgG binding of ^{125}I-insulin and provided the maximal inhibition of the binding activity for bovine insulin in the test system. — Very recently FEDERLIN and VELCOVSKY (1974) reported the measurement of insulin-specific JgE-antibodies using insulin-sepharose and the radio immunosorbent-test (Rist).

c) Histological Examinations

Little is known about the morphological changes in the skin during a state of delayed allergy to insulin. HAGEN and HAGEN (1962) studied the skin lesions of patients histologically by successive biopsies. Initially they found perivascular infiltrations of the "round cell" type and 3—4 weeks later, a granulomatous inflammation.

FEDERLIN (1971) also observed perivascular lymphocytic infiltrates resembling those of the tuberculin-type reaction in a few patients shortly after the onset of the clinical symptoms (Fig. 5). Other patients with longer-lasting allergic symptoms of the delayed type showed granulomatous inflammatory changes, thus confirming the findings of HAGEN and HAGEN in their studies of the same patients. — RENOLD *et al.* (1969) examined the skin of insulin-sensitized sheep after intradermal injections of an antigen test dose. They found perivascular mononuclear cell infiltrations and, using immunofluorescent techniques no indications of the presence of humoral antibodies.

5. Pathogenesis and Classification

On the basis of the pathogenetic mechanisms which are discussed in section 4 b d, β, insulin allergy can be classified according to the scheme of COOMBS and GELL (1968) (Fig. 6). The local or generalized reactions of the immediate type resemble type I reaction. Circulating antigen (= insulin) combines with reaginic antibody fixed on mast cells, which results in liberation of histamine and other vasoactive amines. Complement is not involved. — The true delayed allergic reaction represents type IV reaction. Here sensitized lymphocytes react with antigen (= insulin at the injection site) without the participation of humoral antibodies. — Type III reaction due to immune complexes, i.e. Arthus reaction or serum sickness-like syndromes, may occur in the classical sense only in rare cases (see I.C.). It is not known whether skin reactions which do not fulfill the criteria of a type IV reaction because of different time relations, represent mild Arthus phenomena. Finally, type II reaction caused by so-called cytotoxic antibodies has as yet not been proven to exist in insulin allergy. One might only speculate whether these antibodies could play a role in lipodystrophy, though this lesion is also associated with the delayed type allergy (see below). —

6. Concepts of Etiology

a) Immunogenicity of Insulin and the Role of Proinsulin and Insulin-Related Proteins

For a long time no immunogenic properties were attributed to insulin itself. Up to the present this question remains controversial. In the past hormones were not regarded as antigens due to their species-unspecific biological activity. Furthermore compared with other proteins insulin is a small molecule.

Greater insight was achieved with the determination of the chemical structures of different insulins by SANGER (1960). Those mammalian insulins whose structures have been determined demonstrate that the molecules differ in the amino

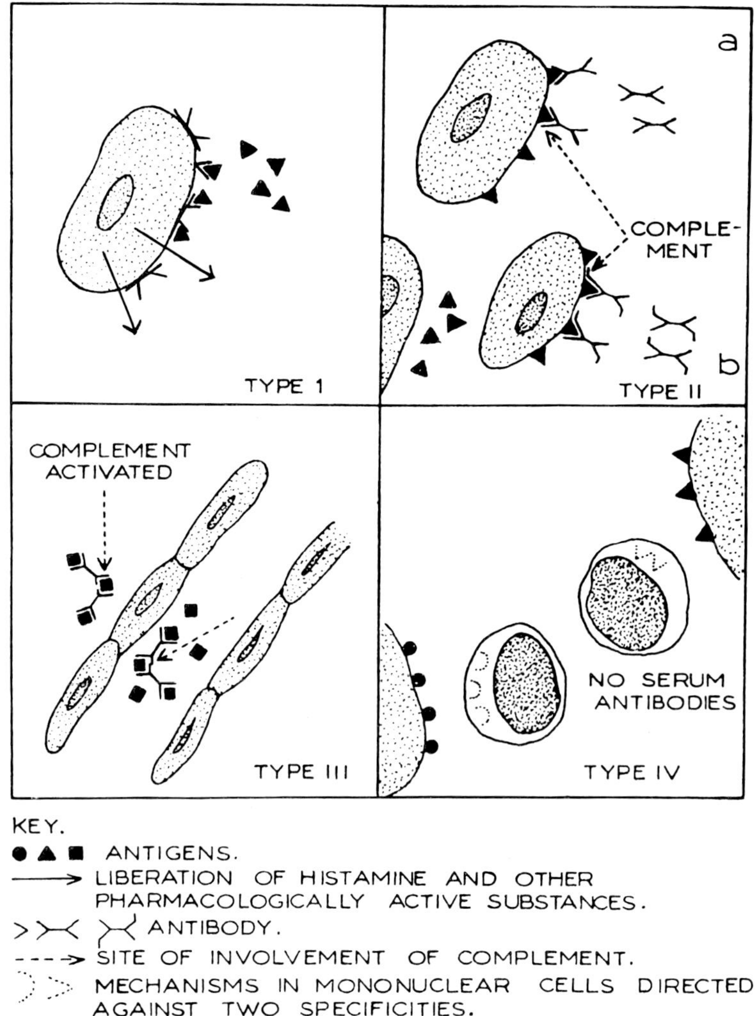

Fig. 6. Classification of allergic reactions according to COOMBS and GELL (1968). Type I. Free antigen reacting with antibody passively sensitizing (allergizing) cell surface. Type II. Antibody reacting with (a) cell surface or (b) with antigen or hapten which becomes attached to cell surface: complement plays a major destructive role. Type III. Antigen and antibody reacting in antigen excess forming complexes which, possibly with the aid of complement, are toxic to cells. Type IV. Specifically modified mononuclear cells (actively allergized cells) reacting with allergen or antigen deposited at a local site

acid sequence at positions 4, 8, 9, 10 of the A chain and positions 3, 29, 30 of the B chain (Fig. 7). It became clear that porcine insulin differs to a lesser degree in its chemical structure to human insulin than bovine because of its variance in only one amino acid (alanin instead of thyreonin at position 30 of the B chain). For a long while it was assumed that antibody production in human diabetics was elicited because of these differences in primary structure. BERSON and YALOW (1963), however, showed that also porcine insulin effected antibody production in diabetics even when the terminal amino acid was separated from the molecule. Somewhat

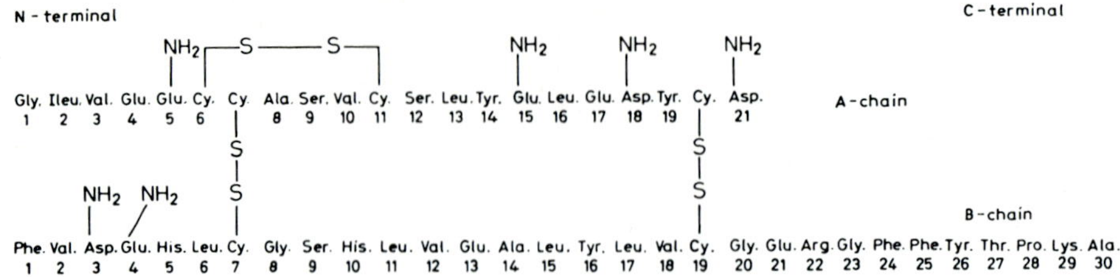

Sequence of aminoacids of insulin from different species

	A-chain				B-chain		
	4	8	9	10	3	29	30
Cattle	Glu	Ala	Ser	Val	Asp.NH_2	Lys	Ala
Sheep	Glu	Ala	Gly	Val	Asp.NH_2	Lys	Ala
Horse	Glu	Thr	Gly	Ileu	Asp.NH_2	Lys	Ala
Pig	Glu	Thr	Ser	Ileu	Asp.NH_2	Lys	Ala
Whale	Glu	Thr	Ser	Ileu	Asp.NH_2	Lys	Ala
Dog	Glu	Thr	Ser	Ileu	Asp.NH_2	Lys	Ala
Man	Glu	Thr	Ser	Ileu	Asp.NH_2	Lys	Thr
Rabbit	Glu	Thr	Ser	Ileu	Asp.NH_2	Lys	Ser
Rat	Asp	Thr	Ser	Ileu	Lys	Lys	Ser

Fig. 7. Sequence of amino acids of ox insulin and variations in different species

later, an unexpected immunogenicity of insulin was demonstrated in cattle and sheep (Renold *et al.*, 1964; Renold *et al.*, 1969). Subcutaneous injections of homologous insulin produced antibody response and severe lesions of the islets of Langerhans. The explanation was sought in differences of the spatial configuration of endogenous secreted insulin and extracted hormone. Other reasons of antibody production against insulin were seen in "impurities" (Brunfeldt, 1966) or in deamidation (Berson and Yalow, 1966) of acid insulins which may occur during prolonged storage in the cold. Since it is recognized that proteins which are less readily soluble possess stronger immunologic properties than more soluble proteins, suspicion even fell upon the acidity of injectable insulin (Deckert, 1966). The hormone in this preparation precipitates within the tissue at the injection site. Clinicians have repeatedly mentioned that antibody production leading to increased requirement of insulin or allergy to insulin is somewhat more frequent in patients treated with acid solutions of insulin than in those trated with neutral insulin. Nevertheless it is very difficult to draw binding conclusions because species differences of these insulins often interfere with the observations. In order to overcome such problems, animal experiments were performed. Perings (1973) immunized guinea pigs daily with small amounts of insulin. Skin tests were used as the parameter for the immune response. He found that immunogenicity of the different insulins was slightly higher in acid compared with neutral, in intermediate compared with rapid and in slow compared with intermediate insulins. The main finding was that insulins with delayed absorption were more immunogenic than those with rapid absorption. This was to be expected because the processing of antigen by macrophages is enhanced when antigen is in a particular form or slowly liberated from a depot.

After the discovery by Steiner (1967) of proinsulin as the precursor of the hormone, interest was again focused on "impurities" as the main cause of antibody production against the injected insulin. Extending their studies of the biosynthesis of insulin by islet-cell tumors, Steiner and his co-workers (Steiner and Oyer, 1967; Steiner *et al.*, 1967) demonstrated that insulin is formed from a precursor of higher molecular weight (proinsulin), which consists of a single polypeptide chain (see Fig. 8) beginning with the N terminal of the B chain and continuing through the so-called "connecting peptide" to the N terminal of the A chain. The task of proinsulin in the cell appears to be to facilitate the formation of disulfide bonds (STEINER and CLARK, 1968). It can be found in small amounts in the serum of normal and obese subjects (MELANI *et al.*, 1970a) and in diabetic patients (RUBENSTEIN *et al.*, 1968). Also the C-peptide portion of proinsulin is secreted along with insulin and circulates in the blood. Proinsulin has been identified in insulin preparations from cattle, pig, rat and human pancreas. It amounts to (on the average) about 2% of the total protein of the preparation investigated (STEINER *et al.*, 1968). By further separation studies, SCHLICHTKRULL and his group (SCHLICHTKRULL, 1970) isolated several insulin-related proteins within 3 fractions (fraction a: material from exocrine pancreas, an as yet uncharacterized substance; fraction b: proinsulin, intermediate, dimer (non-convertible fraction); fraction c: insulin, arginin insulin, insulin ester, desamidoinsulin.

On the assumption that only the hormone insulin itself, C-peptide and small amounts of proinsulin are secreted by the B cell, it follows that injection of extracted (crystalline) insulin introduces substances to which the homologous

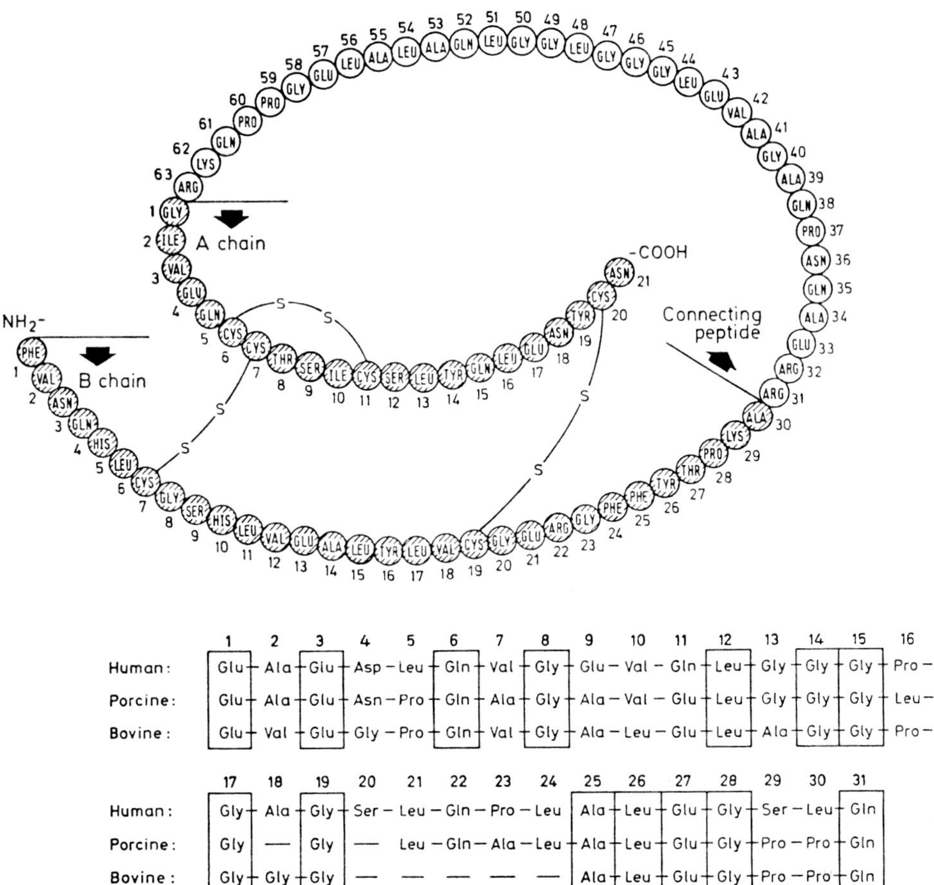

	1	2	3	4	5	6	7	8	9	10	11	12	13	14	15	16
Human:	Glu	Ala	Glu	Asp	Leu	Gln	Val	Gly	Glu	Val	Gln	Leu	Gly	Gly	Gly	Pro
Porcine:	Glu	Ala	Glu	Asn	Pro	Gln	Ala	Gly	Ala	Val	Glu	Leu	Gly	Gly	Gly	Leu
Bovine:	Glu	Val	Glu	Gly	Pro	Gln	Val	Gly	Ala	Leu	Glu	Leu	Ala	Gly	Gly	Pro

	17	18	19	20	21	22	23	24	25	26	27	28	29	30	31
Human:	Gly	Ala	Gly	Ser	Leu	Gln	Pro	Leu	Ala	Leu	Glu	Gly	Ser	Leu	Gln
Porcine:	Gly	—	Gly	—	Leu	Gln	Ala	Leu	Ala	Leu	Glu	Gly	Pro	Pro	Gln
Bovine:	Gly	Gly	Gly	—	—	—	—	—	Ala	Leu	Glu	Gly	Pro	Pro	Gln

Fig. 8. Amino acid sequence of porcine proinsulin (from SHAW and CHANCE, 1968) and primary structures of human, porcine and bovine C-peptides. (From MELANI *et al.*, 1970b)

organism would be expected to have no immunological tolerance. Thus antibody formation to "insulin" may be more directed against the insulin-related proteins than against the essential hormone. This would explain why antibody formation to bovine insulin can be stimulated in cattle (Renold *et al.*, 1964), to porcine insulin in pigs (Brunfeldt and Deckert, 1964), to bovine insulin in sheep (Renold *et al.*, 1965) and even to human insulin in humans (Deckert and Grundahl, 1970). In the heterologous system antibody formation bases on the different primary structure of insulin but may be enhanced by the discrepancy in the chemical structure of proinsulin. Yet immunization studies in guinea pigs showed that the immunogenicity of proinsulin compared with that of insulin was not very different (Wright and Makulu, 1969; Federlin, 1970; Kerp *et al.*, 1970b). On the other hand rabbits immunized with small doses (40 μg) of crystalline ox-proinsulin formed antibodies which were able to bind insulin to a considerably greater extent than was possible in animals immunized with the same dose dose of 4 $\times$ crystallized bovine insulin (Schlichtkrull *et al.*, 1972). Pure monocomponent insulin did not evoke antibody formation in these animals. The a-component was particularly antigenic.

Investigations of the immunogenic role of proinsulin in patients treated with commercial insulin led to contradictory results. Ditschuneit *et al.* (1970) showed preferential binding of the antibodies in serum to proinsulin. Hinke *et al.* (1970) found higher concentrations of antibody-binding sites to insulin than to proinsulin in patients treated with bovine insulin. Further studies by this group and by others (Kumar and Miller, 1973) did not confirm the hypothesis that proinsulin in commercial insulin preparations is the essential stimulus for antibody production (Kerp *et al.*, 1970a; Kerp, 1971) and for increased insulin requirement.

In the meantime, greater importance of the immunogenicity of crystalline insulin has been attributed to the so-called a-component, i.e. substances from the exocrine part of the pancreas. The concept is that some of the a-component contain immuno-reactive insulin-like sites inducing antibodies which also react with the hormone (Schlichtkrull, 1974). While Schlichtkrull and his group studied rabbits, Wright and Gingerich (1973) using guinea pigs reported completely different results. They concluded that either the antibodies induced by the a-component differ from those induced by insulin but crossreact weakly with the hormone, or that insulin is more immunogenic than the a-component in guinea pigs.

In general it is agreed that purification of crystalline insulin from the different "impurities" reduces or even abolishes immunogenicity of the injected hormone. Thus in attempts to treat patients with allergy to commercially available insulin, Galloway and Root (1972) found that the "single component" insulin of porcine origin (Root *et al.*, 1972) containing 99 % pure insulin was usually but not always superior to "single peak" insulin containing 99% insulin-like material (comprised of "pure" insulin, desamidoinsulin, arginine insulin, esterified insulin) and 1% noninsulin.

A great part of what was called "allergy to insulin" in the past may actually have been allergy against impurities; nevertheless there is evidence — at least for neutralizing antibodies — that the pure hormone can be also immunogenic (Fankhauser and Michl, 1973; Czyzyk *et al.*, 1974). Therefore, species differences which still exist, i.e., porcine insulin is less immunogenic in man than bovine, will also play a role in the future.

Finally, there are other factors independent of source of insulin, pH, additives etc., which may enhance immunogenicity of insulin. Superficial injections which do not reach the subcutaneous area increase the tendency toward allergic responses. An even more important factor is the interruption of insulin therapy for any reason whatsoever. In such cases, the initial period of exposure may serve to sensitize the individual while the second course of therapy represents an anamnestic response (GOLDSTEIN, 1971). —

b) Antigenic Determinants of the Insulin Molecule

Several studies have been concerned with the antigenic determinants, i.e. the sites of insertion of antibodies. WILSON (1969) demonstrated that guinea pig antibodies to bovine insulin reacted with determinants within the region A_{10-16}, B_{1-8}, B_{23-30}.

The situation has become more complicated since the discovery of proinsulin and insulin-related proteins. KERP (1971) concluded from experiments in guinea pigs that one half of the total concentration of antibodies with high affinity inserted specifically at the insulin part of the proinsulin molecule. The other half of this type of antibody found its specific insertion on the C-chain of proinsulin. Antibodies with low affinity were found to be specific only for the insulin part of the molecule.

Studies in diabetics disclosed that the last 8 amino acids of the B chain carry antigenic determinants (PATTERSON *et al.*, 1973). Porcine desoctapeptide insulin was less inhibitory to the reaction of antibody against bovine insulin than against porcine insulin. Furthermore inhibition of the bovine insulin — anti-insulin reaction by A and B chains of bovine insulin was minimal, indicating the importance of the insulin molecule in its entirety, thus providing the antigenic determinants against which the human antibodies are directed.

It must also be taken into account that antigenic determinants of insulin may differ in respect to the antibody type, for example IgG or IgE (see section VII.). —

7. Relationship to Insulin Resistance

The simultaneous occurrence of insulin allergy and insulin resistance has been repeatedly reported since the beginning of insulin therapy (GLASSBERG *et al.*, 1927; RUDY, 1931; GOLDNER and RICKETTS, 1942; SHERMAN, 1950; ENGBRING *et al.*, 1962). Exact figures regarding the frequency of incidence are not available, but it seems to be not too rare. SHIPP *et al.* (1965) examined the details in cases with insulin resistance and found that in one third of 34 cases insulin allergy preceded insulin resistance. It is not known from all cases described what type of allergy developed, but it seems that both immediate and delayed allergic reactions were observed. Very close relationships were described in detail by KERP *et al.* (1965), FREI *et al.* (1965) and FEDERLIN *et al.* (1966). Here, the first symptoms were marked delayed allergic reactions which in one case were even followed by immediate type allergy finally resulting in insulin resistance. Recently DOLOVICH *et al.* (1970) and PATTERSON *et al.* (1973) described in detail several cases of simultaneous occurrence of insulin allergy of the immediate type and insulin resistance. The latter found marked differences between reactivity of IgE antibodies with the different insulins, more so than with IgG antibodies. This indicates different antigenic determinants at the insulin molecule for both types of antibodies.

A relationships between allergy of the delayed type and production of humoral antibodies was also found in experimental animals. HEINEMANN *et al.* (1969) observed that antibody titer was highest in those animals whose "delayed hypersensitivity" against insulin was most pronounced (tested by migration inhibition test with peritoneal macrophages).

8. Relationship to Lipodystrophy

Despite the fact that the real cause of lipodystrophy is still unknown, evidence is being accumulated which favors at least partially immunological factors. Histological examinations of affected skin regions have revealed inflammatory changes [perivascular infiltrates consisting mainly of lymphocytes, eosinophils (Poulsen, 1967; Federlin, 1972)] similar to those observed in delayed allergic reactions. Furthermore lipoatrophy is frequently preceded by local allergy of the delayed type (Kerp and Kasemir, 1973), or at least by "dermal reactions", as stated by Paley as early as 1953.

9. Treatment

a) Delayed Allergic Reaction

The occurrence of mild allergic reactions raises the question of whether the injections are made deeply enough, i.e. into the subcutaneous tissue, since a superficial injection increases the tendency to allergy; apart from that, most cutaneous reactions which do not exceed a moderate degree of intensity tend to regress spontaneously. Therefore the best method in treating this type of allergy consists simply of continuing the administration. This spontaneous desensitization may take several weeks. Only in rare cases does the intensity of the reaction increase, leading to great discomfort and eventually also to retarded absorption of insulin. In such cases it is necessary to change the insulin preparation to one from another species. Furthermore it is recommended that intradermal skin tests be performed in order to detect allergic reactions which are directed against additives of the insulin charges. Because evidence exists that the allergy may be caused by impurities (see 6.), change to chromatographically purified insulin might be successful if "commercial" insulin was used previously (Galloway and Root, 1972; Kerp and Kasemir, 1973; Bruni *et al.*, 1973; Korp and Levett, 1973; Federlin, 1972). A change to insulin from another species is necessary only if allergic symptoms continue. In most cases this means a change from beef to pig insulin, although the reversed situation may occur (Burkart *et al.*, 1963; Federlin *et al.*, 1966).

In the case of cross reactivity between different species as alternate methods, the injection of small amounts of antihistamines along with insulin is recommended (Goldstein, 1971) as well as hydrocortisone (2 mg along with insulin, according to Cockel and Mann, 1967). According to the author's own experience, which corresponds to that reported in the literature, local delayed allergy to insulin, in almost all instances, could be controlled by one of these measures. More complications arise with the immediate type allergy to insulin.

b) Immediate Allergic Reactions

The more severe local or generalized immediate allergic responses to insulin require completely different management because of serious dangers such as anaphylactic shock. Here continuation of therapy which was recommended for the delayed allergic reaction may be fatal. Skin tests using very small amounts (0.04 U) may clarify doubtful cases.

The following scheme is recommended:

α) Hypoglycemic agents

Sudden interruption of exogenous insulin and use of endogenous insulin by giving oral hypoglycemic agents with or without starvation especially in obese diabetics.

β) Change of insulin

If exogenous insulin is required, a skin test will indicate whether chromatographically purified insulin of the same or of another species will be tolerated, although there is no absolute parallelism between skin test and tolerance of therapeutic doses. Because of the frequent occurrence of cross reactions, the continuation of therapy, also with purified insulin of another species, may not be possible due to preformed antibodies. In such cases oral or parenteral administration of steroids in greater amounts (50—100 mg/day) may become necessary for a few days. The high daily catabolic rate of IgE (70% according to WALDMAN *et al.*, 1973) supports the therapeutic measure. Nevertheless also purified insulins may stimulate antibody production (which may be caused either by small amounts of impurities still present or by the pure hormone itself) as observed in one of our own cases (FEDERLIN *et al.*, in prepar.).

γ) Desensitization

Desensitization as a possible treatment has been recommended by several authors and with different techniques, from the early times of insulin therapy up to the present (BAYER, 1934; BAKER, 1936; CORCORAN, 1938; HEROLD, 1938; ULRICH *et al.*, 1939; WOLF, 1962; STROHFELDT, 1969; LIEBERMAN *et al.*, 1971; BLUM *et al.*, 1972). Different time intervals between the single doses were described. The scheme of the Joslin clinic starts with 1/1000 unit of insulin (GOLDSTEIN, 1971). If no reaction occurs, the dose is doubled at each succeeding injection. When no emergency exists, four doses are given daily, i.e. day 1: 1/1000, 1/500, 1/250, 1/125 unit, on day 2: 1/100, 1/50, 1/25, 1/12, day 3: 1/5, 1/2, 1, 2 units. The success of desensitization trials is variable. While the reports from the Joslin clinic (GOLDSTEIN, 1971) and from LIEBERMAN *et al.* (1971) describe tolerance of therapeutic doses in most patients after desensitization, the author's own experiences are less favorable. KERP and KASEMIR (1973) express a warning, because desensitization may lead to insulin resistance. It is noteworthy that also after successful desensitization, allergic reactions may recur; therefore insulin therapy should not be discontinued in an effort to prevent such a possibility. Several attempts were made to change the insulin molecule in order to eliminate antigenic determinants. KREINES (1965) was able to treat patients with immediate allergy against insulin successfully with desalinated insulin, MENCZEL *et al.* (1966), with sulfated insulin. Later KREINES (1971) reported successful treatment with sheep insulin.

δ) Other measures

In extreme cases, the method of DOLGER (1952) using boiled insulin may be tried. The purpose of this procedure (heating at 100° for 30 min) is to destroy antigenic determinants of the insulin molecule but to preserve the biological activity, although LOVELESS (1958) found that the ability of insulin heated to 100° for 1—4 h to induce wheal reactions did not differ from that of unboiled insulin. According to NICHOLS (1955) and our own experiences in one case, it might prove successful. However it is very difficult to obtain enough samples of insulin which fulfill the needed criteria, i.e. it may become necessary to examine different boiled charges of insulin until the wanted insulin is found.

Similar attempts to change the chemical configuration of insulin while preserving its biological activity were reproted recently by KATSILAMBROS (1973). He successfully used phenylated (5% phenol-treated) insulin in 18 patients with insulin allergy and with a history of anaphylactic shock. Formalin-treated insulin did not retain its hypoglycemic effect. —

II. "Cellular" Antibodies and Insulitis

The injection of insulin in man and animals may elicit not only the production of humoral antibodies of different types but may also be associated with the state of delayed hypersensitivity. The underlying principle (basis) for this type of immune response is found in sensitized lymphocytes (T-lymphocytes), which were mentioned briefly in section IV 2 a.

The T-cells are antigen-sensitive and are thought to recognize their surface. The allergic reaction is probably initiated by antigen, which may be associated with or processed by a macrophage, combining with the immunoglobulin-like receptors on the surface of appropriate T-lymphocytes present as memory cells following an earlier sensitization process (ROITT, 1972). The term "cellular" antibodies is not quite correct, because no complete antibodies have as yet been detected on the surface of sensitized lymphocytes. But the term may be used loosely to distinguish this type of immune reaction from humoral antibodies which consist of well-defined immunoglobulins.

Cell-mediated hypersensitivity to insulin is not only known from allergic skin reactions in diabetics or animals but seems to play an important role in experimental insulitis. RENOLD and his group immunized sheep with bovine or porcine insulin in incomplete Freund's adjuvant and produced not only circulating antibodies to insulin but also lymphocytic infiltration of the islets of Langerhans (Fig. 9). Intracutaneous injections of antigen led to pronounced delayed hypersensitivity reactions (FEDERLIN *et al.*, 1968; RENOLD *et al.*, 1969). Chronic insulitis with mononuclear infiltration of the islets was also induced in rabbits (GRODSKY *et al.*, 1966; TORESON *et al.*, 1964), but no skin tests have been performed.

Nevertheless much evidence exists for the assumption that in this type of an autoimmune process as in other similar conditions, sensitized lymphocytes are primarily responsible for the lesions. LEE *et al.* (1969) observed electonmicroscopically in these animals that lymphocytes inserted pseudopods between islet cells,

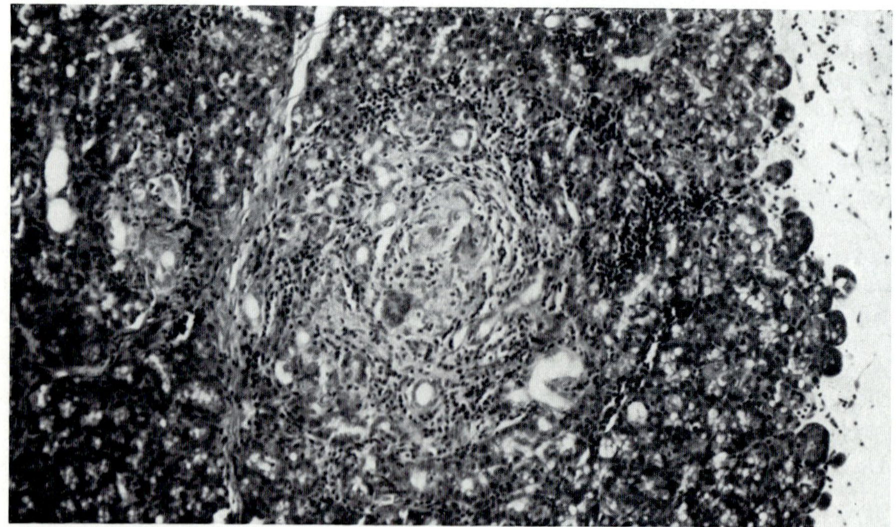

Fig. 9. Lymphocytic infiltration of islets (insulitis) in a sheep immunized with porcine insulin and incomplete Freund's adjuvant. HE-staining

making close contact, and that many beta cells lost their cell membranes, releasing their cytoplasmic contents into the surrounding intercellular spaces. Because immunofluorescent studies of the inflamed area for the demonstration of humoral antibodies produced negative results, it is likely that the infiltrating mononuclear cells were sensitized lymphocytes with cytotoxic activity.

Recently, lymphocytic infiltrates of different degrees in the endocrine and exocrine pancreas (periductulitis, periinsulitis, insulitis) could be induced in mice with once crystallized or chromatographed insulin (FREYTAG *et al.*, 1973; JANSEN and FREYTAG, 1973). The authors suggest that this insulitis, a type of cellular immune reactions, may not be induced by true SANGER insulin but by an antigenically independent antigen contained in crystalline insulin or an antigenically related derivative of insulin. In extension of these studies, relationships between insulitis, intracutaneous skin tests, antibody titer and decreased glucose tolerance were studied in rabbits immunized with bovine insulin (KLÖPPEL *et al.*, 1973). The authors found positive skin reactions to insulin and an insulitis in 30—60% of their animals. Intensity of skin reaction did not in all cases parallel insulitis. Development of a diabetic syndrome seemed to be correlated with high antibody titers to insulin. The authors concluded that insulitis is elicited by an antigen which differs from that which is responsible for a positive skin reaction and circulating antibodies (insulin-like contaminant probably associated with the crude proinsulin fraction). —

Whether lymphocytic insulitis in human diabetics as well as in animals with spontaneous diabetes represents the expression of cell-mediated hypersensitivity against insulin or against another product of the islet tissue or represents the consequence of viral infection must remain open at the present time. —

References

ALLAN, F.N., SCHERER, L.R.: Insulin allergy. Endocrinology **16**, 417 (1932)

ANDREANI, G., CORTI, L.: Allergy to insulin: Statistical study of 1,500 diabetics. J. Amer. med. Ass. **157**, 184 (1955)

ARKINS, J.A., ENGBRING, N.H., LENNON, E.J.: The incidence of skin reactivity to insulin in diabetic patients. J. Allergy **33**, 69 (1962)

BAKER, T.W.: A clinical survey of 108 consecutive cases of diabetic coma. Arch. intern. Med. **58**, 373 (1936)

BARTELHEIMER, H.: Insulinbedingte Hautnekrosen bei einem Diabetiker. Schweiz. med. Wschr. **82**, 573 (1952)

BAYER, L.M.: Desensitization to insulin allergy. J. Amer. med. Ass. **102** (1934)

BERMONT, A.: Sensibilité du derme aux préparations d'insuline. Thèse, 3ième partie, Nancy, 1967

BERSON, S.A., YALOW, R.S.: Antigens in insulin. Determination of specificity of porcine insulin in man. Science **139**, 844 (1963)

BERSON, S.A., YALOW, R.S.: Deamidation of insulin during storage in frozen state. Diabetes **15**, 875 (1966)

BLUM, H.J., TEMPE, D., DE LA HARPE, F., MANTZ, J.M., STEPHAN, F.: Allergie a l'insuline et cuve de desensibilisation accélérée chez deux diabétiques. J. Méd. **2**, 125 (1972)

BOULIN, R., LAPRESLE, CL., GUÉNIOT, M., LAPRESLE, J.: Périartérite noueuse apparue chez un diabetique quelques mois après une période d'insulino-résistance sévère. Presse méd. **63**, 1433 (1955)

BRUNFELDT, K. (1966) cited by DEVLIN (1968)

BRUNFELDT, K., DECKERT, T.: Antibodies in the pig against pig insulin. Acta endocr. (Kbh.) **47**, 367 (1964)

BRUNI, B., ALBERTO, M. DE, OSEDA, M., RICCI, C., TURCO, G.L.: Clinical trial with Monocoponent Lente Insulins. Diabetologia **9**, 492 (1973)

BURKART, F., HARTMANN, G., FANKHAUSER, S., KOLLER, F.: Insulinresistenz und Insulinallergie. Schweiz. med. Wschr. **93**, 1247 (1963)

CAWLEY, M.J., BROWNE, D.S.: Insulin resistance and thrombocytopenic purpura occurring in the same patient. Brit. J. clin. Pract. **24**, 169 (1970)

CLARK, C., MUNOZ, J.: Delayed hypersensitivity to insulin and its component polypeptide chains. J. Immunol. **105**, 574 (1970)
COCKEL, R., MANN, S.: Insulin allergy treated by low dosage hydrocortisone. Brit. med. J. **3**, 722 (1967)
CONSTAM, G.R.: Thrombocytopenic purpura as a probable manifestation of insulin allergy. Report of a case. Diabetes **5**, 121 (1956)
COOMBS, R.R.A., GELL, P.G.H.: Diagnostic and analytical in vitro methods. In: Clinical aspects of immunology, p. 3 (Eds. P.G.H. GELL, R.R.A. COOMBS). Oxford and Edinburgh: Blackwell Scientific Publications 1968
CORCORAN, A.C.: Rapid desensitization in case of hypersensitivitness to insulin. Amer. J. med. Sci. **196**, 359 (1938)
CZYZYK, A., LAWECKI, J., ROGALA, H., MIEDZINSKA, E., POPIK-HANKIEWICZ, A.: Serum levels of insulin binding antibodies in diabetic patients treated with monocomponent insulin. Diabetologia **10**, 233—236 (1974)
DAHL, L. (1950) cited by HANSEN, Allergie 1957
DAWEKE, H.: Schwierigkeiten bei der Insulinbehandlung, insbesondere beim labilen Diabetes, bei Insulinallergie und Insulinresistenz. Therapiewoche **1**, 20 (1968)
DECKERT, T.: Personal communication (1966)
DECKERT, T., GRUNDAHL, E.: The antigenicity of pig insulin. Diabetologia **6**, 15 (1970)
DEVLIN, J.G.: Hormone resistance and hypersensitivity. Clinical aspects of immunity, p. 672 (Eds. P.G.H. GELL, R.R.A. COOMBS). Oxford and Edinburgh: Blackwell Scientific Publications 1968
DITSCHUNEIT, H., HINZ, M., FAULHABER, J.D.: Vergleichende quantitative Untersuchungen über Antikörper gegen Proinsulin und Insulin im Blut bei insulinbehandelten Diabetikern. 1. Tagg. Ges. Immunol. Freiburg, 1969, Europ. J. Immunol. 1970, p. 12
DOLGER, H.: Denaturated insulin. A simplified, rapid means of treatment to allergy to insulin complicating diabetic ketosis. N.Y. J. Med. **52**, 2023 (1952)
DOLOVICH, J., SCHNATZ, J.D., REISMAN, R.E., YAGI, Y., ARBESMAN, C.E.: Insulin allergy and insulin resistance. J. Allergy **46**, 127 (1970)
ENGBRING, N.H., ARKINS, J.A., LENNON, E.J.: Insulin allergy and insulin resistance. J. Allergy **33**, 62 (1962)
FANKHAUSER, S., MICHL, J.: Two years experience with a new monocomponent insulin in diabetic patients. VIII. Congress of the Int. Diab. Fed., Brussels, 1973, Nr. 280, p. 130, Abstracts, Amsterdam: Excerpta Medica
FAULK, W.P., TOMSOVIC, E.J., FUDENBERG, H.H.: Insulin resistance in juvenile diabetes mellitus. Immunologic studies. Amer. J. Med. **49**, 133—139 (1970)
FEDERLIN, K.: Untersuchungen über die Antigenität von Insulin, Proinsulin and verwandten Proteinen am Meerschweinchen mit der passiven kutanen Anaphylaxie. Proinsulin and verwandte Proteine, Monokompanentinsulin. Arbeitsgespräch Novo. Mainz 1970
FEDERLIN, K.: Immunopathology of Insulin. Monographs on Endocrinology, Vol. 6. Berlin-Heidelberg-New York: Springer 1971
FEDERLIN, K.: 50 Jahre Insulin. Dtsch. med. J. **23**, 612 (1972)
FEDERLIN, K., HEINEMANN, G., GIGLI, I., DITSCHUNEIT, H.: Antigenbindung durch zirkulierende Leukozyten bei der verzögerten lokalen Insulinallergie. Dtsch. med. Wschr. **91**, 814 (1966)
FEDERLIN, K., GIGLI, J.: Immunzytologische Aspekte der Antikörperbildung gegen Insulin. In: Allergie und Immunitätsforschung. II. p. 47 (Ed. by A. HEYMER, W. GRONEMEYER). Stuttgart: F.K. Schattauer 1968
FEDERLIN, K., RENOLD, A.E., PFEIFFER, E.F.: Antigen-binding leucocytes in patients and in insulinsensitized animals with delayed insulin allergy. Immunopathology Vth Symposium, p. 107 (Ed. by P.A. MIESCHER, P. GRABAR). Basel/Stuttgart: Schwabe & Co. Pubs. 1968a
FEDERLIN, K., KRIEGBAUM, D., FLAD, H.D.: Lymphocytentransformation in vitro bei verschiedenen Formen der Insulinallergie. Therapiewoche **45**, 2042 (1968b)
FEDERLIN, K., KRIEGBAUM, D., FLAD, H.D.: Experimentelle Untersuchungen zur verzögerten Insulinallergie. Verh. dtsch. Ges. inn. Med. **75**, 708 (1969)
FEDERLIN, K., JONATHA, E.M., SCHRÖDER, K.E., PFEIFFER, E.F.: Cellular immunity and delayed hypersensitivity reactions to insulin in diabetic patients. In: Immunity and the Autoimmunity in Diabetes mellitus. Francqui Foundation Coloquium (Ed. by P. BASTENIE) Brussels. Amsterdam: Excerpta Medica 1974, p. 99
FREI, P.C., CRUCHAUD, S., VANOTTI, A.: Allergie a l'insuline de type cellulaire. Rev. franç. Étud. clin. biol. **10**, 1083 (1965)
FEDERLIN, K., VELCOVSKY, H.G.: JgE-Antikörper bei Patienten mit Insulinallergie. Verh. dtsch. Ges. Inn. Med. **80**, 1613 (1974)

Freytag, G., Jansen, F.K., Klöppel, G.: Immune reactions to fractions of crystalline insulin. I. Significance of lymphocytic infiltrates in the endocrine and exocrine pancreas of mice. Diabetologia **9**, 185 (1973)

Galloway, J.A., Root, M.A.: New forms of Insulin. Diabetes **21**, Suppl. 2, 637 (1972)

Gelfand, M.L., Fabrykant, M., Ashe, B.: Sensitivity tests to insulin in patients with local skin lesions from insulin. Soc. exp. Biol. Med. **86**, 258 (1954)

Glassberg, B., Somogyi, M., Taussig, A.E.: Diabetes mellitus. Report of a case refractory to insulin. Arch. intern. Med. **40**, 676 (1927)

Goldner, M.G., Ricketts, H.T.: Insulin allergy. Report of a case with generalized symptoms. J. clin. Endocr. **2**, 595 (1942)

Goldstein, H.H.: Allergy and diabetes. In: Joslin's diabetes mellitus. 11th Edition (Ed. by A. Marble, P. White, R.F. Bradley, L.P. Krall). Philadelphia: Lea and Febiger 1971

Grodsky, G.M., Feldmann, R., Toreson, W.E., Lee, J.C.: Diabetes mellitus in rabbits immunized with insulin. Diabetes **15**, 579 (1966)

Hagen, H., Hagen, W.: Experimentelle Untersuchungen über die Hautverträglichkeit von Insulinpräparaten. Ärztl. Forsch. **XIII**, 578 (1959)

Halpern, B., Ky, N., Amache, N.: Diagnosis of drug allergy in vitro with the lymphocyte transformation test. J. Allergy **40**, 168 (1967)

Hagen, H., Hagen, W.: Experimental studies on cutaneous tolerance to insulin preparations. Med. Welt **24**, 1375 (1962)

Hagen, H., Hagen, W., Heinsen, H.A., Olters, E., Scheffler, H.: Experimentelle Untersuchungen über die Hautverträglichkeit von Insulinpräparaten. Dtsch. med. Wschr. **83**, 1480 (1958).

Hansen, K.: Arzneimittel-Allergie. In: Allergie, p. 395. Stuttgart: G. Thieme 1957

Heinemann, G., Kriegbaum, D., Federlin, K.: Untersuchungen über „zellständige" und humorale Antikörper bei der Insulinallergie. I. Donausymposion über Diabetes mellitus, p. 397. Wien 27./28. 6. 1969. Wien: Verlag der Wiener Med. Akademie 1970

Herold, A.A.: Insulin allergy. Report of severe case with successful desensitization. New Orleans med. surg. J. **91**, 163 (1938)

Hinke, H., Steinhilber, S., Schmidt, D., Kerp, L.: Quantitative Untersuchungen zur Antikörperbindung von Rinderinsulin und Rinderproinsulin in Seren insulinbehandelter Diabetiker, p. 375. 76. Verh. Dtsch. Ges. Inn. Med. München: J.F. Bergmann 1970

Jansen, F.K., Freytag, G.: Immune reactions to fractions of crystalline insulin. II. May periinsulitis be produced by an antigen different from true Sanger-insulin? Diabetologia **9**, 191 (1973)

Jones, T.D., Mote, J.R.: Phase of foreign protein sensitization in human beings. New Engl. J. Med. **210**, 120 (1934)

Joslin, E., Gray, H., Root, R.: Insulin in hospital and home. J. metab. Res. **2**, 651 (1922)

Katsilambros, L.: Treatment of insulin allergy and insulin resistance with phenylated and formolated insulin. VIII. Congress Int. Diab. Fed. Brussels, 1973. Abstracts, Nr. 280, p. 132. Amsterdam: Excerpta Medica 1973

Kern, R.A., Langer, P.H.: Protamine and allergy: Nature of local reactions after injections of protamine zinc insulin; induction of sensitivity to insulin by injections of protamine zinc insulin. J. Amer. med. Ass. **113**, 198 (1939)

Kerp, L.: Quantitative data concerning the localisation of antibody binding sites on insulin and proinsulin molecules. Int. Arch. Allergy **41**, 216—218 (1971)

Kerp, L., Kasemir, H.: Praxis und Theorie der Arzneimittelallergien. Kurzmonographie, Sandoz, Nr. 9, 1973

Kerp, L., Steinhilber, S., Kieling, F., Creutzfeldt, W.: Klinische und experimentelle Untersuchungen zur Insulinallergie und Insulinresistenz. Dtsch. med. Wschr. **90**, 806 (1965)

Kerp, L., Steinhilber, S., Kasemir, H.: Besitzt die Proinsulinverunreinigung kommerzieller Insulinpräparate Bedeutung für die Stimulierung von Insulinantikörpern? Klin. Wschr. **48**, 884 (1970a)

Kerp, L., Steinhilber, S., Schmidt, D.D.: Vergleichende Analyse der gegen Rinderproinsulin und Rinderinsulin gebildeten Antikörper. FEBS Letters **8**, 157 (1970b)

Kloeppel, G., Altenaehr, E., Jansen, F.K., Freytag, G.: Relations between insulitis, intracutaneous skin reaction, antibody titer and decreased glucose tolerance in rabbits immunized with bovine insulin. VIII. Congr. Int. Diab. Fed. Brussels, Nr. 280, p. 132. Abstracts. Amsterdam: Excerpta Medica 1973

Korp, W., Levett, R.E.: Erfahrungen mit Monokomponenten-Insulin. Wien. klin. Wschr. **85**, 326 (1973)

Kreines, K.: The use of various insulins in insulin allergy. Arch. intern. Med. **116**, 167 (1965)

Kreines, K.: Use of sheep insulin in insulin allergy. Diabetes **20**, 774 (1971)

KUMAR, D., MILLER, L.V.: Studies on the antibodies in insulin treated diabetic patients. VIII. Congr. Int. Diab. Fed. Brussels, Nr. 280, p. 132. Abstracts. Amsterdam: Excerpta Medica 1973

LAYTON, L.L., LEE, S., YAMANAKA, E.: Allergen testing on monkeys passively sensitized by Hay Fever and Asthma Reagins of Human Sera. Nature (Lond.) **193**, 988 (1962)

LEE, C.L., GRODSKY, G.M., CAPLAN, J., CRAW, L.: Experimental immune diabetes in the rabbit. Amer. J. Path. **57**, 597 (1969)

LIEBERMAN, P., PATTERSON, R., METZ, R., LUCENA, G.: Allergic reactions to insulin. J. Amer. med. Ass. **215**, 1106 (1971)

LOVELESS, M.H.: Immunologic studies of insulin in man. Effect of heat on allergenicity. Diabetes **7**, 278 (1958)

MARBLE, A.: Allergy and diabetes. In: JOSLIN, E.P., ROOT, H.F., WHITE, P., MARBLE, A.: The treatment of diabetes mellitus, 10. Edition. p. 395. Philadelphia: Lea & Febiger 1959

McDEVITT, H.O.: Delayed hypersensitivity to insulin in guinea pigs. Fed. Proc. **23**, 259 (1964)

MELANI, F., RUBENSTEIN, A.H., STEINER, D.F.: Human serum proinsulin. J. clin. Invest. **49**, 497 (1970a)

MELANI, F., RUBENSTEIN, A.H., OYER, P.E., STEINER, D.F.: Identification of proinsulin and C-peptide in human serum by a specific immuno-assay. Proc. nat. Acad. Sci. (Wash.) **67**, 148 (1970b)

MENCZEL, J., LEVEY, M., BENTWICH, Z.: Insulin resistant diabetes treated with sulfated insulin. Israel J. med. Sci. **2**, 754 (1966)

MILLER, R.: Tödliche anaphylaktische Reaktion nach Insulininjektion. Med. Welt 1962, 2735

NICHOLS, M.N.: Insulin allergy: case report with response to boiled insulin. J. Pediat. **46**, 314 (1955)

PALEY, R.G.: Lipodystrophy following insulin injections. Metabolism **2**, 201 (1953)

PALEY, R.G., TUNBRIDGE, R.E.: Dermal reactions to insulin therapy. Diabetes **1**, 22 (1952)

PATTERSON, R., ROBERTS, M., PRUZANSKY, J.J.: Comparison of reaginic antibodies from three species. J. Immunol. **102**, 466 (1969)

PATTERSON, R., MELLIES, C.J., ROBERTS, M.: Immunologic reactions against insulin. II. IgE anti-insulin, insulin allergy and combined IgE and IgG immunologic insulin resistance. J. Immunol. **110**, 1135 (1973)

PERINGS, E.: Round table Conference on Immunology of diabetes. (unpublished) 8th Kongress German Diabetes Assoc. (1973)

PORTER, R.D., HARTMANN, C.R.: Arthus reactions from insulin. Association with lupus erythematosus cell phenomena. J. Amer. med. Ass. **214**, 1884 (1970)

POULSEN, J.E.: Insulin. Desirable and undesirable effects. Acta med. scand. Suppl. **476**, 91 (1967)

PRAUSNITZ, C., KÜSTNER, H.: Studien über die Überempfindlichkeit. Zbl. Bakt. **86**, 160 (1921)

RENOLD, A.E., SOELDNER, J.S., STEINKE, J.: Immunological studies with homologous and heterologous pancreatic insulin in the cow. Ciba Foundation Colloq. Endocr. Vol. 15, p. 122. London: Churchill 1964

RENOLD, A.E., STEINKE, J., SOELDNER, J.S., GONET, A.E., LECOMPTE, P.: Insulite experimentale chez la genisse. Fourth Internat. Symposium on Immunopathology, p. 349 (Eds. MIESCHER, GRABAR). Basel: Benno Schwabe 1965

RENOLD, A.E., GONET, A.E., VECCHIO, D.: Immunopathology of the endocrine pancreas. In: Textbook of Immunopathology. (Eds. P.A. MIESCHER, H.J. MÜLLER-EBERHARD). Vol. II, p. 959. New York-London: Grune and Stratton 1969, p. 595

ROITT, I.M.: Essential immunology, p. 123. Oxford-London-Edinburgh: Blackwell 1972

ROOT, M., CHANCE, R., GALLOWAY, J.: Immunogenicity of insulin. Diabetes **21**, Suppl. 2, 657—660 (1972)

RUBENSTEIN, A.H., CHO, S., STEINER, D.F.: Evidence for proinsulin in human urine and serum. Lancet **1968 I**, 353

RUDY, A.: Urticaria and insulin resistance with reference to the relation of the skin to carbohydrate metabolism. New Engl. J. Med. **204**, 791 (1931)

SANGER, F.: Chemistry of insulin. Brit. med. Bull. **16**, 183 (1960)

SCHEFFLER, H.: Lokalisierte allergische Hautreaktionen mit Pigmentablagerung nach Insulininjektion, p. 1409. Medizinische 1955

SCHIRREN, G.C.: Ein ungewöhnlicher Fall von lokaler Insulinanaphylaxie. Hautarzt **4**, 531 (1953)

SCHLICHTKRULL, J.: Monocomponent insulin and its clinical implications. Francqui Foundation Colloquium "Immunity and Autoimmunity in diabetes mellitus." Brussels, 1974, p. 29

SCHLICHTKRULL, J.: Proinsulin und verwandte Proteine. Chemische und biologische Untersuchungen, p. 14, 70. Tagg. Dtsch. Ges. Inn. Med. München: J.F. Bergmann 1970

SCHLICHTKRULL, J., BRANGE, J., CHRISTIANSEN, A.H., HALLUND, O., HEDING, L.G., JØRGENSEN, K.H.: Clinical aspects of insulin-antigenicity. Diabetes **21**, Suppl. 2, 649 (1972)
SHAW, W.N., CHANCE, R.E.: Effect of porcine proinsulin in vitro on adipose tissue and diaphragm of the normal rat. Diabetes **17**, 737 (1968)
SHERMAN, W.B.: A case of coexisting insulin allergy and insulin resistance. J. Allergy **21**, 49 (1950)
SHIPP, J.C., CUNNINGHAM, R.W., RUSSELL, R.O., MARBLE, A.: Insulin resistance: Clinical features, natural course and effects of adrenal steroid treatment. Medicine **44**, 165 (1965)
STEINER, D.F.: Evidence for a precursor in the biosynthesis of insulin. Trans. N.Y. Acad. Sci., Series II, **30**, 60 (1967)
STEINER, D.F., OYER, P.: The biosynthesis of insulin and a probable precursor of insulin by a human islet cell adenoma. Proc. nat. Acad. Sci (Wash.) **57**, 473 (1967)
STEINER, D.F., CUNNINGHAM, D., SPIGELMAN, L., ATEN, B.: Insulin biosynthesis: Evidence for a precursor. Science **157**, 697 (1967)
STEINER, D.F., CLARK, J.L.: The spontaneous reoxidation of reduced beef and rat proinsulins. Proc. nat. Acad. Sci. (Wash.) **60**, 622 (1968)
STEINER, D.F., HALLUND, O., RUBENSTEIN, A., CHO, S., BAYLISS, C.: Isolation and properties of proinsulin, intermediate forms and other minor components from crystalline bovine insulin. Diabetes **17**, 725 (1968)
STROHFELDT, P.: Insulinallergie und Insulinresistenz. In: H. ROBBERS. Praktische Diabetologie, S. 114. München: Werk-Verlag Dr. Banaschewski 1969
TORESON, W.E., FELDMAN, R., LEE, J.C., GRODSKY, G.M.: Pathology of diabetes mellitus produced in rabbits by means of immunization with beef insulin. Amer. J. clin. Path. **42**, 531 (1964)
TUFT, L.: Insulin hypersensitivitiness-Immunologic considerations and case reports. Amer. J. med. Sci. **176**, 707 (1928)
ULRICH, H., HOOKER, S.B., SMITH, H.H.: Allergic reaction to insulin. Report of a case. New Engl. J. Med. **221**, 522 (1939)
WALDMANN, T.A., POLMAR, S.H., TERRY, W.: Cited by PATTERSON, MELLIES and ROBERTS (1973)
WALKER, S.E.: Cited by MICHEL (1961). U.S. Vet. Bur. Med. Bull. **2**, 2700 (1926)
WENIG, K.H., CALAP, J.: Auslösung allergischer Phaenomene durch Insulin-Präparate. Münch. med. Wschr. **10**, 345 (1971)
WILSON, S.: The antigenic loci in insulin. Proc. 6th Int. Diab. Fed. Stockholm, 1967. Ed. J. ÖSTMAN. Amsterdam: Excerpta Medica Foundation, p. 403, 1969
WOLF, A.J.: Insulin allergy. Texas J. Med. **58**, 499 (1962)
WRIGHT, P.H., MAKULU, D.R.: Some immunological properties of insulin and proinsulin. Diabetes **18**, Suppl. 339 (1969) Abstr.
WRIGHT, P.H., GINGERICH, R.L.: Immunogenicity of insulin in guinea pigs. VIII. Congr. Int. Diab. Fed. Brussels, Nr. 280, p. 137. Abstracts. Amsterdam: Excerpta Medica 1973

B. Insulin-Binding Antibodies of Serum and Insulin Resistance

Lothar Kerp, Helmut R. Henrichs and Hans Kasemir

With 5 Figures

Insulin is an *effective antigen* which can bring about a specific immune response both in a variety of animal species and in man. The reaction of the organism comprises the formation of immunologically competent cells and the production of antigen-specific antibodies of different immunoglobulin classes. Both the various manifestations of insulin allergy and the neutralization of insulin through binding to antibodies depend on this reaction. The *immunogenicity* of insulin characterizes the properties that are responsible for inducing the formation of insulin-specific immune cells and of insulin antibodies. *The antigen specificity* of insulin represents the properties of the molecule that are responsible for the binding of insulin to immune cells or to antibodies. The specific suppression of the immune reactions against insulin, which is produced by administration of the insulin antigen in very high or in very low doses, is called *immuntolerance.*

Two years after the first clinical work on insulin by BANTING *et al.* (1922) and before the first preparation of crystalline insulin by ABEL (1926), FALTA (1924) described a patient with insulin-insensitive diabetes mellitus. An insulin allergy with generalized urticaria was reported by TUFT in 1928. In the same year DEPISCH and HASENÖHRL reported a case of insulin resistance in which an insulin-weakening serum factor was detected by animal experiments. The immunogenicity of insulin in man was confirmed by further observations of insulin allergy and insulin resistance (BERNE and WALLERSTEIN, 1950; SMELO, 1948; and others), by the occurrence of insulin-neutralizing antibodies (BANTING *et al.*, 1938; BERSON *et al.*, 1956; BURROWS *et al.*, 1957; COLWELL and WEIGER, 1956; DE FILLIPS and JANNACCONE, 1952; GLEN and EATON, 1938; KAYE *et al.*, 1955; LERMAN, 1944; MARSH and HAUGAARD, 1952; SEHON *et al.*, 1955; SHERMAN, 1950; SKOM and TALMAGE, 1958a, b; WEIGER and COLWELL, 1956; WELSH *et al.*, 1956; and others), and occasionally by the detection of precipitating (LERMAN, 1944; MOLONEY and APRILE, 1959; STEIGERWALD *et al.*, 1960; TUFT, 1928; and others), complement-binding (STEIGERWALD and SPIELMANN, 1956; WASSERMANN *et al.*, 1940; and others) or agglutinating antibodies (ARQUILLA and STAVITSKY, 1956a, b; CANNON and MARSHALL, 1941; GOLDNER and RICKETTS, 1942; and others).

Even before the elucidation of the structure of insulins from different animal species, it was demonstrated by immunological methods that the insulins from different species differ immunologically. Observations of WILLIAMS (1933) gave the first evidence of species-specific insulin antigenicity. In two cases of allergy-dependent gastrointestinal symptoms following administration of porcine insulin, WILLIAMS was able to induce positive skin reactions only by using porcine insulin and not bovine insulin. Investigations by LEWIS (1937) confirmed the species-specificity of insulin antigens and showed that bovine and porcine insulin, although immunologically related, are not identical. A comparison between human insulin and foreign insulin by LOWELL (1942) demonstrated that human insulin remained metabolically effective in a patient with resistance against a mixture of bovine and porcine insulin. The existence of immunological differences between insulin from different species has been confirmed in animal experiments (BERNSTEIN *et al.*, 1938; WASSERMANN and MIRSKY, 1942; MOLONEY and COVAL, 1955; ARQUILLA and STAVITSKY, 1956b).

The postulate of the immunogenicity of insulin was opposed on the grounds that the insulin molecule is too small to be effective as an immunogen (CLUTTON *et al.*, 1938a, b; GUTFREUND, 1952; HAUROWITZ, 1950; JORPES, 1949; SANGER *et al.*, 1955; SCHWARZ and KOLLER, 1949; SHERRILL and LAWRENCE, 1950). This objection was refuted by the demonstration that polypeptides with an even smaller molecular weight than insulin exert an immunogenic activity (ARNON and SELA, 1960; SELA and ARNON, 1960a, b; SELA and HAUROWITZ, 1958). On the other hand, it has been assumed in recent years that it is not primarily monomeric insulin that evokes insulin-specific immune responses, but associated substances of higher molecular weight that possess structural portions of insulin antigenicity.

I. Methods for the Determination of Insulin Antibodies

1. Determination by Inhibition of Insulin Effects

a) Inhibition of Insulin Effects in Animals

Mainly in earlier studies on insulin resistance, insulin-binding antibodies were assayed in the whole animal by inhibition of insulin effects. These methods are in principle based on a comparison of the blood sugar-lowering effect of insulin in the presence and in the absence of serum to be tested.

BANTING *et al.* (1938) were the first to utilize the inhibition of insulin-dependent hypoglycemic convulsions in the mouse (mouse convulsion test) for the antibody determination. Fasting mice are injected with 0.25 ml of the test serum or a serum dilution contemporaneously with a certain insulin quantity (approximately 0.05 IU) which, given without serum, induces convulsions in 90—100% of the mice.

A further experimental procedure which uses intact test animals is based on the neutralization of their endogenous insulin by injection of antibody-containing serum.

MOLONEY and COVAL (1955) were the first to demonstrate that guinea-pig anti-insulin serum, given intraperitoneally to white mice, induces a rise in the blood sugar up to 21 h after beginning of the experiment. Rise in blood sugar, acetonuria, and weight loss have been observed following intravenous and intraperitoneal administration of the anti-insulin serum to mice over a period of 3 days. WRIGHT (1959a), ARMIN *et al.* (1960a, b) and ROBINSON and WRIGHT (1961) demonstrated that guinea pig anti-insulin serum induces hyperglycemia in rabbits, rats, and cats, its degree and duration being dependent upon the dosage of the antiserum. A rise in blood sugar could be produced by a single injection of guinea pig anti-insulin serum in dogs, pigs and sheep as well, but not in the guinea pig (ARMIN *et al.*, 1960a; MOLONEY and COVAL, 1955).

b) Inhibition of Insulin Effects in Isolated Tissue

Methods for insulin determination by means of isolated tissue preparations (rat diaphragm, fat pads, or isolated fat cells from the epididymal fat organ of the rat) were adapted for the detection of insulin-binding antibodies. These techniques are appropriate for detecting insulin antagonists by their inhibitory effect on the insulin-like activity. However, it is difficult to distinguish between hormones with insulin-antagonist activity (thyroid hormone, growth hormone, adrenocorticotropic hormone, glucocorticoids, adrenalin, noradrenalin, glucagon), insulin-binding proteins, and antibodies or as yet unknown insulin antagonists.

PERLMUTTER and GREEP (1948) used glycogen synthesis in the *rat diaphragm* as a parameter of insulin activity. Many authors utilized the stimulating effect of insulin on the glucose uptake by the rat diaphragm (BORNSTEIN, 1953; BORNSTEIN and PARK, 1953; DAVIDSON and GOODNER, 1966; GEMMIL, 1941; KRAHL *et al.*, 1959; RANDLE, 1954, 1956, 1957, 1960; VALLANCE-OWEN *et al.*, 1955, 1958a, 1958b; VALLANCE-OWEN and HURLOCK, 1954; VALLANCE-OWEN and LILLEY, 1961; VALLANCE-OWEN and LUKENS, 1957; WILLEBRANDS *et al.*, 1958; WRIGHT, 1959b). Some investigators worked with the less sensitive index of glycogen production in muscle (FIELD and STETTEN, JR., 1956a, b; FIELD *et al.*, 1957; MARSH and HAUGAARD, 1952).

ANTONIADES and SIMON (1972), BEIGELMAN and ANTONIADES (1958), FROESCH *et al.* (1963), LYNGSØE (1962), MARTIN *et al.* (1958), RAMSEIER *et al.* (1961), RENOLD *et al.* (1957, 1960), SLATER *et al.* (1961) and WINEGARD and RENOLD (1958a, 1958b) used insulin effects on carbohydrate metabolism in adipose tissue to measure insulin activity in *epididymal fat tissue of the rat.*

In this substrate various parameters of the carbohydrate metabolism may be determined: (1) glucose uptake by the adipose tissue and glucose disappearance in the incubation medium, respectively (HASSELBLATT and SCHMIETA, 1961); (2) net gas exchange (CO_2 production, O_2 consumption) (RAMSEIER *et al.*, 1961); (3) oxidation of glucose-1-^{14}C to $^{14}CO_2$ (GLIEMANN, 1969; MARTINI and HAHN, 1967; PFEIFFER and DITSCHUNEIT, 1962).

c) Inhibition of Insulin Degradation and Elimination

Observations by Elgee *et al.* (1953, 1954), Williams *et al.* (1953), Welsh *et al.* (1956) and Berson *et al.* (1956) showed that ^{131}I-insulin disappeared significantly more slowly from the blood of insulin-treated persons than from that of untreated persons. Further investigations demonstrated a parallelism between insulin retention *in vivo* and a protective effect of the sera on insulin degradation by rat liver homogenates *in vitro* (Welsh *et al.*, 1956). Yalow and Berson (1957) demonstrated that both the prolonged half-life of ^{131}I-insulin in the serum of insulin-treated patients and the inhibition of insulin degradation observed in the presence of such sera (Berson *et al.*, 1956; Yalow and Berson, 1957) are due to the binding of insulin to acquired insulin-binding antibodies. These investigations offer two possibilities for indirect determination of insulin-binding antibodies:

1. Determination of the insulin retention *in vivo* after intravenous administration of insulin (Berson *et al.*, 1956; Bolinger *et al.*, 1964; Elgee *et al.*, 1953; Følling and Norman, 1972; Haugaard *et al.*, 1954; Horino *et al.*, 1967; McAdams *et al.*, 1967; Menzel *et al.*, 1971; Orskov and Christensen, 1969; Palumbo *et al.*, 1972; Stimmler, 1967; Tomasi *et al.*, 1967; Welsh *et al.*, 1956; Williams *et al.*, 1953).

2. Determination of insulin degradation by liver slices or homogenates *in vitro* in presence of sera of insulin-treated patients (Berson *et al.*, 1956; Narahara and Williams, 1964; Welsh *et al.*, 1956). Both methods, however, are of little value for quantitative estimation of insulin-binding antibodies.

2. Determination of Insulin-Binding Antibodies by Immunological Tests

a) Serologic Methods

Serologic methods for the detection of insulin antibodies are based on precipitation, agglutination, hemolysis or complement binding as a result of an antigen-antibody reaction. It is a disadvantage of these methods that antigen and antibody can combine without such secondary reactions, in particular, if soluble antigen-antibody complexes are involved, as is the case with insulin (Boyd, 1956). Therefore it is doubtful whether serologic techniques are appropriate to determine total insulin antibody concentration.

Several working groups were able to detect *precipitating antibodies* by testing of the sera of insulin-resistant diabetics, of patients with insulin allergies and of insulin-treated experimental animals (Birkinshaw *et al.*, 1962; Ceska, 1968; Corcos and Ovary, 1965; Ezrin and Moloney, 1959; Feinberg, 1954; Hirata and Blumenthal, 1962a, 1963; Horino *et al.*, 1967; Jones and Cunliffe, 1961; Karr *et al.*, 1931; Lerman, 1944; Lockwood and Prout, 1965; Moloney and Aprile, 1959; Patterson *et al.*, 1964; Penchev *et al.*, 1965; 1968; Renold *et al.*, 1966; Smelo, 1947; Steigerwald *et al.*, 1960; Tuft, 1928). Precipitation was lacking in other cases (Arquilla and Stavitsky, 1956a; Berne and Wallerstein, 1950; Berson and Yalow, 1964a, 1965; Ditschuneit *et al.*, 1963; Lachnit and Wiedemann, 1961; Moloney and Coval, 1955; Steigerwald and Spielmann, 1956; Wasserman *et al.*, 1940).

Wasserman *et al.*, (1940), Steigerwald and Spielmann (1956), Rausch-Stroomann and Sauer (1953), Pav *et al.* (1963), Van de Wiel and Van de Wiel-Dorfmeyer (1964), Chetty and Watson (1965) employed a *complement-binding* or *complement consumption test*, for detection of insulin antibodies. Mancini *et al.* (1964, 1965) found insulin antibodies in diabetics with and without insulin treatment by means of the *immunofluorescent technique*.

Cannon and Marshall (1941), Goldner and Ricketts (1942), Moinat (1958) and Pal *et al.* (1969a, b) reported the *agglutination* of insulin-coated collodion particles by sera of insulin-resistant patients.

Arquilla and Stavitsky (1956a, b), Stavitsky and Arquilla (1953) and Stavitsky (1954) succeeded in detecting antibodies against insulin in insulin-treated rabbits as well as in insulin-resistant diabetics by *hemagglutination* and by *hemolysis*. The insulin antigen was attached to rabbit or sheep erythrocytes via a diazo bridge. The pretreated erythrocytes were agglutinated by anti-insulin sera or subjected to hemolysis in the presence of complement.

Brinckerhoff and Rose (1969), Devlin (1966), Moinat (1958), Patterson *et al.* (1964), Scecsey *et al.* (1963), Scheiffarth and Frenger (1956), Scheiffarth *et al.* (1959), and Steigerwald and Spielmann (1956) also employed a hemagglutination technique. In the indirect hemagglutination test according to Boyden (1951), the insulin antigen is adsorbed to sheep erythrocytes after pretreatment with tannic acid.

b) Passive Antibody Transfer

Loveless (1956) transferred serum of an insulin-allergic patient at several sites into the skin of a healthy recipient. The threshold dose necessary for the induction of an immediate allergic reaction is determined by injection of increasing doses of bovine insulin into the sites of serum application. Insulin along with antibody-containing serum is then injected into prepared sites of the skin. The threshold dose of insulin will increase with increasing antibody titer of the serum tested. This method is no longer employed because of the danger of hepatitis inoculation.

In the very sensitive technique of *passive cutaneous anaphylaxis (PCA)* used by Ovary (1958, 1959) for the detection of IgG antibodies, the serum to be tested first is injected intracutaneously into guinea pigs. Several hours after injection of the serum the antigen, together with a dye, is injected intravenously. A local antigen-antibody reaction enhances the permeability of blood vessels and extravasation of the dye is observed in the presence of antibodies. The extension of the erythematous areola is quantitatively indicative of the antibody titer. This method has been widely used by e.g. Oakley *et al.* (1959), Ditschuneit *et al.* (1962), Wilson *et al.* (1966, 1967).

3. Detection of Insulin Antibodies by Direct Measurement of Insulin-Antibody Binding

Insulin was radioactively labeled for the first time by Kallee in 1952. Since labeled insulin with a limited degree of iodination is bound by antibodies such as unlabeled insulin (see p. 617), it is possible to measure the insulin antibody binding directly. Various procedures have been recommended for the separation of antibody-bound and free insulin fractions.

a) Electrophoresis

Electrophoretic techniques may be utilized for determination of the binding of labeled low-molecular-weight ligands by serum proteins. It must, however, be taken into account that measurements obtained by electrophoresis cannot be absolute since the concentration of proteins, as well as of bound and free ligands, depends on the progress of the separation because, especially in the case of easily dissociable complexes, concentration equilibria are changing throughout the electrophoretic migration period.

Berson *et al.* (1956), Berson and Yalow (1957 and later), Burrows *et al.* (1957), Ensinck *et al.* (1964), Feldman *et al.* (1963), Freedlender *et al.* (1964), Grodsky and Forsham (1958), Koenig *et al.* (1956), Morse (1959), Morse and Heremans (1962), Sehon *et al.* (1955) used *paper electrophoresis* for the detection of insulin-binding antibodies. ^{131}I-labeled insulin remains detectable at the site of application after electrophoresis on paper. On application of ^{131}I-insulin together with serum of subjects not treated with insulin, nearly the total insulin radioactivity is found at the site of application. However, in the presence of sera containing insulin-binding antibodies, some or all the ^{131}I-insulin migrates with the γ- or β-globulin fraction. By means of this technique Berson *et al.* (1956) were able to plot insulin antibody-binding curves and to determine the concentration of antibody-binding sites and the association constants for complex formation between specific antibodies and the insulin antigen.

Electrophoretic methods were modified by changing the supporting material to avoid unspecific insulin absorption. Følling and Norman (1972), Hirata and Blumenthal (1962), Kallee *et al.* (1963a, b), Lohss and Kallee (1961), Melani *et al.* (1965), Pfeiffer *et al.* (1965), Prout *et al.* (1963) and others worked with *agar gel* as substrate; Grüneklee *et al.* (1971), Kerp (1963), Weiger and Colwell (1956) used *cellulose acetate film, acrylamide gel* or *starch gel.* A *polyacrylamide disc gel electrophoresis* for determination of insulin antibodies was described by Ditzov *et al.* (1971), by Heideman, Jr. (1964), by Ramachandran *et al.* (1969) as well as by Sirakov and Ditzov (1973).

Further procedures for the detection of insulin antibodies are based on gel filtration or *anion and cation exchange chromatography* in column and paper techniques (Abdel Wahab and El Kinawi, 1965; Chao *et al.*, 1965; Følling and Norman, 1972; Horwitz *et al.*, 1964; Horino and Blumenthal, 1966; Mitchell and Bradford, 1963; Striebel *et al.*, 1962).

Because it offers the possibility of a specific identification of immunoglobulins, many authors use *radioimmunoelectrophoresis* for the determination of insulin antibodies. The technique for the separation of protein fractions was pointed out by Grabar (1959). Localization and quantitative determination of the I-labeled insulin is carried out by autoradiography or by quantitative procedures for the measurement of isotopes. According to Miller and Owen (1960), this method was employed by many investigators to confirm the presence of insulin antibodies (Clausen *et al.*, 1963; Devlin and O'Donovan, 1965; Dolovich *et al.*, 1970; Følling and Norman, 1972; Geerling and Sirek, 1965; Kerp and Kasemir, 1968; Menzel *et al.*, 1971; Morse and Heremans, 1962; Palumbo *et al.*, 1965; Patterson *et al.*, 1964; Prout *et al.*, 1963; Randle and Taylor, 1958; Starzynska *et al.*, 1967; Starzynska, 1969; Yagi *et al.*, 1962; and others).

Christiansen (1970) modified the method of radioimmunoelectrophoresis, using agar gel as support for the electrophoresis. The gel contains γ-globulin from rabbits immunized against human γ-globulin. The detection of antibody-bound ^{125}I-insulin is carried out by autoradiography or by determination of the radioactivity of a cut-out pherogram. Root *et al.* (1972), Schlichtkrull *et al.* (1970, 1972) and Serrano-Rios *et al.* (1973a, b) adopted this modification.

The *crossed antigen-antibody electrophoresis* method seems appropriate to exclude too high results — as obtained by the method of Christiansen (1970) — with respect to the unspecific insulin binding to albumin, to α-2-macroglobulin and to β-lipoprotein (Schlichtkrull *et al.*, 1972a).

The *radioimmunodiffusion technique* according to Ouchterlony (1958, 1962) was also used for the detection of insulin-binding antibodies (Dolovich *et al.*, 1970; Menzel *et al.*, 1971; Menzel and Ziegler, 1970b).

b) Ultracentrifugation

Ultracentrifugation techniques for the investigation of insulin-antibody binding were employed for the first time in 1956 by Berson *et al.* and later by Kerp (1963), Chao *et al.* (1965), Geerling and Sirek (1965), Grodsky (1965) and Følling and Norman (1972). An ultracentrifugation technique for quantitative investigation of protein-ligand complexes was indicated by Kerp *et al.* in 1962. This technique was later used for the determination of insulin-antibody binding. Antibody-bound insulin sediments quantitatively in the gravitational field of the ultracentrifuge in the course of 8 h at 100,000 *g*. A concentration gradient for free insulin develops in the gravitational field of the centrifuge, which has to be checked before each analysis in the absence of antibodies. The concentration of free insulin in the sediment can be calculated from the concentration of insulin in the supernatant. The concentration of antibody-bound insulin in the sediment results from the total insulin concentration in the sediment, reduced by the calculated concentration of free insulin in the sediment (Fig. 1). If, at constant antibody concentration, the concentration of the added insulin varies, a hyperbolic binding curve is obtained on plotting bound versus applied insulin up to saturation of antibody-binding sites. The concentration of antibody-binding sites and the strength of binding are determined from this curve by appropriate transformation (see p. 602). The ultracentrifugation method has the advantage that the constant equilibrium of the antigen-antibody binding reaction is not disturbed by the separation procedure. The law of mass action is strictly applicable only to this state.

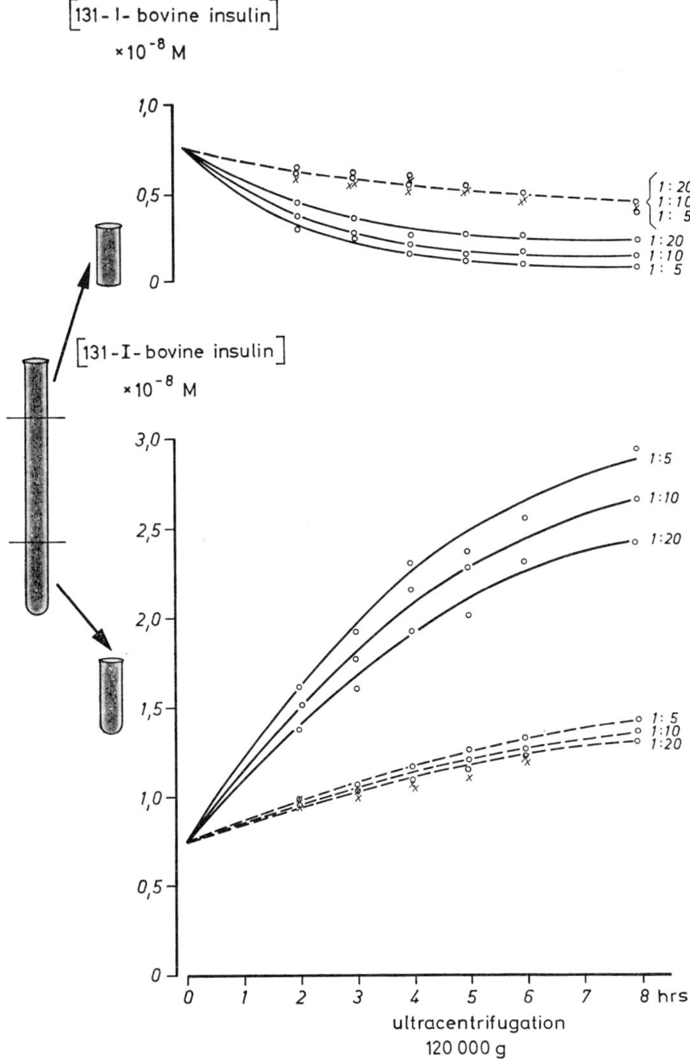

Fig. 1. Behavior of insulin-binding antibodies during ultracentrifugation (120000 g, 8 h). Sedimentation pattern of 131-I-bovine insulin in antibody-containing serum (○——○) compared to normal serum (○-----○). The decrease of the 131-I-insulin concentration in the supernatant as well as the increase of the 131-I-insulin concentration in the sediment fraction drops with further dilution of the antiserum. (The sedimentation pattern of 131-I-insulin in control experiments in buffer without serum is indicated by x)

c) Precipitation of Insulin-Protein Complexes

Precipitation methods with determination of the protein-bound ligand in the precipitate are also used to measure insulin-protein binding. As regards the quantitative evaluation of the measurements, it has been objected that the presence of a ligand in the precipitate does not prove that a binding to the native protein existed prior to the precipitation (DAVIS, 1948) and that the binding capacity of a protein for ligands can be altered by precipitation and denaturation (BENNHOLD, 1938; DAVIS, 1948; and others).

GORDIS from BERSON's group described in 1960 a technique for the precipitation of antibody-bound insulin with *sodium chloride-saturated 76% ethyl alcohol* in 0.01 mol/l potassium hydroxide solution. Methods of GRODSKY and FORSHAM (1960) as well as of KARAM *et al.* (1963) are based on salt precipitation with *sodium sulfate*. Such precipitation methods are somewhat questionable because of the highly alkaline pH and high ion concentration, since neither condition is optimum for antigen-antibody complex formation. The determination of insulin-binding antibodies carried out by HEDING (1965, 1966) and by WELBORN *et al.* (1967) is based on *alcohol precipitation* of the insulin-antibody complex. As a method for the detection of insulin-binding antibodies, STEINKE (1972) recommended precipitation with *polyethylene glycol*, as suggested by DESBUQUOIS and AUERBACH (1971) for the separation of free and antibody-bound peptide hormones.

With reference to the technique indicated by FEINBERG (1954) for the detection of soluble antigen-antibody complexes, SKOM and TALMAGE (1956a, b, 1958a, b) developed a method for the detection of antibodies by *double antibody precipitation*. Anti-insulin sera are incubated with ^{131}I-insulin, then the γ-globulin fraction is precipitated with an antihuman γ-globulin serum from rabbits. The portion of ^{131}I-insulin bound to γ-globulins can be determined by measuring the radioactivity in the precipitate and in the supernatant.

This assay principle is based on methods for the detection of insulin by GOETZ *et al.* (1963), by HALES and RANDLE (1963), and by MORGAN and LAZAROW (1962, 1963). DECKERT and GRUNDAHL (1970) as well as KUMAR and MILLER (1973a, b) employed analogous techniques for the detection of insulin-binding antibodies.

ANDERSEN *et al.* (1972) used a modification of the immunoprecipitation technique in which anti-insulin serum from guinea pig is precipitated with rabbit antiserum against guinea pig serum and is equilibrated with trace amounts of I-labeled insulin. The addition of a serum of unknown antibody content reduces the radioactivity of the immune precipitate in proportion to the antibody content of the sample.

d) Adsorption Techniques

Adsorption techniques for the measurement of the protein binding of I-labeled insulin are based on the fact that free rather than protein-bound insulin is bound to suitable adsorbents.

MITCHELL and O'ROURKE (1959) and MITCHELL *et al.* (1959) determined the ^{131}I-insulin binding of various sera by adsorption of the non-protein-bound insulin portion to the anion exchange resin *Amberlite* IRA 400. The antibody-containing serum sample is incubated with ^{131}I-insulin and subsequently brought together with the anion exchanger. The radioactivity remaining on the anion exchange resin after separation is indicated in % of the initial activity as the "resin index". The disadvantage of this technique is that serum proteins and insulin compete for binding sites on the resin, which means that the "resin index" depends on the protein concentration of the serum tested. Thus, antibody-containing and antibody-free sera show an average difference of only 7% in ^{131}I-insulin binding to the resin.

MEADE and KLITGAARD (1962), MELANI *et al.* (1965), DITSCHUNEIT and FEDERLIN (1966) as well as JANSEN (1971c) also utilize Amberlite adsorption of free insulin. The suitability of Dowex cation exchangers for the separation of free and bound insulin was investigated by HORWITZ *et al.* (1964) and MELANI *et al.* (1965).

The adsorption of insulin on *dextran-coated charcoal* was used by HERBERT *et al.* (1965) for the first time and later by LEV-RAN *et al.* (1972), HILDEBRANDT *et al.* (1968) and SEBRIAKOVA and LITTLE (1973) as method of separating free and bound insulin for the detection of insulin-binding antibodies.

ZINDER *et al.* (1961) chose *erythrocytes* for adsorption of free insulin by analogy with the procedure indicated by CRISPELL *et al.* (1956) for the detection of thyroxine- and triiodothyronine-binding plasma proteins. A disadvantage of this technique is the application of a biological adsorbent, the adsorption capacity of which must be subject to variations. Furthermore, insulin-binding proteins are adsorbed to the surface of the erythrocytes too, which can falsify the results.

A technique in which the *rat diaphragm* is used as an adsorbent is equally vague (STADIE *et al.*, 1949; NEWERLY and BERSON, 1957). Not only insulin antibodies but also other proteins (NEWERLY and BERSON, 1957) inhibit the adsorption of insulin to the musculature of the diaphragm.

BERSON *et al.* (1956) observed a marked adsorption of free insulin to *cellulose*. Various separation methods for the detection of insulin antibodies are based on this fact (DENDRINOS *et al.*, 1961; KERP and STEINHILBER, 1963; KERP *et al.*, 1966; KÜHNAU, JR., 1968; LOCKWOOD and PROUT, 1965; WRIGHT, 1965; WRIGHT and MALAISSE, 1966; and others).

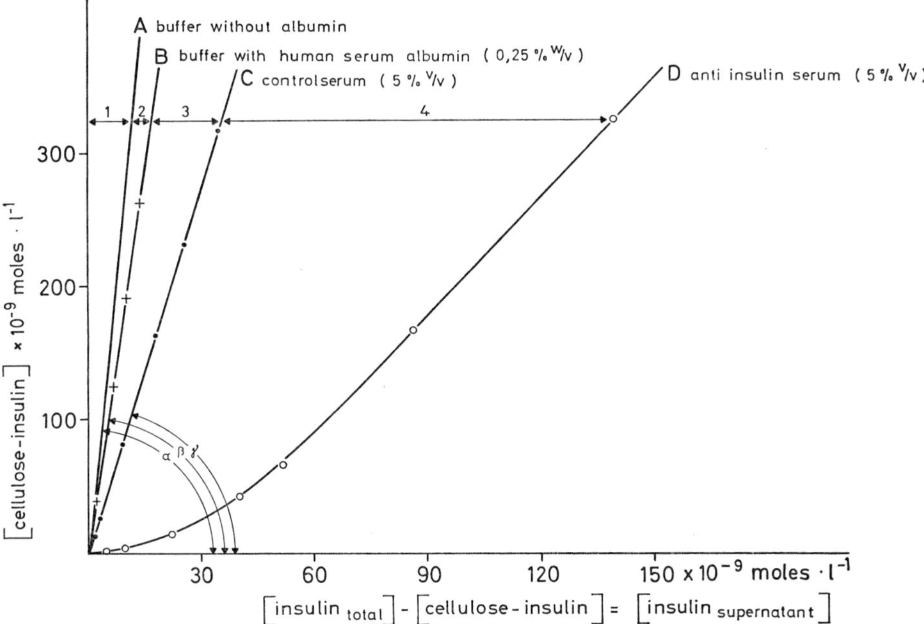

Fig. 2. Determination of insulin-binding antibodies by means of differential adsorption to cellulose powder. The adsorption of labeled insulin to the adsorbent varies with the presence of buffer (A), human serum albumin (B), human normal serum (C) or anti-insulin serum (D) and is characterized by the respective isotherms (for details see text). Intercept 1 stands for the free insulin concentration, intercept 4 stands for the concentration of antibody-bound insulin

The procedure indicated by KERP and STEINHILBER (1963) for the detection of insulin-binding antibodies by differential adsorption is also based on insulin adsorption by cellulose powder (KERP *et al.*, 1966, 1968).

When I-labeled insulin is in binding equilibrium with serum proteins, such as albumin and the other serum protein fractions, possibly including specifically binding antibodies and an adsorbent, it is possible to measure protein-bound and free insulin provided the isotherms for the unspecific insulin adsorption are known. With the insulin concentration increasing from 0.64×10^{-9} mol/l to 1.29×10^{-6} mol/l, the proportion of free and antibody-bound insulin is determined from the isotherms measured in the adsorption system for the adsorption of I-labeled insulin to the cellulose powder (a) in an albumin-free phosphate buffer, (b) in an albumin-containing (0.25%) phosphate buffer, (c) in an albumin-containing (0.25%) phosphate buffer with added anti-insulin serum. The proportion of free and antibody-bound insulin in the binding equilibrium is calculated from the measured results (Fig. 2).

Insulin-antibody binding curves are obtained by this technique. The data are transferred into the coordinate system indicated by SCATCHARD *et al.* (1957) for calculating association constants and maximum concentration of antibody binding sites.

4. Calculation of Quantitative Parameters of Insulin-Antibody Binding at Equilibrium

The binding of insulin to serum antibodies is inadequately described by a single parameter, e.g. as insulin binding in percent of the quantity applied, or in the form of a titer. Such single parameters fail to take into account the maximum concentration of the binding sites and the strength of the insulin-antibody binding. Furthermore, in judging the strength of binding, it is important to know whether the insulin-antibody binding can be described by a single association constant or whether the antibodies are heterogeneous in regard to their strength of binding. If, a technique permits the determination of very low concentrations of free insulin besides the antibody-bound insulin at equilibrium, binding curves can be plotted. The plotting of the transformed data in the coordinate system according to SCATCHARD *et al.* (1957) with the abscissa [antibody-insulin] and the ordinate [antibody-insulin]/[insulin$_{\text{free}}$] (Fig. 3), enables the calculation of the association constant k and the maximal concentration of the antibody-binding sites [Ak′] of the anti-insulin serum. [Ak′] does not directly designate the concentration of insulin-binding antibodies but the product of the number of binding sites per antibody molecule and of the molar concentration of the antibodies.

The concave shape of the binding curve in Fig. 3b shows that at least two antibody-binding sites, Ak_1 and Ak_2, which differ in their affinity for the insulin antigen, are involved in the insulin binding. The corresponding association constants are

$$k_1 = \frac{[Ak_1 - \text{insulin}]}{[\text{insulin}_{\text{free}}]\,[Ak_{1\,\text{free}}]} \qquad k_2 = \frac{[Ak_2 - \text{insulin}]}{[\text{insulin}_{\text{free}}]\,[Ak_{2\,\text{free}}]}$$

The maximum concentration of binding sites of an anti-insulin serum $[Ak_1'] + [Ak_2']$ is obtained from the intersection on the abscissa of the extrapolation curve. The respective concentration values of the antibody-binding sites $[Ak_1']$ and $[Ak_2']$ are obtained from the abscissa intersection points of the asymptotes approaching the extrapolation curve. After calculation of $[Ak_1]$ and $[Ak_2]$ the association constants k_1 and k_2 can be determined from the intersection points on the ordinate of the extrapolation curve ($k_1\,[Ak_1'] + k_2\,[Ak_2']$) and of the asymptotes ($k_1\,[Ak_1']$ and $k_2\,[Ak_2']$), respectively. The asymptotes of the extrapolation curves are constructed graphically. This calculation corresponds to a modification of the Scatchard plot and of the curve extrapolation of BERSON and YALOW (1959a).

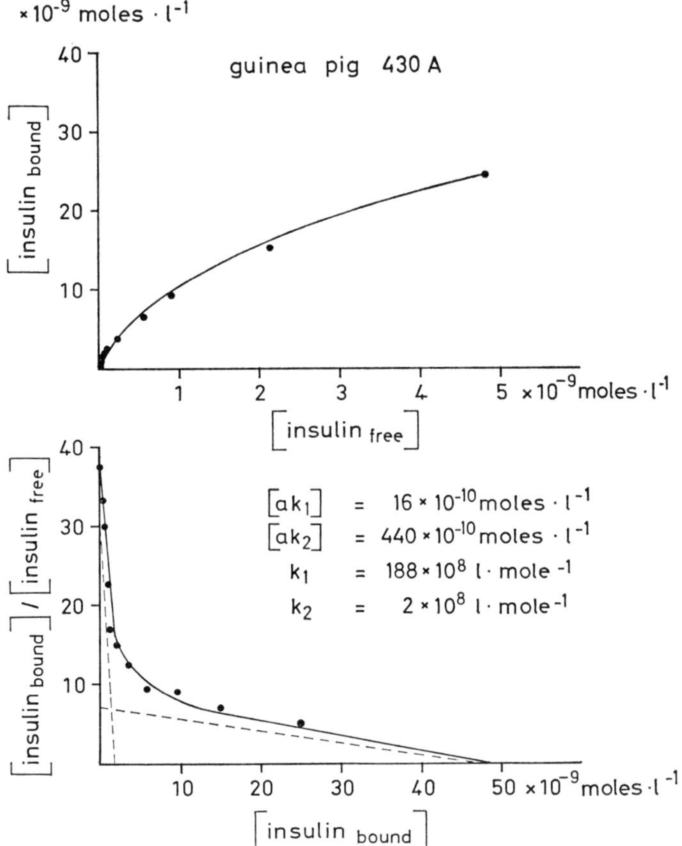

Fig. 3. Antibody binding of 131-I-bovine insulin in guinea pig anti-insulin serum (cellulose differential adsorption technique). a) binding curve, linear plot (top), b) binding curve, extrapolated and transformed according to SCATCHARD *et al.* (1957). The quantitative parameters of insulin-antibody binding were calculated using the asymptotes as described in the text (bottom)

The *free binding energy* $-\Delta F^\circ$ can be computed from the association constants according to the formula

$$-\Delta F^\circ = R T \ln k$$

where R denotes the gas constant, T the absolute temperature, and k the association constant.

The antibody-binding capability of modified as against unmodified insulin can be detected by comparing independently determined binding curves, or from *displacement* curves, which result from antigen competition for the antibody-binding sites. The displacement of insulin from antibody-binding sites by a modified antigen in equimolar concentration is a measure of the antigenic reactivity of the modified substance. According to KABAT (1971), the inhibition of antigen-antibody binding by a modified antigen is proportional to its free binding energy. The inhibitory effect of the modified antigen on both main components of the antibody can be seen from the shift of the extrapolation curve, and the free binding energy can be calculated as indicated above.

A particular problem of quantitative insulin-antibody determination is *interference from unlabeled insulin antigen* contained in the sample with the added labeled insulin antigen. Because of this interference, an apparent reduction of the serum antibody content is observed following injection of insulin (MICHEL, 1959). The injected insulin combines with the circulating antibodies, thereby reducing the concentration of the free antibody binding sites. Depending on the binding strength, insulin is then released from this complex (HARWOOD, 1960; FANKHAUSER and GOETZ, 1961). SCHADE and WEHNER (1969) found a marked reduction of insulin-binding capacity in insulin-immunized guinea pigs 90 min after the administration of insulin, and the maximum reduction of approximately 28% after 3—4 h. Even 9 h after injection of insulin, the initial value of the insulin-binding capacity was not yet reached. The relation of the free insulin-binding capacity to the saturated binding capacity in undiluted serum samples can be compared with that of the visible to the invisible portion of a "floating iceberg" (JAYARAO *et al.* 1969). KARAM *et al.* (1969b) succeeded in extracting between 15 and 3000 μU/ml of bound insulin from the serum of noninsulin-resistant patients with low antibody titer even 42 days after cessation of insulin therapy. In 4 patients with antibody-dependent insulin resistance, the total insulin concentration in the fasting serum was even higher, i.e. between 8000 and 12000 μU/ml.

In order to reduce the interference of the free antibody-binding capacity with the unknown insulin content of the samples, administration of exogenous insulin should be avoided for as long as possible prior to the antibody determination. In certain cases the total insulin-antibody binding capacity has to be determined by additional measures. It is possible to measure the "masked" insulin-antibodies by removing the free insulin by adsorption on charcoal (JAYARAO *et al.*, 1969) or on cellulose followed by cleavage of the insulin-antibody complex, for example, by acid treatment at pH 2—3 and subsequent antibody determination. Otherwise, the values of the free binding capacity ought to be corrected by the amount of bound insulin. For the determination of bound insulin, HEDING and NIELSEN (1967), HEDING (1969), and FØLLING and NORMAN (1972) proposed the differential determination of free and acid ethanol-extractable insulin.

II. Chemical-Physical Properties of Insulin Antibodies

1. Classification in Regard to Serum Protein Fractions

The first attempts to localize insulin-neutralizing antibodies in the serum protein fractions were made with *insulin-resistant patients*. DE FILLIPS and JANNACCONE reported in 1952 that the γ-globulins isolated by salt precipitation from the serum of an insulin-resistant patient inhibit the blood sugar-lowering effect of insulin in rats to the same extent as does whole serum from these patients. This finding was confirmed by COLWELL and WEIGER (1956). It was also shown by electrophoresis that the insulin antibodies of patients with antibody-dependent insulin resistance are located in the γ-globulin region (BERSON *et al.*, 1956, 1957; BURROWS *et al.*, 1957; MITCHELL, 1960; SEHON *et al.*, 1955). LOVELESS and CANN (1953, 1955), CANN and LOVELESS (1954), and LOWELL (1942, 1944b) were able to detect antibodies in the sera of patients with insulin resistance and insulin allergy in both the γ- and β-globulin fractions by means of electrophoresis. MILLER and OWEN (1960) and HARRIS-JONES *et al.* (1963), using the method of immunoelectrophoresis, found two insulin antibodies separated from each other in the serum of insulin-resistant patients in the zones of the γ- and β-globulins.

In insulin-treated but *not insulin-resistant diabetics* BERSON *et al.* (1956), GRODSKY and FORSHAM (1958) and HARRIS-JONES *et al.* (1963) found ^{131}I-insulin in the γ-globulin fraction after paper-electrophoretic serum fractionation. BURROWS *et al.* (1957), however, found that in the presence of such sera ^{131}I-insulin remained at the site of application of the paper electrophoresis. Their findings were confirmed by RANDLE and TAYLOR (1958) with column electrophoresis on ethanolized cellulose, as well as by MITCHELL (1960), who used electrophoresis on cation-exchange paper. The different results probably depend on differences in the strength of adsorption of insulin to the electrophoretic supporting material; if there is strong adsorption of insulin to the support, antibodies with a relatively weak binding capacity can escape detection. With especially weak adsorption of insulin, for example, to acetyl cellulose as support, insulin antibodies were regularly found in the γ-globulin fraction (KERP, 1963).

In *rabbit and guinea pig* insulin-binding antibodies could be demonstrated in the γ-globulin fraction (MORSE, 1959; KERP, 1963), in the guinea pig additionally in the β-globulin fraction (MORSE, 1959; YAGI *et al.*, 1962a, 1962b; KERP, 1963). The faster migrating component of these guinea pig antibodies later was found to belong to the γ_1-globulins and the component migrating more slowly to the γ_2-globulins. γ_1- and γ_2-insulin antibodies exhibit different structures of the Fc fragments and different biological properties. A passive cutaneous anaphylaxis reaction can be evoked only by intradermal injection of antibodies of the γ_1-globulin class (OVARY *et al.*, 1963). Only γ_2-antibodies lead to hemolysis of sensitized erythrocytes with complement consumption (BLOCH *et al.*, 1963).

BRUCCHIERI and GRASSO (1967) found guinea-pig insulin antibodies in the region of the γ-, β_3- and β_2-globulins. After immunization with bovine insulin only 2 and after immunization with porcine insulin 3 electrophoretically identifiable antibody types — including an IgM-globulin — were detectable.

Insulin antibodies are detectable in all immunoglobulin classes by means of *immunoelectrophoresis*. An isolated occurrence in the *IgG or IgM class* or a common occurrence in both immunoglobulin classes are described by CHRISTIANSEN (1970), CHRISTIANSEN and VØLUND (1971), CUNLIFFE (1965), DECKERT (1964), DEVLIN (1966), DEVLIN and O'DONOVAN (1965, 1966), DOLOVICH *et al.* (1970), FØLLING and NORMAN (1972), HORINO *et al.* (1966), KERP and KASEMIR (1968), MORSE and HEREMANS (1962), PALUMBO *et al.* (1965), PATTERSON *et al.* (1973a), SAMOLS and JONES (1965), STARZYNSKA and DEPOWSKA (1967), YAGI *et al.* (1963) and others. The distribution to these immunoglobulin classes can be determined quantitatively by ultracentrifugal analyses. HORINO and BLUMENTHAL (1966) found in the guinea pig during the initial phase of immunization 9.5% of the insulin antibodies in the 19S and 90.7% in the 7S globulin region.

Before the finding by the working group of ISHIZAKA (1966a, b) that the antibodies (reagins) responsible for immediate allergic reactions of the anaphylactic type (e.g. urticaria, Quincke's edema) occur in the IgE-immunoglobulin class, and before proof was furnished by DOLOVICH *et al.* (1970), LIEBERMAN *et al.* (1971) and PATTERSON *et al.* (1973b) that in case of insulin allergies of the anaphylactic type the insulin-specific antibodies belong to the IgE class, the reaginic activity of the insulin antibodies was thought to reside in the IgA class. Such IgA insulin antibodies were first described by YAGI *et al.* (1963) and later by CERASI *et al.* (1966), CORCOS and OVARY (1965), HORINO *et al.* (1966), PALUMBO *et al.* (1965), PATTERSON *et al.* (1969), STARZYNSKA (1969), YAGI *et al.* (1963) and others. IgA insulin antibodies were detected relatively seldom, for example, 5 times in 50 insulin-treated diabetics (FAULK *et al.*, 1971).

IgD insulin antibodies were detected by DEVEY *et al.* (1970) in 3 of 6 diabetics with additional IgG insulin antibodies (red blood cell-linked antigen—antiglobulin reaction). An insulin allergy with urticaria and gastrointestinal symptoms has been observed in one of these cases.

Most of the specific insulin antibodies belong to the *IgG class*.

2. Two Main Components of Insulin Antibodies of IgG Class

Two main components of insulin antibodies are found in the *IgG class* (BERSON and YALOW, 1959a; DITSCHUNEIT and FEDERLIN, 1966; GRODSKY and FORSHAM, 1961; KERP *et al.*, 1965; KERP *et al.*, 1966; KÜHNAU and GRIMM, 1971; LEV-RAN *et al.*, 1972 etc.; ROSSELIN *et al.*, 1965; YAGI *et al.*, 1962a). They can be identified from the analysis of insulin-antibody complex formation at reaction equilibrium and from the determination of the reaction velocities. Proof has been provided that all antibody-containing sera from patients or corresponding IgG-globulin fractions (KERP *et al.*, 1966) as well as the sera of insulin-immunized guinea pigs (YAGI *et al.*, 1962; KERP *et al.*, 1970a) contain two main components of insulin-binding antibodies. The main components of the antibodies differ in the strength of binding the insulin antigen. In insulin-treated diabetics the association constant for the high-affinity antibody component k_1 reaches the order of magnitude of $10^{9-10}\,l \times mol^{-1}$. The association constant k_2 of low-affinity antibody component is in the range of 10^7—$10^8\,l \times mol^{-1}$. 10% of the insulin antibody-binding sites within the IgG class belong to the high-affinity antibody component Ak_1 and 90% to the low-affinity antibody component Ak_2. The free binding energies calculated from the association constants are for $-\Delta F°_1$ in the range 12—13 kcal $\times$ mol^{-1} and for $-\Delta F°_2$ 10 kcal $\times$ mol^{-1} (KERP *et al.*, 1966).

The reaction rates of antibody complex formation can be determined in systems with high antibody dilution. The association rate is at 37° in the range of 2—500 $\times$ 10^5 l/mol antibody/min (BERSON and YALOW, 1959a). By the association rates of the complex formation it can also be shown that the sera of insulin-treated diabetics contain at least two antibody components, a rapidly and a slowly binding one (KÜHNAU and GRIMM, 1971; LEV-RAN *et al.*, 1972). The antigen-antibody complexes dissociate *in vitro* with half-lives of minutes up to many hours or even days, depending upon the binding energy of the individual antibody (BERSON and YALOW, 1959a). The different properties of both IgG-antibody components are reported in Table 1.

Table 1. *Properties of the IgG insulin antibody main components*

Antibody component	Ak_1	Ak_2
Relative share of total insulin binding capacity in serum	10%	90%
Strength of complex formation with insulin	high	low
Determinant regions on the insulin molecule when tested with isolated chains	B-chain	A-chain
Insulin neutralizing effect	existent	?
Alteration by partial insulin immun tolerance	marked	unimportant

Corresponding to the different affinity for insulin, the binding to the higher-affinity antibody component prevails at low serum insulin concentrations, whereas the lower-affinity antibody component is involved in the binding of insulin at higher insulin concentrations.

The antibody main components are probably antibodies which are directed against different antigen-determinant regions of the insulin molecule. This is in agreement with the findings of BERSON and YALOW (1959b) that the antibody main components of the serum of patients possess a different strength in binding insulins from various species. Also in guinea pigs the main components of insulin antibodies are directed against different determinant regions. Isolated A chains of insulin are prevalently bound by the low-affinity component, whereas derivatives or partial sequences of the B chain of insulin are preferentially bound by the high-affinity antibody main component (see p. 609).

III. Influence of the Insulin Molecule on its Binding to Insulin Antibodies of Serum

1. Effect of Species Differences on Insulin Immunology

Different amino acids occur in 29 out of 53 positions in the primary structures of all insulins analyzed to date (SMITH, 1972). Human insulin and bovine and porcine insulin used therapeutically in man differ only in the positions A^8—A^{10} and B^{30} (BEHRENS and BROMER, 1958; NICOL and SMITH, 1960; SANGER, 1958, 1959).

The question as to whether bovine insulin, which differs from human insulin in the amino acids at positions A^8—A^{10} and B^{30}, or porcine insulin which differs from human insulin only in the amino acid at position B^{30}, possesses a stronger *immunogenicity* has not yet been unequivocally answered. ANDERSEN (1973a), BERSON and YALOW (1966b), DEVLIN and DUGGAN (1969), FANKHAUSER and MICHL (1971, 1973), KERP (1973) and KÜHNAU, JR. (1968) reported that bovine insulin stimulates antibody formation more strongly than porcine insulin. DECKERT (1965), FANKHAUSER and MORELL (1968), HURN *et al.* (1969) and SCHLICHTKRULL (1970) found the immunogenicity of porcine and bovine insulin to be equipotent in man. ANDERSEN (1973b) observed a distinct predominance of the immunogenicity of bovine insulin only when comparing neutral insulin solutions from beef and pig, but not when using protamine insulin preparations.

Species dependent differences have also been observed in regard to the *antigenicity* of insulin. WRIGHT *et al.* (1967) found marked differences in cross-reactions between insulins from beef, pig, rat, man or codfish in binding to bovine insulin antibodies from guinea pig: the bovine insulin used for immunization was the most strongly bound, cod insulin the weakest. WILSON and FALKMER (1964) as well as FALKMER and WILSON (1967) investigated the binding of 19 different insulins to guinea-pig antibodies against bovine, chicken and cod insulin: most of the insulins from mammals, birds and amphibians resemble bovine insulin in their behavior. The insulins from catfish, cartilaginous fishes and from *Ciona intestinalis* (tunicates) were more analogous to chicken insulin, and insulins from the sea scorpion and other bony fishes were more similar to cod insulin.

The investigations of VARANDANI (1967) demonstrate that differences in antigen specificity extend also to isolated sulfonated insulin A chains. Sulfonated A chains of bovine insulin are more strongly bound by guinea-pig antibodies against bovine insulin than are sulfonated A chains of porcine insulin.

Human insulin, bovine and porcine insulin, too, differ in antigen specificity (BURROWS *et al.*, 1957; GRODSKY and FORSHAM, 1960, 1961; YALOW and BERSON, 1960, 1961a). As a rule, human insulin is more weakly bound than bovine insulin while human insulin, porcine insulin and rabbit insulin are equally bound by guinea-pig antibodies against porcine insulin (YALOW and BERSON, 1961; POTTER *et al.*, 1973).

Guinea-pig insulin holds an exceptional position with regard to its antigenicity, possibly because its primary structure differs markedly from that of other mammalian insulins. Guinea-pig insulin is not neutralized by antibodies of sheep against porcine insulin nor by antibodies of guinea pigs against bovine or porcine insulin (MOLONEY and COVAL, 1955). Accordingly, BERSON and YALOW (1966b) required approximately 2000 times higher concentrations of guinea-pig insulin as compared to porcine insulin in order to obtain an equal displacement of labeled porcine insulin from binding to antibodies against porcine insulin. According to investigations of DAVIDSON *et al.* (1968, 1969), only the insulins from the coypu (nutria) and the capybara (*Capybara carpincho* or *Hydrochoerus hydrochoerus*) cannot be neutralized in their biological effects by antibodies of guinea pigs against beef, chicken or cod insulin.

From the clinical point of view, the antigen reactivity of therapeutically used insulins toward the insulin antibodies that form in insulin-treated diabetics is of special interest. In comparisons between the binding of bovine and porcine insulin to insulin antibodies of patients treated with a mixture of bovine and porcine insulin, in most cases the binding of bovine insulin prevails regardless of the relative species proportions within the mixture of insulin preparation used (BERSON and YALOW, 1959b; DEVLIN and BRIEN, 1965; DEVLIN *et al.*, 1967; DEVLIN and DUGGAN, 1969; FANKHAUSER, 1969; FELDMAN *et al.*, 1963; KASEMIR *et al.*, 1968; KÜHNAU, JR., 1968; LEV-RAN *et al.*, 1971; ROSSELIN *et al.*, 1965; SOELDNER and STEINKE, 1965). In single cases, an even stronger binding of bovine insulin as compared to porcine insulin by antisera of patients treated with pig insulin has been reported (ANDERSEN, 1973a). Compared with bovine or porcine insulin, bonito and tuna-fish insulin is hardly bound at all by human antibodies against mixed bovine-porcine insulin (BURRILL *et al.*, 1969; DAVIDSON *et al.*, 1969; WILSON and DIXON, 1961; YALOW and BERSON, 1964).

The first quantitative surveys of complex formation by different insulins with antibodies of patients treated with a mixture of porcine and bovine insulin were done by BERSON and YALOW (1959b). These investigators showed that the insulins from beef, sheep, pig and horse differ in the strength of binding of the antigen-antibody complexes formed. The binding capacity proved to be nearly equal for the insulins from different species.

YALOW and BERSON (1964) later showed in comparative investigations of bovine and fish insulin that species-dependent differences in antigenicity can affect not only the binding strength but also the concentration of the antibody-binding sites. Also, in anti-insulin sera from diabetics treated with mixed bovine-porcine insulin, the concentrations of antibody-binding sites are higher for the binding of bovine insulin than for the binding of porcine insulin. Again, bovine insulin is more strongly bound, at least to the high-affinity antibody component Ak_1, than porcine insulin (KASEMIR *et al.*, 1968).

Initially BERSON and YALOW (1959b) and BURNETT (1961) traced the different immunogenicity and antigenicity of insulins from different species back to differences in the primary structure. Accordingly, the amino acids at positions A8, A9, A10 and B30 differing from human insulin would constitute antigen-determinant groups for the therapeutically used insulins from beef and pig. The larger non-differing molecule moieties were considered to be immunologically neutral. From this hypothesis one would expect the immunogenicity of porcine insulin in man to be based on the different amino acid in position B30. Experimentally, however, after cleavage of alanine at position B30, porcine insulin entered unchanged into an antigen-antibody binding with antisera from patients treated with porcine insulin (BERSON and YALOW, 1963). This finding is in accordance with the observation that whale insulin (ISHIHARA *et al.*, 1958) and porcine insulin (BEHRENS and BROMER, 1958) can be distinguished immunologically (BERSON and YALOW, 1961a) in spite of the fact that they have an identical amino acid sequence (HARRIS *et al.*, 1956).

2. Effects of Chemical Modifications on the Antibody Binding of Insulin

a) Insulin Chains and Chain Fragments

WILSON *et al.* (1962) demonstrated that an insulin which consists of an A chain of bovine insulin and a B chain of cod insulin is neutralized by guinea-pig antibodies against bovine insulin in the biological effect on the isolated mouse diaphragm.

However, the biological effect of an insulin composed of the A chain of cod insulin and the B chain of bovine insulin is not affected by these antibodies. Thus the authors inferred the location of antigen-determinant groups in the A chain of the insulin molecule.

Investigations with isolated A and B chains and with chain fragments supported this concepts only in part. Rabbits and guinea pigs produce chain-specific antibodies on immunization with A and B chains of insulin (BLACKARD, 1967; KERP *et al.*, 1967c; MEEK *et al.*, 1968; ORSETTI *et al.*, 1972; VARANDANI, 1967; WILSON *et al.*, 1967; YAGI *et al.*, 1965). Antibodies from guinea pig against sulfonated A chains of bovine insulin form complexes only with isolated A chain but not with intact bovine insulin, whereas antibodies against isolated B chains of insulin enter into antibody binding not only with isolated B chains but also with intact bovine insulin (KERP *et al.*, 1967c; PRESSMAN *et al.*, 1965; TOUBER *et al.*, 1970; VARANDANI, 1967; YAGI *et al.*, 1965). WILSON *et al.* (1967) however, detected a weak cross-reaction of antibodies against A chain with insulin, which was confirmed by TOUBER *et al.* (1970) for insulin and proinsulin.

According to BERSON and YALOW (1959b) as well as SURMACZYNSKA and METZ (1969), human antibodies against bovine insulin do not bind isolated A and B chains of bovine insulin at all. In contrast, YAGI *et al.* (1965) at least found a binding of isolated B chain by antibodies of guinea pig against bovine insulin. This latter finding is in agreement with observations by PRESSMAN *et al.* (1965), KERP *et al.* (1967c) and VARANDANI (1967).

Finally, contrary to YAGI *et al.* (1965), KERP *et al.* (1967a, b) demonstrated that ^{131}I-insulin can be displaced from the binding to guinea-pig antibodies against bovine insulin by sulfonated B chains of bovine insulin. Isolated sulfonated A chain exhibited no displacement effect. On immunization of pigs with porcine insulin, ^{131}I-porcine insulin was also displaced from the antibody binding by the isolated B chain of porcine insulin.

Analogous findings were made on investigation of the insulin immune reaction of the delayed type in the migration inhibition test (KRIEGBAUM and FEDERLIN, 1970; FEDERLIN, 1971). Only isolated B chain of bovine insulin induced on addition to the chamber medium a significant migration inhibition of the macrophages from guinea pigs immunized with bovine insulin.

The conclusion was drawn from these findings that the antigen-determinant groups of insulin, if represented by isolated chains, are preferentially located in the region of the B chain. Approximately one third of the high-affinity antibody binding sites contained in an anti-bovine insulin serum from the guinea pig find insertion sites in the region of the B chain of insulin, whereas the insertion sites of only about 3% of these high-affinity antibody binding sites are located in the region of the A chain. Conversely, approximately one third of the total concentration of the low-affinity antibody binding sites enter into complex formation with the A chain, whereas the B chain does not possess insertion sites for these antibody components (KERP *et al.*, 1970c).

The testing of chain fragments for antigen reactivity toward antibodies from the guinea pig against bovine insulin by means of the passive cutaneous anaphylaxis showed that the amino acid sequences A 10—21 and B 1—8 are potential antigen-determinant groups. Insignificant antigenic determinants were found in the regions A 1—9 and B 24—30. The peptides $(B\ 2—8)_2$, B 9—14 and $(B\ 17—23)_2$ were inactive (WILSON *et al.*, 1967).

KERP *et al.* (1967c, 1968a, 1969a,b, 1971a) investigated the displacement of bovine insulin from the binding to guinea pig antibodies against bovine insulin by synthetic fragments of the A and B chains in order to localize determinant groups in circumscribed molecular regions.

It was shown that the amino acid sequence $(B\ 17—30)_2$ effects a displacement of bovine insulin from the insulin-antibody binding. The partial sequences $(B\ 1—8)_2$, B 11—16 and B 21—30 were ineffective (KERP *et al.*, 1970b). The investigation with anti-insulin sera of diabetics demonstrated that also the sequence $(B\ 1—8)_2$, in addition to the sequence $(B\ 17—30)_2$, induced a displacement of bovine insulin from the binding to the high-affinity antibody component (KERP *et al.*, 1969b).

The macrophages of guinea pigs of the Pirbright-white strain immunized with bovine insulin showed a migration inhibition in the presence of the B chain sequence B 11—16, as was demonstrated by investigations of KRIEGBAUM and FEDERLIN (1970) and FEDERLIN (1971). The chain fragments B 24—30, B 21—30, B 23—30, $(B\ 17—20)_2$ and $(B\ 1—8)_2$ did not inhibit the migration.

Summarizing, it may be said that the antigen-determinant regions of the insulin molecule, as far as they are represented by isolated chains and by fragments of these chains, are primarily located in the region of the B chain. Isolated A chains seem to possess determinant regions for the antibody component with lower affinity and, furthermore, for insulin antibodies of the IgG class which are detectable by passive cutaneous anaphylaxis.

In investigations with isolated chains and chain fragments of insulin it has to be taken into account that only positive findings can be utilized for a localization of antigen-determinant regions for the following reasons: firstly, the portion of a chain is only recognizable as a determinant group or as a part of a determinant group if the spatial configuration is the same or at least similar to the corresponding portion of the chain in the intact insulin molecule. Secondly, the portion of a chain which is involved in the binding of antibodies is only detectable if its contribution to the total standard free energy of binding is measurably large. A complete determinant group has to extend at least to 5 or 6 (ARNON *et al.*, 1965), 7 (ATASSI, 1973; GILL, 1973) or more (BROWN, 1962) amino acids. According to concepts gained from X-ray spectrum analyses of the spatial configuration of insulin (HODGKIN, 1972), it may also be assumed that antigen-determinant groups consist of adjacent portions of both chains. This would explain the fact that only part of the insertion sites of insulin antibodies is recovered in experiments with isolated chains.

b) Insulin Modifications with Intact Spatial Configuration

Any loss of integrity of the insulin molecule will significantly reduce the binding to specific insulin antibodies (ARQUILLA and BROMER, 1967; BERSON and YALOW, 1959b; CORCOS and OVARY, 1965; WILSON *et al.*, 1967; YAGI *et al.*, 1965). For an analysis of antigen-determinant groups by means of molecular modifications it is therefore necessary to carry out molecule modifications in such a way that the spatial configuration remains virtually intact. Immunologic investigations have been performed on insulin analogs with shortened or prolonged chains, on insulin analogs with altered amino acid sequence, and on other insulin derivatives.

α) Analogs of insulin with shortened chains

Des-Gly^{A1} insulin

Des-Gly^{A1} insulin is semisynthetically obtained by modification of the isolated A chain of insulin and by recombination with the natural B chain (BRANDENBURG *et al.*, 1971a; WEINERT *et al.*, 1969).

CD spectra of the substance indicate marked structural changes as compared to insulin. The biological *in vivo* activity to lower blood sugar in fasted rats corresponds to 10% of the effect exerted by intact insulin. The biological *in vitro* activity measured by glucose oxidation of isolated fat cells amounts to 2 and 10%, respectively, of the effect of comparative insulin (BRANDENBURG *et al.*, 1971a).

Different data on the antibody binding of des-Gly^{A1} insulin have been presented. The minimum concentration of des-Gly^{A1} insulin to obtain a precipitation with guinea-pig anti-insulin sera in the agar immunodiffusion test is 25 μg/ml, corresponding to 12.5 μg/ml of intact bovine insulin (WILSON, 1971).

Approximately 100-fold higher concentrations of des-Gly^{A1}-bovine insulin than of bovine insulin are required in order to prevent hemagglutination of insulin-loaded erythrocytes in the presence of insulin antibodies (WILSON, 1971). In the experimental procedure of the passive cutaneous anaphylaxis, the extension of the erythema on application of des-Gly^{A1} insulin as an antigen is less than 20% of that of to insulin.

By means of a double-antibody method the antibody binding is reduced to 30 and 20%, respectively (BRANDENBURG *et al.*, 1971a). The free binding energies for the binding of des-Gly^{A1} insulin to the high-affinity antibody component show a reduction to 67% in comparison with intact bovine insulin. The free binding energy for the binding to the low affinity antibody component is unaltered in comparison to nonmodified insulin (KERP *et al.*, 1972).

Des-Gly^{A1}-des-Phe^{B1} insulin

This insulin analog without the N-terminal amino acids of both chains was prepared by BRANDENBURG and OOMS (1968) as well as by AFRICA and CARPENTER (1968, 1970). It possesses a blood sugar-lowering effect of only 7% in the fasting rat, 3% on the isolated adipose tissue, and 1.6% on the isolated fat cells of the rat (BRANDENBURG *et al.*, 1971a).

BRANDENBURG *et al.* (1971a) discuss whether the residual biological activity of this substance may be attributed to the existence of incompletely split intermediate products with biological activity.

The binding of des-Gly^{A1}-des-Phe^{B1} insulin to insulin antibodies amounts to 25% in the agar immunodiffusion test, to 1.6% in the hemagglutination inhibition test and to 6.4% in the complement fixation test as compared to insulin (WILSON, 1971). In order to obtain a 50% displacement of labeled insulin from the binding to insulin antibodies, a 6-fold quantity of the substance is required in comparison to insulin (BRANDENBURG *et al.*, 1971a). KERP *et al.* (1972) found the antibody binding of des-Gly^{A1}-des-Phe^{B1} insulin measured as free binding energy $-\Delta F°$ for binding to guinea-pig anti-bovine-insulin serum to be reduced to 70% at the high-affinity antibody component and to 49% at low-affinity antibody component as compared to insulin.

Des-(Gly^{A1}, Ile^{A2}, Phe^{B1}, Val^{B2}) insulin

The cleavage of two N-terminal amino acids, respectively, from both insulin chains leads to a nearly complete loss of biological activity. The residual effect on isolated fat cells is less than 0.2% in comparison with intact insulin (BRANDENBURG *et al.*, 1971a).

The antibody binding of des-(Gly^{A1}, Ile^{A2}, Phe^{B1}, Val^{B2}) insulin measured by the displacement of ^{131}I-labeled insulin from the binding to antibodies from the guinea pig was 2% in comparison to bovine insulin (BRANDENBURG *et al.*, 1971a).

Des-Phe^{B1} insulin

WEBER and WEITZEL (1968) described the preparation of this insulin analog by combination of a modified B chain, obtained by Merrifield synthesis, with a natural A chain of bovine insulin. BRANDENBURG (1969) obtained des-Phe^{B1} insulin by reaction of insulin with phenylisothiocyanate and subsequent treatment of the derivatives with trifluoroacetic acid. Preparation of des-Phe^{B1} insulin by selective protection of the amino groups at Gly^{A1} and Lys^{B29} by BOC (tertiary butyloxycarbonyl acid) and subsequent Edman degradation was described by GEIGER *et al.* (1971).

Des-Phe^{B1} insulin has the same crystallization properties as insulin (ZAHN *et al.*, 1972) and possesses a CD spectrum differing only slightly from that of insulin (BRANDENBURG *et al.*, 1971a). The biological activity corresponds to that of insulin. The blood sugar reduction amounts to 90% in the fasting rat (BRANDENBURG *et al.*, 1971a) and to 97 ± 5% in the rabbit

(Kerp *et al.*, 1974) as compared to the effect of intact insulin. The *in vitro* activity tested in the rat fat pad amounts to 110% in comparison to the effect of insulin (Brandenburg *et al.*, 1971a); the *in vitro* activity measured in isolated fat cells adds up to 89 ±9% compared to that of bovine insulin (Kerp *et al.*, 1974). Des-Phe^{B1} insulin synthesized by Weber and Weitzel (1968) possesses a biological activity in the mouse convulsion test and in the fat pad assay which does not differ from that of the corresponding hybrid insulins from synthetic A and natural B chains.

The binding of des-Phe^{B1}-bovine insulin to specific insulin receptors of isolated fat cells is 78—102% in comparison to insulin (Gliemann and Gammeltoft, 1973; Henrichs *et al.*, 1974).

The binding of des-Phe^{B1} insulin to antibodies of the guinea pig against bovine insulin corresponds to that of intact insulin in the agar immunodiffusion test and in the hemagglutination inhibition test (Wilson, 1971). Brandenburg *et al.* (1971a) also did not find changes in the antibody binding after splitting off Phe^{B1}. The free energy of antibody binding of des-Phe^{B1} insulin amounts to 77% for the high-affinity component of antibodies and to 48% for the low-affinity component of antibodies (Kerp *et al.*, 1974) as compared to bovine insulin. From these latter investigations it may be concluded that the antibody binding of des-Phe^{B1} insulin is markedly reduced without significant impairment of the biological activity in comparison to unmodified bovine insulin.

Des-(Phe-Val)$^{B1-2}$ *insulin*

Analogous to the preparation of des-Phe^{B1} insulin from a synthetic modified B chain and a natural A chain of insulin, Weber and Weitzel (1968) synthetized des-(Phe-Val)B^{1-2} [Ala^{B4}]-hybrid insulin with the additional substitution of glutamine^{B4} by L-alanine. Geiger (1971) as well as Geiger and Langner (1973) obtained des-(Phe-Val)$^{B1-2}$ insulin by repetition of the Edman degradation which yielded des-Phe^{B1} insulin.

The biological effect of des-(Phe-Val)$^{B1-2}$ [Ala^{B4}]-hybrid insulin on isolated tissue and in the mouse convulsion test corresponds to the effect of a corresponding hybrid insulin from a synthetic A chain and a natural B chain (Weber and Weitzel, 1968).

Kerp *et al.* (1974) reportet for des-(Phe-Val)$^{B1-2}$-bovine insulin (Geiger and Langner, 1973) an effect of 95 ±5% on the blood sugar reduction in the rabbit and an effect of 86 ±3.5% on the stimulation of the glucose oxidation of isolated fat cells as compared to bovine insulin.

The binding of des-(Phe-Val)$^{B1-2}$ insulin to antibodies of guinea pigs against bovine insulin corresponds to 6.25% in the agar immunodiffusion test, to 3% in the hemagglutination inhibition test and to 3.2% in the complement fixation test as compared to intact insulin. By means of passive cutaneous anaphylaxis, the compound produced an erythema of 20 mm compared to an erythema of 30 mm on application of insulin as an antigen (Wilson, 1971).

The free energy for the binding of the modified compound to bovine insulin antibodies from guinea pigs in their high-affinity component amounts to 76% (in comparison to that of bovine insulin) and is reduced to 0% in their low affinity component (Kerp *et al.*, 1974).

Des-(Phe-Val-Asn)$^{B1-3}$-[*Pyr*^{B4}] *insulin*

To synthesize this insulin analog Geiger (1971) as well as Geiger and Langner (1973) repeated the Edman degradation of des-(Phe-Val)$^{B1-2}$ insulin with protection of the functional amino groups at A_1 and B_{29}. Contrary to des-Phe^{B1}- and des-(Phe-Val)$^{B1-2}$ insulin, this substance is hardly crystallizable. This can be indicative of a spatial configuration deranged by the modification (Kerp *et al.*, 1974). The biological activity of the substance amounts to 68% in the fat cell test and to 70% measured by the blood sugar-lowering effect in the rabbit in comparison to bovine insulin.

The binding to guinea-pig antibodies against bovine insulin measured as free binding energy at the high-affinity antibody component is reduced to 68% and completely abolished at the low-affinity component of antibodies (Kerp *et al.*, 1974).

Des-Ala^{B30} *insulin*

The C-terminal alanine of the A chain of insulin can be split off by mild hydrolysis with carboxypeptidase A without affecting the CD spectrum of insulin (ARQUILLA *et al.*, 1972). The biological effect of the substance corresponds to that of insulin (HARRIS and LI, 1952; NICOL, 1960; SLOBIN and CARPENTER, 1966).

The primary structures of human and porcine insulin differ in position B30 only; alanine constitutes the C terminus of the B chain for porcine insulin, whereas threonine forms the C terminus of the B chain for human insulin. A diminution or suppression of the immunogenicity and antigenicity of porcine insulin was expected in man by the removal of alanine^{B30}. Nevertheless, BERSON and YALOW (1963) could not prove a reduction in the antibody binding of des-Ala^{B30} insulin to antibodies against porcine insulin from diabetics.

Des-Ala^{B30}*-des-Asp*^{A21} *insulin*

Like des-Ala^{B30} insulin, this substance is prepared from insulin by hydrolysis with carboxypeptidase (SLOBIN and CARPENTER, 1963a, b). This insulin derivative differs significantly from native insulin in its UV and CD spectra (BRUGMAN and ARQUILLA, 1973; MORRIS *et al.*, 1970a). The biological activity of des-Ala^{B30}-des-Asp^{A21} insulin is reduced to approximately 4% in the mouse convulsion test as compared to insulin (ARQUILLA *et al.*, 1969). It has no biological effect on isolated adipose tissue and on isolated diaphragm (SURMACZYNSKA *et al.*, 1969).

The binding of des-Ala^{B30}-des-Asp^{A21} insulin to insulin antibodies in the immune-hemolysis test, depending on the guinea pig strain under test, measured between 1 and approximately 20% of that of unmodified bovine insulin (ARQUILLA and BROMER, 1967; BRUGMAN and ARQUILLA, 1973). SURMACZYNSKA *et al.* (1969) found complete abolition of the binding to antibodies.

Desoctapeptide^{B23-30} *insulin*

Desoctapeptide insulin is obtained by controlled trypsin digestion of insulin (BROMER and CHANCE, 1967; CARPENTER and YOUNG, 1959; YOUNG and CARPENTER, 1961). CD spectra of desoctapeptide^{B23-30} insulin showed a distinct difference in comparison to insulin (ARQUILLA *et al.*, 1969; BRUGMAN and ARQUILLA, 1973; MERCOLA *et al.*, 1967). A biological activity is not measurable in the mouse convulsion test (ARQUILLA and BROMER, 1967; CARPENTER, 1966; YOUNG and CARPENTER, 1961) nor in the adipose tissue or hemidiaphragm test (SURMACZYNSKA *et al.*, 1969).

BERSON and YALOW (1961b, 1963) and YALOW and BERSON (1961b) investigated the antibody binding of desoctapeptide^{B23-30} insulin. Antibodies of patients who received mixed bovine-porcine insulin enter into a markedly lower binding with desoctapeptide $^{B23-30}$ beef insulin than with intact bovine insulin. ARQUILLA *et al.* (1969) needed, depending on the guinea pig strain under test, a 200—4000-fold higher concentration of desoctapeptide $^{B23-30}$ insulin than of unmodified bovine insulin in order to obtain a 50% inhibition in the immune-hemolysis inhibition test. Investigations of SURMACZYNSKA *et al.* (1969) did not prove binding of desoctapeptide $^{B23-30}$ insulin to guinea-pig antibodies.

β) Insulin analogs with prolonged chains

Arg-Gly^{A1} *insulin*

Arg-Gly^{A1} insulin is prepared by a semisynthetic procedure from the S sulfonate of the A chain after reaction with N-carboxyanhydride of the arginine hydrobromide and combination with the B chain of insulin (WEINERT *et al.*, 1969, 1971). The substance is easily crystallizable. Arginyl insulin is a potential intermediate product on conversion of pro-insulin to insulin. The substitution of the arginyl residue at position Gly^{A1} reduces the biological activity to 59% in the mouse convulsion test and the stimulation of the glucose oxidation of isolated fat cells to 68% as compared to the nonsubstituted insulin.

The binding of Arg-Gly^{A1} insulin to insulin antibodies was 40% in relation to bovine insulin, as was determined by BRANDENBURG *et al.* (1971a) by means of the double-antibody technique. In the agar immunodiffusion test and in the hemagglutination inhibition test WILSON (1971) found the Arg-Gly^{A1} insulin binding to insulin antibodies from the guinea pig to be reduced to 50% of unmodified insulin.

Lys-Arg-Gly^{A1} insulin

An elongation of the N-terminal A chain of insulin with Lys-Arg (GATTNER, 1970) was obtained by further elongation of the Arg-Gly^{A1}-A chain with a lysyl residue. The product was combined with natural B chain. The biological effect of the compound in the mouse convulsion test amounts to 20% of the insulin effect.

ZAHN *et al.* (1972) found by means of the double-antibody method that the binding of Lys-Arg^{A1} insulin to antibodies is 34% of that of insulin. In the agar immunodiffusion test the minimal precipitation concentration corresponds to 25% and in the hemagglutination inhibition test to 6% of that of insulin (WILSON, 1971). In passive cutaneous anaphylaxis Lys-Arg^{A1} insulin produced an erythematous areola of 22 mm and of 12 mm on application of bovine insulin antibodies from the guinea pig and of chicken insulin antibodies from the guinea pig, respectively, in comparison to 30 and 13 mm, respectively, on application of bovine insulin as an antigen (WILSON, 1971).

Monoarginine insulin (Arg^{31} at position Ala^{B30})

Monoarginine insulin (Arg^{31} at position Ala^{B30}) is contained in insulin preparations extracted from the pancreas or results *in vitro* from treatment of proinsulin with trypsin. Monoarginine insulin can be isolated by chromatography on DEAE-cellulose and Sephadex or by polyacrylamide disc gel electrophoresis (CHANCE, 1971). Monoarginine insulin possesses 66% of the effect of porcine insulin in the mouse convulsion test.

Measured by the alcohol precipitation technique of HEDING (1965, 1966), the binding of monoarginine insulin to porcine insulin antibodies from guinea pig corresponds to 67% as compared to porcine insulin (CHANGE, 1971).

Diarginine insulin (Arg^{31}-Arg^{32} at position Ala^{B30})

Like monoarginine, diarginine insulin can be isolated from extracted insulins by gel chromatography or it can be obtained by tryptic hydrolysis of proinsulin or proinsulin intermediates (CHANCE, 1971). Diarginine insulin possesses 62% of the effect of porcine insulin in the mouse convulsion test.

The binding of diarginine insulin to guinea-pig antibodies against porcine insulin is 80% of the binding of porcine insulin (CHANCE, 1971).

Proinsulin intermediates

Split proinsulin, cleaved between Leu^{54}-Ala^{55}, desdipeptide proinsulin with Lys^{62} and Arg^{63} removed, and desnonapeptide proinsulin with B$^{55-63}$ removed are proteins, which can be isolated from pancreas extract. The biological activity determined in the mouse convulsion test was 20%, 58% and 62% respectively, in comparison to the effect of porcine insulin.

The antibody binding of these derivatives to porcine insulin antibodies of the guinea pig is 45%, 61% and 61%, respectively (CHANCE, 1971).

γ) Insulin analogs with varied primary structure

Modifications in position A 1

Des-Gly^{A1}-A chain reacted with activated esters of butyloxycarbonyl amino acids after combination with natural B chain to yield insulin analogs with glutamyl^{A1}, leucyl^{A1}, prolyl^{A1}, or acetyl^{A1} substitution for Gly^{A1}. The biological activity of glutamyl^{A1}, leucyl^{A1} and prolyl-^{A1} insulin modifications corresponds to that of insulin (BRANDENBURG *et al.*, 1970). In contrast, the modification to acetyl^{A1} or desamino^{A1} insulin leads in the fat-cell test to a loss of activity amounting to 15% in comparison with insulin (BRANDENBURG *et al.*, 1971a; ZAHN *et al.*, 1972).

The binding of desamino^{A1} insulin to insulin antibodies as measured by the double-antibody method is according to ZAHN *et al.* (1972) 40% and according to BRANDENBURG *et al.* (1973) 30% of that of the comparative insulin. The marked alteration of the biological and immunological properties by these modifications in position A1 is probably a result of conformational changes affecting the entire molecule. These conformational changes were demonstrated by CD-spectrum analyses (BRANDENBURG *et al.*, 1971a).

Desamido insulin

The desaminated form of insulin which contains asparaginic acid instead of asparagine at position A^{21} results from mild acid treatment of insulin and can be removed from insulin preparations by appropriate chromatographic techniques. The biological effect of the substance corresponds to that of porcine insulin in the mouse convulsion test (SLOBIN and CARPENTER, 1963b; CHANCE, 1971).

An antibody binding of 80% to porcine insulin antibodies from the guinea pig in comparison to porcine insulin was reported for desamido insulin by means of the alcohol precipitation technique (CHANCE, 1971).

Gly^{B1}-acetyl^{B29} insulin

This substance with amino acid variation in position B1 and acetylation of Lys^{B29} possesses a biological *in vitro* activity of 35% and an antibody binding of 25% in comparison to unchanged insulin (ZAHN *et al.*, 1972).

δ) Insulin derivatives

Since insulin possesses 3 primary amino groups, 6 carboxyl groups and 4 tyrosine residues, which means a variety of functional groups, mixtures of different reaction products mostly result from reactions with reagents of limited selectivity. The nonhomogeneity of those products complicates the characterization of their biological or immunological properties. Some homogeneous insulin derivatives were also obtained and investigated (survey by BRANDENBURG *et al.*, 1971a,b).

Acetyl insulins

Acetyl insulins were prepared according to LINDSAY and SHALL (1971) or to BRANDENBURG *et al.* (1972b) either via intact insulin with protection of free functional groups and subsequent reaction with acetic anhydride or by recombination of previously acetylated chains with the respective matching chain. The acetylation affects the N-terminal amino groups at positions A1 and B1 as well as the ε-amino group of Lys^{B29}. Biologically, the derivatives with acetylation of an unselected NH_2-group exhibited full insulin activity in the mouse convulsion test in contrast to acetoacetyl- or thiazolidine-carbonyl derivatives, as demonstrated by investigations of LINDSAY and SHALL (1971). Acetylation reduces the biological activity by specific substitution at position Gly^{A1} but not at positions Phe^{B1} or Lys^{B29}.

ZAHN *et al.* (1972) found a marked diminution of the biological activity *in vitro*, whereas the activity *in vivo* measured by the blood sugar reduction in the rat was equal to that of insulin. The loss of activity *in vitro* was dependent upon degree and location of acetylation. Acetyl-Gly^{A1} insulin showed 40%, acetyl^{B29} insulin 75% and diacetyl^{B1,B29} insulin 85% of the insulin effect in the fat cell test. The discrepancy between *in vivo* and *in vitro* findings seems to be the result of an enzymatic deacetylation under *in vivo* conditions (BRANDENBURG *et al.*, 1972b).

According to earlier investigations, acetylation does not affect the immunological properties of insulin (GRODSKY *et al.*, 1959; KITAGAVA *et al.*, 1960). In the investigations of ZAHN *et al.* (1972), however, the binding of monoacetyl insulins to insulin antibodies was gradually diminished. The antigen reactivity of acetyl^{A1} insulin corresponded to 47%, of acetyl^{B29} insulin to 85% and of diacetyl-^{B1,B29} insulin to 30% of that of comparative insulin. LINDSAY and SHALL (1971) observed for Phe^{B1} acetyl insulin a markedly reduced affinity for insulin antibodies of the guinea pig.

Sulfated insulins

Sulfated insulins are synthesized by reaction of insulin with sulfuric acid under controlled conditions (MOLONEY *et al.*, 1964). The biological activity is reduced to 95—30% of the insulin effect according to the degree of sulfation (THOMAS, 1971).

The binding of sulfated insulins to bovine insulin antibodies diminishes with increasing sulfate content of the derivatives (THOMAS, 1971). In the hemagglutination inhibition test the antibody binding of sulfated insulin corresponds to 0.3% or less, as compared to insulin (WILSON, 1971). Due to their low antibody binding, sulfated insulins were used for the treatment of antibody-dependent insulin resistance (ARNOTT and LITTLE, 1965; LITTLE and ARNOTT, 1966; MOLONEY *et al.*, 1964; SCHREIBER and ROTTENHÖFER, 1968). Also the immunogenic activity of bovine insulin in man is reduced by sulfation, as shown by a study of PLAUTZ and LITTLE (1970). The authors treated 18 diabetics with sulfated bovine insulin and for comparison 17 diabetics with commercial bovine Lente insulin. The mean insulin antibody titers in the first group after 3, 6, 9 and 12 months amounted to 10, 8, 2 and 11 μU/ml compared with 678, 4329, 3663 and 482 μU/ml in the group treated with nonsulfated insulin.

Maleyl and succinyl insulins

Maleyl insulins from the beef are obtained by reaction of bovine insulin with maleyl anhydride in dimethyl sulfoxide (MOLONEY and TIRPAK, 1969; MOLONEY and JACKSON, 1973). According to the reaction conditions, different maleyl residues are introduced per insulin molecule. In the mouse convulsion test the biological effect of a maleyl insulin batch with 14 maleyl residues is 4% of that of standard insulin (MOLONEY and JACKSON, 1973).

The binding of M5-maleyl insulin to insulin antibodies is reduced to approximately 0.3% in the hemagglutination inhibition test (WILSON, 1973; WILSON *et al.*, 1973). Along with incomplete Freund's adjuvant, maleyl insulin from the beef exerts only a weak immunogenic effect in guinea pigs. An insulin immuntolerance in regard to the formation of antibodies may be produced in guinea pigs with maleyl as well as with succinyl insulin from beef (MOLONEY and TIRPAK, 1969; MOLONEY and EVANS, 1971; MOLONEY and JACKSON, 1973; WILSON, 1973).

Nitro insulins

Mono-, di- and trinitro insulins are obtained by the reaction of tetranitromethane or p-nitrophenyl acetate with insulin (BOESEL and CARPENTER, 1970; BRANDENBURG *et al.*, 1971a, 1972a; LINDSAY and SHALL, 1971; MORRIS *et al.*, 1970b). They can be isolated by DEAE-Sephadex chromatography. With increasing nitration, the formation of derivatives primarily affects the tyrosyl residue at position A 14, subsequently the tyrosines at positions A 14 and A 19, and then B 16 and B 26.

The binding of mononitro insulin to insulin antibodies is 40%, of dinitro insulin 30% and of trinitro insulin 20% of that of the comparative insulin (BRANDENBURG *et al.*, 1971a).

Iodinated insulins

Numerous techniques have been indicated for the iodination of insulin, especially with radioactively labeled iodine (for surveys see KALLEE, 1952, 1969; ROTH, 1973; ZAHN and KLOSTERMEYER, 1969).

The iodination concerns the tyrosyl residues at positions A8, A14, A19, B16, B26 and B27 of the insulin molecules to various degrees. Histidine residues are usually not involved in the iodination (KALLEE, 1969). BRUNFELDT *et al.* (1968) found that the biological activity of iodinated insulins is limited *in vivo* (blood sugar-lowering effect in the rabbit and mouse convulsion test) and *in vitro* (fat-cell test) in proportion to the degree of iodination, which is in accordance with old findings of JENSEN *et al.* (1932). ^{125}I-insulin with 0.5 or less iodine atoms per molecule which was purified by disc electrophoresis in 15% acrylamide gel did not show any biological effect *in vitro* in investigations of BROMER and ARQUILLA (1967) with the aid of the fat-pad assay. LAMBERT *et al.* (1972) found that their ^{125}I-monoiodine insulin preparation had lost the capacity to stimulate the glucose uptake in isolated rat diaphragm, but that it was bound to plasma insulin receptors like unlabeled insulin. Further data on the relationship of biological effect and degree of iodination are contained in the survey by KALLEE (1969). The loss of biological activity is dependent both on the degree of iodination and on the chemical conditions of the iodination reaction (ROTH, 1973). It is possible that spontaneous intermolecular cross linkages to insulin dimers with reduced biological activity play an important role (CSORBA and GATTNER, 1970). Furthermore, the position of the iodine-substituted tyrosyl residues is of significance for the biological activity. KRAIL *et al.* (1971) detected by means of the fat-cell test that the biological *in vitro* effect of a monoiodine insulin obtained semisynthetically in the form of p-iodine-phenylalanine^{B1} insulin amounts to 65% in comparison to unlabeled insulin. A tyrosine iodination at positions A19 and B16 led to the abolition of the biological insulin activity in investigations of GARATT *et al.* (1972).

The binding to insulin antibodies, too, is affected in a different manner by degree and technique of iodination as well as by the location of the substituent. IZZO *et al.* (1964) did not observe an influence of the iodination on the antibody binding of insulin. ARQUILLA *et al.* (1965, 1966, 1968, 1969), however, reported a marked reduction of the antigen reactivity in the immune-hemolysis inhibition test, which was partly dependent on the degree of iodination and partly on the preparation technique. Inhibition of the antigen reactivity was still observed on minimal iodination of 0.55 to 0.03 iodine atoms/insulin molecule. BRUNFELDT *et al.* (1968) also detected a distinct restriction of the binding to porcine insulin antibodies from the guinea pig in the double-antibody technique, which is dependent on the degree of iodination of insulin.

The antigen reactivity of a ^{131}I-bovine insulin with a degree of iodination of approximately one iodine atom per insulin molecule was unchanged in comparison to intact bovine insulin, as shown in investigations of KERP *et al.* (1966). The data-points of the insulin antibody binding were located on a common adsorption isotherm in the differential cellulose adsorption technique, independent of the mixture ratio of labeled and unlabeled insulin.

Cyanoethyl insulins

Cyanoethyl insulins are obtained by reaction of insulin with acrylonitrile (BOSSHARD *et al.*, 1969). Derivatives are formed at the site of amino groups and, to a varying extent, at the histidine residues at positions B5 and B10 of the insulin molecule. Depending on the degree of cyanoethylation, the biological effect of bovine insulin is reduced to 50—20% in the mouse convulsion test and in isolated epididymal fat pads of the rat. Blocking of both histidyl residues lowers the residual biological activity to only 1.5%. It follows that histidine^{B5} is probably of particular significance for the biological activity.

The binding of the derivatives to insulin antibodies varies according to the degree of derivative formation. The binding of cyanoethyl insulin with a residual histidine content of 50% to guinea pig antibodies against porcine insulin corresponds to the binding of unmodified porcine insulin. The evaluation of the findings is difficult since the acrylonitrile reaction can simultaneously block α- and ε-amino groups in addition to the histidyl residues (BOSSHARD *et al.*, 1969).

Fluorescein insulin conjugates

Insulin undergoes reaction with fluorescein isothiocyanate to form fluorescein conjugates at positions Phe^{B1}, Gly^{A1} and Lys^{B29} (ARQUILLA *et al.*, 1966, 1969; BROMER *et al.*, 1966, 1967; MERCOLA *et al.*, 1972).

The loss of biological activity correlates with the degree of conjugation. The antibody binding is dependent on the degree of conjugation, as is shown in Table 2 (ARQUILLA *et al.*, 1969; ARQUILLA, 1967).

Table 2. *Biological activity and antigen reactivity of fluorescein insulin conjugates*

Biological effect (Mouse convulsion test and fat pad assay)		Antigen reactivity (50% inhibition of the immune hemolysis)		
		Strain: 13	Strain: 2	Mixed breed
Monoconjugate	40%	0.09 μg	0.22 μg	0.25 μg
Diconjugate	4%	0.16 μg	0.81 μg	1.81 μg
Triconjugate	0%	1.3 μg	7050.0 μg	223.5 μg

(according to ARQUILLA and BROMER, 1967)

Phenylthiocarbamyl (PTC) insulins

PTC insulins are obtained by the reaction of insulin with the Edman reagent phenylisothiocyanate. PTC substitution is observed at positions B1 or A1, and B1 or A1, B1 and B29.

The PTC substitution leads, analogous to modifications by other monofunctional substituents, to a loss of biological activity that increases with the number of substituents.

KERP *et al.* (1972) found the antibody binding of mono-PTC insulin to bovine insulin antibodies from the guinea pig to be the same as that of bovine insulin. The free binding energy between di-PTC insulin and the low-affinity antibody component is 100% and the high-affinity antibody component 84% in comparison to bovine insulin.

Carbamyl and methylcarbamyl insulins

LINDSAY *et al.* (1972) obtained carbamyl and methylcarbamyl derivatives of insulin by reaction of insulin with potassium cyanate and methylisothiocyanate. The substitution affects the *a*-amino groups of the N-terminal amino acids of both chains of the insulin molecule. The biological activity of the derivatives corresponds to that of insulin.

The binding of bovine insulin to antibodies of the guinea pig is significantly reduced by the carbamyl and methylcarbamyl substitution at positions Gly^{A1} and Phe^{B1} (LINDSAY *et al.*, 1972).

ε) Cross-linked insulins

Insulin derivatives with intra- or intermolecular cross linkages of non-peptide nature are obtained by bifunctional reagents such as m-phenylene-diisothiocyanate or aliphatic dicarbonic acids (BRANDENBURG *et al.*, 1971a, 1972a).

The spatial fixation of the N-terminal amino acids effects a drastic loss of activity and a marked reduction of the binding of this insulin modification to insulin antibodies. CD spectra of A1-B1-PBC insulin indicate significant configurational changes of the molecule. In contrast, CD spectra of insulin derivatives which entered into an A1-B29 cross linkage via dicarbonic acids correspond approximately to a noncross-linked insulin with acetyl residues at positions A1 and B29 (BRANDENBURG *et al.*, 1972a).

Furthermore, BRANDENBURG synthesized an insulin derivative with a Phe^{B1}-$Phe^{B1'}$ cross-linkage, leading to a homologous dimer configuration. The biological activity of the compound in the rat fat-pad assay is about 20% in comparison to monomeric insulin.

The antibody binding of the insulin dimer is reduced to about 50% of unmodified insulin (BRANDENBURG *et al.*, 1971a).

ζ) Insulin with partially cleaved disulfide bridges

An electrochemical reduction of insulin under certain conditions leads to the cleavage of the interchain A7-B7 (GATTNER, 1970), or intrachain A6-A11 disulfide bridges. The selective cleavage of the disulfide bridge A7-B7 is also obtained by sulfitolysis (BUSSE and GATTNER,

1973). CD spectra of insulin derivatives with cleaved intrachain or interchain disulfide bridges are similar to each other, but drastically different from insulin (BRANDENBURG *et al.*, 1972a; BRANDENBURG and WOLLMER, 1973). The biological activity of the A7-B7-di-S-insulin-sulfonate is reduced to 4—10% in the rat hypoglycemia test and to 15% in the mouse convulsion test (BUSSE and GATTNER, 1973).

The antibody binding of A7-B7-di-S-insulin sulfonate is 5—12% in passive cutaneous anaphylaxis in guinea pig (BUSSE and GATTNER, 1973), 50% in the agar immunodiffusion test, and 6% in the hemagglutination inhibition test (WILSON, 1971) as compared to insulin.

As an insulin derivative lacking the intrachain disulfide bridge A6-A11, KATSOYANNIS *et al.* (1973) synthesized Ala^{A6-A11} sheep insulin by substitution of the cysteines at positions A6 and A11 by alanines. The biological activity of this derivative without the intrachain cyclic system is approximately 10% of that of comparative insulin in the mouse convulsion test.

The antibody binding of Ala^{A6-A11} insulin is reduced to the same extent as the biological activity in comparison to sheep insulin.

In conclusion, modifications of the insulin molecule mostly lead to a reduction in the antibody binding which is primarily dependent on the localization and, to a lesser degree, on the specific kind of modification. Modifications of the insulin molecule by amino acid substitution, by elongation or shortening of the chains, or by derivative formation at the chain termini show that changes in the insulin molecule at the C-terminal B chain, N-terminal B chain, C-terminal A chain and N-terminal A chain in the aforesaid order effect an increasing reduction of the antigenicity. This order corresponds to the different significance of the termini of the chains for maintenance of the spatial configuration of insulin. The substitutions of functional groups with formation of acetyl, acetoacetyl, sulfate, maleyl, succinyl, nitro, iodinated, cyanoethyl, fluorescein, PTC, carbamyl and methylcarbamyl insulins lead to various degrees of reduction of antibody binding. A systematic dependence on the kind of substitution is not as yet recognizable. Cross-linkages by covalent binding of the insulin chains lead to significant losses of antibody binding, if associated with conformational changes. A cleavage of intrachain or interchain disulfide bridges results in corresponding losses of biological activity as well as antibody binding.

The binding of modified insulins to insulin antibodies only permits conclusions relative to the localization of antigenic determinants if their spatial configuration is also taken into account. Spatial configuration may be studied indirectly by analysis of biological activity *in vivo* or *in vitro*, or by the binding to insulin receptors (FREYCHET, 1973; GLIEMANN and GAMMELTOFT, 1973; GAMMELTOFT and GLIEMANN, 1973; HENRICHS *et al.*, 1974), or directly by X-ray analysis (BLUNDELL *et al.*, 1971a, b, 1972; HODGKIN, 1972) and by CD spectra (ETTINGER and TIMASHEFT, 1971).

If a localized chemical modification of the molecule influences both the biological activity and the antibody binding of insulin to the same extent, it cannot be excluded that the modification may have caused an alteration in spatial configuration of the molecule as well. A dissociating effect after a modification with a diminution of antigenicity and the biological activity remaining unchanged indicates that the modification may have directly affected an antigen determinant region of the molecule.

Therefore, it must not be concluded from the marked reduction of antibody binding which followed the modifications at positions Gly^{A1} or Asp^{A21}, that these positions in themselves must be included in antigenic determinant regions. In contrast, it may be inferred from the findings with modifications in the N-terminal region of the B chain of insulin that an antigen-determinant group, or portions of the latter, has to be located in this molecule region. Modifications that involve the N-terminal B chain by chain shortening or derivative formation lead to a relatively vigorous reduction of the antibody binding, whereas the biological activity of insulin is insignificantly impaired by these modifications.

IV. Insulin Antibodies in Man

1. Without Previous Insulin Treatment

The question whether insulin antibodies can occur in man without previous insulin treatment is of interest in regard to the pathophysiology of diabetes mellitus. The demonstration of spontaneously occurring insulin antibodies would be an argument in favor of the autoimmunogenesis of diabetes mellitus. PAV *et al.* (1963) were the first to report the occurrence of insulin antibodies in persons not treated with insulin. By means of a complement consumption method, insulin antibodies were detected in 40% of the control persons and in 34.4% of the diabetics. These findings were confirmed by VAN DE WIL and by VAN DE WIL-DORFMEYER (1964). With the same method CHETTY and WATSON (1965) proved an "antibody-like activity" in 26% of non-diabetics and in 78% of diabetics without prior insulin treatment. The passive hemagglutination reaction according to BOYDEN (1951) was positive for insulin for 58 out of 62 non-diabetics with various chronic diseases. SCHEIFFARTH *et al.* (1959) by substituting liver extract for insulin proved the positive hemagglutination reaction to be unspecific and not appropriate for the detection of insulin-binding antibodies. PAL *et al.* (1969a, b) by means of a hemagglutination technique according to MOINAT (1958) detected insulin antibodies in 58% of diabetics under treatment with oral antidiabetic drugs and in 50% of untreated diabetics. Spontaneously occurring insulin antibodies also were demonstrated by BERNS *et al.* (1965) with the aid of a complement consumption method, by MANCINI *et al.* (1965) by means of an immunofluorescence technique, and by PENCHEV *et al.* (1968) by precipitation according to OUDIN. The latter study was repeated by means of a disc-electrophoretic separation of free and antibody-bound ^{125}I-insulin (DITZOV *et al.*, 1971). The frequency of antibody-positive sera in diabetics not treated with insulin was then diminished from 33.3% to 18.7%.

With the exception of some newer reports mentioned below, insulin antibodies without previous insulin treatment were not detected with radioimmunological methods by BERSON *et al.* (1956), BURROWS *et al.* (1957), CHAO *et al.* (1965), DECKERT (1967), KALANT *et al.* (1958), KERP (1963), KUMAR and MILLER (1973b), SKOM and TALMAGE (1958) and others. BERSON and YALOW (1965) support the view that any proof of insulin antibodies indicates a previous exogenous insulin administration, even if such a therapy is not evident from the patients history.

Several cases of an "*insulin auto-immune syndrome*" (HIRATA *et al.*, 1973) were recently reported. The patients develop hyperglycemic episodes alternating with postprandial hypoglycemic attacks. Circulating insulin antibodies detected in the serum of these patients could not be traced back to an earlier insulin treatment (FØLLING and NORMAN, 1972; HIRATA and ISHIZU, 1972; HIRATA *et al.*, 1973; OHNEDA *et al.*, 1973). The detection of insulin antibodies cannot be doubted in the cases reported so far.

FØLLING and NORMAN (1972) detected insulin antibodies in a 42-year-old male patient *in vitro* by gel filtration, preparative ultracentrifugation, agar electrophoresis and immunoelectrophoresis. Insulin elimination from blood and insulin sensitivity were diminished *in vivo*. The free insulin binding capacity of the patient's serum amounted to several units/l. More than 7U/l insulin were released by acid cleavage of the insulin-antibody complex. The serum insulin concentration increased by 2.3 U/l after an oral glucose load. The specificity of the antibodies for human and porcine insulin was higher than for bovine insulin. The antibodies exhibited a striking homogeneity upon agar electrophoresis and immunoelectrophoresis. A monoclonal origin of these antibodies was therefore discussed.

Two patients of HIRATA and one patient of OHNEDA, who demonstrated this syndrome, were subjected to partial pancreatectomy. A β-cell hyperplasia or increase in the number of islets of Langerhans was found.

The insulin-neutralizing effect of the antibodies was considered the reason for the hyperglycemic states. The postprandial hypoglycemia was ascribed to insulin secretion by maximally stimulated intact β-cells far exceeding the saturation of the antibody-binding capacity.

2. After Insulin Treatment

The *frequency* with which insulin-binding antibodies are demonstrated in serum after insulin treatment varies considerably (see Table 3).

Table 3. *Insulin-binding antibodies in serum after insulin treatment of diabetic patients*

Authors	Method of antibody determination	Number of patients tested	Percentage of antibody-positiv cases
WELSH *et al.* (1956)	131-I-insulin retention *in vivo*	56	80
BERSON *et al.* (1956)	paper electrophoresis	31	81
ARQUILLA and STAVITSKY (1956a)	hemagglutination	13	46
BERSON and YALOW (1957)	131-I-insulin retention *in vivo*, paper electrophoresis	9	100
SKOM and TALMAGE (1958b)	immunoprecipitation	37	76
MOINAT (1958)	hemagglutination	96	74
SCHEIFFARTH *et al.* (1959)	hemagglutination	110	25
PROUT and KATIMS (1959)	131-I-insulin retention *in vivo*	6	67
ROBINSON *et al.* (1961)	hemagglutination	45	4.7
ENGLESON and NILSSON (1962)	hemagglutination	39	13
YAGI *et al.* (1963)	immunoelectrophoresis	18	80
FANKHAUSER (1963a)	immunoprecipitation	100	27
PAV *et al.* (1963)	complement consumption	154	32
KERP (1963)	cellulose adsorption	216	55
STARCYNSKA and DEPOWSKA (1967)	immunoelectrophoresis	—	100
HÜRTER and KÜHNAU, JR. (1970)	cellulose adsorption	64	95
PAL *et al.* (1969b)	hemagglutination	46	98
SCHWEIZER (1970)	cellulose adsorption	450	63
CHRISTIANSEN (1971)	immunoelectrophoresis	—	100
DITZOV *et al.* (1971)	disc electrophoresis	50	58
ANDERSEN (1972)	immunoprecipitation	51	76

The divergence of findings may, for instance, be ascribed to the different sensitivity of the methods used or to the different composition of the patient groups in regard to age, duration of treatment, daily requirement of insulin, or type of insulin administered. The frequency of occurrence of insulin-binding antibodies moreover depends on the origin of applied insulin, on the degree of purity and the pharmaceutical preparation of insulin. To judge from experience to date, it has to be taken into account that most of the patients develop insulin-binding antibodies under insulin treatment, though sometimes it is necessary to repeat antibody estimations several times to detect antibody production. Insulin antibodies of IgM class are found only transiently at the beginning of the insulin treatment (DEVLIN, 1966; HORINO *et al.*, 1966; YAGI *et al.*, 1963).

The *time interval* from initiation of insulin therapy up to the occurrence of insulin antibodies ranges through 2 (DEVLIN, 1966), 6 and 35 days (BERSON and YALOW, 1959; DOLOVICH *et al.*, 1970; KALLEE, 1963a). But even after years of insulin therapy, insulin antibodies can appear for the first time (HÜRTER and KÜHNAU, 1970). On therapy with porcine monospecies insulin, ANDERSEN (1972) observed the first antibody formation after 1—3 months. A maximum of antibody concentration was reached after 4—9 months.

After termination of administration of insulin, insulin antibodies are detectable over a long period of time. In cases investigated by KARAM *et al.* (1969a) insulin could be detected for more than 18 months after termination of the insulin therapy. From the fall in insulin antibody titer the mean half-life of insulin antibodies was estimated to be 18—20 days (Karam *et al.*, 1969a; Plautz and Little, 1970). Thus the half-life corresponds to that of other immunoglobulins.

Jørgensen *et al.* (1966), Kodejszko *et al.* (1963), Kodejszko (1964), Meier and Yerganian (1961), Moloney and Coval (1955), Spellacy and Goetz (1963), Starzynska *et al.* (1969) demonstrated insulin-binding antibodies in *newborns of insulin-treated diabetic mothers.* Corresponding findings — even in the fetus — were made in animal experiments (Meade, 1963; Starzynska *et al.*, 1969; Thorell, 1966a, b). These antibodies are transferred across the placenta, as was shown by passive immunization of guinea pigs (Thorell, 1966a). According to investigations of Thorell (1966a, 1966b) and Starzynska *et al.* (1969), IgM antibodies do not penetrate the placenta in contrast to IgG antibodies. In the amniotic fluid of pregnant guinea pigs immunized with insulin, the concentration of insulin antibodies was approximately 1/100 of their plasma concentration. After parturition the plasma insulin antibodies of the new born guinea pig disappeared with a mean half-life of 8 days (Thorell, 1966a). Spellacy and Goetz (1963) calculated a half-life of 25 days for insulin antibodies of infants of diabetic mothers.

Hürter and Kühnau (1970) did not find a correlation between the formation of antibodies and the *age at the beginning of insulin therapy* in the age group between 2 and 16 years (n = 64). Also Welsh *et al.* (1956), Lev-Ran *et al.* (1971) as well as Moinat (1958) did not observe correlations between the age of the patients at the beginning of the treatment and the formation of antibodies. Andersen (1972), however, showed in 43 adult diabetics that antibody formation is more pronounced in younger patients after initiation of insulin therapy than in older patients.

In the initial phase the antibody formation is positively correlated with the *duration of insulin therapy.* Lev-Ran *et al.* (1971) did not find a correlation between the duration of insulin treatment and the occurrence of insulin antibodies, when the initial phase was not taken into account. At first, the antibody-binding capacity of insulin mostly increases rapidly during insulin treatment, as was shown by Schlichtkrull *et al.* (1972) and Kerp (1973) in adults and by Hürter and Kühnau (1970) in diabetic children. Through the course of a longer lasting insulin treatment the antibody binding capacity is subjected to marked variations (Kerp, 1973). Waldhäusl *et al.* (1972) did not see any correlation between an insulin-binding capacity of more than 100 μg/l serum and the duration of insulin treatment.

The antibody formation is increased by *other factors*: by infections (Andersen, 1972), tuberculosis (Penchev *et al.*, 1968) or pregnancy (Palumbo *et al.*, 1964).

a) Insulin-Binding Antibodies and Insulin Requirement

Many authors did not find a correlation between insulin requirement and the concentration or the titer of insulin-binding antibodies in insulin-sensitive patients in contrast to patients with insulin resistance (Berson and Yalow, 1959a; Christiansen *et al.*, 1971; Engleson and Nielson, 1962; Kalant *et al.*, 1958; Korp and Levett, 1973; Levett and Korp, 1972; Loveless and Cann, 1955; Moinat, 1958; Mowbray *et al.*, 1971; Palumbo *et al.*, 1964; Rosselin *et al.*, 1965; Scheiffarth *et al.*, 1967; Skom and Talmage, 1958b; Waldhäusl *et al.*, 1972; Welsh *et al.*, 1956; Yagi *et al.*, 1963). Other investigators, however, observed a positive correlation between the daily dose of insulin and the antibody concentration also for insulin-sensitive patients (Andersen, 1972; Berson and Yalow, 1964b; Colwell and Weiger, 1956; Deckert, 1965; Fankhauser, 1963b; Fankhauser and Montadon, 1963; Harris-Jones *et al.*, 1963; Horino *et al.*, 1959;

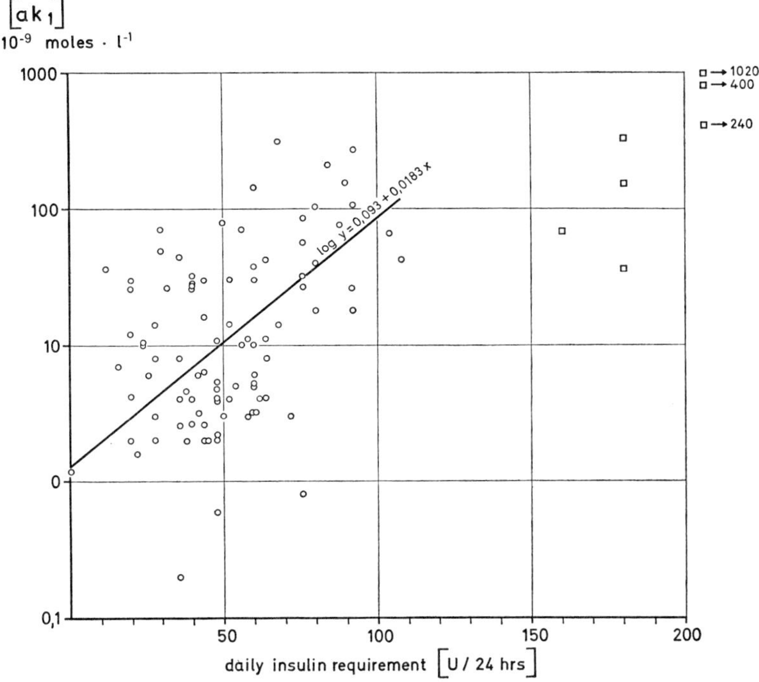

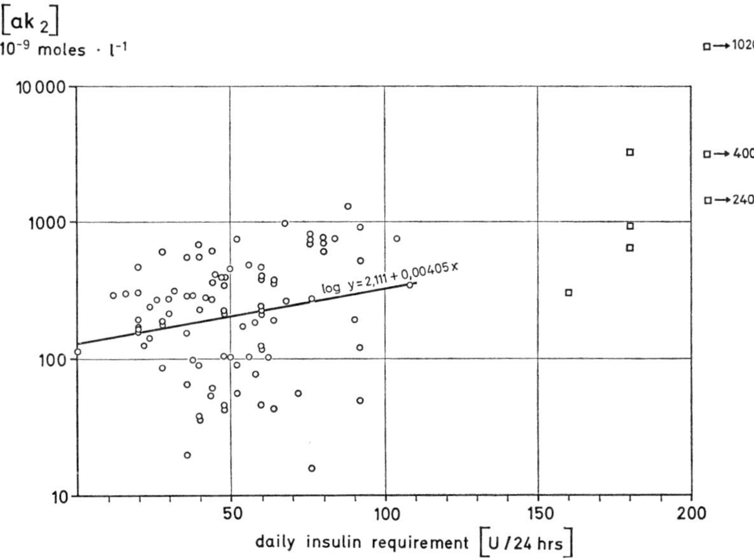

Fig. 4a and b. Daily insulin requirement (U per 24 h) and concentration of antibody-binding sites for insulin in insulin-treated diabetics. (○ insulin-sensitive diabetics, $n = 91$; □ insulin-resistant diabetics, $n = 7$). a) binding to high-affinity antibody binding sites (Ak_1), $r = 0.605$; $p < 0.0005$ (top); b) binding to low-affinity antibody binding sites (Ak_2), $r = 0.33$; $p < 0.005$ (bottom). (Data from KERP and KASEMIR, 1968)

HÜRTER and KÜHNAU, 1970; KERP, 1965; KERP et al., 1968b; KÜHNAU, 1968; KÜHNAU and MEYER, 1967; MEYER, 1968; PAL et al., 1969b; PROUT and KATIMS, 1960; ROSSELIN et al., 1965; SCÈCSEY et al., 1963; STRUWE et al., 1970). A quantitative analysis of 91 anti-insulin sera of patients with balanced metabolic state without insulin resistance, which was carried out by KERP et al. (1968b) showed a positive correlation between the daily insulin requirement and the concentration of the antibody binding sites (Fig. 4a,b). However, relationships between the strength of the insulin-antibody binding and the daily insulin requirements could not be proved (DITSCHUNEIT and FEDERLIN, 1966; KERP et al., 1968b).

LEV-RAN et al. (1973) examined 50 insulin-treated diabetics with a daily insulin requirement between 20 and 100 U. The free serum insulin in the fasting state, independent of the insulin amount bound to antibodies, was found to be 58±5 μU/ml. The total insulin concentration was 1900±125 μU/ml. Though the insulin binding capacity is only partially saturated with 2—40%, free insulin close to the physiological concentration is available in the plasma.

b) Insulin-Binding Antibodies and the Quality of Metabolic Control in Diabetics

It is not easy to answer the question whether insulin antibodies affect the quality of metabolic control in diabetics by insulin therapy because of the difficulty of measuring the quality of metabolic control. KERP (1963), PALUMBO et al. (1972) and KORP and LEVETT (1973) did not observe a difference in the frequency of antibody occurrence between patients adjusted in "stable" and "labile" manner. An inversely proportional relation, however, was found between the antibody titer of the individual sera and the quality of adjustment (DIXON et al., 1972; KERP, 1963; LEV-RAN et al., 1973). ANDERSEN (1972) found a positive correlation between the regulation index of diabetes mellitus and the antibody titers in patients under 25 years of age. He did not observe this dependence in older patients and in the total collective of his study.

WALDHÄUSL et al. (1972) did not see a relation between fasting blood sugar or glucosuria and antibody-binding capacity of insulin in the sera of patients. FANKHAUSER and GOETZ (1961) as well as FANKHAUSER (1963c) found a decrease in the tendency toward ketosis in diabetics as the insulin-binding antibodies increased. Such findings were considered to be indicative of a stabilizing effect of insulin antibodies on the metabolic state of diabetics (FANKHAUSER, 1969; DIXON et al., 1972).

Insulin-binding antibodies also protect against the danger of hypoglycemia on acute administration of insulin. This antibody effect for instance is shown by the fact that, after injection of bovine insulin into guinea pigs with insulin immuntolerance, more fatalities occurred than after insulin administration to animals with antibodies against bovine insulin (MOLONEY and TIRPAK, 1969). Insulin antibodies also seem to be a protection against the development of hypoglycemia in diabetic patients (KRAUTWALD, 1971; WELSCH et al., 1956). Investigations of PALUMBO et al. (1972) do not show this interrelation between the antibody content of the sera and the insulin tolerance of patients. A decrease in the insulin binding to antibodies is possibly responsible for delayed spontaneous hypoglycemia, which is occasionally observed on remission of a phase of insulin resistance (BERSON and YALOW, 1957c, 1958; HARWOOD, 1960; PAL et al., 1969b).

c) Acute Effects of Insulin Antibodies on Metabolic Processes

Acute effects of a passive immunization with insulin antibodies can be demonstrated in animals by looking at numerous insulin-dependent metabolic parameters. For example, elevation of the blood sugar in anesthetized (ARQUILLA et al.,

1962) or unanesthetized rats (SAMAAN and FRAZER, 1964), as well as hyperglycemia and ketonemia in sheep and cows (CUNNINGHAM *et al.*, 1963) have been observed. Insulin deficiency also becomes evident through the parameters of hepatic fatty acid and protein synthesis, of glycolysis, of the tricarbonic acid cycle or the concentration of pyridine nucleotides in rats (KALKHOFF and KIPNIS, 1966; KALKHOFF *et al.*, 1966). Insulin deficiency was found by COHEN *et al.* (1969) in fetal sheep and by BALASSE *et al.* (1972) in dogs after administration of insulin antisera. The arterial concentration of blood sugar, free fatty acids, glycerol, triglycerides and of the very-low-density lipoproteins in dogs increased two-fold and that of the ketone bodies increased fourfold, as compared to the initial concentration.

Insulin-neutralizing effects of insulin antibodies are also detectable *in vitro*, e.g. by the glucose uptake or glucose oxidation of isolated diaphragms, of epididymal fat pads, of isolated fat cells or by the formation of glycogen in the musculature. PECK (1971) demonstrated that the insulin-dependent incorporation of pyridine ribonucleotides into bone cells is inhibited by insulin antibodies. BEIGELMANN and HOLLANDER (1965) were able to suppress the enhancing effect of insulin on the electrical resting potential in the fatty tissue of rats by insulin antibodies. HAHN and ZIEGLER (1971) as well as ZIEGLER *et al.* (1972c) showed that insulin antibodies stimulate the insulin secretion of isolated Langerhans' islets of mice.

Insulin remains longer in the organism in the presence of insulin antibodies (BERSON *et al.*, 1956; BECK, 1966; BOLINGER *et al.*, 1964; BUTTERFIELD *et al.*, 1963; HORINO *et al.*, 1967; MC ADAMS *et al.*, 1967; ORSKOV and CHRISTIANSEN, 1969; SCOTT *et al.*, 1958; SRIVASTAVA *et al.*, 1971; STIMMLER, 1967; TOMASI *et al.*, 1967; WILLIAMS *et al.*, 1968; PALUMBO *et al.*, 1972). In rats antibody-bound insulin is predominantly found in the liver (80%) and in the spleen. In contrast, in non-immunized animals insulin is prevalently found in the kidneys (GINGERICH *et al.*, 1971).

The antibody binding protects insulin against degradation, as was proved *in vivo* in the mouse (BECK *et al.*, 1966) and *in vitro* in experiments on liver insulinase (YALOW and BERSON, 1957) and glutathione-insulin transhydrogenase (VARANDANI and TOMIZAWA, 1965).

d) Chronic Effects of Insulin-Binding Antibodies on Metabolic Processes

Insulin neutralization by antibodies leads to increasing insulin requirement. This causes increased insulin secretion in non-diabetic test animals, as demonstrated immunohistologically *in vivo* by BURKLE *et al.* (1971) and *in vitro* by HAHN and ZIEGLER (1971) as well as by ZIEGLER *et al.* (1972). LOGOTHETOPOULOS (1965) as well as LOGOTHETOPOULOS and BELL (1966) observed in mice under treatment with guinea pig anti-insulin sera a rapid persistent degranulation of the β-cells with swelling of the Golgi apparatus. These findings are in agreement with those made in rats (LACY and WRIGHT, 1965; LOGOTHETOPOULOS *et al.*, 1965). GRODSKY *et al.* (1966) observed also in rabbits actively immunized with bovine insulin a degranulation of β-cells besides serious signs of β-cell damage and of lymphocytic infiltrations.

A persistence of insulin antibodies leads in test animals to an "immune diabetes" (ARMIN *et al.*, 1960b; ARQUILLA *et al.*, 1973; FREYTAG, 1972; GOFF *et al.*, 1973; GRODSKY *et al.*, 1966; HIRATA and BLUMENTHAL, 1962b; KITAGAWA *et al.*, 1960; LEE *et al.*, 1969; MOLONEY and COVAL, 1955; MOLONEY and GOLDSMITH, 1957; ROBINSON and WRIGHT, 1961; SAMAAN and FRAZER, 1964; SCHÖFFLING, 1966; WRIGHT, 1959a, 1961). This can be induced by active as well as by passive immunization (FREYTAG and KLOEPPEL, 1971; FREYTAG, 1972; KLOEPPEL *et al.*, 1973).

V. Antibody-Dependent Insulin Resistance

Suppression or diminution of insulin effects characterize the state of insulin resistance. Antibody-induced insulin resistance in insulin-dependent diabetics leads to an enhancement of their insulin deficiency. The requirement of foreign insulin is therefore of critical importance for the diagnosis of insulin resistance.

On the basis of early investigations by ROOT (1929) and MARTIN *et al.* (1941), insulin resistance is defined as the requirement of foreign insulin of a non-acidotic patient exceeding (150—) 200 units per day over at least a 48-h period. In children insulin resistance is assumed if the doses are higher than 1 unit/kg/day (MURTHY *et al.*, 1969). Since insulin resistance is a matter of clinical diagnosis, daily doses of insulin may be chosen on arbitrary establishment of a resistance limit dose, which induces "therapeutic problems" (FEDERLIN *et al.*, 1971). DAWEKE (1966), DITSCHUNEIT and FEDERLIN (1966) as well as FEDERLIN *et al.* (1971) accept an insulin requirement of more than 100 units per day as insulin resistance.

Observations of insulin resistance as well as of insulin allergies were made for the first time by FALTA in 1924.

DEPISCH and HASENÖHRL (1928) as well as GLEN and EATON (1938) detected in the serum of an insulin-resistant patient a factor which suppressed the effect of insulin.

1. Pathogenesis

Under continuous treatment with insulin, insulin-binding antibodies are formed in almost all patients (see p. 621). In patients with insulin resistance insulin binding capacities are higher, sometimes extremely higher than in insulin-nonresistant patients (ARQUILLA and STAVITSKY, 1956a; BERSON *et al.*, 1956; BERSON and YALOW, 1959c, 1964b; DITSCHUNEIT and FEDERLIN, 1966; ENGLESON and NILSON, 1962; KERP *et al.*, 1965; KERP and KASEMIR, 1968; MORSE, 1961; OAKLEY *et al.*, 1967; PROUT and KATIMS, 1959; ROSSELIN *et al.*, 1965; SKOM and

Table 4. *Insulin antibody binding in serum of insulin-resistant and of insulin-nonresistant diabetics (unselected cases). The quantitative parameters of insulin antibody binding were analysed using the cellulose differential adsorption technique* (KERP *et al., 1966)*

Patient	$[Ak_1]$ $\cdot 10^{-9}$ Mol/l	k_1 $\cdot 10^9$ l/Mol	$[Ak_2]$ $\cdot 10^{-9}$ Mol/l	k_2 $\cdot 10^9$ l/Mol	Insulin requirement U/day
with insulin resistance					
Bac	36	26	660	0.28	180
Rix	144	92.1	3216	0.52	180
Hub	312	13.5	940	0.97	180
Dro	68	8.4	304	0.44	160
Ko	384	5.2	1400	0.15	240
Dil	940	7.6	19260	0.08	1020
Hay	776	7.0	3800	0.15	400
without insulin resistance					
May	0.2	177.0	20	0.12	36
Rei	2.0	27.0	166	0.08	20
Kin	2.6	17.5	560	0.02	36
Nan	1.6	43.5	126	0.20	22
Sce	6.0	16.7	272	0.18	26
Wei	2.0	23.2	180	0.14	28
Pfa	4.2	17.0	308	0.16	20
Zip	14.0	14.0	608	0.31	28
Hag	84.0	1.9	820	0.07	76
Hin	10.0	16.7	102	0.31	56
Tie	40.0	1.9	700	0.05	80

TALMAGE, 1958b; STEIGERWALD and SPIELMANN, 1956; YALOW and BERSON, 1964). Table 4 contains the values of insulin binding parameters of unselected diabetics with and without insulin resistance. KASEMIR *et al.* (1968) demonstrated the special importance of high-affinity antibody component Ak_1 for the insulin resistance.

The significance of insulin antibodies in the pathogenesis of this kind of insulin resistance is underlined by studying the course of an insulin resistance (see Table 5).

Table 5. *Insulin-antibody binding in serum during insulin resistance (a) and after remission of insulin resistance (b) in two patients (data from* KERP *et al. 1965)*

	Maximal insulin binding $[Ak_1]+[Ak_2]$ U/l	Calculated amount of antibody bound insulin *in vivo** U/l	Insulin requirement U/24 h
Patient 1 (a)	6580	1000	> 200
(b)	117.5	34.7	44
Patient 2 (a)	5410	680	> 1710
(b)	189	43.9	76

* Concentration of free insulin in serum set to 10 U/l

The concentration of the binding sites of insulin antibodies during the phase of resistance was found to be 5—8-fold higher for Ak_1 and 30—80 fold higher for Ak_2 in two patients than after remission of the resistance (KERP *et al.*, 1965). Similar findings were made by BERSON and YALOW (1958), FIELD (1962), LERMAN (1944), PROUT and KATIMS (1960), SHIPP *et al.* (1961), OAKLEY and CUNLIFFE (1968) as well as by GRÜNEKLEE *et al.* (1970). OAKLEY and CUNLIFFE (1968) were able to

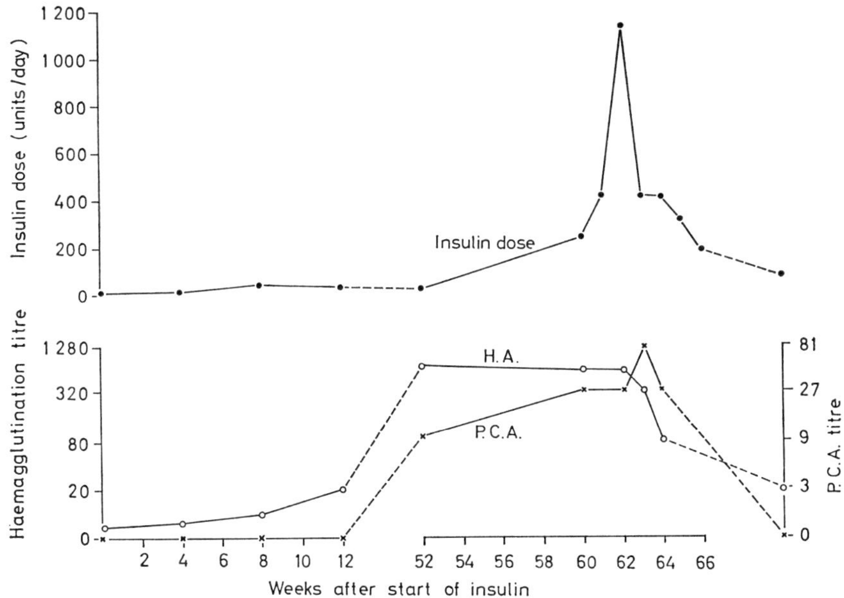

Fig. 5. A case of insulin resistance in which the rise in antibody titers preceded an increase in insulin dose. (From OAKLEY and CUNLIFFE, 1968)

describe a case of insulin resistance, where determinations of insulin antibodies in patients' serum were carried out from the beginning of insulin therapy. Already prior to the rise in insulin requirement the insulin antibody titer was rising; thereafter the clinical picture of insulin resistance developed (Fig. 5). Similar case reports were given by Grüneklee *et al.* (1970) and Dolovich *et al.* (1970).

In contrast to the binding capacity, the association constants of insulin antibodies from sera of patients vary only insignificantly between the phases of resistance and of remission (Kerp *et al.*, 1965).

2. Frequency of Occurrence

Up to 1948, 54 cases of insulin resistance (Smelo, 1948) and for the time from 1950 to 1961 (Shipp *et al.*, 1961) 59 cases were compiled from literature. According to observations in the Joslin Clinic, in 1961 insulin resistance was found in 0.1% of all insulin-treated diabetics (Shipp *et al.*, 1961). In agreement with Morcos *et al.* (1965) and Daweke (1968), Federlin *et al.* (1971) too expect a frequency of insulin resistance of 0.1% in insulin-treated diabetics; however, they point to the possibility of regional differences. It is noteworthy that Deckert (1964) did not observe a single case of insulin resistance among approximately 3000 diabetics in Scandinavia, which is possibly a consequence of the application of porcine insulin preparations, whereas insulin resistance during this time was not as rare on predominant application of a mixture of bovine and porcine insulin in the Anglo-Saxon countries and in Germany (Field, 1962; Ditschuneit and Federlin, 1966; Guthrie *et al.*, 1967; Oakley and Cunliffe, 1968). 3.6% out of 1089 patients of Ditschuneit and Federlin (1966) needed more than 100 U insulin/day. Menzel *et al.* (1971) found among 7927 insulin-dependent diabetics after hospitalization 16 patients (14 female and 2 male patients) or 0.2% with an insulin requirement exceeding 100 units/day.

3. Clinical Picture

Antibody-dependent insulin resistance is equally found in men and women. According to Oakley *et al.* (1967), a certain predominance of insulin resistance is observed in patients over 50 years of age. Among the insulin-resistant patients of Shipp *et al.* (1965) 75% were older than 40 years. But cases of insulin resistance in children have also been described (Guthrie *et al.*, 1967; Khurana *et al.*, 1973). Insulin resistance develops predominantly in the first year after insulin therapy. In 3 out of 41 cases of Oakley and Cunliffe (1968) antibody-dependent insulin resistance developed within a few weeks, in 12 cases within 1 to 6 months and in 50% of the cases within the first year after initiation of insulin therapy. Antibody-dependent insulin resistance frequently developed in patients if insulin therapy was resumed after an interruption of therapy.

Insulin allergies are reported of different frequency before the beginning of the phase of resistance. Oakley and Cunliffe (1968) did not find insulin allergies more frequently in patients with insulin resistance than in patients without resistance. In contrast, Shipp *et al.* (1961) observed insulin allergies in almost one third, Brucart (1963) even in two thirds of the insulin-resistant patients. Conversely, in 6 out of 16 patients with insulin allergies an antibody-dependent insulin resistance developed (Fankhauser and Diacon, 1966).

In 19 out of 60 cases of insulin resistance (31%) a generalized urticaria was found after administration of insulin. Only in 5 out of 142 (3.5%) diabetics without insulin resistance did a generalized urticaria occur after injection of insulin (Kerp *et al.*, 1965). Four out of 7 patients of Kerp with clear manifestation of antibody-dependent insulin resistance showed local allergic reactions of the delayed type (tuberculin type) towards the tenth day of insulin treatment. Several days later the insulin resistance became manifest. Two of these patients between the local allergic reaction of delayed type and the phase of insulin resistance developed an urticarial reaction of the immediate type around the injection site, and on the following day a generalized urticaria with a rise of temperature up to 38.5° C. In both female patients major deviations in carbohydrate metabolism were not recognizable during the urticarial exanthema. Only on remission of the allergy-dependent symptoms did insulin resistance develop, with a rise in blood sugar, increasing glucosuria and acetonuria.

For a *reliable diagnosis* of antibody-dependent insulin resistance, quantitative determination of insulin-binding antibodies in the serum of the patients is required.

In general, the *prognosis* of antibody-dependent insulin resistance is favourable on adequate treatment. Nevertheless, a diabetic coma can develop in the course of an antibody-dependent insulin resistance (see DAWEKE and BACH, 1963) and even fatalities have been reported (PFEIFFER, 1966).

4. Therapy

Due to the rare occurrence of antibody-dependent insulin resistance, comparative therapeutic studies are not available.

Cases of spontaneous disappearance of insulin resistance have been reported (AXELROD *et al.*, 1947; FIELD *et al.*, 1961; DAWEKE and BACH, 1963), which can be misinterpreted as therapeutic successes.

In case of antibody-dependent insulin resistance, therapy aims at maintaining the metabolic equilibrium and avoiding ketoacidosis.

It is a principle of therapy to attempt the reduction of the insulin requirement of insulin-resistant patients. This can be achieved e.g. by a successful *reduction in body weight*. In addition, the inhibition or elimination of insulin *antagonists* can effect a reduction in the dosage of insulin from foreign sources. The favourable effect of α-methyl-dopa (MEYTHALER and WEILER, 1964; MEYTHALER and KOTLORZ, 1965) in 2 cases of insulin resistance was interpreted as an inhibition of catecholamine effects. Analogously, NADEL (1958) employed reserpine. DITSCHUNEIT *et al.* (1971) were able in a case of severe insulin resistance to reduce the daily requirement of several thousand units of insulin per day by hypophysectomy to 100 units per day for a period of 6 months.

Another principle in the treatment of insulin resistance consists in influencing the immunological processes which lead to insulin neutralization by insulin-binding antibodies. Since insulin antibodies in case of antibody-dependent insulin resistance do not always enter into cross-reactions with endogenous human insulin, it has been attempted to apply *sulfonylureas* alone or in addition to insulin therapy in order to stimulate the endogenous insulin. BARRET and BOSHELL (1962), BOSHELL *et al.* (1962), CREUTZFELDT and SCHLAGINTWEIT (1957), CREUTZFELDT and SÖLING (1960), DITURI (1954), DUNCAN *et al.* (1957), FRIEDLANDER (1957), FRIEDLANDER and BRYANT (1959) and SEGRE (1962) reported successes of this therapy. Four out of 10 insulin-resistant patients of BARRET and BOSHELL (1962) responded to the addition of 3 g of tolbutamide. Onset of action was observed after 2—12 weeks. Three out of four successfully treated patients were overweight. According to BARRET and BOSHELL (1962), the administration of sulfonylurea gave propromising results in patients with recent-onset diabetes, in clearly overweight patients, in cases of short duration of insulin resistance and in cases of not too high insulin requirement. Sulfonylureas however do not always exert a favorable influence on the antibody-dependent insulin resistance (BARRET and BOSHELL, 1962; DAWEKE and BACH, 1962, 1963; EZRIN and MOLONEY, 1959; OAKLEY and CUNLIFFE, 1968).

It seems that tolbutamide does not affect the antibody binding of insulin directly. A release of insulin from antibody binding in the presence of increasing tolbutamide concentrations was not detectable *in vitro* (KERP *et al.*, 1963). HASSELBLATT and SCHMIETA however had demonstrated in 1961 by means of rat epididymal fat pad assay that antibody-bound insulin recovers some of its biological activity in the presence of tolbutamide.

In favorable cases antibody-dependent insulin resistance can be treated by *discontinuing the administration of insulin* from foreign sources. A marked reduction of high insulin antibody titers and normalization of the metabolic disturbance was reported by KARAM *et al.* (1969) and JACOTOT *et al.* (1973) in cases of antibody-dependent insulin resistance after termination of administration of exogenous insulin. In most cases of antibody-dependent insulin resistance a discontinuation of the treatment with foreign insulin is not possible because metabolic derangement will develop.

The insulin requirement can increase to several 100 or 1000 units per day (survey by WOLFF 1968). SMELO (1947) described the case of a young female patient who had to inject a total of 1.25 million units of insulin (approximately 50 g) in the course of 4 years. This corresponds to an average administration of 850 units daily. TUCKER *et al.* (1964) reported an insulin requirement of 177,500 units per day. Even under insulin treatment at such a high dosage level, a remission of the antibody-dependent insulin resistance can be induced in some of the patients (AXELROD *et al.*, 1947; FIELD *et al.*, 1961; DAWEKE and BACH, 1963; OAKLEY and CUNLIFFE, 1968).

SHIPP *et al.* (1961), DAWEKE and BACH (1963), FANKHAUSER (1963) and GRÜNEKLEE *et al.* (1970) inaugurated the iv. administration of high insulin doses for the treatment of insulin resistance. Previously, FRIEDLANDER (1957) as well as FRIEDLANDER and BRYANT (1959) had described the remission of a case of insulin resistance on intravenous administration of insulin together with simultaneous treatment with tolbutamide.

In the course of *intravenous high dose treatment* doses of several hundred units of insulin are administered by i.v. injection or infusion (MÜLLER, 1967). After saturation of the free binding sites of the insulin antibodies additional, unbound insulin can become metabolically effective. Findings in animal experiments made by JANSEN (1971a, b, c), MOLONEY and JACKSON (1973) and WILSON *et al.* (1973) also suggest that the high-dosage intravenous insulin therapy may induce a high dose tolerance or immune-deviation.

Since the insulin-neutralizing IgG antibodies have a long persistence with half-life of approximately 18 days, the intravenous administration of insulin must be continued over a sufficient period of time. Interruption of treatment after 8 days led to a relapse in one case of GRÜNEKLEE *et al.* (1970).

In case of proven dependence on foreign insulin, it is possible to substitute one insulin preparation by *insulin* from another animal *species*. BEEUWKES *et al.* (1956), BERSON and YALOW (1966), BOSHELL *et al.* (1964), BOULET *et al.* (1959), COHEN (1972), DEROT and RATHERY (1960), DEVLIN *et al.* (1966), FANKHAUSER (1964), FANKHAUSER and MORELL (1967), FELDMAN *et al.* (1963), GOLDMAN and KAYE (1962), JENSEN *et al.* (1929), KERP (1965), KISSEL and DEBRY (1960), KHURANA *et al.* (1973), KREUTZER *et al.* (1956), KÜHNAU and VON STRITZKY (1963), MICHEL

(1962), SOELDNER and STEINKE (1965) and others recommended a shift from mixed bovine-porcine insulin to pure porcine insulin. Therapeutic successes have also been achieved by a shift from monospecies bovine to monospecies porcine insulin (FANKHAUSER and MORELL, 1967; KÜHNAU and VON STRITZKY, 1963; MICHEL, 1962). In case of therapeutic failure of porcine insulin, there are limited possibilities for further shifts to insulins from other species, Bonito insulin has attained some limited importance in this indication (YAMAMOTO *et al.*, 1960; YALOW and BERSON, 1964; GRÜNEKLEE *et al.*, 1970).

Chemically modified insulins too have been applied for the treatment of antibody-dependent insulin resistance. Of interest are those insulin modifications, the immunological properties of which are more reduced than their biological properties.

Des-Ala^{B30}*-porcine insulin* was employed for the treatment of antibody-dependent insulin resistance due to its primary structure, which is identical with human insulin (AKRE *et al.*, 1964; BOSHELL *et al.*, 1964; KUMAR and MILLER, 1970). The effect of the shift to des-Ala^{B30} insulin on the insulin requirement approximately corresponded to a shift from mixed to monospecies insulin from the pig. KUMAR and MILLER (1970) were even able to reduce the mean daily insulin requirement of 5 out of 14 patients with antibody-dependent resistance against porcine insulin by a shift to des-Ala^{B30} insulin from 770 units of porcine insulin to 88 units of des-Ala^{B30}-porcine insulin. Des-Ala^{B30} insulin is more weakly bound to insulin antibodies of insulin-resistant patients than bovine and porcine insulin, but it is more strongly bound than human insulin (KUMAR and MILLER, 1970).

MOLONEY *et al.* (1964), ARNOTT and LITTLE (1965), LITTLE and ARNOTT (1966), SCHREIBER and ROTTENHÖFER (1968) and DAVIDSON (1972) reported a successful therapy of insulin resistence with sulfated insulins. In one case of GRÜNEKLEE *et al.* (1970), however, the treatment with sulfated insulin induced a metabolic derangement associated with ketoacidosis. KATSILABROS (1972) described a favorable effect of phenylated insulin (commercial insulin: phenol 5% = 1:1) on antibody-dependent insulin resistance.

Only few reports are available in regard to the effect of *chromatographically purified insulins* on antibody-dependent insulin resistance.

Over 5 weeks TANTILLO *et al.* (1973) measured no decrease of insulin antibody titer or a diminution of the insulin requirement in an insulin-resistant patient with a daily insulin requirement of 400 units of standard insulin after a shift to chromatographically purified insulin (SPI). PFEIFFER (1971) reported a case in which insulin resistance could be extinguished by the administration of chromatographically purified insulin. The insulin requirement dropped as a consequence of the shift from 800 units per day (regular) to 80 units per day of SCI insulin. WALDHÄUSL *et al.* (1972) treated a group of 9 patients with chromatographically purified insulin who showed an antibody-binding capacity of more than 100 μg/l of serum. As a result of the shift, the insulin binding capacity was reduced in all patients and the insulin requirement in 5 out of 9 patients was diminished. CRABTREE *et al.* (1971) examined 4 patients with a history of antibody-dependent insulin resistance. Chromatographed insulin (SCI) from man, pig, beef and non-chromatographed bovine insulin was administered to these patients over a period of one week, each. The determination of a "resistance index" from the mean blood sugar value and the daily dose of insulin showed for the chromatographed insulins from man and pig advantages in comparison to bovine insulin; chromatographed and non-chromatographed bovine insulin, however, could not be distinguished from each other by means of the "resistance index".

Corticosteroids and ACTH have been applied for the treatment of antibody-dependent insulin resistance. Therapeutic successes have been reported by COLLENS and BANOWITCH (1955), BERSON and YALOW (1958), BRUCART (1963), COLWELL and WEIGER (1956), DITSCHUNEIT *et al.* (1962), EZRIN and MOLONEY (1959), FAULK *et al.* (1970), FIELD and WOODSON (1959), FIELD (1962), FRIEDLANDER (1957), FRIEDLANDER and BRYANT (1959), KERP *et al.* (1965), KLEEBERG *et al.* (1956), KÜHNAU and SAUER (1970), MERIMEE (1965), MICHEL (1965), OAKLEY *et al.* (1959, 1967), OAKLEY and CUNLIFFE (1968), PALUMBO *et al.* (1964), PROUT and KATIMS (1960), SHIPP *et al.* (1961, 1965), ZAROWITZ (1972) and others. In the case of severe insulin resistance reported by COLLENS and BANOWITCH (1965), cortisone induced a decrement of the daily dose of insulin from 1000 to 200 units. An even more pronounced reduction of the insulin requirement from 11,400 units to 100 units per day was induced by ACTH treatment in a case of insulin resistance associated with hemochromatosis (COLWELL and WEIGER, 1956). OAKLEY and CUNLIFFE (1968) observed in 16 patients with antibody-dependent insulin resistance an immediate response to prednisone. Other authors described cases in which steroid therapy did not effect an improvement in insulin resistance (DAWEKE and BACH, 1963; FIELD *et al.*, 1961; KAYE *et al.*, 1955; LOVELESS and CANN, 1955).

OAKLEY and CUNLIFFE (1968) recommended a *prednisone dose* of 30 mg daily which should be increased to 45 mg in case of non-responsiveness. Higher initial doses of 50 mg (DITSCHUNEIT, 1968) or 100 mg (KERP, 1965) have been proposed. At the beginning of steroid therapy the insulin requirement frequently increases and drops after 24—48 h. This rapid onset of action was repeatedly observed. After stabilization of the insulin requirement, the administration of corticoids should be continued over a longer period of time (FIELD, 1963). Attempting to omit the steroids earlier, MERIMEE (1965) observed a recurrence of antibody-dependent insulin resistance; an immediate remission was observed on readministration of prednisone. The steroid treatment often may be discontinued after 3 months.

The mode of action of steroids on antibody-dependent insulin resistance has not as yet been clarified. The rapid onset of steroid activity and the low effective doses argue against inhibition of the biosynthesis of IgG antibodies to insulin. In accordance with what has been said, some authors reported therapeutic successes with steroids even without detectable decrease of the insulin antibody titers (FIELD and WOODSON, 1959; MERIMEE, 1965; OAKLEY *et al.*, 1967; PALUMBO *et al.*, 1964). A slight reduction of the insulin-binding capacity under steroid treatment was found by KANTOR and BERKMAN (1967). BERSON and YALOW (1958), BRUNFELDT and DECKERT (1964), FIELD (1962), MERIMEE (1965), PROUT and KATIMS (1959), SHIPP *et al.* (1961) and ZAROWITZ (1972), however, observed an decrease of the insulin antibody titer, which was parallel to the clinical effect of the steroid treatment. It is conceivable that steroids affect the antigen-antibody binding.

KÜHNAU and SAUER (1970) showed that under treatment with 6-methylprednisolone (Urbason) the avidity of insulin antibodies for the insulin antigen, which is characterized by the rate of antigen-antibody complex formation, decreased in two cases of antibody-dependent insulin resistance. The binding capacity of the sera was decreased under steroid therapy in one case and was unchanged in a second case. Due to the findings made, the authors assume that the favorable effect of 6-methylprednisolone on antibody-dependent insulin resistance is primarily based on a reduction of the avidity of newly formed insulin antibodies.

In experiments on guinea pigs KERP *et al.* (1967c) did not find a decrease in the antibody titers on administration of 0.5—10 mg of prednisolone per kg. Even higher antibody titers than in control animals without prednisolone were observed during or after insulin immunization in guinea pigs treated with prednisolone or ACTH. On application of very high, catabolically active doses of prednisolone, Makulu and Wright (1971) found a distinctly diminished insulin antibody formation in guinea pigs which received 20 mg/kg of prednisolone over a period of 30 days.

Under therapy with the alkylating compound *N-Lost*, Friedlander and Bryant (1959) as well as Geller *et al.* (1951) observed a remission of insulin resistance. In contrast, Alavi *et al.* (1971) reported the occurrence of antibody-dependent insulin resistance in a patient during steroid and N-Lost therapy with spontaneous remission after discontinuation of this therapy.

Merimee (1965) investigated the effect of *6-mercaptopurine* (150 mg daily) on antibody-dependent insulin resistance. In both cases investigated, no effect of 6-mercaptopurine was observed, whereas subsequent treatment of these patients with prednisone (30 mg daily) induced a rapid suppression of insulin resistance. The treatment of insulin resistance with 200 mg of azathioprine daily in a case of Grüneklee *et al.* (1970) was also unsuccessful. The therapy even led to a deterioration of the metabolic state. It is possible, however, that this case of insulin resistance is not caused by antibodies. By administration of azathioprine over a longer period of time at a dosage of 5 mg/kg/day, Kühnau and Bläker (1971) were able to treat otherwise refractory insulin resistance in a 10-year-old girl successfully.

Under therapy with the antimetabolite *5-fluorouracil* (6.48 g/2 weeks), Zarowitz (1972) observed in a female patient who had been subjected to total pancreatectomy because of an adenocarcinoma the remission of antibody-dependent insulin resistance as evidenced by by the insulin requirement and the titer of insulin-binding antibodies.

In individual cases therapeutic successes were obtained with *epsilon-aminocaproic acid* (Weise and Rolle, 1964; Grüneklee *et al.*, 1970). The mode of action of epsilon-aminocaproic acid on antibody-dependent insulin resistance is not yet fully explored.

References

Abdel-Wahab, M.F., El-Kinawi, S.A.: Preparation of I-131-labelled insulin and isolation by gelfiltration. Int. J. appl. Radiat. **16**, 668 (1965)

Abel, J.J.: Crystalline insulin. Proc. nat. Acad. Sci. (Wash.) **12**, 132 (1926)

Africa, B., Carpenter, F.H.: Preparation and characterization of diphenylthiocarbamyl insulin and des Gly^{A1}-des Phe^{B1}-insulin (bovine). Biochemistry (Wash.) **9**, 1962 (1970)

Africa, B., Carpenter, F.H.: Di-phenylthio-carbamoyl-insulin and des Gly^{A1}-des Phe^{B1}-insulin. Fed. Proc. **27**, 766 (1968)

Akre, P.R., Kirtley, W.R., Galloway, J.A.: Comparative hypoglycemic response of diabetic subjects to human insulin or structurally similar insulins of animal source. Diabetes **13**, 135 (1964)

Alavi, J.A., Sharma, B.K., Pillay, V.K.G.: Steroid induced diabetic ketoacidosis. Amer. J. med. Sci. **262**, 15 (1971)

Andersen, O.O.: Insulin antibody formation. I. The influence of age, sex, infections, insulin dosage and regulation of diabetes. Acta endocr. (Kbh.) **71**, 126 (1972)

Andersen, O.O., Brunfeldt, K., Abildgard, F.: A method for quantitative determination of insulin antibodies in human plasma. Acta endocr. (Kbh.) **69**, 195 (1972)

Andersen, O.O.: Insulin antibody formation. II. The influence of species differences and method of administration. Acta endocr. (Kbh.) **72**, 33 (1973a)

Andersen, O.O.: Antibodies to proinsulin in diabetic patients treated with porcine insulin preparations. Acta endocr. (Kbh.) **73**, 304 (1973b)

Antoniades, H.N., Simon, J.D.: Neutralization of the biological activity of human serum bound insulin by potent insulin antisera. Diabetes **21**, 930 (1972)

Armin, J., Grant, R.T., Wright, P.H.: Acute insulin deficiency provoked by single injection of anti-insulin serum. J. Physiol. (Lond.) **153**, 131 (1960a)

ARMIN, J., GRANT, R.T., WRIGHT, P.H.: Experimental diabetes in rats produced by parenteral administration of anti-insulin serum. J. Physiol. (Lond.) **153**, 146 (1960b)
ARNON, R., SELA, M.: Studies on the chemical basis of the antigenicity of proteins. 2. Antigenic specificity of polystyrosyl gelatins. Biochem. J. **75**, 103 (1960)
ARNON, R., SELA, M., YARON, A., SOBER, H.A.: Polylysine-specific antibodies and their reaction with oligolysines. Biochemistry (Wash.) **4**, 948 (1965)
ARNOTT, J.H., LITTLE, J.A.: Sulfated insulin in mild, moderate, severe and insulin-resistant diabetes mellitus. Diabetes **14**, 440 (1965)
ARQUILLA, E.R., STAVITSKY, A.B.: The production and identification of antibodies from diabetic patients and their use in assaying insulin. J. clin. Invest. **35**, 458 (1956a)
ARQUILLA, E.R., STAVITSKY, A.B.: Evidence for the insulin-directed specificity of rabbit anti-insulin serum. I. clin. Invest. **35**, 467 (1956b)
ARQUILLA, E.R., ALEXANDER, J.D., PTACEK, E.D., LOOSLI, E.S.: Studies on insulin neutralization by antisera from various species. I. Methodology and assay of insulin with intact anesthetized rats. Diabetes **11**, 412 (1962)
ARQUILLA, E.R., OOMS, H., FINN, J.: Relative combination of guinea pig insulin antibodies with crystalline insulin and I-125 insulin. Diabetes **14**, 449 (1965)
ARQUILLA, E.R., OOMS, H., FINN, J.: Genetic differences of combining sites of insulin antibodies and importance of c-terminal portion of the A chain to biological and immunological activity of insulin. Diabetologia **2**, 1 (1966)
ARQUILLA, E.R.: Relationships between A and B chains, necessary for antigenic determinants and the biologic activity of insulin. VI. Congress International Diabetes Federation, Stockholm (1967)
ARQUILLA, E.R., BROMER, W.W.: Conformation of antigenic determinants on insulin and biological activity of insulin, Proc. 6th Congr. Int. Diabetes Federation, Stockholm. Excerpta Medica, Int. Congr. Ser. **172**, 28 (1967)
ARQUILLA, E.R., OOMS, H., MERCOLA, K.: Immunological and biological properties of iodoinsulin labelled with one or less atoms of iodine per molecule. J. clin. Invest. **47**, 474 (1968)
ARQUILLA, E.R., BROMER, W.W., MERCOLA, D.A.: Immunology, conformation and biological activity of insulin. Diabetes **18**, 193 (1969)
ARQUILLA, E.R., MILES, P.V., MORRIS, J.W.: Immunochemistry of insulin. In: Handbook of Physiology; Endocrine Pancreas, p. 160. Baltimore: Williams and Wilkins Co. 1972. Cited by BRUGMAN and ARQUILLA (1973)
ARQUILLA, E.R., GOFF, J., GOFF, M., BRUGMAN, T.: The induction of experimental diabetes with insulin antibodies against a restricted determinant. Diabetes **22**, Suppl. 1, 306 (1973)
ATASSI, M.Z.: Antigenic structure of proteins inferred from myoglobin as the first protein whose antigenic structure has reached completion. In: Specific receptors of antibodies, antigens and cells. 3rd Int. Convoc. Immunol. Buffalo, N.Y., 1972, p. 118. Basel: Karger 1973
AXELROD, A.R., LOBE, S., ORTEN, J.M., MYERS, G.B.: Insulin resistance. Ann. intern. Med. **27**, 555 (1947)
BALASSE, E.D., BIER, D.M., HAVEL, R.J.: Early effects of anti-insulin serum on hepatic metabolism of plasma free fatty acids in dogs. Diabetes **21**, 280 (1972)
BANTING, F.G., BEST, C.H., COLLIP, J.B., CAMPBELL, W.R., FLETCHER, A.A.: Pancreatic extracts in the treatment of diabetes mellitus. Canad. med. Ass. J. **12**, 142 (1922)
BANTING, F.G., FRANKS, W.R., GAIRNS, S.: Anti-insulin activity of serum of insulin treated patients. Amer. J. Psychiat. **95**, 562 (1938)
BARRET, J.C., BOSHELL, B.R.: Tolbutamide in the therapy of insulin resistance. Diabetes **11**, Suppl. 35 (1962)
BECK, L.V., ZAHARKO, D.S., ROBERTS, N., KING, C.: On insulin I-131-metabolism in mice modifying effects of anti-insulin serum and of total insulin dosage. Diabetes **15**, 336 (1966)
BECK, H.: Über Insulin bindende Gammaglobuline. A) Schwundrate von 131-J-Rinderinsulin und 125-J-Kaninchen-Gammaglobulin aus dem Serum insulinsensibilisierter Kaninchen. B) Versuche zur Reindarstellung von Insulin bindenden Gammaglobulinen mit Hilfe von Rivanol und Surfen. Dissertation Tübingen 1966
BEEUWKES, H., HOLLMAN, E.C.M.J., KREUTZER, H.H.: Specifiske antistoffen tegen runderinsuline. Ned. T. Geneesk. **100**, 3600 (1956)
BEHRENS, O.K., BROMER, W.W.: Biochemistry of the protein hormones. Ann. Rev. Biochem. **27**, 57 (1958)
BEIGELMAN, P.M., ANTONIADES, H.N.: Insulinlike activity of human plasma constituents. IV. Insulin levels of normal human serum and plasma. Metabolism **7**, 269 (1958)
BEIGELMAN, P.M., HOLLANDER, P.B.: Effect of insulin and insulin antibody upon rat adipose tissue membrane resting electrical potential. Acta endocr. (Kbh.) **50**, 648 (1965)
BENNHOLD, H.: Die Vehikelfunktion der Bluteiweißkörper. In: Die Eiweißkörper des Blutplasmas. H. BENNHOLD, E. KEYLIN, S. RUSZNYAK, Hrsg. Leipzig: Steinkopf 1938

BERNE, R.M., WALLERSTEIN, R.S.: The role of antibodies in insulin resistance. Report of a case. J. Mt Sinai Hosp. **17**, 102 (1950)

BERNS, A.W., CURRY, M.C., BLUMENTHAL, H.T.: An evaluation of the complement consumption technic for insulin antibody. Fed. Proc. **24**, 243 (1965)

BERNSTEIN, C., KIRSNER, J.B., TURNER, W.J.: Studies on anaphylaxis with insulin. J. Lab. clin. Med. **23**, 938 (1938)

BERSON, S.A., YALOW, R.S., BAUMAN, A., ROTHSCHILD, M.A., NEWERLY, K.: Insulin J-131 metabolism in human subjects. Demonstration of insulin binding globulin in circulation of insulin treated subjects. J. clin. Invest. **35**, 170 (1956)

BERSON, S.A., YALOW, R.S.: Kinetics of reaction between insulin and insulin binding antibody. J. clin. Invest. **36**, 873 (1957a)

BERSON, S.A., YALOW, R.S.: Ethanol fractionation of plasma and electrophoretic identification of insulin binding antibody. J. clin. Invest. **36**, 642 (1957b)

BERSON, S.A., YALOW, R.S.: Studies with insulin binding antibodies. Diabetes **6**, 402 (1957c)

BERSON, S.A., YALOW, R.S.: Insulin antagonists, insulin antibodies and insulin resistance. Amer. J. Med. **25**, 155 (1958)

BERSON, S.A., YALOW, R.S.: Quantitative aspects of the reaction between insulin and insulin-binding antibodies. J. clin. Invest. **38**, 1996 (1959a)

BERSON, S.A., YALOW, R.S.: Species specificity of human anti-beef-, pork insulin serum. J. clin. Invest. **38**, 2017 (1959b)

BERSON, S.A., YALOW, R.S.: Recent studies on insulin-binding antibodies. Ann. N.Y. Acad. Sci. **82**, 338 (1959c)

BERSON, S.A., YALOW, R.S.: Immunochemical distinction between insulins with identical aminoacid sequences from different mammalian species (pork and sperm whale insulins). Nature (Lond.) **191**, 1392 (1961a)

BERSON, S.A., YALOW, R.S.: Immunologic aspects of insulin. Amer. J. Med. **31**, 882 (1961b)

BERSON, S.A., YALOW, R.S.: Antigens in insulin. Determinants of specificity of porcine insulin in man. Science **139**, 844 (1963)

BERSON, S.A., YALOW, R.S.: Bound insulin — fact, fancy or phantasy. Proceed. II. Intern. Congr. Endocrinol., London, p. 332 (1964a)

BERSON, S.A., YALOW, R.S.: The present status of insulin antagonists in plasma. Diabetes **13**, 247 (1964b)

BERSON, S.A., YALOW, R.S.: Some current controversies in diabetes research. Diabetes **14**, 549 (1965)

BERSON, S.A., YALOW, R.S.: Insulin in blood and insulin antibodies. Amer. J. Med. **40**, 676 (1966)

BIRKINSHAW, V.J., RANDALL, S.S., RISDALL, P.C.: Formation of precipitin lines between insulin and anti-insulin serum produced in sheep and in guinea pigs. Nature (Lond.) **193**, 1089 (1962)

BLACKARD, W.G.: Radioimmunoassay of the A chain of insulin. Diabetes **16**, 681 (1967)

BLOCH, K., KOURILSKY, F., OVARY, Z.N., BENACERRAF, B.: Properties of guinea pig 7-s-antibodies. III. Identification of antibodies involved in complement fixation and hemolysis. J. exp. Med. **117**, 965 (1963)

BLUNDELL, T.L., DODSON, G.G., DODSON, E.J., HODGKIN, D.C., VIJAYAN, M.: X-ray analysis and the structure of insulin. Recent Progr. Hormone Res. **27**, 1 (1971a)

BLUNDELL, T.L., CUTFIELD, J.F., CUTFIELD, S.M., DODSON, E.J., DODSON, G.G., HODGKIN, D.C., MERCOLA, D.A., VIJAYAN, M.: Atomic positions in rhombohedral 2-zinc insulin crystals. Nature (Lond.) **231**, 506 (1971b)

BLUNDELL, T.L., CUTFIELD, J.F., CUTFIELD, S.M., DODSON, E.J., DODSON, G.G., HODGKIN, D.C., MERCOLA, D.A.: 3-dimensional atomic structure of insulin and its relationship to activity. Diabetes **21**, Suppl. 492 (1972)

BOESEL, R.W., CARPENTER, F.H.: Crosslinking during the nitration of bovine insulin with tetranitromethane. Biochem. biophys. Res. Commun. **38**, 678 (1970)

BOLINGER, R.E., MORRIS, J.H., MCKNIGHT, F.G., DIEDERICH, D.A.: Disappearance of I-131-labeled insulin from plasma as a guide to management of diabetes. New Engl. J. Med. **270**, 767 (1964)

BORNSTEIN, J.A.: Insulin reversible inhibition of glucose utilisation by serum lipoprotein fractions. J. biol. Chem. **205**, 513 (1953)

BORNSTEIN, J.A., PARK, C.R.: Inhibition of glucose uptake by the serum of diabetic. J. biol. Chem. **205**, 503 (1953)

BOSHELL, B.R., BARRETT, J.C., BARR, J.H.C., JR.: Insulin resistance, a clinical and experimental study. J. Med. Ass. Ga **51**, 51 (1962)

BOSHELL, B.R., BARRETT, J.C., WILENSKY, A.S., PATTON, T.B.: Insulin resistance. Response to insulin from various animal sources including human. Diabetes **13**, 144 (1964)

BOSSHARD, H.R., JØRGENSEN, K.H., HUMBEL, R.E.: Preparation and properties of cyanoethylated insulin. An insulin derivative with blocked amino- and imidazole-groups. Europ. J. Biochem. **9**, 353 (1969)

BOULET, P., MITROUZE, J., BARJON, P., SCHMOUKER, Y.: Utilité de l'insuline de porc dans les traitments de diabètes rebelles à l'insuline de boeuf (à propos de 2 cas recents). Diabète (Le Raincy) **5**, 177 (1959)

BOYD, W.C.: Fundamentals of immunology. III. Edition, p. 37 (Interscience Publishers, Inc. N.Y. 1956)

BOYDEN, S.V.: The adsorption of proteins on erythrocytes treated with tannic acid and subsequent hemagglutination by antiprotein sera. J. exp. Med. **93**, 107 (1951)

BRANDENBURG, D., OOMS, H.A.: Des glycine^{A1}- des phenylalanin^{B1} insulin and related insulin derivatives. In: Proceedings, Intern. Symposium on Protein and peptide Hormones Liège, 1968, ed. M. MARGOULIES. Excerpta Medica Int. Congr. Ser., **161**, 482 (1968)

BRANDENBURG, D.: Des-Phe^{B1}-Insulin, ein kristallines Analogon des Rinderinsulins. Hoppe-Seylers Z. physiol. Chem. **350**, 741 (1969)

BRANDENBURG, D., BIELA, M., HERBERTZ, L., ZAHN, H.: Chemical modifications at the amino group of insulin chains and their influence on biological activity of the hormone. Diabetologia **6**, 38 (1970) (abstr.)

BRANDENBURG, D., GATTNER, H.-G., WEINERT, M., HERBERTZ, L., ZAHN, H., WOLLMER, A.: Structure function studies with derivatives and analogs of insulin and its chains. In: Proc. VII. Congr. Intern. Diabetes Federation, Buenos Aires 1970, Int. Congr. Ser. Excerpta Medica **231**, 363 (1971a)

BRANDENBURG, D., GATTNER, H.-G., HERBERTZ, L., KRAIL, G., WEINERT, M., ZAHN, H.: Semisynthetic insulin analogues. Biochem. J. **125**, 51 (1971b)

BRANDENBURG, D., BUSSE, W.D., GATTNER, H.-G., ZAHN, H., WOLLMER, A., GLIEMANN, J., PULS, W.: Structure function studies with chemically modified insulins. In: Proc. 11th Europ. Peptide Symposium, Reinhardsbrunn Castle (1972a), eds. HANSON, H., JAKUBKE, H.-D.

BRANDENBURG, D., GATTNER, H.-G., WOLLMER, A.: Darstellung und Eigenschaften von Acetyderivaten des Rinderinsulins. Hoppe-Seylers Z. physiol. Chem. **353**, 599 (1972b)

BRANDENBURG, D., WOLLMER, A.: The effect of a non-peptide interchain crosslink on the reoxidation of reduced insulin. Hoppe-Seylers Z. physiol. Chem. **354**, 613 (1973)

BRINCKERHOFF, C.E., ROSE, N.R.: Characteristics of some „natural" autoantibodies in rabbits. J. Immunol. **102**, 682 (1969)

BROMER, W.W., BERNS, A.W., KNAPP, S., ARQUILLA, E.R.: The preparation and properties of fluoresceinthiocarbamyl insulins. Diabetes **15**, 523 (1966)

BROMER, W.W., SHEEHAN, S.K., BERNS, A.W., ARQUILLA, E.R.: Preparation and properties of fluoresceinthiocarbamyl insulins. Biochemistry (Wash.) **6**, 2378 (1967)

BROMER, W.W., CHANCE, R.: Preparation and characterization of desoctapeptide-insulin. Biochim. biophys. Acta (Amst.) **133**, 219 (1967)

BROWN, R.K.: Studies on the antigenic structure of ribonuclease. III. Inhibition by peptides of antibody to performic acid-oxidized ribonuclease. J. biol. Chem. **237**, 1162 (1962)

BRUCART, F., HARTMANN, G., FANKHAUSER, S., KOLLER, F.: Insulinresistenz und Insulinallergie. Schweiz. med. Wschr. **93**, 1247 (1963).

BRUCCHIERI, A., GRASSO, S.: Immunoelectrophoretic identification of antiinsulin antibodies in guinea pigs. Boll. Soc. ital. Biol. sper. **43**, 1108 (1967)

BRUGMAN, T.M., ARQUILLA, E.R.: Circular dichroic and immunologic studies of structure relationship of insulin and derivatives. Biochemistry (Wash.) **12**, 727 (1973)

BRUNFELDT, K., DECKERT, T.: The antigenic properties of pig insulin. Acta endocr. (Kbh.) **47**, 353 (1964)

BRUNFELDT, K., HANSEN, B.A., JØRGENSEN, K.R.: The immunological reactivity and biological activity of iodinated insulin. Acta endocr. (Kbh.) **57**, 307 (1968)

BURKLE, P.A., HAMM, G., HUBER, V., FEDERLIN, K.: Immunohistological demonstration of insulin in islets of Langerhans after stimulation of insulin secretion by glucose sulfonylureas and insulin antibodies. Diabetologia **7**, 423 (1971)

BURNET, F.M.: The new approach to immunology. New Engl. J. Med. **264**, 24 (1961)

BURRILL, K., KARAM, J.K., CHING, K.N., GRODSKY, G.M., FORSHAM, P.H.: The use of fish insulin: A simple test to evaluate the role of insulin antibodies in insulin resistance. Diabetes **18**, 344 (1969) (abstr.)

BURROWS, B.A., PETERS, T., LOWELL, F.D., TRAKAS, T.N., REILLY, P.: Physical binding of insulin by gammaglobulins of insulin resistant subjects. J. clin. Invest. **36**, 393 (1957)

BUSSE, W.D., GATTNER, H.-G.: Selective cleavage of one disulfide bond in insulin. Preparation and properties of insulin-A7-B7-di-S-sulfonate. Hoppe-Seylers Z. physiol. Chem. **354**, 147 (1973)

BUTTERFIELD, W.J.H., GARRATT, C.J., WHICHELOW, M.J.: Peripheral hormone action: Studies on the clearence and effect of (131 I)-iodo-insulin in the peripheral tissues of normal, acromegalic and diabetic subjects. Clin. Sci. **24**, 331 (1963)

CANN, J.R., LOVELESS, M.H.: Distribution of sensitizing antibody in human serum proteins, fractionated by electrophoresis convection. J. Immunol. **72**, 270 (1954)

CANNON, P., MARSHALL, C.E.: Studies on insulin allergy. Amer. J. Path. **17**, 442 (1941)

CARPENTER, F.H., YOUNG, J.D.: Isolation of desoctapeptide insulin. Fed. Proc. **18**, 201 (1959)

CARPENTER, F.H.: Relation of structure to biological activity of insulin as revealed by degradative studies. Amer. J. Med. **40**, 750 (1966)

CERASI, E., HOGEMAN, O., LUFT, R., PORATH, J., ROOVETTE, A.: Insulin antibodies: description of specific serum protein localisation in a patient with insulin resistant diabetes. Diabetologia **2**, 45 (1966)

CESKA, M.: Detection of insulin precipitating antibodies. Nature (Lond.) **217**, 356 (1968)

CHANCE, R.E.: Chemical, physical, biological and immunological studies on porcine proinsulin and related polypeptides. Proc. 7th Congr. Intern. Diabetes Federation, Buenos Aires, 1970. Excerpta Medica Int. Congr. Ser. **231**, 292 (1971)

CHAO, P.J., KARAM, J.H., GRODSKY, G.M.: Insulin I-131 binding in serum from normal and diabetic subjects by ultracentrifugation and gelfiltration. Diabetes **14**, 27 (1965)

CHETTY, M.P., WATSON, K.C.: Antibody-like activity in diabetic and normal serum measured by complement consumption. Lancet **1965** I, 67

CHRISTIANSEN, A.H.: A new method for determination of insulin binding immunoglobulin in insulin treated diabetic patients. Horm. Metab. Res. **2**, 187 (1970)

CHRISTIANSEN, A.H., RASMUSSEN, S.M., VØLUND, A.: Levels of insulin-binding immunoglobulin in diabetics compared to clinical data. Diabetologia **7**, 474 (1971) (abstr.)

CHRISTIANSEN, A.H., VØLUND, A.: Studies on insulin-binding serum proteins in normals and diabetics applying immunoelectrophoresis. Diabetologia **7**, 475 (1971)

CLAUSEN, J., GJEDDE, F., JØRGENSEN, K.: Insulin binding proteins in human serum. *In vitro* experiments. Proc. Soc. exp. Biol. (N.Y.) **112**, 778 (1963)

CLUTTON, R.F., HARINGTON, C.R., YUILL, M.E.: Studies in synthetic immunochemistry. II. Serological investigation of 0-ß-glucosidotyrosyl derivatives of proteins. Biochem. J. **32**, 1111 (1938)

CLUTTON, R.F., HARINGTON, C.R., YUILL, M.E.: Studies in synthetic immunochemistry. III. Preparation and antigenic properties of thyroxyl derivatives of proteins and physiological effects of their antisera. Biochem. J. **32**, 1119 (1938)

COHEN, N.M., DINWIDDY, G., ALEXANDER, D.P., BRITTON, H., NIXON, D.A.: The effect of anti-insulin serum in the fetal sheep and young lamb. Diabetologia **5**, 201 (1969)

COHEN, S.S.: Pork vs beef insulin in control of diabetes mellitus. A case study. Amer. J. Hosp. Pharm. **29**, 874 (1972)

COLLENS, W.S., BANOWITCH, M.M.: Insulin resistance. Report of a case with requirement up to 7840 units in 24 hours. Metabolism **4**, 355 (1955)

COLWELL, A.R., WEIGER, R.W.: Inhibition of insulin action by serum gamma globulin. J. Lab. clin. Med. **47**, 844 (1956)

CORCOS, J.M., OVARY, Z.: Biological properties of guinea pig anti-insulin antibodies. Proc. Soc. exp. Biol. (N.Y.) **119**, 142 (1965)

CRABTREE, R.E., YOUNG, E.C., GALLOWAY, J.A., RODDA, B.E.: The use of highly purified "single component" insulins in insulin resistance. Diabetes **20**, Suppl. 1, 352 (1971) (abstr.)

CREUTZFELDT, W., SCHLAGINTWEIT, S.T.: Kasuistischer Beitrag zur Wirkung der Sulfonylharnstoffe bei einigen Sonderformen der Zuckerkrankheit. (Steroiddiabetes, Diabetes bei Haemochromatose, Diabetes renalis and Diabetes mit hochgradiger Insulinresistenz.) Dtsch. med. Wschr. **82**, 1539 (1957)

CREUTZFELDT, W., SÖLING, D.: Orale Diabetestherapie und ihre experimentellen Grundlagen. Ergebn. inn. Med. Kinderheilk. **15**, 1 (1960)

CRISPELL, K.R., KAHANA, S., HYER, H.: The effect of plasma on the *in vitro* uptake or binding by human red cells of radioactive labeled l-thyroxin and l-triiodothyronine. J. clin. Invest. **35**, 121 (1956)

CSORBA, T.S., GATTNER, H.-G.: Cross-linking of insulin induced by iodination. Horm. Metab. Res. **2**, 305 (1970)

CUNLIFFE, A.C.: In Colloquium on the Immunology of Insulin. London (1965). Cited by DEVLIN and O'DONOVAN (1966)

CUNNINGHAM, N.F., PATTERSON, D.S.P., WRIGHT, P.H.: Acute insulin deficiency provoked in sheep and cows by single injections of antiinsulin serum. J. Physiol. (Lond.) **169**, 137 (1963)

Davidson, J.K., Haist, R.E.: Failure of guinea pig antibody to beef insulin to neutralize pancreatic and serum guinea pig insulin activity *in vitro*. Canad. J. Physiol. Pharmacol. **43**, 373 (1965)

Davidson, M.B., Goodner, C.J.: Assay of insulin antagonism by serial incubation of paired rat hemidiaphragms. Diabetes **15**, 380 (1966)

Davidson, J.K., Zeigler, M., Haist, R.E.: Failure of guinea pig antibody to beef insulin to neutralize coypu (nutria) insulin. Diabetes **17**, 8 (1968)

Davidson, J.K., Zeigler, M., Haist, R.E.: Failure of guinea pig antibodies to beef insulin, chicken insulin, and cod insulin to neutralize capybara insulin. Diabetes **18**, 212 (1969)

Davidson, J.K.: contribution during discussion. Diabetes **21**, Suppl. 2, 648 (1972)

Daweke, H., Bach, I.: Neue Erkenntnisse in der Behandlung der chronischen Insulinresistenz und experimentelle Untersuchungen zu ihrer Genese. Klin. Wschr. **41**, 257 (1963)

Daweke, H., Bach, I.: Zur Therapie und Genese der chronischen Insulinresistenz. In: Fortschritte der Diabetesforschung. Düsseldorf 1962, p. 43. Stuttgart: G. Thieme 1963

Daweke, H.: Klinik der Insulinresistenz. Dtsch. med. Wschr. **91**, 974 (1966)

Daweke, H.: Schwierigkeiten der Insulinbehandlung, insbesondere bei labilem Diabetes, bei Insulinallergie and Insulinresistenz. Therapiewoche **18**, 20 (1968)

Deckert, T.: Insulin antibodies. Inaugural Dissertation Kopenhagen, Munksgaard (1964)

Deckert, T.: Insulin antibodies. Rep. Steno Hosp. (Kbh.) **12**, 11 (1965)

Deckert, T.: Autoimmunological aspects of diabetes mellitus. Acta med. scand. Suppl. **478** (1967)

Deckert, T., Grundahl, E.: The antigenicity of pig insulin. Diabetologia **6**, 15 (1970)

De Fillips, V., Jannaccone, A.: Insulin neutralizing activity of gamma globulins derived from the serum of an insulin-resistant patient. Lancet **1952** I, 1191

Dendrinos, G.J., Prout, T.E., Odak, V.V.: A simplified technic for measurement of insulin binding globulin. 43. Ann. Meeting of the Endocr. Soc. N.Y. City, Abstract No. 65 (1961)

Depisch, F., Hasenöhrl, R.: Experimentelle Untersuchungen über die Insulinresistenz beim Diabetes mellitus. Z. ges. exp. Med. **58**, 110 (1928)

Derot, M., Rathery, M.: Sur un cas de diabète sensible à l'insuline de porc. Diabète (Le Raincy) **8**, 65 (1960)

Desbuquois, S., Auerbach, G.D.: Use of polyethylene glycol to separate free and antibody bound peptide hormones in radioimmunoassay. J. clin. Endocr. **33**, 732 (1971)

Devey, M., Carter, D., Sanderson, C.J., Coombs, R.R.A.: IgD antibody to insulin. Lancet **1970 II**, 7686, 1280

Devlin, J.G., Brien, T.G.: Relationship between differential antibody binding capacity and clinical requirements of beef and pork insulin. Metabolism **14**, 1034 (1965)

Devlin, J.G., O'Donovan, D.K.: Association of acute local reactions to insulin with an insulin binding gamma IgM antibody. J. clin. Path. **18**, 356 (1965)

Devlin, J.G.: Evidence for the existence of an IgM immunoglobulin to insulin. Irish J. med. Sci. **6**, 507 (1966)

Devlin, J.G., O'Donovan, D.K.: Preferential beef/pork insulin-binding capacity. Radioimmunoelectrophoretic and chromatographic data in patients with dermal reactions to insulin. Diabetes **15**, 790 (1966)

Devlin, J.G., Brien, T., Stephenson, N.: Effect of alteration of species source of insulin on insulin-antibody levels. Lancet **1966 II**, 883

Devlin, J.G., Brien, T., Stephenson, N.: Relationship between antibody and insulin dose. Brit. med. J. **1967 I**, 542

Devlin, J.G., Duggan, M.: Antibody studies in patients on mixed bovine/porcine insulins. Diabetologia **5**, 192 (1969)

Ditschuneit, H., Kapp, H., Pfeiffer, E.F.: Nachweis und klinische Bedeutung von Insulinantikörpern bei Insulinresistenz. 9. Symposium Dtsch. Ges. Endokrin. S. 186. Berlin- Göttingen-Heidelberg: Springer 1962

Ditschuneit, H., Schmidt, H., Roadi, A., Pfeiffer, E.F.: Beitrag zum Problem der Insulin Antikörper bei Diabetikern mit hohem Insulinbedarf. Verh. dtsch. Ges. inn. Med. **69**, **435** (1963)

Ditschuneit, H., Federlin, K.: Beitrag zur Pathogenese der Insulinresistenz. Dtsch. med. Wschr. **91**, 853 (1966)

Ditschuneit, H.: Die Behandlung der immunologisch bedingten Insulinresistenz. Rundtischgespräch: Therapieprobleme bei Insulinresistenz. 74. Kongr. Dtsch. Ges. Inn. Med., Wiesbaden 1968

Dituri, B.: Insulin resistant diabetes after total pancreatectomy. Report of a case. New Engl. J. Med. **251**, 13 (1954)

Ditzov, S., Penchev, J., Andreev, D., Sirakov, L., Tarkolev, N.: Insulin-binding antibodies in insulin treated and untreated diabetic patients. Diabetologia **7**, 477 (1971) (abstr.)

DIXON, K., EXON, P.D., HUGHES, H.R.: Insulin antibodies in aetiology of labile diabetes. Lancet **1972 I**, 7746—343

DOLOVICH, J., SCHNATZ, J.D., REISMAN, R.E., YAGI, J., ARBESMAN, C.E.: Insulin allergy and insulin resistance. J. Allergy **46**, 127 (1970)

DUNCAN, G.G., LEE, C.T., YOUNG, J.K.: Clinical experiences with the sulfonylurea compounds. Ann. N.Y. Acad. Sci. **71**, 233 (1957/58)

ELGEE, N.J., WILLIAMS, R.H., LEE, N.D., WONG, T., HOGNESS, I.R.: Studies of radioactive insulin. Diabetes **2**, 370 (1953)

ELGEE, N.J., WILLIAMS, R.H., LEE, N.D.: Distribution and degradation studies with insulin-J-131. J. clin. Invest. **33**, 1252 (1954)

ENGLESON, G., NILSSON, S.B.: Insulin antibodies in juvenile diabetes. Acta paediat. (Uppsala) **51**, 433 (1962)

ENSINCK, J.W., COOMBS, G.J., WILLIAMS, R.H., VALLANCE-OWEN, J.: Studies *in vitro* of the transport of the A and B chains of insulin in serum. J. biol. Chem. **239**, 3377 (1964)

ESKIND, J.B., FRANKLIN, W., LOWELL, F.C.: Insulin resistant diabetes mellitus associated with hemochromatosis. Ann. intern. Med. **38**, 1295 (1953)

ETTINGER, M.J., TIMASHEFF, S.N.: Optical activity of insulin. I. On the nature of the circular dichroism bands. Biochemistry (Wash.) **10**, 824 (1971)

EZRIN, C., MOLONEY, P.J.: The antigenicity of insulin. J. clin. Invest. **38**, 1002 (1959)

FALKMER, S., WILSON, S.: Comparative aspects of the immunology and biology of insulin. Diabetologia **3**, 519 (1967)

FALTA, W.: Über einen insulinrefraktären Fall von Diabetes mellitus. Klin. Wschr. **3**, 1315 (1924)

FANKHAUSER, S., GOETZ, F.C.: Zur Bedeutung der Insulinantikörper für das klinische Verhalten des Diabetes mellitus. Helv. med. Acta **28**, 496 (1961)

FANKHAUSER, S.: Zur Pathophysiologie des Diabetes. Schweiz. med. Wschr. **93**, 1515 (1963a)

FANKHAUSER, S.: In: Symp. Internat. sul. Diabete, Modena (1963b). Cited by MORCOS *et al.* (1965)

FANKHAUSER, S.: Insulinantikörper und Ketosetendenz bei Diabetes mellitus. Helv. med. Acta **30**, 500 (1963c)

FANKHAUSER, S., MONTADON, A.: Immunologic aspect of the insulin treatment. Rev. méd. Suisse. rom. **83**, 33 (1963)

FANKHAUSER, S.: Zur Klinik und Therapie der Insulinresistenz. Praxis **53**, 185 (1964)

FANKHAUSER, S., DIACON, CH.: Die Bedeutung der Insulinantikörper bei Komplikationen der Insulintherapie. Helv. med. Acta **33**, Suppl. 46, 164 (1966)

FANKHAUSER, S., MORELL, B.: Beobachtungen über das Verhalten von Insulin-Antikörpern bei Patienten mit Insulinresistenz unter Behandlung mit Corticosteroiden. VI. Congr. Int. Diab. Fed., Stockholm (1967)

FANKHAUSER, S., MORELL, B.: Antigenicity of different insulin preparations in psychiatric and diabetic patients. Diabetologia **4**, 389 (1968) (abstr.)

FANKHAUSER, S.: Neuere Aspekte der Insulintherapie. Schweiz. med. Wschr. **99**, 414 (1969)

FANKHAUSER, S., MICHL, J.: New possibilities to avoid the formation of insulin-antibodies in diabetic patients. Diabetologia **7**, 478 (1971) (abstr.)

FANKHAUSER, S., MICHL, J.: Die Antigenität verschiedener Depotinsuline bei Diabetikern. 2. Int. Donausymposium über Diabetes mellitus, Budapest (1971)

FANKHAUSER, S., MICHL, J.: Zwei Jahre Erfahrungen mit Monocomponent-Insulin bei Diabetikern. 3. Int. Donausyposium über Diabetes mellitus, Salzburg (1973)

FAULK, W.P., TOMSOVIC, E.J., FUDENBERG, H.H.: Insulin resistance in juvenile diabetes mellitus. Amer. J. Med. **49**, 133 (1970)

FAULK, W.P., KARAM, J.H., FUDENBERG, H.H.: Human anti-insulin antibodies. J. Immunol. **106**, 1112 (1971)

FEDERLIN, K., KRIEGBAUM, D., HEINEMANN, G., FLACH, H.D., PFEIFFER, E.F.: Experimental studies in animals on the antigenicity of insulin, of A and B chains and of fragments of synthetic insulin in terms of delayed immunoreactivity to insulin. Diabetologia **6**, 44 (1970) (abstr.)

FEDERLIN, K.: Untersuchungen über die Antigenität von Insulin, Proinsulin und verwandten Proteinen am Meerschweinchen mit der passiven kutanen Anaphylaxie. Proinsulin und verwandte Proteine, Monokomponentinsulin. Arbeitsgespräch Novo. Mainz (1970) cited in Immunopathology of Insulin, p. 29. Berlin-Heidelberg-New York: Springer 1971

FEDERLIN, K.: Immunopathology of insulin. Monographs on Endocrinology, Vol. 6, p. 3. Berlin-Heidelberg-New York: 1971

FEDERLIN, K., DITSCHUNEIT, H., PFEIFFER, E.F.: Insulinallergie und Insulinresistenz. In: Handbuch des Diabetes mellitus. Hrsg. E.F. PFEIFFER, Band II, S. 1141. München: J.F. Lehmann 1971

FEINBERG, R.: Detection of non-precipitating antibodies coexisting with precipitating antibodies using I-131 labeled antigen. Fed. Proc. **13**, 493 (1954)

FELDMAN, R., GRODSKY, G.M., KOHOUT, F.W., MCWILLIAMS, N.B.: Immunologic studies in a diabetic subject resistant to bovine insulin but sensitive to porcine insulin. Amer. J. Med. **35**, 411 (1963)

FIELD, J.B., STETTEN, D., JR.: Studies on humoral insulin antagonism associated with diabetic acidosis. Amer. J. Med. **21**, 339 (1956a)

FIELD, J.B., STETTEN, D., JR.: Studies on humoral antagonist in diabetic acidosis. Diabetes **5**, 391 (1956b)

FIELD, J.B., TIETZE, F., STETTEN, D., JR.: Further characterization of an insulin antagonist in the serum of patients in diabetic acidosis. J. clin. Invest. **36**, 1588 (1957)

FIELD, J.B., WOODSON, M.L.: Studies on the circulating insulin inhibitor found in some diabetic patients exhibiting chronic insulin resistance. J. clin. Invest. **38**, 3 (1959)

FIELD, J.B., JOHNSON, P., HERING, B.: Insulin resistant diabetes associated with increased endogenous plasma insulin followed by complete remission. J. clin. Invest. **40**, 1672 (1961)

FIELD, J.B.: Insulin resistance in diabetes. Ann. Rev. Med. **13**, 249 (1962)

FIELD, J.B.: Studies on steroid treatment of chronic insulin resistance. Diabetes **11**, 165 (1962)

FIELD, J.B.: Chronic insulin resistant diabetics. Geriatrics **18**, 846 (1963)

FØLLING, J., NORMAN, N.: Hyperglycemia, hypoglycemic attacks, and production of anti-insulin-antibodies without previous known immunization. Immunological and functional studies in a patient. Diabetes **21**, 814 (1972)

FREEDLENDER, A.E., REES, S.R., SOELDNER, J.S. (introduced by RENOLD, A.E.): Some physical-chemical variables affecting insulin migration *in vitro*. I. Electrophoresis. Proc. Soc. exp. Biol. (N.Y.) **115**, 21 (1964)

FREYCHET, P.: Insulin-receptor interaction: Some recent developments. Symposium: Chemie des Insulins and Proinsulins, Aachen (1973)

FREYTAG, G., KLÖPPEL, G.: Contribution to the immunopathology of experimental insulitis. Diabetologia **7**, 479 (1971) (abstr.)

FREYTAG, G.H.: Immunpathologie des Diabetes mellitus. Veröffentlichungen aus der Morphologischen Pathologie, Heft 88. Stuttgart: Gustav Fischer 1972

FRIEDLANDER, E.O.: Use of tolbutamide in insulin-resistant diabetes. Report of a case. New Engl. J. Med. **257**, 11 (1957)

FRIEDLANDER, E.O., BRYANT, M.D.: Idiopathic insulin-resistant diabetes mellitus. Report of a case associated with insulin allergy. Amer. J. Med. **26**, 139 (1959)

FROESCH, E.R., BÜRGI, H., RAMSEIER, E.B., BALLY, P., LABHART, A.: Antibody suppressible and nonsuppressible insulinlike activities in human serum and physiological significance. J. clin. Invest. **42**, 1816 (1963)

GAMMELTOFT, S., GLIEMANN, J.: Binding and degradation of 125-I-labelled insulin by isolated rat fat cells. Biochim. biophys. Acta (Amst.) **320**, 16 (1973)

GARATT, C.J., HARRISON, D.M., WICKS, M.: The effect of iodination of particular tyrosine residues on the hormonal activity of insulin. Biochem. J. **126**, 123 (1972)

GATTNER, H.-G.: A partially reduced insulin with full hypoglycaemic action. 8. Int. Congr. Biochem., Interlaken (1970). Cited by ZAHN *et al.* (1972)

GEERLING, H., SIREK, O.V.: Alpha-2-macroglobulin and the question of a protein carrier for insulin in human serum. Canad. J. Physiol. Pharmacol. **43**, 885 (1965)

GEIGER, R.: Selective chemical modifications of insulin. Hoppe-Seylers Z. physiol. Chem. **352**, 7 (1971)

GEIGER, R., LANGNER, D.: Insulin-analoga mit N-terminal verkürzter B-Kette; selectiver Edman-Abbau an der B-Kette des Insulins. Hoppe-Seylers Z. physiol. Chem. **354**, 1285 (1973)

GELLER, W., LA DUE, J.S., GLASS, C.B.J.: Insulin resistant diabetes precipitated by cortisone and reversed by nitrogen mustard. A.M.A. Arch. Int. Med. **87**, 124 (1951)

GEMMIL, C.L.: Effects of glucose and of insulin on metabolism of isolated diaphragm of the rat. Bull. Johns Hopk. Hosp. **68**, 329 (1941)

GILL, III. T.J.: Antigenic determinants on synthetic polypeptides. In: Specific receptors of antibodies, antigens and cells. 3rd Int. Convoc. Immunol., Buffalo, N.Y., 1972, pp. 136—169. Basel: Karger 1973

GINGERICH, R.L., CARTER, G.A., MAKULU, D.R., WRIGHT, P.H.: The fate of insulin/antibody complexes in rats. Diabetes **20**, 356 (1971)

GLEN, A., EATON, J.C.: Insulin antagonism. Quart. J. Med. **7**, 271 (1938)

GLIEMANN, J.: Insulinlike activity of dilute human serum by isolated adipose cell method. Diabetes **14**, 643 (1969)

GLIEMANN, J., GAMMELTOFT, S.: Insulin receptors in fat cells. Symposium Chemie des Insulins und Proinsulins, Aachen (1973)

GOETZ, F.C., GREENBERG, B.Z., ELLS, J., MEINERT, C.: A simple immunoassay for insulin: application to human and dog plasma. J. clin. Endocr. **23**, 1237 (1963)

GOFF, J., GOFF, M., BRUGMAN, T., ARQUILLA, E.R.: The induction of experimental diabetes with insulin antibodies against a restricted determinant. Excerpt. Medica, Int. Congr. Ser. **280**, 131 (1973)

GOLDMAN, A.S., KAYE, R.: Insulin resistance in a diabetic child. Diabetes **11**, 122 (1962)

GOLDNER, M.G., RICKETTS, H.T.: Insulin allergy. A report of eight cases with generalized symptoms. J. clin. Endocr. **2**, 595 (1942)

GORDIS, E. (introduced by BERSON, S.A.): Detection of insulin-binding antibodies and separation of free and antibody-bound insulin by a rapid chemical procedure. Proc. Soc. exp. Biol. (N.Y.) **103**, 542 (1960)

GRABAR, P.: Immunoelectrophoretic analysis. In: Methods of biochemical analysis. New York: Interscience Publishers, Inc. 1959

GRODSKY, G.M., FORSHAM, P.H.: Binding mechanism for insulin in "insulin resistant" sera. Fed. Proc. **17**, 234 (1958)

GRODSKY, G.M., PENG, C.T., FORSHAM, P.H.: Effect of modification of insulin on specific binding in insulin resistant sera. Arch. Biochem. **81**, 264 (1959)

GRODSKY, G.M., FORSHAM, P.H.: An immunochemical assay of total extractable insulin in man. J. clin. Invest. **39**, 1070 (1960)

GRODSKY, G.M., FORSHAM, P.H.: Comparative binding of beef and human insulin to insulin antibodies produced in man and guinea pigs. J. clin. Invest. **40**, 799 (1961)

GRODSKY, G.M.: Production of autoantibodies to insulin in man and rabbits. Diabetes **14**, 396 (1965)

GRODSKY, G.M., FELDMAN, R., TORESON, W.E., LEE, J.C.: Diabetes mellitus in rabbits immunized with insulin. Diabetes **15**, 579 (1966)

GRÜNEKLEE, D., TAKAISHI, T., DAWEKE, H.: Insulin Resistenz. Diagnostische und therapeutische Probleme. Münch. med. Wschr. **27**, 1278 (1970)

GRÜNEKLEE, D., HESSING, J., DAWEKE, H., HERBERG, L., GRIESS, F.A.: Insulin resistance without circulating antibodies, evidence for an antagonist? Diabetologia **7**, 482 (1971) (abstr.)

GUTFREUND, H.: The reversible dissociation of insulin and its minimum molecular weight. Biochem. J. **50**, 564 (1952)

GUTHRIE, R.A., MURTHY, D.Y.N., WOLMACK, W.: Insulin resistance in diabetes on juveniles. A case report in a child and a review of the literature. Pediatrics **40**, 642 (1967)

HAHN, H.J., ZIEGLER, M.: Influence of isolated insulin antibodies on the insulin secretion *in vitro*. Diabetologia **7**, 483 (1971) (abstr.)

HALES, C.N., RANDLE, P.J.: Immunoassay of insulin with insulin-antibody precipitate. Biochem. J. **88**, 137 (1963)

HARRIS, J.I., LI, C.H.: The biological activity of enzymatic digests of insulin. J. Amer. chem. Soc. **74**, 2945 (1952)

HARRIS, J.I., SANGER, F., NAUGHTON, M.A.: Species differences in insulin. Arch. Biochem. **65**, 427 (1956)

HARRIS-JONES, J.M., MILLER, H., OWEN, G.: Insulin binding antibodies in relation to insulin therapy. J. clin. Path. **16**, 120 (1963)

HARWOOD, R.: Insulin binding antibodies and "spontaneous" hypoglycemia. New Engl. J. Med. **262**, 979 (1960)

HASSELBLATT, A., SCHMIETA, J.: Aktivierung von gebundenem Insulin durch Tolbutamid. Klin. Wschr. **39**, 910 (1961)

HAUGAARD, N., VAUGHAN, M., HAUGAARD, E.S., STADIE, W.C.: Studies of radioactive injected labeled insulin. J. biol. Chem. **208**, 549 (1954)

HAUROWITZ, F.: Chemistry and biology of proteins, 1st ed. New York: Academic Press 1950

HEDING, L.G.: Ethanol precipitation as a substitute for the double-antibody reaction in a simplified insulin immunoassay method. Diabetologia **1**, 76 (1965) (abstr.)

HEDING, L.G.: A simplified insulin radioimmunoassay method. Conference on problems connected with the preparation and use of labelled proteins in tracer studies, Pisa (1966)

HEDING, L.G., NIELSEN, A.V.: Determination of free and antibody bound immunoreactive insulin in serum from insulin treated diabetic patients. Excerpta Medica, Int. Congr. Ser. **140**, 114 (1967)

HEDING, L.G.: Determination of free and antibody-bound insulin in insulin treated diabetic patients. Horm. Metab. Res. **1**, 145 (1969)

HEIDEMAN, M.L., JR.: Separation of (^{131}I) Insulin-antibody complexes and of antibodies by disc electrophoresis in polyacrylamide gels. Biochemistry (Wash.) **3**, 1108 (1964)

HENRICHS, H.R., SCHWALD, A., KASEMIR, H., BURMEISTER, P., KERP, L.: Der Einfluß einer Abspaltung von Aminosäuren am N-terminalen Ende der B-Kette auf die spezifische Bindung von Rinderinsulin an Fettzellrezeptoren. 9. Kongr. Dtsch. Diabetes Ges., Travemünde (1974)

HERBERT, V., LAU, K.S., GOTTLIEB, C.W., BLEICHER, S.J.: Coated charcoal immunoassay of insulin. J. clin. Endocr. **25**, 1375 (1965)

HILDEBRANDT, H.E., AMMON, J., PFEIFFER, E.F.: Ergebnisse einer Bestimmung der Konzentration von Antikörpern gegen Insulin mit Hilfe zweier verschiedener radioimmunologischer Methoden. In: Nebenschilddrüse und endokrine Regulation des Calciumstoffwechsels. Hrsg. J. KRACHT. Berlin-Heidelberg-New York: Springer 1968

HIRATA, Y., BLUMENTHAL, H.T.: Precipitation of insulin with the sera of insulin treated guinea pigs and rabbits. J. Lab. clin. Med. **60**, 194 (1962a)

HIRATA, Y., BLUMENTHAL, H.T.: Blood sugar and anti-insulin serum levels of activity and passively immunized rabbits. Diabetes **11**, Suppl. 26 (1962b)

HIRATA, Y., BLUMENTHAL, H.T.: Demonstration of a precipitating insulin-binding antibody in the sera of insulin-treated guinea pigs and rabbits. J. Lab. clin. Med. **62**, 683 (1963)

HIRATA, Y., ISHIZU, H.: Elevated insulin-binding capacity of serum proteins in a case with spontaneous hypoglycemia and mild diabetes not treated with insulin. Tohoku J. exp. Med. **107**, 277 (1972)

HIRATA, Y., ISHIZU, H., ITO, J.: A new syndrome: insulin autoimmune syndrome. Excerpta Medica, Int. Congr. Ser. **280**, 131 (1972)

HODGKIN, D.C., MERCOLA, D.A.: In: Handbook of Physiology, sect. 7, vol. I, p. 139. Baltimore, Md.: Waverly 1972. Cited by BRUGMAN et ARQUILLA (1973)

HODGKIN, D.C.: The structure of insulin. Diabetes **21**, 1131 (1972)

HORINO, M., HIRATA, Y., SATO, T., ITO, M., SHIROUZU, H., MAKINO, N.: Studies on insulin antibodies. Folia endocr. (Japan) **35**, 330 (1959)

HORINO, M., YU, S.Y., BLUMENTHAL, H.T.: Studies on experimental insulin immunity. I. Dynamics of insulin immunity in the guinea pig. Diabetes **15**, 812 (1966)

HORINO, M., SHIU, Y.Y., BLUMENTHAL, H.T.: Studies on experimental insulin immunity. II. The organ distribution of insulin in immune rabbits. Diabetes **16**, 402 (1967)

HORWITZ, F., ALP, H., RECANT, L.: Observations on cationic exchange resins in relation to insulin binding. J. Lab. clin. Med. **64**, 942 (1964)

HURN, B.A.L., FARRANT, P.C., YOUNG, B.A., GRAHAME, A.: Insulin-binding antibody and hormone dosage in non-resistant diabetes. Postgrad. Med. Suppl. 819 (1969)

HÜRTER, P., KÜHNAU, J., JR.: Die Aktivität zirkulierender Insulinantikörper bei kindlichen Diabetikern. Helv. paediat. Acta **25**, 154 (1970)

HÜRTER, P., KÜHNAU, J., Jr.: Insulinantikörper bei diabetischen Kindern unter verschiedenen Monospezies-Insulinen. 7. Kongr. dtsch. Diabetes-Gesellschaft, Bad Nauheim, abstr. 28 (1972)

ISHIHARA, Y., SAITO, T., ITO, Y., FUJINO, M.: Structure of sperm- and sei-whale insulin and their breakdown by whale pepsin. Nature (Lond.) **181**, 1468 (1958)

ISHIZAKA, K., ISHIZAKA, T., HORNBROOK, M.M.: Physicochemical properties of human reagenic antibody. IV. Presence of a unique immunoglobulin as a carrier of reagenic activity. J. Immunol. **97**, 75 (1966a)

ISHIZAKA, K., ISHIZAKA, T., HORNBROOK, M.M.: Physicochemical properties of reagenic antibody. V. Correlation of reagenic activity with γE-globulin antibody. J. Immunol. **97**, 840 (1966b)

IZZO, J.L., RONCONE, A., IZZO, M.J., BALE, W.F.: Relationship between degree of iodination of insulin and its biological, electrophoretic, and immunochemical properties. J. biol. Chem. **239**, 3749 (1964)

JACOTOT, B., NAVARRO, N., DELPLANQUE, B., LE PARCO, J.-C., BEAUMONT, J.-L.: Diabète gras, insulino-résistance et anticorps anti-insuline. Nouv. Presse méd. **2**, 1121 (1973)

JANSEN, F.K.: The ability of monocomponent insulin or 1× crystallized insulin in the development of immunological tolerance in mice. Diabetologia **7**, 485 (1971a) (abstr.)

JANSEN, F.K.: Hochdosis und Niedrigdosistoleranz mit kristallinem Insulin und ihre zeitliche Entstehung. 6. Kongr. dtsch. Diabetes-Gesellschaft, Düsseldorf, abstr. 8 (1971b)

JANSEN, F.K.: Tolerance to high and low doses of natural crystalline insulin. Diabetologia **7**, 290 (1971c)

JAYARAO, K., KARAM, J.H., FAULK, W.P., GRODSKY, G.M., FORSHAM, P.H.: Measurement of "masked" insulin antibodies in insulin resistance. Diabetes **18**, Suppl. 1, 324 (1969)

JAYARAO, K., KARAM, J.H., FAULK, W.P., GRODSKY, G.M., FORSHAM, P.H.: "Masked" insulin antibodies in insulin resistance. Effectiveness of fish insulin in therapy. 29th Annual Meeting Amer. Diabetes Ass., New York (1969)

JENSEN, H., WINTERSTEINER, O., GEILING, E.M.K.: Studies on crystalline insulin. VIII. The isolation of crystalline insulin from fish islets (cod and pollock) and from the pig's pancreas. The activity of crystalline insulin and further remarks on its preparation. J. Pharmacol. exp. Ther. **36**, 115 (1929).

JENSEN, H., SCHOCK, E., SOLLERS, E.: Studies on crystalline insulin. XVI. The action of ammonium hydroxide and of iodine on insulin. J. biol. Chem. **98**, 93 (1932)

JONES, V.E., CUNLIFFE, A.G.: A precipitating antibody to insulin. Nature (Lond.) **192**, 136 (1961)

JØRGENSEN, K.H., DECKERT, T., PEDERSEN, L.M., PEDERSEN, J.: Insulin, insulin antibodies and glucose in plasma of newborn infants of diabetic women. Acta endocr. (Kbh.) **52**, 154 (1966)

JORPES, J.E.: Recrystallized insulin for diabetic patients with insulin allergy. Arch. intern. Med. **83**, 363 (1949)

KABAT, E.: Einführung in die Immunchemie und Immunologie, S. 71. Berlin-Heidelberg-New York: Springer 1971

KALANT, N., GOMBERG, C., SCHUCKER, R.: The effect of insulin binding antibodies on insulin sensitivity. Lancet **1958 II**, 614

KALKHOFF, R.K., HORNBROOK, K.R., BURCH, H.B., KIPNIS, D.M.: Studies on the metabolic effects of acute insulin deficiency. II. Changes in hepatic glycolytic and Krebs-cycle intermediates and pyridine nucleotides. Diabetes **15**, 451 (1966)

KALKHOFF, R.K., KIPNIS, D.M.: Studies on the metabolic effects of acute insulin deficiency. I. Mechanism of impairment of hepatic fatty acid and protein synthesis. Diabetes **15**, 443 (1966)

KALLEE, E.: Über 131J-signiertes Insulin. I. Mitteilung (Nachweis). Z. Naturforsch. **7b**, 661 (1952)

KALLEE, E., WILMANNS, W., WEISS, G.: Geschwindigkeit der Neubildung insulinbindender γ-Globuline. Z. Naturforsch. **18b**, 1124 (1963a)

KALLEE, E., DEBIASI, S., D'ADDABBO, A.: Studies on I-131 labelled insulin. VI. Immunological experiments on the binding of 131-I-insulin to serum proteins of normal, analbuminemic, and insulin-treated subjects. Acta isotop. **3**, 239 (1963b)

KALLEE, E.: Die Inselzellhormone: Radiojodiertes Insulin. In: Handbuch des Diabetes mellitus. Vol. I, p. 247. Hrsg. E.F. PFEIFFER. München: J.F. LEHMANNS 1969

KANTOR, F.S., BERKMAN, P.M.: Steroid amelioration of immunogenic insulin-resistant diabetes: a proposed mechanism. Yale J. Biol. Med. **40**, 46 (1967)

KARAM, J.H., GRODSKY, G.M., FORSHAM, P.H.: Excessive insulin response to glucose in obese subjects, as measured by immunochemical assay. Diabetes **12**, 197 (1963)

KARAM, J.H., GRODSKY, G.M., FORSHAM, P.H.: Insulin resistant diabetes with autoantibodies induced by exogenous insulin. Successful treatment by insulin withdrawal. Diabetes **18**, 445 (1969a)

KARAM, J.H., LEVIN, S.R., LECHARNY, B., GRODSKY, G.M., FORSHAM, P.H.: Circulating insulin levels in insulin treated diabetics. Diabetes **18**, 361 (1969b) (abstr.)

KARR, W.G., FREIDER, W.A., SEULL, C.W., PETTY, O.H.: Certain immunologic studies in insulin sensitivity. Amer. J. med. Sci. **181**, 293 (1931)

KASEMIR, H., PAULUS, U., STEINHILBER, S., KERP, L.: Comparative quantitative studies on insulin antibody formation by beef and pork insulin. Diabetologia **4**, 395 (1968) (abstr.)

KASEMIR, H., KERP, L., STEINHILBER, S., STRUWE, F.: Auswirkungen insulinbindender Antikörper auf den Insulinbedarf und den Verlauf des Diabetes mellitus. In: 2. Intern. Donausymp. Diab. mell. Budapest, Hrsg.: J. MAGYAR, A. BERNINGER, S. 399. Verlag der Wiener Mediz. Akademie 1971

KATSILABROS, L.: Treatment of insulin allergy and insulin resistance with phenylated insulin. Israel J. med. Sci. **8**, 893, 897 (1972)

KATSOYANNIS, P.G., OKADA, Y., ZAHNT, C.: Synthesis of a biologically active insulin analog lacking the intrachain cyclic system. Biochemistry (Wash.) **12**, 2516 (1973)

KAYE, M., MCGARDY, E., ROSENFELD, I.: Accquired insulin resistance. A case report. Diabetes **4**, 133 (1955)

KERP, L., STEINHILBER, S.: Verbesserte Ultrazentrifugenmethodik zur quantitativen Untersuchung von Protein-Liganden Komplexen. Klin. Wschr. **40**, 540 (1962)

KERP, L.: Insulinbindende Antikörper. Habilitationsschrift, Freiburg (1963)

KERP, L., CREUTZFELDT, W., STEINHILBER, S.: Wird die Insulin-Antikörperbindung durch Tolbutamid *in vitro* beeinflußt? In: Fortschritte der Diabetesforschung 1962, Düsseldorf. Stuttgart: G. Thieme 1963

KERP, L., STEINHILBER, S.: Quantitativer Nachweis insulinbindender Proteine durch Differentialadsorption. Protid. biol. Fluids **11**, 455 (1963)

KERP, L., STEINHILBER, S., KIELING, F., CREUTZFELDT, W.: Klinische und experimentelle Untersuchungen zur Insulinallergie und Insulinresistenz. Dtsch. med. Wschr. **90**, 806 (1965)

KERP, L.: Insulin als Antigen. Dtsch. med. Wschr. **90**, 841 (1965)
KERP, L., STEINHILBER, S., KASEMIR, H.: Ein Verfahren zum Nachweis insulinbindender Antikörper durch Differentialadsorption. Klin. Wschr. **44**, 560 (1966)
KERP, L., KIELING, F., STEINHILBER, S.: Zur Lokalisation der Antikörper-Bindungsstellen an heterologen Insulinmolekülen. Naturwissenschaften **54**, 167 (1967a)
KERP, L., KIELING, F., KASEMIR, H.: Zur Lokalisation von Antikörperbindungsstellen an homologen Insulinmolekülen. Naturwissenschaften **54**, 368 (1967b)
KERP, L., SIHLER, K., RAJU, S., BERNING, E., STEINHILBER, S.: Influence of prednisolone and ACTH on the formation of insulin-binding antibodies. Int. Arch. Allergy **31**, 195 (1967c)
KERP, L., KASEMIR, H., KIELING, F., KEIDERLING, W.: Spezifität der gegen isolierte A- und B-Ketten und gegen intaktes Insulin gebildeten Antikörper. Naturwissenschaften **54**, 589 (1967c)
KERP, L., KASEMIR, H.: Klinische und experimentelle Untersuchungen zur Pathogenese der Insulinresistenz. Allergie u. Asthma **14**, 200 (1968)
KERP, L., KASEMIR, H., KIELING, F., STEINHILBER, S.: Zur Lokalisation von Antikörper-Bindungsstellen am Insulinmolekül. Verh. dtsch. Ges. inn. Med. **74**, 552 (1968a)
KERP, L., KASEMIR, H., KIELING, F.: Insulinbindende Antikörper und Insulinbedarf bei Diabetikern. Klin. Wschr. **46**, 376 (1968b)
KERP, L., KASEMIR, H., STEINHILBER, S., KIELING, F.: Untersuchungen zur Lokalisation der Insertionsstellen insulinbindender Antikörper am Insulinmolekül. Protid. biol. Fluids **16**, 265 (1969a)
KERP, L., KASEMIR, H., KIELING, STEINHILBER, S.: Localisation of antibody-binding sites on insulin molecules. Int. Arch. Allergy **36**, 143 (1969b)
KERP, L., STEINHILBER, S., SCHMIDT, D.D.: Vergleichende Analyse der gegen Rinderproinsulin und Rinderinsulin gebildeten Antikörper. FEBS Letters **8**, 157 (1970a)
KERP, L., STEINHILBER, S., KASEMIR, H.: Quantitative Ergebnisse zur Lokalisation determinanter Gruppen am Insulinmolekül. Naturwissenschaften **57**, 196 (1970b)
KERP, L.: Quantitative data concerning the localization of antibody binding sites on insulin and proinsulin molecules. Int. Arch. Allergy **41**, 216 (1971a)
KERP, L.: Experimentelle Untersuchungen zur antikörperbedingten Insulinneutralisation. In. 2. Intern. Donausymp. Diab. mell. Budapest, Eds.: J. MAGYAR, A. BERNINGER, S. 89. Verlag der Wiener Mediz. Akademie 1971b
KERP, L., STEINHILBER, S., KASEMIR, H., BRANDENBURG, D.: Zur Antikörperbindung von Insulinmolekülen mit Modifikationen an den Aminosäuren A^1 und B^1. 4. Tagg. Ges. Immunologie, Bern (1972)
KERP, L.: Klinisch vergleichende Untersuchungen zur Immunogenität chromatographisch gereinigter mit nicht chromatographierten Insulinen von Rind und Schwein. 8. Kongr. Dtsch. Diabetes Ges., München, Round table (1973)
KERP, L., STEINHILBER, S., KASEMIR, H., HAHN, J., HENRICHS, H.R., GEIGER, R.: Changes in the immunospecificity of bovine insulin due to splitting off the amino acids B_1, B_2 and B_3. Diabetes **23**, 651 (1974)
KHURANA, R.C., BARNETT, D.M., BRADLEY, R.F., MARBLE, A.: Insulin resistance in children with diabetes mellitus. Diabetes **22**, Suppl. 1, 289 (1973)
KISSEL, P., DEBRY, G.: Efficacité de l'insuline de porc chez trois diabétiques traités sans succès par l'insuline de boeuf. Bull. Soc. méd. Hôp. Paris 344 (1960)
KITABCHI, A.E.: The biological and immunological properties of porc and beef insulin, proinsulin and connecting peptides. J. clin. Invest. **49**, 979 (1970)
KITAGAWA, M., OUVUE, K., KAMURA, Y., ANAI, M., YAMAMURA, Y.: Immunochemical studies of insulin. II. The specificity of insulin neutralizing antibody and experimental diabetes. J. Biochem. (Tokyo) **48**, 438 (1960)
KLEEBERG, J., DIENGOTT, D., GOTTFRIED, J.: A case of insulin resistance treated with corticotrophin. J. clin. Endocr. **16**, 680 (1956)
KLÖPPEL, G., ALTENAEHR, E., JANSEN, F.K., FREYTAG, G.: Relations between insulitis, intracutaneous skin reaction, antibody titer and decreased glucose tolerance in rabbits immunized with bovine insulin. Excerpta Medica, Int. Congr. Ser. **280**, 132 (1973)
KODEJSZKO, E.: Investigation upon insulin resistance. Excerpta Medica, Int. Congr. Ser. **74**, 73 (1964)
KODEJSZKO, E., SENIOW, S., NIEDŹWIEDZKA: Badania nadn opornosćia na insuline. XXII. Zjazd. Tow. Int. Polsk. Pol. Arch. Med. Wewnet. **33**, 1071 (1963). Cited by STARZYNSKA *et al.* (1969)
KOENIG, V.L., WEIGER, R.W., SOWINSKI, R.: Electrophoretic analysis of sera from a patient with hemochromatosis and diabetes resistant to insulin. J. Lab. clin. Med. **47**, 862 (1956)
KORP, W., LEVETT, R.E.: Erfahrungen mit Monokomponenten-Insulin. Wien. klin. Wschr. **85**, 326 (1973)

KRAHL, M.E., TIDBALL, M.E., BREGMAN, E.: Preparation and antiinsulin activity of lipoprotein from rat serum. Proc. Soc. exp. Biol. (N.Y.) **101**, 1 (1959)

KRAIL, G., BRANDENBURG, D., ZAHN, H.: (B_1-p-Jodphenylalanin)Insulin, ein einheitliches Monojodinsulin. Hoppe-Seylers Z. physiol. Chem. **352**, 1595 (1971)

KRAUTWALD, D.: Auswirkungen insulinbindender Antikörper auf das Verhalten des Blutzuckers nach iv. Insulininjektion beim Menschen. Dissertation Freiburg (1971)

KREUTZER, H.H., MOORS, J.J., VERHILLE, R.: Specificke resistentic tegen rinder-insuline. Ned. T. Geneesk. **100**, 3598 (1956)

KRIEGBAUM, D., FEDERLIN, K.: Tierexperimentelle Untersuchungen zur verzögerten Immunreaktion gegenüber Insulin, A- und B-Kette sowie Insulinbruchstücken. Diabetologia **6**, 78 (1970) (abstr.)

KÜHNAU, J., JR., VON STRITZKY, A.: Mit Schweineinsulin erfolgreich behandelte Insulinresistenz bei Diabetes mellitus. Mitteilung über 2 Fälle. Schweiz. med. Wschr. **93**, 914 (1963)

KÜHNAU, J., JR., MEYER, H.-W.: Über die Bedeutung insulinneutralisierender Antikörper für die Insulintherapie bei Diabetes mellitus. Excerpta Medica, Int. Congr. Ser. **140**, 77 (1967)

KÜHNAU, J., JR.: Die Bedeutung humoraler Insulinantikörper für die Insulinansprechbarkeit bei Diabetes mellitus und die Konsequenzen für die Therapie. Habilitationsschrift, Hamburg (1968)

KÜHNAU, J., JR.: Development and characteristics of humoral insulin antibodies in man treated with species-homogeneous insulin of cow and pig. Diabetologia **4**, 395 (1968) (abstr.)

KÜHNAU, J., JR., SAUER, H.: Effekt von 6-methyl-prednisolon (Urbason) auf die antikörperbedingte Insulinresistenz bei Diabetes mellitus. Diabetologia **6**, 78 (1970) (abstr.)

KÜHNAU, J., JR., BLÄKER, F.: Besserung der antikörperbedingten Insulinresistenz eines diabetischen Kindes unter Azathioprin-Therapie. 6. Kongr. dtsch. Diabetes Gesellschaft Düsseldorf 1971

KÜHNAU, J., JR., GRIMM, B.: Die Beziehungen zwischen Aktivitätseigenschaften neutralisierender Insulinantikörper und dem Insulinbedarf bei Diabetes mellitus. In: 2. Intern. Donausymp. Diab. mell. Budapest, Hrsg.: J. MAGYAR, A. BERNINGER, Verlag der Wiener Mediz. Akademie 1971

KUMAR, D., VON MILLER, L.: Pork insulin resistance treated with desalaninated insulin. Diabetes **19**, 392 (1970) (abstr.)

KUMAR, D., VON MILLER, L.: Proinsulin-specific antibodies in human sera. Diabetes **22**, 361 (1973a)

KUMAR, D., VON MILLER, L.: Prevalence of proinsulin-specific antibodies in diabetic patients. Horm. Metab. Res. **5**, 1 (1973b)

KUMAR, D., VON MILLER, L.: Studies on the antibodies in insulin treated diabetic patients. Excerpta Medica, Int. Congr. Ser. **280**, 133 (1973c)

LACHNIT, V., WIEDEMANN, G.: Untersuchungen bei Insulinallergie. Z. Immun.-Forsch. **122**, 216 (1961)

LACY, P.E., WRIGHT, P.H.: Allergic interstitial pancreatitis in rats injected with guinea pig anti-insulin serum. Diabetes **14**, 634 (1965)

LAMBERT, B., SUTTER, B.C.J., JAQUEMIN, C.: Effect of iodination on the biological activity of insulin. Horm. Metab. Res. **4**, 149 (1972)

LEE, J.C., GRODSKY, G.M., CAPLAN, J., GRAW, L.: Experimental immune diabetes in the rabbit. Amer. J. Path. **57**, 597 (1969)

LERMAN, J.: Insulin resistance: The role of immunity in its production. Amer. J. med. Sci. **207**, 354 (1944)

LEVETT, R.E., KORP, W.: Der Tagesinsulinbedarf des juvenilen Diabetikers. Bedeutung des gebundenen Insulins und der IgG-Insulinantikörper. 7. Kongr. dtsch. Diabetes Gesellschaft, Bad Nauheim (1972) (abstr. 26)

LEV-RAN, A., JOSHUA, H., MANNHEIMER, S.: Insulin antibodies in diabetes. Israel J. med. Sci. **7**, 1035 (1971)

LEV-RAN, A., RATT, L., LAOR, J.: Some characteristics of insulin antibodies in non resistant diabetes. Israel J. med. Sci. **8**, 905 (1972)

LEV-RAN, A., RATT, L., GERSHT, N.: Free and total insulin and insulin binding capacity in serum of insulin treated non resistant diabetics. Excerpta Medica, Int. Congr. Ser. **280**, 134 (1973)

LEWIS, J.H.: The antigenic properties of insulin. J. Amer. med. Ass. **108**, 1336 (1937)

LIEBERMAN, P., PATTERSON, R., METZ, R., LUCENA, G.: Allergic reactions to insulin. J. Amer. med. Ass. **215**, 1106 (1971)

LINDSAY, D.G., SHALL, S.: The acetylation of insulin. Biochem. J. **121**, 737 (1971)

LINDSAY, D.G., LOGE, O., LOSERT, W.: Carbamyl and methylthiocarbamyl insulins. Biochim. biophys. Acta (Amst.) **263**, 658 (1972)

LITTLE, J.A., ARNOTT, J.H.: Sulfated insulin in mild, moderate, severe and insulin-resistant diabetes mellitus. Diabetes **15**, 457 (1966)
LOCKWOOD, D.H., PROUT, T.E.: Antigenicity of heterologous and homologous insulin. Metabolism **14**, 530 (1965)
LOGOTHETOPOULOS, J.: Cytological and autoradiographic studies of the islets of mice injected with insulin antibodies. Diabetes **14**, 449 (1965)
LOGOTHETOPOULOS, J., DAVIDSON, J.K., HAIST, R.E., BEST, C.H.: Degranulation of beta cells and loss of pancreatic insulin after infusions of insulin antibody or glucose. Diabetes **14**, 493 (1965)
LOGOTHETOPOULOS, J., BELL, E.G.: Histological and autoradiographic studies of the islets of mice injected with insulin antibody. Diabetes **15**, 205 (1966)
LOHSS, F., KALLEE, E.: Immunological detection of the binding of 59-Fe ascorbinate, 131-I-thyroxine and 131-I-insulin to serum proteins. In: Protid. biol. Fluids **8**, 142 (1961)
LOVELESS, M., CANN, J.R.: Distribution of allergic and "blocking" activity in human serum proteins fractionated by electrophoresis convection. Science **117**, 105 (1953)
LOVELESS, M.H., CANN, J.R.: Distribution of "blocking" antibody in human serum protein fractioned by electrophoresis convection. J. Immunol. **74**, 329 (1955)
LOVELESS, M.: A means of estimating circulating insulin in man. Quart. Rev. Allergy **10**, 374 (1956)
LOWELL, F.C.: Evidence for the existence of two antibodies for crystalline insulin. Proc. Soc. exp. Biol. (N.Y.) **50**, 167 (1942)
LOWELL, F.C.: Immunological studies in insulin resistance. I. Report of a case exhibiting variations in resistance and allergy to insulin. J. clin. Invest. **23**, 225 (1944a)
LOWELL, F.C.: Immunological studies in insulin resistance. II. The presence of a neutralizing factor in the blood exhibiting some characteristics of an antibody. J. clin. Invest. **23**, 233 (1944b)
LYNGSØE, J.: Insulin-like activity in serum determined by the epididymal fat pad method. II. The values in undiluted and diluted serum from diabetic patients determined before and after the ingestion of glucose. Acta med. scand. **172**, 41 (1962)
MAKULU, D.R., WRIGHT, P.: Immune response to insulin in guinea pigs. Metabolism **20**, 770 (1971)
MANCINI, A.M., CONSTANZI, G., ZAMPA, G.A.: Human insulin antibodies detected by immunofluorescent technique. Lancet **1964** I, 726
MANCINI, A.M., ZAMPA, G.A., VECCHI, A., CONSTANZI, G.: Histoimmunological technics for detecting anti-insulin antibodies in human sera. Lancet **1965** I, 1189
MARSH, J.B., HAUGAARD, N.H.: The effect of serum from insulin resistant cases on the combination of insulin with the rat diaphragm. J. clin. Invest. **31**, 107 (1952)
MARTIN, P.W., MARTIN, H.E., LYSTER, R.W., STROUSE, S.: Insulin resistance. A critical survey of the literature with the report of a case. J. clin. Endocr. **1**, 387 (1941)
MARTIN, D.B., DAGENAIS, Y.M., RENOLD, A.E.: An assay for insulin-like activity using rat adipose tissue. Lancet **1958** II, 76
MARTINI, O., HAHN, J.: Messung von Insulinaktivität an isolierten Fettzellen. Hoppe-Seylers Z. physiol. Chem. **348**, 1461 (1967)
MCADAMS, G.B., KNOX, K.R., WILCOX, D.S.: The initial, rapid phase disappearance of intravenous radio-insulin in diabetes. J. nucl. Med. **8**, 173 (1967)
MEADE, R.C., KLITGAARD, H.M.: A simplified method for immunoassay of human serum insulin. J. nucl. Med. **3**, 407 (1962)
MEADE, R.C.: Placental transfer of insulin binding antibodies in the guinea pig. Amer. J. Physiol. **205**, 845 (1963)
MEEK, J.C., DOFFING, K.M., BOLINGER, R.E.: Radioimmunoassay of insulin A and B chains in normal and diabetic human plasma. Diabetes **17**, 61 (1968)
MEIER, H., YERGANIAN, D.: Spontaneous diabetes mellitus in the offspring of diabetic parents. Diabetes **10**, 12 (1961)
MELANI, F., DITSCHUNEIT, H., BARTELT, K.M., FRIEDRICH, H., PFEIFFER, E.F.: Über die radioimmunologische Bestimmung von Insulin im Blut. Klin. Wschr. **43**, 1000 (1965)
MENZEL, R., ZIEGLER, M.: Fehlende immunogene Wirkung exogenen Insulins bei Hunden nach langsamer Adaptation an Insulin. Experientia (Basel) **26**, 906 (1970a)
MENZEL, R., ZIEGLER, M.: Nachweis von zirkulierenden Insulinantikörpern beim Hund. Endokrinologie **56**, 334 (1970b)
MENZEL, R., KNOSPE, S., ZIEGLER, M., WILKE, W., MICHAEL, R.: Failure of appearance of insulin antibodies in dogs adapted to bovine-porcine insulin. Diabetologia **7**, 386 (1971)
MERCOLA, D., MORRIS, J., ARQUILLA, E.R., BROMER, W.: The ultraviolet circular dichroism of bovine insulin and desoctapeptide insulin. Biochim. biophys. Acta (Amst.) **133**, 224 (1967)
MERCOLA, D.A., MORRIS, J.W.S., ARQUILLA, E.R.: Use of resonance interaction in the study of the chain folding of insulin in solution. Biochemistry (Wash.) **11**, 3860 (1972)

MERIMEE, T.J.: Insulin resistance. Study of effect of 6-mercaptopurine. Lancet **1965 I**, 69
MEYER, H.W.: Über die Bindung von Rinder- und Schweineinsulin durch zirkulierende Antikörper im Serum von Diabetikern. Med. Welt **19**, 1758 (1968)
MEYTHALER, F., WEILER, K.: Durchbrechung der Insulinresistenz mittels Alphamethyldopa. Klin. Wschr. **42**, 590 (1964)
MEYTHALER, F., KOTLORZ, H.: Insulinresistenz. Ärztl. Forsch. **19**, 241 and 325 and 379 (1965)
MICHEL, H.: Beitrag zur Serologie der Insulin-Antikörper bei Insulin-Resistenz. In: Diabetes mellitus. III. Kongr. Int. Diabetes Fed. (1958), p. 608. Stuttgart: G. Thieme 1959
MICHEL, H.: Insulinallergie und Insulinresistenz. Internist **3**, 728 (1962)
MICHEL, H.: Behandlung des Diabetes mellitus bei Insulinresistenz und Insulinallergie. Dtsch. med. Wschr. **90**, 2211 and 2212 (1965)
MILLER, H., OWEN, G.: Immunoelectrophoresis of insulin-binding antibodies. Nature (Lond.) **188**, 70 (1960)
MITCHELL, M.L., O'ROURKE, M.E.: Differential resin binding of insulin in sera from insulin responsive and resistant diabetic subjects. 41st Meeting of the Endocrine Soc., Atlantic City, N.Y., 1959, abstr. No. 83, progr. p. 58
MITCHELL, M.L., WHITEHEAD, W.O., O'ROURKE, M.E.: Differential resin binding of insulin in serum. Endocrinology **65**, 322 (1959)
MITCHELL, M.L.: Abnormal insulin-binding fractions demonstrated by the electrophoresis on ion-exchange paper of sera from diabetic patients. J. clin. Endocr. **20**, 1319 (1960)
MITCHELL, M.L., BRADFORD, A.H.: Measurement of insulin binding by resin paper *in vitro*. Diabetes **12**, 257 (1963)
MOINAT, P.: A quantitative estimation of antibodies to exogenous insulin in diabetic subjects. Diabetes **7**, 462 (1958)
MOLONEY, P.J., COVAL, M.: Antigenicity of insulin. Diabetes induced by specific antibodies. Biochem. J. **59**, 179 (1955)
MOLONEY, P.J., APRILE, M.A.: On the antigenicity of insulin: Flocculation of insulin-antiserum. Canad. J. Biochem. **37**, 793 (1959)
MOLONEY, P.J., APRILE, M.A., WILSON, S.: Sulfated insulin for treatment of insulin-resistant diabetics. J. New Drugs **4**, 258 (1964)
MOLONEY, P.J., TIRPAK, A.E.: Immuntolerance to ox insulin induced in the adult guinea pig Canad. med. Ass. J. **100**, 573 (1969)
MOLONEY, P.J., EVANS, M.A.: Immuntolerance to insulin and Freund's adjuvant. Canad. J. Biochem. **49**, 865 (1971)
MOLONEY, P.J., JACKSON, S.G.: Specific immunosuppression of antibody response to ox insulin: Effect of adjuvant and dosage of maleyl insulin. Canad. J. Biochem. **51**, 421 (1973)
MORCOS, R.H., ABD EL NABY, S., DITSCHUNEIT, H., PFEIFFER, E.F.: Über die Ursache der Insulinresistenz bei der Insulinschocktherapie in der Psychiatrie. Med. Klin. **60**, 1073 (1965)
MORGAN, C.R., LAZAROW, A.: Immunoassay of insulin using a two-antibody system. Proc. Soc. exp. Biol. (N.Y.) **110**, 29 (1962)
MORGAN, C.R., LAZAROW, A.: Immunoassay of insulin. Two antibody system, plasma insulin levels of normal, subdiabetic and diabetic rats. Diabetes **12**, 115 (1963)
MORRIS, J.W.S., MERCOLA, D.A., MILES, P.V., ARQUILLA, E.R.: The role of Asn A–21 in the conformation of insulin. Fed. Proc. **29**, 313 (1970a)
MORRIS, J.W.S., MERCOLA, D.A., ARQUILLA, E.R.: Preparation and properties of 3-nitro-tyrosine insulins. Biochemistry (Wash.) **9**, 3930 (1970b)
MORSE, J.H. (introduced by BERSON, S.A.:) Rapid production and detection of insulin binding antibodies in rabbits and guinea pigs. Proc. Soc. exp. Biol. (N.Y.) **101**, 722 (1959)
MORSE, J.H.: Correlations of insulin requirements with the concentration of insulin binding antibody in two cases of insulin resistance. J. clin. Endocr. **21**, 533 (1961)
MORSE, J.H., HEREMANS, J.F.: Immunoelectrophoretic analysis of human insulin antibody and its papain produced fragments. J. Lab. clin. Med. **59**, 891 (1962)
MOWBRAY, R.R. DE, TURNER, J.J., GARNER, S.D., BRUCK, E., NYE, L., TRIGGS, S.: Comparative requirements of bovine and porcine insulin. Diabetologia **7**, 476 (1971) (abstr.)
MÜLLER, L.: Zur Therapie der Insulinresistenz. Med. Klin. **62**, 1916 (1967)
MURTHY, D.Y.N., GUTHRIE, R.A., WOMACK, W.N., JACKSON, R.L.: Insulin binding in children with diabetes mellitus. Pediatrics **43**, 558 (1969)
NADEL, M.B.: Reserpin in cholinergischer Behandlung und cholinergischer Insulintherapie von Diabetes mellitus. Wien. klin. Wschr. **70**, 193 (1958)
NARAHARA, H.T., WILLIAMS, R.H.: The reaction of rabbit antibeef insulin serum with heterologous and homologous insulin preparations. Diabetes **13**, 22 (1964)
NEWERLY, K., BERSON, S.A.: Lack of specificity of insulin I^{131}-binding by isolated rat diaphragm. Proc. Soc. exp. Biol. (N.Y.) **94**, 751 (1957)

NICOL, D.S.H.: The biological activity of pure peptides obtained by enzymatic hydrolysis of insulin. Biochem. J. **75**, 395 (1960)
NICOL, D.S.H.W., SMITH, L.F.: Amino-acid sequence of human insulin. Nature (Lond.) **187**, 483 (1960)
OAKLEY, W., FIELD, J.B., SOWTON, G., RIGBY, B., CUNLIFFE, A.C.: Action of prednisone in insulin resistant diabetes. Brit. med. J. **1959** II, 1601
OAKLEY, W.G., JONES, V.E., CUNLIFFE, A.C.: Insulin resistance. Brit. med. J. **1967 II**, 134
OAKLEY, W.G., CUNLIFFE, A.C.: Insulin resistance. In: Clin. Diabetes and its Biochemical Basis. Eds.: W.G. OAKLEY, D.A. PYKE, K.W. TAYLOR, p. 722. Oxford: Blackwell Scientific Publ. 1968
OHNEDA, A., MATSUDA, K., ISHII, S., CHIBA, M., YAMAGATA, S.: Hypoglycemia and production of antibodies to insulin without previous treatment of insulin. Excerpta Medica, Int. Congr. Ser. **280**, 135 (1973)
ORSETTI, A., BALI, J.P., SERRE, A., MIROUZE, J.: Insulin immunology and synthesis. Diabetologia **8**, 62 (1972) (abstr.)
ORSKOV, H., CHRISTENSEN, N.J.: Plasma disappearance rate of injected human insulin in juvenile diabetic, maturity onset diabetic and nondiabetic subjects. Diabetes **18**, 653 (1969)
OVARY, Z.: Immediate reactions in the skin of experimental animals provoked by antibody-antigen interaction. Progr. Allergy **5**, 459 (1958)
OVARY, Z.: Passive cutaneous anaphylaxis in the guinea pig: Degree of reaction as a function of the quantity of antigen and antibody. Int. Arch. Allergy **14**, 18 (1959)
OVARY, Z., BENACERRAF, B., BLOCH, K.: Identification of antibodies involved in passive cutaneous and systematic anaphylaxis. J. exp. Med. **117**, 951 (1963)
OUCHTERLONY, O.: Diffusion in gel methods for immunological analysis. I. Progr. Allergy **5**, 1 (1958)
OUCHTERLONY, O.: Diffusion in gel methods for immunological analysis. II. Progr. Allergy **6**, 30 (1962)
PAL, S., CHATURVEDY, V.C., MEHROTA, R.M.L., GUPTA, N.N., SIRCAR, A.R.: Insulin "auto-antibodies" in diabetes mellitus. Indian J. med. Sci. **23**, 598 (1969a)
PAL, S., GUPTA, N.N., MEHROTA, R.M.L., SIRCAR, A.R., CHATURVEDI, V.C.: Insulin antibodies in diabetes mellitus. Indian J. med. Res. **57**, 573 (1969b)
PALUMBO, P.J., MOLNAR, G.D., TAUXE, W.N.: Serum protein binding of exogenous insulin in menstruating and pregnant diabetic patients. Diabetes **13**, 634 (1964)
PALUMBO, P.J., TAUXE, W.N., GREENBERG, B., GOETZ, F.C., MOLNAR, G.D.: Serum protein binding of insulin by chromatoelectrophoresis and immunoprecipitation technics. Amer. J. clin. Path. **43**, 532 (1965)
PALUMBO, P.J., TAYLOR, W.F., MOLNAR, G.D., TAUXE, W.N.: Disappearance of bovine insulin from plasma in diabetic and normal subjects. Metabolism **21**, 787 (1972)
PATTERSON, R., COLWELL, J.A., GREGOR, W.H., CARY, E.: Avian anti-insulin serum: A comparison of its immunologic and biologic activity with that of guinea pig and rabbit antisera. J. Lab. clin. Med. **64**, 399 (1964)
PATTERSON, G.R., LUCENA, G., METZ, R., ROBERTS, M.: Reaginic antibody against insulin. Demonstration of antigenic distinction between native and extracted insulin. J. Immunol. **103**, 1061 (1969)
PATTERSON, R., O'ROURKE, J., ROBERTS, M., SUSZKO, J.: Immunologic reactions against insulin. I. IgG antiinsulin and insulin resistance. J. Immunol. **110**, 1126 (1973a)
PATTERSON, R., MELLIES, C.J., ROBERTS, M.: Immunologic reactions against insulin. II. IgE antiinsulin, insulin allergy and combined IgE and IgG immunologic insulin resistance. J. Immunol. **110**, 1135 (1973b)
PAV, J., JEŹKOVÁ, Z., SKRHA, F.: Insulin antibodies. Lancet **1963 II**, 221
PECK, W.A.: Regulation of pyrimidine ribonucleoside incorporation in isolated bone cells. Stimulation by insulin and by 2,3-dihydroxy-1,4-dithiobutane (dithiotreitol). J. biol. Chem. **246**, 4439 (1971)
PENCHEV, J., ANDREEV, D., DITZOV, S.: Insulin-precipitierende Antikörper bei insulinbehandelten und unbehandelten Diabetikern und mit Insulin immunisierten Meerschweinchen. Acta diabet. Lat. **2**, 454 (1965)
PENCHEV, J., ANDREEV, D., DITZOV, S.: Insulin-precipitating antibodies in insulin treated and untreated diabetic patients. Diabetologia **4**, 164 (1968)
PERLMUTTER, M., GREEP, R.O.: The uptake of glucose and the synthesis of glycogen by the isolated diaphragm of normal and pituitectomized rats. J. biol. Chem. **174**, 915 (1948)
PFEIFFER, E.F., DITSCHUNEIT, H.: Aktuelle Probleme der Diabetestherapie. Dtsch. med. Wschr. **87**, 2290 (1962)
PFEIFFER, E.F., MELANI, F., DITSCHUNEIT, H.: Radioimmunologische Bestimmung des Insulins. Bull. schweiz. Akad. med. Wiss. **21**, 276 (1965)

PFEIFFER, E.F.: Die Insulinresistenz. Dtsch. med. Wschr. **91**, 314 (1966)
PFEIFFER, E.F., DITSCHUNEIT, H., FEDERLIN, K.: Die Inselzellhormone: Die Immunologie des Insulins. In: Handbuch des Diabetes mellitus, Band 1, S. 155. Hrsg.: E.F. PFEIFFER u. Mitarb. München: J.F. Lehmanns Verlag 1969
PFEIFFER, E.F.: contribution during discussion. Diabetes **21**, Suppl. 2, 660 (1971)
PLAUTZ, M., LITTLE, J.A.: An immunoassay for insulin antibodies in humans: Their development in diabetics treated with sulfated or Lente insulin. Diabetes **19**, Suppl. 1, 371 (1970) (abstr.)
POTTER, D.E., MORATINOS, J., ELLIS, S.: Rabbit and human insulins: Similar cross-reactivities with antibodies to porcine insulin. Experientia (Basel) **29**, 1144 (1973)
PRESSMAN, D., YAGI, Y., MAIER, P.: Antibodies against the component polypeptide chains of bovine Insulin. Science **147**, 617 (1965)
PROUT, T.E., KATIMS, R.B.: The effect of insulin-binding serum globulin on insulin requirement. Diabetes **8**, 425 (1959)
PROUT, T.E., KATIMS, R.B.: Relationship between serum binding globulin and insulin requirement. Bull. Johns Hopk. Hosp. **106**, 119 (1960)
PROUT, T.E., ODAK, V.V., DENDRINOS, G.J., LOCKWOOD, D.H.: The insulin carrying protein of normal human serum. Diabetes **12**, 144 (1963)
RAMACHANDRAN, S., RITCHIE, D., WAGLE, S.R.: Studies on the measurement of insulin antibodies in controlled and resistant human diabetic patients by polyacrylamid gel electrophoresis. Proc. Soc. exp. Biol. (N.Y.) **131**, 796 (1969)
RAMSEIER, E.B., FROESCH, E.R., BALLY, P., LABHART, A.: Seruminsulinbestimmung am Fettgewebe *in vitro*: Beeinflussung durch andere Hormone. "Freie" und "gebundene" Insulinaktivität. 4. Kongr. Intern. Diab. Fed., Genf (1961). Ed. Méd. Hyg., Vol. I, p. 64 J
RANDLE, P.J.: Assay of plasma insulin activity by the rat-diaphragm method. Brit. med. J. **1954 I**, 1237
RANDLE, P.J.: The assay of insulin *in vitro* by means of the glucose uptake of the isolated diaphragm. J. Endocr. **14**, 82 (1956)
RANDLE, P.J.: Insulin in blood. Ciba Found. Coll. Endocrin. **11**, 115 (1957)
RANDLE, P.J., TAYLOR, K.W.: Insulin in protein fractions of serum from healthy people and from insulin treated diabetics. Lancet **1958 II**, 996
RANDLE, P.J.: Insulin antagonism in plasma. In: Diabetes, ed. R.H. WILLIAMS, p. 257. New York: Hoeber 1960
RAUSCH-STROOMANN, J.G., SAUER, H.: Zur Frage der Insulinresistenz durch Antikörperbildung. Klin. Wschr. **31**, 551 (1953)
RENOLD, A.E., WINEGRAD, A.J., MARTIN, D.B.: Diabète sucré et tissue adipeux. Helv. med. Acta **24**, 322 (1957)
RENOLD, A.E., BEIGELMAN, P.M., WILLEBRANDS, A.F., GROEN, J., MARTIN, D.B., DAGENAIS, Y.M., BERSON, S.A., YALOW, R.S., KRAHL, M.E., ANTONIADES, H.N.: Insulin like activity and antiinsulin factors in human plasma. In: Hormones in Human Plasma, ed. H.N. ANTONIADES. Boston, Mass.: Little, Brown & Company 1960
RENOLD, A.E., STEINKE, J., SOELDNER, J.S., ANTONIADES, H.N., SMITH, R.E.: Immunological response to the prolonged administration of heterologous and homologous insulin in cattle. J. clin. Invest. **45**, 702 (1966)
ROBINSON, B.H.B., WRIGHT, P.H.: Guinea pig antiinsulin serum. J. clin. Physiol. **155**, 302 (1961)
ROOT, H.F.: Insulin resistance and bronze diabetes. New Engl. J. Med. **201**, 201 (1929)
ROOT, M.A., CHANCE, R.E., GALLOWAY, J.A.: Immunogenicity of insulin. Diabetes **21**, 657 (1972)
ROSSELIN, G., TCHOBROUTSKY, G., ASSAN, R., LELLOUCH, L., DOLAIS, J., DÈROT, M.: Etude quantitative d'anticorps humains anti-insulines animales par la méthode radio-immunologique de BERSON et YALOW. Diabetologia **1**, 33 (1965)
ROTH, J.: Peptide hormone-binding to receptors: A review of direct studies *in vitro*. Metabolism **22**, 1059 (1973)
SAMAAN, N. FRAZER, R.: Effect of circulating antibody to insulin on serum levels of insulin-like activity in rats, guinea pigs and a diabetic patient. Brit. med. J. **1964 II**, 482
SAMOLS, E., JONES, V.: Insulin resistance and the relationship of human antibodies to insulin when measured by three different methods. Diabetologia **1**, 75 (1965) (abstr.)
SANGER, F., THOMPSON, E.O.P., KITAI, R.: The amide groups of insulin. Biochem. J. **59**, 509 (1955)
SANGER, F.: Chemistry of insulin. Science **129**, 1340 (1959)
SANGER, F.: Structure of insulin. In: Les Prix Nobel en 1958, p. 134. Stockholm 1959
SCATCHARD, G., COLEMAN, J.S., SHEN, A.L.: Physical chemistry of protein solutions. VII. The binding of some small anions to serum albumin. J. Amer. chem. Soc. **79**, 12 (1957)

SCÈCSEY, G., BRETAN, M., BIKICH, G., KAMMERER, L.: Der Nachweis von Insulin-Antikörpern bei Zuckerkranken durch passives Hämagglutinationsverfahren. Z. Immun.-Forsch. **125**, 253 (1963)

SCHADE, U., WEHNER, H.: Der Einfluß von Insulin auf die Insulinbindungskapazität des Serums insulinsensibilisierter Kaninchen. Klin. Wschr. **47**, 438 (1969)

SCHEIFFARTH, F., FRENGER, W.: Die Verwendbarkeit der passiven oder indirekten Haemagglutinationsreaktion nach BOYDEN beim Nachweis von Antikörpern. Blut **2**, 102 (1956)

SCHEIFFARTH, F., FRENGER, W., MÖCKEL, G.: Serologische Studien über das Wesen der Insulin-Antikörper. Dtsch. med. Wschr. **84**, 177 (1959)

SCHEIFFARTH, F., WEIST, F., WARNATZ, H., SCHNELL, K.: Das Vorkommen von Insulinantikörpern und die Beeinflussung dieser Insulineiweißbindung durch Sulfonylharnstoff und Glycodiazin. Med. Pharmacol. Exp. (Basel) **17**, 17 (1967)

SCHLICHTKRULL, J., BRANGE, J., EGE, H., HALLUND, O., HEDING, L.G., JØRGENSEN, K., MARKUSSEN, J., STAHNKE, P., SUNDBY, F., VØLUND, A.: Proinsulin und verwandte Proteine. 4. Kongr. dtsch. Diabetes Gesellschaft, Ulm (1969a). Diabetologia **6**, 80 (1970) (abstr.)

SCHLICHTKRULL, J., BRANGE, J., EGE, H., HALLUND, O., HEDING, L.G., JØRGENSEN, K.H., MARKUSSEN, J., STAHNKE, P., SUNDBY, F., VØLUND, A.: Proinsulin and related proteins. 5th Ann. Meeting Europ. Ass. Study of Diabetes, Montpellier (1969b). Diabetologia **6**, 63 (1970) (abstr.)

SCHLICHTKRULL, J., BRANGE, J., HALLUND, O., CHRISTIANSEN, Aa.H., HEDING, L.G., JØRGENSEN, K.H.: Hochgereinigtes Insulin zu therapeutischen Zwecken. 8. Jahresversammlung Schweiz. Diab. Ges., Lausanne (1972a). Sonderdruck abstracta diabetologica

SCHLICHTKRULL, J., BRANGE, J., CHRISTIANSEN, Aa.H., HALLUND, O., HEDING, L.G., JØRGENSEN, K.H.: Clinical aspects of insulin-antigenicity. Diabetes **21**, Suppl. 649 (1972b)

SCHÖFFLING, K.: Insulinstoffwechsel des pankreaslosen Hundes. 12. Symp. dtsch. Ges. Endokr., Wiesbaden (1966), p. 200. Berlin-Heidelberg-New York: Springer 1967

SCHREIBER, F., ROTTENHÖFER, H.: Insulinresistenz und Granulosazelltumor. Verlaufsbeobachtung bei einer 63jährigen Frau. Verh. dtsch. Ges. inn. Med. **74**, 1225 (1968)

SCHWARZ, E., KOLLER, F.: Verwendung von gereinigten (umkristallisierten) Insulinpräparaten bei Zuständen von Insulinallergie. Schweiz. med. Wschr. **79**, 936 (1949)

SCHWEIZER, R.: Insulinbehandlung und Insulinantikörper. Dissertation Freiburg (1970)

SCOTT, G.W., PROUT, T.E., WEAVER, J.A., ASPER, S.P.: A comparison of the behavior of insulin and insulin labeled with I-131 in serum. Diabetes **7**, 38 (1958)

SEBRIAKOVA, M., LITTLE, J.A.: A method for the determination of plasma insulin antibodies and its application in normal and diabetic subjects. Diabetes **22**, 30 (1973)

SEGRE, E.J.: Diabetes mellitus with insulin resistance: report of a case successfully treated with tolbutamid. Metabolism **11**, 562 (1962)

SEHON, A.H., KAYE, M., MCGARRY, E., ROSE, B.: Localization of an insulin-neutralizing factor by zone electrophoresis in a serum of an insulin-resistant patient. J. Lab. clin. Med. **45**, 765 (1955)

SELA, M., HAUROWITZ, F.: Serological properties of poly-L-tyrosine derivatives. Experientia (Basel) **14**, 91 (1958)

SELA, M., ARNON, R.: Studies on the chemical basis of the antigenicity of proteins. 1. Antigenicity of polypeptidyl gelatins. Biochem. J. **75**, 91 (1960a)

SELA, M., ARNON, R.: Studies on the chemical basis of the antigenicity of proteins. 3. The role of rigidity in the antigenicity of polypeptidyl gelatins. Biochem. J. **77**, 394 (1960b)

SERRANO-RÍOS, M., MALO, J., OYA, M., LARRODERA, L., HAWKINS, F., ESCOBAR, F.: Failure to find Ig-G-insulin antibodies in Down's syndrome. Horm. Metab. Res. **5**, 57 (1973a)

SERRANO-RÍOS, M., SANROMAN COS GAYON, C., SORDO, M.T., RODRIGUEZ-MINÓN, J.L.: Insulin secretion in Down's syndrome. Diabetologia **9**, 50 (1973b)

SHERMAN, W.B.: A case of coexisting insulin allergy and insulin resistance. J. Allergy **21**, 49 (1950)

SHERRILL, J.W., LAWRENCE, R., JR.: Insulin resistance: mechanisms involved and influence of infection and refrigeration. U.S. Armed Forces med. J. **1**, 1399 (1950)

SHIPP, J.C., RUSSELL, R.O., STEINKE, J., MITCHELL, M.L., HADLEY, W.B.: Insulin resistance with high levels of circulating insulin-like activity demonstrable *in vitro* and *in vivo*. Diabetes **10**, 1 (1961)

SHIPP, J.C., CUNNINGHAM, R.W., RUSSELL, R.O., MARBLE, A.: Insulin resistance: clinical features, natural course and effect of adrenal steroid treatment. Medicine **44**, 165 (1965)

SIRAKOV, L.M., DITZOV, S.P.: Quantitative determination of insulin-binding antibodies in human serum Clin. chim. Acta **45**, 145 (1973)

SKOM, J.H., TALMAGE, D.W.: In: Proc. centr. Soc. clin. Res. **29**, 80 (1956a). Cited by STAVITSKY and ARQUILLA (1958)

SKOM, J.H., TALMAGE, D.W.: Nonprecipitating insulin-binding antibodies. J. Lab. clin. Med. **48**, 943 (1956b)

SKOM, J.H., TALMAGE, D.W.: Nonprecipitating insulin antibodies. J. clin. Invest. **37**, 783 (1958a)

SKOM, J.H., TALMAGE, D.W.: The role of nonprecipitating antibodies in diabetes. J. clin. Invest. **37**, 787 (1958b)

SLATER, J.D.H., SAMAAN, N.A., FRASER, R., STILLMAN, D.: Immunologic studies with circulating insulin. Brit. med. J. **1961 I**, 1712

SLOBIN, L.J., CARPENTER, F.H.: Action of carboxypeptidase-A on bovine insulin: Preparation of desalanine-desasparagine-insulin. Biochemistry (Wash.) **2**, 16 (1963a)

SLOBIN, L.J., CARPENTER, F.H.: The labile amide in insulin: Preparation of desalanine-desamido-insulin. Biochemistry (Wash.) **2**, 22 (1963b)

SLOBIN, L.J., CARPENTER, F.H.: Kinetic studies on the reaction of carboxypeptidase-A on bovine insulin and related model peptides. Biochemistry (Wash.) **5**, 499 (1966)

SMELO, L.S.: Lack of response to insulin. Report of a patient treated with five thousand units per twenty-four hours. Sth. med. J. (Bgham, Ala.) **40**, 333 (1947)

SMELO, L.S.: Insulin resistance. Proc. Amer. Diab. Ass. **8**, 75 (1948)

SMITH, L.F.: Amino acid sequences of insulin. Diabetes **21**, Suppl. 2, 457 (1972)

SOELDNER, J.S., STEINKE, J.: Insulin resistance. Med. Clin. N. Amer. **49**, 939 (1965)

SPELLACY, W.N., GOETZ, F.C.: Insulin antibodies in pregnancy. Lancet **1963 I**, 222

SRIVASTAVA, M.C., SONKSEN, P.H., TOMKINS, C.V., NABARRO, J.D.N.: Studies on the metabolism of monocomponent-human insulin in man. 7th Ann. Meeting Europ. Ass. Study of Diabetes, Southampton (1971). Diabetologia **8**, 68 (1972) (abstr.)

STADIE, W.C., HAUGAARD, N., HILLS, A.G., MARSH, J.B.: Hormonal influence on the chemical combination of insulin with rat muscle (diaphragm). Amer. J. med. Sci. **218**, 275 (1949)

STARZYNSKA, R., DEPOWSKA, B.: The immunological consequences of insulin therapy. Acta diabet. lat. **4**, 550 (1967)

STARZYNSKA, R., SENIOW, S., KODEJSZKO, E., KOWALSKI, H., STARZYNSKI, S., DEPOWSKA, B.: Studies on the transport of insulin antibodies across the placenta to the fetus and their effects on the fetal pancreatic islet system. Acta diabet. lat. **6**, 573 (1969)

STARZYNSKA, R.: Insulin allergy. Clinical and immunological effects of specific desensitization. Acta diabet. lat. **6**, 796 (1969)

STAVITSKY, A.B., ARQUILLA, E.R.: Estimation of insulin and antibodies to insulin *in vitro* by hemagglutination and hemolysis of insulin-treated red cells and inhibition of these reactions. Fed. Proc. **12**, 461 (1953)

STAVITSKY, A.B.: Micromethods for the study of proteins and antibodies. I. Procedure and general applications of hemagglutination and hemagglutination-inhibition reactions with tannic acid and protein treated red blood cells. J. Immunol. **72**, 360 (1954)

STEIGERWALD, D., SPIELMANN, W.: Nachweis von Insulinantikörpern bei Diabetikern mit Insulinresistenz im Haemagglutinationstest und Coombstest. Klin. Wschr. **34**, 80 (1956)

STEIGERWALD, H., SPIELMANN, W., FRIES, H., GREBE, S.T.: Neuere Untersuchungen über die Antigenwirkung des Insulins. Klin. Wschr. **38**, 973 (1960)

STEINKE, J.: A new screening test of circulating antibodies to insulin using polyethylene glycol. Diabetes **21**, Suppl. 1, 379 (1972)

STIMMLER, L.: Disappearance of immunoreactive insulin in normal and adult-onset diabetic subjects. Diabetes **16**, 652 (1967)

STRUWE, F.E., STEINHILBER, S., TEUSCHER, V., KERP, L.: Diabetesverlauf, Insulinbedarf und insulinbindende Antikörper bei Kindern. 5. Kongr. dtsch. Diabetes-Gesellschaft, Bad Godesberg, 1970, Nr. 46

SURMACZYNSKA, B., METZ, R.: Hormonal and immunological properties of insulin fragments. 1. The individual peptide chains. Endocrinology **85**, 368 (1969)

SURMACZYNSKA, B., METZ, R., BARRETT, R., LUCENA, G.: Hormonal and immunological properties of insulin fragments. 2. Products obtained by enzymatic hydrolysis. Endocrinology **85**, 577 (1969)

TANTILLO, J.J., KARAM, J.H., BURRILL, K.C., JONES, M.A., GRODSKY, G.M., FORSHAM, P.H.: Antigenicity of "single peak" insulin preparations in diabetics. Diabetes **22**, Suppl. 1, 293 (1973)

THOMAS, J.H.: Electrophoresis of (^{35}S)-sulfated insulin. Horm. Metab. Res. **3**, 207 (1971)

THORELL, J.I.: Placental transfer of insulin 131-I in guinea pigs immunized against insulin. Acta endocr. (Kbh.) **52**, 276 (1966b)

THORELL, J.I.: Insulin antibodies in pregnant guinea pigs and their offspring. Acta endocr. (Kbh.) **52**, 255 (1966a)

TOMASI, T., SLEDZ, D., WALES, J.K., RECANT, L.: Insulin half-life in normal and diabetic subjects. Proc. Soc. exp. Biol. (N.Y.) **126**, 315 (1967)

TOUBER, J.L., STOLL, R.W., ENSINCK, J.W., WILLIAMS, R.H.: Immunological studies of the A and B chains of insulin. Diabetes **19**, 409 (1970)

Tucker, W.R., Klink, D., Goetz, F., Zalme, E., Knowles, H.C., Jr.: Insulin resistance and acanthosis nigricans. Diabetes **13**, 395 (1964)

Tuft, L.: Insulin hypersensitiviness; immunologic consideration and case reports. Amer. J. med. Sci. **176**, 707 (1928)

Vallance-Owen, J., Hurlock, B., Please, N.W.: Plasma insulin activity in diabetes mellitus measured by the rat diaphragm technique. Lancet **1955 II**, 583

Vallance-Owen, J., Dennes, E., Campbell, P.H.: Insulin antagonism in plasma of diabetic patients and normal subjects. Lancet **1958 II**, 336 (a)

Vallance-Owen, J., Dennes, E., Campbell, P.H.: The nature of insulin-antagonist associated with plasma albumin. Lancet **1958 II**, 696 (b)

Vallance-Owen, J., Hurlock, B.: Estimation of plasma insulin activity by the rat diaphragm method. Lancet **1954 I**, 68 u. 983

Vallance-Owen, J., Lilley, M.D.: Further studies on insulin antagonism associated with plasma albumin. IVe Congr. Fed. int. du Diabète, Genève (1961), abstr. No. 179

Vallance-Owen, J., Lukens, F.D.W.: Studies on insulin antagonism in plasma. Endocrinology **60**, 625 (1957)

Van de Wiel, Th.W.M., Van de Wiel-Dorfmeyer, H.: Insulin antibodies. Lancet **1964 I**, 561

Varandani, P.T., Tomizawa, H.H.: Studies on action of glutathion-insulin transhydrogenase on antibody bound insulin. Biochim. biophys. Acta (Amst.) **97**, 498 (1965)

Varandani, P.T.: Studies on the nature of antigenicity of A and B chains of bovine insulin. Biochemistry (Wash.) **6**, 100 (1967)

Waldhäusl, W.K., Frisch, H., Haydl, H.: Vorkommen und Bedeutung von Insulinantikörpern bei Diabetikern und ihre Beeinflussung durch Monocomponenteninsulin. 7th Ann. Meeting Europ. Ass. Study of Diabetes, Madrid (1972)

Wasserman, P., Broh-Kahn, R.H., Mirsky, I.A.: The antigenic properties of insulin. J. Immunol. **38**, 213 (1940)

Wasserman, P., Mirsky, J.A.: Immunological identity of insulin from various species. Endocrinology **31**, 115 (1942)

Weber, V., Weitzel, G.: Struktur und Wirkung von Insulin. V. Synthetische B-Ketten mit variierter Sequenz. Hoppe-Seylers Z. physiol. Chem. **349**, 1431 (1968)

Weiger, R.W., Colwell, A.R.: The inhibition of insulin action by serum gamma globulin. Clin. Res. Proc. **4**, 123 (1956)

Weinert, M., Brandenburg, D., Zahn, H.: Peptidsynthesen mit der Insulin A-Kette. Hoppe-Seylers Z. physiol. Chem. **350**, 1556 (1969)

Weinert, M., Kircher, K., Brandenburg, D., Zahn, H.: Kristallisiertes Arginyl ^{A1}-insulin. Hoppe-Seylers Z. physiol. Chem. **352**, 719 (1971)

Weise, H., Rolle, J.: Zur Therapie des Diabetes mellitus mit herabgesetzter Insulinempfindlichkeit. Arzneimittel-Forsch. **14**, 1266 (1964)

Welborn, T.A., Richards, R., Fraser, T.R.: Simple test for insulin antibodies in sera using I-131-insulin and ethanol precipitation. Brit. med. J. **1967 I**, 719

Welsh, G.W., Henley, E.D., Williams, R.H., Cox, R.S.: I^{131}-Insulin metabolism in man. Plasmabinding distribution and degradation. Amer. J. Med. **21**, 324 (1956)

Willebrands, A.F., v. d. Geld, H., Groen, J.: Determination of serum insulin using the isolated rat diaphragm. The effect of serum dilutions. Diabetes **7**, 113 (1958)

Williams, J.R.: A second case of gastro-intestinal allergy due to insulin. J. Amer. med. Ass. **100**, 658 (1933)

Williams, R.H., Elgee, N.J., Lee, N.D., Hobness, J.R., Wong, T.: Insulin metabolism Trans. Ass. Amer. Physiol. **66**, 137 (1953)

Williams, R.F., Gleason, R.E., Soeldner, J.S.: The half-life of endogeneous serum immunoreactive insulin in man. Metabolism **17**, 1025 (1968)

Wilson, S., Dixon, G.H.: A comparison of cod and bovine insulin. Nature (Lond.) **191**, 876 (1961)

Wilson, S., Dixon, G.H., Wardlow, A.C.: Resynthesis of cod insulin from its polypeptide chains and the preparation of cod-ox hybrid insulins. Biochim. biophys. Acta (Amst.) **62**, 483 (1962)

Wilson, S., Falkmer, S.: Comparative immunology of insulin. Excerpta Medica, Int. Congr. Ser. **74**, 174 (1964)

Wilson, S., Aprile, M.A., Sasaki, L.: Passive cutaneous anaphylaxis induced in guinea pigs by insulins and their component chains. Canad. J. Biochem. **44**, 989 (1966)

Wilson, S., Aprile, M.A., Sasaki, L.: The antigenic loci of insulin. Canad. J. Biochem. **45**, 1135 (1967)

Wilson, S.: The antigenic loci in insulin. 6th Congr. Int. Diab. Fed., Stockholm (1967). In: J. Östman, ed., Excerpta Medica Foundation Amsterdam (1969), p. 403

WILSON, S.: Insulin und modifizierte Insuline. Arbeitstagung 11.—13. 5. 1971, Düsseldorf (1971)
WILSON, S.: The immune response to insulin at the submolecular level. Symp.: Chemie des Insulins und Proinsulins, Aachen (1973)
WILSON, S., JAKUS, C.M., LOGAN, L.: Induction of tolerance to insulin at the molecular and submolecular levels. Excerpta Medica, Int. Congr. Ser., No. **280**, 136 (1973) (abstr.)
WINEGARD, A.J., RENOLD, A.E.: Studies on rat adipose tissue *in vitro*. I. Effects of insulin on the metabolism of glucose, pyruvate and acetate. J. biol. Chem. **233**, 267 (1958a)
WINEGARD, A.J., RENOLD, A.E.: Studies on rat adipose tissue *in vitro*. II. Effects of insulin on the metabolism of specifically labeled glucose. J. biol. Chem. **233**, 273 (1958b)
WOLFF, G.: Insulinresistenz. Med. Welt 1139 (1968)
WRIGHT, P.H.: Production of acute insulin deficiency by administration of insulin antiserum. Nature (Lond.) **183**, 829 (1959a)
WRIGHT, P.H.: The effect of insulin antibodies on glucose uptake by the isolated rat diaphragm. Biochem. J. **71**, 633 (1959b)
WRIGHT, P.H.: The production of experimental diabetes by means of insulin antibodies. Amer. J. Med. **31**, 892 (1961)
WRIGHT, P.H.: Guinea pig anti-insulin serum (GPAIS). Diabetes **14**, 449 (1965)
WRIGHT, P.H., MALAISSE W.J.: A simple method for the assay of guinea pig anti-insulin serum. Diabetologia **2**, 178 (1966)
WRIGHT, P.H., MALAISSE, W.J., RENOLDS, J.J.: Assay of partially neutralized guinea pig anti-insulin serum. Endocrinology **81**, 226 (1967)
YAGI, J., MAIER, P., PRESSMAN, D.: Two different anti-insulin antibodies in guinea pig antisera. J. Immunol. **89**, 442 (1962a)
YAGI, Y., MAIER, P., PRESSMAN, D.: Immunoelectrophoretic identification of guinea pig anti-insulin antibodies. J. Immunol. **89**, 736 (1962b)
YAGI, Y., MAIER, P., PRESSMAN, D., ARBESMAN, C.E., REISMAN, R.E., LENZNER, R.A.: Multiplicity of insulin-binding antibodies in human serum. Presence of antibody in gamma-1-, beta-$_{2A}$-, and beta$_{2M}$-globulins. I. Immunol. **90**, 760 (1963)
YAGI, Y., MAIER, P., PRESSMAN, D.: Antibodies against the component polypeptide chains of bovine insulin. Science **147**, 617 (1965)
YALOW, R.S., BERSON, S.A.: Apparent inhibition of liver insulinase activity by serum and serum fractions containing insulin binding antibodies. J. clin. Invest. **36**, 648 (1957)
YALOW, R.S., BERSON, S.A.: Plasma insulin concentration in non-diabetic and early diabetic subjects. Determination by a new sensitive immunoassay technic. Diabetes **9**, 254 (1960)
YALOW, R.S., BERSON, S.A.: Immunological specificity of human insulin: application to immunoassay of insulin. J. clin. Invest. **40**, 2190 (1961a)
YALOW, R.S., BERSON, S.A.: Immunologic aspects of insulin. Amer. J. Med. **31**, 882 (1961b)
YALOW, R.S., BERSON, S.A.: Reaction of fish insulin with human insulin antiserum. Potential value in the treatment of insulin resistance. New Engl. J. Med. **270**, 1171 (1964)
YAMAMOTO, M., KOTAKI, A., OKUYAMA, T., SATAKE, K.: Studies on insulin. I. Two different insulins from Langerhans islets of Bonitofish. J. Biochem. **48**, 84 (1960)
YOUNG, J.D., CARPENTER, F.H.: Isolation and characterization of products formed by the action of trypsin on insulin. J. biol. Chem. **236**, 743 (1961)
ZAHN, H., KLOSTERMEYER, H.: Die Inselzellhormone: Chemie, Struktur und Synthese von Insulin. In: Handbuch des Diabetes mellitus, Band I, Ed.: E.F. PFEIFFER. München: J.F. Lehmanns Verlag 1969
ZAHN, H., SCHMIDT, G.: Synthese der Insulinsequenz $(B17—30)_2$ als symmetrisches Disulfid und der Insulin-B-Kette als polymeres Disulfid. Liebigs Ann. Chem. **731**, 101 (1970)
ZAHN, H., BRANDENBURG, D., GATTNER, H.-G.: Molecular basis of insulin action. Contributions of chemical modifications and synthetic approaches. Diabetes **21**, Suppl. 2, 468 (1972)
ZAROWITZ, H.: Postpancreatectomy insulin-resistant diabetes mellitus. N. Y. St. J. Med. **72**, 3005 (1972)
ZIEGLER, M., HAHN, H.J., KLATT, D.: Influence of isolated insulin antibodies on the insulin secretion of the islets of Langerhans *in vitro*. Diabetologia **8**, 148 (1972)
ZINDER, J.I., BERGER, S., GOLDSTEIN, M.S.: *In vitro* red blood cell uptake of radio-insulin. Simple method for detecting insulin antibodies. Proc. Soc. exp. Biol. (N.Y.) **107**, 345 (1961)

Determination and Preparations of Insulin

A. Radioimmunoassay of Insulin

HANS DITSCHUNEIT and JENS-DIETER FAULHABER

With 6 Figures

I. Introduction

Biological methods of determining insulin are relatively tedious, liable to disruption, and subject to a high degree of error. They are therefore unsuitable for the routine determination of insulin in blood and other body fluids. The search for more accurate and simpler methods of measuring insulin also took into consideration the immunogenic and antigenic properties of the insulin molecule. ARQUILLA and STAVITSKY (1956) were the first to attempt to measure the insulin in the blood quantitively with the aid of the antibodies induced by the immunogenic properties of insulin. In this method the parameter used for unknown quantities of insulin is inhibition of the agglutination of erythrocytes loaded with insulin and pretreated with bidiazobenzidine by means of insulin antibodies. This process, however, is neither very sensitive nor accurate, the minimum insulin concentration measurable being about 25 mU/ml.

The method of radioimmunoassay described by YALOW and BERSON (1959, 1960) has been adopted for experimental research and in hospitals over the last few years. The principle of this method is also used to determine many other polypeptide hormones. It is called "radioimmunoassay" because radioactively labeled insulin and other hormones are used.

The specificity of the radioimmunoassay of insulin is very high as the following observations show:

i) After pancreatectomy, the insulin in the blood of animals and humans falls to an undeterminable level (GOLDBERG and EGDAHL, 1961; SCHÖFFLING, 1966).

ii) Recovery of serum insulin is complete.

iii) Dilution of the serum produces a proportional fall in determinable insulin content.

iv) Cysteine destroys both determinable blood insulin and crystalline insulin.

v) Crystalline insulin precipitates in the ultracentrifuge in the same way as immunologically measurable serum insulin.

vi) Both serum and crystalline insulin bind to cellulose and Amberlite.

vii) Both serum and crystalline insulin react with insulin antibodies.

In addition to its greater sensitivity and accuracy, radioimmunoassay is distinguished by simplicity. One assistant can carry out several hundred measurements daily, which is one of the reasons why it is widely used in hospitals. The original procedure as described by YALOW and BERSON involved some technical difficulties, but these were eliminated by various modifications, and now-a-days simple ready-to-use test packs are on the market. These modifications are based mainly on various separation techniques for free and antibody-bound insulin (MORGAN and LAZAROV, 1962, 1963; HALES and RANDLE, 1963; MEADE and KLITGAARD, 1962; MELANI *et al.*, 1965; HERBERT *et al.*, 1965; HEDING, 1965).

II. Principles of the Radioimmunological Method

BERSON and YALOW (1959) observed that I^{131}-labeled insulin was not irreversibly bound to insulin antibodies and that the complex did not precipitate. They also discovered that the antigenic properties of insulin are unchanged by labeling with I^{131}. The law of mass action applies to this antigen — antibody reaction of insulin as it does to other antigens. If the concentration of the I^{131}-insulin and antibodies is constant while that of the unlabeled insulin is variable, the ratio of the antibody-bound (B) to free (F) I^{131}-insulin (B/F) is a function of the unmarked insulin

$$\left[I^{131}\text{-insulin}\right] + \left[\begin{matrix}\text{Insulin}\\ \text{antibodies}\end{matrix}\right] \rightleftharpoons \left[\begin{matrix}I^{131}\text{-insulin —}\\ \text{antibody complex}\end{matrix}\right]$$

$$+$$

$$\left[\text{unlabeled insulin}\right]$$

$$\upharpoonleft\downharpoonright$$

$$\left[\begin{matrix}\text{unlabeled insulin —}\\ \text{antibody complex}\end{matrix}\right]$$

The biological and immunological properties of insulin are situated in different parts of the molecule. Immunological and biological assays therefore give identical values only when the insulin molecule is intact. Any alteration in a biological or immunological property will produce discrepancies in the biological and immunological values. Immunologically measurable insulin does not necessarily correlate with the biological effect of the hormone and vice versa.

The immunological determinants of insulin are located at the carboxyl end of the B chain and in positions 8—10 of the A chain. WILSON *et al.* (1962) showed that hybrid insulin with a bovine A chain and a codfish B chain reacts much more strongly with antiserum to bovine insulin than does insulin with a codfish A chain and a bovine B chain.

Dog, pig and whale insulin have identical amino-acid sequences. Human, pig, cow, sheep, rabbit, and rat insulin and that of other animals differ in their amino-acid structures and therefore react differently with an anti-insulin serum. Certain antibodies, however, can also differentiate between insulins with identical amino-acid sequences. This shows that not only the primary structure, but also the tertiary structure determine the antigenic properties of the insulin molecule (Berson and Yalow, 1959).

In general, bovine insulin antibodies in guinea pigs do not react as strongly with human and porcine insulin as with bovine insulin. Moreover, the intensity of the reaction of human and porcine insulin antibodies to bovine insulin antibodies also differs. However, porcine insulin in guinea pigs reacts with human insulin in almost the same way as with porcine insulin. This is a great advantage of the radioimmunoassay of insulin: in order to determine insulin in human blood, it is not absolutely necessary to immunize guinea-pigs with human insulin; it is possible to use porcine insulin, which is easier to obtain.

To obtain an exact measurement of an unknown sample it is always necessary to make sure that the insulin contained reacts with the antibody used in the same intensity as the insulin employed to draw up the standard curve. On the other hand, other binding constants may apply to the I^{131}-insulin employed simply as tracer. However, in order to keep the variables as low as possible, it is advisable to ensure that the insulin for the immunization, for drawing up the standard curve, and for the I^{131}-insulin tracer is from the same species as the insulin to be assayed. In human assays, however, it is possible to use porcine insulin for the production of antibodies, the standard curve and the tracer without introducing important errors.

In the original technique of Yalow and Berson free insulin is separated from antibody-bound insulin by paper electrophoresis. The antibody-bound insulin migrates with the gamma-globulins, whilst the free insulin remains at the starting point. The radioactivity of both parts, which can be measured in various ways, is used to draw up a standard curve. In the method described below, which we have used as a routine method for many years, separation is simplified by using Amberlite CG 400 to which free insulin binds (Meade and Klitgaard, 1962; Melani *et al.*, 1965).

Labeling insulin with I^{131} according to the original method of Baumann *et al.* (1950) and Yalow and Berson (1960) requires I^{131}-activities of 30—80 mCi and therefore special safety measures. Nowadays, insulin and all the other proteohormones that are determined radioimmunologically are more easily labeled by Greenwood and Hunter's (1963) method using ^{131}iodide and chloramine T. I^{125} can be used instead of I^{131}; its much longer half-life of 60 days gives it many advantages. The various methods are described below.

III. Methods of Radioimmunoassay of Insulin

1. Materials

Antisera. Sera containing antibodies are obtained from guinea pigs by immunization with highly purified monocomponent porcine insulin (25—27 U/mg, Novo, Copenhagen). Four subcutaneous injections of 1 ml of an emulsion composed of the following are given to the guinea pigs at weekly intervals: 0.5 ml insulin solution (40 U/ml in 0.03 *N* HCl) 0.5 ml Bacto-adjuvant complete (Difco Laboratories, Detroit, USA). The serum is obtained 8—10 days after the final injection and cooled to —20° C. Precipitating guinea-pig anti-gamma-globulin sera can be obtained from Behring-Werke, Marburg/Lahn, West Germany, or Sylvana Company, Millburn, New Jersey, USA.

Sephadex. Sephadex G-25 and G-75 (Pharmacia, Uppsala, Sweden) are allowed to swell according to the directions and then poured into columns. They are equilibrated with 0.07 *M* Veronal sodium buffer and saturated with 1 ml of a 2% albumin solution.

Ion Exchanger. Amberlite CG 400 I (Serva, Heidelberg) is used. Before use, the chlorine ions of the amber must be substituted by OH ions. This is done by allowing 8 times the amount (v/v) of 2 *M* sodium hydroxide to react for 2 h and then washing the amber over a frit with distilled water until the pH of the washings falls below 8. The ion exchanger is then allowed to dry in air or in an incubator (50° C) and kept closed.

Charcoal. Charcoal (Norit "A", Amend Drug and Chemical Company Inc., New York) is suspended in a buffer solution (5 g/100 ml) consisting of 1.472 g/l sodium barbiturate and 0.972 g/l sodium acetate and adjusted to pH 7.4 with 0.1 *N* HCl. The charcoal suspension is mixed with Dextran buffer solution in the ratio 1:1 (v/v), shaken briefly and stored at +4° C. Dextran buffer solution contains 0.5 g Dextran 80 (Pharmacia Inc., Uppsala, Sweden) in 100 ml of the above buffer.

Cellulose Powder. Before use the cellulose powder (cellulose powder MN 300, Machrey, Nagel & Co., Germany) is washed for 2 h in distilled water (1:10, v/v), then in alcohol (96%) and once more in distilled water; the cellulose is dried in an incubator, crushed finely and stored at room temperature.

I^{125}, I^{131}. For iodization ^{131}I or ^{125}I (2—4 mCi iodide in 0.05 ml NaOH, Radiochemical Centre, Amersham, England) is used.

Measuring Apparatus. Radioactivity is measured with a normal gamma-spectrometer.

2. Insulin Labeling

a) Principles

In 1963 Greenwood and Hunter described a simple method of labeling growth hormone; this is now generally used for insulin and many other polypeptide hormones. The advantage of this method is that a specific activity of 100—400 mCi/mg hormone can be obtained with a relatively small total activity. With this method ^{131}iodide is oxidized by chloramine T to I^{131} or I^{125}, which binds to the tyrosyl radicals of the hormone.

During labeling, radiation and chemical reactions produce radioactive degradation products; these impede the assay and must therefore be removed by purification.

The biological and immunological properties of insulin are changed by iodization. The biological activity falls with the rising number of iodine atoms per insulin molecule. If more than two of the four tyrosyl residues present in the insulin molecule are occupied by iodine, the hormone is biologically inactive (Rosa *et al.*, 1966). According to the investigations of Arquilla *et al.* (1966), the biological activity falls to zero when only 1 tyrosyl residue is occupied by iodine. The immunological properties are also thought to be affected, even by this small degree of iodization. This slight influence does not affect the subsequent test, since the labeled hormone acts only as tracer. What determines the specificity and accuracy of the method is that the unlabeled insulin of the standard solution and that of the sample to be assayed react similarly with the antibodies used, and both compete with the labeled insulin to bind to the antibody molecules with the same intensity. With $I^{125}/^{131}$-insulin special care should be taken to see that no degradation products are included; they bind unspecifically to the serum proteins, thus interfering with the assay.

b) Method of Labeling Insulin

With a micropipet the following are dropped one after the other into tubes containing 2—4 mCi ^{131}iodide or ^{125}iodide in 0.05 ml NaOH:

i) 0.025 ml phosphate buffer (0.05 *M*, pH 7.5)
ii) 0.004 mg insulin in 0.025 ml HCl (0.03 *N*)
iii) 0.1 mg chloramine T in 0.025 ml phosphate buffer (0.05 *M*, pH 7.5); shake for 10—20 sec
iv) 0.24 mg sodium bisulphite in 0.1 ml phosphate buffer (0.05 *M*, pH 7.5)
v) 2.0 mg potassium in 0.2 ml phosphate buffer (0.05 *M*, pH 7.5)

The contents of the tube are poured on to a Sephadex column (G-25) (0.8—1.0, 10—12 cm) equilibrated before use with 0.07 *M* Veronal sodium buffer (pH 8.6), saturated with 1—1.5 ml of a 2% albumin solution and eluted with 0.07 *M* Veronal buffer. The radioactivity measured in the 1 ml fractions gives 2 peaks; the first contains the iodized hormone and the second low-molecular products and free iodine (Fig. 1).

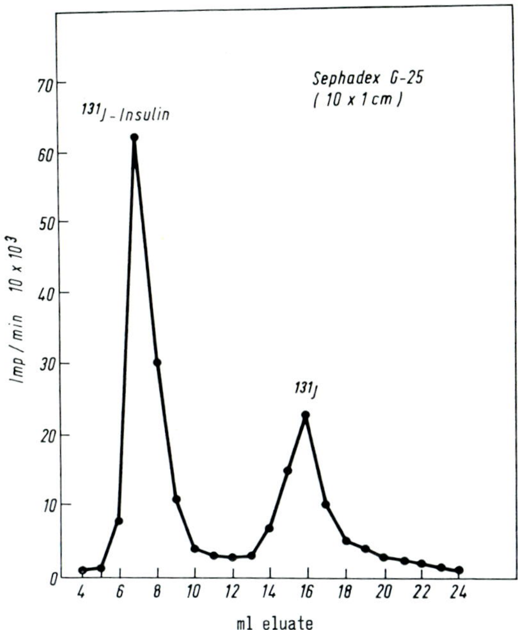

Fig. 1. Separation of ^{131}I-insulin from ^{131}I by column chromatography

c) Purification of Iodine-Labeled Insulin

Only freshly purified labeled insulin should be used for the assay of insulin. Purification removes all the radioactively labeled degradation products, which are bound unspecifically to serum proteins and thus affect the determination of the B/F ratio. For reliable results, the amount of radioactivity unspecifically bound by serum proteins must be less than 10%. Iodine-labeled insulin stored for several days at +4° C or cooled to —20° C must be repurified before use.

This is done by incubating 0.2—0.3 ml labeled insulin (first peak of the eluant after labeling) with 0.2—0.3 ml human serum (Melani *et al.*, 1966). Iodine acetamide (0.5%) must be added beforehand to protect the hormone and bromphenol blue (0.01%) to identify the protein fraction later. The batch is held at +4° C for 15 min and the labeled insulin is then separated from the serum protein over a Sephadex column (G-75), equilibrated before use with 0.07 *M* Veronal sodium buffer and saturated with 1 ml of a 2% albumin solution. The radioactive degradation products bound to the serum proteins appear first in the eluant, followed by the purified labeled insulin. After purification the degradation products account for approx. 3—5% of the total radioactivity (Fig. 2).

3. Separation of Free Insulin from Antibody-Bound Labeled Insulin by Means of Amberlite

Insulin is adsorbed by the anion exchangers Dowex 1 and Amberlite. Amberlite is better suited for insulin assay than Dowex 1. If the insulin is in albumin solution, the Amberlite, which is in the Cl form, must be converted to the OH form.

The following solutions are pipetted into 10 ml tubes one after the other:

1 ml of standard solutions of crystalline porcine or human monocomponent insulin, the concentration being such that the final concentration of the solutions amounts to 2.5, 5.0, 10.0, 25.0 and 50.0 μU/ml;

1 ml of each of the serum samples to be measured is pipetted (diluted 1:10) into another tube;

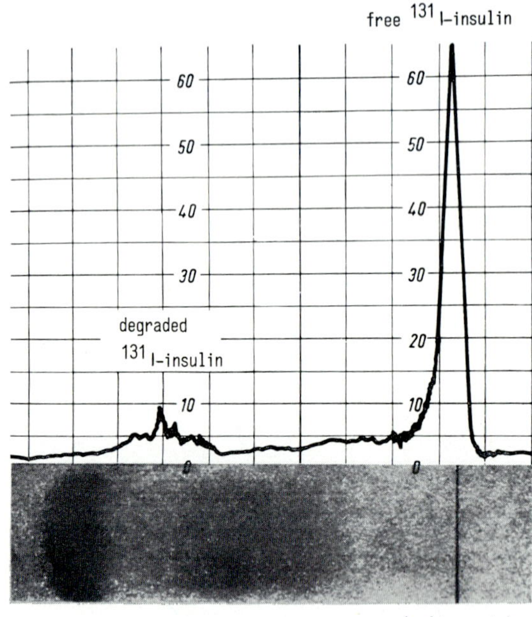

Fig. 2. Paper electrophoresis of normal serum with unpurified ^{131}I-insulin

1.0 buffer solution with 4—8 μU iodine-insulin and antiserum is added. The dilution of the antiserum is tested beforehand. All the solutions are prepared with Veronal sodium buffer (0.1 *M*, pH 8.6), 2% albumin, 0.5% iodine acetamide, and 0.01% merthiolate.

The batches are stored for 3 days at +4°C before the total activity of the individual tubes is measured. Than 200 mg amberlite (OH form) is added and the tubes are shaken for 40 min. The Amberlite, to which the free hormone is bound, is removed by means of a centrifuge and 1.0 ml of the supernatant is measured for radioactivity. The radioactivity in the supernatant corresponds to half the insulin bound to the antibodies. The free insulin value is obtained by subtracting the bound insulin ($^1/_2$ B$\times$2) from the total activity. The free insulin value can also be obtained by determining the radioactivity in the Amberlite; this, however, necessitates washing the Amberlite twice.

The adsorption capacity of 200 mg Amberlite is sufficient to adsorb completely more than the total of 100 μU insulin contained in one batch (Fig. 3). Accurate weighing of the Amberlite is therefore not necessary; it can simply be measured in a measuring beaker.

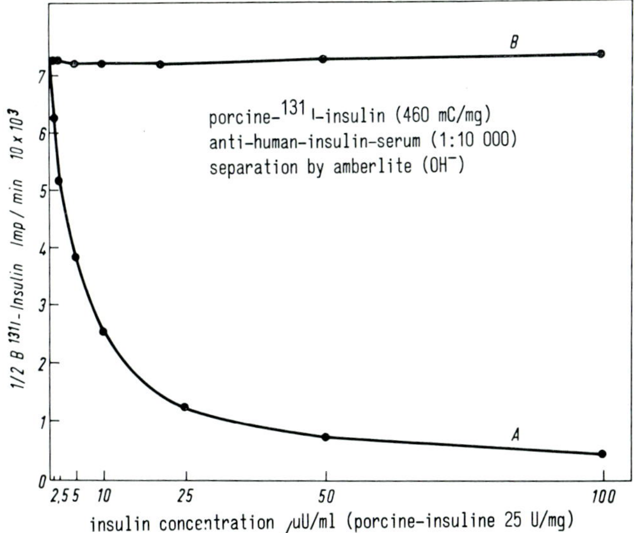

Fig. 3. Typical standard curve for insulin concentrations 0—100 μU/ml (curve A). 200 mg Amberlite removes all the standard insulin (curve B)

4. Sensitivity and Accuracy of the Radioimmunoassay of Insulin

a) Serum Dilution and Antiserum Used

The method must be at least sensitive enough to measure accurately the very low insulin concentrations contained in serum samples diluted 1:10. Higher serum concentrations cannot be used as they change the immunological properties of insulin with the result that they bind unspecifically to serum proteins and not to antibodies. Thus, with the method described the values for free insulin are too high and consequently the B/F ratio is too small. This process of degradation, partly due to reduction of the SS bridges, is largely eliminated by diluting the serum and adding iodine acetamide (Berson and Yalow, 1964).

The sensitivity of the method is also determined by the antiserum used. Adding the smallest amounts of insulin must displace the labeled insulin from its antibody and shift the B/F ratio considerably.

The graph of the B/F ratio will then show a sharp fall, depending on the amount of standard insulin added. Sharp falls in the standard curves are achieved with very few antisera. The curves must usually be taken from a number of sera. The antibody concentration in the serum is of less importance. Although sera with high antibody titres can be greatly diluted, they are often useless for insulin assay, as the standard curves produced are too flat (Fig. 4).

The desirable property of antisera is determined by the energy of the antigen-antibody binding. Antigens and antibodies react according to the law of mass action:

$$[AG] + [AK] \underset{K_2}{\overset{K_1}{\rightleftharpoons}} [AGAK]$$

$$K = \frac{k}{k_1} = \frac{[AGAK]}{[AG] \times [AK]}$$

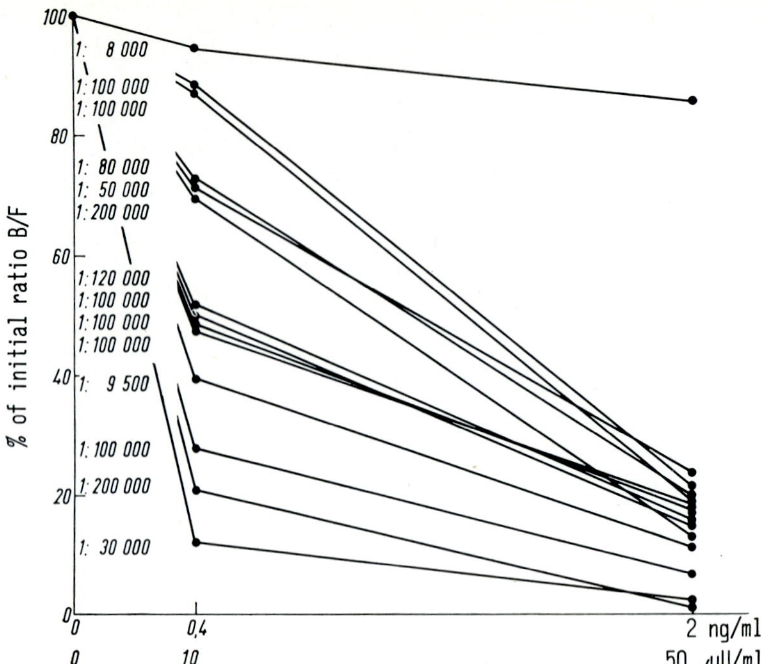

Fig. 4. Insulin concentration

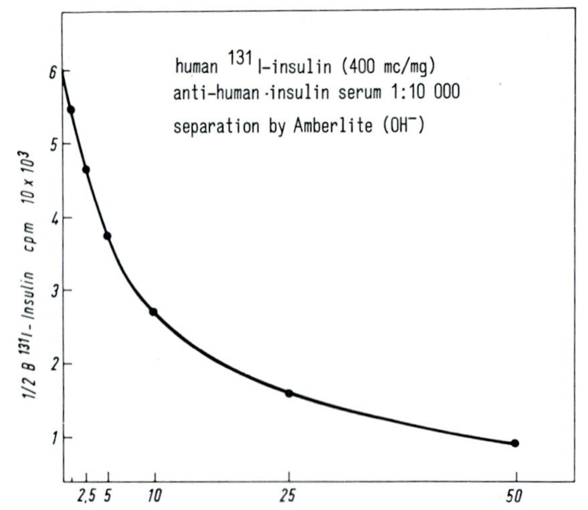

Fig. 5. Insulin concentration in μU/ml (human insulin 23.5 U/mg)

K stands for the equilibrium constant and k and k_1 for the velocity constants of the two reactions. The equilibrium constant K is based on the standard free exchange of energy (ΔF°) of the reaction, and both ΔF° and K are inversely proportional to the temperature of the reaction. The standard free exchange of energy (ΔF°), which induces the formation of the antigen-antibody complex, is responsible for the initial fall of the B/F in the standard curve and thus determines the sensitivity of the method. The methodological work involved in evaluating the result can be reduced by drawing a graph of the recorded impulses corresponding to the bound insulin, and not of the B/F ratio (Fig. 5).

According to HALES and RANDLE (1963) the relation is linear if the ratio of the antibody-bound impulses without added standard insulin (R_0) to the bound impulses with added standard insulin is plotted on the ordinate. The quantity of iodine-labeled insulin corresponds to the intersection of the extended straight line with the abscissa. If the concentration of labeled insulin is known, the unknown serum concentration can theoretically be calculated even without the standard curve.

For example, 5 μU/ml I^{131}-insulin gives:

$$\text{Serum insulin } (\mu\text{U/ml}) = \frac{5 \times R_0 - 1)}{R_S}$$

R_0 = bound radioactivity of the blank (I^{131}-insulin + antibody)

R_S = bound radioactivity of the serum sample (I^{131}-insulin + antibody + serum).

b) Concentration of Radioactively Labeled Insulin

The sensitivity of the method is also determined by the amount of labeled insulin added to all the samples. It should not be more than 5 μU/ml. The smaller the amount, the more sensitive the method. The use of small concentrations, however, requires high specific activities and a high degree of purification.

The initial B/F ratio is determined by the amount of iodine-labeled insulin at a constant antiserum dilution. Experience has shown that this should be approx. 1.5—2.0 so that about 60—70% of the added iodine-labeled insulin is bound. Higher degrees of binding are unfavorable as they affect the accuracy.

With small amounts of iodine-labeled insulin, a favorable initial binding ratio, and an antiserum with high energy values, the accuracy amounts to more than 99% (MELANI, 1968). This high degree of accuracy can never be obtained by biological assay (DITSCHUNEIT and FAULHABER, 1971).

5. Serum Insulin Assays

The fasting serum insulin concentration lies between 5 and 25 μU/ml (0.2—1 μg/ml). In order to keep insulin degradation by the serum at a low level, the serum is diluted with buffer solution in a 1:10 ratio. The method must therefore have a sensitivity of at least 0.5 μU/ml (0.02 μg/ml). If this is not sufficient and a more concentrated serum has to be used, the accuracy diminishes as a result of increasing degradation. Degradation products caused by radiation or other chemical reactions associated with labeling can be removed by column chromatography. Degradation by serum proteins during the 3-day incubation period will be reflected in the assay and the B/F ratio will be too low. As a result the final result will turn out too high.

The 5—6% of impurities remaining after the purification of iodine-labeled insulin will be adsorbed from the buffer solution by the amber. Albumin (2—4%) must therefore be added to the standard solution so that these impurities remain in the supernatant as they do in the serum samples (Fig. 6).

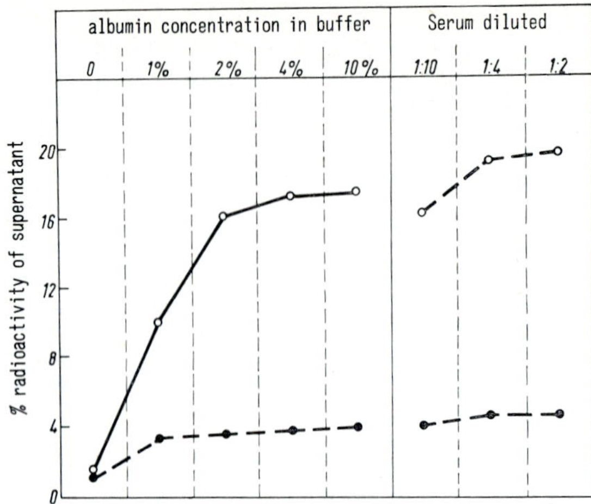

Fig. 6. O——O ^{131}I-insulin before purification on Sephadex G-75; ● - - - - ● ^{131}I-insulin after purification on Sephadex G-75

The following checks are always necessary for every batch for insulin assay:

i) Buffer check:

4—6 μU $I^{131/125}$-insulin
\+ buffer (2% albumin)

ii) Serum check:

4—6 μU $I^{131/125}$-insulin
\+ serum (1:10)
\+ buffer (2% albumin).

After 3 days' incubation the radioactivity in the supernatant should be less than 10% of the total activity.

The insulin employed to draw up the standard curve and the serum insulin must react identically with the antiserum used. When human insulin is taken as the standard, the absolute values of dilutions of a human serum sample must lie on the standard curve. Then the correlation of serum dilution and insulin values will give a corresponding straight line. Similar results are obtained with most antisera if porcine insulin is used instead of human insulin. The antiserum, which is then often used for many months, should always be tested accordingly.

Cooling the serum to —20° C does not affect the insulin content. Serum samples can therefore be deep frozen and stored for 1 year or longer without changing the values (MELANI *et al.*, 1971).

6. Other Methods of Separation

a) General Survey

Free and antibody-bound insulin can also be separated by precipitating the antibody-bound insulin with the aid of a guinea-pig globulin antibody after the reaction and equilibration have been completed. The precipitate can be drawn off by means of a centrifuge or a filter. This method, described by MORGAN and LAZAROV (1963) and HALES and RANDLE (1963), is widely used.

It is also possible to adsorb insulin by means of small particles of charcoal coated with Dextran. Since antibody-bound insulin is not adsorbed it is possible to use the charcoal particles together with Dextran for the radioimmunoassay of insulin (Herbert *et al.*, 1965). This method is also frequently employed. The coating of active charcoal is technically simple and it is easily removed with a centrifuge.

Cellulose is another good means of adsorbing free insulin. It is also easily activated, can be stored for a long time and may be drawn off with a centrifuge in a simple manner. Kerp *et al.* (1966) used cellulose to determine insulin antibodies, where there is also the problem of separating free insulin from antibody-bound insulin. Cellulose can also be employed in the radioimmunoassay of insulin (Melani *et al.*, 1971).

Melani (1971) showed that all these methods produce almost identical values (Table 1). As all four methods are about equally difficult, none is recommended more than the others. They are all suitable for routine investigations.

Table 1. *Insulin concentration ($\mu U/ml$) in three serum samples determined with three different techniques. All values are the mean of triplicate determinations*

		Amberlite CG-400	Charcoal coated with Dextran	Cellulose Powder	Double Antibody Method
Serum	1.	18	26	16	20
1:4	2.	16	24	18	19
Serum	3.	88	96	86	88
1:10	4.	104	108	98	100
Serum	5.	164	176	170	168
1:20	6.	210	218	204	216

b) Double-Antibody Method

Our experience has shown that this method, based on the reports of Morgan and Lazarov (1963), can easily be used for routine investigations as follows:

1.0 ml standard solution or serum sample (diluted 1:10)
0.1 ml $I^{131}/^{125}$-insulin (4—8 μU),
0.1 ml guinea-pig anti-insulin serum
are incubated for 48 h at +4°C.
0.1 ml anti-guinea-pig gamma globulin serum (from rabbits or sheep),
0.1 ml normal guinea-pig serum (diluted 1:400)
are incubated for 48 h at +4°C or for 20 h after the addition of small amounts of heparin.
The mixture is centrifuged and the radioactivity of the sediment (antibody-bound insulin) measured.

c) Separation with Charcoal and Dextran

The charcoal is coated with Dextran according to Herbert *et al.* (1965). The method is described on p. 658.

The following solutions are pipetted into the incubation tubes one after the other:

2 ml standard solution or unknown serum samples (diluted 1:10) (the standard solutions contain insulin such that the final concentrations amount to 2.5, 5, 10, 25 and 50 μU/ml).

2.0 ml $I^{131}/^{125}$-insulin (4—8 μU) + antibody serum diluted accordingly.

After 3 days' incubation at +4°C, 2 ml charcoal coated with Dextran is added, shaken, and centrifuged; the radioactivity of 2.0 ml supernatant is determined.

All the solutions are prepared with Veronal sodium buffer (0.1 *M*, pH 8.6, 1% albumin, 0.5% iodine acetamide and 0.01% merthiolate).

d) Cellulose Powder

The cellulose is prepared according to the method of Kerp *et al.* (1966) described on p. 658.

1.0 ml buffer + $I^{131}/^{125}$-insulin + anti-insulin serum

1.0 ml standard insulin solutions (final concentration 2.5—50 μU/ml) or serum samples (diluted 1:10)

Are incubated for 2 days at +4°C; 150 mg cellulose powder is adden, shaken, and centrifuged and the radioactivity of the bound insulin in 1.0 ml supernatant is measured.

The solutions are prepared with Veronal sodium buffer (0.1 *M*, pH 8.6, 0.5% albumin, 0.5% iodine acetamide, 0.01% merthiolate).

7. Use of Insulin Receptors for Assay Purposes

Radioimmunoassay covers only the part of the insulin molecule that reacts immunologically. This is not the same as the biological determinant of the hormone and therefore the values are theoretically not necessarily a measure of the biological action of the hormone. Many observations, however, seem to indicate (cf. p. 656) that the immunological value is also practically a parameter of the action of the hormone. Nevertheless, there have been numerous attempts to exploit the biological effect for quantitative assays. As biological methods, the evaluation of metabolic effects in intact animals and tissue slices *in vitro* showed inadequate sensitivity, accuracy, and practicability. There have recently been attempts to use insulin receptors, which are located on the cell membrane, for quantitative assays. These receptors have a high specificity and the methods based on them promise to be highly sensitive and sufficiently accurate. The first attempts with insulin receptors were described by CUATRECASAS (1971).

CUATRECASAS *et al.* showed that I^{131}-labeled insulin is also bound by these receptors. It is therefore possible to use insulin receptors instead of the insulin antibodies employed in radioimmunoassays.

However, radioactive insulin suitable for radioimmunoassay may not be quite suitable for receptor studies. A high proportion of the labeled hormone may have a reduced affinity for cell receptors, an increased affinity for nonspecific sites, or reduced survival during incubation *in vitro* as was demonstrated for glucagon (RODBELL *et al.*, 1971), human chorionic gonadotropin (REICHENBERGER and REICHERT, 1972) and human luteinizing hormone (LEE and RYAN, 1971). The reason is excess exposure to the oxidizing agent chloramine T, or the reducing agent metabisulfite, or a higher degree of labeling than one I atom per molecule.

For a $^{125}/^{131}I$-labeled hormone with high specific radioactivity suitable for hormone receptor studies one should label only a small fraction (10% or less) of the molecules with one I atom of iodine, followed by chemical separation of the uniodized molecules (FREYCHET *et al.*, 1971). Another possibility is to label directly with only 0.2—0.8 of an I atom per molecule of hormone under special conditions, followed by a classic purification step. This last can be done by the following modifications to the original chloramine-T method:

i) the concentrations of the reactants are maximized by reducing the volume as much as possible;

ii) only a small volume of concentrated $H_2PO_4^-$ is taken for neutralization of the $Na^{125}I$-NaOH;

iii) the amount of ^{125}iodide must be 2—5 times greater than the amount it is intended to incorporate;

iv) chloramine-T is added in multiple small additions, depending on the results of the continously measured degree of iodination;

v) the amount of metabisulfite is limited to twice that of the chloramine-T added.

The residual reactive iodine is bound to albumin, which can readily be removed. One obtains a superior iodoinsulin with these modifications of the original chloramine-T method than with the standard procedure (ROTH, 1974).

The specific receptors for insulin are found in a variety of tissues including hepatocytes, adipocytes, or purified plasma membrane fractions of either of these cells. Circulating and cultured human lymphocytes also contain specific binding sites for insulin and hence provide a highly satisfactory tissue for the radioreceptor assay (GAVIN *et al.*, 1972).

When a tracer of ^{125}I-insulin is incubated with cultured human lymphocytes binding occurs. The percentage of a given amount of the tracer bound is a function of cell concentration. The binding reaction is time- and temperature-dependent. Binding of the labeled hormone is inhibited by as little as 0.1 ng/ml ($\sim$2.5 μU/ml) unlabeled insulin. The sensitivity is thus quite sufficient for insulin in blood or other biological fluids.

Competitive inhibition of the reversible ^{125}I-insulin receptor binding occurs with the addition of insulin or of insulin-like substances. The ability of an insulin preparation to inhibit the binding of ^{125}I-insulin is directly proportional to the potency of that preparation to stimulate glucose oxidation in fat cells. Proinsulin, for example, has only about 20% the potency of insulin in both the receptor assay and the glucose-oxidation assay. By contrast, the radioimmunoassay may distinguish very well insulins of equal biologic potency (beef, pork or human insulins) but very poorly insulin preparations of different biologic activity. Thus, somatomedin, a substance with insulin-like effects but a very poor reaction with insulin antibodies, is able to compete with insulin for biologic receptors (Hintz *et al.*, 1972). The same ability has been demonstrated for nonsuppressible insulin-like substances.

The separation of receptor-bound insulin from free insulin may be effected by centrifugation or filtration on Millipore filters. The centrifugation method of Rodbell *et al.* (1971) is particularly convenient. When the receptor is soluble, gel filtration can be used (Gavin *et al.*, 1972).

IV. Assay of Proinsulin and C-Peptide

1. Proinsulin Assay

Proinsulin has a high species specificity due to the unusual amino-acid composition of C-peptide. Proinsulin antibodies are therefore also highly species-specific and demonstrate hardly any cross-reactions with proinsulins from other species. Radioimmunoassay of human proinsulin can therefore only be carried out by using antiserum to human proinsulin. Antiproinsulin serum also frequently reacts with insulin and C-peptide, and conversely insulin antisera react with proinsulin. Therefore ^{131}/^{125}I-insulin can be used as a tracer to determine a proinsulin with a corresponding antiproinsulin serum and proinsulin from the same species as the standard (Rubenstein *et al.*, 1969).

When measuring serum proinsulin, the cross-reaction with insulin and C-peptide necessitates prior separation of proinsulin, insulin and C-peptide (Rubenstein *et al.*, 1968). In order to do this, insulin and proinsulin must be extracted from the serum with acid ethanol and separated on 1×50 cm columns of Bio-Gel p-30 with 3 *M* acetic acid. During gel filtration 2 peaks occur, which react immunologically. The fraction eluted first contains proinsulin and the other insulin (Melani *et al.*, 1970). Proinsulin is measured with a proinsulin antiserum, with proinsulin as the standard, and insulin or proinsulin as the tracer. The insulin in the second peak can be measured in the usual way.

In healthy subjects the proinsulin content amounts to 0.05—0.4 ng/ml, or 5—48% of total insulin. The oral administration of glucose increases insulin and proinsulin but the percentage increase of proinsulin is less than that of insulin (Melani *et al.*, 1971).

In adipose subjects with hyperinsulinemia the absolute proinsulin concentration is elevated. The ratio of insulin to proinsulin in the fasting serum and after glucose loading in these patients, however, corresponds to that of normal persons. In diabetes mellitus the ratio of proinsulin to insulin is also normal (Melani *et al.*,

1971). Nevertheless, an increase of proinsulin in the blood has been found in islet adenomas (GOLDSMITH *et al.*, 1969; LAZARUS, TANASE and RECANT, 1969; MELANI *et al.*, 1970, 1971). In this disease stimulation with tolbutamide did not increase proinsulin as much as insulin (MELANI *et al.*, 1970).

2. C-Peptide

In the pancreatic extract of cattle and humans C-peptide and insulin have the same molar concentration. C-peptide is secreted by the β cells in the same molar ratio as insulin (CLARK *et al.*, 1969; RUBENSTEIN *et al.*, 1969a). The amino-acid sequences vary greatly from species to species. Human, bovine and porcine C-peptides differ, for example, in 50% of their amino acids. Due to this large difference in the primary structure, the antisera are highly specific. Therefore, proinsulin antiserum reacts weakly with the insulin of the same species, but not at all with the insulin from other species. Thus, only an antiserum which reacts specifically to human C-peptide or proinsulin can be used in the radioimmunoassay of C-peptide in humans.

C-peptide is obtained from hydrochloric pancreas extract by means of purification with gel filtration over Sephadex G-50, cation exchanger chromatography on carboxymethylcellulose, and paper electrophoresis in 30% formic acid and pyridine glacial acetic acid. To produce the antiserum, immunization of guinea-pigs is carried out. The C-peptide is coupled to rabbit albumin treated with carbodiimide HCl and injected together with Freund's adjuvant on four occasions (MELANI *et al.*, 1970). Human C-peptide which has been tyrosinized and labeled with $I^{131}/^{125}$ is used as the tracer. The antiserum thus obtained also reacts with human proinsulin. The competitive displacement of the tracer by proinsulin is only half as much as that by C-peptide. However, radioimmunoassay of serum C-peptide requires prior separation of the C-peptide from proinsulin by means of gel filtration. Thus the C-peptide appears to be distinctly separated from the proinsulin in a characteristic position.

The fasting serum concentration of C-peptide is somewhat higher than that of insulin, namely 1.2 ± 0.2 ng/ml and 0.19 ± 0.03 ng/ml respectively (HOWITZ *et al.*, 1973). In the oral glucose tolerance test the C-peptide concentration (5.8 ± 1.01 ng/ml) was higher than that of insulin (only 1.5 ± 4.3 ng/ml). C-peptide reached its peak 15 min after insulin.

The half-life of C-peptide is 11.1 min against 4.8 min for insulin. Accordingly higher production rates of the liver were measured, namely 132 ± 22 pg/ml/min for C-peptide and 28 ± 4 pg/ml/min for insulin. Therefore the adsorption of insulin by the liver is greater than that of C-peptide.

Radioimmunoassay of C-peptide is very important in determining the endogenic secretion of insulin in diabetics receiving insulin. In these patients the antibody content in the blood makes radioimmunoassay very difficult, and only an assay of the C-peptide can give an accurate idea of endogenic insulin secretion.

References

ARQUILLA, E.R., OOMS, H.A., FINN, J.: Genetic differences of combining sites of insulin antibodies and importance of C-terminal portion of the A chain to biological and immunological activity of insulin. Diabetologia **2**, 1—13 (1966)

ARQUILLA, E.R., STAVITSKY, A.B.: The production and identification of antibodies to insulin and their use in assaying insulin. J. clin. Invest. **35**, 458—466 (1956)

BAUMANN, A., ROTHSCHILD, M.A., YALOW, R.S., BERSON, S.A.: Distribution and metabolism of ^{131}I-labeled human serum albumin in congestive heart failure with and without proteinuria. J. clin. Invest. **34**, 1359—1368 (1955)

Berson, S.A., Yalow, R.S.: Species-specifity of human antibeef, pork insulin serum. J. clin. Invest. **38**, 2017—2025 (1959)

Berson, S.A., Yalow, R.S.: Immunoassay of protein hormones. In: The Hormones, Vol. IV, p. 557—630. New York-London: Academic Press 1964

Clark, J.L., Cho, S., Rubenstein, A.H., Steiner, D.F.: Isolation of a proinsulin-connecting peptide fragment (C-peptide) from bovine and human pancreas. Biochem. biophys. Res. Commun. **35**, 456—461 (1969)

Cuatrecasas, P.: Properties of the insulin receptor of isolated fat cell membranes. J. biol. Chem. **246**, 7265 (1971)

Ditschuneit, H., Faulhaber, J.D.: Die biologische Bestimmung der insulinähnlichen Serumaktivität (ILA). In: Handbuch des Diabetes mellitus, Bd. II, p. 41—68 (Ed. E.F. Pfeiffer). München: J.F. Lehmanns Verlag 1971

Freychet, P., Roth, J., Neville, D.M., Jr.: Monoiodoinsulin: Demonstration of its biological activity and loading to fat cells and liver membranes. Biochem. biophys. Res. Commun. **43**, 400 (1971)

Gavin, J.R., Archer, J.A., Lesniak, M.A., Gordon, P., Roth, J.: Hormone-receptor interactions of circulating cells: Studies in normal and pathologic states in man. J. clin. Invest. **51**, 35a (1972)

Goldberg, H.L., Egdahl, R.H.: Studies suggesting the extra-pancreatic production of substances with insulin-like activity. Fed. Proc. **20**, 190 (1961)

Goldsmith, S.J., Yalow, R.S., Berson, S.A.: Significance of human plasma insulin Sephadex fractions. Diabetes **18**, Suppl. 1, 340 (1969)

Greenwood, F.C., Hunter, W.M., Glover, J.S.: The preparation of ^{131}I-labeled human growth hormone of high specific radioactivity. Biochem. J. **89**, 114—123 (1963)

Hales, C.N., Randle, P.J.: Immuno assay of insulin with insulin antibody precipitate. Biochem. J. **88**, 137—146 (1963)

Heding, L.G.: Ethanol precipitation as a substitute for the double antibody reaction in a simplified insulin immunoassay method. First Ann. Meeting of Europ. Ass. Diabetes, Montecatini 1965

Herbert, V., Lau, K.S., Gottlieb, C.W., Bleicher, S.J.: Coated charcoal immunoassay of insulin. J. clin. Endocrinol. **25**, 1375—1384 (1965)

Hintz, R.L., Clemmons, D.R., Underword, L.E., Van Wyk, J.J.: Competitive binding of somatomedin to the insulin receptors of adipocytes, chondrocytes and liver membranes. Proc. nat. Med. Sci. **69**, 2351 (1972)

Kerp, L., Steinhilber, S., Kasemir, H.: Ein Verfahren zum Nachweis insulinbindender Antikörper durch Differenzialadsorbtion. Klin. Wschr. **44**, 560—567 (1966)

Lazarus, N.R., Tanese, T., Recant, L.: Proinsulin and insulin synthesis and release by human human insulinoma. Diabetes **18**, Suppl. 1, 340 (1966)

Leidenberger, F., Reichert, C.E., Jr.: Studies on the uptake of human chorionic gonadotropin and its subunits by rat testicular homogenates and interstitial tissue. Endocrinology **91**, 135 (1972)

Lee, C.Y., Ryan, R.J.: The uptake of human luteinizing hormone(HLH) by slices of luteinized rat ovaries. Endocrinology **89**, 1515 (1971)

Meade, R.C., Klitgaard, H.M.: A simplified method for immunoassay of human serum insulin. J. nucl. Med. **3**, 407—416 (1962)

Melani, F., Ryan, W.G., Rubenstein, A.H., Steiner, D.F.: Proinsulin secretion by a pancreatic beta-cell adenoma. New Engl. J. Med. **283**, 713—719 (1970)

Melani, F., Rubenstein, A.H., Steiner, D.F.: Human serum proinsulin. J. clin. Invest. **49**, 497 (1971)

Melani, F., Steiner, D.F.: Proinsulin and C-peptide in human serum. 4th Capri Conference. Acta diab. lat. **7**, Suppl. 1, 107—121 (1970)

Melani, F., Ditschuneit, H., Bartelt, K.M., Friedrich, H., Pfeiffer, E.F.: Über die radioimmunologische Bestimmung von Insulin im Blut. Klin. Wschr. **43**, 1000—1007 (1965)

Melani, F., Bartelt, K.M., Friedrich, H., Pfeiffer, E.F.: Die Jod^{131}-Markierung von Insulin, ACTH und STH mit hoher spezifischer Aktivität zur Anwendung in der radioimmunologischen Methode. Z. klin. Chem. **4**, 189—195 (1966)

Melani, F.: Das immunologisch meßbare Insulin im Blut. Habilitationsschrift, Universität Ulm, 1968

Morgan, C.R., Lazarow, A.: Immunoassay of insulin using a two-antibody system. Proc. Soc. exp. Biol. (N.Y.) **110**, 29—32 (1962)

Morgan, C.R., Lazarow, A.: Immunoassay of insulin: two-antibody system. Plasma insulin levels of normal, subdiabetic and diabetic rats. Diabetes **12**, 115—126 (1963)

Rodbell, M., Kraus, H.M.J., Pohl, S.L., Birnbaumer, L.: The glucagon-sensitive adenyl cyclase system in plasma membranes of rat liver. III. Binding of glucagon: Method of assay and specificity. J. biol. Chem. **246**, 1861 (1971)

Rosa, U., Massaglia, A., Pennisi, G.F., Rossi, C.A., Cozzani, I.: Correlation of chemical changes due to iodination with insulin biological activity. In: Labelled Proteins in Tracer Studies. European Atomic Energy Community EURATOM; Brussels, October 1966

Roth, J.: Peptide hormone binding to receptors: A review of direct metabolism. 1974, in press

Rubenstein, A.H., Cho, S., Steiner, D.F.: Evidence for proinsulin in human urine and serum. Lancet **I**, 1353—1355 (1968)

Rubenstein, A.H., Clark, J.L., Melani, F., Steiner, D.F.: Secretion and circulation of the proinsulin C-peptide. Nature (Lond.) **224**, 697—701 (1969a)

Rubenstein, A.H., Steiner, D.F., Cho, S., Lawrence, A.W., Kirstens, L.: Immunological properties of bovine proinsulin and related fractions. Diabetes **18**, 598 (1969b)

Schöffling, K.: Der Insulinstoffwechsel des pankreaslosen Hundes. 12. Symp. Dtsch. Ges. Endokr., S. 200—214, Wiesbaden, 21.—23. April 1966

Wilson, S., Dixon, G.H., Wardlaw, A.C.: Resynthesis of cod insulin from its polypeptide chains and the preparation of cod-ox "hybrid" insulins. Biochim. biophys. Acta (Amst.) **62**, 483—489 (1962)

Yalow, R.S., Berson, S.A.: Assay of plasma insulin in human subjects by immunological methods. Nature (Lond.) **21**, 1648—1649 (1959)

Yalow, R.S., Berson, S.A.: Immunoassay of endogenous plasma insulin in man. J. clin. Invest. **39**, 1157—1175 (1960)

B. The Biological Assay of Insulin-Like Serum Activity (ILA)

JENS-DIETER FAULHABER and HANS DITSCHUNEIT

With 3 Figures

I. Introduction

Determination of insulin activity in fluids with the aid of biological methods is still of great importance today. Insulin immunoassays (cf. p. 655) have not completely superseded biological assays despite their much higher sensitivity and greater accuracy. Certain scientific questions still require determination of the biological activity of insulin from body fluids and other media, as recently demonstrated with the discovery of proinsulin (STEINER, 1967). Both the immunological and biological methods can determine substances in the blood that are not structurally identical with the pancreatic insulin molecule, the structure of which was clarified by SANGER and TUPPY (1951). The use of the terms "insulin-like activity" (ILA) for the biological value and "immunologically measurable insulin" (IMI) for the immunological result takes this fact into account.

With the aid of insulin antibodies ILA was separated into two components, one inhibited by insulin antibodies *in vitro*, the other not. This produced the terms "suppressible" and "nonsuppressible" ILA (SLATER *et al.*, 1961; RAMSEIER *et al.*, 1962; FROESCH *et al.*, 1963), whilst SAMAAN *et al.* (1963) chose the terms "atypical" and "typical" ILA. Both forms of insulin bear a certain relationship to the "free" and "bound" insulin components in the blood postulated by ANTONIADES *et al.* (1961) on the basis of column chromatography. On the other hand, the "little" and "big" insulins described by ROTH *et al.* (1968) are more like insulin and proinsulin. LYNGSOE (1967) gives a detailed survey of the various forms of insulin.

II. Principle and Survey of Insulin Bioassays

1. In-Vivo Methods

In-vivo methods are based on the hypoglycemic effect of insulin in intact animals, where there is a linear relationship between the logarithm of the insulin dose and the fall in blood sugar. The methods listed in Table 1 are based either on measurements of the fall in blood sugar in fasting rabbits, as used in the pharmaceutical industry to standardize insulin preparations (BANTING *et al.*, 1922), or on effecting hypoglycemic spasms in mice by insulin injections (FRASER, 1923; HEMMINGSEN and KROGH, 1926; TREVAN and BOOCK, 1926). However, neither method is sensitive enough to determine serum insulin quantitatively, as blood insulin concentrations are about one thousandth the amount that can influence blood sugar in animals. In rats and mice the low insulin concentration in the blood can be determined from the fall in blood sugar only after the anti-insulin endocrine glands (pituitary and adrenals) have been removed and the β cells destroyed with alloxan.

By removing only the adrenal medulla and pituitary GELLHORN, FELDMAN and ALLEN (1941) were able to increase the sensitivity of the test animal to 300 μU/100 g body weight in rats: 130-g rats were hypophysectomized 1 week after removal of the adrenal medulla, and insulin or human blood, resp. were injected into the abdominal cavity. 2.5 h after the intake of food, insulin activities of 200 μU/ml were measured in the blood of nondiabetic persons.

ANDERSON *et al.* (1947) increased the sensitivity by using hypophysectomized and alloxan-diabetic rats in which the adrenal medulla had also been removed (ADH rats). The adrenal medulla of weaned animals was removed. When the animals weighed 225—250 g, diabetes was produced with the aid of alloxan (12 mg/100 g body weight) and the pituitary excised 10 days later. After 1—2 weeks tests can be carried out on these animals, which are then used for up to 10 tests. The smallest significantly hypoglycemic insulin dose is around 125 μU.

BORNSTEIN (1950) achieved a further increase in sensitivity by total adrenalectomy (ADHA rats) instead of simple removal of the medulla. After fasting for 1 h these highly sensitive animals received subcutaneous injections of insulin, and the blood sugar was determined 60 min later. This method raises the sensitivity to 50 μU, and BORNSTEIN and LAWRENCE (1951) measured blood insulin levels of 190—290 μU/ml in obese maturity-onset diabetics 2 h after oral glucose loading.

BEIGELMAN, GOETZ, ANTONIADES and THORN (1956) used hypophysectomized and alloxan-diabetic rats to assay insulin activity in the various protein fractions of the serum. The animals were given glucose orally before the experiment, then intraperitoneal injections of insulin in 5% human albumin. The dose-activity relationship showed a linear correlation between fall in blood sugar and the logarithm of the insulin dose in the range 2.5—10 mU. The addition of albumin increased insulin sensitivity.

Anderson, Wherry, Bates and Cornfield (1957) used hypophysectomized mice treated with alloxan. There was a linear regression between the reduction of the blood sugar and the dose logarithm 20 min after intravenous injection of 250—4,000 μU insulin per 25 g body weight.

Table 1. *In-vivo methods of measuring blood insulin*

Species and preparation	Index of the insulin activity	Sensitivity (μU)	Authors
Hypophysectomized rats with the adrenal medulla removed	Fall in blood sugar after injection of intraperitoneal insulin	300	Gellhorn *et al.* (1941)
Hypophysectomized alloxan-diabetic rats with the adrenal medulla removed	Reduction in blood sugar after intravenous injection of insulin and prior treatment with oral glucose	125	Anderson *et al.* (1947)
Hypophysectomized adrenalectomized alloxan-diabetic rats (ADHA-rats)	Reduction in blood sugar after subcutaneous injection of insulin	50	Bornstein (1950)
Hypophysectomized alloxan-diabetic rats	Reduction in blood sugar after intraperitoneal injection of insulin and prior treatment with oral glucose	2,500	Beigelman *et al.* (1956)
Intact mice	Reduction in blood sugar after intraperitoneal injection of insulin	1,000	Beigelman (1958)
Hypophysectomized alloxan-diabetic mice	Reduction in blood sugar 20 min after intravenous injection of insulin	250	Anderson *et al.* (1957)
Adrenalectomized alloxan-diabetic mice under Nembutal anesthesia	Reduction in blood sugar after intravenous injection of insulin	1,000	Baird and Bornstein (1959)
Intact rats	Increase in diaphragm glycogen content after intraperitoneal injections of insulin	100	Rafaelsen (1961)

Baird and Bornstein (1959) assayed the insulin activity in plasma extracts using adrenalectomized and alloxan-diabetic mice. The linear range between the logarithm of the insulin dose and the blood sugar fall was 1,000—4,000 μU/25 g body weight.

Rafaelsen (1961) described a modified *in-vivo* technique using intact rats which was sufficiently sensitive to assay insulin in the blood. The parameter of the insulin activity was the concentration-dependent increase in the glycogen content of the diaphragm after intraperitoneal injection of insulin or body fluids containing insulin. 100 μU clearly raised the glycogen content of the diaphragm; 10,000 μU achieved the greatest effect, increasing the glycogen content by 200—400%, while the blood sugar remained constant. Intravenous administration of 10,000 μU insulin per 100 g body weight, however, produced an increase of 25% of the glycogen content and a barely determinable fall in blood sugar.

A mean insulin activity of 166 μU/ml was assayed in the undiluted serum of 12 nondiabetic fasting subjects. A mean of 583 μU/ml was found in the serum of 6 insulinoma patients. Growth hormone, glucagon, desoxycorticosterone and acetylsalicylic acid increased the diaphragm glycogen only at much higher doses than insulin.

RAFAELSEN, LAURIS and RENOLD (1965) modified this technique by injecting the insulin intraperitoneally together with a tracer dose of U–^{14}C glucose and determining the incorporation of labeled carbon into the glycogen of the diaphragm and the epididymal adipose tissue. This method is very suitable for distinguishing the various forms of insulin in the blood and their different effects on muscle and adipose tissue.

2. In-Vitro Methods

The *in-vitro* methods shown in Table 2 are those most widely used, as they are relatively simple, the material being the isolated diaphragm and epididymal adipose tissue of rats.

Experiments have been made with other tissues, e.g. pigeon flight muscles (KREBS and EGGELSTON, 1938), mouse melanoma tissue (WOODS *et al.*, 1953), lactating mammary glands of rats (BALMAIN *et al.*, 1954), or embryo chick hearts (LESLIE and PAUL, 1954). However, these tissues are difficult to obtain and are usually less sensitive. As with the *in-vivo* techniques, the insulin content is assessed by comparing the effects of a standard insulin dose with those of a serum sample. This comparison is by its very nature doubtful and is discussed on p. 676.

Table 2. *In-vitro methods of measuring insulin in the blood*

Incubation technique Type of tissue	Parameter of the insulin effect	Sensitivity (Serum levels) (μU/ml)	Authors
Hemidiaphragms from rats weighing 80—100 g and fasted for 24 h, 200 mg/100 ml glucose buffer after Gey and Gey. Incubation: 90 min, 4 hemidiaphragms per vessel. Serum dilution 1:6.25	Glucose uptake/100 mg wet weight	5—500 (60—600*) seasonal fluctuations	GROEN *et al.* (1952)
Hemidiaphragms of rats weighing 120—150 g fasted for 24 h, 300 mg/100 ml glucose buffer after Gey and Gey. Incubation: 90 min, 1 hemidiaphragm per vessel. Undiluted plasma	Glucose uptake/10 mg dry weight/hour	10 (40—80*) (600—800**)	VALLANCE-OWEN and HURLOCK (1954)
Hemidiaphragms of rats weighing 100—150 g fasted for 18—24 h, 250 mg/100 ml glucose buffer after Gey and Gey. Incubation: 180 min, 6 hemidiaphragms per vessel. Plasma dilution 1:4	Glucose uptake/g wet weight/hour	100 (9,000—22,000**)	RANDLE (1954)
Hemidiaphragms of rats weighing 110 g fasted for 24 h, 150 mg/100 ml glucose buffer after Gey and Gey. Incubation: 90 min, 1 hemidiaphragm per vessel. Serum dilution 1:10	Glucose uptake/hemidiaphragm	30 (900—4,600*)	WILLEBRANDS *et al.* (1958)
Hemidiaphragms of rats weighing 100—150 g fasted for 18—24 h, 7.5 mg/100 ml 1-^{14}C glycine, 250 mg/100 ml glucose buffer after Gey and Gey. Incubation: 120 min, 2 hemidiaphragms per vessel. Plasma dilution 1:4	1-^{14}C glycine incorporation into the diaphragm protein	50 (2,000—10,000**)	MANCHESTER *et al.* (1959)

Table 2 (continued)

Incubation technique Type of tissue	Parameter of the insulin effect	Sensitivity (Serum levels) (μU/ml)	Authors
Epididymal adipose tissue of non-fasted rats, bicarbonate buffer after Krebs and Henseleit, 100—300 mg adipose tissue per vessel	Net CO_2 production	10	BALL *et al.* (1959)
Epididymal adipose tissue of non-fasted rats, weighing 200—260 g, 300 mg/100 ml 1-^{14}C glucose bicarbonate buffer after Krebs and Henseleit, 70—170 mg adipose tissue per vessel. Serum dilution 20:1	$^{14}CO_2$ pro duction per 100 mg wet weight $\times$120 min	10 (33—940*)	RENOLD *et al.* (1960)
Epididymal adipose tissue of non-fasted rats, weighing 120—150 g, 250 mg/100 ml 1-^{14}C glucose bicarbonate buffer after Krebs and Henseleit, 80—150 mg adipose tissue per vessel. Serum dilution 1:2. Radioactivity assay with a liquid scintillation counter	$^{14}CO_2$ pro duction per 100 mg wet weight $\times$180 min	10 (135—680*)	DITSCHUNEIT *et al.* (1962)

* fasting ** after glucose

a) Rat-Diaphragm Method

During the search for the mechanism of action of insulin GEMMILL (1940) and GEMMILL and HAMMANN (1941) showed that insulin raises the glycogen content and glucose utilization of rat diaphragm incubated in a phosphate buffer solution containing glucose. There was a quantitative relation between the insulin concentration of the medium and its effect on the glucose metabolism of the diaphragm (STADIE and ZAPP, 1947; KRAHL and PARK, 1948). The diaphragms of young rats were particularly sensitive to insulin (WILLEBRANDS *et al.*, 1950).

The method of insulin assay in human plasma developed by GROEN *et al.* (1952) is based on these observations. Here the effect of various standard insulin solutions on the glucose uptake of the diaphragm *in vitro* is compared with that of unknown serum samples. The authors fasted 80—100 g rats for 24 h and then bisected the diaphragms. One half was incubated alone for 90 min at 37° C in a buffer containing glucose (200 mg/100 ml), the other together with a known quantity of insulin or the serum sample to be assayed, which was diluted with buffer in the ratio 1:6.25. The difference in the glucose uptake of the diaphragm halves in the various incubation media served as the parameter of the insulin activity. With crystalline insulin there were clear dose-activity relations for a range of 5—5,000 μU/ml. The sensitivity of the diaphragm exhibited seasonal fluctuations, declining in the summer months.

The levels measured by the rat diaphragm method lay between 60 and 600 μU/ml in the serum of nondiabetic animals. In severe diabetic ketoacidosis the levels were not, or were hardly measurable, whilst an islet-cell adenoma, which was confirmed operatively, gave levels 4—5 times higher. The observation that in pancreatectomized dogs the insulin activities fell below measurable levels and that the insulin effect of serum samples was eliminated by cysteine and glutathione (DUVIGNEAUD *et al.*, 1931) indicated that the metabolic effect determined was caused by insulin.

Modifications of this method with the aim of improving the accuracy of the assays were described by VALLANCE-OWEN and HURLOCK (1954), RANDLE (1954), and WILLEBRANDS *et al.* (1958). The main details are shown in Table 2. All these authors used the glucose uptake of the diaphragm from the incubation medium as the parameter of insulin activity. Differences in the methods include the incubation period, the number of hemidiaphragms incubated, the serum concentration and the correlation of the measurements with the standard insulin concentration.

Table 2 shows that the serum insulin activities yielded by the various methods differ greatly. WILLEBRANDS *et al.* (1958) suggested that a "dilution phenomenon" was one of the possible reasons for this. The serum insulin activity is intensified by dilution because it eliminates insulin inhibitors more rapidly (RANDLE, 1957). The observation by HILL (1959) that crystalline insulin is strongly adsorbed to glass walls but that this can be prevented by gelatin, is also significant in this connection. According to CUNNINGHAM (1962), with insulin concentrations between 100 and 1,000 μU/ml, up to 80% is lost in this way. As human serum albumin also prevents insulin adsorption (WISEMAN and BALTZ, 1961), an unknown serum sample will give values which are too high if the corresponding standard insulin curves are plotted without the addition of albumin or gelatin.

The degradation of insulin by proteolytic enzymes of the material, as demonstrated by PIAZZA *et al.* (1959), may also account for some of the very divergent results obtained by various workers. The greatest proteolysis was demonstrated in the *in-vitro* methods with diaphragms. Apparently most of the proteolytic activity passes into the medium from the edges of the cuts in the tissue and the extent of the insulin degradation is determined by the number of incubated hemidiaphragms. When adipose tissue is used, degradation is minimal.

As PIAZZA *et al.* (1959) showed, insulin degradation is inhibited by plasma factors. The inhibitory effect is correlated with the plasma concentration of the incubation medium. Effective insulin degradation is therefore determined by the plasma concentration used in the test system and the number of hemidiaphragms incubated. As it is exactly in this respect that the usual diaphragm methods (RANDLE, 1954; GROEN *et al.*, 1952; VALLANCE-OWEN and HURLOCK, 1954) vary greatly, this could explain the divergent measurements. These factors must also cause distortion compared with the standard curve plotted in pure buffer medium and with known insulin concentrations, as the inhibitory effects of the plasma would not be used to full advantage, thus producing an overestimate of serum insulin activity.

Moreover, the low proteolytic activity of the adipose tissue might account for its high insulin sensitivity in *in-vitro* experiments. This assumption is supported by the findings of RAFAELSEN *et al.* (1965) that with the Rafaelsen technique (see p. 674 and 673) diaphragms and epididymal adipose tissue did not differ as regards insulin sensitivity *in vivo*.

Insulin also greatly stimulates amino acid incorporation into muscle protein (SINEX *et al.*, 1952; KRAHL, 1953; MANCHESTER and YOUNG, 1958). The incorporation of ^{14}C glycine into the protein of the isolated rat diaphragm was therefore used by MANCHESTER *et al.* (1959) as the parameter in a bioassay on the isolated diaphragm. The sensitivity of this method is around 50 μU/ml. The insulin content of the blood corresponds to that obtained from carbohydrate metabolism of the diaphragm.

PERLMUTTER *et al.* (1952) used the increase in glycogen content in the diaphragm as the parameter for an insulin assay. According to VILLAR-PALASI and LARNER (1961) and MOODY and FELBER (1966), glycogen synthesis is very specifically enhanced by insulin. However, on account of the low sensitivity of the methods of glycogen assay employed at that time, the authors were unable to determine the insulin activities in the blood. JESSUP and WIBERG (1961) were the first to make this method highly sensitive and accurate. They divided the diaphragms into eight equal parts, thus reducing the biological fluctuations of the material itself, and assayed the free glycogen with anthrone reagent after VAN DER VIES (1957). A glucose concentration of 200 mg/100 ml and an incubation of 90 min achieved the greatest insulin effect on glycogen synthesis. Storing the diaphragm sections in ice-cold buffer solution until incubated, as described by GROEN *et al.* (1952) and VALLANCE-OWEN and HURLOCK (1954), slightly decreased glucose uptake and glycogen deposition (JESSUP and WIBERG, 1961 b).

From the specificity criteria recognized in the assessment of insulin bioassay there is no doubt that the rat diaphragm method is a very specific test for insulin.

i) Cysteine and glutathione destroy serum insulin activity (GROEN *et al.*, 1952; RANDLE, 1954; VALLANCE-OWEN and HURLOCK, 1954).

ii) Addition of insulin antibodies to the incubation medium neutralizes serum insulin activity (MANCHESTER *et al.*, 1959).

iii) Blood flowing from the pancreas via the pancreaticoduodenal vein contains much more insulin activity than that from the femoral artery (METZ, 1960).

iv) Serum insulin activity completely disappears from the blood of pancreatectomized cats (VALLANCE-OWEN and LUKENS, 1957). In the serum of pancreatectomized dogs the activity is undeterminable or less than 10% of the initial value. These findings of GROEN *et al.* (1952) could not, however, be confirmed later (SCHÖFFLING *et al.*, 1965).

The extent to which the remaining hormones circulating in the blood promote or inhibit the insulin activity determined in the rat diaphragm was investigated for glucose uptake and glycogen. The ILA of growth hormone on glucose uptake could only be demonstrated in phosphate buffer and in concentrations far above the physiological hormon concentration in serum (RANDLE and WHITNEY, 1957). Corticotropin exhibited no effect (RANDLE, 1957). The inhibition of insulin activity by cortisol and glucagon, discovered by STADIE *et al.* (1951) and SNEDECOR *et al.* (1955), respectively, was also demonstrated only by using doses far above the physiological serum concentrations.

Adrenalin and noradrenalin (WALAAS and WALAAS, 1956) inhibit glucose uptake and glycogen synthesis of the isolated rat diaphragm in physiological concentrations. This observation emphasizes that the insulin activity in the serum cannot be completely equated with the crystalline insulin used as the standard.

b) Rat-Adipose-Tissue Method

As with the rat-diaphragm method, the use of adipose tissue to assay serum insulin activity was based on biochemical investigations of the effect of insulin on adipose tissue (KRAHL, 1951; HAUGAARD and MARSH, 1952; WINEGRAD and RENOLD, 1958a and b). The isolated rat epididymal adipose tissue proved to be a very good material. Its metabolism is very sensitive to insulin, it is branched and arranged in pairs so that the tissue of one animal can be used for several assays. It is easily accessible and can therefore be removed without damaging the tissue, which is essential for optimal insulin activity (WINEGRAD and RENOLD, 1958a).

Insulin acts on a number of metabolic parameters in adipose tissue. It stimulates glucose uptake (KRAHL, 1951), glycogen synthesis (CAHILL *et al.*, 1959), glucose oxidation and lipid synthesis (WINEGRAD and RENOLD, 1958b; CAHILL *et al.*, 1959). Under the action of insulin the respiratory quotient, also rises above 1, which is relatively easy to demonstrate by the manometric technique (BALL *et al.*, 1959).

Each of these insulin-dependent metabolic processes can be used to make a quantitative assay of insulin. As with the rat-diaphragm method, the simplest method technically is the determination of glucose uptake from the incubation medium (BEIGELMAN, 1960; HUMBEL, 1959). The accuracy of this method, however, suffers from the large margin of error of the glucose assay, which, with a glucose content of 300 mg/100 ml, cannot be reduced to less than 1—2%, or in absolute terms 3—6 mg/100 ml, even with very exact working. As the glucose concentration minus the basal effect is reduced by only 20—30 mg/100 ml when 1,000 μU/ml crystalline insulin is added to the incubation medium, the margin of error of the method is about 25%, due entirely to the inaccuracy of the glucose assay. This makes the method unsuitable for a quantitative investigation.

According to JEANRENAUD and RENOLD (1959) glucose oxidation and the incorporation of glucose carbon into fatty acids gives the most favorable dose-activity relation. Since, however, carbon dioxide production from radioactively marked glucose can be more easily detected, MARTIN *et al.* (1958) developed a method which has become popular and on which most insulin bioassays are still based. Since insulin stimulates mainly the anaerobic breakdown of glucose by way of the pentose-phosphate cycle (MILSTEIN, 1956; WINEGRAD and RENOLD, 1958b) in the reaction series of which the first carbon atom of the glucose is split off as carbon dioxide, $1\text{-}^{14}C$ glucose is added to the incubation medium and the $^{14}CO_2$ formed is measured as parameter of the insulin activity. The optimal incubation conditions were by set up RENOLD *et al.* (1960), with an incubation time of 2 h with Krebs-Ringer bicarbonate buffer solution as the incubation medium. Basal metabolism of the incubated tissue is slightly inhibited in phosphate buffer. The glucose concentration of the incubation medium should amount to 300 mg/100 ml to achieve an optimal insulin effect. In view of the adsorption of insulin to the glass walls of the incubation vessels, demonstrated by HILL (1959), gelatin or albumin (100—200 mg/100 ml) is added. Rats weighing 220—260 g are best, since the adipose tissue from smaller rats is often not sufficient. The weight of the individual pieces of fat should be between 70 and 170 mg. Under these conditions the smallest effective amount of insulin is 10 μU/ml. The dose-activity relation is a linear relation between 30 and 500 μU/ml, obtained by correlating the logarithms of the insulin concentration and those of the radioactive carbon dioxide formed, measured as radioactivity/min and mg fat, respectively.

Reduced glutathione and cysteine completely neutralize the activity of crystalline insulin and serum. Insulin antibodies also inhibit the effect of crystalline insulin, but only partially that of serum. Adrenalin has a positive effect on glucose uptake, glucose oxidation, and glyceride-glycerol synthesis. The addition of up to 18 μg/l adrenalin to the incubation medium does not interfere with direct glucose oxidation by way of the pentose-phosphate shunt. Other hormones, such as growth hormone, corticotropin, prolactin, glucocorticoids, glucagon and triiodothyronine do not affect the result in physiological concentrations, either (DITSCHUNEIT *et al.*, 1961; CAHILL *et al.*, 1960; WINEGRAD *et al.*, 1959).

LEONARDS *et al.* (1962) chose glycogen synthesis of the rat epididymal adipose tissue as the parameter of insulin activity. Without insulin, almost no incorporation of labeled glucose into the glycogen fraction is recorded, whereas the smallest insulin concentrations produce a considerable rise. This effect is due to the specific activation of UDP-glucose-glycogen transglucosylase by insulin, as established by VILLAR-PALASI and LARNER (1961). In the experiment non-fasting rats weighing 200—250 g were used. Fat weighing 40 mg gives the best metabolic activity; greater weights produce less activity. The effect of insulin on glycogen synthesis in the adipose tissue of rats fasted for 48 h is greatly reduced. With 20—160 μU/ml insulin there is a linear relation between the logarithm of the insulin concentration and ^{14}C radioactivity in the glycogen of adipose tissue. Adrenalin and glucagon have no effect in physiological concentrations of 0.01 mmol/ml and 0.01 μg/ml respectively. Serum insulin activity is also completely inhibited by cysteine in this procedure, but it persists for many days after pancreatectomy and is not fully neutralized by insulin antibodies (LEONARDS *et al.*, 1962).

c) Rat-Fat-Cell Method

The large margin of error of insulin bioassays with isolated tissue sections is due mainly to the differing sensitivity of the various tissue particles. The use of aliquots of a cell suspension of the material produced from several adipose pieces from various animals therefore promised a considerable increase in accuracy. Consequently, GLIEMANN (1965) used a preparation of isolated fat cells as described by RODBELL (1964) for insulin assay. Besides the expected improvement in the accuracy of such a method, there was also an increase in insulin sensitivity up to 0.25—1.0 μU/ml insulin (GLIEMANN, 1967a). $^{14}CO_2$ production from 1–^{14}C glucose was again used as the parameter of insulin activity. Adrenalin, oxytocin, ACTH and TSH do not affect glucose oxidation in physiological concentrations. Adjusting the pH to alkalinity and raising the ion strength of the buffer increases carbon dioxide production in the absence of insulin without affecting the metabolism of insulin-stimulated cells.

At a dilution of 1:100 serum insulin activity in the blood of non-diabetic fasting subjects was between 20 and 70 μU/ml and was only partly inhibited by the addition of insulin antibodies. Thirty to 60 min after oral glucose loading suppressible serum insulin activity rose to 32—97 μU/ml (GLIEMANN, 1967b). Nonsuppressible serum insulin activities of 50—60 μU/ml were measured in all samples. This fraction remained unchanged during a glucose tolerance test. Suppressible serum insulin activity corresponded to insulin values assayed according to HALES and RANDLE (1963).

III. Practical Execution of Insulin Bioassays

1. In-Vivo Methods (Glycogen Synthesis of the Rat Diaphragm in Situ)

a) Experimental Animals

RAFAELSEN (1964a, b) used male and female albino rats weighing 80—120 g. The rats were fasted for 18 h before the experiment began, but were allowed free access to water. It is recommended that each batch contains rats of both sexes.

b) Method

Each substance is tested on a group of 4 rats. The material is dissolved in physiological saline and injected with a fine needle into the peritoneal cavity to the right of the navel. A control group receives 1 ml of physiological saline. The standard curve is obtained by injecting another 3 groups with respectively 100, 1,000, and 10,000 μU crystalline insulin/100 g body weight. The animals are killed by a blow on the back of the neck after 180 min, decapitated, and the diaphragms excised.

c) Analytic Methods

To determine the glycogen content, each diaphragm is placed immediately after removal in a test tube (12×100) containing 0.5 ml 30% KOH and boiled for 10—15 min in a water bath until the tissue is completely dissolved. The glycogen is precipitated in a previously cooled solution of 0.2 ml 2% Na_2SO_4 and 5 ml ethyl alcohol, centrifuged at 3,000 rpm, dissolved in 1 ml distilled water, and precipitated once more in 5 ml ethyl alcohol. The precipitated glycogen is hydrolyzed with 2 ml 0.6 n HCl for 2.5 h in a water bath at 100°C. The medium is neutralized by the usual methods and the glucose is determined quantitatively.

d) Calculation

The insulin content of an unknown serum sample is read off from the calibration curve plotted with known insulin concentrations, correlating the logarithms of dose and activity.

e) Norms

A mean of 186 μU/ml was measured in the serum of 11 fasting nondiabetics, individual levels ranging between 0 and 420 μU/ml. In 6 patients in whom an operation confirmed islet-cell adenoma, fasting levels were around 583 μU/ml, the lowest being 145 and the highest 1,520 μU/ml (RAFAELSEN, 1964b).

f) Interference

Intraperitoneal injections of human (100 μg/ml) and bovine (10 μg/ml) growth hormone, glucagon (1 μg/ml), desoxycorticosterone (10 μg/ml) and acetylsalicylic acid (10 μg/ml) increase diaphragm glycogen while adrenalin (1 μg/ml) reduces it. The minimum doses used (given in brackets) are much higher than physiological blood levels and these substances are hence not expected to influence the measurements.

2. In-Vitro Methods

Of the various *in-vitro* methods, the rat-diaphragm and adipose-tissue methods are the most popular; the former has many variations. The method used by us and described below is based on that of VALLANCE-OWEN and HURLOCK (1954). The parameter of insulin activity, however, is not glucose uptake from the incubation medium, as originally described, but glycogen synthesis by the hemidiaphragm. According to VILLAR-PALASI and LARNER (1961) and MOODY and FELBER (1966), glycogen synthesis is a metabolic process specifically stimulated by insulin, whereas glucose uptake is affected by the osmolarity of the medium (KUZUYA *et al.*, 1965) and by certain amino acids and hormones (RANDLE, 1957).

When rat epididymal adipose tissue is used, the method proposed by MARTIN *et al.* (1958) has generally prevailed. A modification devised by DITSCHUNEIT *et al.* (1962) makes the method simpler and more accurate. It is described below.

a) Determination of Insulin Activity from Glycogen Synthesis of the Isolated Rat Diaphragm

α) Experimental animals

Male rats weighing 130—150 g and fasted for 4 h before the experiment commences are used. Wet weight of the incubated diaphragms is between 80 and 120 mg.

β) Materials

Buffer solution after GEY and GEY (1936): 7.0 g NaCl, 0.370 g KCl, 0.170 g $CaCl_2$, 0.070 g $MgSO_4 \times 7\ H_2O$, 0.210 g $Mg\ Cl_2 \times 6H_2O$, 0.150 g $NaHPO_4 \times 2H_2O$, 0.030 g KH_2PO_4, 2.270 g $NaHCO_3$, 3.0 g glucose to 1,000 ml distilled water.

U-^{14}C *glucose:* dissolve in physiological saline to a final concentration of 0.1 mCi/ml.

Standard insulin solution: crystalline bovine or porcine insulin with a specific activity of 25—28 μ/mg.

The standard solution is prepared with n/300 HCl (50 μ/ml).

γ) Method

The hemidiaphragms are incubated in small cylindrical glass vessels (Braun, Melsungen) with 2 ml buffer solution containing glucose (300 mg/100 ml) and 0.05 ml U-^{14}C glucose (5 μCi) is added to each batch. Each value is determined three times. In addition to the assay of basal glycogen synthesis in buffer solution, the activities of 250, 500, and 1,000 μU/ml insulin are measured for each batch and a calibration curve is plotted from these values.

The rats are killed by a blow on the back of the neck; no large amounts of blood should pass into the thorax and abdominal cavity. The abdomen is opened, and the diaphragm excised *in toto* close to the thorax wall with curved scissors and placed in ice-cold buffer solution without glucose. The edges are trimmed with small scissors in the buffer solution and the pieces of fat and connective tissue removed. The diaphragms are cut in half and placed in the incubation vessels, which are gassed briefly with carbogen (95% O_2 and 5% CO_2) and closed with a rubber cap. They are incubated at 37.5° C in a Warburg V85 apparatus and shaken.

δ) Analytic methods

After 90 min incubation, the diaphragms are removed and the glycogen assayed by the method described in section III.1.C. The dry glycogen is dissolved in 0.2 ml distilled water and 0.1 ml is mixed with BRAY's (1960) scintillator solution and the radioactivity determined in the liquid scintillation counter.

ε) Calculation

A graph of the activity of 250, 500 and 1,000 μU/ml of crystalline insulin is plotted in the semilogarithmic coordinate system (Fig. 1) and the insulin concentration of the unknown sample is read off from the calibration curve.

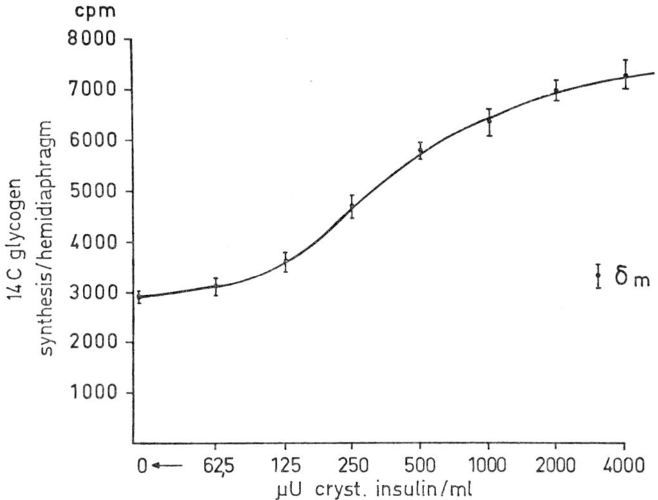

Fig. 1. Effect of crystalline insulin (0—4,000 μU/ml) on the incorporation of U-^{14}C glucose into glycogen of the isolated rat diaphragm (KLÖR, 1968)

b) Determination of the Insulin Activity from $^{14}CO_2$ Production of Isolated Rat Epididymal Adipose Tissue

α) Experimental animals

Non-fasting male rats weighing 120—150 g are killed by a blow on the back of the neck and decapitated. A total of 6 pieces of epididymal adipose tissue is carefully removed from the three-piece appendages close to the base.

β) Materials

Krebs-Ringer bicarbonate buffer solution (KRB) after KREBS and HENSELEIT (1932) is a mixture of 4.0 ml 0.15 *M* KCl, 3.0 ml 0.110 *M* $CaCl_2$, 1.0 ml 0.154 *M* $MgSO_4$, 1.0 ml 0.154 *M* KH_2-PO_4, 100.0 ml 0.154 *M* NaCl gassed with carbogen (95% O_2 and 5% CO_2), with 21.0 ml 0.154 *M* $NaHCO_3$ and 260 mg gelatin or albumin added. The pH is adjusted while gassing once more until a pH of 7.4 is reached. Glucose is added to prepare two KRB-G buffer solutions with 250 and 500 mg/100 ml glucose, respectively.

1-^{14}C *glucose solution:* 1-^{14}C glucose is dissolved in KRB-G to give a final concentration of 0.25 μCi/ml.

Standard insulin solutions: from the standard solution of 50 U/ml insulin fresh insulin solutions containing 50 and 500 μU/ml are prepared daily with KRB-G-250.

γ) Method

Each unknown serum sample is assayed at least twice, preferably four times. For every batch, the effect of 500 and 50 μU/ml crystalline insulin is determined four times to plot the calibration curve. The serum samples are diluted with KRB-G-500 and KRB in the ratio 1:2, the two buffer solutions being added such that the final glucose concentration is 250 mg/100 ml. 0.1 ml 1-^{14}C glucose is pipetted into each incubation tube. The total incubation volume is 2.0 ml. Glass tubes (Braun, Melsungen) are used for incubation. Fat pieces from many rats are stored in buffer solution and distributed so as to give 100 mg fatty tissue in every batch; this is done with sensitive, directly indicating scales. Each tube is briefly gassed once more with carbogen and closed with a rubber cap. The tubes are incubated and shaken at 37.5°C for 180 min in the Warburg V85 apparatus at a frequency of 80/min and an amplitude of 3 cm.

δ) Analytic methods

After incubation 0.2 ml of hyamine hydroxide is injected into the plastic containers attached to the caps and 0.3 ml 10% sulphuric acid into the incubation medium by means of a fine needle, thus keeping the system airtight. Within 1 h the carbon dioxide is completely adsorbed by the hyamine hydroxide and the

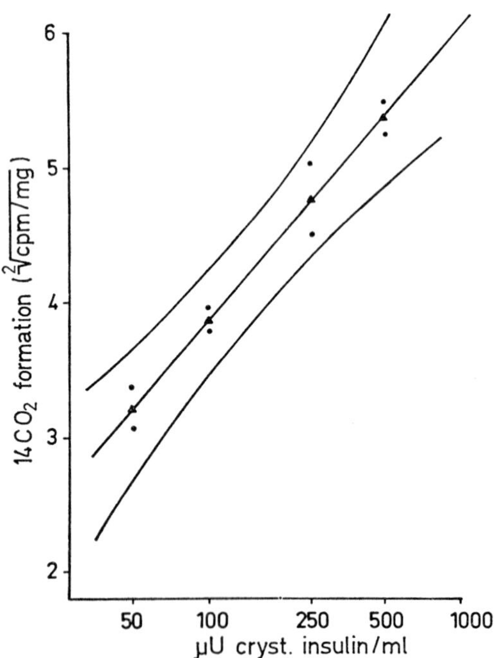

Fig. 2. Effect of insulin on $^{14}CO_2$ formation from 1-^{14}C glucose. The hyperbolae embrace the confidence limits (DITSCHUNEIT, FAULHABER and PFEIFFER, 1962)

incubation tubes can be opened. The plastic containers are removed and placed complete with the adsorption medium in the counting tubes filled with 10.0 ml of BRAY's (1960) scintillator liquid. They are closed, shaken vigorously and the radioactivity determined in the liquid scintillation counter.

ε) Calculation

The counts per min are correlated with the corresponding fat weights (mg) and the square roots of these figures used with the logarithms of the insulin concentrations. The dose-activity relation from 50—500 μU/ml is almost linear so that a calibration curve can be plotted with these two insulin concentrations alone to determine the unknown serum insulin activities (Fig. 2).

δ) Norm

Levels of 135—680 μU/ml were found in the serum of 15 fasting nondiabetics.

IV. Forms of ILA in the Blood and their Significance: Conclusions

All the available methods for the quantitative assay of insulin in blood or other biologic fluids are indirect procedures. They are based on certain insulin-like biologic or immunologic activities in the solutions to be tested. Quantitative determination is carried out by comparing the biologic or immunologic activities with those of crystalline insulin.

1. Immunologic and Biologic ILA

Substances with insulin-like properties have been obtained from the blood, but it has not yet been possible to purify them to the extent that they can be definitely identified as insulin by chemical methods. MARTIN *et al.* (1958) therefore called the value measured by the adipose-tissue method "insulin-like activity" (ILA); this term found general approval and was soon used for the values obtained with the rat-diaphragm method, too.

When comparing the properties of immunologic serum with those of crystalline insulin, it is not legitimate to equate the insulin-like compounds in the serum with insulin. FROESCH *et al.* (1967) logically call the insulin value obtained by immunoassay "immunologic insulin-like activity" and the value determined biologically "biologic insulin-like activity". It depends on the circumstances which of the two principles is better in biologic media. Both have advantages and disadvantages. However, they do not preclude, but to a certain extent supplement each other; therefore both methods have to be employed in particular situations.

In an immunoassay where antibodies are to react specifically with the substance to be assayed, the same substance must be used to form antibodies. Ideally, with an insulin immunoassay, either the insulin extracted from the serum should be employed for immunization, or its chemical identity with the insulin extracted from the pancreas ascertained. So far, it has not been possible to meet these stringent requirements. The immunologic method also involves difficulties in interpretation because insulin antibodies react with biologically inactive fragments of the insulin molecule. YALOW and BERSON (1960), for example, showed that an insulin molecule which has lost 10 amino acids from the B chain and is completely inactive biologically can still react with insulin antibodies.

With biologic methods the specific metabolic effect for the material to be investigated is the main problem. In the case of the insulin assay of the blood, no concrete evidence has been produced. There are also large differences between the biologic serum insulin activity and the immunologic effect on it. For example, much of the biological activity in rat adipose tissue is not inhibited by insulin antibodies, thus indicating that the reaction of insulin antibody with the substance responsible for the biologic activity differs from the reaction of crystalline insulin. The serum factor is probably also responsible for the great discrepancy between biologic and immunologic values. Thus, with the immunologic method only about 10—20 μU/ml was found in the serum of fasting nondiabetics (YALOW and BERSON, 1960; SAMOLS and MARKS, 1963; HALES and RANDLE, 1963; MELANI *et al.*, 1965; LYNGSOE, 1965), whereas with the biologic diaphragm method it was 30—150 μU/ml (VALLANCE-OWEN and HURLOCK, 1954; WRIGHT, 1957, 1960; SELTZER and SMITH, 1959; SELTZER, 1961; SHAW and SHUEY, 1963; ANTONIADES and GUNDERSEN, 1961; ANTONIADES *et al.*, 1962) and with the adipose-tissue method 50—500 μU/ml (STEINKE *et al.*, 1961; LYNGSOE, 1962; DITSCHUNEIT, 1963).

Moreover, the proportion of biologic activity inhibited by insulin antibodies does not correspond at all to the immunologic value. Our own experience has shown that in adipose tissue 50—60% of the activity is inhibited by adding insulin antibodies — a much higher proportion than would be expected from the immunoassay.

In Houssay dogs, which have had first the pituitary and then the pancreas removed, the IMI disappeared from the blood immediately, while the ILA could still be detected up to the end of the experiment, more than 100 days later (SCHÖFFLING, 1966). Surprisingly, the remaining ILA in adipose and muscle tissue was inhibited by antibodies to the same extent as the biologic serum insulin activity in the normal dog; similar results were obtained with insulin activity extracted from animal serum. Similar discrepancies were also found between immunologically measurable hormone concentration and immunologic inhibition of hormone activity in the serum or plasma as regards ACTH. PFEIFFER (1966) pointed out the inadequate correlation between immunologic neutralization of the biologic activity and the antigenetic reactivity of certain protein hormones (insulin, ACTH). Gradually, the complex activity of antibodies against protein hormones seems to be receiving the attention that has long been given to the field of enzyme research (MICHAELI *et al.*, 1967).

The differences between ILA and IMI values become clinically significant in certain diseases. Very high fasting ILA values have been recorded in comparative ILA and IMI determinations in obese patients with and without incipient disorders of glucose metabolism, and they changed only slightly on intravenous glucose loading. On the other hand, the fasting IMI in obese patients gave only moderately increased concentrations, and rose reactively several 100% above the basal values (PFEIFFER, 1968). Clearly, only the IMI reflects the functional hyperinsulinism of obese patients, whereas the ILA remains neutral and takes no recognizable part in the regulation of blood sugar or nutrients.

SÖNKSEN *et al.* (1965) reported good correlation between suppressible ILA and the immunological measurement. FROESCH *et al.* (1969) obtained similar results in comparative investigations in rats. Nevertheless, these authors were only able to inhibit the ILA of human serum samples with insulin antibodies by 7% (FROESCH *et al.*, 1963). On the other hand in obese hyperglycemic mice STAUFFACHER *et al.* (1967) found that the values which could be inhibited by antibodies were 3—4 times higher than those determined immunologically, even when they used mouse insulin, as the standard. These findings indicate that the ILA substance in the serum that reacts with insulin antibodies is more than the amount that can be effective in the competitive displacement of crystalline insulin from the antibody binding in the immunologic method.

Moreover, *in vitro* investigations produced findings which cast doubt on the identity of immunologically measurable and suppressible activity. On incubation of rabbit pancreas sections, higher values were measured with the biologic method on isolated rat adipose tissue than with the immunologic method in the incubation media (Fig. 3). After glucose stimulation of insulin secretion, both values rose, but the biologic, value went much higher than the immunologic value. On the other hand, the addition of antibodies completely suppressed the biologic value (DITSCHUNEIT *et al.*, 1966). This observation shows that after glucose stimulation of insulin secretion too, substances are secreted which react with insulin antibodies, but not in the same way as the crystalline insulin used as the standard in the assay. So far there have been no investigations into the nature of these substances, or the various insulin antibody preparations.

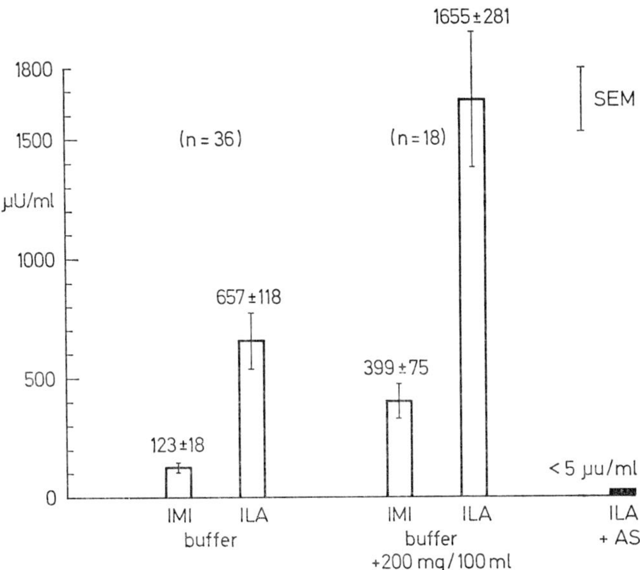

Fig. 3. Secretion of insulin from isolated rabbit pancreas sections (with and without the addition of glucose) compared in immunologic (IMI) and biologic (ILA) insulin assays. Complete neutralization of the ILA occurs when insulin antiserum is added

2. Nonsuppressible Insulin-like Activity (NSILA)

Great efforts are being made to identify the nonsuppressible insulin-like activity (NSILA) in the serum, but they have so far not been very successful. The investigations of FROESCH *et al.* (1967) clearly show that NSILA does not interfere with acute blood sugar regulation and bears no relationship to the insulin produced in the β cells. This form of ILA is not changed by pancreatectomy (FROESCH *et al.*, 1967).

The NSILA fractions were divided into two components by physicochemical methods (JACOB *et al.*, 1968; BÜRGI *et al.*, 1966). One component contains approximately 90% of the total NSILA and consists of a large protein with a molecular weight of 100,000—150,000.

It is precipitated by hydrochloric acid alcohol and inactivated by heat. Because it can be precipitated, it was termed NSILA-P. The other component is about 5—10% of the total NSILA and has a molecular weight of 6,000—10,000. This substance is heat-resistant and soluble in hydrochloric acid alcohol, and was therefore called NSILA-S by BÜRGI *et al.* (1966). The soluble fraction of NSILA has many insulin-like properties. In adrenalectomized rats it reduces the blood sugar and free fatty acids for a longer period than insulin, since unlike insulin it is not activated by the liver. NSILA-S stimulates the incorporation of ^{14}C glucose into the diaphragm glycogen to a greater extent than insulin, while both substances have the same effect in adipose tissue. According to the investigations of OELZ *et al.* (1970) NSILA-S seems to have a special affinity for the muscle cell membrane.

3. Bound Insulin

The total fraction of nonsuppressible ILA is similar in certain respects to the "bound insulin" described by ANTONIADES *et al.* (1958). In numerous publications since 1958 ANTONIADES and coworkers have attempted to substantiate the hypothesis that insulin circulates in the blood in both biologically active and inactive forms (ANTONIADES, 1965a, b, 1966, 1967; ANTONIADES *et al.*, 1961; ANTONIADES *et al.*, 1962; ANTONIADES and GERSHOFF, 1966; ANTONIADES *et al.*, 1965). The bound form is said to be produced in the liver and other extrapancreatic tissues from the free active insulin secreted by the pancreas. In the fasting state insulin is mainly bound and activated by an increase in blood sugar. The two forms can be separated on cation exchange resins, the bound form being adsorbed to the resin. After elution, it can be concentrated to 3,000 times by means of hydrochloric acid alcohol. Because it binds to cation-exchange resin, ANTONIADES assumes that bound insulin comprises pancreas insulin and a basic protein. Its molecular weight is said to be between 40,000 and 60,000 and it is inactivated by glutathione. On electrophoresis the bound insulin migrates with the β- and γ-globulins, and the free insulin with the α1-globulins/albumins. *In vitro* bound insulin is active only in isolated adipose tissue and is not inhibited by antibodies. In the isolated diaphragm it can be activated by an extract from adipose tissue. *In vivo*, bound insulin has a hypoglycemic effect in adrenalectomized and hypophysectomized rats by stimulating glycogenesis in the muscles and lipogenesis in adipose tissues.

Unlike the NSILA described by FROESCH and co-workers, most of the bound insulin is said to disappear from the blood of pancreatectomized rats. This is considered to be an indication that bound insulin originates in the peripheral blood from pancreatic insulin.

Bound insulin in the rat diaphragm is activated by adding adipose tissue extract. According to ANTONIADES *et al.* (1965) the extract also has a hypoglycemic effect in insulin-sensitive adrenalectomized rats due to activation of the bound insulin in the periphery.

4. Synalbumin

Insulin-like substances were also demonstrated in the albumin fraction precipitated from the serum with hydrochloric acid alcohol (DITSCHUNEIT, 1966, 1967, 1968a, b, 1969; DITSCHUNEIT *et al.*, 1968). In this fraction VALLANCE-OWEN found the much-discussed insulin antagonist synalbumin (VALLANCE-OWEN *et al.*, 1958a, b; VALLANCE-OWEN, 1961). The insulin-like fraction that can be precipitated with hydrochloric acid alcohol contains a substance which, when injected intraperitoneally, has a metabolic action in muscle and adipose tissues, but which cannot be inhibited by insulin antibodies. The lack of suppression by antibodies has also been demonstrated *in vitro* on isolated adipose tissue and fat cells (DITSCHUNEIT, 1966,

1967). The ILA also extends to the antilipolytic action, as has been shown in isolated fat cells (DITSCHUNEIT, 1966, 1967). This insulin-like substance is accumulated by column chromatography with Dowex-50. On electrophoresis it migrates with the β- and γ-globulins, and therefore bears a certain similarity to "bound insulin". As already mentioned, it is detectable for a long time in hypophysectomized and pancreatectomized dogs, and is therefore probably not related to pancreatic insulin. POFFENBARGER *et al.* (1968) showed that the ILA of the bound insulin, precipitated albumin, and nonsuppressible insulin is the same compound. It is present in the serum in relatively high concentrations, but does not play an active part in controlling the blood sugar, and its physiological significance is so far unknown. Structurally, it is certainly different from insulin and, as far as is known, it is not secreted by any specific organ. A large part of the activity in all insulin bioassays is due to this compound; the currently undeterminable magnitude should therefore be attributed to the insulin-like activities measured by biologic methods.

References

ANDERSON, E., LINDER, E., SUTTON, V.: A sensitive method for the assay of insulin in blood. Amer. J. Physiol. **149**, 350 (1947)

ANDERSON, E., WHERRY, F., BATES, R.W., CORNFIELD, J.: A method for assay of insulin using alloxan diabetic hypophysectomized mouse. Proc. Soc. exp. Biol. (N.Y.) **94**, 321 (1957)

ANTONIADES, H.N., BEIGELMAN, P.M., TRANQUADA, R.B., GUNDERSEN, K.: Studies on the state of insulin in blood: free insulin and insulin complexes in human sera and their *in vitro* biological properties. Endocrinology **69**, 46 (1961)

ANTONIADES, H.N.: Extrapancreatic regulation of insulin activity in human beings. 5. Congr. Internat. Diab. Fed., Toronto. Amsterdam: Excerpta Medica Found. 1965

ANTONIADES, H.N.: Bound insulin and tissue resistance to insulin. Lancet **2**, 159 (1965b)

ANTONIADES, H.N.: Rat serum "bound" insulin: *In vivo* biologic effects in rats. Diabetes **15**, 889 (1966)

ANTONIADES, H.N.: Bound insulin: Further purification and *in vivo* biologic activity in rats. Vox Sang. (Basel) **13**, 49 (1967)

ANTONIADES, H.N., BEIGELMAN, P.M., PENNELL, R.B., THORN, G.W., ONCLEY, J.L.: Insulin-like activity in human plasma constituents. III. Elution of insulin-like activity from cation resin. Metabolism **7**, 266 (1958)

ANTONIADES, H.N., BEIGELMAN, P.M., TRANQUADA, R.B., GUNDERSEN, K.: Studies on the state of insulin in blood: free insulin and insulin complexes in human sera and their *in vitro* biological properties. Endocrinology **69**, 46 (1961)

ANTONIADES, H.N., BOUGAS, J.A., PYLA, H.M.: Studies on the state of insulin in blood: Examination of splenic, portal and peripheral blood serum of diabetic and non-diabetic subjects for free insulin and insulin complexes. New Engl. J. Med. **267**, 218 (1962)

ANTONIADES, H.N., GERSHOFF, S.N.: Inhibitory effects of bound insulin on insulin uptake by isolated tissues. Diabetes **15**, 655 (1966)

ANTONIADES, H.N., GUNDERSEN, U.: Studies on the state of insulin in blood: Materials and methods for the estimation of free and bound insulin in sera. Endocrinology **70**, 95 (1962)

ANTONIADES, H.N., HUBER, A.M., GERSHOFF, S.N.: Bound insulin: *in vivo* and *in vitro* biologic activity. Diabetologia **1**, 195 (1965)

BAIRD, C.W., BORNSTEIN, J.: Assay of insulin-like activity in the plasma of normal and diabetic human subjects. J. Endocr. **19**, 74 (1959)

BALL, E.G., MARTIN, D.B., COOPER, O.: Studies on the metabolism of adipose tissue. I. The effect of insulin on glucose utilization as measured by the manometric determination of carbon dioxide output. J. biol. Chem. **234**, 774 (1959)

BALMAIN, J.H., COX, C.P., FOLLEY, S.J., MCNAUGHT, M.L.: Bioassay of insulin *in vitro* by manometric measurements on slices of mammary glands. J. Endocr. **11**, 269 (1954)

BANTING, F.G., BEST, C.H., COLLIP, J.B., MACLEOD, J.J.R., NOBLE, E.C.: The effect of pancreatic extract (insulin) on normal rabbits. Amer. J. Physiol. **62**, 162 (1922)

BEIGELMAN, P.M.: Bioassay for insulin-like activity utilizing glucose uptake by rat epididymal adipose tissue. Metabolism **9**, 580 (1960)

BEIGELMAN, P.M., GOETZ, F.C., ANTONIADES, H.N., THORN, G.W.: Insulin-like activity of human plasma constituents. I. Description and evaluation of biologic assay for insulin-like activity. Metabolism **5**, 35 (1956)

Bornstein, J.: A technique for the assay of small quantities of insulin using alloxan-diabetic, hypophysectomized, and adrenalectomized rats. Aust. J. exp. Biol. med. Sci. **28**, 87 (1950)

Bornstein, J., Lawrence, R.D.: Two types of diabetes mellitus with and without available plasma insulin. Brit. med. J. **1**, 732 (1951)

Bray, G.A.: A simple, efficient liquid scintillator for counting aqueous solutions in a liquid scintillation counter. Analyt. Biochem. **1**, 297 (1960)

Bürgi, H., Müller, W.A., Humbel, R.E., Labhart, A., Froesch, E.R.: Nonsuppressible insulin-like activity of human serum. I. Physicochemical properties, extraction and partial purification. Biochim. biophys. Acta (Amst.) **121**, 349 (1966)

Cahill, G.F., Leboeuf, B., Renold, A.E.: Studies on rat adipose tissue *in vitro*. III. Synthesis of glycogen and glycerid-glycerol. J. biol. Chem. **234**, 2540 (1959)

Cahill, G.F., Leboeuf, B., Flinn, R.B.: Studies on rat adipose tissue *in vitro*. VI. Effect of epinephrine on glucose metabolism. J. biol. Chem. **235**, 1246 (1960)

Cunningham, N.F.: The insulin activity of bovine and ovine blood plasma. I. Biological assay of insulin using the isolated rat diaphragm. J. Endocr. **25**, 35 (1962)

Ditschuneit, H., Ziegler, R., Pfeiffer, E.F.: Über die Bestimmung von Insulin im Blute am epididymalen Fettanhang der Ratte mit Hilfe markierter Glukose. Die Wirkung von menschlichem und bovinem Wachstumshormon und anderen Stoffwechselhormonen auf den Kohlenhydratstoffwechsel des isolierten Rattenfettgewebes. Klin. Wschr. **39**, 426 (1961)

Ditschuneit, H., Faulhaber, J.-D., Pfeiffer, E.F.: Verbesserung der Methode zur Bestimmung von Insulin im Blut mit Hilfe radioaktiver 1-^{14}-C-Glucose und dem epididymalen Rattenfettgewebe. Atompraxis **8**, 172 (1962)

Ditschuneit, H.: Die biologische und klinische Bedeutung der Insulinwirkung von Blut- und Bluteiweißfraktionen. Vergleichende Untersuchungen an Stoffwechselgesunden, Diabetikern und Prädiabetikern. Habilitationsschrift, Universität Frankfurt/Main, 1963

Ditschuneit, H.: Insulinantagonisten. Tagung der Dtsch. Ges. f. Endokrinologie, Wiesbaden 1966, S. 83. Berlin-Göttingen-New York: Springer 1967

Ditschuneit, H.: Die hormonale Regulation der Lipogenese unter besonderer Berücksichtigung von Diabetes und Fettsucht. Acta diabet. lat. **5**, 364 (1968a)

Ditschuneit, H.: Die hormonelle Regulation von Lipolyse und Lipogenese des Fettgewebes. Therapiewoche **18**, 2015 (1968b)

Ditschuneit, H.: Definition and criteria of prediabetes. 6th Congr. Internat. Diab. Fed. Stockholm, 1967, p. 479. Amsterdam: Excerpta Medica Found. 1969

Ditschuneit, H., Faulhaber, J.-D., Petruzzi, E.N.: Weitere Untersuchungen zur Charakterisierung und Identifizierung der im „Synalbumin" enthaltenen Substanz mit lipogenetischen und antilipolytischen Eigenschaften. 3. Kongr. Dtsch. Diab. Ges., Göttingen, 7.—8. 6. 1968

Ditschuneit, H., Beyer, J., Melani, F., Schöffling, K., Telib, M., Pfeiffer, E.F.: Vergleich zwischen biologischer und radio-immunologischer Insulinbestimmung. Proc. of the Conference on problems connected with the preparation and use of labelled proteins in tracer studies. S. 335, Pisa, 1966

Fraser, D.T.: White mice and the assay of insulin. J. Lab. clin. Med. **8**, 425 (1923)

Froesch, E.R., Bürgi, H., Müller, W.A., Humbel, R.E., Jakob, A., Labhart, A.: Nonsuppressible insulin-like activity of human serum: purification, physicochemical and biological properties, and its relation to total serum ILA. Recent Progr. Hormone Res. **23**, 565 (1967)

Froesch, E.R., Bürgi, H., Ramseier, E.B., Bally, P., Labhart, A.: Antibody-suppressible and nonsuppressible insulin-like activities in human serum and their physiologic significance. An insulin assay with adipose tissue of increased precision and specificity. J. clin. Invest. **42**, 1816 (1963)

Froesch, E.R., Jakob, A., Labhart, A.: Suppressible and non-suppressible ILA of human serum. 6. Congr. Intern. Diab. Fed. Stockholm, 1967, p. 157. Amsterdam: Excerpta Medica Found. 1969

Gellhorn, E., Feldman, J., Allen, A.: Assay of insulin on hypophysectomized, adrenodemedullated and hypophysectomized-adrenodemedullated rats. Endocrinology **29**, 137 (1941)

Gemmill, C.L.: The effect of insulin on the glycogen content of isolated muscles. Bull. Johns Hopk. Hosp. **66**, 232 (1940)

Gemmill, C.L., Hamman, L.: The effect of insulin on glycogen deposition and on glucose utilization by isolated muscles. Bull. Johns Hopk. Hosp. **68**, 50 (1941)

Gey, G.O., Gey, M.K.: The maintenance of human normal cells and tumor cells in continuous culture. I. Preliminary report: Cultivation of mesoplastic tumors and normal tissue and notes on methods of cultivation. Cancer **27**, 45 (1936)

Gliemann, J.: Insulin-like activity of dilute human serum assayed by an isolated adipose cell method. Diabetes **14**, 643 (1965)

GLIEMANN, J.: Assay of insulin-like activity by the isolated fat cell method. I. Factors influencing the response to crystalline insulin. Diabetologia **3**, 382 (1967a)

GLIEMANN, J.: Assay of insulin-like activity by the isolated fat cell method. II. The suppressible and nonsuppressible insulin-like activity of serum. Diabetologia **3**, 389 (1967b)

GROEN, J., KAMMINGA, C.E., WILLEBRANDS, A.F., BLICKMAN, J.R.: Evidence for the presence of insulin in blood serum. A method for an approximate determination of the insulin content of blood. J. clin. Invest. **31**, 97 (1952)

HALES, C.N., RANDLE, P.J.: Immunoassay of insulin with insulin-antibody precipitate. Biochem. J. **88**, 137 (1963)

HAUGAARD, N., MARSH, J.B.: Effect of insulin on the metabolism of adipose tissue from normal rats. J. biol. Chem. **194**, 33 (1952)

HEMMINGSEN, A.M., KROGH, A.: The biological standardisation of insulin, including reports on the preparation of the international standard and the definition of the unit. (Publication of the League of Nations III, Health, III. 7, C.H. 398, p. 40). League of Nations Health Organisation, Genf, 1926

HILL, J.B.: The adsorption of I^{131}insulin to glass. Endocrinology **65**, 515 (1959)

HUMBEL, R.E.: Messung der Serum-Insulin-Aktivität mit epididymalem Ratten-Fettgewebe *in vitro*. Experientia (Basel) **15**, 256 (1959)

JAKOB, A., HAURI, CH., FROESCH, E.R.: Nonsuppressible insulin-like activity in human serum. III. Differentiation of two distinct molecules with nonsuppressible ILA. J. clin. Invest. **47**, 2678 (1968)

JEANRENAUD, B., RENOLD, A.E.: Studies on rat adipose tissue *in vitro*. IV. Metabolic patterns produced in rat adipose tissue by varying insulin and glucose concentrations independently from each other. J. biol. Chem. **234**, 3082 (1959)

JESSUP, D.C., WIBERG, G.S.: Insulin bioassay using glycogen deposition in a single rat diaphragm. Diabetes **10**, 201 (1961a)

JESSUP, D.C., WIBERG, G.S.: Effects of incubation conditions on the *in vitro* assay method for insulin. Canad. J. Biochem. **39**, 1381 (1961b)

KLÖR, H.-U.: Vergleichende Untersuchungen über die insulin-ähnliche Wirkung (ILA) von Serumeiweißfraktionen am isolierten Diaphragma und am isolierten epididymalen Fettgewebe der Ratte. Dissertation, Universität Ulm, 1968

KRAHL, M.E., PARK, C.R.: The uptake of glucose by the isolated diaphragm of normal and hypophysectomized rats. J. biol. Chem. **174**, 939 (1948)

KREBS, H.A., EGGLESTON, L.V.: Effect of insulin on oxidations in isolated muscle tissue. Biochem. J. **32**, 913 (1938)

KREBS, H.A., HENSELEIT, K.: Untersuchungen über die Harnstoffbildung im Tierkörper. Z. physiol. Chem. **210**, 33 (1932)

KUZUYA, N., SAMOLS, E., WILLIAMS, R.H.: Stimulation by hyperosmolarity of glucose metabolism in rat adipose tissue and diaphragm *in vitro*. J. biol. Chem. **240**, 2277 (1965)

LEONARDS, J.R., LANDAU, B.R., BARTSCH, G.: Assay of insulin-like activity with rat epididymal fat pad. J. Lab. clin. Med. **60**, 552 (1962)

LESLIE, I., PAUL, J.: The action of insulin on the composition of cells and medium during culture of chick heart explants. J. Endocr. **11**, 110 (1954)

LYNGSOE, J.: The insulin-like activity in serum determined by the rat epididymal fat method. I. Normal values in undiluted and diluted serum, and the effect of ingestion of glucose. Acta med. scand. **171**, 365 (1962)

LYNGSOE, J.: Serum insulin. A review. Acta med. scand. **179**, Suppl. 441, 1 (1965)

MANCHESTER, K.L., YOUNG, F.G.: The effect of insulin on incorporation of amino acids into protein of normal rat diaphragm *in vitro*. Biochem. J. **70**, 353 (1958)

MANCHESTER, K.L., RANDLE, P.J., YOUNG, F.G.: An insulin assay based on the incorporation of labelled glycine into the protein of isolated rat diaphragm. J. Endocr. **19**, 259 (1959)

MARTIN, D.B., RENOLD, A.E., DAGENAIS, Y.M.: An assay for insulin-like activity using rat adipose tissue. Lancet **1958 II**, 76

MELANI, F., DITSCHUNEIT, H., BARTELT, K.M., FRIEDRICH, H., PFEIFFER, E.F.: Über die radioimmunologische Bestimmung von Insulin im Blut. Klin. Wschr. **43**, 1000 (1965)

METZ, R.: The effect of blood glucose concentration on insulin output. Diabetes **8**, 89 (1960)

MILSTEIN, S.W.: Oxidation of specifically labelled glucose by rat adipose tissue. Proc. Soc. exp. Biol. (N.Y.) **92**, 632 (1956)

MOODY, A.J., FELBER, J.P.: Effect of insulin on the formation of glycogen by the mouse diaphragm in the presence and absence of glucose. Diabetes **15**, 492 (1966)

OELZE, O., JAKOB, A., FROESCH, E.R.: Nonsuppressible insulin-like activity (NSILA) of human serum. V. Hypoglycaemia and preferential metabolic stimulation of muscle by NSILA-S. Europ. J. clin. Invest. **1**, 48 (1970)

PERLMUTTER, M., WEISENFELD, S., MUFSON, M.: Bio-assay of insulin in serum using the rat diaphragm. Endocrinology **50**, 442 (1952)

POFFENBARGER, P.L., ENSINCK, J.W., HEPP, D.K., WILLIAMS, R.H.: The nature of human serum insulin-like activity (ILA) characterization of ILA in serum and serum fractions obtained by acid-ethanol extraction and adsorption chromatography. J. clin. Invest. **47**, 301 (1968)

RAFAELSEN, O.J.: Action of insulin and other substances on glycogen synthesis of rat diaphragm *in vivo*. p. 625. In: 4. Congr. de la Fédérat. Intern. du Diabète, Med. Hyg. (Genf) 1961

RAFAELSEN, O.J.: Glycogen content of rat diaphragm after intraperitoneal injection of insulin and other hormones. Acta physiol. scand. **61**, 314 (1964a)

RAFAELSEN, O.J.: Insulin-like activity of human serum determined by glycogen increase of diaphragm after intraperitoneal injection into the intact rat. Acta physiol. scand. **61**, 323 (1964b)

RAFAELSEN, O.J., LAURIS, V., RENOLD, A.E.: Localized intraperitoneal action of insulin on rat diaphragm and epididymal adipose tissue *in vivo*. Diabetes **14**, 19 (1965)

RAMSEIER, E.B., FROESCH, E.R., BALLY, P., LABHART, A.: Serum-Insulinbestimmung am Fettgewebe *in vitro*: Beeinflussung durch andere Hormone, „freie" und „gebundene" Insulinaktivität. Med. Hyg. **20**, 643 (1962)

RANDLE, P.J.: Assay of Plasma Insulin Activity by the Rat-Diaphragm Method. Brit. med. Bull. **1954 I**, 1237

RANDLE, P.J.: Insulin in blood. Ciba Found. Collog. Endocrinol. **11**, 115 (1957)

RANDLE, P.J., WHITNEY, J.E.: *In vitro* effect of growth hormone on the glucose uptake of isolated rat diaphragm. Nature (Lond.) **179**, 472 (1957)

RENOLD, A.E., MARTIN, D.B., DAGENAIS, Y.M., STEINKE, J., NICKERSON, R.J., SHEPS, M.C.: Measurement of small quantities of insulin-like activity using rat adipose tissue. I. A proposed procedure. J. clin. Invest. **39**, 1487 (1960)

RODBELL, M.: Metabolism of isolated fat cells. I. Effects of hormones on glucose metabolism and lipolysis. J. biol. Chem. **239**, 375 (1964)

ROTH, J., GORDON, P., PASTAN, I.: "Big insulin": a new component of plasma insulin detected by immunoassay. Proc. nat. Acad. Sci. (Wash.) **61**, 138 (1968)

SAMAAN, N., FRASER, R., DEMPSTER, W.J.: The "typical" and "atypical" forms of serum insulin. Diabetes **12**, 339 (1963)

SAMOLS, E., MARKS, V.: Insulin assay in insulinomas. Brit. med. J. **5329**, 507 (1963)

SANGER, F., TUPPY, H.: The amino-acid sequence in the phenylalanyl chain of insulin. I. The identification of lower peptides from partial hydrolysates. Biochem. J. **49**, 463 (1951)

SCHÖFFLING, K., BEYER, J., ALTHOFF, P., WALTER, A., DITSCHUNEIT, H., MELANI, F., DITSCHUNEIT, H.H., AMMON, J., PFEIFFER, E.F.: Weitere Untersuchungen über das Verhalten der beiden Insulinaktivitäten und des immunologisch nachweisbaren Insulins am hypophysektomierten und pankreatektomierten Hunde. Diabetologia **1**, 77 (1965)

SELTZER, H.S., SMITH, W.L.: Plasma insulin activity after glucose; an index of insulogenic reserve in normal and diabetic man. Diabetes **8**, 417 (1959)

SELTZER, H.S., SMITH, W.L.: Exhaustion of insulogenic reserve in maturity-onset diabetics during prolonged and continuous hyperglycemic stress. p. 650. IV. Kongr. Intern. Diab. Fed., Ed. Medicine u. Hygiene, Genf 1961

SHAW, W.N., SHUEY, E.W.: The presence of two forms of insulin in normal human serum. Biochemistry (Wash.) **2**, 286 (1963)

SHORT, A.L., WRIGHT, F.E., WHITNEY, J.E.: Effect of anaerobiosis and cell poisons on glucose uptake of hemidiaphrams and epididymal fat pads *in vitro*. Diabetes **14**, 128 (1965)

SINEX, F.M., MACMULLEN, J., HASTINGS, A.B.: Effect of insulin on incorporation of ^{14}C amino acids into protein of rat diaphragm. J. biol. Chem. **198**, 615 (1952)

SLATER, J.D.H., SAMAAN, N.A., FRASER, R., STILLMAN, D.: Immunologic studies with circulating insulin. Brit. med. J. **1**, 1712 (1961)

SNEDECOR, J.G., DE MEIO, R.H., PINCUS, I.J.: Reduction by glucagon of glycogen deposition effect of insulin in rat diaphragm. Proc. Soc. exp. Biol. (N.Y.) **89**, 396 (1955)

SÖNKSEN, P.H., ELLIS, J.P., LOWY, C., RUTHERFORD, A., NABARRO, J.D.N.: Plasma insulin: A correlation between bioassay and immunoassay. Brit. med. J. **5455**, 209 (1965)

STAUFFACHER, W., LAMBERT, A.E., VECCHIO, D., RENOLD, A.E.: Measurements of insulin activities in pancreas and serum of mice with spontaneous (obese and New Zealand obese) and induced (gold thioglucose) obesity and hypoglycemia with consideratious on the pathogenesis of the spontaneous syndrome. Diabetologia **3**, 230 (1967)

STADIE, W.C., ZAPP, J.A.: The effect of insulin upon synthesis of glycogen by rat diaphragm *in vitro*. J. biol. Chem. **170**, 55 (1947)

STADIE, W.C., HAUGGARD, N., MARSH, J.B.: Combination of epinephrine and 2,4-dinitrophenol with muscle of the normal rat. J. biol. Chem. **188**, 173 (1951)

STEINER, D.F., OYER, P.E.: The biosynthesis of insulin and a probable precursor of insulin by a human islet-cell adenoma. Proc. nat. Acad. Sci. (Wash.) **57**, 473 (1967)

STEINKE, J., CAMERINI-DAVALOS, R., MARBLE, A., RENOLD, A.E.: Elevated levels of serum ILA as measured with adipose tissue in early untreated diabetes and prediabetes. Metabolism **10**, 707 (1961)

TREVAN, J.W., BOOCK, R.: The biological standardisation of insulin including reports on the preparation of the international standard and the definition of the unit. (Publication of the League of Nations III, Health, III. 7, C.H. 398, p. 47). League of Nations Health Organisation, Genf, 1926

VALLANCE-OWEN, J., HURLOCK, B.: Estimation of plasma-insulin by the rat-diaphragm method. Lancet **1954 I**, 68

VALLANCE-OWEN, J., LUKENS, F.D.W.: Studies on insulin antagonism in plasma. Endocrinology **60**, 625 (1957)

VALLANCE-OWEN, J., LILLEY, M.D.: An insulin antagonist associated with plasma albumin. Lancet **1**, 804 (1961)

VALLANCE-OWEN, J., DENNES, E., CAMPBELL, P.N.: The nature of the insulin antagonist associated with plasma albumin. Lancet **2**, 696 (1958b)

VALLANCE-OWEN, J., DENNES, E., CAMPBELL, P.N.: Insulin antagonism in plasma of diabetic patients and normal subjects. Lancet **2**, 336 (1958a)

DU VIGNEAUD, V.A., FITCH, A., PEKAREK, E., LOCKWOOD, W.W.: The inactivation of crystalline insulin by cysteine and glutamine. J. biol. Chem. **94**, 233 (1931)

VILLAR-PALASI, C., LARNER, J.: Insulin treatment and increased UDPG-glycogen transglucosylase activity in muscle. Arch. Biochem. **94**, 436 (1961)

WALAAS, E., WALAAS, O.: The effect of noradrenaline and adrenochrome on carbohydrate metabolism of rat diaphragm. Biochim. biophys. Acta (Amst.) **20**, 77 (1956)

WILLEBRANDS, A.F., VAN DER GELD, H., GROEN, J.: Determination of serum insulin using the isolated rat diaphragm: The effect of serum dilution. Diabetes **7**, 119 (1958)

WILLEBRANDS, A.F., GROEN, J., KAMMINGA, C.E., BLICKMAN, J.R.: Quantitative aspects of the action of insulin on the glucose and potassium metabolism of the isolated rat diaphragm. Science **112**, 277 (1950)

WINEGRAD, A.I., RENOLD, A.E.: Studies on rat adipose tissue *in vitro*. I. Effects of insulin on the metabolism of glucose, pyruvate and acetate. J. biol. Chem. **233**, 267 (1958a)

WINEGRAD, A.I., RENOLD, A.E.: Studies on rat adipose tissue *in vitro*. II. Effects of insulin on the metabolism of specifically labeled glucose. J. biol. Chem. **233**, 273 (1958b)

WINEGRAD, A.I., SHAW, W.N., LUKENS, F.D.W., STADIE, W.C.: Effects of prolactin *in vitro* on fatty acid synthesis in rat adipose tissue. J. biol. Chem. **234**, 3111 (1959)

WISEMAN, R., BALTZ, B.: Prevention of insulin-I-131 adsorption to glass. Endocrinology **68**, 354 (1961)

WOODS, M., WIGHT, K., HUNTER, J., BURK, D.: Effects of insulin on melanoma and brain metabolism. Biochim. biophys. Acta (Amst.) **12**, 329 (1953)

WRIGHT, P.H.: Plasma-insulin estimation by the rat-diaphragm method. Lancet **2**, 621 (1957)

WRIGHT, P.H.: Plasma-insulin activity in acromegaly and spontaneous hypoglycemia. Lancet **2**, 951 (1960)

YALOW, R.S., BERSON, S.A.: Immunoassay of endogenous plasma insulin in man. J. clin. Invest. **39**, 1157 (1960)

C. Methods for the Standardization of Insulin and the Determination of Blood Glucose Concentration

August W. Forst and Sigurd Hansen

I. Standardization of Insulin

1. Synopsis and Introduction

The following references are relevant to a review of the present topic:

Best, 1938; Burn, 1928; Burn and Bülbring, 1937; Geiling *et al.*, 1937; Bomskow, 1937; De Jongh and Laqueur, 1938; Spanhoff, 1938; Van Eekelen and Van Esveld, 1941; Rausch, 1947; Kaernbach, 1952; Hahn *et al.*, 1956a, b; 1957a, b; Burn *et al.*, 1950; Stewart, 1960; Voldan, 1966; Lacey, 1967; Ashford *et al.*, 1969; Pharmacopoeia Internationalis, 1957/68; Pharmacopoeia Austrica, 1960; Pharmacopoeia Britannica, 1973; European Pharmacopoeia, 1969—1974; Pharmacopoeia Helvetica, 1971; US Pharmacopoeia, 1970; Editorial, 1970; Stein, 1972; WHO, 1973.

Crystallized insulin is not a single pure substance but is made up of varying amounts of insulin and proinsulin (Lubetzki, 1969; Rolando and Torroba, 1972). The dosage of insulin is thus defined, not by weight, but by the biological activity of the particular preparation used. Neither chemical nor physical methods are capable of measuring this activity. Even biological methods, applied *in vitro* to isolated tissues, do not meet all the requirements of insulin standardization. Such procedures are based on the metabolic effects induced by insulin in muscle or adipose tissue, which may per se yield quantitative information. The same is true of the effects of insulin on gas exchange by pigeon breast muscle and slices of mammary gland. Whether and to what extent radioimmunological methods could be applied has not yet been decided.

Thus, even today, insulin is standardized in the whole, intact animal. In order to define the biological activity of insulin, an international unit for insulin was established in 1926 by the League of Nations in Geneva. The international unit is based on the blood sugar-lowering effect of insulin; it has been defined as the amount of insulin that lowers the blood glucose level of a fasting rabbit of 2 kg body weight to 0.045% within 2—4 h. At this blood glucose concentration, the majority of animals exhibited hypoglycemic convulsions (League of Nations, 1926). The official definition of the unit was subject to changes in the following years (GEILING *et al.*, 1937; see also KÜHNE, 1966). The unit of the currently valid Fourth Standard is defined as the amount of insulin that, when injected subcutaneously, lowers the blood glucose of a normal rabbit of 2 kg body weight to 0.064% within 1 h and to 0.045% after 2 h. This activity is present in 0.04167 mg of the Fourth International Standard insulin preparation (BANGHAM and MUSSETT, 1959; STEWART, 1960; LACEY, 1967; PFEIFFER, 1971). When correctly stored, the standard preparation does not lose its biological activity (LACEY, 1968; PINGEL and VOLUND, 1972). The standard is supplied by various international centers (PERRY, 1955).

2. Methods of Standardization

Only two methods are accepted for testing the biological activity of the standard itself, or for comparing the activity of various preparations of insulin with the standard. These are the mouse convulsion test and the blood glucose test on the rabbit. The convulsion test measures the proportion of mice showing hypoglycemic convulsions, and the test on rabbits is based on the degree of the hypoglycemic response. The older literature is reviewed by GEILING *et al.* (1937). Only these two methods are considered reliable enough for incorporation into official pharmacopoeias (SPANNHOFF, 1938; F.D.A.: Insulin Regulations, 1955; VOLDAN, 1966).

a) Mouse Convulsion Test

The subcutaneous injection of small amounts of insulin induces hypoglycemic convulsions in mice; the percentage of animals affected within a given group increases with increasing dose of insulin. The mouse is the most suitable animal species for this test. In principle, little has changed in this now classic method since it was first developed (GEILING *et al.*, 1937): a few improvements to the procedure have been recommended (THOMPSON, 1946; YOUNG and LEWIS, 1947). Tolerance of insulin by inbred animals is one recognized source of error (CHASE *et al.*, 1948). Other factors which may give rise to erroneous results have been pointed out by IRWIN (1943), YOUNG and STEWART (1952), and J. Pharmacy and Pharmacology **4**, 382—391 (1952). The mouse convulsion test requires large number of animals. Details of the procedure itself, of the calculation of data, and statistical evaluation may be found in the papers of BOMSKOW (1937), BURN *et al.* (1950) and in the pharmacopoeias.

b) Hypoglycemic Effect in Rabbits

In principle, it should be possible to measure the activity of insulin preparations not only from normoglycemic but also from hyperglycemic blood glucose levels of diabetic animals (See also Vol. I of this handbook, pp. 159—202 and 203—273). In practice, the blood sugar-lowering effect in normoglycemic rabbits gives the best results (RAUSCH, 1947). The blood-glucose response is subject to biological variations and multiple factors may interfere with the results (EDITORIAL, 1970; HASSELBLATT, 1969). The cross-over test was introduced by MARKS (1925) in an attempt to eliminate such factors. In this test, both the unknown insulin solution and the standard are tested in the same group of animals. The main advantage of the cross-over test, which may be done one, two, or three times, is that it eliminates most of the variability caused by variations in sensitivity between individual animals. The principal procedure of this test remains valid, with some minor modifications. When standardization of insulin is based on measurements of blood glucose, it is important to take into account findings on circadian rhythms in animals (Hrubetz, 1934; Stamm, 1967; Cohn, 1972; Jarret *et al.*, 1972).

Statistical evaluation is discussed in the original literature (Hershey and Lacey, 1936; Walden, 1936; Marks and Pak, 1936; Smith *et al.*, 1944; Lacey, 1941, 1946; Hahn *et al.*, 1957a, 1957b; see also Bomskow, 1937).

Blood glucose estimations are usually done in deproteinized blood samples; some authors believe that this step can be eliminated by diluting the blood sample (Feteris, 1965; Stork and Schmidt, 1968). The literature concerning deproteinization by heavy metals, metalloids, and organic agents, or by dialysis etc., is bulky, comprising over 500 references. Deproteinization may be achieved at acid, neutral or alkaline pH. The procedure of choice depends on the method to be used for glucose estimation and should be quoted in that context. It is important to ensure, that no substances that could interfere with the glucose tests are introduced by the deproteinization procedure (Dische, 1931; Sunderman *et al.*, 1951; Bergmeyer, 1962; Müller, 1965; Strassner and Neubert, 1966; Bürgi *et al.*, 1967; Schmidt, 1971). The same points have to be considered in selecting agents to inhibit clotting or to conserve blood samples (Caneclides *et al.*, 1962; Bergmeyer, 1962; Richterich, 1965; Schmidt, 1971).

c) Standardization of Insulin Preparations with Prolonged Action

The effect of a single injection of insulin may be prolonged by addition of zinc salts, surfen or proteins such as globin or protamine. A detailed discussion of insulin preparations with prolonged action is given in the section by Schlichtkrull *et al.* (this volume). As with normal insulin, the potency of insulin preparations with prolonged action can be measured by comparison with a normal standard preparation (Patel and Rönnmark, 1936). For the duration of action an insulin preparation is measured by injecting it undiluted and determining the blood glucose level for 7 h or, if necessary, even up to 24 h. The assay is performed as a cross-over test, employing a special procedure (Scott and Fisher, 1936; Reiner *et al.*, 1939). A standard prolonged-action insulin preparation may also be used for comparison (Emmens *et al.*, 1952; Lacey, 1952; Miles, 1954).

d) Statistics

The data derived from the biological tests are evaluated according to accepted statistical methods (Linder, 1951; Fisher, 1956; Snedecor, 1959; Lienert, 1962; Weber, 1967). Special problems arising from the evaluation of the insulin assays are discussed in the pharmacopoeias. The mouse convulsion test and the blood glucose test on rabbits are described by the following authors: Irwin, 1943; Young and Stewart, 1952; J. Pharmacy and Pharmacology **4**, 382—391 (1952); Smith *et al.*, 1944; de Jongh *et al.*, 1947; Trnkova *et al.*, 1966; see also Burn *et al.*, 1950.

Guidelines for quality control in laboratory methods are given by Richterich and Colombo (1962) and by Bürgi (1972).

II. Methods of Determining Blood Glucose Concentration

The quantitative determination of glucose in blood is a problem that has been approached in many ways. It has been the subject of over 1000 publications within the last 50 years (see also Bray, 1968).

1. Chemical Methods of Measuring Blood Glucose Concentration

a) Methods Based on Reduction

Methods based on the capacity of glucose to act as a reducing agent have long been used in experiments designed to evaluate the effects of insulin. Compounds containing heavy metals, metalloids, or other inorganic or organic moieties have been employed as substrates for the reduction. The old and by now classic procedures (e.g. those of BERTRAND; AMBARD; BENEDICT; BANG; HAGEDORN-JENSEN, FOLIN-WU, MCLEAN; SHAFFER-HARTMANN; VAN SLYKE) and the methods frequently applied even today (SOMOGYI-NELSON, FRANK-KIRBERGER, HOFFMAN) are described by FONTES and THIVOLLE (1927), BAUDOUIN (1928), DISCHE (1931), GEILING (1937), HINSBERG *et al.* (1953), HINSBERG and LANG (1957), FRIED and HOEFLMAYR (1964), HALLMANN (1966), REINAUER *et al.* (1966), GUBITZ (1967), LORENTZ and LÜDEMANN (1967), and HENRY (1968).

The procedure based on a reaction with a heavy metal makes use of copper, which in its reduced form is bound by neocuproin (2.9-dimethyl-1.10-phenanthroline hydrochloride), to form a red chelate. For this method 0.01—0.03 ml of blood suffices (CAMPBELL and KING, 1963; BITTNER and MCLEARY, 1963; DYGERT *et al.*, 1965).

The well-known method named after CRECELIUS and SEIFERT and based on the reduction of picric acid is now obsolete (CRECELIUS and SEIFERT, 1928; RICHTERICH and LORENZ, 1968). The coupling of glucose to 5-hydroxy-tetralone results in a compound (benzonaphthenedione) which can be measured by its green fluorescence (MOMOSE and OHKURA, 1959; OHKURA *et al.*, 1972). Numerous substances will yield colored compounds when reduced by glucose and may thus be used for colorimetry (Table 1).

Table 1.

Reagent	Color of product of reaction	Special points	Authors
Ammonia molybdate H_2SO_4	blue	kinetic test for glucose in the presence of fructose	PAPA (1962)
o-dinitrobenzene	violet		PERONNET (1951)
3,5-dinitrosalicylic acid	yellow orange red	range of measurement 70 mg/100 ml; stable scale of colors, spectrophotometry	HOSTETTLER, F. *et al.* (1951) SUMNER, J. B. *et al.* (1944) LEE, J. (1954) SCHOUTEN, H. *et al.* (1963) MOHUN, A. F. *et al.* (1962)
3,6-dinitrophthalic acid	orange wine red	stabilization of color by thiosulfate	MOMOSE, F. *et al.* (1960)
2,3,5-triphenyl-tetrazonium-halogenide, water-soluble	formazan: cherry red, insoluble in water	solvents for formazan: isopropanol, 60% acetone, methanol	FAIRBRIDGE, R. A. *et al.* (1951) CHERONIS, N. D. *et al.* (1953) LORENTZ, K. (1966a) LORENTZ, K. *et al.* (1966b) LORENTZ, K. *et al.* (1967)
2,3,4-triphenyl-tetrazoniumsalt (p-anisyltetra-zolium blue), water-soluble	diformazan: blue, insoluble in water	solvent for diformazan: dioxane; suitable for micro- and ultramicro tests	CHERONIS, N. D. *et al.* (1957)

Different methods based on the reductive potency of glucose do not necessarily yield identical data even on the same blood sample. The reducing equivalents other than glucose present in the blood may interfere to a variable extent with the results. The methods that include nonglucose reduction and hence are subject to such interference are listed by WATSON (1962).

b) Formation of Osazone

Glucose reacts as an aldose with phenylhydrazine to yield a yellow product, which is measured at 396 μm. For this method blood samples of 0.05 ml suffice (DENIGES, 1923). The results agree well with those from enzymic tests (STROES *et al.*, 1963).

c) Furfural-Reaction

Another way to get a colored compound from glucose is to form *w*-hydroxymethyl-furfural by heating glucose in concentrated acids. A red color develops when diluted solutions of glucose are heated with concentrated sulfuric acid. The hydroxymethyl-furfural may bind to aromatic compounds (phenols, amines etc.) to form dyes of the triphenylmethane type, a reaction employed in other procedures to determine blood glucose concentration (Table 2).

A critical evaluation of the methods based on the furfural reaction is given by DUNKER *et al.* (1965), GROS and SMREKAR (1967), HANKE and THIELE (1967), SCHÄFER and ELEK (1969) BÜRGI and MITTELHOLZER (1968), and HÄRTEL *et al.* (1969).

2. Enzymic Methods of Determining Glucose

a) Digestion by Microorganisms

The digestion of deproteinized blood samples by yeast (O'MALLEY *et al.*, 1943) is obsolete. Coli bacteria selectively degrade the glucose present in the sample to water and CO_2; the latter is measured to give the amount of "true glucose" (RONA and FABISCH, 1930a, b; VAN SLYKE and HAWKINS, 1929).

b) Reaction with Pure Enzymes

α) Glucose oxidase plus peroxidase

The enzyme glucose oxidase, isolated from *Penicillium notatum*, catalyzes the oxidation of glucose to gluconic acid and hydrogen peroxide (MÜLLER, 1928, 1936; KEILIN and HARTREE, 1948; BERGMEYER, 1962; FREE, 1963; SCHMIDT, 1971). The gluconic acid formed may be determined directly (LIM, 1965). More usually, the hydrogen peroxide formed serves as indicator after being split by either the catalase present in glucose oxidase or by added peroxidase. Both enzymes will catalyze the cleavage of hydrogen peroxide into water and oxygen. The oxygen is then transferred to an agent that can be easily measured in the oxidized form by methods based on colorimetric, electrophotometric, spectrophotometric, manometric, or potentiometric measurements. All such determinations are based on the quantitative measurement of oxygen, which is, however, subject to interference. For this reason enzymic oxidation has been combined with a copper-reducing procedure and the difference has been taken as "true glucose" (NELSON, 1944; FROESCH, RENOLD, MCWILLIAMS, 1956).

Chromogens are oxygen acceptors and are easily measured as o-toluidine and o-dianisidine (3.3'-dimethoxybenzidine) (KESTON, 1956; TELLER, 1956). Stable maximum absorption is obtained with dianisidine (HUGGETT and NIXON, 1957; REALDON, 1958).

Table 2.

Glucose + acid + alcohol	Products of reaction or partner to condensation	Modifications	Automation	Authors
H_2SO_4	*w*-hydroxyfurfural	serum or plasma		Sanchez, J.A. (1935)
		deproteinization		Mendel, B. *et al.* (1926, 1950, 1954)
				Frey, U.R.Th. (1954)
H_2SO_4	phenol			Kellen, J. *et al.* (1961)
H_2SO_4	catechol			Harvey, St.G. *et al.* (1953)
HCl	resorcinol			Glassmann, B. (1926)
H_2SO_4				Barac, G. *et al.* (1947)
H_2SO_4				Schmör, J. (1955)
H_2SO_4	thymol	+ urea		Kraus, P. *et al.* (1961)
60%				Gröger, W.K. *et al.* (1961)
H_2SO_4	orcinol			Ruppert, F. (1955)
H_2SO_4 77.5%	indole			Dische, Z. *et al.* (1926)
glacial	aniline	+ thiourea		Lorentz, K. (1963)
acetic		to raise sensitivity;		Lorentz, K. *et al.* (1967)
acid		test in 0.02 ml of blood		Richterich, R. *et al.* (1962)
	aniline 0.5%	without	+	Dunker, S. *et al.* (1965)
		deproteinization		Gros, M. *et al.* (1967)
				Simon, K. (1968)
				Simon, K. *et al.* (1968)
glacial acetic acid	p-bromoaniline	+ thiourea		Deckert, T. (1967)
glacial	2-aminobiphenyl	deproteinization		Athanail, G. *et al.* (1958)
acetic		plus elevated		Forsell, O.M. *et al.* (1959)
acid		pressure		
		+ boric acid		Shibata, S. (1961)
		+ borip acid and NaF		Shibata, S. *et al.* (1962)
glacial acetic acid	m-aminophenol	range: 50—600 mg/100 ml		Ek, J. *et al.* (1958)
	p-aminobenzoic acid	range: 50—1200 mg/100 ml		Ek, J. *et al.* (1958)
glacial	p-aminosalicylic			Ek, J. *et al.* (1957)
acetic	acid			Reisz, G.Z. (1966)
acid				

Table 2 (continued)

Glucose + acid + alcohol	Partner to condensation	Modifications	Automation	Authors
glacial acetic acid	o-toluidine color generated: green			HULTMAN, E. (1959)
		prolonged boiling time; aging of color allowed		DUBOWSKI, K.M. (1962)
			+	ZENDER, R. (1963 u. 1965)
			+	WENK, R.E. *et al.* (1969)
				FRIED, R. *et al.* (1964)
		deproteinization		HOEFLMAYER, J. *et al.* (1965)
				AHLERT, G. *et al.* (1964)
			+	KREUTZ, F.H. (1966)
			+	LEYBOLD, K. (1968)
				HENKEL, E. *et al.* (1968)
		+ thiourea to stabilize color		HYVÄRINEN, A. *et al.* (1962)
				HYVÄRINEN, A. *et al.* (1963)
		+ thiourea		AHLERT, G. *et al.* (1964)
		+ deproteinization		AHLERT, G. *et al.* (1965)
		without deproteinization		RUSSEL, S. *et al.* (1964)
		technical improvements		BORMAN, U. *et al.* (1967)
			+	SCHÜTZ, W. (1968)
				MÖBIUS, H.M. *et al.* (1971)
		test for serum or plasma	+	SUDDUTH, N.C. *et al.* (1970)
		+ thiourea + borate to improve sensitivity		GOODWIN, J.F. (1968)
		+ technical improvements		FRINGS, CH.S. *et al.* (1970)
50% acetic acid				BRAUN, H. *et al.* (1965)
				BRAUN, H. (1967a, b, c)
		test in serum or plasma + borate		LÜSS, K. (1967)
			+	MOOREHEAD, W.R. *et al.* (1970)
				WINCKERS, P.L.M. *et al.* (1971)
glacial acetic acid + 40 vol% H_2O		+ borate		YEE, H. *et al.* (1971)
acetic acid + citric acid		+ thiourea in ethylenelglycol-monomethylether		HÄRTEL, A. and H. LANG (1969)
malonic acid + glyoxylic acid + methanol				HÄRTEL, A., R. HELGER and H. LANG (1969)

Table 2 (continued)

Glucose + acid + alcohol	Partner to condensation	Modifications	Automation	Authors
glyoxylic acid + benzyl alcohol		thiourea in hexamethylphosphortriamide		De Haan, J.B. *et al.* (1969)
citric acid + methoxyethanol		proteins do not precipitate		Richter, M.D. (1970)
H_2SO_4	anthrone	glucose in general		Dreywood, R. (1946)
		adapted to blood glucose		Motegi, K. (1949)
		deproteinization		Kapuscinski, V. *et al.* (1953)
		deproteinization plus additional heat		Zipf, R.E. *et al.* (1952)
		deproteinization plus thiourea		Roe, J.H. (1955)
				Hinsberg, K. *et al.* (1957)
		test in 0.05 ml of blood		Nugent, M.A. *et al.* (1958)
		test in 0.02 ml of blood		Richterich, R. (1965)
		simultaneous determination together with fructose		Wenke, M. *et al.* (1954)
		determination together with ketone bodies		Hansen, O. (1960)

Numerous procedures have been suggested to improve both the stability of the color reagent and the sensitivity of the method (SAIFER and GERSTENFELD, 1958; SAIFER *et al.*, 1958; SCHMIDT, 1959; KRÄTSCHEL, 1964; THYBUSCH, 1971). The glucose oxidase method permits one to measure glucose and urea nitrogen in the same sample (BUTLER, 1961); it is, moreover, capable of detecting minute amounts of glucose (BÜCHNER and KRÄTZSCHMAR, 1964; MATTENHEIMER, 1966). The indicator may be stabilized by additives, such as polyvinyl pyrrolidone (Kollidon 25), gum ghatti (PÜTTER and STRUFE, 1967; GUIDOTTI *et al.*, 1961), or collidine buffer, or by keeping the probes in an ice bath in the dark (FEINSMITH, 1962).

Factors which are released from erythrocytes and hence may interfere with the test can be excluded by using plasma instead of whole blood. The sensitivity, stability, and accuracy of the test are improved by dilution of the plasma sample, by addition of glycerol to the enzyme, and by adding the enzyme in excess (BÜRGI *et al.*, 1967a; CAWLEY, 1959; WASHKO and RICE, 1961; MEITES and BOHMAN, 1963). Generally, as little as 0.02 ml plasma is taken for one test (KINGSLEY and GETCHELL, 1960; LENZ and PASSANNANTE, 1970).

The glucose oxidase reaction is sensitive to changes in pH and exposure to light (WEIBEL and BRIGHT, 1971; ÅBERG, 1967). The reaction may be accelerated by adding mutarotase and thus stimulating mutarotation of α- to β-glucose (MIWA *et al.*, 1972).

All agents present in the probe which are capable of reducing hydrogen peroxide or oxidizing the chromogen indicator employed in the test will interfere with the reliability of the enzymic method. The significance of such effects may be judged from comparison with a blank without glucose oxidase (HJELM and VERDIER, 1963). Dissolving the enzymes and the technique of deproteinization constitute further sources of possible error, which may be eliminated by applying special methods (RICHTERICH and COLOMBO, 1962; CHRISTENSEN, 1967). The test employ ing o-dianisidine has been adapted to the autoanalyzer. It is yielding reliable data and permits continuous determination of blood glucose levels (HILL and KESSLER, 1961; JOHANNSSON and EKMARK, 1962; ASROW, 1969; SPATHIS, 1970). To save peroxidase, the inhibiting NaF present in blood samples may be removed as MgF_2 prior to dialysis (DISCOMBE, 1963). The autoanalyzer is capable of running glucose tests in the micro range (KINGSLEY and GETCHELL, 1960; GETCHELL *et al.*, 1964; SAIFER and ROBIN, 1965; ROBIN and SAIFER, 1965). A special microtechnique permits two separate measurements with only 0.025 ml of blood (FAULKNER, 1965).

The combination of enzyme and chromogen for blood glucose estimation was first used by KESTON (1956) with o-toluidine. The technique has been modified and adapted to the autoanalyzer (MIDDLETON and GRIFFITHS, 1957; WINCEY and MARKS, 1961; MARKS and LLOYD, 1963; MIDDLETON, 1964, 1968).

Besides o-toluidine and o-dianisidine, other agents that proved suitable as chromogens are o-anisidine (BEACH and TURNER, 1958) 3.3-dimethoxy benzidine (CAMPBELL and KRONFELD, 1961), 2.6-dichlorobenzene-indophenone (CLARK and TIMMS, 1968), 2.6-dichlorobenzophenone-indophenole (DOBRICK, 1958), and 4-aminophenazone plus phenol (TRINDER, 1969). In this mixture sulfonated 2.4-dichlorophenol may replace the phenol (BARHAM and TRINDER, 1972), as may D,L-adrenaline (TRINDER, 1969), guaiacum plus acetone (MORLEY *et al.*, 1968), potassium ferrocyanide (MÜLLER, 1971), or 3-methyl-2-benzothiazolinonhydrazone + N,N-dimethylaniline (GOCHMAN and SCHMITZ, 1972).

When 44 chromogens were tested for solubility, autoxidation, inhibiting effects on the enzyme, etc., the ammonia salt of 2.2'-azino-di-3-ethylbenzene-thiazoline-sulfonic acid-6 (ABTS) exhibited optimal properties. This acid is four times as sensitive as o-dianisidine (Gawehn *et al.*, 1970; Wielinger, 1970; Werner *et al.*, 1970; Deuser and Sitzmann, 1972). When ABTS is used in automated tests, deproteinization is mandatory (Schläger *et al.*, 1971). The test combination "blood glucose-GOD-Perid" (Boehringer, Mannheim) contains ABTS. It has been compared with the above-mentioned methods by Sharp (1972).

Hydrogen peroxide and oxidative enzymes may be measured by fluorescence employing homovanillinic acid (3-methoxy-4-hydroxy phenylacetic acid) (Guibault *et al.*, 1967). With this fluorimetric method the glucose concentration in 1 μl of plasma can be determined (Phillips and Elevitch, 1968).

β) Glucose oxidase without peroxidase

The hydrogen peroxide formed by the glucose oxidase reaction may be measured by the formaldehyde formed in the presence of methanol and catalase. Formaldehyde reacts with chromotropic acid (1,8-dihydroxy-2,7-naphthaline disulfonic acid) to yield a stable blue product (Sunderman and Sunderman, 1961). It may also be combined with acetyl acetone and ammonia acetate to form a yellow compound, diacetyl-dihydrolutidine (Ikawa and Obara, 1965). To eliminate any lack of specificity of the peroxidase-chromogen system, the hydrogen peroxide may be titrated directly (Otomo, 1963; Tammes and Nordshow, 1968).

Another approach to the measurement of hydrogen peroxide is based on the formation of iodine from iodide and subsequent iodometry by different methods (Malmstadt and Pardue, 1961, 1962; Ware and Marbach, 1965, 1968; Thompson, 1966; Aw, 1969; Simon *et al.*, 1968). The triiodide formed by oxidation of iodide in the presence of molybdate is measured by spectroscopy (Malmstadt and Hadjiioannou, 1962; Mikac-Dević *et al.*, 1972); vanadate may also be employed to catalyze the reaction (Härtel *et al.*, 1968; Härtel, 1968). The procedure is critically evaluated by Köhler and Blaufeld (1969).

When the enzyme glucose oxidase is bound to a polystyrole and thus added in a form not soluble in water, the hydrogen peroxide formed by oxidation of glucose may be measured by colorimetry when acid KI solution is added (Hornby *et al.*, 1970).

When the oxygen taken up by the glucose-oxidase reaction is measured directly by polarography, any release of oxygen from the hydrogen peroxide formed must be prevented. This is achieved by two reducing reactions which proceed simultaneously. Hydrogen peroxide is reduced by iodide in the presence of molybdate. Ethanol is added to capture any oxygen released by catalase in acetoaldehyde. The direct measurement of the oxygen taken up is independent of the use of chromogens (Kadish *et al.*, 1968; Skerry, 1970; Stevens, 1971; Kipping, 1972).

The enzyme glucose oxidase may be fixed to a water-insoluble carrier and thus used repeatedly. The measurement is done by an electrode sensitive to oxygen. A highly economical procedure makes use of a recirculating system (Bergmeyer and Hagen, 1972). Any catalase that may be present is suppressed by sodium azide (Okuda and Okuda, 1969).

γ) Hexokinase plus glucose-6-phosphate-dehydrogenase

The enzyme hexokinase catalyzes the phosphorylation of glucose, a reaction that consumes ATP. The resulting glucose-6-phosphate is oxidized by a second enzyme, glucose-6-phosphate dehydrogenase, to 6-phosphogluconic acid while NADP is reduced. The amount of NADPH thus formed may be measured in a photometer. The reaction is highly specific (SLEIN, 1962; BARTHELMAI and CZOK, 1962).

The method is convenient as test kits are commercially available (SCHMIDT, 1961, 1963, 1973; MATTENHEIMER, 1966).

STORK and SCHMIDT (1968) use 5 μl capillary blood; when the sample is diluted with water, deproteinization is not required (SITZMANN and ESCHLER, 1970). NEELY (1972) compares his own hexokinase-glucose-6-phosphate-dehydrogenase method with the glucose oxidase-peroxidase procedure.

Addition of 3% N-ethylmaleinimide and Triton X 100 does accelerate the enzymic reaction following deproteinization by perchloric acid (STORK and SCHMIDT, 1968).

The same procedure serves to stabilize the concentration of glucose in the sample (HAECKEL, 1970; HAECKEL and HAECKEL, 1972). HARDING and HEINZEL (1969) developed the first fully automatic hexokinase method, which was further simplified by FÜHR and STARY (1971), WIDDOWSON and PENTON (1972) and YEE (1972). The method is applicable to the autoanalyzer without deproteinization when the test agents of BOEHRINGER (Mannheim) are used in three separate solutions and the measuring is done by fluorimeter (DUNSBACH, 1971). More than 100 glucose estimations of deproteinized blood samples can be carried out in an hour with a specially designed automated analyzer (RICHTERICH and DAUWALDER, 1971).

The hexokinase reaction may also be measured by a colorimetric procedure, when the NADPH formed is allowed to reduce phenazine methosulfate. The reduced salt of phenazine is subsequently oxidized by the colorless iodine tetrazolium chloride to the corresponding red formazan derivative (CARROL *et al.*, 1970; WRIGHT *et al.*, 1971).

It is difficult to free the enzymes hexokinase and glucose-6-phosphate dehydrogenase from contaminating hexose-phosphate isomerase to a residual content of 0.05% or under, which is considered acceptable. Higher purity and higher specifity are achieved by enzymes with similar activity but which are easier to purify, namely the acyl-phosphate-glucose-6-phosphate transferases (BERGMEYER and MOELLERING, 1966). SHARP *et al.* (1972) made a check of how sulfonylureas affect glucose determinations by enzymic methods.

References

ÅBERG, B.: Interference of light on the determination of low glucose concentrations with glucose oxidase. Acta physiol. scand. **71**, 186—193 (1967)

AHLERT, G., HOFER, E., HOFFMANN, W., BESTVATER, G.: Die Bestimmung des Blutzuckers mit o-Toluidin im Vergleich zur enzymatischen Methode. Dtsch. Gesundh.-Wes. **19**, 2256—2259 (1964)

AHLERT, G., HOFER, E., BESTVATER, G.: Zur Blutzuckerbestimmung mit dem o-Toluidin-Eisessig-Reagens. Dtsch. Gesundh.-Wes. **20**, 349—353 (1965)

ASHFORD, W.R., CAMPBELL, J., DAVIDSON, J.K., FISHER, A.M., HAIST, R.E., LACEY, A.H., LIN, B., MARTIN, J.M., MORLEY, N.H., RASTOGI, K.S., STORVICK, W.O.: A consideration of methods of insulin assay. Diabetes **18**, 828—833 (1969)

ASROW, G.: Semiautomated enzymic micromethods for blood glucose and lactic acid on a single filtrate. Analyt. Biochem. **28**, 130—138 (1969)

ATHANAIL, G., CABAUD, P.G.: Simplified colorimetric method for the true blood glucose. J. Lab. clin. Med. **51**, 321—324 (1958)

AW, S.E.: An enzymatic method for glucose estimation using the starch-iodine chromogen. Clin. chim. Acta **26**, 235—238 (1969)

BANGHAM, D.R., MUSSETT, M.V.: The Fourth International Standard for Insulin. Bull. Wld Hlth Org. **20**, 1209—1220 (1959)

BARAC, G., DELVENNE, J.: Nouvelle technique de dosage de la glycémie. Bull. Soc. Chim. biol. (Paris) **29**, 1094—1097 (1947)

Barham, D., Trinder, P.: An improved colour reagent for the determination of blood glucose by the oxidase system. Analyst **97**, 142—145 (1972)

Barthelmai, W., Czok, R.: Enzymatische Bestimmungen der Glukose in Blut, Liquor und Harn. Klin. Wschr. **40**, 585—589 (1962)

Baudouin, A.: Le dosage des matières réductrices du sang. Bull. Soc. Chim. biol. (Paris) **10**, 977—1049 (1928)

Beach, E.F., Turner, J.J.: An enzymatic method for glucose determination in body fluids. Clin. Chem. **4**, 462—475 (1958)

Bergmeyer, H.U.: Methoden der enzymatischen Analyse. 1. Aufl. Weinheim: Verlag Chemie 1962

Bergmeyer, H.U., Bernt, E., Schmidt, F., Stork, H.: D-glukose. Bestimmung mit Hexokinase und Glukose-6-phosphat-dehydrogenase. In: Bergmeyer, H.U. Methoden der enzymatischen Analyse, 2. Aufl., Bd. II, S. 1163—1190. Weinheim: Verlag Chemie 1970

Bergmeyer, H.U., Hagen, A.: Ein neues Prinzip enzymatischer Analyse. Z. analyt. Chem. **261**, 333—336 (1972)

Bergmeyer, H.U., Moellering, H.: Enzymatische Glukosebestimmung mit Acylphosphat: D-glucose-6-phosphotransferase. Clin. chim. Acta **14**, 74—82 (1966)

Best, C.H.: Die Standardisierung von Insulin. Abderhalden Hdb. d. biol. Arbeitsmethoden, Abt. V, Teil 3, B, p. 513—527 (1938)

Bittner, D.L., McLeary, M.L.: The cupric phenanthroline chelate in the determination of monosaccharides in the whole blood. Amer. J. clin. Path. **40**, Abstr. 423—424 (1963)

Bomskow, C.: Methodik der Hormonforschung. Die Auswertungsverfahren des Insulins am gesunden Tier, p. 643—657. Leipzig: Thieme 1937

Bormann, U., Kienholz, M.: Zur Technik und Durchführung der Blutzuckerbestimmung mit der o-Toluidin-Methode. Ärztl. Lab. **13**, 519—521 (1967)

Braun, H.: Blutzuckerbestimmung mit o-Toluidin unter Verwendung des Pulfrich Photometers. Dtsch. Gesundh.-Wes. **22**, 254—255 (1967a)

Braun, H.: o-Toluidin in 50% Essigsäure zur Blutzuckerbestimmung. Ärztl. Lab. **13**, 177—180 (1967b)

Braun, H.: o-Toluidin in 50% Essigsäure zur Blutzuckerbestimmung. Ärztl. Lab. **13**, 518—519 (1967c)

Braun, H., Hofmann, J.: Methodisches zur Blutzuckerbestimmung mit o-Toluidin. Dtsch. Gesundh.-Wes. **20**, 2271—2276 (1965)

Bray, W.E.: Clinical Laboratory Methods. 7. Edn. Clin. Chem. **6**, 299—308. St. Louis: Moosby Co. 1968

Büchner, M., Krätzschmar, K.: Beiträge zur Ultramikroanalyse im Kliniklaboratorium, I. Mitt. Ultramikrobestimmung von Gesamtbilirubin und Blutzucker. Dtsch. Gesundh.-Wes. **19**, 881—884 (1964)

Bürgi, W.: Die Zuverlässigkeit klinisch-chemischer und hämatologischer Laboratoriumsanalysen. Schweiz. med. Wschr. **102**, 367—374 (1972)

Bürgi, W., Mittelholzer, M.L.: Die Spezifität der o-Toluidin-Methode zur Blutzuckerbestimmung. Hinweis auf die Toxicität von o-Toluidin. Praxis (Bern) **57**, 1135—1138 (1968)

Bürgi, W., Richterich, R., Mittelholzer, M.L.: Der Einfluß der Entweißung auf die Resultate von Serum- und Plasma-Analysen. Klin. Wschr. **45**, 83—86 (1967a)

Bürgi, W., Richterich, R., Mittelholzer, M.L., Monstein, S.: Die Glukoseconzentration im kapillären und venösen Plasma bei direkter enzymatischer Bestimmung. Schweiz. med. Wschr. **97**, 1721—1725 (1967b)

Büttner, H., Hansert, E., Stamm, D.: Auswertung, Kontrolle und Beurteilung von Meßergebnissen. In: Bergmeyer, H.U.: Methoden der enzymatischen Analyse. 2. A., Bd. I, p. 281—329. Weinheim: Verlag Chemie 1970

Burn, J.H.: Methods of Biological Assay, p. 53—64. London: Oxford Univ. Press 1928

Burn, J.H., Bülbring, E.: Biologische Auswertungsmethoden, p. 62—81. Berlin: Springer 1937

Burn, J.H., Finney, D.J., Goodwin, L.G.: Biological Standardization, p. 26—176 (Statistical analysis); 194—214 (Insulin). London: Oxford Univ. Press 1950

Butler, T.J.: The determination of blood glucose and urea nitrogen on a simple microsample. Amer. J. med. Technol. **27**, 205—213 (1961)

Campbell, D.M., King, E.J.: Colorimetric determination of glucose in 20 μl of blood. J. clin. Path. **16**, 173—174 (1963)

Campbell, L.A., Kronfeld, D.S.: Estimation of low concentrations of plasma glucose using glucose oxidase. Amer. J. vet. Res. **22**, 587—589 (1961)

Caneclides, R.M., Chantal Tomlinson, S.M. de: A comparison of anticoagulants and or preservatives affecting blood glucose. Amer. J. med. Technol. **28**, 195—201 (1962)

CARROLL, J., SMITH, N., BABSON, A.L.: A colorimetric serum glucose determination using hexokinase and glucose-6-phosphate dehydrogenase. Biochem. Med. **4**, 171—180 (1970)

CAWLEY, L.P., SPEAR, F.E., KENDALL, R.: Ultra chemical analysis of blood glucose with glucose oxidase. Amer. J. clin. Path. **32**, 195—200 (1959)

CHASE, H.B., GUNTHER, M.S., MILLER, J., WOLFFSON, D.: High insulin tolerance in an inbred strain of mice. Science **107**, 297—299 (1948)

CHERONIS, N.D., SKUPP, S.: Glucose in blood. Chem. Engin. News **31**, 874 (1953)

CHERONIS, N.D., ZYMARIS, M.C.: The microdetermination of reducing sugars in blood by means of p-anisyl-tetrazolium blue. Mikrochim. Acta 769—783 (1957)

CHRISTENSEN, N.J.: Notes on the glucose-oxidase method. Scand. J. clin. Lab. Invest. **19**, 379—384 (1967)

CLARK, A., TIMMS, B.G.: Reduced 2,6-dichlorophenol-indophenol as a replacement for o-toluidine in the enzymatic determination of blood glucose. Clin. chim. Acta **20**, 352—354 (1968)

COHN, C., JOSEPH, D.: Feeding habits and daily rhythms in tissue glycogen in the rat. Proc. Soc. exp. Biol. (N.Y.) **137**, 1303—1306 (1972)

CRECELIUS, W., SEIFERT: Ein neues Blutzuckercolorimeter nach Crecelius-Seifert. Münch. med. Wschr. **75**, 1301—1302 (1928)

DECKERT, T.: Method for determining glucose in plasma, cerebrospinal fluid and urine by means of p-bromaniline. Scand. J. clin. Lab. Invest. **20**, 217—223 (1967)

DENIGES, G.: Dosage clinique du sucre hématique par colorimétrie et réductrimétrie. Bull. Soc. Pharm. Bordeaux **61**, 8—17 (1923)

DEUSER, K.H., SITZMANN, F.C.: GOD-Perid-Methode zur Blutzuckerbestimmung. Med. Klin. **67**, 1406—1409 (1972)

DISCHE, Z.: Bestimmung der Kohlehydrate im Blute. Mikrochemie **10**, 129—187 (1931)

DISCHE, Z., POPPER, H.: Über eine neue kolorimetrische Mikrobestimmungsmethode der Kohlehydrate in Organen und Körpersäften. Biochem. Z. **175**, 371—411 (1926)

DISCOMBE, G.: An inexpensive method for the estimation of true glucose in blood and other fluids by the Autoanalyzer. J. clin. Path. **16**, 170—172 (1963)

DOBRICK, L.A.: Screening method for glucose of serum utilizing glucose oxidase and indophenol indicator. J. biol. Chem. **231**, 403—409 (1958)

DREYWOOD, R.: Qualitative test for carbohydrate material. Ind. Engin. Chem. Anal. Ed. **18**, 499 (1946)

DUBOWSKI, K.M.: An o-toluidine method for body-fluid glucose determination. Clin. Chem. **8**, 215—235 (1962)

DUNKER, S., AMMON, J., DISCHUNEIT, H., PFEIFFER, E.F.: Blutzuckerbestimmung mit dem Auto-Analyzer unter Verwendung von Anilin-Eisessig. Internat. Technicon Sympos. Frankfurt/M., Okt. 1965, p. 617

DUNSBACH, F.: Fluorometrische Bestimmung der Glukose im Blut nach der Hexokinase-Methode mit dem Auto-Analyzer, Technicon. Sympos. 71, Frankfurt/M., 1971, Sep. No. 956

DYGERT, ST., DON FLORIDA, L.H.LI., THOMA, J.A.: Determination of reducing sugar with improved precision. Analyt. Biochem. **13**, 367—374 (1965)

EDITORIAL: These 52 factors can affect blood glucose levels. J. Amer. med. Ass. **214**, 2272 (1970)

VAN EEKELEN, M., VAN ESVELD, L.W., BEUS, J. DE: Een onderzoek naar het aantal eenheden, het stikstof en zinkgehalte en de pH van handelspraeparaten. Ned. T. Geneesk. **85**, 3676—3682 (1941)

EK, J., HULTMAN, E.: A new method for determining aldosaccharides. Scand. J. clin. Lab. Invest. **9**, 315—316 (1957)

EK, J., HULTMAN, E.: Determination of glucose and laevulose in body fluids. Nature (Lond.) **181**, 780—781 (1958)

EMMENS, C.W., GRAY, J.A.B., MILES, A.A., PERRY, W.L.M.: The preparation and testing of the provisional British Standard for globin zinc insulin. J. Pharm. Pharmacol. **4**, 382—391 (1952)

EMMENS, C.W. *et al.*: The preparation and testing of the provisional British standard for Globin Zinc insulin. J. Pharm. Pharmacol. **4**, 382—391 (1952)

European Pharmacopoeia, Vol. III (in press 1975). Biological Assay of Insulin

FAHLEN, M., ODÉN, A., BJÖRNTORP, P., TIBBLIN, G.: Seasonal influence on insulin secretion in man. Clin. Sci. **41**, 453—458 (1971)

FAIRBRIDGE, R.A., WILLIS, K.J., BOOTH, R.G.: The direct colorimetric estimation of reducing sugars and other reducing substances with tetrazolium salts. Biochem. J. **49**, 423—427 (1951)

FAULKNER, D.E.: An automated micro-determination of blood glucose using the Autoanalyzer. Internat. Technicon Sympos. Automation in der Analyt. Chemie Frankfurt/M., 1965, p. 976

FDA: Insulin regulations. U.S. Dep. Health and Welfare, F.D.A., 29. XI. 1955
Feinsmith, E. M.: Die enzymatische Bestimmung der Blutglukose. Clin. chim. Acta **7**, 58—64 (1962)
Feteris, W. A.: A serum glucose method without protein precipitation. Amer. J. med. Technol. **31**, 17—21 (1965)
Fisher, R. A.: Statistical methods for research workers. Edinburgh: Oliver and Boyd 1941
Fisher, R. A.: Statistische Methoden für die Wissenschaft. Übers. von Dora Lucka. Edinburgh: Oliver and Boyd 1956
Fontès, G., Thivolle, L.: Recherches expérimentales sur le microdosage des substances glucidiques réductrices du sang. Bull. Soc. Chim. biol. (Paris) **9**, 353—423; 441—445 (1927) (Lit.)
Forsell, O. M., Palva, J. P.: A rapid method for the true blood glucose estimation. Scand. J. clin. Lab. Invest. **11**, 409 (1959)
Free, A. H.: Enzymatic determination of glucose. Advanc. clin. Chem. **6**, 67—96 (1963)
Frey, U. R. Th.: Untersuchungen mit der Blutzuckerbestimmungsmethode nach Mendel-Hoagland. Helv. med. Acta **21**, 1—19 (1954)
Fried, R., Hoeflmayr, J.: Eine kolorimetrische Methode zur Blutzuckerbestimmung mit o-Toluidin. Ärztl. Lab. **10**, 59—62 (1964)
Frings, Ch. S., Ratliff, Ch. R., Dunn, R. T.: Automated determination of glucose in serum or plasma by direct o-toluidine-procedure. Clin. Chem. **16**, 282—284 (1970)
Froesch, E., Renold, A. E., McWilliams, N. B.: Specific enzymatic determination of glucose in blood and urine, using glucose oxidase. Diabetes **5**, 1—6 (1956)
Führ, J., Stary, E.: Vollmechanisierte Glukosebestimmung mit der Hexokinase-G-6-PDH-Methode. Technicon Sympos. 71, Frankfurt/M., 1971, Sep. no. 960
Gawehn, K., Wielinger, H., Werner, W.: Screening von Chromogenen für die Blutzuckerbestimmung nach der GOD/POD-Methode. Z. anal. Chem. **252**, 222—224 (1970)
Geiling, E. M. K., Jensen, H., Farrar, G. E.: Insulin, V. Standardization of insulin. Dieses Hdb. Erg. Werk, Bd. V, 218—222 (1937)
Gerritzen, F.: The duration of the action of different insulins. Brit. med. J. **1952 I**, 249—250
Gerritzen, F.: The classification of various insulins. Brit. med. J. **1953 II**, 1030—1031
Gerritzen, F.: Über die Wirkungsdosen eines Zink-Protamin-Insulins. Münch. med. Wschr. **96**, 493—494 (1954)
Getchell, G., Kingsley, G. R., Schaffert, R. R.: Direct automated determination of glucose by a glucose oxidase-peroxidase system. Clin. Chem. **10**, 540—548 (1964)
Glassmann, B.: Eine Vereinfachung meiner colorimetrischen Mikromethode zur Bestimmung des freien Blutzuckers. Z. physiol. Chem. **158**, 113—138 (1926)
Gmeiner, G.: Die Fehlermöglichkeiten der täglichen Labordiagnostik. Med. Mschr. **3**, 190—195 (1949)
Gochman, N., Schmitz, J. M.: Application of a new peroxide indicator reaction to the specific, automated determination of glucose with glucose oxidase. Clin. Chem. **18**, 943—950 (1972)
Goodwin, J. F.: Simultaneous direct estimation of glucose and xylose in serum. Clin. Chem. **14**, 825—826 (1968)
Gröger, W. K. L.: Determination of sugars in biological media with thymol in sulfuric acid. Clin. chim. Acta **6**, 866—873 (1961)
Gros, M., Smrekar, M.: An aniline-acetic acid method for body fluid glucose determination. Clin. chim. Acta **17**, 518—519 (1967)
Gubitz, H.: Allgemeine Betrachtungen zur Blutzuckerbestimmung. Dtsch. Apoth.-Ztg. **107**, 1307—1311 (1967)
Guibault, G. G., Kramer, D. N., Hackley, E.: New substrate for fluorometric determination of oxidative enzymes. Analyt. Chem. **39**, 271 (1967)
Guidotti, C., Colombo, J. P., Foa, P. F.: Enzymic determination of glucose. Stabilization of color developed by oxidation of o-anisidine. Analyt. Chem. **33**, 151—153 (1961)
De Haan, J. B., Roth, M.: A new medium for the aldohexose-o-toluidine reaction: direct microdetermination of blood glucose. Z. klin. Chem. **7**, 624—626 (1969)
Haeckel, R.: The rapid, enzymatic determination of glucose in hemolysates. Z. klin. Chem. **8**, 480—482 (1970)
Haeckel, R., Haeckel, H.: Die Bestimmung der Glucosekonzentration in 20 Mikroliter Kapillarblut, Liquor und Urin nach der Hexokinasemethode mit dem Endpunktautomaten 5030 (Eppendorf). Z. klin. Chem. **10**, 453—461 (1972)
Härtel, A.: Ein neuer Redoxkatalysator für die Blutzuckerbestimmung mit Glukoseoxidase. Ärztl. Lab. **14**, 183—185 (1968)
Härtel, A., Fabel-Schulte, K., Lang, H., Rick, W.: Ein neuer Redoxkatalysator für die Blutzuckerbestimmung mit Glukoseoxydase. Z. klin. Chem. **6**, 34—37 (1968)
Härtel, A., Helger, R., Lang, H.: Die Blutzuckerbestimmung mit der o-Toluidin-Methode ohne Eisessig. Z. klin. Chem. **7**, 14—17 (1969)

Härtel, A., Lang, H.: Blutzuckerbestimmung mit o-Toluidin. Ärztl. Lab. **15**, 60—61 (1969)

Hahn, J., Hohlweg, W., Rückert, A., Seel, H.: Insulin und Insulinlösungen. II. Bestimmungsmethoden. Pharmazie **12**, 35—38 (1957a)

Hahn, J., Hohlweg, W., Rückert, A., Seel, H.: Insulin und Insulinlösungen, II. Teil: Bestimmungsmethoden. Pharm. Zentralh. **96**, 63—67 (1957b)

Hahn, J., Hohlweg, W., Seel, H.: Insulin und Insulinlösungen. Pharmazie **11**, 88—91 (1956a)

Hahn, J., Hohlweg, W., Seel, H.: Weitere Vorschläge für den Nachtrag zum DAB 6, Insulin und Insulinlösungen. Pharm. Zentralh. **95**, 134—138 (1956b)

Hallmann, L.: Klinische Chemie und Mikroskopie, 10. Aufl., S. 541—543; 589—590. Stuttgart: Thieme 1966

Hanke, G., Thiele, H.J.: o-Toluidin in 50%iger Essigsäure zur Blutzuckerbestimmung. Ärztl. Lab. **13**, 517 (1967)

Hansen, O.: A micromethod for simultaneous determination of glucose and lactone bodies in blood and glycogen and ketone bodies in the liver. Scand. J. clin. Lab. Invest. **12**, 18—24 (1960)

Harding, U., Heinzel, G.: Vollautomatische Bestimmung des Blutzuckers nach der Hexokinasemethode. Z. klin. Chem. **7**, 640—643 (1969)

Harvey, St. C., Higby, V.: A microcolorimetric method for the determination of glucose. Tex. Rep. Biol. Med. **11**, 489—493 (1953)

Hasselblatt, A.: Pharmakologische Ausschaltung vegetativer Störungen der Blutzuckerhomöostase. Pfeiffer, E. F. Hdb. Diabetes mellitus, Bd. I, p. 877—893. München: J. F. Lehmann 1969/1971

Henkel, E., Delbrück, A.: Automatisierte Blutzuckerbestimmung mit o-Toluidin. Vergl. Untersuchung mit dem Hexokinase-Zwischenferment-Test. Ärztl. Lab. **14**, 458—463 (1968)

Henry, R.J.: Clinical Chemistry, Principles and Technics. New York: Harper (Hoeber) 1968

Hershey, J., Lacey, A.H.: Comparison, as regards unit value, between the original international insulin standard and the proposed new standard. Quart. Bull. Hlth Org. L. o. N. **5**, 589—598 (1936)

Hjelm, M., de Verdier, C.H.: A methodological study of the enzymatic determination of glucose in blood. Scand. J. clin. Lab. Invest. **15**, 415—428 (1963)

Hill, J.B., Kessler, G.: An automated determination of glucose utilizing a glucose oxidase-peroxidase system. J. Lab. clin. Med. **57**, 970—980 (1961)

Hinsberg, K.: Blut, Organische Bestandteile, Kohlenhydrate, Glukose. Hoppe-Seyler-Thierfelder: Hdb. physiol. pathol. chem. Analyse, p. 65—75. Berlin: Springer 1953

Hinsberg, K., Lang, K.: Bestimmung der Glukose, Medizinische Chemie, für den klinischen und theoretischen Gebrauch. 3 edn., p. 346—355. München: Urban u. Schwarzenberg 1957

Hoeflmayr, J., Fried, R.: Vereinfachte klinisch-chemische Laboratoriumsbestimmungen (photometrische Methoden). Ther. d. Gegenw. **104**, 74—76, Lit. p. 363 (1965)

Hornby, W.E., Filippusson, H., McDonald, A.: The preparation of glucose oxidase chemically attached to polystyrene and its use in the automated analysis of glucose. FEBS Letters **9**, 8—10 (1970)

Hostettler, F., Borel, E., Deuel, H.: Reduction von 3,5-dinitrosalicylsäure durch Zucker. Helv. chim. Acta **34**, 2132—2139 (1951)

Hrubetz, M.C.: Diurnal variation in blood sugar level of the rat. Proc. Soc. exp. Biol. (N.Y.) **32**, 217 (1934)

Huggett, A., St. G., Nixon, D.A.: Enzyme determination of blood glucose. Biochem. J. **66**, 12 P (1957)

Hultman, E.: Rapid specific method for the determination of aldosaccharides in body fluids. Nature (Lond.) **183**, 108—109 (1959)

Hyvärinen, A., Nikkilä, E.A.: Specific determination of blood glucose with o-toluidine. Clin. chim. Acta **7**, 140—143 (1962)

Hyvärinen, A., Nikkilä, E.A.: Blutzuckerbestimmung mit o-Toluidin. Clin. Chem. **9**, 234—235 (1963)

Ikawa, S., Obara, T.: Determination of blood glucose by means of glucose-oxidase-catalase system (in Japanese). Jap. J. clin. Path. **13**, 197—200 (1965)

Irwin, J.O.: The error of the biological assay of insulin by the mouse convulsion test. Quart. J. Pharm. **16**, 352—362 (1943)

Jarrett, H.J., Baker, I.A., Keen, H., Oakley, N.W.: Diurnal variation in oral glucose tolerance: blood sugar and plasma insulin levels, morning, afternoon and evening. Brit. med. J. **1972 I**, 199—201

Johannsson, St., Ekmark, J.: Automatik blodsockerbestämmig med anvendande av ett färdigberett glykoseoxidasereagens. Svenska Läk.-Tidn. **59**, 3028—3031 (1962)

De Jongh, S.E., Laqueur, E.: Eichung von Insulin. Abderhalden Hdb. d. biol. Arb. Meth., Abt. V, Teil 3, B. h. 9, p. 1475—1492 (1938)

De Jongh, S.E., Lens, J., Spanhoff, R.W.: On the standardization of insulin by means of the rabbit test. Arch. int. Pharmacodyn. **74**, 63—82 (1947)

Kadish, A.H., Litle, R.L., Sternberg, J.C.: A new and rapid method for the determination of glucose by measurement of rate of oxygen consumption. Clin. Chem. **14**, 116—131 (1968)

Kaernbach, K.: Über Insulin. Mitteilungen aus der Insulinabteilung der VVB Pharma Schering. Chem. Techn. **4**, 99—107 (1952) (Lit.)

Kapuscinski, V., Zak, B.: Use of perchloric acid filtrate and stabilized anthrone for determination of serum glucose. Amer. J. clin. Path. **23**, 784—788 (1953)

Keilin, D., Hartree, E.F.: Properties of glucose oxidase (Notatin). Biochem. J. **42**, 221—229 (1948)

Kellen, J., Vajkova, M.: Blutzuckerbestimmung mit Phenol-Schwefelsäure. Z. ges. inn. Med. **16**, 188 (1961)

Keston, A.S.: Specific colorimetric enzymatic analytical reagents for glucose. Abstr. of papers of the 129th meeting of the Amer. chem. Soc., Texas, April 1956. Div. of Biol. chem., p. 31, C—32 C

Kingsley, G.R., Getchell, G.: Direct ultramicro glucose oxidase method for determination of sugar in biological fluids. Clin. Chem. **6**, 466—475 (1960)

Kipping, D.: Erfahrungen mit einer polarographischen Blutglukosebestimmung. Z. med. Lab.-Techn. **13**, 53—57 (1972)

Köhler, P., Blaufeld, H.: Über weitere Modifikationen der enzymatischen Blutzuckerbestimmung mittels Glukoseoxidase. Z. med. Lab.-Techn. **10**, 102—104 (1969)

Krätschel, B.: Hinweis zur enzymatischen Blutzuckerbestimmung mit Testbestecken. Z. med. Lab.-Techn. **5**, 307—308 (1964)

Kraus, P., Simane, Z.: Eine verbesserte Methode zur Blutzuckerbestimmung mit Thymol-Schwefelsäure-Reagens. Klin. Wschr. **39**, 309 (1961)

Kreutz, F.H.: Blood glucose determination with an automated o-toluidine reaction. Enzym. biol. clin. **6**, 258 (1966)

Kühne, P.: Die I. E. Insulin als unzulänglich erwiesen. Med. Tribune **1**, 11 (1966); Parm. Ztg. (Frankfurt) **111**, 1914—1915 (1966)

Lacey, A.H.: The rabbit method of insulin assay. Endocrinology **29**, 866—876 (1941)

Lacey, A.H.: Further observation on the rabbit method of insulin assay. Endocrinology **39**, 344—357 (1946)

Lacey, A.H.: A comparison of preparation of NPH insulin. J. Pharmacol. **105**, 196—202 (1952)

Lacey, A.H.: The unit of insulin. Diabetes **16**, 198—200 (1967)

Lacey, A.H.: International insulin standards. Diabetes **17**, 705—707 (1968)

League of Nations: Insulin Committee of the University of Toronto: Report. League of Nations III, Health III, **7**, 24—33 (1926)

League of Nations: Report on the international Insulin standard, League of Nations III, Health III, **7**, 34—35 (1926)

Lee, J.: A quick and simple method for blood-sugar estimation. Brit. med. J. **1954 II**, 1087—1088

Lenz, P.H., Passannante, A.J.: Rapid glucose oxidase-peroxidase ultramicro method for determination of blood glucose. Clin. Chem. **16**, 427—430 (1970)

Leybold, K.: Automatisierung der Glukosebestimmung mit o-Toluidin. Z. klin. Chem. **6**, 51—52 (1968)

Lienert, G.A.: Methoden der Biostatistik. Meisenheim a.d. Glan: A. Hain 1962

Lim, F.: Automatic micro glucose determination with a 60-second direct-reading analyser. Clin. Chem. **11**, Abstr. 792 (1965)

Linder, A.: Statistische Methoden für Naturwissenschaftler, Mediziner und Ingenieure, 2. Aufl. Basel: S. Birkhäuser 1951

Lorant, M.: Aufgaben der Abteilung für biologische Standards des öffentlichen Gesundheitsdienstes der USA. Med. Klin. **66**, 99—100 (1971)

Lorentz, K.: Blutzucker-Schnellbestimmung mit Anilin-Eisessig. Z. klin. Chem. **1**, 127—128 (1963)

Lorentz, K.: Blutzuckerbestimmung mit Triphenyltetrazoniumchlorid (TTC) als Schnell- und Ultramikromethode. Clin. chim. Acta **13**, 660—665 (1966)

Lorentz, K., Hoffmeister, H.: Untersuchungen über den Einfluß der Wasserstoffionenconzentration auf die Spezifität der TTC-Reaktion. Mikrochim. Acta **1966**, 1062—1067

Lorentz, K., Lüdemann, C.: Vergleichende Blutzuckerbestimmung mit enzymatischen und kolorimetrischen Verfahren. Dtsch. med. J. **18**, 420—422 (1967)

Lubetzki, J.: L'hétérogénéité de l'insuline. La Pro-Insuline. Presse méd. **77**, 995—996 (1969)

LÜSS, K.: Zur Blutzuckerbestimmung mit o-Toluidin-Reagenz. Dtsch. Gesundh.-Wes. **22**, 227—228 (1967)

MALMSTADT, H.V., HADJIIOANNOU, S.I.: New automatic spectrophotometric rate method for selective determination of glucose in serum, plasma or blood. Analyt. Chem. **34**, 452—455 (1962)

MALMSTADT, H.V., PARDUE, H.L.: Quantitative analysis by automatic potentiometric reaction rate method. Analyt. Chem. **33**, 1040—1047 (1961)

MALMSTADT, H.V., PARDUE, H.L.: Specific enzymatic determination of glucose in blood, serum or plasma by an automatic potentiometric reaction rate method. Clin. Chem. **8**, 606—615 (1962)

MARKS, H.P.: The biological assay of insulin preparations in comparison with a stable standard. Brit. med. J. **1925**, 1102—1104

MARKS, H.P.: The biological assay of insulin preparations in comparison with a stable standard. League of Nations III, Health III, **7**, 57—71 (1926)

MARKS, H.P., PAK, C.: Evaluation of the new international standard insulin by the rabbit and mouse methods of assay. Quart. Bull. Hlth Org. L. o. N. **5**, 631—651 (1936)

MARKS, V., LLOYD, K.: The enzymatic measurement of glucose by autoanalysis. Proc. Ass. clin. Biochem. **2**, 176—179 (1963)

MATTENHEIMER, H.: Mikromethoden für das klinische und biochemische Laboratorium, 2. Aufl., p. 109. Berlin: W. de Gruyter 1966

MAXWELL, L.C., BISCHOFF, F.: Augmentation of the physiological response to insulin. Amer. J. Physiol. **112**, 172—175 (1935)

MEITES, S., BOHMAN, N.: Evaluation of an ultramicromethod for blood glucose determination. Amer. J. Technol. **29**, 327—331 (1963)

MENDEL, B., BAUCH, M.: Eine colorimetrische Mikromethode zur quantitativen Bestimmung des Blutzuckers in 8 Minuten. Klin. Wschr. **5**, 1329—1330 (1926)

MENDEL, B., HOAGLAND, P.L.: Rapid determination of blood sugar; a simple method. Lancet **1950 II**, 16—17

MENDEL, B., KEMP, A., MYERS, D.K.: A colorimetric micromethod for the determination of glucose. Biochem. J. **56**, 639—646 (1954)

MIDDLETON, J.E.: Experience with a glucose oxidase method for estimating glucose in blood and C.S.F. Brit. med. J. **1959 I**, 824—826

MIDDLETON, J.E.: Colorimetric estimation of glucose. Brit. med. J. **1964 II**, 384—385

MIDDLETON, J.E.: Preparation and investigation of a stabilized glucose oxidase-peroxidase reagent for estimating glucose, using o-toluidine with an alkylaryl sulphonate and polyethylene glycol. Clin. chim. Acta **22**, 433—437 (1968)

MIDDLETON, J.E., GRIFFITHS, W.J.: Rapid colorimetric micromethod for estimating glucose in blood and C.S.F. using glucose oxidase. Brit. med. J. **1957 II**, 1525—1527

MIKAC-DEVIĆ, D., STANKOVIĆ, H., WÜRTH, G.: Manual and automated determination of glucose in blood with glucose oxidase and molybdate/iodide as redox catalyst. Z. klin. Chem. **10**, 372—373 (1972)

MILES, A.A.: Biological specification and biological standards in the British Pharmacopoeia. Nature (Lond.) **173**, 433—434 (1954)

MIWA, I., OKUDA, J., MAEDA, K., OKUDA, G.: Mutarotase effect on colorimetric determination of blood glucose with β-D-glucose oxidase. Clin. chim. Acta **37**, 538—540 (1972)

MÖBIUS, H.M., MICKLAUSCH, H., BEIER, A.: Über eine Pipettier- und Absaugvorrichtung zur Vereinfachung der Blutzuckerbestimmung nach der o-Toluidin Methode. Z. med. Lab.. Techn. **12**, 307—311 (1971)

MOHUN, A.F., COOK, I.J.: An improved dinitrosalicylic acid method for determining blood and cerebrospinal fluid sugar level. J. clin. Path. **15**, 169—180 (1962)

MOMOSE, T., INABA, A., MUKAI, Y., WATANABE, M.: Organic analysis XXIII. Determination of blood sugar and urine sugar with 3,6-dinitrophthalic acid. Talanta **4**, 33—37 (1960)

MOMOSE, T., OHKURA, Y.: Organic analysis XX. Microestimation of blood sugar with 5-hydroxy-1-tetralone. Talanta **3**, 151—154 (1959)

Monopolies and Restrictive Practices Commission: Report on the suply of insulin. London: HMSO 1952

MOOREHEAD, W.R., SASSE, E.A.: An automated micromethod for determination of serum glucose, with an improved o-toluidine reagent. Clin. Chem. **16**, 285—290 (1970)

MORLEY, G., DAWSON, A., MARKS, V.: Manual and autoanalyzer methods for measuring blood glucose using guaiacum and glucose oxidase. Clin. Biochem. **5**, 42—45 (1968)

MOTEGI, K.: A new quantitative determination of blood sugar. J. Japan biochem. Soc. **21**, 40—41 (1949)

MÜLLER, D.: Studien über ein neues Enzym. Glykoseoxidase. I. u. II. Biochem. Z. **199**, 136—170 (1928); **205**, 111—143 (1929)

MÜLLER, D.: Die Glukoseoxidase. Ergebn. Enzymforsch. **5**, 259—272 (1936)

Müller, G.: Über die Hemmung der enzymatischen Glukosebestimmung mit Glukoseoxidase und Peroxidase durch Glutathion. Dtsch. Z. Verdau.- u. Stoffwechselkr. **25**, 70—76 (1965)

Müller, H.: Enzymatische Bestimmung von D. Glukose mit Glukoseoxidase. Stärke **23**, 314—319 (1971)

Neeley, W.E.: Simple automated determination of serum or plasma glucose by hexokinase/glucose-6-phosphate dehydrogenase method. Clin. Chem. **18**, 509—515 (1972)

Nelson, N.: A photometric adaption of Somogyi's method for the determination of glucose. J. biol. Chem. **153**, 375—380 (1944)

Nugent, M.A., Fleming, D.G.: A micromethod for blood sugar using anthrone. Amer. J. med. Technol. **24**, 8—10 (1958)

Ohkura, Y., Watanabe, Y., Momose, T.: Fluorometric determination of glucose in cerebrospinal fluid and blood by the revised 5-hydroxy-1-tetralone method. Biochem. Med. **6**, 97—104 (1972)

Okuda, J., Okuda, G.: A rapid polarographic microdetermination of glucose with glucose oxidase. Clin. chim. Acta **23**, 365—367 (1969)

O'Malley, E., Conway, E.J., Fitzgerald, O.: Microdiffusion methods. Blood glucose. Biochem. J. **37**, 278—281 (1943)

Otomo, M.: The spectrophotometric determination of titanium with hydrogen peroxide and xylenolorange. Bull. chem. Soc. Japan **36**, 1577—1581 (1963)

Papa, I.J., Mark, H.B., Reilley, C.N.: Simultaneous spectrophotometric determination of fructose and glucose mixtures by differential reaction rates. Analyt. Chem. **34**, 1443—1446 (1962)

Patel, R.P., Rönnmark, B.: The action of Protamine Insulin in rabbits in relation to its standardisation. Quart. J. Pharm. **9**, 679—683 (1936)

Peronnet, M., Hugonnet, J.: Nouvelle méthode colorimétiique de dosage du glucose dans les liquides biologiques. Ann. pharm. franç. **9**, 397—407 (1951)

Perry, W.L.M.: Work on biological standards: International standards. Pharm. J. **174**, 6 (1955)

Pfeiffer, E.F. *et al.*: Handb. Diabetes mellitus. Bd. 1. Pathophysiologie, Bd. 2. Klinik. München: J. F. Lehmann 1971

Pharmacopoeia Austriaca, Edn. IX: p. 107. Biologische Wertbestimmung von Insulin; p. 112. Beurteilung der Depotwirkung. Wien 1960

Pharmacopoeia Britannica, 1973

Pharmacopoeia Helvetica, Vol. 1, p. 219; 221 (1971). Biologische Wertbestimmung von Insulin-Präparaten

Pharmacopoeia Internationalis, 1 edn. (1957), p. 296—300, Anl. 13: Biologische Wertbestimmung für Insulin-Injektionslösungen. Anl. 14: Bestimmung der durch Zink-Protamin-Insulin-Injektionssuspensionen bedingten Verlängerung der Insulinwirkung, p. 300—303 2. edn. 1968

Phillips, R.E., Elevitch, F.R.: An enzymatic fluorometric method for the determination of glucose in plasma. Amer. J. clin. Path. **49**, 622—626 (1968)

Pingel, N., Volund, A.: Stability of pharmaceutical insulin preparations. 6. Ann. Meet. Europ. Ass. for the Study of Diabetes. Diabetes **21**, 805—813 (1972)

Pütter, J., Strufe, R.: Eine Verbesserung der enzymatischen Bestimmung von H_2O_2. Anwendung auf die Glukosebestimmung. Clin. chim. Acta **15**, 159—163 (1967)

Purich, D.L., Fromm, H.J., Rudolph, F.B.: The hexokinases: Kinetic, physical and regulatory properties. Advanc. Enzymol. **39**, 249—362 (1973)

Rausch, L.: Über die Entwicklung und Brauchbarkeit von Insulin-Eichungsmethoden. Pharmazie **2**, 149—154 (1947)

Realdon, A.M.: Determinazione enzimatica del glucosio nel sangue e nell'urina. Boll. chim. farm. **97**, 560—566 (1958)

Reinauer, H., Hollmann, S.: Bestimmungsmethoden von D-Glukose und niedermolekularen Kohlenhydraten. In: D-Glukose und verwandten Verbindungen, ed. H. Bartelheimer *et al.*, p. 71—86. Lit.: 150—157. Stuttgart: Enke 1966

Reiner, L., Searle, D.S., Lang, E.H.: On the hypoglycemic activity of globin insulin. J. Pharmacol. exp. Ther. **67**, 330—340 (1939)

Reisz, G.Z.: Eine photometrische Methode zur Blutzuckerbestimmung. Z. med. Lab.-Techn. **7**, 53—54 (1966)

Richter, M.D.: Zur Bestimmung von Glukose mit o-Toluidin ohne Eisessig. Dtsch. Gesundh.-Wes. **25**, 1493—1496 (1970)

Richterich, R., Colombo, J.P.: Vereinfachte enzymatische Bestimmung der Blutglukose mit 20 Mikroliter Blut. Klin. Wschr. **40**, 1208—1211 (1962)

Richterich, R.: Klinische Chemie. Theorie und Praxis. Frankfurt/M.: Akad. Verl. Ges. 1965

Richterich, R., Lorenz, E.: Die Blutzuckerbestimmung nach Crecelius-Seifert, eine obsolete Labormethode. Praxis (Bern) **57**, 100—101 (1968)

RICHTERICH, R., DAUWALDER, H.: Zur Bestimmung der Plasmaglukosekonzentration mit der Hexokinase/Glukose-6-phosphat-Dehydrogenase-Methode. Schweiz. med. Wschr. **101**, 615—618 (1971)

ROBIN, M., SAIFER, A.: Determination of glucose in biologic fluids with an automated enzymatic procedure. Clin. Chem. **11**, 840—845 (1965)

ROE, J.H.: The determination of sugar in blood and spinal fluid with anthrone reagent. J. biol. Chem. **212**, 335—343 (1955)

ROLANDO, R.L., TORROBA, D.: Heterogenicity of the fourth international standard for insulin by gel-chromatography on Sephadex. Experientia (Basel) **28**, 1169 (1972)

RONA, P., FABISCH, W.: Untersuchungen über den Blutzucker. I. Untersuchungen über den sogenannten Eiweißzucker im Blute. Biochem. Z. **217**, 1—33 (1930a)

RONA, P., FABISCH, W.: Untersuchungen über den Blutzucker. II. Biochem. Z. **227**, 205—220 (1930b)

ROOTH, G., CARLSTRÖM, S.: Diurnal variations in blood glucose, 3-hydroxybutyrate, acetoacetate, plasma free fatty acids and glycerol in diabetics. Acta med. scand. **191**, 559—563 (1972)

RUPPERT, F.: Über die Orcinmethode zur Bestimmung des Blutzuckers und die Frage ihrer Hexosespezifität. Ärztl. Lab. **1**, 13—20 (1955)

RUSSEL, S., BRYANT, M., MORRISON, D.B.: A rapid blood glucose method. Clin. Chem. **10**, Abstr. 641 (1964)

SAIFER, A., GERSTENFELD, S.: The photometric microdetermination of blood glucose with glucose oxidase. J. Lab. clin. Med. **51**, 448—460 (1958)

SAIFER, A., GERSTENFELD, S., ZYMARIS, M.C.: Rapid system of microchemical analysis for the clinical laboratory. Clin. Chem. **4**, 127—141 (1958)

SAIFER, A., ROBIN, M.: Determination of glucose in biological fluids with an automated enzyme procedure. Sympos. Automation in Analytical Chemistry, Frankfurt/M. 1965, p. 944 (1966)

DE SAINT RAT, L., RONFAUT, J.: Sur le dosage de petites quantités de sucres réducteurs dans les liquides de l'organisme. Bull. Soc. Pharmacol. **27**, 289—293 (1920)

SANCHEZ, J.A.: A new color reaction of the hexoses and polyhexoses and its application for the colorimetric determination of glucose in blood. Sem. méd. (B. Aires) **1935 II**, 914—917

SCHÄFER, L., ELEK, S.: Blutzuckerbestimmung mit dem o-Toluidinreagens. Vergleichende Untersuchungen zwischen der Originalmethode von Hultman und der Modifikation von Lüss. Ärztl. Lab. **15**, 391—398 (1969)

SCHLÄGER, R., STUHLMANN, I., KATTERMANN, R.: Einfluß des Enteiweißungsmittels auf die Blutzuckerbestimmung mit der Glukoseoxidase-Peridmethode. Z. klin. Chem. **9**, 178—179 (1971)

SCHMIDT, F.H.: Die Bestimmung der Glukose im Blut mit Hilfe von Enzymreaktionen. Röntgen- u. Lab.-Prax. **12**, L75—L79 (1959)

SCHMIDT, F.H.: Die enzymatische Bestimmung von Glukose und Fructose nebeneinander. Klin. Wschr. **39**, 1244—1247 (1961)

SCHMIDT, F.H.: Enzymatische Methoden zur Bestimmung von Blut- und Harnzucker unter Berücksichtigung von Vergleichsuntersuchungen mit klassischen Methoden. Internist (Berl.) **4**, 554—559 (1963)

SCHMIDT, F.H.: Methoden der Harn- und Blutzuckerbestimmung. In: Hdb. Diabetes Mellitus, ed. E. F. PFEIFFER, p. 913—921; 922—946. München: J. F. Lehmann 1971

SCHMIDT, F.H.: Blutglukosewerte im Capillarblut von Erwachsenen unter Verwendung der Hexokinase Methodik. Klin. Wschr. **51**, 520—522 (1973)

SCHMÖR, J.: Blutzuckerbestimmung mit Thymol-Schwefelsäure. Klin. Wschr. **33**, 449—450 (1955)

SCHOUTEN, H., GITERSON, A.: Blood, urine and liquor sugar. Clin. chim. Acta **8**, 802—803 (1963)

SCHÜTZ, W.: Die Bestimmung des Blutzuckers mit o-Toluidin im Autoanalyzer. Ärztl. Lab. **14**, 500—507 (1968)

SCOTT, D.A., FISHER, A.M.: Studies on insulin with protamine. J. Pharmacol. exp. Ther. **58**, 78—92 (1936)

SHARP, P.: Interference in glucose oxidase-peroxidase blood glucose methods. Clin. chim. Acta **40**, 115—120 (1972)

SHARP, P., RILEY, C., COOK, J.G.H., PINK, P.J.F.: Effect of two sulphonylureas on glucose determinations by enzymic methods. Clin. chim. Acta **36**, 93—98 (1972)

SHIBATA, S.: An ultramicro-colorimetric method for the determination of plasma glucose with o-aminobiphenyl, circumventing deproteinization. Bull. Yamaguchi med. Sch. **8**, 209—214 (1961); CA **57**, 7542d (1962)

SHIBATA, S., MISHIMA, SH.: Improved technique of o-aminobiphenyl method for the determination of glucose in blood. Bull. Yamaguchi med. Sch. **9**, 13—17 (1962); CA **58**, 10500a (1963)

Simon, R.K.: Eine neue Schnellbestimmung des Blutzuckers ohne Enteiweissung. Med. Mschr. **22**, 36 (1968)

Simon, R.K., Christian, G.D., Purdy, W.C.: The coulometric determination of glucose in human serum. Clin. Chem. **14**, 463—476 (1968)

Sitzmann, F.C., Eschler, P.: Enzymatische Bestimmung der Blutglukose mit einer modifizierten Hexokinasemethode. Med. Klin. **65**, 1178—1183 (1970)

Skerry, D.: Rapid determination of plasma glucose by measurement of oxygen consumption. Clin. Biochem. **3**, 319—326 (1970)

Slein, M.W.: D-Glukose-Bestimmung mit Hexokinase und D-Glukose-6-phosphat-Dehydrogenase. In: Bergmeyer, H.U.: Methoden der enzymatischen Analyse, p. 117—123. Weinheim: Verlag Chemie 1962

Van Slyke, D.D., Hawkins, J.A.: A gasometric method for determination of reducing sugars, and its application to analysis of blood and urine. J. biol. Chem. **79**, 739—767 (1928)

Van Slyke, D.D., Hawkins, J.A.: Gasometric determination of fermentable sugar in blood and urine. J. biol. Chem. **83**, 51—70 (1929)

Smith, K.W., Marks, H.P., Fieller, C.E., Broom, W.A.: An extended cross-over design and its use in insulin assay. Quart. J. Pharm. **17**, 108—117 (1944)

Snedecor, G.W.: Statistical methods. Ames, Iowa: Iowa State College Press. Reprinting 1959

Spanhoff, R.W.: Die biologischen Eichungen in der Pharmakopoe, insbesondere das Eichen von Insulin. Dutch Pharm. Weekbl. **75**, 190—202 (1938)

Spathis, G.S.: Continous monitoring of blood sugar in Brittle Diabetes. Diabetologia **6**, 586—592 (1970)

Sudduth, N.C., Widish, J.R., Moore, J.L.: Automation of glucose measurement using o-toluidine reagent. Amer. J. clin. Path. **53**, 181—189 (1970)

Sumner, J.B., Sisler, E.B.: A simple method for blood sugar. Arch. Biochem. **4**, 333—336 (1944)

Sunderman, F.W., Fuller, J.B.: A modification of the Benedict method for measuring blood glucose. Amer. J. clin. Path. **21**, 1077—1084 (1951)

Sunderman, F.W., MacFate, R.P., Evans, G.T., Fuller, J.B.: Symposium on blood sugar. Amer. J. clin. Path. **21**, 901—934 (1951)

Sunderman, F.W., Jr., Sunderman, F.W.: Measurement of glucose in blood, serum and plasma by means of glucose oxidase-catalase enzyme system. Amer. J. clin. Path. **36**, 75—91 (1961)

Stamm, D.: Tagesschwankungen der Normalbereiche diagnostisch wichtiger Blutbestandteile. Verh. dtsch. Ges. inn. Med. **73**, 982—989 (1967)

Stein, P.: 50 Jahre Insulin. Schweiz. Rdschau Medizin (Praxis) **61**, 443—450 (1972)

Stevens, J.F.: Determination of glucose by an automatic analyser. Clin. chim. Acta **32**, 199—201 (1971)

Stewart, G.A.: Insulin. Methods of insulin assay. Brit. med. Bull. **16**, 196—201 (1960)

Stork, H., Schmidt, F.H.: Mitteilung über eine enzymatische Schnellmethode zur Bestimmung des Blutzuckers in 5 μl Capillarblut ohne Enteiweissung und ohne Zentrifugation. Klin. Wschr. **46**, 789—790 (1968)

Strassner, W., Neubert, R.: Ein Beitrag zur Blutzuckerbestimmung mit o-Toluidin. Dtsch. Gesundh.-Wes. **21**, 1735—1738 (1966)

Stroess, J.A.P., Zondag, H.A., Cornelissen, P.J.H.C.: Some experience with a colorimetric method for the determination of glucose in biological fluids. Clin. chim. Acta **8**, 152—154 (1963)

Tammes, A.R., Nordshow, C.D.: An approach to specificity in glucose determinations. Amer. J. clin. Path. **49**, 613—621 (1968)

Teller, J.D.: Direct quantitative, colorimetric determination of serum or plasma glucose. Abstr. Papers 130th meeting. Amer. Chem. Soc., Div. biol. Chem., Atlantic City, Sep. 1956, p. 69 C

Thompson, R.E.: Biological assay of insulin. Objective determination of the quantitative response of mice. Endocrinology **39**, 62 (1946)

Thompson, R.H.: Colorimetric glucose oxidase method for blood glucose. Clin. chim. Acta **13**, 133—135 (1966)

Thybusch, D.: Enzymatische Mikrobestimmung der Blutglukose mit dem Fermokognost-Blutzucker-Testbesteck. Z. med. Labortechn. **12**, 249—254 (1971)

Trnková, M.M., Voldan, M., Fialowá, M., Srámkova, J., Sinkulowá, E.: Vergleich des ein- und zweidosigen Auswertungsverfahrens von Insulin. Arzneimittel-Forsch. **16**, 89—91 (1966)

Trinder, P.: Determination of glucose in blood using glucose oxidase with an alternative oxygen acceptor. Ann. clin. Biochem. **6**, 24—27 (1969)

TRINDER, P.: Determination of blood glucose using an oxidase-peroxidase system with a noncarcinogenic chromogen. J. clin. Path. **22**, 158—161 (1969)

U.S. Pharmacopoeia, 18 edn. (1970), Insulin Assay, p. 329—336; 882—884

VOLDAN, M.: Standardisierung von Insulin und seine Eingliederung in die Arzneibücher (Czech.). Čs. Farm. **15**, 447—451 (1966)

WALDEN, G.B.: Comparison of the old international insulin standard with the new crystalline standard (Rabbit method). Quart. Bull. Hlth Org. L. o. N. **5**, 629—630 (1936)

WARE, A.G., MARBACH, E.P.: Application of glucose oxidase method to serum. Clin. Chem. **11**, 792 (1965)

WARE, A.G., MARBACH, E.P.: Glucose in serum and cerebrospinal fluid by direct application of a glucose oxidase method. Clin. Chem. **14**, 548—554 (1968)

WASHKO, M.E., RICE, E.E.: Determination of glucose by an improved enzymatic procedure. Clin. Chem. **7**, 542—545 (1961)

WATSON, D.: Reducing substances other than glucose in blood. Clin. chim. Acta **7**, 145—146 (1962)

WEBER, E.: Grundriss der biologischen Statistik, 6 edn. Stuttgart: G. Fischer 1967

WEIBEL, M.K., BRIGHT, H.I.: The glucose oxidase mechanism. Interpretation of the pH dependence J. biol. Chem. **246**, 2734—2744 (1971)

WENK, R.E., CRENO, R.J., LOOK, V., HENRY, J.B.: Automated micro measurement of glucose by means of o-toluidine. Clin. Chem. **15**, 1162—1170 (1969)

WENKE, M., LABSKA, J.: Differential determination of levulose and dextrose in single samples of 0.1 ml of blood. Čas. Lék. čes. **93**, 23—25 (1954); CA **48**, 12862e (1954)

WERNER, W., REY, H.G., WIELINGER, H.: Über die Eigenschaften eines neuen Chromogens für die Blutzuckerbestimmung nach der GOD/POD-Methode. Z. analyt. Chem. **252**, 224—228 (1970)

WHO: International standards and units for biological substances. WHO Chronicle **27**, 323—324 (1973)

WIDDOWSON, G.M., PENTON, J.R.: Determination of serum or plasma glucose on the "Autoanalyzer II" by use of the hexokinase reaction. Clin. Chem. **18**, 299—300 (1972)

WIELINGER, H.: GOD-Perid-Methode, ein neues überlegenes Verfahren zur enzymatischen Blutzuckerbestimmung. Krankenhausarzt **43**, 390—391 (1970)

WINCEY, C., MARKS, V.: A micro method for measuring glucose using the Autoanalyzer and glucose-oxidase. J. clin. Path. **14**, 558—559 (1961)

WINCKERS, P.L.M., JACOBS, P.: A simple automated determination of glucose in body fluids using an aqueous o-toluidine-acetic acid reagent. Clin. chim. Acta **34**, 401—408 (1971)

WRIGHT, R.W., RAINWATER, J.C., TOLLE, L.D.: Glucose assay systems: Evaluation of a colorimetric hexokinase procedure. Clin. Chem. **17**, 1010—1015 (1971)

YEE, H.Y.: Automated hexokinase procedure for assaying glucose in urine, serum, or plasma. Clin. Chem. **18**, 1416—1419 (1972)

YEE, H., JENEST, E.S., BOWLES, P.R.: Modified manual or automated o-toluidine system for determining glucose in serum, with an improved aqueous reagent. Clin. Chem. **17**, 103—107 (1971)

YOUNG, D.M., LEWIS, A.H.: Detection of hypoglycemic reactions in the mouse assay for insulin. Science **105**, 368—369 (1947)

YOUNG, D.M., REID, D.B.W., ROMANS, K.C.: A comparison of three methods for the assay of commercial insulin preparations. Canad. J. Res., Sect. E **28**, 19—22 (1950)

YOUNG, D.S.: High-pressure column chromatography of carbohydrates in the clinical laboratory. Amer. J. clin. Path. **53**, 803—810 (1970)

YOUNG, P.A., STEWART, G.A.: The distribution of error in mouse insulin assays. J. Pharm. Pharmacol. **4**, 169—180 (1952)

ZENDER, R.: Une micro-méthode automatique pour l'analyse quantitative des aldohexoses dans les liquides biologiques par l'-o-toluidine. Clin. chim. Acta **8**, 351—358 (1963)

ZENDER, R.: Micro-analyse automatique des aldohexoses dans les liquides biologiques par l'-o-toluidine. Clin. chim. Acta **11**, 88—91 (1965)

ZIPF, R.E., WALDO, A.L.: Spectrophotometric analysis of carbohydrates and study of anthrone reagent. J. Lab. clin. Med. **39**, 497—502 (1952)

D. The Isolation of Insulin from the Pancreas

Wolfgang Burgermeister, Franz Enzmann and Hans-Hermann Schöne

I. General Aspects of Insulin Isolation

1. The Need for Insulin and How It Is Satisfied

The extraction and purification of insulin are among the most carefully executed procedures used to prepare a protein. One encounters all the problems involved in the extraction of any complex natural product.

Until now, bovine and porcine pancreata have been the only source of insulin. The possibility also exists of using sheep and even horse or goat pancreata in countries where they are more plentiful. At the present time, however, it is difficult to calculate the world supply of pancreata and, thus, of insulin. Current estimates are based on the projected number of animals which will be slaughtered for food. With proper perspective, one may assume that only 20—30% of all insulin resources are being utilized at the present time. The insulin requirement is expected to double within the next 10 years. This figure is also relatively uncertain, since such factors as diagnosis, increased inheritance of diabetes, the standard of living, current schools of thought (recently there has been a greater tendency to prescribe insulin) and the purity of the insulin play an important role. It may be assumed from these two estimates of use and requirement that it will be possible to satisfy the insulin requirements for at least the next ten and probably the next 20 years using natural sources. This time is then available to develop a chemically synthesized insulin which is commercially acceptable. According to the technical progress of peptide synthesis, this goal is not unreasonable.

The number of diabetics in West Germany amounts to 1 or 2% of the population (Entmacher and Marks, 1965; Gsell, 1968; Mehnert *et al.*, 1968). Approximately one third of these are dependent on insulin. The mean daily insulin dose is 40 units; that is, 1.6 mg. More than 100 kg of insulin per year are required in Germany. These figures are similar in other highly developed countries, taking the number of people into consideration. Japan, however, is an exception, in that the insulin requirement is only one thenth to one fifth that of West Germany.

2. Properties of the Pancreas Influencing Isolation

In the extraction of insulin, one must consider the natural conditions under which insulin is present in the pancreas. The most important characteristic is that 99% of the pancreatic tissue consists of exocrine tissue and only 1% of islet tissue. This means quantitatively that in one kilogram of bovine pancreas 40 g of proteolytic enzymes are in close association with 100 mg of insulin. Although proteases such as trypsin, chymotrypsins, elastase, carboxypeptidases, etc. are present as inactive precursors, investigations have shown that a partial activation of the proteases cannot be avoided despite careful handling of the pancreata. The degree of activation depends on the care taken in the treatment of the pancreata.

The following is a description of how the pancreas may be properly handled (LINDNER, 1956): The pancreas must be removed as fast as possible after the death of the animal and then rapidly frozen and stored at temperatures between —20 and —25° C.

This temperature must be maintained until the insulin is to be extracted. Temperature between —5 to —10° C are not sufficient for storage over a period of several weeks. Proteolysis becomes manifest not only by lesser insulin yields but also by difficulties in the preparation of insulin so that eventually additional purification steps must be taken. Examples will be given later concerning the extraction of insulin from human pancreata. A proof of the proteolysis is the appearance of insulin degradation products which may significantly disturb separation and crystallization.

The insulin content of pancreata of fully grown animals of different species does not vary significantly. The content ranges from 1000—4000 units per kg, or 40—160 mg. Differences observed among the various species seem to stem from the condition of the pancreas and the age of the animal, rather than from variation in the species. The insulin content may be markedly higher in young animals. This has been particularly well investigated in calves. Insulin contents of 10,000 I.U. (= 400 mg) per kg have been found in calves with up to 40,000 I.U. per kg in the fetal calf pancreas.

The extraction procedure must be modified depending on the preservation condition and insulin content of the pancreata. The fat content, which is particularly high in pork and sheep glands, also requires additional steps in the purification process.

3. Properties of Insulin Influencing Isolation

Conditions which are contradictory to insulin's protein properties must be avoided during the isolation procedure (KLOSTERMEYER and ZAHN, 1971). Although insulin is heat-sensitive, it can be subjected to rapid heating under special conditions. For example, at the isoelectric point it can be heated up to 90°. At pH-values above 10, the disulfide bonds are broken. Oxidizing and reducing agents have the same effect. As a result, the biological activity is destroyed and reactivation is not possible. In a strong acidic solution insulin is converted to an insoluble, inactive form, fibrillar insulin. In this case, renaturation is possible (WAUGH, 1944, 1948).

Acid causes additional changes in insulin's structure. The insulin molecule contains three asparagines and three glutamines. Depending on the acidity of the medium, particularly in the presence of organic solvents, cleavage of single acid amide bonds and release of ammonia occur. The Asp-A21 is especially sensitive. Insulin which has lost one or two acid amide groups maintains its full biological activity. Due to the manufacturing conditions employed (see below), all commercial insulins — including insulin which has been recrystallized several times — contain desmonoamido- and desdiamido insulin. Porcine insulin is more easily deaminated than bovine insulin (CHRAMBACH and CARPENTER, 1960; CARPENTER and CHRAMBACH, 1962; SLOBIN and CARPENTER, 1963; SUNDBY, 1962; MIRSKY and KAWAMURA, 1966; BERSON and YALOW, 1966).

Chromatographic methods of purification are complicated by the solubility properties of insulin. Insulin is difficult to dissolve between pH 4.0 and 7.0 with the minimum solubility at pH 5.3—5.4. The range of poor solubility can be extended in the presence of bivalent cations and of salts and is reduced in the presence of organic solvents such as alcohols and ketones. The insulins from different species show slight differences in solubility.

The crystallization of insulin represents an efficient purification step (SCOTT, 1934; SCHLICHTKRULL, 1958). It also has limitations, however. Due to the largely homogeneous tertiary structure of insulin and its precursors, derivatives and degradation products, crystallization cannot be used to separate these molecules. Even multiple recrystallization cannot prevent the accompanying proteins from being incorporated into the crystal lattice structure of insulin (MIRSKY and KAWAMURA, 1966; BLUNDELL *et al.*, 1972; STEINER, 1973).

4. Methods of Detecting Impurities

With the improved specificity and sensitivity of detection methods, progress in the purification of insulin has also been achieved. Chromatographic and electrophoretic methods have contributed more than biological and radioimmunological methods to characterizing insulin. Heterogeneity of highly purified insulin preparations was demonstrated even before the discovery of proinsulin. These findings were made using countercurrent distribution (HARFENIST and CRAIG, 1951, 1952), partition chromatography (CARPENTER and HESS, 1956), ion exchange chromatography (COLE, 1960), starch gel electrophoresis (BARRET *et al.*, 1962), paper electrophoresis (SUNDBY, 1962) and polyacrylamide gel electrophoresis (MIRSKY and KAWAMURA, 1966).

High-molecular weight impurities are detectable by means of paper chromatography (LIGHT and SIMPSON, 1956a) and gel chromatography (DAVOREN, 1962) while countercurrent distribution and partition chromatography are used to detect desamido insulins. Ion exchange chromatography is used to detect insulins of different ionic charges. At present, the most efficient method is polyacrylamide gel electrophoresis, particularly when used after gel and ion exchange chromatography (CHANCE, 1970, 1971; STEINER *et al.*, 1968; NOLAN *et al.*, 1971).

II. Methods of Insulin Isolation

Since v. Mehring's and Minkowsky's discovery that depancreatized dogs show symptoms of diabetes, numerous investigations have been made to extract insulin from the pancreas. An important success was achieved in 1922 by BANTING and BEST who used acidic aqueous ethanol to extract insulin. Further developments in insulin preparation were the first crystallization of insulin by ABEL (1926), and the discovery by SCOTT (1934) that crystallization requires zinc ions. Starting with this basic knowledge, further efforts have been directed toward two goals: to improve the insulin yield and its purity. These aims were thought to have been reached in the sixties. Then the discovery of proinsulin by STEINER (1967) promoted the use of chromatographic methods for the purification of insulin. Chromatography is the most effective method of obtaining pure insulin.

1. Extraction and Precipitation

The procedure published by ROMANS *et al.* (1940) should be mentioned first among the methods for the recovery of insulin by extraction and precipitation. The pancreas glands are extracted with 70% aqueous ethanol made acidic with hydrochloric acid. During the subsequent adjustment of the pH to 8, the precipitate formed is centrifuged off. The ethanol is then removed under vacuum at pH 2—3. The precipitated fat is removed by filtration, and the insulin is precipitated from the solution by adding 25% sodium chloride. Another precipitation with 15% sodium chloride follows and an isoelectric precipitation at pH 5—5.4. The crude insulin is then crystallized in an acetate buffer containing zinc ions and acetone. The biological activity of the insulin crystals is 22—24 I.U. per mg. From 1 kg of beef pancreas, 1750—2000 I.U. of crystalline insulin are obtained[1].

Extensive efforts have been made to improve the individual steps of the classical purification procedure. MAXWELL and HINKEL (1950, 1951) replace hydrochloric acid with phosphoric and oxalic acids. This facilitates processing the precipitates from the pancreas, and increases insulin yields to 3100—3400 I.U. HOMAN (1950) and also ROMANS (1954) alter the ethanol concentration (ROMANS also changes the pH to 5.2) and add various salts (particularly sodium chloride). They obtain yields of 2600—3700 I.U.. In the preparation of small quantities of pancreas, RANDALL (1964) removes the ethanol by extraction with ether to avoid alcohol distillation. The yield by his procedure is 1750—3500 I.U. MEYER CLUWEN (1961) uses aromatic hydrocarbons or higher aliphatic alcohols. HOEK (1961) avoids distillation and extraction by precipitating the crude insulin with zinc ions from the original extract which had been diluted with H_2O to about 30% ethanol content at pH 6—8. He obtains 3750—4250 I.U. ROMANS (1954) distills the solution to a 30% ethanol concentration and removes the fat and residual alcohol by extraction with hydrocarbons.

Using crystallization, PETERSEN and SCHLICHTKRULL (1952) obtain especially well-formed crystals by adding sodium chloride in higher concentrations. JACKSON (1970) crystallizes in the absence of zinc in a range of pH from 7.2—10 and obtains 2600—4600 I.U. He also uses higher sodium chloride concentrations.

The method published by RANDALL in 1964 is appropriate for isolating insulin from small amounts of pancreas. He precipitates the crude insulin from the solution with picric acid. The insulin can be easily separated from the picric acid by dissolving it in aqueous acetone and then precipitating out the insulin by raising the acetone concentration. WAUGH (1950) isolates insulin from solutions by causing the formation of fibrillar insulin.

Insulin extracted by various methods frequently still contains small amounts of proteolytic enzymes. HOMAN and EVERTZEN (1957) remove these enzymes from aqueous-organic solvents through precipitation at slightly acidic pH in the presence of small amounts of alkali ions.

Some of the efforts are aimed at simultaneous isolation of insulin and the enzymes. LAUTENSCHLÄGER and LINDNER (1943) treat the pancreata with aqueous-organic solvents at pH 8.0—8.5, whereby insulin is extracted yielding 2000 I.U. The gland residues may then be used for pancreatin extraction. KÖLLENSPERGER *et al.* (1971) subject the pancreas glands to lyophilization and subsequent defatting with a lipid solvent. They then extract the insulin with aqueous ethanol (60—80%) in the presence of 1—5% sodium chloride. In both instances the subsequent steps in the purification process are not changed.

---

1 For purpose of comparability, yield data in the following text always refer to the quantity of crystalline insulin obtained from 1 kg of beef pancreas.

2. Adsorption to Ion Exchangers

Ion exchange has often been used to adsorb insulin directly from the crude pancreatic extract. The concentration of the crude extract by evaporation and the separation of fat can thus be avoided. The crude extract is either stirred with the ion exchanger (batch-wise procedure) or is passed over an ion exchange column. The insulin is subsequently eluted from the exchanger with a suitable solvent. It is isolated in the usual manner by precipitation with sodium chloride and then further purified.

According to the procedure of JORPES *et al.* (1956), insulin is adsorbed from the aqueous-alcoholic pancreatic extract by alginic acid at pH 4.8 and eluted with 0.3 N HCl. ANTONIADES *et al.* (1960) bind insulin to Dowex 50 at pH 6.6. KATKOVSKI *et al.* (1965) bind insulin at pH 3.5 to a sulfonic acid exchanger based on polystyrol. The resin is washed with ethanol to remove fatty material also adsorbed by the exchanger. The elution of insulin is achieved with aqueous ammonia containing 20% acetone. SMITH *et al.* (1966) use CM (= carboxymethyl)-cellulose at pH 4.1—6.3 for adsorption. After the exchanger is washed with ethanol, the insulin is eluted with 0.1 N hydrochloric acid and purified using picrate precipitation, isoelectric precipitation and, finally, crystallization. The yields (3100—4700 I.U.) are 11—47% higher than in RANDALL's (1964) isolation procedure.

Anion exchangers may be employed in a similar manner. Insulin is adsorbed by DEAE (= diethylaminoethyl)-cellulose from crude extracts adjusted from pH 5.5—8 (VOLINI and MITZ, 1959). Elution is carried out with 0.1 N hydrochlorid acid.

3. Table: Yield of Insulin Obtained Using Different Methods

Some data of insulin yields obtained using various isolation methods are compiled in the following table. When comparing the data one must consider that uncontrolled factors such as the age of the animal and the preserved condition of the gland may also influence the yields.

Table 1

Animal	Yield of crystalline from 1 kg of pancreas [I.U.]	Biological activity [I.U./mg]	Method of isolation	References
beef	1750—2000	22—24	a	ROMANS *et al.* (1940)
beef	2000		b	LAUTENSCHLÄGER AND LINDNER (1943)
beef	3100—3400		a	MAXWELL and HINKEL (1950)
beef	2800—3500		a	HOMAN (1950)
calf	10400		a	HOMAN (1950)
beef	2600—3700		a	ROMANS (1954)
beef	3750—4250	25	a	HOEK (1961)
beef	1750—3500	21—23	c	RANDALL (1964)
beef	3100—4700		d	SMITH *et al.* (1966)
beef	2600—4600	23—24	a	JACKSON (1970)
pork	2400—2750	23—25	a	JACKSON (1970)

a: Extraction and precipitation.
b: As a, with simultaneous isolation of insulin and pancreatic enzymes.
c: As a, small-scale preparation.
d: Adsorption to ion exchanger.

III. Insulin Purification Using Chromatographic Methods

Efforts to purify insulin were aided by the development of chromatography. Earlier, characterization of insulin's structure and chemical properties had been of primary interest, but most recently attention has been focused on the preparative aspects of isolation.

1. Paper Chromatography

Paper chromatography was the first chromatographic technique used to separate insulin. 1-butanol-acetic acid-water and 2-butanol-1% aqueous acetic acid, respectively, are used as solvent systems in which insulin and related proteins cover approximately the same distance. Other pancreatic proteins remain, for the most part, at the application site.

Paper chromatographic separation of insulin is frequently applied in the analytical field (ROBINSON and FEHR, 1952; LIGHT and SIMPSON, 1956a; GRODSKY and TARVER, 1956; FENTON, 1959; TAYLOR *et al.*, 1962), but occasionally this method is also used for the preparative recovery of insulin from small quantities of crude insulin. LIGHT and SIMPSON (1959b) reported an isolation of ^{14}C-labelled insulin by repeated paper chromatography and subsequent use of paper electrophoresis for further purification. TAYLOR *et al.* (1961) described the isolation of insulin from crude pancreatic extracts of different species. TAYLOR and SMITH (1964) mention purification of a crude insulin preparation from rat using paper chromatography. Rat insulin, however, is composed of two different molecules which must then be separated by paper electrophoresis.

2. Gel Chromatography

Gel chromatography (see FISCHER, 1971) makes efficient separation of insulin from proteins of a higher molecular weight possible. Precipitated or crystallized crude insulin is usually chosen as the starting material. In the eluate, high-molecular weight foreign proteins appear first (the a-component mentioned by STEINER *et al.*, 1967) followed by insulin-related substances with longer amino acid sequences, such as proinsulin and intermediate insulins (the b-component). After the appearance of these protein, insulin is eluted together with desamido insulins and other derivatives of equal molecular size (the c-component).

DAVOREN (1962) prepared insulin from a single cat pancreas using the method of ROMANS *et al.* (1940). After precipitation with sodium chloride, the crude insulin is fractioned in 1 M acetic acid on a Sephadex G-50 column. HUMBLE (1963) uses Sephadex G-75 and a more acidic elutrient (5 M acetic acid/0.15 M NCl) to purify crude insulin prepared according to JEPHCOTT (1931). EPSTEIN and ANFINSEN (1963) apply crude insulin isolated according to PETTINGA (1958) to a Sephadex G-50 column in a weak alkaline solution (0.2 M ammonium hydrogen carbonate, pH 7.8).

Gel chromatography has now become a routine step in the purification of insulin (comp. MIRSKY *et al.*, 1963; WANG and CARPENTER, 1965; KIMMEL and POLLOCK, 1967; JACKSON *et al.*, 1969; WEITZEL *et al.*, 1969; SHAPCOTT and O'BRIEN, 1970). Further application in combination with ion exchange chromatography is discussed below.

3. Ion Exchange Chromatography

Proteins can be fractionated by an ion exchanger (comp. RYBÁK *et al.*, 1966) depending on the ionic charge. Ion exchange chromatography can thus be used to isolate insulin from accompanying proteins of similar molecular weight, a separation which gel chromatography does not achieve. For example, arginine insulin and the insulin ester, when present in certain buffers, have stronger positive charges than insulin, while the desamido insulins have more negative electrical charges.

a) Cation Exchangers

BOARDMAN (1956) separates insulin in an acetate buffer of pH 3.4 on an exchange resin containing sulfonic acid groups. He obtains a clear separation of crude insulin, but only a barely detectable fractionation of crystalline insulin into two components which are not further described.

COLE (1960) and MENDIOLA and COLE (1960) use the resin Amberlite IRC-50 which contains carboxyl groups, and a phosphate buffer of pH 6.0 with 8 M urea. Insulin is separated into 3 components, one of which is identified as desamido insulin. The addition of 8 M urea results in a desaggregation of the insulin, and thus improves chromatographic separation. DILLON and ROMANS (1966) using the same method fractionate insulin into pure insulin, desmonoamido- and desdiamido insulin, as well as carbamylated insulin.

A number of authors have reported the use of CM-cellulose for the purification of insulin. YAMAMOTO *et al.* (1960) fractionate crystallized bonito insulin in an acetate buffer at pH 4. Elution with a formic acid gradient leads to the separation of bonito insulin I and II.

SMITH (1964) uses a citrate buffer (pH 3—3.4) and elutes the column with a sodium chloride gradient. Bovine and porcine insulins appear together in the eluate. DILLON and ROMANS (1967) select a citrate buffer of pH 5—5.5 and add 7 M urea. At pH 5.38 a good separation of desamido insulins is obtained whereas at pH 5.5 these are eluted together. Further application of CM-cellulose for the purification of insulin under similar conditions is described by NEUMANN and HUMBEL (1969) and by RUTTENBERG (1972).

The purification of insulin by gel chromatography with subsequent ion exchange chromatography on CM-cellulose is described by HUMBEL and CRESTFIELD (1965) as well as by NEUMANN *et al.* (1969).

b) Anion Exchangers

THOMPSON and O'DONNELL (1960) describe a technique for the purification of insulin on DEAE-cellulose. In this process insulin is fractionated using 0.01 M tris-HCl buffer at pH 7.4. The buffer contains 8 M urea and 0.001 M EDTA (ethylenediamine tetraacetate). Desamido insulin is separated only when urea is present and is eluted after insulin. The influence of temperature, pH-value and ionic strength on the elution behavior of insulin is investigated by the same authors (O'DONNELL and THOMPSON, 1960).

BROMER *et al.* (1967), BROMER and CHANCE (1967), LEVY and CARPENTER (1967), and CHANCE *et al.* (1968) separate insulin and its derivatives using the same chromatographic method, but mostly with DEAE-Sephadex, the dextran equivalent. In order to obtain especially pure insulin preparations, KIMMEL *et al.* (1968) and ZIMMERMANN *et al.* (1972) employ this procedure after the insulin has been subjected to gel chromatography. GRANT and REID (1968) combine chromatography on Sephadex G-75, DEAE-Sephadex, and CM-cellulose.

KRISHCHENKO (1969) describe the separation of bovine and porcine insulin on TEAE (= triethylaminoethyl)-cellulose in a phosphate buffer — initial pH 7.6 — using a complex ionic strength- and pH gradient.

SCHLICHTKRULL *et al.* (1972) use QAE (= quaternary aminoethyl)-Sephadex and a tris-HCl buffer in 60% aqueous ethanol to purify crystallized insulin. Some of the associated proteins appear before insulin and some after, the major fraction contains a very pure insulin. MARKUSSEN and SUNDBY (1972) use QAE-Sephadex under similar conditions to purify NaCl precipitated insulin.

IV. Special Purification Processes

1. Countercurrent Distribution and Partition Chromatography

HARFENIST and CRAIG (1952) and HARFENIST (1953) describe attempts to carry out countercurrent distribution of crystalline and amorphous insulin. The separation of desamido insulin takes place in a 2-butanol-1% aqueous dichloracetic acid system. DOSCH *et al.* (1971) purify commercial insulin by countercurrent distribution in a butanol-pyridine-0.5% acetic acid system (5:3:11). The content of proinsulin and intermediate insulins is thereby reduced from 11% (beef) and 3.5% (pork), to approximately 1% for both types. Desamido insulins separate out, with the exception of a small desmonoamido insulin residue.

PORTER (1953) employs the column partition chromatography technique. He applies ethylene glycol ether on silane-treated silica gel (hyflo-super-cel) as the stationary phase and phosphate buffer as the mobile phase (pH 7.6 and 3, respectively). A good separation of the foreign proteins is obtained with crude insulin preparations. Five-times recrystallized insulin appears homogeneous in his system. CARPENTER and HESS (1956), and also CARPENTER (1958), use 2-butanol-0.1 N HCl as a partition system. Untreated hyflo-super-cel serves as a solid support for the stationary aqueous phase. Crystallized insulin separates into two components. Later, CHRAMBACH and CARPENTER (1960) succeeded in separating 4 components corresponding to insulin and various deamidation products by using 1-butanol, 2-butanol-0.1 N HCl, and another silica gel preparation (micro-cel and celite). YOUNG and CARPENTER (1961) report separation of insulin and desoctapeptide insulin in a similar system.

2. Electrophoresis

The preparative electrophoresis of commercial insulin is described by TIMASHEFF *et al.* (1953) as well as by TIMASHEFF and KIRKWOOD (1953). The authors are able to separate a heterogeneous, less active component from insulin in an apparatus designed by Tiselius. ZIEGLER and LIPPMANN (1968) use agar gel electrophoresis for the preparative separation of insulin and glucagon. HINZ *et al.* (1970) separate insulin and proinsulin on a microscale by elution from a polyacrylamide gel.

V. Table: Isolation of Insulin from Different Species

The following table is a compilation of various studies containing detailed methods for the isolation of certain insulins. These studies explain laboratory procedures which, for the most part, are carried out with small quantities of pancreas (~ 50 g) or with single glands. The specific methods used have already been described.

Species	*Author*
Man	MIRSKY *et al.* (1963); SMITH (1964); KIMMEL and POLLOCK (1967); JACKSON *et al.* (1969); SHAPCOTT and O'BRIEN (1970).
Cow, Pig	PETTINGA (1958); RANDALL (1964); SMITH (1964).
Whale	EGOROVA *et al.* (1967).
Dog	PETTINGA (1958); SMITH (1964).
Cat	DAVOREN (1962).
Rabbit	MENDIOLA and COLE (1960); SMITH (1964).
Guinea pig	ZIMMERMANN *et al.* (1972).
Rat	MALLORY *et al.* (1964); TAYLOR and SMITH (1964); SMITH (1964).
Mouse	MARKUSSEN (1971)
Chicken	SMITH (1964); KIMMEL *et al.* (1968).
Turkey	WEITZEL *et al.* (1969)
Duck	MARKUSSEN and SUNDBY (1973).
Angler fish	HUMBEL (1963); HUMBEL and CRESTFIELD (1965); NEUMANN *et al.* (1969).
Bonito	YAMAMOTO *et al.* (1960); NEUMANN and HUMBEL (1969).
Cod	GRANT and REID (1968).

VI. Isolation of Insulin Analogs and the C-Peptide

For a discussion of the isolation of insulin to be complete, insulin analogs and the C-peptide must also be included. STEINER and OYER (1967), STEINER *et al.* (1967), and STEINER (1967) have done studies which, by demonstrating the presence of proinsulin, give a key to the explanation of the various bands obtained when purified insulin is subjected to electrophoresis, as particularly observed by MIRSKY and KARAMURA (1966). Although the separation of the C-peptide from insulin is possible without much difficulty due to its different primary and tertiary structures, the insulin analogs accompany the insulin throughout crystallization. In this case, separation is possible only by utilizing the often subtile differences in molecular weight and electrical charge. One should therefore realize that hardly any of the products recovered in this manner satisfy the high purity and identity standard required of insulin.

For the isolation of porcine proinsulin, CHANCE *et al.* (1968) and CHANCE (1970, 1972) run crystalline porcine insulin through DEAE-cellulose columns in a tris buffer of pH 8.1 in the presence of 7 M urea. HORINO *et al.* (1972) prepare a crude proinsulin by repeated gel chromatography of insulin on Bio-Gel P30 and then purify it on DEAE-cellulose. For the preparation of bovine proinsulin, SCHMIDT and ARENS (1968), STEINER *et al.* (1968) as well as NOLAN *et al.* (1971) use fractions enriched with proinsulin which had been obtained from gel chromatography of insulin on Sephadex G-50. SCHMIDT and ARENS (1968) then extract proinsulin by ion exchange chromatography on DEAE-Sephadex A-25 in a tris buffer of pH 7.5 in the presence of 7 M urea. STEINER *et al.* (1968) and NOLAN *et al.* (1971) separate the crude proinsulin on CM-cellulose at pH 5.5 in the presence of 7 M urea into an "acidic" and a "basic" fraction; then the proinsulin is separated from the "basic" fraction on DEAE-cellulose at pH 7.4 in the presence of 7 M urea. SUNDBY and MARKUSSEN (1972) isolate both types of rat proinsulin by chromatography on QAE-Sephadex A-25 at pH 7.4 in the presence of 60% ethanol, and then separate them by means of polyacrylamide gel electrophoresis at pH 5.4.

The preceding methods used by CHANCE (1970, 1972), by STEINER *et al.* (1968) and NOLAN *et al.* (1971) are appropriate for further isolation of proinsulin and insulin analogs from pig and cow extracts. Porcine insulin preparations contain partially cleaved proinsulin (the Leu_{54}—Ala_{55} bond is cleaved), desdipeptide proinsulin (Lys_{62}, Arg_{63} are missing), desnonapeptide proinsulin (amino acids 55—63 are missing), diarginine insulin (B_{31} = Arg, B_{32} = Arg), and monoarginine insulin (B_{31} = Arg). A mixture of two desdipeptide proinsulins (in the intermediate insulin form I Lys $_{59}$ and Arg $_{60}$ are missing; in the intermediate insulin form II Arg_{31}, Arg_{32} are missing) is present in bovine insulin preparations.

For the preparation of bovine C-peptide, STEINER *et al.* (1971) extract insulin from the pancreas and separate the C-peptide and insulin on CM-cellulose at pH 5 in 7 M urea. SUNDBY and MARKUSSEN (1970) utilize the ability of proinsulin to remain dissolved at acidic pH in 15% sodium chloride solution for separation. In both cases, as in the subsequent studies, further purification steps are required. Following similar procedures, SUNDBY and MARKUSSEN (1970) isolate porcine C-peptide, MARKUSSEN *et al.* (1971) and OYER *et al.* (1971) human C-peptide, PETERSEN *et al.* (1972) monkey-, sheep- and dog C-peptide, and SUNDBY and MARKUSSEN (1972) the two rat C-peptides.

References

ABEL, J.J.: Crystalline insulin. Proc. nat. Acad. Sci. (Wash.) **12**, 132 (1926)

ANTONIADES, H.N., RENOLD, A.E., DAGENAIS, Y.M., STEINKE, J.: Preliminary observations on state of insulin in human and bovine pancreas. Proc. Soc. exp. Biol. (N.Y.) **103**, 677 (1960)

BANTING, F.G., BEST, C.H.: The internal secretion of the pancreas. J. Lab. clin. Med. **7**, 465 (1922)

BARRETT, R.J., FRIESEN, H., ASTWOOD, E.B.: Characterization of pituitary and peptide hormones by electrophoresis in starch gel. J. biol. Chem. **237**, 432 (1962)

BERSON, S.A., YALOW, R.S.: Desamidation of insulin during storage in frozen state. Diabetes **15**, 875 (1966)

BLUNDELL, T., DODSON, G., HODGKIN, D., MERCOLA, D.: Insulin. The structure in the crystal and its reflection in chemistry and biology. Advanc. Protein Chem. **26**, 279 (1972), New York-London: Academic Press, especially, p. 371 ff

BOARDMAN, N.K.: An improved ion-exchange reagent. British Patent 871541 (1956)

BOARDMAN, N.K.: Chromatography of insulin on a celite-sulfonic acid ion-exchange resin. J. Chromatogr. **2**, 398 (1959)

BROMER and CHANCE 1967

BROMER, W.W., SHEEHAN, S.K., BERNS, A.W., ARQUILLA, E.R.: Preparation and properties of fluoresceinthiocarbamyl insulins. Biochemistry **6**, 2378 (1967)

CARPENTER, F.H.: Partition column chromatography of insulin in 2-butanol-aqueous acid systems. Arch. Biochem. **78**, 539 (1958)

CARPENTER, F.H., CHRAMBACH, A.: Amide content of insulin fractions isolated by partition column chromatography and countercurrent distribution. J. biol. Chem. **237**, 404 (1962)

CARPENTER, F.H., HESS, G.P.: The theory and use of elution analysis in the partition column chromatography of insulin between 2-butanol and dichloroacetic acid, hydrochlorid acid solvent systems. J. Amer. chem. Soc. **78**, 3351 (1956)

CHANCE, R.E.: Chemical, physical, biological, and immunological studies on porcine proinsulin and related polypeptides. Proc. of the VII. Congress of the Internat. Diabetes Fed., Buenos Aires, 1970; Excerpta Medica Internat. Congress Series, No. 231, p. 292—305

CHANCE, R.E.: Amino acid sequences of proinsulin and intermediates. Diabetes **21**, Suppl. 2, 461 (1972)

CHANCE, R.E., ELLIS, R.M., BROMER, W.W.: Porcine proinsulin: characterization and amino acid sequence. Science **161**, 165 (1968)

CHRAMBACH, A., CARPENTER, F.H.: Partition column chromatography of insulin: production and separation of transformation products. J. biol. Chem. **235**, 3478 (1960)

COLE, R.D.: The chromatography of insulin in urea-containing buffer. J. biol. Chem. **235**, 2294 (1960)

DAVOREN, P.R.: The isolation of insulin from a single cat pancreas. Biochim. biophys. Acta (Amst.) **63**, 150 (1962)

DILLON, W.W., ROMANS, R.G.: Heterogeneity of insulin. I. Isolation of a chromatographically purified, high-potency insulin and some of its properties. Canad. J. Biochem. **44**, **1171** (1966)

DILLON, W.W., ROMANS, R.G.: Heterogeneity of insulin. II. Chromatography of insulin on carboxymethyl cellulose in urea containing buffers. Canad. J. Biochem. **45**, 221 (1967)
DOSCH, R., WERNER, J.P., PUCHINGER, H., WACKER, A.: Reinigung von Insulin durch Gegenstromverteilung. Arzneimittel-Forsch. **21**, 1422 (1971)
EGOROVA, L.N., SABASHNIKOVA, G.P., MROCHKOV, K.A., KOVALENKO, I.P., KATKOVSKII, S.B., GASANOV, S.G., FREDRIKOVA, L.S., VASILEVSKII, B.S.: U.S.S.R. Patent 277 188 (1967)
EGOROVA, L.N., SABASHNIKOVA, G.P., MROCHKOV, K.A., KOVALEKO, I.P., KATKOVSKII, S.B., GASANOV, S.G., FREDRIKOVA, L.S., VASILEVSKII, B.S.: Chem. Abstr. **74**, 61331 h (1971)
ENTMACHER, P.S., MARKS, H.H.: Diabetes in 1964. A world survey. Diabetes **14**, 212 (1965)
EPSTEIN, C.J., ANFINSEN, C.B.: The use of gel filtration in the isolation and purification of beef insulin. Biochemistry **2**, 461 (1963)
FENTON, E.L.: A method for the assay of insulin by paper chromatography. Biochem. J. **71**, 507 (1959)
FISCHER, L.: An Introduction to gel chromatography. Amsterdam: North Holland Publ. Comp. 1971
GRANT, P.T., REID, K.B.M.: Isolation and partial amino acid sequence of insulin from the islet tissue of cod (gadus callarias). Biochem. J. **106**, 531 (1968)
GRODSKY, G., TARVER, H.: Paper chromatography of insulin. Nature (Lond.) **177**, 223 (1956)
GSELL, O.: Epidemiologie des Diabetes. Dtsch. med. Wschr. **93**, 2446 (1968)
HARFENIST, E.J.: The amino acid compositions of insulins isolated from beef, pork, and sheep glands. J. Amer. chem. Soc. **75**, 5528 (1953)
HARFENIST, E.J., CRAIG, L.C.: Countercurrent distribution of insulin. J. Amer. chem. Soc. **73**, 877 (1951)
HARFENIST, E.J., CRAIG, L.C.: Countercurrent distribution studies with insulin. J. Amer. chem. Soc. **74**, 3083 (1952)
HINZ, M., KATSILAMBROS, N., PFEIFFER, E.F.: Determination of insulin and proinsulin after separation by continuous flow elution from polyacrylamide electrophoresis. Horm. Metab. Res. **2**, 123 (1970)
HOEK, S.: Verfahren zur Gewinnung von Insulin aus Pankreasextrakt. Deutsche Auslegeschrift Nr. 1 492 044 (1961)
HOMAN, J.D.H.: Verfahren zur Gewinnung von Insulin aus insulinhaltigen Organen im Wege der Extraktion. Deutsche Patentschrift Nr. 876143 (1950)
HOMAN, J.D.H., EVERTZEN, A.A.: Verfahren zur Herstellung protaminasefreier Insulinpräparate. Deutsche Auslegeschrift Nr. 1036469 (1957)
HORINO, M., KABAYASHI, K., ARIYOSHI, K.: Isolation of porcine proinsulin from crystalline porcine insulin. Endocr. jap. **19**, 579 (1972)
HUMBEL, R.E.: Isolation of insulin from the fish, lophius piscatorius, by gel filtration. Biochem. biophys. Res. Commun. **12**, 333 (1963)
HUMBEL, R.E., CRESTFIELD, A.M.: Isolation and partial structure analysis of insulin from the separate islet tissue of lophius piscatorius (anglerfish). Biochemistry **4**, 1044 (1965)
JACKSON, R.L.: Verfahren zur Isolierung und Reinigung von Insulin. Deutsche Auslegeschrift Nr. 2018588 (1970)
JACKSON, R.L., SHUEY, E.W., GRINNAN, E.L., ELLIS, R.M.: Preparation and partial characterization of crystalline human insulin. Diabetes **18**, 206 (1969)
JEPHCOTT, C.M.: Extraction of insulin and stability of various preparations. Trans. roy. Soc. Can., Sect. V **25**, 183 (1931)
JORPES, E., MUTT, V., RASTGELDI, S.: Verfahren zur Gewinnung von Insulin. Deutsche Patentschrift Nr. 1043584 (1956)
JORPES, E., MUTT, V., RASTGELDI, S.: A new principle for large scale production of insulin. Acta chem. scand. **14**, 1777 (1960)
KATKOVSKI, S.B., SHVARTS, S.I., GLAZYAN, I.G.S., GLAZYAN, E.G.S., GITTERMAN, E.B.T., FEDOTOVA, A.S.T., ZALIKHOVSKY, A.B., SAMSONOV, G.V., TUGUNOV, S.S., DMITRIENKO, L.V.: A method of preparing crystalline insulin. British Patent 1054523 (1965)
KIMMEL, J.R., POLLOCK, H.G.: Studies of human insulin from nondiabetic and diabetic pancreas. Diabetes **16**, 687 (1967)
KIMMEL, J.R., POLLOCK, H.G., HAZELWOOD, R.L.: Isolation and characterization of chicken insulin. Endocrinology **83**, 1323 (1968)
KLOSTERMEYER, H., ZAHN, H.: Struktur, Eigenschaften und Synthese des Insulins. In: Handbuch d. exper. Pharmakologie, XXXII/1, p. 273. (Ed. E. DÖRZBACH). Berlin-Heidelberg-New York: Springer 1971
KÖLLENSPERGER, G.F., GÖDICKE, V., SCHULTZE, H.: Verfahren zur Gewinnung von Insulin und Pankreatin. Deutsche Offenlegungsschrift Nr. 2146275 (1973)
KRISHCHENKO, V.P.: Cellulose ion exchangers for separation of proteins. Dokl. Vses. Akad. Sel'skokhoz. Nauk **1969**, 5, 34

Lautenschläger, C.L., Lindner, F.: Verfahren zur gleichzeitigen Gewinnung von Fermentpräparaten neben dem blutzuckersenkenden Hormon aus Bauchspeicheldrüsen. Deutsche Patentschrift Nr. 745284 (1942)

Levy, D., Carpenter, F.H.: The synthesis of triaminoacyl-insulins and the use of the t-butyloxycarbonyl group for the reversible blocking of the amino groups of insulin. Biochemistry **6**, 3559 (1967)

Light, A., Simpson, M.V.: Paper chromatography of insulin. Nature (Lond.) **177**, 225 (1956a)

Light, A., Simpson, M.V.: The paper chromatographic isolation of ^{14}C-labeled insulin from calf pancreas slices. Biochim. biophys. Acta (Amst.) **20**, 251 (1956b)

Lindner, F.: Chemie und Biochemie des Insulins. In: Insulin und Insulintherapie, p. 17. München-Berlin: Verlag Urban u. Schwarzenbach 1956

Mallory, A., Smith, G.H., Taylor, K.W.: The incorporation of tritium-labeled amino acids into insulins in rat pancreas in vitro. Biochem. J. **91**, 484 (1964)

Markussen, J.: Mouse insulins — separation and structure. Int. J. Protein Res. **3**, 149 (1971)

Markussen, J., Sundby, F.: Duck insulin: isolation, crystallization and amino acid sequence. Int. J. Peptide Protein Res. **5**, 37 (1973)

Markussen, J., Sundby, F., Smyth, D.G., Ko, A.: Preparation of human C-peptide. Horm. Metab. Res. **3**, 229 (1971)

Maxwell, L.C., Hinkel, W.P.: Preparation of insulin from pancreas glands. U.S.A. Patent 2595278 (1950)

Maxwell, L.C., Hinkel, W.P.: Preparation of insulin from pancreas glands. U.S.A. Patent 2674560 (1951)

Mehnert, H., Sewering, H., Reichstein, W., Vogt, H.: Früherfassung von Diabetikern in München 1967/68. Dtsch. med. Wschr. **93**, 2044 (1968)

Mendiola, L., Cole, R.D.: On the chromatographic isolation of insulin from laboratory animals. J. biol. Chem. **235**, 3484 (1960)

Meyer Cluwen, A.H.: Verfahren zur Herstellung von Insulin aus Pankreasdrüsen. Deutsche Auslegeschrift Nr. 1174451 (1961)

Mirsky, I.A., Jinks, R., Perisutti, G.: The isolation and crystallization of human insulin. J. clin. Invest. **42**, 1869 (1963)

Mirsky, A., Kawamura, K.: Heterogeneity of crystalline insulin. Endocrinology **78**, 1115 (1966)

Neumann, P., Humbel, R.E.: Isolation of a single component of fish insulin from a bonito-tuna-swordfish insulin mixture and its complete amino acid sequence. Int. J. Protein Res. **125**, 1 (2), (1969)

Neumann, P.A., Koldenhof, M., Humbel, R.E.: Amino acid sequence of insulin from the angler fish (lophius piscatorius). Hoppe-Seylers Z. physiol. Chem. **350**, 1286 (1969)

Nolan, C., Margolish, E., Peterson, J., Steiner, D.F.: The structure of bovine proinsulin. J. biol. Chem. **246**, 2780 (1971)

O'Donnell, I.J., Thompson, E.O.P.: The effect of temperature on the chromatography of insulin on DEAE-cellulose. Aust. J. biol. Sci. **13**, 69 (1960)

Oyer, P.E., Cho, S., Peterson, J.D., Steiner, D.F.: Studies on human proinsulin. Isolation and amino acid sequence of the human pancreatic C-peptide. J. biol. Chem. **246**, 1375 (1971)

Petersen, K., Schlichtkrull, J.: Improvements in or relating to a process for the production of crystalline insulin. Danish Patent 733740 (1952)

Peterson, J.D., Nehrlich, S., Oyer, P.E., Steiner, D.F.: Determination of the amino acid sequence of the monkey, sheep, and dog proinsulin C-peptides by a semi-micro Edman degradation procedure. J. biol. Chem. **247**, 4866 (1972)

Pettinga, C.W.: Insulin. Biochem. Preparations **6**, 28 (1958)

Porter, R.R.: Partition chromatography of insulin and other proteins. Biochem. J. **53**, 320 (1953)

Randall, S.S.: The small-scale preparation of crystalline insulin. Biochim. biophys. Acta (Amst.) **90**, 472 (1964)

Robinson, F.A., Fehr, K.L.A.: Estimation of protamine and insulin in protamine-zinc-insulin. Biochem. J. **51**, 298 (1952)

Romans, R.G.: The preparation and chemistry of crystalline insulin. Recent Progr. Hormone Res. **10**, 241 (1954)

Romans, R.G., Scott, D.A., Fisher, A.M.: Preparation of crystalline insulin. Ind. Engng. Chem. **32**, 908 (1940)

Ruttenberg, M.A.: Human insulin: Facile synthesis by modification of porcine insulin. Science **177**, 623 (1972)

Rybák, M., Brada, Z., Hais, I.M.: Säulenchromatographie an Cellulose-Ionenaustauschern. Jena: VEB Gustav Fischer Verlag 1966

Schlichtkrull, J.: Insulin crystals. Dissertation. Kopenhagen: Munsgaard Publ. 1958

SCHLICHTKRULL, J., BRANGE, J., CHRISTIANSEN, A.H., HALLUND, O., HEDING, L.G., JORGENSEN, K.H.: Clinical aspects of insulin-antigenicity. Diabetes **21**, Suppl. 2, 649 (1972)

SCHMIDT, D.D., ARENS, A.: Proinsulin vom Rind. Isolierung, Eigenschaften und seine Aktivierung durch Trypsin. Hoppe-Seylers Z. physiol. Chem. **349**, 1157 (1968)

SCOTT, D.A.: Crystalline insulin. Biochem. J. **28**, 1592 (1934)

SHAPCOTT, D., O'BRIEN, D.: A method for the isolation of insulin from single human pancreas. Diabetes **19**, 831 (1970)

SLOBIN, L.I., CARPENTER, F.H.: The labile amide in insulin: preparation of dealanine-deamido-insulin. Biochemistry **2**, 22 (1963)

SMITH, L.F.: Isolation of insulin from pancreatic extracts using carboxymethyl and diethylaminoethyl celluloses. Biochim. biophys. Acta (Amst.) **82**, 231 (1964)

SMITH, G.H., THOMAS, D., HALL, A.H.: Verfahren zur Gewinnung von Insulin. Deutsche Auslegeschrift Nr. 1617937 (1966)

STEINER, D.F.: Evidence for a precursor in the biosynthesis of insulin. Trans. N.Y. Acad. Sci. (1967), 60

STEINER, D.F.: Cocrystallization of proinsulin and insulin. Nature (Lond.) **243**, 528 (1973)

STEINER, D.F., CHO, S., OYER, P.E., TERRIS, S., PETERSON, J.D., RUBENSTEIN, A.H.: Proinsulin C-peptide from bovine pancreas. J. biol. Chem. **246**, 1365 (1971)

STEINER, D.F., CUNNINGHAM, D., SPIGELMAN, L., ATEN, B.: Insulin biosynthesis: evidence for a precursor. Science **157**, 697 (1967)

STEINER, D.F., HALLUND, O., RUBENSTEIN, A., CHO, S., BAYLISS, C.: Isolation and properties of proinsulin, intermediate forms, and other minor components from crystalline bovine insulin. Diabetes **17**, 725 (1968)

STEINER, D.F., OYER, P.E.: The biosynthesis of insulin and a probable precursor of insulin by a human islet cell adenoma. Proc. nat. Acad. Sci. (Wash.) **57**, 473 (1967)

SUNDBY, F.: Separation and characterization of acid-induced insulin transformation products by paper electrophoresis in 7 M urea. J. biol. Chem. **237**, 3406 (1962)

SUNDBY, F., MARKUSSEN, J.: Preparative method for the isolation of C-peptides from ox and pork pancreas. Horm. Metab. Res. **2**, 17 (1970)

SUNDBY, F., MARKUSSEN, J.: Rat proinsulins and C-peptides. Isolation and amino-acid compositions. Europ. J. Biochem. **25**, 147 (1972)

TAYLOR, K.W., HUMBEL, R.E., STEINKE, J., RENOLD, A.E.: The paper chromatography of insulin from ox pancreas, human pancreas and the isolated islet tissue of the N. American toadfish (opsanus tau). Biochim. biophys. Acta (Amst.) **54**, 391 (1961)

TAYLOR, K.W., SMITH, G.H.: The purification of insulins in crude extracts of rat pancreas by two-dimensional chromatography and electrophoresis on paper. Biochem. J. **91**, 491 (1964)

TAYLOR, K.W., SMITH, G.H., GARDNER, G.: Paper-chromatographic methods for the identification of insulin in extracts of rat pancreas. Biochem. J. **82**, 2 P (1962)

THOMPSON, E.O.P., O'DONNELL, I.J.: The chromatography of insulin on DEAE-cellulose in buffers containing 8 M urea. Aust. J. biol. Sci. **13**, 393 (1960)

TIMASHEFF, S.N., BROWN, R.A., KIRKWOOD, J.G.: The fractionation of insulin by electrophoresis-convection. J. Amer. chem. Soc. **75**, 3121 (1953)

TIMASHEFF, S.N., KIRKWOOD, J.G.: Electrophoresis-convection applied to the complexed insulin-protamine system. J. Amer. chem. Soc. **75**, 3124 (1953)

VOLINI, M., MITZ, M.A.: Insulin recovery process. U.S.A. Patent 3069323 (1959)

WANG, S., CARPENTER, F.H.: A compositional assay for insulin applied to a search for "proinsulin". J. biol. Chem. **240**, 1619 (1965)

WAUGH, D.F.: A fibrous modification of insulin. J. Amer. chem. Soc. **66**, 663 (1944)

WAUGH, D.F.: Regeneration of insulin from insulin fibrils by the action of alkali. J. Amer. chem. Soc. **70**, 1850 (1948)

WAUGH, D.F.: Purifying insulin by seeding with unclumped fibrils of insulin. U.S.A. Patent 2648622 (1950)

WEITZEL, G., OERTEL, W., RAGER, K., KEMMLER, W.: Insulin vom Truthuhn. Hoppe-Seylers Z. physiol. Chem. **350**, 57 (1969)

YAMAMOTO, M., KOTAKI, A., OKUYAMA, T., SATAKE, K.: Studies on insulin. I. Two different insulins from Langerhans islet of bonito fish. J. Biochem. (Tokyo) **48**, 84 (1960)

YOUNG, J.D., CARPENTER, F.H.: Isolation and characterization of products formed by the action of trypsin on insulin. J. biol. Chem. **236**, 743 (1961)

ZIEGLER, M., LIPPMANN, H.G.: Quantitative elektrophoretische Trennung von Insulin und Glukagon. Naturwissenschaften **55**, 181 (1968)

ZIMMERMAN, A.E., KELLS, D.I.C., YIP, C.C.: Physical and biological properties of guinea pig insulin. Biochem. biophys. Res. Commun. **46**, 2127 (1972)

E. Insulin Preparations with Prolonged Effect

JOERGEN SCHLICHTKRULL, MARIANNE PINGEL, LISE G. HEDING, JENS BRANGE and KLAUS H. JØRGENSEN

With 38 Figures

I. Introduction

1. History

For more than a decade (1922—1936) following the discovery of insulin (BANTING and BEST, 1922), unmodified, short-acting insulin, Ordinary Insulin (OI), was the only preparation available. In the treatment of diabetes with this type of insulin, one injection daily may be adequate in some patients, but in the majority of cases control is significantly improved by increasing the number of injections to two, three or four daily. The stress and discomfort of multiple daily injections prompted numerous attempts to prolong the subcutaneous absorption of insulin (BEST, 1937; COLWELL *et al.*, 1942; WEITZEL, 1949; TRETENHAHN, 1959; JACKER, 1965). The introduction of protamine insulin (HAGEDORN *et al.*, 1936) and Protamine Zinc Insulin (PZI) (SCOTT and FISHER, 1936) marked a turning point. Smoother control was obtained with fewer injections. It was soon realized, however, that the absorption, and hence the blood sugar-lowering effect of PZI was stretched so far as to be insufficient during the daytime after the morning injection (LAWRENCE and ARCHER, 1937). An intermediary timing of action was obtained by adding OI to the syringe (CAMPBELL *et al.*, 1936; LAWRENCE and ARCHER, 1937; BERTRAM, 1938; GRAHAM, 1938; ULRICH, 1941; COLWELL *et al.*, 1942; COLWELL, 1947; PECK, 1946; SPRAGUE, 1949; IZZO, 1952), or by administration of Globin Insulin (BAUMAN, 1939; REINER *et al.*, 1939), Surfen Insulin (LAUTENSCHLÄGER *et al.*, 1937; UMBER, 1938; UMBER *et al.*, 1938), Iso-insulin (HALLAS-MØLLER and HEY, 1944; HALLAS-MØLLER, 1945; HEY, 1945) or NPH (Neutral Protamine Hagedorn) (KRAYENBÜHL and ROSENBERG, 1946). The Lente insulins (Semilente, Lente and Ultralente) were developed to meet the timing requirements with one daily injection in the morning (HALLAS-MØLLER *et al.*, 1952a, b). The Lente insulins contain no organic additives to slacken the insulin absorption. The suspended crystalline (Ultralente) or amorphous (Semilente) insulin-zinc complex is practically insoluble at neutral reaction, the former being absorbed very slowly (as PZI), the latter much quicker, though not as quickly as OI. Rapitard is a suspension of pure rhombohedral beef-insulin crystals in a neutral solution of pork insulin, its biphasic action meeting the therapeutic requirement irrespective of whether it is administered in one or two daily injections (SCHLICHTKRULL *et al.*, 1961).

The presence of small amounts of protein contaminants in crystalline insulin was demonstrated by MIRSKY and KAWAMURA (1966) using disc electrophoresis. Later, STEINER *et al.* (1968) fractionated crystalline insulin by gel filtration chromatography according to molecular weight into the high-molecular-weight (mol. wt. $> 15{,}000$) a-component, the b-component and the c-component, the latter containing in addition to the true Sanger insulin i.a. desamido-insulins, arginine-insulins and ethyl esters of insulin (SCHLICHTKRULL *et al.*, 1970). An insulin preparation made from the c-fraction (mol. wt. $= 6000$) is referred to as single peak insulin (SPI) (ROOT *et al.*, 1972) or *chromatografisch gereinigtes* insulin. Removal of both the higher-molecular-weight contaminants (a- and b-components) and the impurities having the same molecular weight as insulin results in the monocomponent (MC) insulin (SCHLICHTKRULL *et al.*, 1970) or the single-component insulin (SCI) (ROOT *et al.*, 1972).

2. Pharmaceutical Chemistry

The insulin protein is practically insoluble in water at its isoelectric point, pH $= 5.4$, but dissolves readily on addition of HCl to a pH of 3. At the neutral reaction relevant to the subcutaneous matrix, the soluble, negatively charged insulin molecules may combine with positively charged organic molecules, resulting in the precipitation of insoluble compounds such as protamine or surfen insulin compounds. The pharmaceutical preparation may contain the precipitate in suspension (PZI, NPH) or the precipitate may be formed in the tissue (Globin Insulin, Surfen Insulin, PZI in acid solution). The precipitates formed *in vivo* are more readily absorbed. The insolubility may also be obtained by combining the insulin with a small amount of zinc ions (e.g., 2% by weight of the insulin protein), but in this case, the delay in absorption will be significant only if the insulin is injected in the form of a suspension (the Lente insulins) (SCHLICHTKRULL, 1958, p. 82). Certain buffer anions, such as the phosphate in PZI and NPH, would destroy the insulin-zinc complex, while acetate, actually used, does not. If the particles are crystals of beef insulin they may contain as little as 0.8% of zinc (which is insufficient for the precipitation of pork insulin at pH 7.0) and still be very slowly absorbable (Rapitard) (SCHLICHTKRULL *et al.*, 1965a).

3. Absorption

The subcutaneous form of administration is preferred. Intramuscular injections may be used (and have been used, e.g., in cases with skin allergy), but the absorption is then likely to be quicker and of shorter duration. Recent observations of the absorption of OI have shown even greater differences between various subcutaneous regions, absorption being faster from the trunk regions than from the limb regions (BINDER *et al.*, 1967). Because of the obvious methodological difficulties, very little has been published about the subcutaneous absorption of the various insulins (see BINDER, 1969).

Using tracer insulin, it has been estimated in terms of an average of values from many patients and many injections that the absorption of the injected insulin follows the course shown in Table 1.

Table 1. *Time in hours after injection when the indicated fraction of the dose is absorbed from the subcutaneous tissue (*BINDER *et al., 1967;* BINDER, *1969)*

Insulin	Per cent of dose absorbed		
	25%	50%	75%
Actrapid	1.50	2.75	4.50
Ordinary	2	3.75	5.75
Semilente	5	8	12
Lente	10	20	40
Ultralente	20	40	>55
Rapitard	6	15	40

4. Timing

The timing of action has been studied in rabbits, guinea pigs, depancreatized dogs, healthy students and diabetics both with stable and unstable blood sugar, using either strictly controlled conditions or conditions simulating the ordinary way of life. Despite the many attempts to characterize the timing of action, results that have clinical relevance and value are meager and inexact. It is customary to classify the different insulins by means of idealized time-action curves with no well-defined clinical counterpart. The timing may also be characterized in a table by means of time figures and words describing a blood sugar curve following the injection. First, there is "the time of onset or first action", followed later by the time of "maximum action", "maximal effect" or "peak of activity". Then, as the blood sugar rises, there is the "residual action", which terminates the "time of activity". The length of the whole period is called the "duration of activity or action". If the duration of activity is relatively long, the preparation is said to be "slow acting" (e.g. PZI, Ultralente), and if it is short, we have a "rapidly acting preparation" (OI, Actrapid). There are, in between, preparations with an "intermediate speed of action" or "intermediate action" (Globin Insulin, Surfen Insulin, NPH, Semilente, Monotard, Lente, Rapitard). The timetables vary somewhat from author to author. Examples are given in Tables 2 and 3.

Unfortunately, the confusing picture of the timing of action is a true reflection of the situation. The 24-hour time course of the blood sugar following the morning injection of a constant dose of an insulin preparation shows day-to-day variations that in the labile cases may be so great as to render average curves useless. Less labile cases will show patterns that may, however, change in time, e.g., depending on the diet and physical exercise, and vary from one patient to another. The timing of action of an insulin preparation is, therefore, of a statistical nature and linked to the nature of the diabetic population in question and its life conditions.

Table 2. *The timing of action of various insulin preparations (1:* ELLENBERG *and* RIFKIN, *1962; 2:* TRAISMAN *and* NEWCOMB, *1965; 3:* JACKER, *1969; 4:* NITSCH, *1968; 5:* MEHNERT, *1966; 6:* PETRIDES, *1965; 7:* DÖRZBACH *and* MÜLLER, *1971; 8:* MALINS, *1970; 9:* BRESSLER *and* GALLOWAY, *1971; 10:* OAKLEY *et al., 1968; 11:* ROBBERS, *1969; 12:* DANOWSKI, *1964; 13:* JOSLIN *et al., 1959; 14:* LILLY, *1967; 15:* MARBLE, *1971)*

Insulin preparations	Insulin activity (hours) Onset 1	2	3	4	Maximum 1	2	3	4	5	6	7	8	9	10	11
Actrapid			0.5				1–2		0.5–1		0.5–1	4–8		4–8	0.5–3
Ordinary, regular, soluble or crystalline insulin	0.5	0.5–1	0.5	0.5	2–4	3–4	1–2	1–2	1–2		1–2	4–8	2–4	4–8	{1–4 1–2 1–3
Komb-insulin			1	–1			1.5–4	2–4	1.5–4	1.5–4	1.5–4				1.5–4
Semilente	1	0.5–0.75	1–2	1–2	6–10	5–7	5–10	3–6	3–4	3	3–4	8–12	2–4	8	3–5
HG-insulin									3–7	3–7	3–7				2–3
Depot-insulin (Surfen)			1	1–1.5			3–6	3–6	2–6	2–6	2–6				2–6
Globin	2–4	1–2	1		6–12	8–10	3–5					8–16		8	
PZI (solution)			1	2–4			2–4	4–7	3–6	4–6					4–7
Rapitard			0.5	0.5			6–8	3–6	1.5–6	3–5	1.5–6 biphas.	4–24			1.5–8
NPH	2–4	0.5–1	2		8–12	7–11	6–12		4–7	4–6	4–7	8–16	6–12	8–12	6–12
Long insulin			1	1			3–8	4–8	3–8	3–8	3–8				3–8
Monotard*															
Lente	2–4	1–1.5	1–2	2–4	8–12	14–18	7–15	6–12	4–8	6–8	4–8	4–24	6–12		6–8
PZI (suspension)	3–6	6–8	4–5		14–20	10–18	8–15		5–8	6–8	5–8	10–24	14–24		10–16
Ultralente	8	5–8	2	3–6	16–24	22–26	16–18	6–18	6–10		6–10	10–24	18–24		6–10 6–10

Table 2 (continued)

Insulin preparations	Insulin activity (hours) Duration 1	2	3	4	5	6	7	8	9	10	11	12	13	14	15
Actrapid			–6		5 (4–6)		5 (4–6)	6–12		8–12	6–8				
Ordinary, regular, soluble or crystalline insulin	6–8	6	5–7	6–8	7 (6–8)		7 (6–8)	6–12	5–7	8–12	6–8	6–12	5–7	5–7	5–7
Komb-insulin			9–14	9–14	11 (9–14)	9–14	11 (9–14)				9–14				
Semilente	12–16	12–18	12–16	10–16	12 (9–14)	12	12 (9–14)	12–16	12–16	12–16	8–14	12–16	12–18	12–16	12–16
HG-insulin					14 (12–16)	12–16	14 (12–16)				12–16				
Depot-insulin (Surfen)			10–14	10–18	13 (10–16)	10–16	13 (10–16)				10–16				
Globin	12–20	24	10–14					12–24		12–16		18–32	18–20	18–24	12–18
PZI (solution)			10–14	18–24	13 (12–16)	16–20					18–24				
Rapitard			14–22	12–18	13 (10–14)	16	13 (10–14)	18–24			14–16				
NPH	18–20	24–28	16–24		16 (14–18)	16–20	16 (14–18)	12–24	24–28	12–24	18–24	18–32+	26–30	24–28	18–24
Long insulin			18–26	18–26	24 (18–26)	18–26	24 (18–26)				18–26				
Monotard*															
Lente	28–32	28–32	24	24	20 (18–22)	20–28	20 (18–22)	24–30	24–28		20–28	18–36	26–30	24–28	18–24
PZI (suspension)	24–36	24–36 –72	–30		24 (22–26)	20–28	24 (22–26)	24–30	36+	24–30	20–30 24–30	36+	36	36+	24–36
Ultralente	36+	36–96	30	24–32	26 (22–28)		26 (22–28)	24–30	36+	24–30	22–30	36++	36+	36+	24–36

* Timing approx. like NPH and Lente.

Table 3. *The timing of action of various insulin preparations* (LAWRENCE, *1960*)

Insulin preparation	Dose	Insulin activity (hours) Maximum	Duration
Soluble	to 10 units	2—4	5—6
	to 20 units	3—6	6—8
	to 40 units+	6—9	9—12
Semilente, Globin, NPH	to 20 units	5—8	6—8
	to 40 units	8—12	10—16
	40—60 units+	10—? 20	16—? 24
PZI (suspension), Ultralente	to 20 units	5—8	12
	to 30 units	8—12	18—20
	to 40 units+	18—24	24+

Experimental models using nonclinical conditions, e.g., animal assays, may be used for the pharmacological control of constancy of a preparation, e.g., from one batch to another, or during its shelf-life until the date of expiry.

The complexity of the timing concept and its severe limitations in practice stimulated the development of another concept, the M-value (SCHLICHTKRULL *et al.*, 1965b), which stands for the lack of blood sugar control in the period of observation of a patient (5—7 days). The M-value is obtained from a formula in which the 6 or 7 daily blood sugar values are inserted. The formula was devised so as to imitate the clinical evaluation of the data. The effectiveness of different treatments in diabetics can be compared by means of the M-values. The validity of such comparisons is limited by the lack of an established definition for calculation of the quality of the results pertaining to a group or a population rather than to a single case.

5. Mixtures

Insulin therapy may often call for a stronger initial effect along with the delayed action provided by most modified insulins, such as PZI, NPH and Lente. In such cases it is customary to supplement by administering OI either in a separate injection, or, more often, by mixing it with the modified insulin in the syringe immediately before use. A Lente preparation can be premixed with any other insulin of the Lente trilogy at any ratio, and the mixture can be kept in the vial until used. As a rule, one should avoid mixing quick-acting with modified insulin of another brand if their pH and buffer characteristics are at variance.

6. Stability

The biological potency of insulin is reduced during storage according to a first-order reaction

$$P(t) = P_0 \cdot \exp(-kt),$$

where k follows the Arrhenius equation

$$k = \exp(\alpha - \beta/T),$$

P_0 is the original potency, P the potency after t months of storage at T° Kelvin, α and β are the constants characteristic of the various insulin preparations (PINGEL and VØLUND, 1972).

Table 4 shows how long the various preparations can be stored at the various temperatures until they lose 2% of their biological potency. The figures are inter- and extrapolation values derived from the formula, with the constants α and β having been determined experimentally (accumulated data on stability during storage). It is noteworthy that Actrapid (neutral OI) can be stored two to three times as long as the acid OI.

Table 4. *Duration in months of storage of various insulin preparations at various temperatures until their biological potency is reduced by 2% (*Pingel *and* Vølund, *1972)*

Insulin preparation	Storage temperature 4°C	15°C	25°C	40°C
Insulin Injection (OI-acid)	222	27	4.5	0.4
Neutral Insulin Injection (Actrapid)	433	62	12	1.2
Biphasic Insulin Injection (Rapitard)	258	36	6.6	0.7
Insulin Zinc Suspension (Lente)	427	40	5.4	0.3

Insulin deteriorates when exposed to light. Therefore, insulin preparations should be stored in the dark (for instance, in the cardboard box). One should avoid exposing insulin to freezing, not that freezing affects its biological potency, but it may affect the appearance (flakes) and the timing of action of the turbid, long-acting preparations. Therefore, when insulin is stored in a refrigerator, it should be borne in mind that the temperature may be different in the various sections of the refrigerator (sides, cooling unit) and that it may swing from time to time. The temperature of choice is 4°C, but storage temperatures up to 15°C are in order. One must heed the warning against exposure to heat even for shorter periods of time (for instance, exposure to strong sunlight in a car).

7. Immunological Side Effects

The daily injection of commercial insulin preparations may cause different immunological side effects, such as allergy, local lipodystrophy, increased dose requirement (possibly resistance, that is to say, the patient's requirement rising to more than 100 U/day) and the formation of antibodies against insulin and some of the protein contaminants.

The allergic reactions disappear, or are reduced, in most cases upon transfer to a preparation purified by several recrystallizations (Jorpes, 1949, 1950; Heiskell *et al.*, 1959). It is probable that the contaminating proteins present in some preparations cause the formation of antibodies of the γE-class in the patients. Cases have been reported where allergy against recrystallized insulin preparations disappeared upon transfer to MC insulin (Andreani *et al.*, 1972; Korp and Levett, 1973). Although allergy is not as frequent today as it was in the early days of insulin therapy, Boos (1969) estimated that between 5 and 10% of all diabetics would have allergy associated with the insulin treatment, and Lieberman *et al.* (1971) found that 40% of diabetic patients showed positive intracutaneous reaction to insulin. The allergic reactions may be enhanced by the presence of additives such as protamine in PZI (Kern and Langer, 1939), or directed against surfen in Surfen Insulin (Scheffler, 1955; Scheffler and Hagen, 1956; Schirren and Sauer, 1956; Hagen *et al.*, 1958; Daweke, 1968).

Lipodystrophy is a common side effect; up to 58% of all patients have been reported to suffer from these changes in the subcutaneous fatty tissue (Paley, 1953; Bermont, 1967), the atrophies being 4—5 times as frequent as the hypertrophies. Its pathogenesis is unknown, but an immunological reaction in the fatty tissue has been suggested (Kerp, 1963; Teuscher, 1974), and lipodystrophy is significantly more frequent in patients with allergy or a positive intracutaneous test. Cases of severe lipoatrophy have been cured or alleviated considerably by switching the patient to MC insulin (Teuscher, 1974; Andreani *et al.*, 1972; Korp and Levett, 1973).

Until the introduction of the radioimmunological techniques for the determination of e.g., insulin antibodies in the blood (Berson *et al.*, 1956), insulin antibodies had only been detected in a few cases of insulin resistance (LOWELL, 1944; LERMAN, 1944). But BERSON and YALOW (1963) found this side effect in virtually every person that has been continuously treated with commercial insulin for three to four months. The circulating antibodies bind a portion of the injected insulin, and the timing of action of an insulin preparation may be changed by the formation of a circulating antibody-insulin depot slowly releasing free insulin into the blood. Some types of antibodies were suggested to exert a buffering effect on changes in the free insulin concentration (DIXON *et al.*, 1972). On the other hand, hypoglycemia has been observed in patients with circulating antibodies — even several days after withdrawal of insulin — and related to the release of insulin from antibody complexes (PAL *et al.*, 1969; MOLNAR *et al.*, 1972; HARWOOD, 1960; DITSCHUNEIT and FEDERLIN, 1966).

Only weak positive correlation has been found between the daily insulin dose and the serum insulin antibody levels measured by the radioimmunological techniques (HARRIS-JONES, 1963; KERP *et al.*, 1968; PAL *et al.*, 1969). DEVLIN and BRIEN (1965) and DEVLIN *et al.* (1966, 1967) have shown, however, that in some patients treated with less than 100 U of an ox insulin preparation a significant reduction of the daily dose could be achieved after a changeover to pork insulin (e.g., 76→40, 30→16 and 66→44 U/day). This clearly demonstrates that antibodies may lead to an increased daily insulin requirement. ANDREANI *et al.* (1972) noticed that patients treated with conventional insulin preparations for years showed a fall in the antibody level and a drop in the insulin requirement within a few months of changeover to MC insulin.

With some epidemiological variation of incidence (up to 3.6%) (DITSCHUNEIT and FEDERLIN, 1966), insulin resistance (that is when the dose requirement permanently exceeds 100 U/day) may develop in the course of treatment and become aggravated (SMELO, 1948; SHIPP *et al.*, 1965; DAWEKE, 1966; KATSILAMBROS, 1972). Some cases of resistance cannot be explained by the presence of large amounts of insulin antibodies (DAWEKE and BACH, 1963; DAVIDSON and EDDLEMAN, 1950; PRESLAND and TODD, 1956; LEONARDS and MARTIN, 1959; STEINKE and SOELDNER, 1965), but a reduction of the dose is possible in about 50% of cases by transferring the patient to a pork insulin preparation (BEEUWKES *et al.*, 1956; KREUTZER *et al.*, 1956; CANIVET *et al.*, 1961; GOLDMAN and KAYE, 1962; FELDMAN *et al.*, 1963; KÜHNAU and STRITZKY, 1963; AKRE *et al.*, 1964; BOSHELL *et al.*, 1964; DEVLIN and BRIEN, 1965; FALUDI and MEHBOD, 1965; FANKHAUSER and DIACON, 1966; BERSON and YALOW, 1966). A drastic reduction of the dose has been described after transfer to MC insulin (PFEIFFER, 1972).

Commercial insulin preparations induce, in addition to insulin antibodies, the formation of other types of antibodies. For instance, the proinsulin contaminant induces antibodies both against insulin and against the C-peptide part of the molecule in about 80% of insulin-treated diabetics (KUMAR and MILLER, 1973a, b). The high-molecular-weight fraction, the a-component (consisting of a series of pancreatic proteins), was shown to induce the formation of antibodies against non-insulin-like sites as well as against insulin-like sites (SCHLICHTKRULL *et al.*, 1974) whereas this was not the case in patients treated with highly purified insulin.

In insulin-treated diabetics, binding of fluorescein-insulin and of anti-ox insulin serum to kidney tissue was demonstrated by BERNS *et al.* (1964) and BURKHOLDER (1965), respectively, whereas THOMSEN (1972) and WESTBERG and MICHAEL (1972) could not detect any such binding.

Numerous experiments in animals have shown that injections of commercial insulin cause insulin antibodies in guinea pigs and rabbits, and renal impairment

(WEHNER *et al.*, 1969, 1970; GRIEBLE, 1960). Isolated a- plus b-components were shown, moreover, to induce kidney changes in rabbits whereas no such changes were observed with MC insulin (WEHNER *et al.*, 1973), but the relevance of these findings to diabetes therapy and vascular complications is hypothetic.

II. Insulin Preparations

1. PZI and NPH

a) Protamine Insulin

Protamine insulin was invented by HAGEDORN and his associates (1936). The idea was to combine the insulin with some basic group in order to bring the isoelectric zone of the combination closer to the pH of the tissue fluid than that of insulin hydrochloride. Kyrin, histones, globines and protamines were tried but only the latter group showed promise in effecting precipitation of the insulin. The mono-protamines containing as basic group arginine, only, were the most effective precipitants, lowering the solubility of insulin at pH 7.4 to 0.1—0.5 unit/ml (HAGEDORN *et al.*, 1936). The precipitated protamine-insulin contained about 10% (by weight) of protamine. An acid solution of protamine insulin exhibited the same timing of action as OI, but when injected in suspension, the compound did not show the sharp peak effect of OI 3 or 4 h after the injection, and the effect was more prolonged, roughly twice as long as that of OI (HAGEDORN *et al.*, 1936). The dissolution before absorption was explained by the enzymatic degradation of protamine observed when protamine insulin was added to serum or serum dilutions (HAGEDORN, 1938, 1946; BANG, 1946a, b). Since the neutral suspension was not stable, it was necessary to resort to preparing a vial with an acid solution of protamine and insulin and another one with a phosphate buffer. The patient would then make enough suspension to last him for some days, by injecting buffer into the vial with the acid solution of protamine insulin.

b) PZI

The stability problem with protamine insulin was solved by SCOTT and FISHER, who used a surplus of protamine and added a zinc salt in small quantities (2 mg Zn/1000 units) (SCOTT and FISHER, 1936). The action of the PZI proved to be much more prolonged. Depending on the dose, it may last for up to 72 h (COLWELL, 1947). A prolongation of effect is also obtained when the preparation is injected in unbuffered acid solution (MITTENZWEI, 1956; JACKER, 1965). The neutral PZI suspension was the one, however, to become most widely used. The long duration of action gave hope that one daily injection of this insulin would be sufficient, but it soon became evident (1937) that PZI must be used in combination with a supplementary dose of OI to ensure sufficient action during the day after the morning injection (LAWRENCE and ARCHER, 1937) and to reduce the incidence of the sneaking low blood sugars in the night and early in the morning (NEUHOFF and RABINOVITCH, 1938; LESCHER, 1938). The supplementary dose of OI may be given either as a separate injection or mixed with PZI in the syringe. The latter method requires a larger ratio of OI:PZI (WAUCHOPE, 1940). A large series of clinical trials were undertaken with the aim of finding the best PZI combination for use in one morning injection. Various mixing ratios were recommended, such as 1.5:1 (ULRICH, 1941), 2:1 (COLWELL *et al.*, 1942; COLWELL, 1944) and 3:1 (COLWELL *et al.*, 1942). A ready-made modified PZI with a 25% content of dissolved OI was suggested for general use (MCBRYDE *et al.*, 1943a, b, 1944), but, as the preparation proved to be unstable (PECK and SCHECHTER, 1944), the idea was abandoned.

c) NPH

The stability problems encountered with the PZI modifications were resolved by crystallizing the protamine-zinc-insulin precipitate under specific conditions. The crystalline NPH insulin was invented by KRAYENBÜHL and ROSENBERG in HAGEDORN's laboratory (KRAYENBÜHL and ROSENBERG, 1946). Insulin was crystallized for the first time by ABEL (1926). In 1934, SCOTT discovered that the rhombohedral insulin crystals as prepared by Abel contained zinc, and that no crystals were formed unless either Zn or certain other metals (Cd, Co, Ni) were present (SCOTT, 1934). [Much later, it was shown that insulin may actually crystallize as rhombic dodecahedrons in the total absence of such metal ions (SCHLICHTKRULL, 1958, p. 54).] KRAYENBÜHL and ROSENBERG (1946) prepared a neutral suspension of protamine insulin precipitated under isophane conditions, i.e. no surplus of either protamine or insulin (HAGEDORN *et al.*, 1936). The suspension contained zinc ions, as necessary for insulin crystallization, and phenol or a phenol derivative, preferably a m-derivative such as m-cresol (KRAYENBÜHL and ROSENBERG, 1946). They observed that the amorphous precipitate was gradually transformed into apparently tetragonal, oblong (e.g. 10—20 μ) crystals of protamine insulin containing per insulin molecule the same amount of zinc as the rhombo-

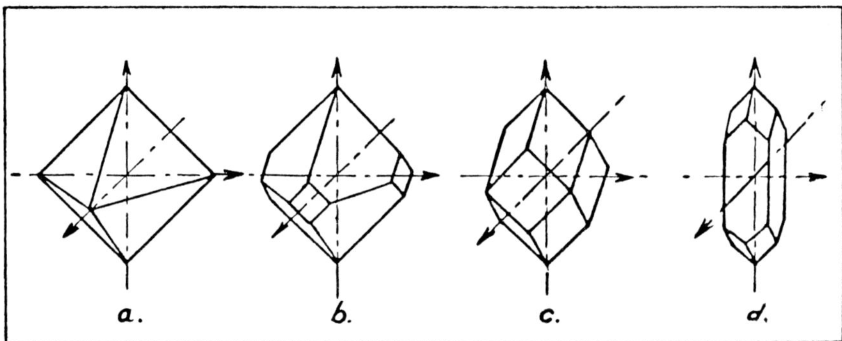

Fig. 1. Models of protamine insulin crystals. (KRAYENBÜHL and ROSENBERG, 1946)

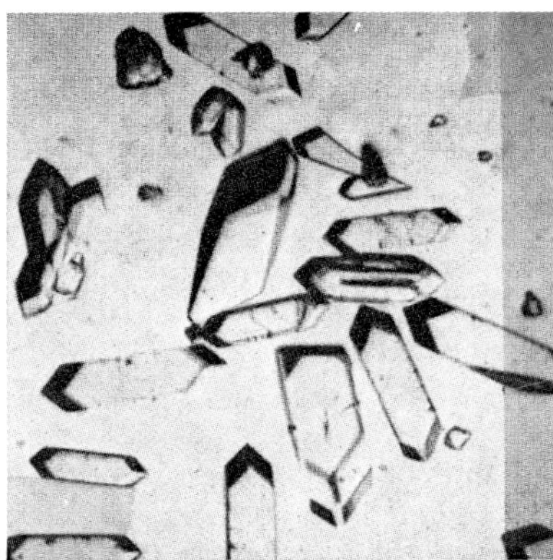

Fig. 2. Protamine insulin crystals. (POULSEN, 1967)

hedral crystals [0.32—0.38% by weight, equivalent to 2 atoms of zinc per 6 of Sanger's insulin monomers (mol. wt. = 5,700)] and about 0.5×10^{-3} mole phenol (or phenol derivative) per gram of protamine insulin (Figs. 1 and 2). Suspensions of this type are stable in the absence of protamine-splitting proteolytic enzymes such as pancreatic enzymes, which may be present in the insulin as impurities (BRITISH PHARMACOPOEIA, 1973, p. 245). NPH insulin, also called "Isophane Insulin", was made available in 1946 to replace the original two-vial system (protamine insulin, buffer) as well as the mixtures of OI and PZI.

For clinical results see: HAGEDORN, 1946; PECK and KIRTLEY, 1950; JAMIESON *et al.*, 1951; BEARDWOOD *et al.*, 1952; DUNCAN, 1952; ESSELIER *et al.*, 1952; PECK *et al.*, 1952; RICKETTS, 1952; BERG *et al.*, 1953; FINEBERG, 1954; HAYES, 1954; MITCHELL, 1955; ZACHAU-CHRISTENSEN, 1958; TRETENHAHN, 1959; FRIEDMAN, 1962; LEBOUC, 1962; AARSETH, 1964; LIPPMANN, 1964; ROMANI, 1965; OAKLEY *et al.*, 1966; BERTRAM *et al.*, 1954; MALINS, 1968; COLWELL, 1970; MOLNAR, 1971; OAKLEY, 1971; MIROUZE *et al.*, 1972.

If OI is added to NPH it stays in solution and provides a stronger initial effect, which is sometimes desirable. Insulin Initard is such a mixture, in which 50% of the insulin occurs in solution (POULSEN, 1967, p. 29). Upon standing, the crystalline, isophane protamine insulin may take up and combine with a surplus of zinc ions and protamine added to the suspension. A crystalline PZI is prepared in this way (POULSEN and KRAYENBÜHL, 1962). Another crystalline PZI is Durasuline (LIBBRECHT, 1968; TUTIN and l'HORTET, 1969; LOEB and DORCHY, 1971), which contains only half the amount of zinc and protamine contained in the older PZI. Ordinary insulin (including Actrapid), NPH and the crystalline PZI may be mixed n th e syringe and practically retain their individual timing of action.

d) Pharmaceutical Composition

Some typical compositions of the insulin preparations containing protamine are given in Tables 5 and 6.

2. Surfen Insulins

In an attempt to substitute protamine by a synthetically produced substance, LAUTENSCHLÄGER *et al.* (1937) found that 1,3-Bis(4-amino-2-methyl-6-quinolyl) urea (surfen) forms a complex with insulin which is sparingly soluble at neutral reaction. The first surfen-insulin preparations (UMBER *et al.*, 1938; UMBER, 1938) were produced as suspensions. Later, it became evident that an acid solution of the surfen-insulin complex such as Depot-Insulin, with 4.2 mg surfen/1000 U, also showed a prolonged action (WEITZEL, 1949; STÖTTER, 1963; MOHNIKE and LIPPMANN, 1964). DÖRZBACH and MÜLLER (1971) explained the prolongation of action of Depot-Insulin by the fact that, because of the neutral reaction relevant to the subcutaneous matrix, the surfen-insulin complex precipitates in the tissue and is then slowly absorbed. A mixture of one part OI and two parts Depot-Insulin (Komb-Insulin) is recommended by BERTRAM (1953) especially for therapy with two daily injections. Chemical and biological studies of the Surfen-Insulin complex (DÖRZBACH, 1950) led to the development of Long-Insulin, which is a suspension of crystalline and amorphous surfen-insulin with 1.2 mg surfen/1000 U and a prolongation of action adequate for therapy with one daily injection (TRETENHAHN, 1959). Depot- and Komb-Insulin are now produced from either crystalline beef insulin or pork insulin purified by gel filtration chromatography (CS). Some typical compositions of the insulin preparations containing surfen are given in Table 6.

Table 5. *Composition of insulin preparations as specified in* British Pharmacopoeia *1973*

Insulin preparation	Retarding substance	Physical state of insulin	pH	Zinc	Buffer	Isotonicum
Neutral Insulin Injection	none	dissolved	6.6—7.7	<0.2 mg/1000 i.u.	0.136% $CH_3COONa,3H_2O$	0.7% NaCl
Insulin Injection . . .	none	dissolved	3.0—3.5	<0.4 mg/1000 i.u.	none	1.45—1.75% glycerol
Insulin Zinc Suspension (Amorphous)	none	amorphous	7.0—7.5	0.00875% (40 i.u./ml) 0.01375% (80 i.u./ml)	0.136% $CH_3COONa,3H_2O$	0.7% NaCl
Globin Zinc Insulin Injection	36—40 mg globin/ 1000 i.u.	dissolved	3.0—3.5	2.5—3.5 mg/1000 i.u.	none	1.45—1.75% glycerol
Biphasic Insulin Injection	none	75% crystalline 25% dissolved	6.6—7.2	0.275—0.375 mg/ 1000 i.u.	0.136% $CH_3COONa,3H_2O$	0.7% NaCl
Isophane Insulin Injection	3—6 mg protamine sulphate/1000 i.u.	crystalline	7.1—7.4	<0.4 mg/1000 i.u.	Na_2HPO_4, $12H_2O$	1.4—1.8% glycerol
Insulin Zinc Suspension	none	60—73% crystalline 27—40% amorphous	7.0—7.5	0.00875% (40 i.u./ml) 0.01375% (80 i.u./ml)	0.136% $CH_3COONa,3H_2O$	0.7% NaCl
Protamine Zinc Insulin Injection	10—17 mg protamine sulphate/1000 i.u.	amorphous and/or crystalline	6.9—7.4	2.0—2.5 mg/1000 i.u.	100—110 mg $Na_2HPO_4,12H_2O$/ 1000 i.u.	1.45—1.75% glycerol
Insulin Zinc Suspension (Crystalline)	none	>85% crystalline <15% amorphous	7.0—7.5	0.00875% (40 i.u./ml) 0.01375% (80 i.u./ml)	0.136% $CH_3COONa,3H_2O$	0.7% NaCl

All the above-mentioned insulin preparations must contain a suitable bactericide except for Isophane Insulin Injection, which is obliged to contain 0.15—0.17% m-cresol and 0.06—0.07% phenol.

Table 6. *Insulin preparations with prolonged action*

Trade name	Retarding substance	Insulin Species	Insulin Purity	Physical state of insulin	pH
Komb-Insulin Hoechst	surfen	beef	cryst.	dissolved	3
Komb-Insulin S (CS) Hoechst	surfen	pork	chromatogr.	dissolved	3
Insulin Novo Semilente (MC)	none	pork	monocomp.	amorphous	7
HG-Insulin Hoechst	human globin	beef	cryst.	dissolved	3
HG-Insulin S Hoechst (CS)	human globin	pork	chromatogr.	dissolved	3
Depot-Insulin Hoechst	surfen	beef	cryst.	dissolved	3
Depot-Insulin S (CS) Hoechst	surfen	pork	chromatogr.	dissolved	3
Deposulin Brunnengräber	protamine	beef	cryst.	dissolved	3
Depot-Insulin Horm	protamine	beef	cryst.	dissolved	3
SP-Depot-Insulin Horm	protamine	pork	cryst.	dissolved	3
Insulin Initard Leo	protamine	pork	cryst.	diss./cryst. (1:1)	7
Insulin Novo Rapitard	none	beef/pork	cryst.	cryst./diss. (3:1)	7
Insulin Retard Leo NPH	protamine	pork	cryst.	crystalline	7
Long-Insulin Hoechst	surfen	pork	cryst.	cryst./amorph. (29:11)	6
Insulin Novo Monotard (MC)	none	pork	monocomp.	cryst./amorph. (7:3)	7
Insulin Novo Lente	none	beef/pork	cryst.	cryst./amorph. (7:3)	7
Insulin Novo Ultralente	none	beef	cryst.	crystalline	7

All the above-mentioned insulin preparations contain methyl-, ethyl- and/or propyl-paraben as bactericide except Depot-Insulin Horm and SP-Depot-Insulin Horm, which contain phenol, and Insulin Initard Leo and Insulin Retard Leo NPH, which contain m-cresol and phenol.

For clinical results see: BERTRAM *et al.*, 1954; DÖRZBACH and LINDNER, 1954; GASSMANN, 1954; PFEIFFER and SCHÖFFLING, 1954; BERTRAM, 1955; SEELEMANN, 1955; SPIESS, 1955; KRAINICK *et al.*, 1958; KRAINICK and STRUWE, 1960; PETRIDES, 1970.

3. The Lente Insulins

a) Introduction

The effect of added zinc ions on the timing of action of insulin solutions was investigated by SCOTT and FISHER (1935). Addition of small amounts, as in PZI, proved to be insignificant, but large quantities (0.4—1 mg/U) definitely prolonged the effect. Because injection of, e.g., 20 mg of zinc per dose probably causes pain and leads to zinc accumulation, the solution has never found clinical application. BISCHOFF and JEMTEGAARD (1937) studied the effect of zinc ions on the timing of action of insulin suspensions. They found that 2 μg Zn/U precipitated the insulin at neutral reaction just as protamine did. However, a prolongation of the effect of the precipitated insulin was obtained only when Zn was added in large quantities as in the case of the solutions. This finding was confirmed by BLATHERWICK *et al.* (1938), who demonstrated the prolonged action of a suspension containing 600 μg Zn/U.

Contrary to the results obtained by these authors, AUBERTIN *et al.* (1939) obtained a prolonged effect with a suspension of amorphous insulin containing only 2—14 μg Zn/U.

A re-investigation of zinc-insulin combinations was initiated by the incidental observation that the phosphate buffer used in PZI eliminated the precipitation of insulin by zinc ions (2 μg/U). Avoiding the phosphate, stable modified PZI pre-

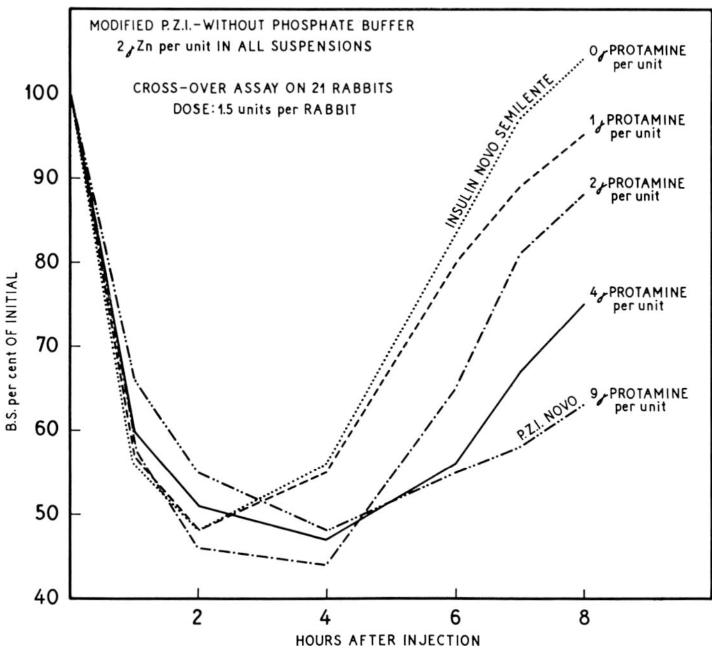

Fig. 3. The timing in rabbits of stable PZI preparations containing no phosphate. (SCHLICHTKRULL, 1958, p. 95)

parations with intermediary action could be prepared simply by reducing the amount of protamine (Fig. 3).

Even in the absence of protamine, some prolongation of action was still observed (Insulin Semilente) but it was inadequate for general use in therapy with one morning injection, only. When, however, the amorphous insulin particles of Semilente were substituted by crystals (Insulin Ultralente) the duration of activity became similar to that of PZI, and the 3:7 mixture (Insulin Lente) was selected for general use in the clinic (HALLAS-MØLLER, 1954a).

b) Chemistry

The solubility of insulin (pork) as a function of the pH is illustrated in Fig. 4. Figure 4E illustrates the concentration of dissolved insulin found in a protamine-zinc-insulin composition adjusted to different pH-values. In the absence of protamine (Fig. 4B), all the insulin is dissolved at neutrality but if the phosphate buffer is not used (Fig. 4D), the solubility is at least as low as in the protamine-zinc-insulin composition. The solubilizing effect of the phosphate is due to precipitation of the zinc ions, as shown in Fig. 5. The hatched area in Fig. 4 represents the pH interval in which the insulin precipitates will crystallize upon standing. At a lower

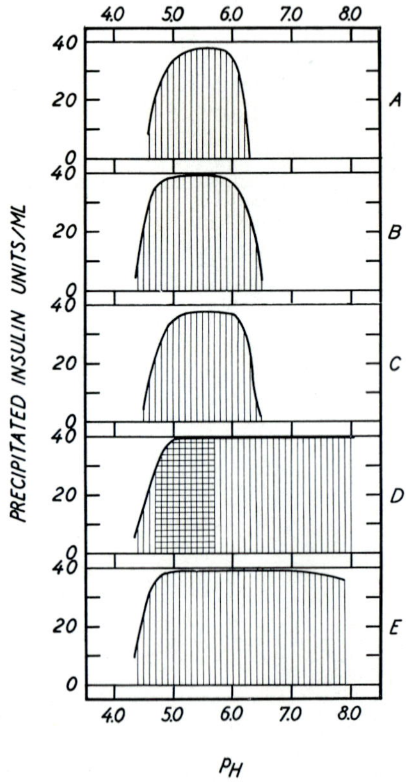

Fig. 4. Precipitation zone of insulin (40 U/ml) in: A. 0.01 M sodium phosphate; B. 0.01 M sodium phosphate with 2 mg of zinc (as chloride)/1000 U; C. 0.01 M sodium acetate; D. 0.01 M sodium acetate with 2 mg of zinc (as chloride)/1000 U; E. 0.01 M sodium phosphate with 2 mg of zinc (as chloride)/1000 U, and 8.5 mg of protamine/1000 U (SCHLICHTKRULL, 1958, p. 61)

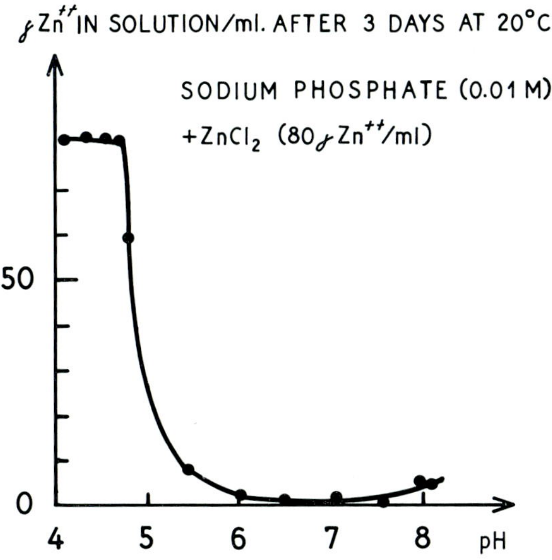

Fig. 5. Solubility of zinc ions in 0.01 M sodium phosphate as a function of pH. (SCHLICHTKRULL, 1958, p. 63)

pH, the insulin binds less than the necessary minimum of 0.35% Zn[1], equivalent to 2 Zn atoms per unit cell containing 6 Sanger units (insulin monomers). At increasing pH, in the right-hand part of the interval, the rate of crystallization decreases progressively, and is almost zero at pH 6, where the amorphous precipitate and the crystals formed contain 0.8% zinc. At pH 7.4, the amorphous precipitate contains about 2.3% zinc and there will be no crystal formation for several years. If, however, the precipitate is allowed to crystallize, e.g. at pH 5.3, and the pH is then readjusted to 7.4, the precipitate will remain crystalline. In the course of neutralization, additional zinc ions are captured to the same extent (2.3%) as in the amorphous insulin particles. The dissolved zinc ions are in a constant flow in and out of the crystal interior, in dynamic equilibrium with the bound zinc ions, as demonstrated with ^{65}Zn (SCHLICHTKRULL, 1958, p. 66). This peculiar behavior resembling that of an ion exchanger resin indicates an open crystal structure with holes and channels permitting the passage of ions. It can be seen in the microscope that even methylene blue may penetrate and stain the crystals. When suspended in water, the crystals contain 40—50% water, which is reduced to 5—10% when the crystals are isolated and air-dried. At the same time, the soft gel-like structure shrinks, cracks and hardens. The residual, more strongly bound water can be removed by further decreasing the humidity by means of vacuum, dessicants or heat.

The zinc content of insulin crystals in suspension (Fig. 4D) is shown in Fig. 6. In the interval $7.0 < \mathrm{pH} < 7.4$, $10 < c_{Zn} < 200$ and $4\,^{\circ}\mathrm{C} < \mathrm{temp.} < 37\,^{\circ}\mathrm{C}$, where c_{Zn} is the concentration (μg/ml) of dissolved zinc ions not bound to insulin, it was found that

$$(c_{Zn,\ \mathrm{bound}})^{4.0} = \mathrm{const.} \cdot c_{Zn}/c_{H^+} \quad \text{and}$$
$$4 \cdot \log(c_{Zn,\ \mathrm{bound}}) = \log c_{Zn} + \mathrm{pH} - 1760/T + 1.60,$$

1 In the present context, the zinc content is expressed in per cent by weight of the air-dried insulin containing approximately 5% water.

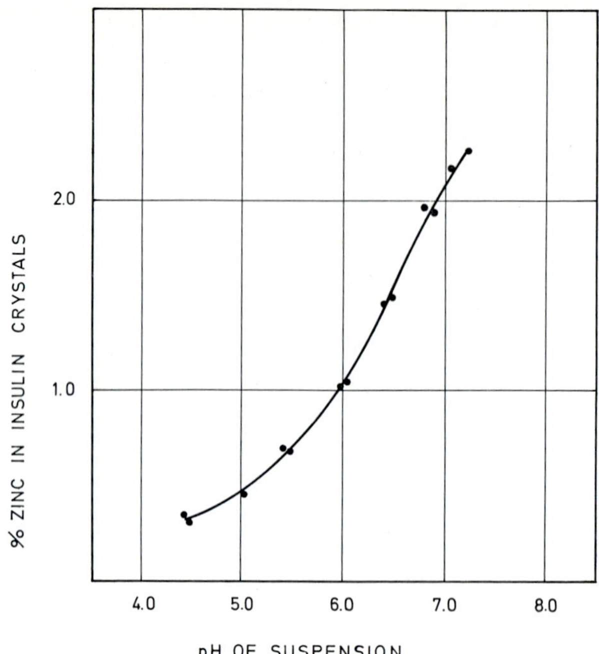

Fig. 6. Zinc content of insulin crystals (40 U/ml) suspended in 0.01 M sodium acetate with 2 mg of zinc (as chloride)/1000 U as a function of pH. (SCHLICHTKRULL, 1958, p. 64)

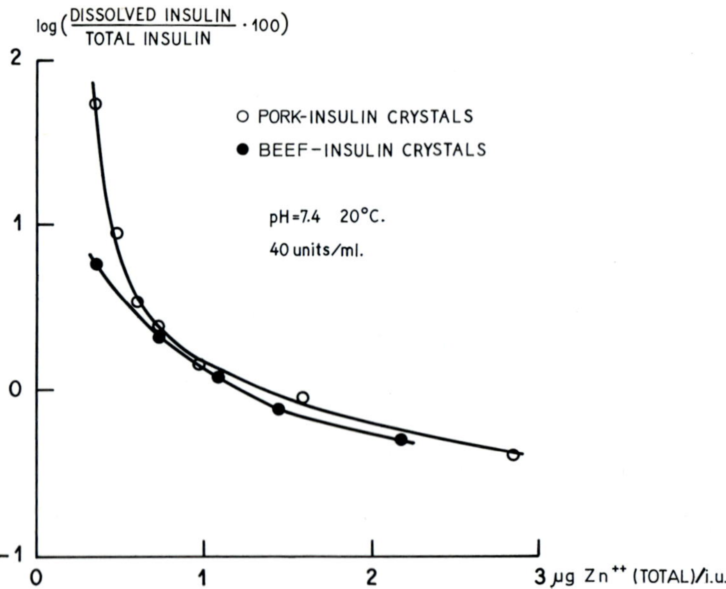

Fig. 7. Solubility of rhombohedral beef and pork insulin crystals (prepared by the sodium chloride-sodium acetate crystallisation method) in 0.01 M sodium acetate, 0.01 M veronal, 0.7% NaCl, as a function of the total concentration of zinc ions. (SCHLICHTKRULL, 1958, p. 65)

where $c_{Zn, bound}$ is the zinc content of the crystals expressed in atoms of zinc per crystallographic unit cell (6 monomers), and T is the temperature (°K) (SCHLICHTKRULL, 1958, p. 71).

The solubility at pH 7.4 depends on the species of insulin and on the concentration of zinc ions as illustrated in Fig. 7. At a concentration of 2.2 μg Zn(total)/U as in the Lente insulins (40 U/ml), less than 0.5% of the insulin is found in solution.

c) Crystallization of Insulin

α) The role of metal ions

ABEL (1926) crystallized insulin from a solution buffered with brucine, pyridine and ammonium acetate. HARRINGTON and SCOTT (1929) obtained better and more reproducible yields by substituting brucine with saponin, which contained the essential zinc ions as found by SCOTT (1934). Having discovered the significance of zinc ions. SCOTT (1934) used, for the first crystallization, a sodium phosphate buffer with an addition of zinc salt, and 15% acetone, which would allow crystallization without concomitant precipitation of insulin in the amorphous state. Co-precipitated zinc phosphate and further proteinacious impurities were removed by recrystallization from a solution of the first crystals in ammonium acetate. When sodium citrate is used, a soluble zinc-citrate complex is formed (PETERSEN, 1945). With this buffer, the crystalline insulin precipitate contains no surplus zinc salts but only the necessary amount of structural zinc (0.35%) together with a corresponding amount of firmly bound citrate.

The zinc ions may be substituted in the crystallization of insulin by Cd^{++}, Co^{++}, Ni^{++} (SCOTT, 1934) or Cu^{++}, Mn^{++}, Fe^{++} (SCHLICHTKRULL, 1956a), but Zn^{++} is used in practice. The structural metal ions (2 atoms/crystallographic unit cell containing 6 monomers) are necessary for the formation of the rhombohedral insulin crystals. However, under conditions in which the insulin protein binds a portion greater than the structural amount, the rate of crystallization will be lower, or there will be no crystallization at all. Formation of rhombohedral insulin crystals containing more than about 0.8% zinc has not been reported (EISENBRAND and WEGEL, 1941). An addition of phenol to the solution renders the crystal structure monoclinic; these crystals contain, in addition to the 2 atoms of structural zinc, 22 moles of phenol per unit cell (SCHLICHTKRULL, 1958, p. 52).

If protamine is also added in the isophane ratio, the crystals will appear to be tetragonal. They will contain, in addition to protamine, at least 2 atoms of structural zinc, 20 moles of phenol (m-cresol) per 6 monomers (see l.c., p. 737, NPH).

In the complete absence of the structural metal ions, the insulin may crystallize, although less readily. The structure is rhombic dodecahedral (SCHLICHTKRULL, 1958, p. 54). This structure was already observed by ABEL *et al.* (1927), who had probably been working with materials free of the structural ions necessary for the formation of rhombohedral crystals.

All the previously mentioned crystallizations take place only at a pH close to or above the isoelectric point of insulin. Crystallization may also take place at acid reaction in the cold. Under such conditions, orthorhombic crystals of, e.g., insulin sulphate (ELLENBOGEN, 1949) or insulin chloride (SUNDBY, 1962) are formed. Binding between insulin and the metal ions, if present, does not take place at the acid reaction, and the unit cell contains one dimer only. This is in agreement with the determinations of molecular size (upon dilution) which is found to be: at acid reaction in HCl — a dimer (MARCKER, 1960a); in acetic acid — a monomer (HEXNER *et al.*, 1961); at alkaline reaction without structural metal ions — a monomer (MARCKER, 1960a); with zinc — a hexamer (MARCKER, 1960b).

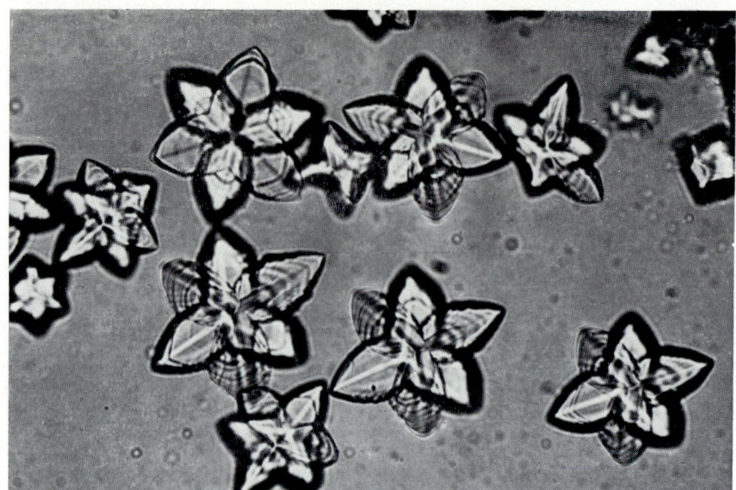

Fig. 8. Twinned beef insulin crystals, "stars". ×250 (Schlichtkrull, 1958, p. 32)

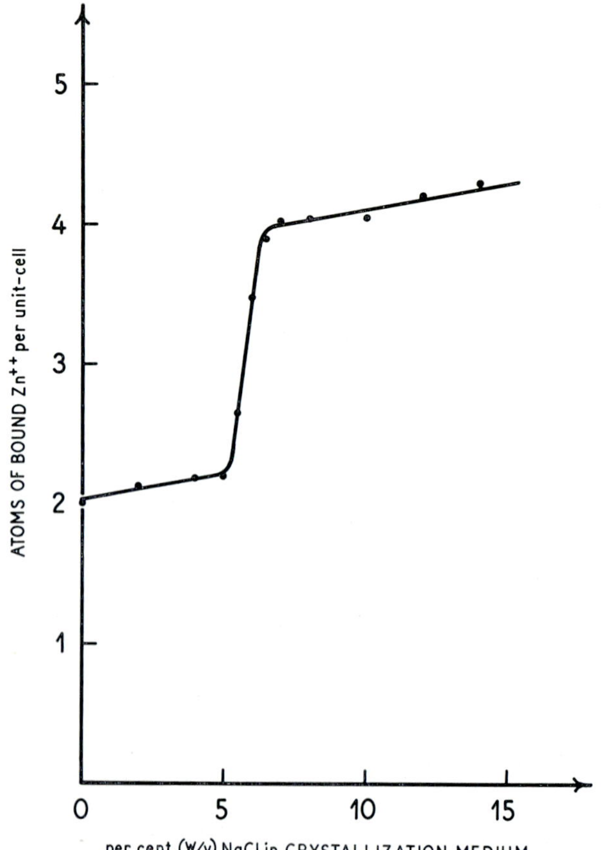

Fig. 9. The zinc content of beef insulin crystals as a function of the NaCl concentration (sodium citrate, pH 6) (Schlichtkrull, 1958, p. 38)

β) The shape and size

The internal rhombohedral structure reveals itself in the appearance of the insulin crystals. The shape, however, displays a variation depending on the species of the insulin. Porcine (and human) insulin forms true rhombohedra, but sheep and beef insulins have a tendency towards what appears to be twin formation, resulting in very peculiar shapes as shown in Fig. 8. The rhombohedral shape, as found in the pharmaceutical preparations, is universally obtained by adding 7% of NaCl to the crystallization medium buffered with sodium acetate. How the chloride ion interferes with the shape and twin formation remains unexplained, but it has been found that, with the concentration of chloride just necessary to avoid distortion, the structural amount of metal rises steeply from 2 to 4 atoms per unit cell as shown in Fig. 9.

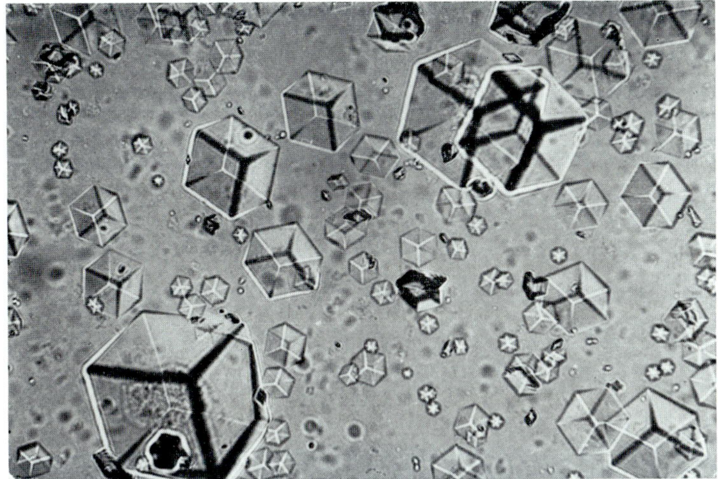

Fig. 10. Beef insulin single crystals formed in the saline-sodium acetate medium. ×250 (SCHLICHTKRULL, 1957b)

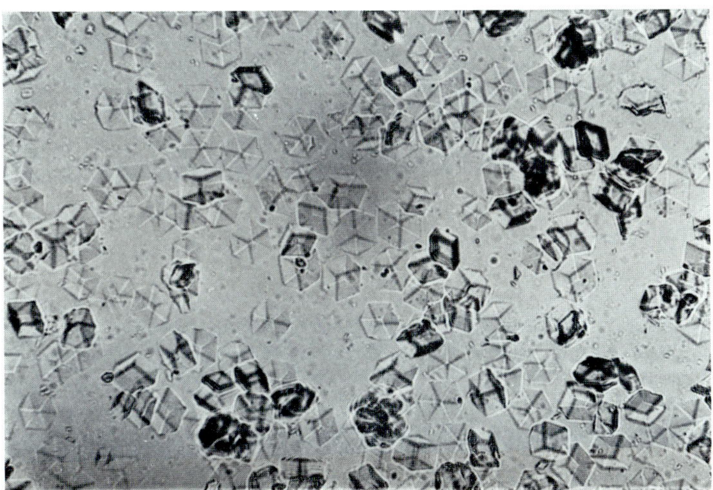

Fig. 11. Monodisperse beef insulin crystals prepared by seeding. ×300 (SCHLICHTKRULL, 1958, p. 51)

In the pharmaceutical preparation of insulin suspensions, not only are the structure and shape held constant but also the distribution of crystal size, since the timing of action is dependent to some extent on the crystal size. For crystallization, a solution is prepared containing 400 units of insulin/ml, 7% of NaCl, 0.1 m of sodium acetate and a quantity of zinc chloride adequate to give a total of 0.8—0.9% of zinc by weight of the insulin. The pH is adjusted to 5.5 (SCHLICHTKRULL, 1956b). At this reaction, most of the insulin is precipitated in the amorphous state, from which it gradually dissolves and then precipitates as crystals (SCHLICHTKRULL, 1957b). Using an India-ink staining technique, it can be shown that the crystals grow only by deposition on three of the faces meeting in an obtuse vertex of the rhombohedron (SCHLICHTKRULL, 1957c). The rate of deposition at room temperature in mm/hour was found to be proportional to the square of the supersaturation, reaching a maximum value of about 0.04 mm/hour for beef insulin (SCHLICHTKRULL, 1957d). If nucleation occurs at one moment only, the crystals will be of the same size, which is determined by the amount of insulin and the number of nuclei. However, a kinetic examination of the crystallization process showed that nuclei are continuously formed by self-reproduction of already existing crystals which sprout nuclei at a rate proportional to the rate of deposition of insulin on the three faces. The result is a highly polydisperse suspension, as shown in Fig. 10. However, the self-nucleation becomes almost insignificant if a predetermined number of nuclei are introduced at the beginning of the crystallization (Fig. 11).

The difference between the distribution of size obtained with spontaneous crystallization and that obtained with seeding is shown in Fig. 12.

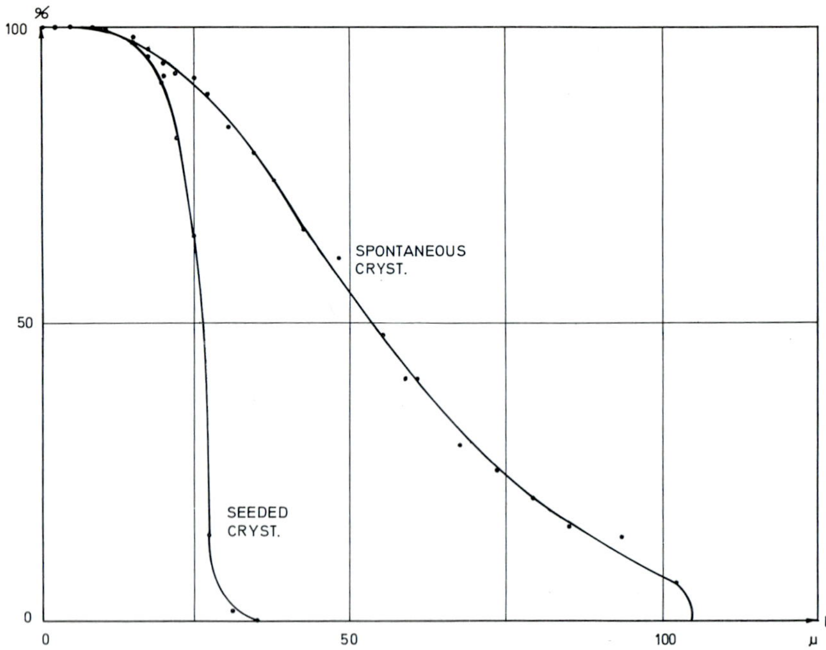

Fig. 12. Cumulative distribution of the size of insulin crystals. (SCHLICHTKRULL, 1957a)

d) Composition

In Semilente, the suspended insulin particles are entirely amorphous, normally of porcine origin, while in Ultralente the particles are approximately 25 μ large rhombohedral beef insulin crystals grown in a solution containing 7% NaCl besides the insulin, zinc and buffer. Insulin Lente is a mixture of 3 parts Semilente and 7 parts Ultralente. Recently, MC Insulin Semilente and Insulin Monotard (3 parts amorphous insulin particles and 7 parts insulin crystals as in Insulin Lente) but made entirely of monocomponent pork insulin has become available (see III. 3., p. 761). The composition of the Lente insulin preparations is given in Tables 5 and 6, p. 739—740.

e) Timing of Action

The blood sugar-lowering effect of the Lente insulins in fasting rabbits is shown in Fig. 13. The experiment was made to check the stability of the insulins. The blood sugar pattern is different in depancreatized dogs, as shown in Fig. 14. The

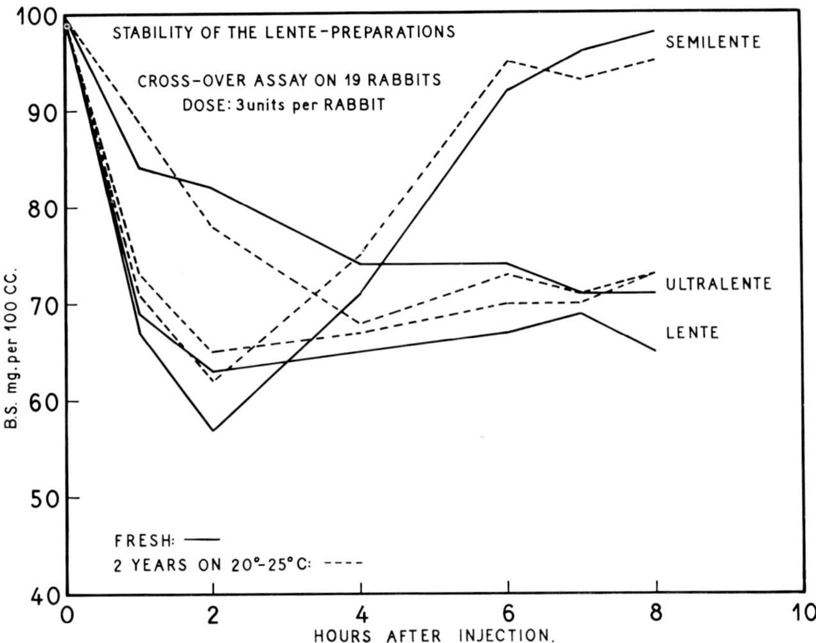

Fig. 13. Rabbit experiments showing the stability of the Lente insulins after 2 years of storage at room temperature. (SCHLICHTKRULL, 1958, p. 96)

insulin was injected at 8 a.m. The results obtained with the dogs indicate that Iso-insulin and Lente possess almost the same timing of action. This is contradicted by the clinical observations. In the dogs, Ultralente is seen to give the best control of the blood sugar, but in the clinic its timing of action is just as inadequate as that of PZI.

The limited clinical relevance of timing estimates observed in animal tests necessitates clinical investigations for characterization and evaluation of the

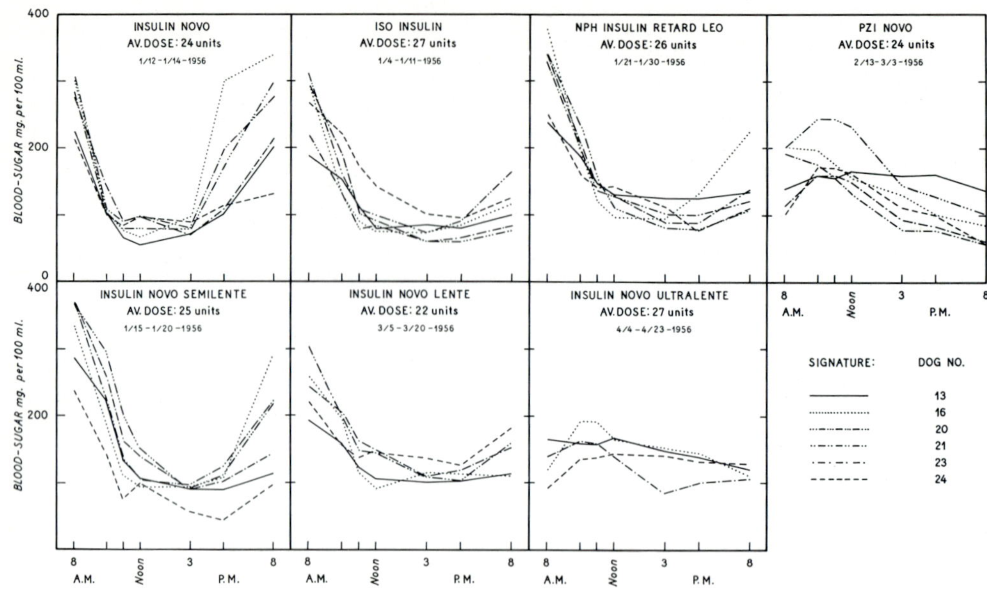

Fig. 14. The action of various insulins in six depancreatized dogs. Each curve is the average blood sugar curve obtained with the preparation indicated, in an individual dog, in the period shown. (Schlichtkrull, 1958, p. 83)

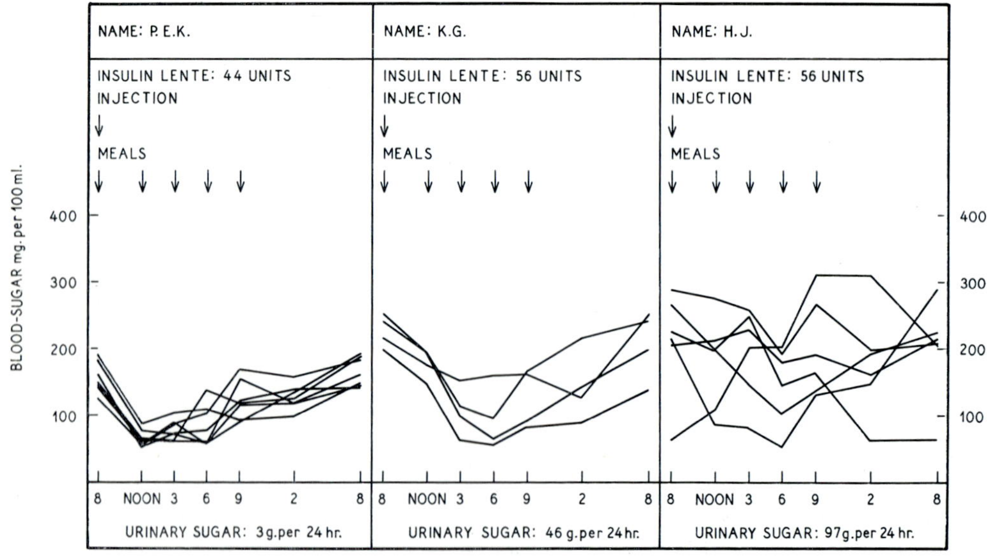

Fig. 15. Scattering of blood sugar values. (Schlichtkrull, 1958, p. 119)

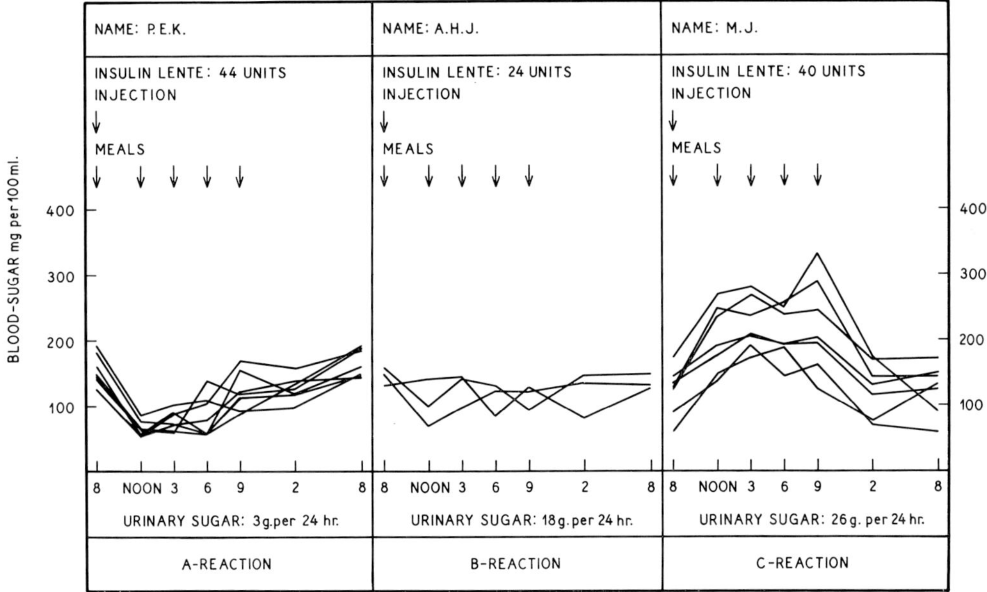

Fig. 16. Types of blood sugar curves. (Schlichtkrull, 1958, p. 118)

timing. Unfortunately, the blood sugar (BS) pattern varies considerably among patients, not only with respect to the scatter, as shown in Fig. 15, but also with respect to the predominant shape, as shown in Fig. 16. Therefore, no intelligible, condensed representation or depiction of the clinical timing is available.

As a compromise, clinical timing has been defined as the distribution of ΔBS values observed in the patients as illustrated in Fig. 17. By arbitrary definition, the ΔBS is said to be positive if the average blood sugar is highest during the day. The 3:7 Semilente/Ultralente ratio in Lente was selected for standard use because the corresponding timing distribution showed no predominance either of the negative or the positive ΔBS values (A- or C-reactions).

f) Clinical Results

For clinical results see:

Drury, 1953; Engleson, 1953; Gerritzen, 1953; Izzo *et al.*, 1953; Jensen, 1953; Lachnit and Ferstl, 1953; Lawrence and Oakley, 1953; Murray and Wilson, 1953; Murray, 1953; Nabarro and Stowers, 1953; Oakley, 1953; Petrides, 1953; Armstrong and Lloyd, 1954; Bertram *et al.*, 1954; Boulin and Nepveux, 1954; Cobley *et al.*, 1954; Colwell, 1954; Constam, 1954; Falk, 1954; Ferguson, 1954; Fitzgerald *et al.*, 1954; Foit and Sirová, 1954; Franzini and Pompili, 1954; Greenhouse, 1954; Hallas-Møller *et al.*, 1954a, b; Holcomb *et al.*, 1954; Lawrence, 1954; Malins and Thorn, 1954; Mangold, 1954; Melton, 1954; Murray, 1954; Oakley, 1954; Paley, 1954; Peck *et al.*, 1954; Sauer, 1954; Stengel and Lassmann, 1954; Venning, 1954; Blöch, 1955; Boller, 1955; Colwell, 1955; Didier, 1955; Grauhan, 1955; Gurling *et al.*, 1955; Haunz, 1955; Hobson, 1955; Kaas, 1955; Kirsch, 1955; Monteiro, 1955; Murray, 1955; Pickert, 1955; Rilliet, 1955; Rouzaud, 1955; Seelemann,

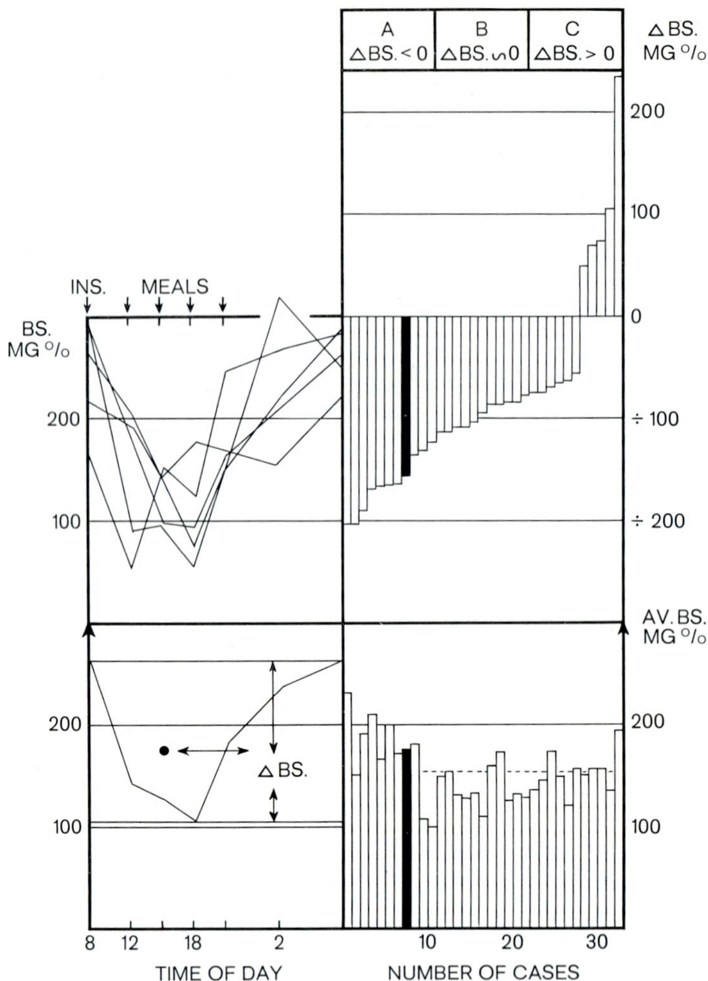

Fig. 17. The distribution of ΔBS observed in 33 patients treated with a preparation of crystalline protamine insulin. The individual blood sugar curves from one arbitrary case are shown in the upper left and the corresponding average blood sugar curve is represented in the lower left figure. The ΔBS-value and the grand average of the blood sugar values are indicated for this patient by the solid columns on the right-hand side of the figure. The columns are arranged in the order given by the magnitude of the ΔBS-values. (SCHLICHTKRULL, 1958, p. 121)

1955; SLAYTON *et al.*, 1955; SPIESS, 1955; SPRAGUE and KILBY, 1955; STOWERS and NABARRO, 1955; SWOBODA and ZWEYMÜLLER, 1955a, b; VOIT and KNICK, 1955; WOLFF and MADDISON, 1955; ZWEYMÜLLER, 1955; DARNAUD *et al.*, 1956; DRURY and GREGG, 1956; IZZO *et al.*, 1956; JENSEN, 1956; JERSILD, 1956a, b; LUSSKY *et al.*, 1956; NEJROTTI and ALBONICO, 1956; PROTAS and KURSTIN, 1956; RECHENBERG, 1956; ROBERTSON, 1956; ROTTMANN and WILLE, 1956; SCHEFFLER and HAGEN, 1956; SCHIRREN and SAUER, 1956; SPENCER and MORGANS, 1956; CONSTAM, 1957; ENGLESON and LEHMANN, 1957; HAGEN, 1957; JOHN, 1957; MARBLE, 1957; MARIGO, 1957; BERNHARD and PICKERT, 1958; BIBERGEIL, 1958; HAGEN *et al.*, 1958; KRAINICK *et al.*, 1958; LANCASTER and MURRAY, 1958;

Rodriguez-Miñón and Garrigues, 1958; Vermeulen and Bekaert, 1958; Baquet, 1959; Eckler and Koch, 1959; Hagen and Hagen, 1959; Newcomb and Traisman, 1959; Oakley, 1959a, b; Rodriguez-Miñón and Garrigues, 1959; Rosenkranz, 1959; Strenger, 1959; Swoboda, 1959; Tretenhahn, 1959; Godon, 1960; Krainick and Struwe, 1960; Rosenkranz, 1960; Spiess and Zschocke, 1960; Sauer, 1961; Friedman, 1962; Hagen and Hagen, 1962; Haunz, 1962; Korp, 1962; Whitehouse *et al.*, 1961; Rosenkranz, 1963; Buchanan and Imrie, 1964; Ferguson *et al.*, 1964; Chaptal *et al.*, 1965; Knick and Folkert, 1965; Gibbs, 1966; Malins, 1968; Nowak *et al.*, 1968; Devlin and Duggan, 1969; Fankhauser, 1969; Aakerblom and Hiekkala, 1970; Colwell, 1970; Fankhauser and Montandon, 1970; Petrides, 1970; Molnar, 1971; Oakley, 1971; Wenig and Calap, 1971; Mirouze *et al.*, 1972; Stowers, 1972; Jersild, 1973.

4. Insulin Rapitard

An insulin preparation, containing 25% ordinary quick-acting insulin in solution and 75% suspended protamine-zinc-insulin particles, was advocated for general use (McBryde, 1943a, b, 1944) but was abandoned because of instability (Peck, 1944, p. 85). In Rapitard, a stable combination of dissolved and slow-acting suspended insulin is obtained by utilization of the species-dependent solubility characteristics of insulin (Fig. 7), as well as the special crystallization methods also used for the preparation of insulin Lente and Ultralente (see 3. c., p. 745).

The composition of Rapitard (Biphasic Insulin Injection) is given in Tables 5 and 6, p. 739—740. The 75% insulin crystals, similar in shape and size to the crystals in Lente, are made entirely of beef insulin, while the 25% dissolved insulin is not entirely of porcine origin. Since the beef insulin crystals are not completely insoluble, a small amount of the dissolved insulin is actually bovine insulin.

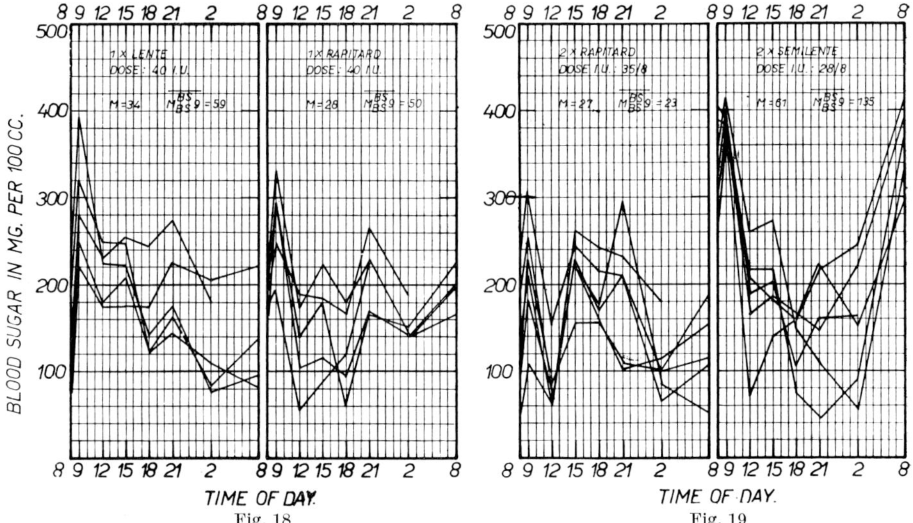

Fig. 18

Fig. 19

Fig. 18. A comparison in one case between the actions of Rapitard and Lente given once daily (Case No. 332). Each period was 5 days of observation. (Schlichtkrull *et al.*, 1965a, p. 110)

Fig. 19. Case 337, showing the most pronounced difference in response (M-value and $M^{BS}9$-value) to Rapitard and Semilente given in two daily injections. (Schlichtkrull *et al.*, 1965a, p. 110)

The course of the subcutaneous absorption of Rapitard is roughly indicated in Table 1. In the first few hours following the injection, the effect of Rapitard is stronger than that of Lente, as shown in Fig. 18. In comparison to Semilente, Rapitard has a stronger initial effect and a longer duration of action, as illustrated in Fig. 19. The timing of action has been evaluated using the M-value method (SCHLICHTKRULL, 1965b). The timing was found to be suitable for therapy with both one and two daily injections. In the relatively few cases calling for a stronger initial effect, Rapitard may be mixed with Actrapid (Neutral Insulin Injection). Recent observations have shown Rapitard and Actrapid to be superior in the treatment of diabetics with lipodystrophy (CRECELIUS, 1967; GLEIZE *et al.*, 1968; WATSON and CALDER, 1971; BLOOM, 1972; WATSON and VINES, 1973).

For clinical results see:

HAGEN and HAGEN, 1962; KINK and STEIGERWALDT, 1962; STRATMANN, 1962; LANG and WALZ, 1963; TRAUMAN and WETZEL, 1964; BRUNI, 1964; GUTSCHE and HASEKI, 1964; LOPEZ and COLOMBO, 1964; BERNARD *et al.*, 1965; CHIMENES and LAURENT, 1965; COLNARD, 1965; DRURY and TIMONEY, 1965; GUIVARCH *et al.*, 1965; KNICK and FOLKERT, 1965; MEHL and DEBRY, 1965; MONTENERRO and COLLETTI, 1965; PIETSCH-BERLIN, 1965; ROMANI, 1965; SCHLICHTKRULL *et al.*, 1965a; STRATMANN, 1965; KAPPELER, 1966; MAKENGO, 1967; SCHLIACK and LOTZ, 1967; CRECELIUS, 1967; DUNCAN, 1967; PYKE, 1967; BRUNI, 1968; DAWEKE, 1968; MALINS, 1968; FEDDER and POMPEN, 1969; AAKERBLOM and HIEKKALA, 1970; WATSON and CALDER, 1971; MIROUZE *et al.*, 1972; STOWERS, 1972; COURT and AMIES, 1973; WATSON and VINES, 1973.

III. Monocomponent Insulin

1. Introduction

The presence of impurities in conventional recrystallized insulin was demonstrated by MIRSKY and KAWAMURA in 1966, using polyacrylamide disc gel electrophoresis. Figure 20 shows such a disc electrophoresis of once-crystallized insulin. The impurities may be fractionated according to molecular size by gel filtration chromatography (STEINER *et al.*, 1968) into the high-molecular-weight (mol. wt.

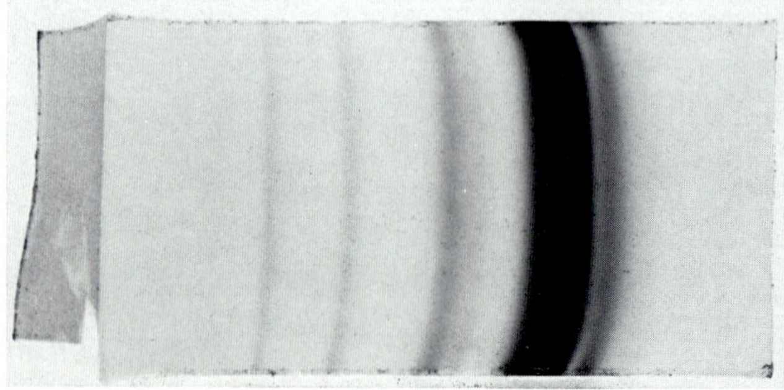

Fig. 20. Disc electrophoresis of once-crystallized pork insulin at pH approx. 8.7. The fastest band moving toward the anode (to the right) is monodesamidoinsulin. The major band contains insulin and the non-convertible insulin dimer. The next band from right to left comprises the proinsulin-intermediates, and the following, very prominent, band contains arginine-insulins (insulin with an arginine in position B_{31} or A_0) and insulin ethyl esters. The fifth band is proinsulin. The remaining bands have not yet been identified (These data were first published in Diabetes, Vol. 21, Suppl. 2, 649, 1972. Reproduced here by courtesy of the Editors.)

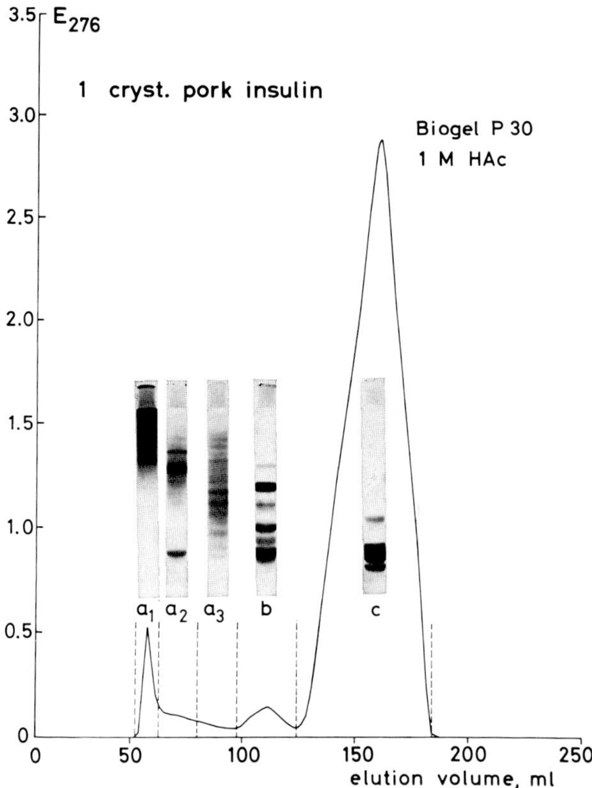

Fig. 21. Gel filtration of once-crystallized pork insulin on Biogel P 30. The disc electrophoreses were carried out after rechromatography of the individual components. The bands of the c-peak are, from top down: arginine-insulins plus insulin ethyl esters, the insulin, and mono-desamidoinsulin. The three most prominent bands of the b-component are, from top down: proinsulin, the intermediates, and the dimer. None of the bands of the a_1, a_2 or a_3-components has been identified, the a_1 containing a series of slowly migrating bands and a smear on the disc electrophoresis. (These data were first published in Horm. Metab. Res., Suppl., Vol. 5, 134, 1974. Reproduced here by courtesy of the Editors.)

Fig. 22. Disc electrophoresis of pork monocomponent (MC) insulin at pH approx. 8.7

> 15,000) a-component, the b-component, containing proinsulin, the intermediates, the dimer, etc. (STEINER and OYER, 1967), and the c-component which comprises, besides the true Sanger insulin, i.a. desamido-insulins, arginine-insulins and insulin ethyl esters. Figure 21 shows a gel filtration pattern of once-crystallized pork insulin on Biogel P 30 in 1 M acetic acid, with the a-component resolved into a_1, a_2 and a_3. Insulin preparations made from the c-component have been referred to as single-peak insulins (SPI) (ROOT *et al.*, 1972). The isolated pure insulin, corresponding to the major component in the c-peak, displays only one band on disc electrophoresis (Fig. 22) and has been termed monocomponent (MC) insulin.

2. Immunogenicity of Components of Crystalline Insulin in Rabbits

In 1963, BERSON and YALOW concluded that almost all the diabetic patients treated with insulin for three to four months will have formed insulin antibodies. Animal experiments revealed later that recrystallized insulin was immunogenic (able to elicit antibodies) in every species tested, including rabbits (GRODSKY, 1965). Immunogenicity of homologous insulin was established in cows (RENOLD *et al.*, 1966), pigs (LOCKWOOD and PROUT, 1962; BRUNFELDT and DECKERT, 1964a) and humans (DECKERT *et al.*, 1972). BRUNFELDT and DECKERT (1964b) found that amorphous insulin was more immunogenic in rabbit than recrystallized insulin, and it was concluded that the impurities function as adjuvants, thereby increasing the amount of insulin antibodies formed (DECKERT, 1964), and that insulin itself functions as an immunogen (FANKHAUSER, 1969; PFEIFFER *et al.*, 1969). The high-molecular-weight pork components isolated from crystalline insulin by gel filtration were found to be highly immunogenic in rabbits (Fig. 23) (SCHLICHTKRULL *et al.*, 1970, 1972, 1974; ROOT *et al.*, 1972). The rabbit was used in the study of

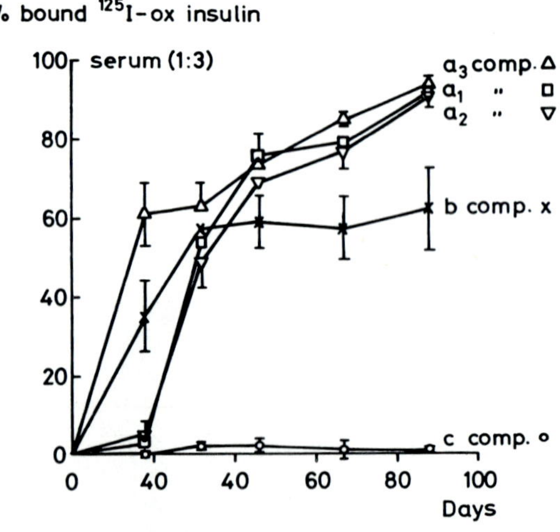

Fig. 23. Groups of 10 rabbits immunized twice weekly with isolated pork components (see Fig. 21), pH 3, 40 μg with Freund's incomplete adjuvant. The ordinate represents the antibody level as determined by the per cent bound ^{125}I-ox insulin in serum diluted 1:3 (SCHLICHTKRULL *et al.*, 1972), the abscissa represents the time of sampling since the start of immunization. Each point and interval represents the mean ± SEM. (These data were first published in Horm. Metab. Res., Suppl., Vol. 5, 134, 1974. Reproduced here by courtesy of the Editors.)

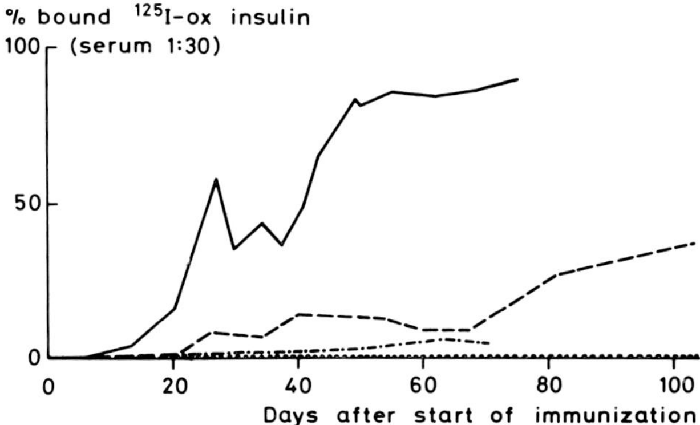

Fig. 24. Groups of 5 rabbits immunized with: —— ox a-component, ----- ox proinsulin, -·-·-·- four-times-crystallized ox insulin and ········· ox MC insulin, three times weekly, pH 7.4, 40 μg without adjuvant. Plotting on the ordinate and the abscissa as in Fig. 23, except that serum was diluted 1:30

immunogenicity of the various components of crystalline insulin (Root *et al.*, 1972; Schlichtkrull *et al.*, 1972) because rabbit insulin — just as pork insulin — differs from human insulin only at position B-30, and rabbit insulin antibodies display insulin binding characteristics that are similar to those of human insulin antibodies (Schlichtkrull *et al.*, 1970). Four-times crystallized ox insulin and components isolated from once-crystallized insulin also induced the formation of insulin antibodies, whereas MC insulin did not (Fig. 24). Thus, it appears that the isolated protein contaminants of crystalline insulin induced the formation of high levels of insulin antibodies in the rabbit whereas the MC insulin was non-immunogenic. Using the same technique in experiments with 3 rabbits per group, Root *et al.* (1972) reported similar results. It has invariably been found that ox components are more immunogenic than the corresponding pork components, e.g., as shown for the a-components in Fig. 25 (Schlichtkrull *et al.*, 1972). Root *et al.* (1972) reported likewise that ox a- and b-components were more immunogenic in rabbits than the pork components.

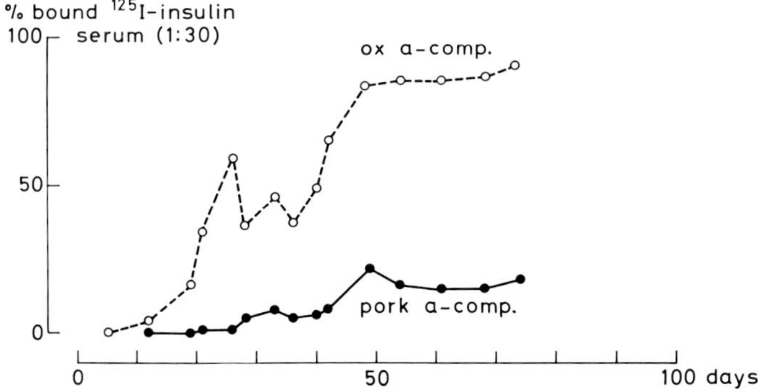

Fig. 25. Groups of 5 rabbits immunized with ox and pork a-component three times weekly, pH 7.4, 40 μg without adjuvant. Plotting on the ordinate and the abscissa as in Fig. 24

Table 7. *Proinsulin-like immunoreactivity (PLI) and insulin-like immunoreactivity (IRI) in isolated pork components (see Fig. 21), as expressed in per cent weight of the fraction. (These data were first published in Horm. Metab. Res., Suppl., Vol. 5, 134, 1974. Reproduced here by courtesy of the Editors)*

Pork components	% PLI	% IRI
a_1	0.1	1
a_2	0.4	2
a_3	2	9
b	49	56
c	0.01	100

The a-component possesses insulin-like immunoreactive sites (Table 7) and is therefore capable of inducing the formation of insulin antibodies. Mixed with MC insulin, the a-component does not apparently exert any adjuvant effect (Fig. 26).

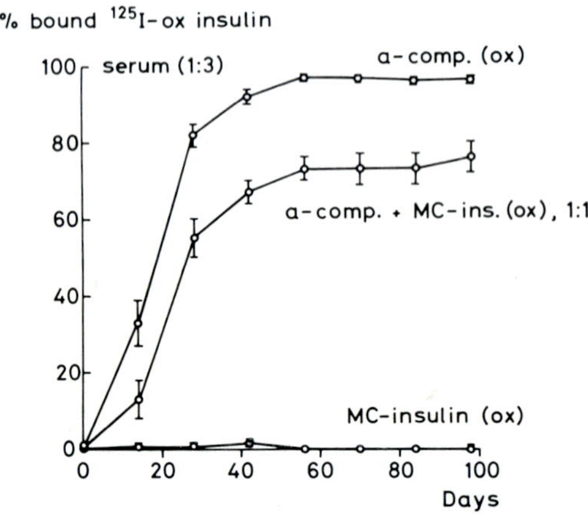

Fig. 26. Groups of 10 rabbits immunized twice weekly with 40 μg of ox a-component, 20 μg of ox a-component + 20 μg of ox MC insulin, and 40 μg ox MC insulin, pH 3, without adjuvant. Ordinate and abscissa as in Fig. 23. Each point and interval represents the mean $\pm$ SEM. (These data were first published in Horm. Metab. Res., Suppl., Vol. 5, 134, 1974. Reproduced here by courtesy of the Editors.)

The immunogenicity of ox and pork insulin preparations of varying purity is shown in Figs. 27, 28 and 29, and it appears that the immunogenicity decreases with increasing purity. However, removal of the a- and b-components by gel filtration on Sephadex G 50 was not sufficient to decrease the immunogenicity significantly below that of five-times-crystallized insulin (Fig. 27).

The IRI- and PLI-containing protein contaminants (see Table 7), e.g., proinsulin and a-component, induce, in addition to insulin antibodies, antibodies against the non-insulin-like sites, which presumably are foreign to the organism. Sera from rabbits immunized with the isolated pork components shown in Fig. 21 were analyzed for the presence of antibodies specific to the C-peptide part of proinsulin (using ^{125}I-labelled pork proinsulin), and the a_1, a_2 and a_3-components (using ^{125}I-a_1, -a_2 and -a_3, respectively) after removal of the insulin antibodies with insulin covalently linked to Sepharose.

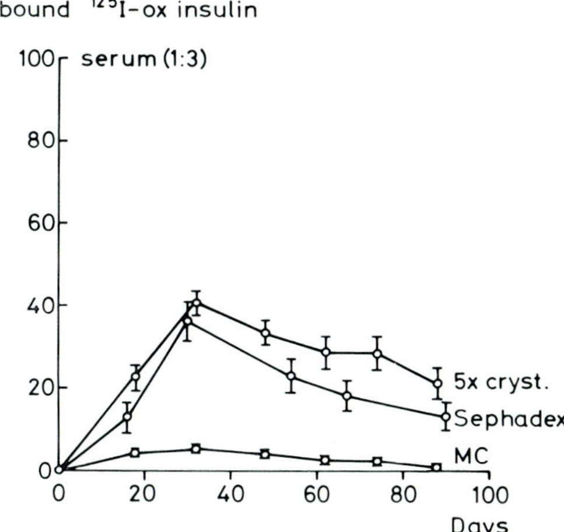

Fig. 27. Rabbits immunized twice weekly with conventional Actrapid made from 5×cryst. pork insulin, Actrapid made from once-crystallized pork insulin purified by chromatography on Sephadex G 50 F and Actrapid made from pork MC insulin; pH 7.4, 20 U with Freund's incomplete adjuvant. Ordinate and abscissa as in Fig. 23. Each point and interval represents the mean ± SEM. (These data were first published in Horm. Metab. Res., Suppl., Vol. 5, 134, 1974. Reproduced here by courtesy of the Editors.)

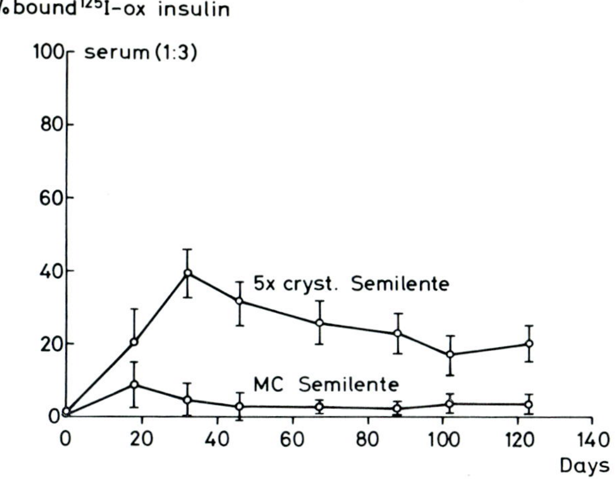

Fig. 28. Groups of 10 rabbits immunized twice weekly with conventional Semilente made from 5×crystallized pork insulin and Semilente made from pork MC insulin; pH 7.4, 20 U with Freund's incomplete adjuvant. Ordinate and abscissa as in Fig. 23. Each point and interval represents the mean ± SEM

Table 8 shows that each component induced more antibodies against itself than against the other contaminants. MC insulin did not induce antibodies against high-molecular-weight proteins (HEDING, unpublished).

The results obtained in rabbits have shown that the high-molecular-weight proteins are immunogenic, as they induce the formation of antibodies against

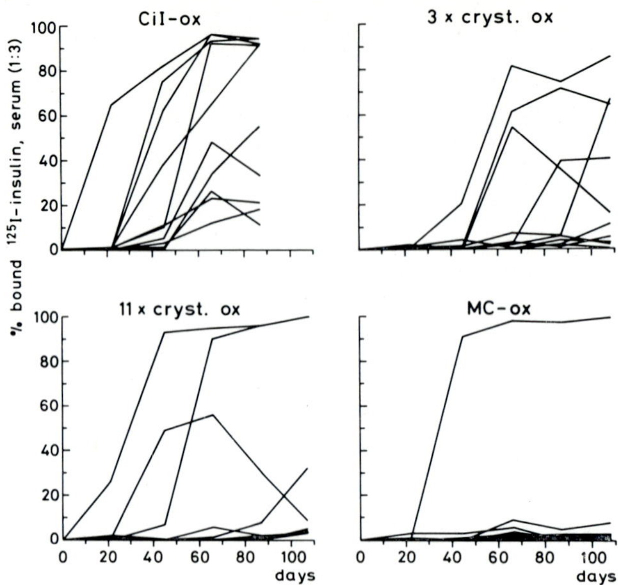

Fig. 29. Groups of 10 rabbits immunized twice weekly with Actrapid made from first crystals (CiI) of ox insulin, 3×crystallized ox insulin, 11×crystallized ox insulin and MC ox insulin, pH 7.4, 4 μg with Freund's incomplete adjuvant. Ordinate and abscissa as in Fig. 23. Each curve represents one rabbit

Table 8. *Determination of antibodies against non-insulin-like sites in rabbits immunized with the high-molecular-weight pork components as shown in Fig. 23. Sera from each group of rabbits (10) were pooled and incubated with insulin coupled to Sepharose to remove insulin antibodies. Then ^{125}I-labelled pork-a_1, -a_2, -a_3 or proinsulin was added to aliquots of the supernatant freed of insulin antibodies. After 24 h of incubation at 4°C, the ^{125}I-a_1, -a_2 and -a_3 bound to antibodies were separated from the complex by double antibody precipitation using anti-rabbit γG pork immunoglobulin (SCHLICHTKRULL et al., 1974). Bound and free ^{125}I-proinsulin were separated using ethanol (HEDING, 1972)*

Immunization components (pig)	Per cent binding of ^{125}I-components (pig)			
	a_1	a_2	a_3	proinsulin
a_1	**40**	22	21	0
a_2	34	**39**	28	16
a_3	27	17	**34**	64
b (proinsulin, etc.)	19	8	18	**100**

insulin-like and non-insulin-like sites. Removal of the a- and b-components and of the contaminants having the same molecular weight as insulin leads to MC insulin preparations with little or no immunogenicity both with regard to insulin antibodies and non-insulin-like antibodies.

3. Preparation and Stability of MC Insulin Preparations

In the preparation of MC insulin, use is made of anion exchange chromatography in an ethanolic medium (JØRGENSEN *et al.*, 1970; SCHLICHTKRULL *et al.*, 1972, 1974). Figure 30 shows the result of the method applied on once-crystallized pork insulin. The presence of ethanol in the eluent ensures such a degree of splitting of the insulin molecules from the contaminating molecules that separation by

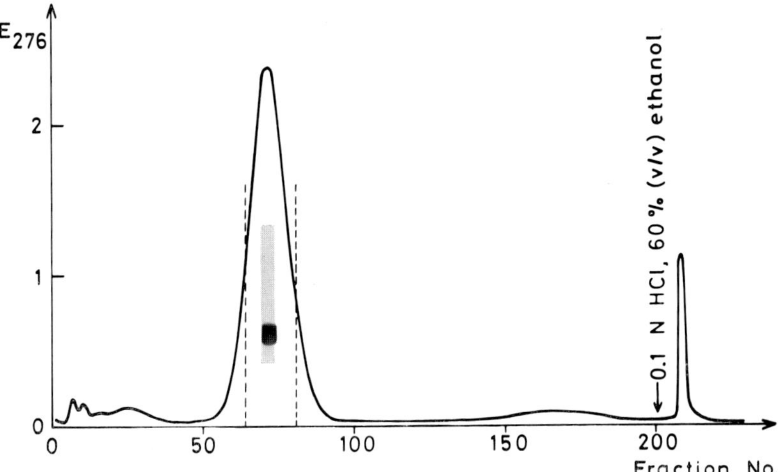

Fig. 30. Anion exchange chromatography of once-crystallized pork insulin at 25 °C. Column material: QAE-Sephadex A-25. Eluent: 0.06 M TRIS, 0.02 N HCl, 0.08 M NaCl, 60% (v/v) ethanol, pH 8.4. Applied sample: 250 mg of once citrate-crystallized pork insulin dissolved in 10 ml of eluent further containing 47 mg of TRIS and 10 mg of disodium ethylenediaminetetraacetate. The undissolved material was removed by centrifugation prior to application. Column size: 2.5×10 cm. Elution rate: 10 ml/h. Fractions of 5 ml were collected at 4 °C. Inserted: Disc electrophoresis of a 0.2 mg sample of insulin crystallized from a pool of the fractions within the broken lines. (These data were first published in Horm. Metab. Res., Suppl., Vol. 5, 134, 1974. Reproduced here by courtesy of the Editors.)

anion exchange chromatography is rendered possible. Insulin showing only one band when analyzed by disc electrophoresis is eluted within the main peak as shown in the figure. Among the c-component impurities the arginine insulins and the ethyl esters of insulin are eluted before, and the desamido-insulins behind the insulin peak. Among the b-component impurities, proinsulin is eluted before, and the intermediates and the non-convertible dimer behind the insulin peak. MC insulin displays a single component not only when analyzed by disc electrophoresis but also when analyzed by gel filtration.

MC insulin is commercially available in the form of the pharmaceutical preparations Actrapid MC and Semilente MC, which possess the same timing of action as conventional Actrapid and Semilente, and, furthermore, as Monotard®, which is a preparation of the Lente type, i.e. consisting of 3 parts of insulin in amorphous state and 7 parts of insulin in crystalline state (see II. 3., p. 749), but in Monotard, the suspended insulin particles — the amorphous as well as the crystalline — are made up entirely of MC pork insulin.

Monotard has the same initial effect as Lente but its duration of action is a little shorter. The timing of action of Monotard is very similar to that of NPH, as shown in subcutaneous absorption studies of Monotard and NPH. Its timing has been shown to be suitable for therapy with both one and two daily injections (BINDER, personal communication).

Like most other polypeptides and proteins, insulin contains asparaginyl and glutaminyl residues, whose side chains are exposed to hydrolytic deamidation. These residues are known to be unstable under storage conditions (MCKERROW and ROBINSON, 1971), especially when the insulin preparation is an acid solution

Table 9. *Formation of deamidation products during 1 year of storage of various MC insulin preparations (*BRANGE, *unpublished)*

Insulin preparation	Per cent deamidation products formed 4°C	15°C
Actrapid MC	2	6
Semilente MC	1.5	5
Monotard (MC)	1	2.5

Table 10. *Formation of dimerization and polymerization products during 1 year of storage of various MC insulin preparations (*BRANGE, *unpublished)*

Insulin preparation	Per cent dimerization and polymerization products formed 4°C	15°C
Actrapid MC	<0.1	0.2
Semilente MC	0.1	0.3
Monotard (MC)	0.2	0.3

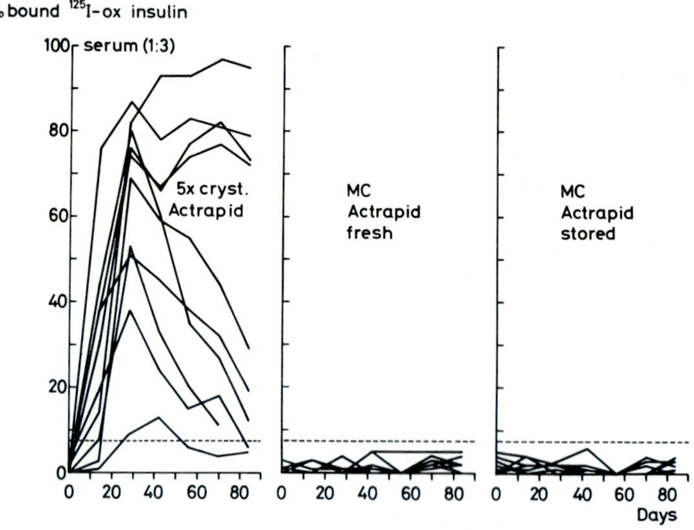

Fig. 31. Groups of 10 rabbits immunized twice weekly with Actrapid made from 5-times-crystallized pork insulin, pork MC insulin (fresh Actrapid preparation) and pork MC insulin (Actrapid preparation stored for 2 years at 25°C); pH 7.4, 20 U with Freund's incomplete adjuvant. Ordinate and abscissa as in Fig. 23. The dotted line represents the antibody detection limit. Each curve represents one rabbit. (These data were first published in Horm. Metab. Res., Suppl., Vol. 5, 134, 1974. Reproduced here by courtesy of the Editors.)

(SUNDBY, 1962; SLOBIN and CARPENTER, 1963). In neutral solution or suspension insulin also undergoes slow deamidation (Table 9). The deamidation products have been shown to possess full or nearly full biological potency (CHANCE, 1972; SØRENSEN, personal communication). Small amounts of dimerization and polymerization products are formed upon storage of pharmaceutical insulin preparations (Table 10).

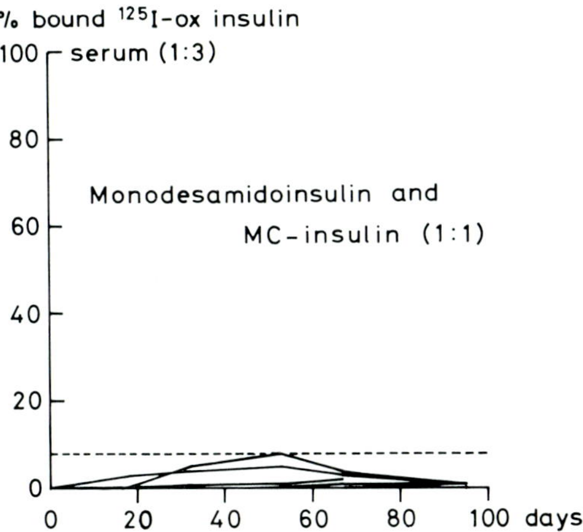

Fig. 32. Group of 9 rabbits immunized twice weekly with Actrapid made from one part Monodesamido-MC insulin (pork) and one part pork MC insulin; pH 7.4, approximately 20 U (total dose) with Freund's incomplete adjuvant. Ordinate and abscissa as in Fig. 23. The dotted line represents the antibody detection limit. Each curve represents one rabbit

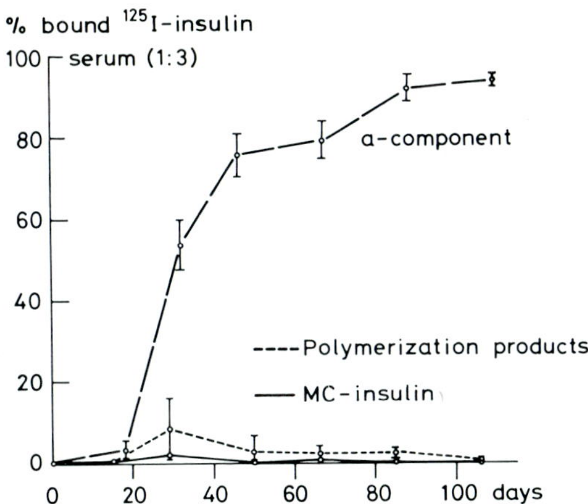

Fig. 33. Groups of 10 rabbits immunized twice weekly with pork a-component, polymerization products isolated from Semilente MC after storage of the preparation for 17 months at 37°C and pork MC insulin; pH 3, 40 μg with Freund's incomplete adjuvant. Ordinate and abscissa as in Fig. 23. Each point and interval represents the mean $\pm$ SEM

The insulin degradation and polymerization products formed upon storage of MC insulin preparations were tested in rabbit immunization experiments and found not to be significantly immunogenic, as shown in Figs. 31—34.

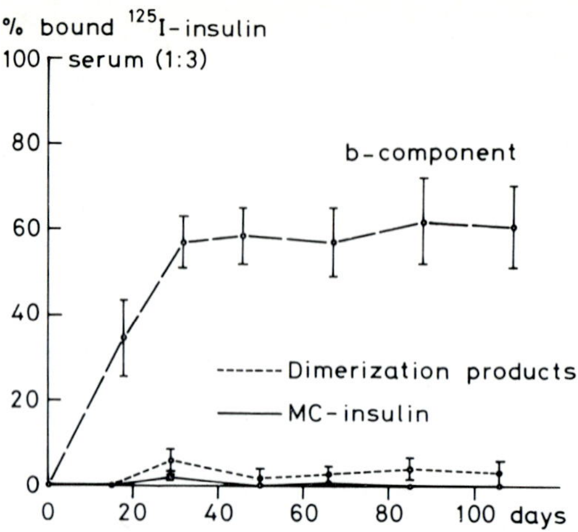

Fig. 34. Groups of rabbits immunized twice weekly with pork b-component (10 rabbits), dimerization products isolated from Monotard MC after storage of the preparation for 15 months at 37°C (19 rabbits) and pork MC insulin (10 rabbits); pH 3, 40 μg with Freund's incomplete adjuvant. Ordinate and abscissa as in Fig. 23. Each point and interval represents the mean ± SEM

4. Clinical Results

a) Insulin Antibodies

Practically all diabetic patients treated with conventional insulins form antibodies (BERSON and YALOW, 1964; DECKERT, 1964). Patients treated exclusively with pork MC insulin preparations (Monotard, MC-Actrapid and MC-Semilente) for about 1 year were found to have low, or undetectable, levels of antibodies, whereas all the patients treated with Lente, Actrapid and Semilente prepared from 5 × crystallized pork insulin showed considerably higher levels (SCHLICHTKRULL *et al.*, 1972; SCHLICHTKRULL *et al.*, 1974; ANDREANI *et al.*, 1972; BRUNI *et al.*, 1973; CZYZYK *et al.*, 1974; FANKHAUSER and MICHL, 1971, 1973; KORP and LEVETT, 1973; MIROUZE *et al.*, 1973). ROOT *et al.* (1972) also showed a difference in the immunogenicity of pork single-component Lente and Lente made from USP pork insulin, whereas single-peak beef/pork insulin did not appear to offer obvious immunologic advantages (TANTILLO *et al.*, 1974).

Figure 35 shows a comparison of antibody levels and total IRI in three groups of patients treated for 1—2 years with conventional Lente (beef + pork), pork Lente and Monotard. In agreement with the findings of BERSON and YALOW (1966), it appears that the conventional Lente, being a mixture of 70% beef and 30% pork insulin, was more immunogenic than pork Lente of corresponding purity.

It has been shown (SCHLICHTKRULL *et al.*, 1972) that immunized rabbits, having a high level of insulin antibodies, exhibited the same rapid drop in antibodies after transfer to MC pork insulin as that seen in animals in which the treatment was discontinued. When patients treated with conventional insulin for years were transferred to Monotard, a drop was observed in the antibody levels in many patients (ANDREANI *et al.*, 1972; KORP and LEVETT, 1973; MIROUZE *et al.*, 1973). ANDREANI *et al.* (1972) showed in a series of 12 patients that the drop in antibody level was accompanied by a significant reduction in the daily insulin dose during the 12 months the patients were followed.

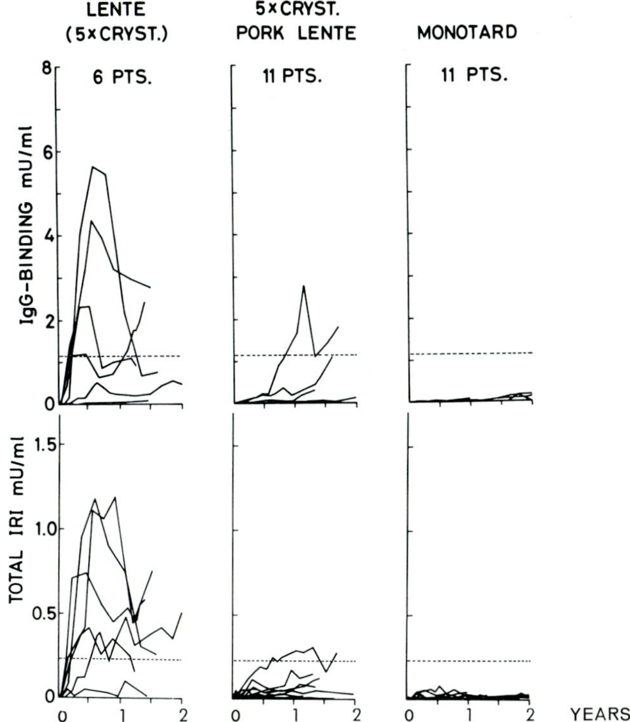

Fig. 35. Levels of insulin antibody and total IRI in diabetics since the beginning of insulin therapy and up to 1—2 years of treatment with either Lente (beef/pork), Lente (pork) or Monotard MC. Binding of ^{125}I-labelled beef insulin to human γG was determined according to Christiansen (1973). (These data were first published in Horm. Metab. Res., Suppl., Vol. 5, 134, 1974. Reproduced here by courtesy of the Editors.)

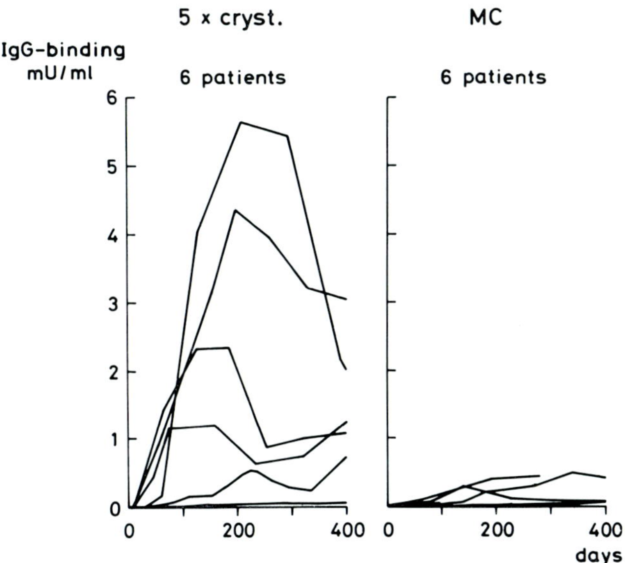

Fig. 36. IgG binding of insulin in sera from diabetic patients since the beginning of insulin therapy and up to 200—400 days of treatment with either conventional Lente (beef/pork 5x cryst.) or Lente (beef/pork) of MC purity (Treatment with insulin was started within a month after diagnosis of diabetes.)

In rabbits, MC insulin (beef) showed less immunogenicity than 5 × crystallized beef insulin, and the same was found to be the case in diabetics (Fig. 36). Lente prepared from beef and pork MC insulin showed lower immunogenicity than the comparable conventional Lente.

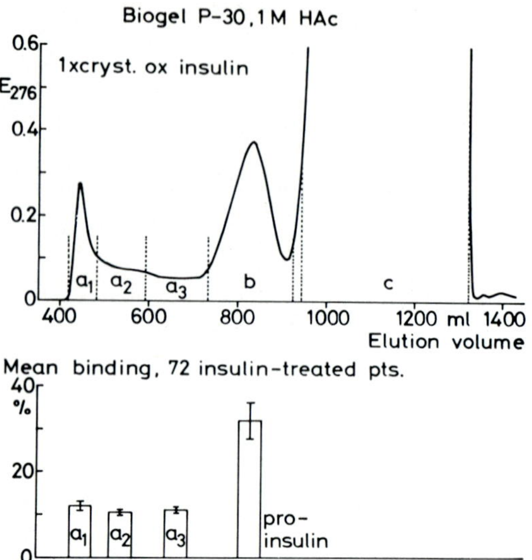

Fig. 37. Antibodies against beef proinsulin and a_1, a_2 and a_3-components (see Fig. 21) in 72 diabetic patients treated with conventional insulin for more than 6 months. Insulin antibodies were removed with insulin coupled to Sephadex before the determinations

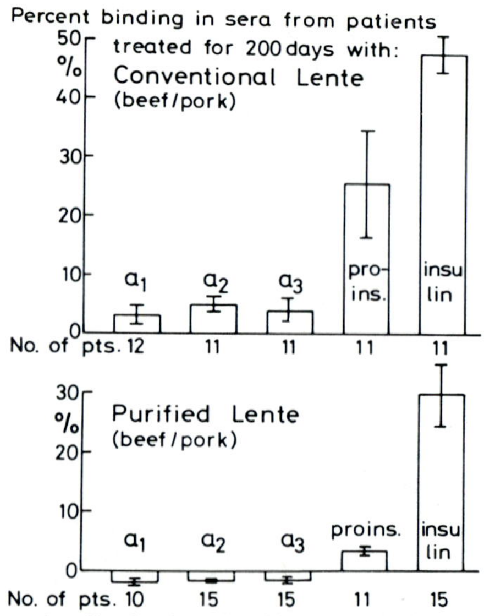

Fig. 38. Antibodies against insulin, beef proinsulin, a_1, a_2 and a_3-components (see Fig. 21) in diabetics after treatment exclusively with either conventional Lente (beef/pork) or Lente (beef/pork) of higher purity. (Treatment with insulin was started within a month after diagnosis of diabetes.) Insulin antibodies were removed with insulin coupled to sepharose before the determination of bound beef proinsulin, a_1, a_2 and a_3-components

b) Antibodies Against Proinsulin and a-Component

The high-molecular-weight protein contaminants have been found to be immunogenic in rabbits with regard to formation of antibodies both against insulin- and non-insulin-like sites (see 2., p. 756—760). Diabetic patients treated with conventional insulin were found to have antibodies against the non-insulin-like sites (Fig. 37), whereas this was not the case in patients treated with a Lente preparation (beef/pork) of higher purity (Fig. 38).

References

Aakerblom, H.K., Hiekkala, H.: Diurnal blood and urine glucose and acetone bodies in labile juvenile diabetics on one- and two-injection insulin therapy. Diabetologia **6**, 130 (1970)

Aarseth, S.: Insulinbehandling (Insulin treatment). T. norske Lægeforen. **4**, 349 (1964)

Abel, J.J.: Crystalline insulin. Proc. nat. Acad. Sci. (Wash.) **12**, 132 (1926)

Abel, J.J., Geiling, E.M.K., Rouiller, C.A., Bell, F.K., Wintersteiner, O.: Crystalline insulin. J. Pharmacol. exp. Ther. **31**, 65 (1927)

Akre, P.R., Kirtley, W.R., Galloway, J.A.: Comparative hypoglycemic response of diabetic subjects to human insulin or structurally similar insulins of animal source. Diabetes **13**, 135 (1964)

Andreani, D., Iavicoli, M., Colletti, A., Menzinger, G., Maltarello, C.: Esperienze nel trattamento del diabete con le insuline di tipo monocomponente (MC) e monospecies (MS). Folia endocr. (Roma) **25**, 516 (1972)

Armstrong, C.N., Lloyd, W.H.: Severe local and general reaction to insulin zinc suspension and soluble insulin. Brit. med. J. **1954 II**, 396

Aubertin, E., Servantie, L., Chassagnette, C.: Action hypoglycémiante chez l'animal normal de l'insuline entrainée par un précipité d'hydrate de zinc. C.R. Soc. Biol. (Paris) **130**, 484 (1939)

Bang, H.O.: Some investigations on the absorption mechanism of protamine insulin. Acta pharmacol. (Kbh.) **2**, 79 (1946a)

Bang, H.O.: Enzymatic break-down of protamine insulin. (Further investigations.) Acta pharmacol. (Kbh.) **2**, 89 (1946b)

Banting, F.G., Best, C.H.: Pancreatic extracts. J. Lab. clin. Med. **7**, 464 (1922)

Baquet, R.: Le traitement du diabète par les insulines lentes. Maroc méd. **38**, 597 (1959)

Bauman, L.: Clinical experience with globin insulin. Proc. Soc. exp. Biol. (N.Y.) **40**, 170 (1939)

Beardwood, J.T., Tittle, C.R., Packer, R.M.: Comparison of diabetic control with NPH and globin insulin. J. Mich. med. Soc. **51**, 1298 (1952)

Beeuwkes, H., Hollman, E.C.M.J., Kreutzer, H.H.: Specifieke Antistoffen Tegen Runderinsuline. (Specific antibody against beef insulin.) Ned. T. Geneesk. **100**, IV, 49, 3610 (1956)

Berg, J.W., Ortmeyer, D.W., Ott, D.L., Jackson, R.L.: Comparison of globin insulin and NPH insulin. Diabetes **2**, 365 (1953)

Bermont, A.: Complications dermatologiques de l'insulinotherapie. Thèse Université de Nancy 1967

Bernard, R., Bernard, C., Laurent, C.: Part respective des critères cliniques classiques et de l'enregistrement glycémique continu par automation dans l'appréciation des indications et des résultats d'une insulinothérapie. Diabète (Le Raincy) **5**, 207 (1965)

Bernhard, H., Pickert, H.: Über praktische Erfahrungen mit Lente-Insulinen in der ambulanten Diabetes-Betreuung. Ärztl. Wschr. **13**, 835 (1958)

Berns, A.W., Owens, C.T., Blumenthal, H.T.: A histo- and immunopathologic study of the vessels and islets of Langerhans of the pancreas in diabetes mellitus. J. Geront. **19**, 179 (1964)

Berson, S.A., Yalow, R.S.: Antigens in insulin determinants of specificity of porcine insulin in man. Science **139**, 844 (1963)

Berson, S.A., Yalow, R.S.: The present status of insulin antagonists in plasma. Diabetes **13**, 247 (1964)

Berson, S.A., Yalow, R.S.: Insulin in blood and insulin antibodies. Amer. J. Med. **40**, 676 (1966)

Berson, S.A., Yalow, R.S., Bauman, A., Rothschild, M.A., Newerly, K.: Insulin-I^{131} metabolism in human subjects: Demonstration of insulin binding globulin in the circulation of insulin treated subjects. J. clin. Invest. **35**, 170 (1956)

Bertram, F.: Über Depotinsuline. Med. Klin. **34**, 1186 (1938)

Bertram, F.: Die Zuckerkrankheit. Stuttgart: G. Thieme 1953

BERTRAM, F.: Erfahrungen mit Long-Insulin „Hoechst". Dtsch. med. Wschr. **80**, 220 (1955)

BERTRAM, F., FELDKIRCHNER, E., MEINECKE, R.: Neue Möglichkeiten einer optimalen Insulintherapie. Dtsch. med. Wschr. **79**, 28 (1954)

BEST, C.H.: The prolongation of insulin action. Symposium on Hormones (Sigma Xi lect.), 362 (1936—1937)

BIBERGEIL, H.: Klinische Untersuchungen über Lente-Insulin. Dtsch. med. Wschr. **83**, 761 and 807 (1958)

BINDER, C., NIELSEN, A., JØRGENSEN, K.: The absorption of an acid and a neutral insulin solution after subcutaneous injection into different regions in diabetic patients. Scand. J. clin. Lab. Invest. **19**, 156 (1967)

BINDER, C.: Absorption of injected insulin. A clinical-pharmacological study. Diss. Copenhagen University 1969

BISCHOFF, F., JEMTEGAARD, L.M.: Divided dosage of insulin. Amer. J. Physiol. **119**, 149 (1937)

BLATHERWICK, N.R., EWING, M.E., BRADSHAW, P.J.: Some effects of zinc and iron salts on the hypoglycemic action of insulin in rats. Amer. J. Physiol. **121**, 44 (1938)

BLOOM, A.: Fat atrophy due to insulin. Brit. med. J. **4**, 366 (1972)

BLÖCH, J.: Neuzeitliche Insulintherapie. Wien klin. Wschr. **67**, 498 (1955)

BOLLER, R.: Zur Klinik des Diabetes mellitus. Wien. klin. Wschr. **67**, 669 (1955)

BOOS, R.: Immunologische Probleme beim Diabetes mellitus. Med. Klin. **64**, 1492 (1969)

BOSHELL, B.R., BARRETT, J.C., WILENSKY, A.S., PATTON, T.B.: Insulin resistance. Response to insulin from various animal sources, including human. Diabetes **13**, 144 (1964)

BOULIN, R., NEPVEUX, F.: Les insulines au zinc à action lente. Presse méd. **62**, 1053 (1954)

BRESSLER, R., GALLOWAY, J.A.: Insulin treatment of diabetes mellitus. Med. Clin. N. Amer. **55**, 861 (1971)

BRITISH PHARMACOPOEIA (1973)

BRUNFELDT, K., DECKERT, T.: Antibodies in the pig against pig insulin. Acta endocr. (Kbh.) **47**, 367 (1964a)

BRUNFELDT, K., DECKERT, T.: The antigenic properties of pig insulin. Acta endocr. (Kbh.) **47**, 353 (1964b)

BRUNI, B.: Un nuovo tipo di insulina ad azione bifasica (Rapitard con Actrapid). (A new type of insulin with biphasic action (rapitard with actrapid).) Minerva med. **55**, 3660 (1964)

BRUNI, B.: Trattamento con insulin bifasica Rapitard dello scompenso diabetico acuto grave, chetoacidosico o imperosmolare. Minerva med. **59**, 5280 (1968)

BRUNI, B., D'ALBERTO, M., OSENDA, M., RICCI, C., TURCO, G.L.: Clinical trial with monocomponent lente insulins. Diabetologia **9**, 492 (1973)

BUCHANAN, K.D., IMRIE, A.H.: Observations on the lente insulins. Scot. med. J. **9**, 89 (1964)

BURKHOLDER, P.M.: Immunohistopathologic study of localized plasma proteins and fixation of guinea pig complement in renal lesions of diabetic glomerulosclerosis. Diabetes **14**, 755 (1965)

CAMPBELL, W.R., FLETCHER, A.A., KERR, R.B.: Protamine insulin in the treatment of diabetes mellitus. Amer. J. med. Sci. **192**, 589 (1936)

CANIVET, J., QUICHAUD, J., MANTEL, O., RAMBERT, P.: Un cas d'insulino-résistance à l'insuline de boeuf par anticorps neutralisants avec sensibilité normale à l'insuline de porc. Bull. Soc. méd. Hôp. (Paris) **77**, 178 (1961)

CHANCE, R.E.: Amino acid sequences of proinsulins and intermediates. Diabetes **21**, Suppl. 2, 461 (1972)

CHAPTAL, J., JEAN, R., GUILLAUMOT, R., MOREL, G.: Association à l'insuline zinc-mixte d'une nouvelle insuline ordinaire d'action rapide étude expérimentale dans le traitement du diabète infantile. Path. et Biol. **13**, 622 (1965)

CHIMENES, H., LAURENT, C.: Diagnostic et traitement de diabètes instables. Diabète (Le Raincy) **3**, 115 (1965)

CHRISTIANSEN, A.H.: Radioimmunoelectrophoresis in the determination of insulin binding to IgG. Methodological studies. Horm. Metab. Res. **5**, 147 (1973)

COBLEY, J.F.C.C., HARRISON, K.S., BLACKETT, R.B., HEWITT, L.E.: Out-patient assessment of the "novo" insulin. Med. J. Aust. **2**, 499 (1954)

COLNARD, C.: Les insulines actrapid et rapitard dans le traitement du diabète sucré de l'adulte (à propos de 65 observations). Thèse Université de Nancy 1965

COLWELL, A.R.: Nature and time action of modifications of protamine zinc insulin. Arch. intern. Med. ad 7, **74**, 331 (1944)

COLWELL, A.R.: Protamine insulin mixtures in the treatment of diabetes mellitus. N.Y. St. J. Med. **47**, 1103 (1947)

COLWELL, A.R.: Insulin zinc suspensions. Diabetes **3**, 162 (1954)

COLWELL, A.R.: Progress report on lente insulin. Diabetes **4**, 419 (1955)

COLWELL, A.R.: Clinical use of insulin. In: ELLENBERG, M., RIFKIN, H.: Diabetes Mellitus: Theory and Practice. McSwan-Hill: 624—637, 1970

Colwell, A.R., Izzo, J.L., Stryker, W.A.: Intermediate action of mixtures of soluble insulin and protamine zinc insulin. Arch. intern. Med. **69**, 931 (1942)

Constam, G.R.: Erfahrungen mit Insulin-Zink-Suspensionen, einer Gruppe von Insulinpräparaten (Lente Insuline) mit verschieden langer Wirkungsdauer. Schweiz. med. Wschr. **84**, 200 (1954)

Constam, G.R.: Insulin-zinc suspensions (lente-insulins) in the treatment of diabetes mellitus. Northw. Med. (Seattle) **56**, 1023 (1957)

Court, J.M., Amies, G.C.: Rapitard insulin in the management of juvenile diabetes. Med. J. Aust. **2**, 5 (1973)

Crecelius, G.: Insulin Novo Rapitard in der ambulanten Diabetesbehandlung. Med. Klin. **62**, 1753 (1967)

Czyzyk, A., Lawecki, J., Rogala, H., Miedzinska, E., Popik-Hankiewicz, A.: Serum levels of insulin-binding antibodies in diabetic patients treated with monocomponent insulin. Diabetologia **10**, 233 (1974)

Danowski, T.S.: Diabetes Mellitus: Diagnosis and Treatment. New York: American Diabetes Association, Inc. 1964

Darnaud, C., Danard, Y., Moreau, G., Didier, E.: Un solution au probléme de l'injection quotidienne unique: L'Insuline zinc "mixte". Diabète (Le Raincy) **4**, 133 (1956)

Davidson, J.K., Eddleman, E.E.: Insulin resistance. Review of the literature and report of a case associated with carcinoma of the pancreas. Arch. intern. Med. **86**, 727 (1950)

Daweke, H.: Klinik der Insulinresistenz. Dtsch. med. Wschr. **91**, 973 (1966)

Daweke, H.: Schwierigkeiten bei der Insulinbehandlung, insbesondere beim labilen Diabetes, bei Insulinallergie und Insulinresistenz. Therapiewoche **18**, 1, 20 (1968)

Daweke, H., Bach, I.: Neue Erkenntnisse in der Behandlung der chronischen Insulinresistenz und experimentelle Untersuchungen zu ihrer Genese. Klin. Wschr. **41**, 257 (1963)

Deckert, T.: Insulin antibodies. Diss. Copenhagen University 1964

Deckert, T., Andersen, O.O., Grundahl, E., Kerp, L.: Isoimmunization of man by recrystallized human insulin. Diabetologia **8**, 358 (1972)

Devlin, J.G., Brien, T.G.: Relationship between differential antibody binding capacity and clinical requirements of beef and pork insulin. Metabolism **14**, 1034 (1965)

Devlin, J.G., Brien, T., Stephenson, N.: Effect of alteration of species source of insulin on insulin-antibody levels. Lancet **1966 II**, 883

Devlin, J.G., Brien, T., Stephenson, N.: Relation between antibody and insulin dose. Brit. med. J. **1**, 542 (1967)

Devlin, J.G., Duggan, M.: Antibody studies in patients on mixed bovine/porcine insulins. Diabetologia **5**, 192 (1969)

Didier, E.: Essai clinique de l'Insuline Zinc Mixte. Diss. Imprimerie Artistique Lavaur (Tarn) 1955

Ditschuneit, H., Federlin, K.: Beitrag zur Pathogenese der Insulinresistenz. Dtsch. med. Wschr. **91**, 853 (1966)

Dixon, K., Exton, P.D., Hughes, H.R.: Insulin antibodies in aetiology of labile diabetes. Lancet **1972 I**, 343

Dörzbach, E.: Über Chemie und Biologie des Surfen-Insulins. Inaug. Diss. Mainz 1950

Dörzbach, E., Lindner, F.: Über ein neues Depot-Insulin mit abgestufter Wirksamkeit (Long-Insulin Hoechst). Dtsch. med. Wschr. **79**, 440 (1954)

Dörzbach, E., Müller, R.: Die Insulintherapie: Die Insulinpräparate. In: Handbuch des Diabetes Mellitus. Vol. II. München: Lehmann's Verlag 1971

Drury, M.I.: The new "lente" insulins. J. Irish med. Ass. **33**, 96 (1953)

Drury, M.I., Gregg, T.: Diabetes mellitus. J. Irish med. Ass. **37**, 159 (1956)

Drury, M.I., Timoney, F.J.: Two new insulins — actrapid and rapitard. J. Irish med. Ass. **57**, 71 (1965)

Duncan, G.G.: Practical use of the various insulins in the management of diabetes mellitus. Metabolism **I**, 101 (1952)

Duncan, L.: New preparations of insulin. Prescribers' J. **6**, 105 (1967)

Eckler, E., Koch, I.: Erfahrungen mit Insulin-Zink-Suspensionen beim kindlichen Diabetes mellitus. Münch. med. Wschr. **101**, 1219 (1959)

Eisenbrand, J., Wegel, F.: Über die Verbindungen von Zink mit Glykokoll, Cystein, Cystin und Glutathion und über die Natur der Bindung zwischen Insulin und Zinc. Hoppe-Seylers Z. physiol. Chem. **268**, 26 (1941)

Ellenberg, M., Rifkin, H.: Clinical Diabetes Mellitus. New York: McGraw-Hill Book Company, Inc. 1962

Ellenbogen, E.: The Determination of the physical-chemical properties of insulin and their application to the equilibrium between insulin of molecular weight 12000 and 36000. Thesis: Harvard University 1949

ENGLESON, G.: Insulin Novo Lente i én daglig injektion vid barn-diabetes. (Insulin Novo Lente in one daily injection in juvenile diabetes.) Nord. Med. **50**, 1008 (1953)
ENGLESON, G., LEHMANN, O.: The "lente" insulins in juvenile diabetes. Acta paediat. (Uppsala) **46**, 317 (1957)
ESSELLIER, A.F., JEANNERET, R.L., KOSZEWSKI, B.J.: Das NPH-Insulin, ein neues Intermediärinsulin. Schweiz. med. Wschr. **82**, 549 (1952)
FALK, W.: Die Behandlung des kindlichen Diabetes Mellitus mit „Insulin Novo Lente". Med. Klin. **49**, 1615 (1954)
FALUDI, G., MEHBOD, H.: Modified pork insulin in the treatment of insulin resistant diabetes. J. Amer. med. Wom. Ass. **20**, 333 (1965)
FANKHAUSER, S.: Neuere Aspekte der Insulintherapie. Schweiz. med. Wschr. **99**, 414 (1969)
FANKHAUSER, S., DIACON, C.: Die Bedeutung der Insulinantikörper bei Komplikationen der Insulintherapie. Helv. med. Acta Suppl. **46**, 164 (1966)
FANKHAUSER, S., MICHL, J.: Die Antigenität verschiedener Depotinsuline bei Diabetikern. Diabetes Mellitus. In: Verhandlungen des II. Internationalen Donau-Symposiums über Diabetes mellitus. Wien: Verlag der Wiener Medizinischen Akademie 1971
FANKHAUSER, S., MICHL, J.: Zwei Jahre Erfahrungen mit Monocomponent-Insulin bei Diabetikern. In: Verhandlungen des III. Internationales Donau-Symposiums über Diabetes mellitus. Wien: Verlag Wilhelm Mandrich 1973
FANKHAUSER, S., MONTANDON, A.: La place de l'insuline porcine dans le traitement du diabète. Rev. méd. Suisse rom. **90**, 287 (1970)
FEDDER, D.G., POMPEN, A.W.M.: Onderzoek naar de bruikbaarheid von Rapitard-insuline. Ned. T. Geneesk. **113**, 239 (1969)
FELDMAN, R., GRODSKY, G.M., KOHOUT, F.W., MCWILLIAMS, N.B.: Immunologic studies in a diabetic subject resistant to bovine insulin but sensitive to porcine insulin. Amer. J. Med. **35**, 411 (1963)
FERGUSON, A.W.: The use of the insulin zinc suspensions in diabetic children. Arch. Dis. Childh. **29**, 436 (1954)
FERGUSON, I.G., BUCHANAN, J., MURRAY, I.: Insulin zinc suspension after ten years. Brit. med. J. **1**, 275 (1964)
FINEBERG, S.K.: Clinical experience with NPH insulin. Amer. J. dig. Dis. **21**, 286 (1954)
FITZGERALD, M.G., THORN, P.A., MALINS, J.M.: Transfer to insulin zinc suspension. Lancet **266**, 187 (1954)
FOIT, R., ŠIROVÁ, S.: Suspense insulinové. (Insulin suspensions.) Čas. Lék. čes. **93**, 1094 (1954)
FRANZINI, P., POMPILI, G.: Osservazioni cliniche su di un nuovo tipo di insulina-ritardo. (Clinical observations with a new type of insulin with retarded action.) Arch. Stud. Fisiopat. Ricambio **19**, I (1954)
FRIEDMAN, G.J.: Available insulins and insulin hypoglycemia. N.Y. St. J. Med. **62**, 527 (1962)
GASSMANN, W.: Klinische Erfahrungen mit Long-Insulin Hoechst. Dtsch. med. J. **5**, 241 (1954)
GERRITZEN, F.: The classification of various insulins. Brit. med. J. **1953 II**, 1030
GIBBS, G.E.: Management of juvenile diabetes. Lancet **86**, 319 (1966)
GLEIZE, J., FRANCOIS, R., PLAUCHU, M.: Contribution à l'étude des lipodystrophies insuliniques. Essai de traitement aux insulines de porc. Diabète (Le Raincy) **16**, 281 (1968)
GODON, C.: Essai clinique des insulines lentes (Suspension insuline-zinc). Rev. méd. Liège **15**, 164 (1960)
GOLDMAN, A.S., KAYE, R.: Insulin resistance in a diabetic child. Report of a case successfully treated with pork insulin. Diabetes **11**, 122 (1962)
GRAHAM, G.: The use of a mixture of ordinary and protamine insulin. Acta med. scand. Suppl. **90**, 54 (1938)
GRAUHAN, G.: Untersuchungen zur Brauchbarkeit der neuen Insulin-Zinc-Suspensionen (Lente-Insuline). Inaug. Diss. Kiel 1955
GREENHOUSE, B.: Lente insulin. Conn. med. J. **18**, 848 (1954)
GRIEBLE, H.G.: Renal lesions induced by heterologous insulin: An example of foreign protein nephritis. J. Lab. clin. Med. **56**, 819 (1960)
GRODSKY, G.M.: Production of autoantibodies to insulin in man and rabbits. Diabetes **14**, 396 (1965)
GUIVARCH, J., RIAHI, M., CHARLIER, M., GOULHEN, M.T., LAURENT, C., ROYER, P.: Traitement du diabète infantile par une nouvelle insuline à action biphasique. Pédiatrie **41**, 384 (1965)
GURLING, K.J., ROBERTSON, J.A., WHITTAKER, H., OAKLEY, W., LAWRENCE, R.D.: Treatment of diabetes mellitus with insulin zinc suspension. Brit. med. J. **1955 I**, 71
GUTSCHE, H., HASEKI, M.: Neue Behandlungsmöglichkeit des unstabilen Diabetes Mellitus (Brittle). Med. Klin. **59**, 824 (1964)
HAGEDORN, H.C.: On the protamine-splitting properties of blood-serum. Skand. Arch. Physiol. **80**, 156 (1938)

HAGEDORN, H.C.: The absorption of protamine insulin. Rep. Steno Hosp. (Kbh.) **1**, 25 (1946)
HAGEDORN, H.C., JENSEN, B.N., KRARUP, N.B., WODSTRUP, I.: Protamine insulinate. J. Amer. med. Ass. **106**, 177 (1936)
HAGEN, H.: Zur Klinik der lokalen Insulinverträglichkeit. Medizinische **47**, 1746 (1957)
HAGEN, H., HAGEN, W.: Experimentelle Untersuchungen über die Hautverträglichkeit von Insulinpräparaten. 2. Mitteilung. Ärztl. Forsch. **13**, 578 (1959)
HAGEN, H., HAGEN, W.: Zur Wahl des Insulin-Präparates. Med. Klin. **57**, 2025 (1962)
HAGEN, H., HAGEN, W., HEINSEN, H.A., OLTERS, E., SCHEFFLER, H.: Experimentelle Untersuchungen über die Hautverträglichkeit von Insulinpräparaten. 1. Mitteilung. Dtsch. med. Wschr. **83**, 1480 (1958)
HALLAS-MØLLER, K.: Chemical and biological insulin studies I and II. Diss. Copenhagen University 1945
HALLAS-MØLLER, K., HEY, A.: Iso-Insulin Novo: Et nyt protraheret virkende insulinpræparat. (A new insulin preparation with prolonged action.) Ugeskr. Læg. **23**, 565 (1944)
HALLAS-MØLLER, K., JERSILD, M., PETERSEN, K., SCHLICHTKRULL, J.: Zinc insulin preparations for single daily injection. J. Amer. med. Ass. **150**, 1667 (1952a)
HALLAS-MØLLER, K., JERSILD, M., PETERSEN, K., SCHLICHTKRULL, J.: The lente insulins. Insulin-zinc suspensions. Dan. med. Bull. **1**, 132 (1954a)
HALLAS-MØLLER, K., JERSILD, M., PETERSEN, K., SCHLICHTKRULL, J.: Insulin trials. Lancet **267**, 975 (1954b)
HALLAS-MØLLER, K., PETERSEN, K., SCHLICHTKRULL, J.: Crystalline and amorphous[1] insulin-zinc compounds with prolonged action. Science **116**, 394 (1952b)
HARINGTON, C.R., SCOTT, D.A.: XLVI. Observations on insulin, part I. Chemical observations. Biochem. J. **23**, 384 (1929)
HARRIS-JONES, J.N., MILLER, H., OWEN, G.: Insulin-binding antibodies in relation to insulin therapy. J. clin. Path. **16**, 120 (1963)
HARWOOD, R.: Insulin-binding antibodies and "spontaneous" hypoglycemia. New Engl. J. Med. **262**, 978 (1960)
HAUNZ, E.A.: Clinical evaluation of lente insulin in one hundred nine diabetic patients. J. Amer. med. Ass. **159**, 1611 (1955)
HAUNZ, E.A.: The current role of insulin in the era of hypoglycemic agents. Amer. Practit. **13**, 3 (1962)
HAYES, D.W.: Insulin preparations in the treatment of diabetes mellitus. J. med. Soc. **106**, 387 (1954)
HEDING, L.G.: Determination of total serum insulin (IRI) in insulin-treated diabetic patients. Diabetologia **8**, 260 (1972)
HEISKELL, C.L., FLORSHEIM, W.H., MEISTER, L.: Electrophoretic distribution of allergenic and hormonal fractions of commercial insulins. Diabetes **8**, 388 (1959)
HEXNER, P.E., RADFORD, L.E., BEAMS, J.W.: Achievement of sedimentation equilibrium. Proc. nat. Acad. Sci. (Wash.) **47**, 1848 (1961)
HEY, A.: Kliniske insulinstudier, Iso-Insulin Novo og Di-Insulin Novo. (Clinical insulin studies, iso-insulin novo and di-insulin novo.) Ugeskr. Læg. **43**, 901 (1945)
HOBSON, Q.J.G.: Diabetes mellitus — current treatment. Med. Press **234**, 470 (1955)
HOLCOMB, B., PAGE, O.C., STEPHENS, J.W.: Lente insulin. Northw. Med. (Seattle) **53**, 239 (1954)
IZZO, J.L.: The design and interpretation of clinical experiments with drugs. A clinical comparison of modified insulins. I. The clinical problem. Biometrics 8, 206 (1952)
IZZO, J.L., GABIGA, A.M., HOFFMASTER, J.: Pharmacologic and clinical studies on two new types of long-acting insulins with special reference to zinc insulin preparations (Novo). Diabetes **2**, 358 (1953)
IZZO, J.L., SUSKIE, A.G., KELLNER, C.: Insulin zinc suspensions. Further studies with emphasis on lente insulin. Amer. J. Med. **20**, 554 (1956)
JACKER, H.J.: Neue Arzneifertigwaren[1]. Überblick über die Depotinsuline. Pharmazie **2**, 39 (1965)
JACKER, H.J.: Antidiabetika. Pharm. Praxis **12**, 270 (1969)
JAMIESON, M., LACEY, A.H., FISHER, A.M.: NPH insulin. Canad. med. Ass. J. **65**, 20 (1951)
JENSEN, B.: Über einen neuen Typus von Verzögerungsinsulinen. Wien. klin. Wschr. **65**, 475 (1953)
JENSEN, B.: Über akute und chronische Insulinschäden bei der Zuckerkrankheit. Wien. klin. Wschr. **68**, 141 (1956)
JERSILD, M.: Une Évaluation clinique des insulines zinc. Diabète (Le Raincy) **4**, 196 (1956a)
JERSILD, M.: Insulin zinc suspension. Four years' experience. Lancet **271**, 1009 (1956b)
JERSILD, M.: Les paramètres d'un équilibre satisfaisant chez les diabétiques. Journées de Diabétologie Hotel-Dieu 1973
JOHN, S.: Die Behandlung des Diabetes mellitus mit Lente Insulin. Medizinische **5**, 190 (1957)

JORPES, J.E.: Recrystallized insulin for diabetic patients with insulin allergy. Arch. intern. Med. **83**, 363 (1949)

JORPES, J.E.: Recrystallized insulin for diabetics with insulin allergy. Acta med. scand. Suppl. **2**, 313 (1950)

JOSLIN, E.P., ROOT, H.F., WHITE, P., MARBLE, A.: The treatment of diabetes mellitus. 10th ed. Philadelphia: Lea & Febiger 1959

JØRGENSEN, K.H., BRANGE, J., HALLUND, O., PINGEL, M.: A method for the preparation of essentially pure insulin. In: International Congress Series No. 209. VII. Congress of the International Diabetes Federation. Abstracts, p. 149. Amsterdam: Excerpta Medica 1970

KAAS, J.: Insulin Lente i ambulant sukkersygepraksis. (Insulin lente in the ambulant treatment of diabetics.) Ugeskr. Læg. **117**, 839 (1955)

KAPPELER, H.J.: Einstellung labiler Diabetiker mit Insulin Rapitard. Schweiz. med. Wschr. **96**, 1450 (1966)

KATSILAMBROS, L.: Treatment of insulin allergy and insulin resistance with phenylated insulin. Israel J. med. Sci. **8**, 893 (1972)

KERN, R.A., LANGNER, P.H.: Protamine and allergy. I. Nature of the local reactions after injections of protamine zinc insulin. II. Induction of sensitivity to insulin by injections of protamine zinc insulin. J. Amer. med. Ass. **113**, 198 (1939)

KERP, L.: Untersuchungen zur klinischen Bedeutung insulin-bindender Antikörper. Allergie- und Immunitätsforsch. **1**, 103 (1963)

KERP, L., KASEMIR, H., KIELING, F.: Insulinbindende Antikörper und Insulinbedarf bei Diabetikern. Klin. Wschr. **46**, 376 (1968)

KINK, R., STEIGERWALDT, F.: Über die Erweiterung der Diabetes-Therapie durch ein neuartiges Depot-Insulin (Rapitard-Insulin). Münch. med. Wschr. **104**, 2056 (1962)

KIRSCH, R.: Vergleichende Prüfung moderner Verzögerungs-Insuline, unter besonderer Berücksichtigung ihrer theoretischen und praktischen Grundlagen. Inaug. Diss. Frankfurt/Main 1955

KNICK, B., FOLKERT, F.: Zur klinischen Einstellbarkeit der verschiedenen Diabetesformen. Münch. med. Wschr. **107**, 83 (1965)

KORP, W.: Zur Therapie des juvenilen Insulinmangeldiabetes mit Insulinzinksuspensionen der Lentereihe. Wien. klin. Wschr. **74**, 453 (1962)

KORP, W., LEVETT, R.E.: Erfahrungen mit Monokomponenten-Insulin. Wien. klin. Wschr. **85**, 326 (1973)

KRAINICK, H.G., STRUWE, F.E.: Zur Situation des kindlichen Diabetes mellitus in Westdeutschland. Dtsch. med. Wschr. **85**, 1632 (1960)

KRAINICK, H.G., STRUWE, F.E., QUINTENZ, R.: Beobachtungen und Erfahrungen aus 11 Ferienlagern für diabetische Kinder (1954—1957). Dtsch. med. Wschr. **83**, 1279 (1958)

KRAYENBÜHL, C., ROSENBERG, T.: Crystalline protamine insulin. Rep. Steno Hosp. (Kbh.) **1**, 60 (1946)

KREUTZER, H.H., MOORS, J.J., VERHILLE, R.: Oorspronkelijke Stukken. Specifieke Resistentie Tegen Runder-Insuline. (Original papers: Specific resistense against beef insulin.) Ned. T. Geneesk. **100**, IV, 49, 3598 (1956)

KÜHNAU, J., VON STRITZKY, A.: Diagnostisch-therapeutische Seite. Mit Schweineinsulin erfolgreich behandelte Insulin-Resistenz bei Diabetes mellitus. Mitteilung über zwei Fälle. Schweiz. med. Wschr. **93**, 914 (1963)

KUMAR, D., MILLER, L.V.: The prevalence of proinsulin-specific antibodies in diabetic patients. Horm. Metab. Res. **5**, 1 (1973a)

KUMAR, D., MILLER, L.V.: Proinsulin-specific antibodies in human sera. Diabetes **22**, 361 (1973b)

LACHNIT, V., FERSTL, A.: Zur Wirkung zusatzfreier Zinkinsuline. Wien. med. Wschr. **103**, 292 (1953)

LANCASTER, W.M., MURRAY, I.: Further experience with the "lente" insulins. Brit. med. J. **1958I**, 1331

LANG, E., WALZ, L.: Über die klinische Wirksamkeit eines neuen Depot-Insulin-Prinzips in der Behandlung des Diabetes mellitus. Med. Welt (Stuttg.) **50**, 2574 (1963)

LAUTENSCHLÄGER, K.L., DÖRZBACH, E., SCHAUMANN, O.: Verfahren zur Herstellung von Präparaten aus dem blutzuckersenkenden Hormon der Bauchspeicheldrüse. D.R.P. 727.888. (1937)

LAWRENCE, R.D.: The new insulin zinc suspensions. Brit. med. J. **1954I**, 518

LAWRENCE, R.D.: The Diabetic Life. 16th Ed. London: J. & A. Churchill Ltd. 1960

LAWRENCE, R.D., ARCHER, N.: Zinc protamine insulin. A clinical trial of the new preparation. Brit. med. J. **1937I**, 487

LAWRENCE, R.D., OAKLEY, W.: A new long-acting insulin. Brit. med. J. **1953I**, 242

LEBOUC, R.: Insuline N.P.H. Gaz. méd. Fr. **69**, 507 (1962)

LEONARDS, J.R., MARTIN, F.I.R.: Insulin insensitivity. A variant of insulin resistance. New Engl. J. Med. **261**, 68 (1959)

LERMAN, J.: Insulin resistance. The role of immunity in its production. Amer. J. med. Sci. **207**, 354 (1944)

LESCHER, F.G.: The modern treatment of diabetes mellitus and the use of zinc protamine insulin. Brit. med. J. **1**, 11 (1938)

LIBBRECHT, L.: Ervaringen met een nieuw insulinpreparaat met verlengde werking. N.P.H. Zink. T. soc. Geneesk. **24**, 639 (1968)

LIEBERMANN, P., PATTERSON, R., METZ, R., LUCENA, G.: Allergic reactions to insulin. J. Amer. med. Ass. **215**, 1106 (1971)

LILLY RES. LAB.: Diabetes Mellitus. 7th Ed. Indianapolis: Eli Lilly Company 1967

LIPPMAN, H.: Über Eigenschaften und Anwendungsmöglichkeiten des NPH-Insulins. Dtsch. Gesundh.-Wes. **19**, 1 (1964)

LOCKWOOD, D.H., PROUT, T.E.: Isoantibodies to insulin. Clin. Res. **10**, 401 (1962)

LOEB, H., DORCHY, H.: Le traitement du diabète infantile par le regime dit "libre" et l'insulinotherapie "adaptèe". Determination clinique d'une association optimum d'insulines. Brux.-méd. **51**, 587 (1971)

LOPEZ, V., COLOMBO, J.P.: Erfahrungen mit Insulin Rapitard bei der Behandlung des juvenilen Diabetes. Schweiz. med. Wschr. **94**, 788 (1964)

LOWELL, F.C.: Immunologic studies in insulin resistance. I. Report of a case exhibiting variations in resistance and allergy to insulin. J. clin. Invest. **23**, 225 (1944)

LUSSKY, R.A., NEWCOMB, A.L., TRAISMAN, H.S.: Lente insulin in diabetic children. Diabetes **5**, 124 (1956)

MAKENGO, P.: Études cliniques du traitement du diabète à l'insuline Rapitard. Thèse Lausanne 1967

MALINS, J.M.: Clinical Diabetes Mellitus. London: Eyre & Spottiswoode 1968

MALINS, J.M.: Insulins and diabetes. Prescribers' J. **10**, 25 (1970)

MALINS, J.M., THORN, P.A.: Lente insulin. Lancet **266**, 372 (1954)

MANGOLD, R.: Klinische Untersuchungen über Insulin-Lente (Zink-Insulin-Suspension mit protrahierter Wirkung). Schweiz. med. Wschr. **84**, 1041 (1954)

MARBLE, A.: Lente insulin in the treatment of diabetes mellitus. Med. Clin. N. Amer. **41**, 485 (1957)

MARBLE, A.: Insulin in the treatment of diabetes. In: Joslin's Diabetes Mellitus. 11th ed. Philadelphia: Lea & Febiger 1971

MARCKER, K.: Association of Zn-free insulin. Acta chem. scand. **14**, 194 (1960a)

MARCKER, K.: The binding of the "structural" zinc ions in crystalline insulin. Acta chem. scand. **14**, 2071 (1960b)

MARIGO, S.: Il trattamento del diabete giovanile instabile con due iniezioni quotidiane di zinco-insulina-lenta. (The treatment of unstable juvenile diabetics with two daily injections of insulin lente.) Clin. ter. **13**, fasc. 4 (1957)

MCBRYDE, C.M., REISS, R.S.: Modified protamine zinc insulin: Comparison with globin zinc insulin and insulin mixtures. J. clin. Endocr. **4**, 469 (1944)

MCBRYDE, C.M., ROBERTS, H.K.: Modified protamine zinc insulin: An improvement on standard protamine zinc insulin. J. Amer. med. Ass. **122**, 1225 (1943a)

MCBRYDE, C.M., ROBERTS, H.K.: A new modified protamine zinc insulin: Comparison with histone zinc insulin, clear, and standard protamine zinc insulins. J. clin. Invest. **XXII**, 791 (1943b)

MCKERROW, J.H., ROBINSON, A.B.: Deamidation of asparaginyl residues as a hazard in experimental protein and peptide procedures. Analyt. Biochem. **42**, 565 (1971)

MEHL, M., DEBRY, G.: Étude expérimentale de l'activité biologique de deux nouvelles insulines, (appréciation des résultats à l'aide du calcul de la valeur M). Diabète (Le Raincy) **13**, 142 (1965)

MEHNERT: Insulintherapie des Diabetes mellitus. Dtsch. med. Wschr. **91**, 1938 (1966)

MELTON, G.: Treatment with insulin zinc suspensions. Brit. med. J. **1954 II**, 448

MIROUZE, J., COLLARD, F., TEISSEIRE, J.: Analyse comparative enregistrement continu des effets hyperglycémiants d'ingestions alimentaires prises à 8, 12, 16 et 19 heures dans le diabete insuliné. Acta diabet. lat. **9**, 972 (1972)

MIROUZE, J., ORSETTI, A., SCHMOUKER, Y., CARTY, E., ALMES, N.: Diabète sucrè. Son traitement par les insulins purifiées monocomposées. La Nouvelle Presse Médicale **2**, 1981 (1973)

MIRSKY, I.A., KAWAMURA, K.: Heterogeneity of crystalline insulin. Endocrinology **78**, 1115 (1966)

MITCHELL, R.E.: Clinical experience with intermediate insulins. Penn. med. J. **58**, 1007 (1955)

MITTENZWEI, H.: Protamin-Zink-Insuline. Insulin und Insulin-Therapie, Urban und Schwarzenberg **55** (1956). (Aus der Wissenschaftlichen Abteilung der Hormon-Chemie München)

MOHNIKE, G., LIPPMANN, H.: Über Depot-Insulin-Hoechst „Klar“. Med. Welt (Stuttg.) **51**, 2750 (1964)

MOLNAR, G.D.: Clinical use of various insulin preparations. In: Diabetes Mellitus. Diagnosis and Treatment. III. Amer. Diab. Ass. 139 (1971) N.Y. 1971 (FAJANS, S.S., SUSSMAN, K.E. Co-editors)

MOLNAR, G.D., TAYLOR, W.F., LANGWORTHY, A.L.: Plasma immunoreactive insulin patterns in insulin-treated diabetics. Studies during continuous blood glucose monitoring. Mayo Clin. Proc. **47**, 709 (1972)

MONTEIRO, J.G.: Tratamento da diabetes com suspensões de insulina-zinco. (Treatment of Diabetes with Insulin-Zinc-Suspension.) Coimbra méd. **1955 II**, 510

MONTENERO, P., COLLETTI, A.: Valutazioni cliniche sui resultati preliminari con una insulina ad azione semiritardata. (A clinical evaluation of preliminary results obtained with an insulin preparation with semiretarded action.) Clin. ter. **33**, 469 (1965)

MURRAY, I.: Insulin zinc suspensions. Brit. med. J. **1953 II**, 1377

MURRAY, I., WILSON, R.: The new insulin — lente, ultralente and semilente. Brit. med. J. **1953 II**, 1023

MURRAY, I.: Insulin-zinc suspensions. Lancet **266**, 623 (1954)

MURRAY, I.: Current therapeutics-XCIV-the newer insulins. Practitioner **175**, 502 (1955)

NABARRO, J.D.N., STOWERS, J.M.: The insulin zinc suspensions. Brit. med. J. **1953 II**, 1027

NEJROTTI, R., ALBONICO, G.: Contributo all'applicazione terapeutica delle sospensioni di insulina-zinco. (The therapeutical use of the lente insulins.) Gazz. med. ital. **115**, 195 (1956)

NEUHOFF, F., RABINOVITCH, S.: Protamine zinc insulin. Clinical observations and comparative analysis of blood sugar curves obtained with use of protamine zinc insulin and with regular insulin. Arch. intern. Med. **62**, 447 (1938)

NEWCOMB, A.L., TRAISMAN, H.S.: Experiences with the lente insulins in diabetic children. Illinois med. J. **115**, 264 (1959)

NITSCH, K.: Insuline und Insulinbehandlung. Beihefte zum Arch. Kinderheilk. 58. Heft. Stuttgart: F. Enke 1968

NOWAK, S., PLANETA-MALECKA, I., MARGOLIS, A., OLSZOWSKA, L., KRZEMIENIÓWA, K.: The activity of various prolonged action insulins in diabetes of children. Pediat. pol. **XLIII**, 585 (1968)

OAKLEY, W.: “Lente” insulin (insulin zinc suspension). Further studies. Brit. med. J. **1953 II**, 1021

OAKLEY, W.: Lente insulin. Lancet **266**, 262 (1954)

OAKLEY, W.: Treatment of diabetes mellitus. I. Insulin: Physiological and therapeutic actions. Brit. med. J. **1959** a **I**, 1291

OAKLEY, W.: Treatment of diabetes mellitus. II. Insulin preparations and therapeutic uses. Brit. med. J. **1959** b **I**, 1407

OAKLEY, W.G.: The management of diabetes over one-third of a century. Postgrad. med. J. 48—53 (January Suppt. 1971)

OAKLEY, W., HILL, D., OAKLEY, N.: Combined use of regular and crystalline protamin (NPH) insulins in the treatment of severe diabetes. Diabetes **15**, 219 (1966)

OAKLEY, W.G., PYKE, D.A., TAYLOR, K.W.: Clinical diabetes and its biochemical basis. Blackwell. Scientific Publications, Oxford 1968

PAL, S., GUPTA, N.N., MEHROTRA, R.M.L., SIRCAR, A.R., CHATURVEDI, U.C.: Insulin antibodies in diabetes mellitus. Indian J. med. Res. **57**, 573 (1969)

PALEY, R.G.: Lipodystrophy following insulin injections. Metabolism **1953 II**, 201

PALEY, R.G.: The design of insulin trials. Insulin-zinc suspension (lente). Lancet **267**, 784 (1954)

PECK, F.B.: Insulin mixtures and modifications. Proc. Amer. diab. Ass. **6**, 273 (1946)

PECK, F.B., KIRTLEY, W.R.: Newer insulins with special reference to NPH insulin. N.Y.St.J. Med. **50**, 2182 (1950)

PECK, F.B., KIRTLEY, W.R., DYKE, R.W., ERNST, C.E.: Present status of insulin-zinc suspensions. Diabetes **3**, 261 (1954)

PECK, F.B., KIRTLEY, W.R., OTTATI, F.C.: Present status of new insulin modifications. Diabetes **1**, 290 (1952)

PECK, F.B., SCHECHTER, J.S.: The newer insulin mixtures. Proc. Amer. diab. Ass. **4**, 57 (1944)

PETERSEN, K.: Method of producing crystalline insulin. U.S.A. Patent 2.626.228 (1945)

PETRIDES, P.: Neue Möglichkeiten der Therapie mit Depot-Insulinen. Medizinische 940 (1953)

PETRIDES, P.: Über den derzeitigen Stand der Diabetes-Behandlung. Klin. Mbl. Augenheilk. **147**, 6. Heft, 777 (1965)

PETRIDES, P.: Insulin-Therapie. Münch. med. Wschr. **112**, 1273 (1970)

PFEIFFER, E.F.: Immunogenicity of insulin. Diabetes **21**, Suppl. 2, 660 (1972)

PFEIFFER, E.F., DITSCHUNEIT, H., FEDERLIN, K.: Die Inselzellhormone: Die Immunologie des Insulins. In: Handbuch des Diabetes mellitus, 1. München: J.F. Lehmanns Verlag 1969

PFEIFFER, E. F., SCHÖFFLING, K.: Therapeutische Erfahrungen. Klinische Prüfung eines neuartigen Verzögerungsinsulins mit 24-Stunden-Wirkung. Schweiz. med. Wschr. **14**, 395 (1954)

PICKERT, H.: Insulin und Insulinwirkungen. II. Fortschr. Med. **73**, 443 (1955)

PIETSCH-BERLIN, R.: Klinische Erfahrungen in der Behandlung des kindlichen Diabetes mellitus mit einem neuen Zwei-Stufen-Insulin und Bewertung der Stoffwechsellage nach der M-Wert-Methode. Inaugural-Dissertation Tübingen 1965

PINGEL, M., VØLUND, A.: Stability of insulin preparations. Diabetes **21**, 805 (1972)

POULSEN, J. E.: Diabetes mellitus. Lectures held in Cairo and Alexandria. Acta endocr. (Kbh.) Suppl. 118, **55** (1967)

POULSEN, J. E., KRAYENBÜHL, C. H.: Slowly acting insulin preparation in crystalline form and method of preparation. U.S.A. Patent 3.060.093 (1962)

PRESLAND, J. R., TODD, C. M.: An investigation of prolonged insulin resistance in a case of diabetes mellitus. Quart. J. Med., New Series **XXV**, 275 (1956)

PROTAS, M., KURSTIN, W.: Clinical results with lente insulin. J. Amer. Geriat. Soc. **IV**, 117 (1956)

PYKE, D. A.: Advances in the treatment of diabetes mellitus. Practitioner **199**, 498 (1967)

RECHENBERG, H. K.: Diabetesbehandlung in der heutigen Praxis. Schweiz. med. Wschr. **86**, 274 (1956)

REINER, L., SEARLE, D. S., LANG, E. H.: On the hypoglycemic activity of globin insulin. J. Pharmacol. exp. Ther. **67**, 330 (1939)

RENOLD, A. E., STEINKE, J., SOELDNER, J. S., ANTONIADES, H. N., SMITH, R. E.: Immunological response to the prolonged administration of heterologous and homologous insulin in cattle. J. clin. Invest. **45**, 702 (1966)

RICKETTS, H. T.: Modern treatment of diabetes mellitus. J. Amer. med. Ass. **150**, 959 (1952)

RILLIET, B.: Nouvelles Insulines. Diabète (Le Raincy) **3**, 86 (1955)

ROBBERS, H.: Insulin-Arten. In: Praktische Diabetologie. München-Gräfelfing: Werk-Verlag 1969

ROBERTSON, J.: Some aspects of diabetes mellitus in childhood. Med. J. Aust. **1956 I**, 218

RODRIGUEZ-MIÑÓN, J. L., GARRIGUES, A.: La insulina lenta. Su manejo propiedades clinicas y equivalencias con otras formas de insulina. (Insulin lente: A clinical evaluation in comparison with other forms of insulin.) Medicamenta (Madr.) **29**, 158 (1958)

RODRIGUEZ-MIÑÓN, J. L., GARRIGUES, A.: La insulina lenta: Algunas particularidades de su manejo. (Insulin lente: Some special therapeutic properties.) Rev. clin. esp. **74**, 226 (1959)

ROMANI, J. D.: Le traitement des diabètes insulino-dépendants de l'adulte par les insulines intermédiaires. Diabète (Le Raincy) **13**, 272 (1965)

ROOT, M. A., CHANCE, R. E., GALLOWAY, J. A.: Immunogenicity of insulin. Diabetes **21**, Suppl. 2, 657 (1972)

ROSENKRANZ, A.: Ergebnisse mehrjähriger Behandlung mit Zink-Insulinen im Kindesalter. 3. Kongress der I.D.F. (1958). „Diabetes Mellitus". Stuttgart: Georg Thieme Verlag 1959

ROSENKRANZ, A.: Zuckerkranke Kinder im Ferienlager. Arch. Kinderheilk. **161**, 218 (1960)

ROSENKRANZ, A.: Dauerbehandlung und Lebensführung beim diabetischen Kind. Pädiat. Prax. **2**, 11 (1963)

ROTTMANN, H., WILLE, F.: Zur Behandlung des Diabetes mit Verzögerungsinsulin. Dtsch. med. Wschr. **81**, 1324 (1956)

ROUZAUD, C.: Recherches sur l'emploi de l'insuline zinc cristallisée. Diabète (Le Raincy) **3**, 21 (1955)

SAUER, H.: Erfahrungen mit Insulin-Zink-Suspensionen. Med. Klin. **49**, 1376 (1954)

SAUER, H.: Erfahrungen mit Insulin-Zink-Suspensionen in der Diabetesbehandlung. Med. Welt (Stuttg.) 287 (1961)

SCHEFFLER, H.: Lokalisierte allergische Hautreaktionen mit Pigmentablagerung nach Insulininjektion. Medizinische **40**, 1409 (1955)

SCHEFFLER, H., HAGEN, H.: Allergische Hautreaktionen nach Insulin in Form der Necrobiosis lipoidica. Med. Klin. **51**, 2128 (1956)

SCHIRREN, C., SAUER, H.: Zur Frage der Insulinallergie. Ärztl. Forsch. **10**, I/175 (1956)

SCHLIACK, V., LOTZ, U.: Erfahrungen mit einem depotkörperfreien Verzögerungs-Insulin. Münch. med. Wschr. **109**, 1328 (1967)

SCHLICHTKRULL, J.: Insulin crystals I. Acta chem. scand. **10**, 1455 (1956a)

SCHLICHTKRULL, J.: Insulin crystals II. Acta chem. scand. **10**, 1459 (1956b)

SCHLICHTKRULL, J.: Insulin crystals IV. Acta chem. scand. **11**, 299 (1957a)

SCHLICHTKRULL, J.: Insulin crystals V. Acta chem. scand. **11**, 439 (1957b)

SCHLICHTKRULL, J.: Insulin crystals VI. Acta chem scand. **11**, 484 (1957c)

SCHLICHTKRULL, J.: Insulin crystals VII. Acta chem. scand. **11**, 1248 (1957d)

SCHLICHTKRULL, J.: Insulin crystals. Chemical and biological studies on insulin crystals and insulin zinc suspensions. Diss. Copenhagen University 1958

SCHLICHTKRULL, J., BRANGE, J., CHRISTIANSEN, A.H., HALLUND, O., HEDING, L.G., JØRGENSEN, K.H.: Clinical aspects of insulin — antigenicity. Diabetes **21**, Suppl. 2, 649 (1972)

SCHLICHTKRULL, J., BRANGE, J., CHRISTIANSEN, AA.H., HALLUND, O., HEDING, L.G., JØRGENSEN, K.H., MUNKGAARD RASMUSSEN, S., SØRENSEN, E., VØLUND, A.: Monocomponent insulin and its clinical implications. Horm. Metab. Res. Suppl. Vol. **5**, 134 (1974)

SCHLICHTKRULL, J., BRANGE, J., EGE, H., HALLUND, O., HEDING, L.G., JØRGENSEN, K., MARKUSSEN, J., STAHNKE, J., SUNDBY, F., VØLUND, A.: Proinsulin and related proteins. 5th Ann. Meeting of The European Association for the Study of Diabetes. Montpellier (1969). Diabetologia **6**, 80 (1970)

SCHLICHTKRULL, J., FUNDER, J., MUNCK, O.: Clinical evaluation of a new insulin preparation. 4e Congrès de la Fédération internationale du Diabète. Genève: Éditions Médecine et Hygiène **I**, 303 (1961)

SCHLICHTKRULL, J., MUNCK, O., JERSILD, M.: Insulin rapitard and insulin actrapid. Acta med. scand. **177**, 103 (1965a)

SCHLICHTKRULL, J., MUNCK, O., JERSILD, M.: The M-value, an index of blood-sugar control in diabetics. Acta med. scand. **177**, 95 (1965b)

SCOTT, D.A.: CCXI. Crystalline insulin. Biochem. J. **28**, 1592 (1934)

SCOTT, D.A., FISHER, A.M.: The effect of zinc salts on the action of insulin. J. Pharmacol. exp. Ther. **55**, 206 (1935)

SCOTT, D.A., FISHER, A.M.: Studies on insulin with protamine. J. Pharmacol. exp. Ther. **58**, 78 (1936)

SEELEMANN, K.: Klinische Erfahrungen mit Insulin Lente (Novo) und Long-Insulin (Hoechst) bei kindlichem Diabetes mellitus. Medizinische 922 (1955)

SHIPP, J.C., CUNNINGHAM, R.W., RUSSELL, R.O., MARBLE, A.: Insulin resistance: Clinical features, natural course and effects of adrenal steroid treatment. Medicine (Baltimore) **44**, 165 (1965)

SLAYTON, R.E., BURROWS, R.E., MARBLE, A.: Lente insulin in the treatment of diabetes. New Engl. J. Med. **253**, 722 (1955)

SLOBIN, L.I., CARPENTER, F.H.: The labile amide in insulin: Preparation of desalanine-desamido-insulin. Biochemistry **2**, 22 (1963)

SMELO, L.S.: Insulin resistance. Proc. Amer. diab. Ass. **8**, 77 (1948)

SPENCER, A.G., MORGANS, M.E.: Lente insulin. Four years' experience. Lancet **271**, 1013 (1956)

SPIESS, H.: Lang wirksame Insuline beim Diabetes mellitus des Kindes. Dtsch. med. Wschr. **80**, 1170 (1955)

SPIESS, H., ZSCHOCKE, D.: Mehrjährige Erfahrungen mit Verzögerungs-Insulinen beim Diabetes mellitus des Kindes. Dtsch. med. Wschr. **85**, 1121 (1960)

SPRAGUE, R.G.: The use of mixtures of protamine zinc and regular insulin. Ann. intern. Med. **31**, 628 (1949)

SPRAGUE, R.G., KILBY, R.A.: Evolution of modified insulins in the treatment of diabetes mellitus, with special emphasis on insulin-zinc suspensions. Amer. J. Med. **19**, 925 (1955)

STEINER, D.F., HALLUND, O., RUBINSTEIN, A., CHO, S., BAYLISS, C.: Isolation and properties of proinsulin, intermediate forms, and other minor components from crystalline bovine insulin. Diabetes **17**, 725 (1968)

STEINER, D.F., OYER, P.E.: The biosynthesis of insulin and a probable precursor of insulin by a human islet cell adenoma. Proc. nat. Acad. Sci. (Wash.) **57**, 473 (1967)

STEINKE, J., SOELDNER, J.S.: Insulin resistance. Differentiation into two types by measurement of serum insulin-like activity in vitro. Diabetes **14**, 432 (1965)

STENGEL, F., LASSMANN, H.: Diabetes im Altersheim und Insulinbehandlung. Wien. klin. Wschr. **66**, 883 (1954)

STÖTTER, G.: Praktische Gesichtspunkte zur Insulinbehandlung. Dtsch. med. J. **14**, 741 (1963)

STOWERS, J.M.: A critical appraisal of insulin treatment. J. roy. Coll. Phycns. Lond. **7**, 69 (1972)

STOWERS, J.M., NABARRO, J.D.N.: Clinical experience of the insulin zinc suspensions. Brit. med. J. **1955 I**, 68

STRATMANN, F.W.: Der klinische Wert von Insulin Novo Rapitard und Actrapid und dessen Objektivierung nach der M-Wert-Methode. (Schlichtkrull). Med. Welt (Stuttg.) **194** (1962)

STRATMANN, F.W.: Beitrag zur Beurteilung der Langzeiteinstellung des Diabetikers. Gastroenterologia (Basel) Suppl. **104**, 181 (1965)

STRENGER, W.: Über die Erfahrung bei diabetischen Kindern nach vierjähriger Anwendung von Lente-Insulin. Wien. med. Wschr. **109**, 347 (1959)

SUNDBY, F.: Separation and characterization of acid-induced insulin transformation products by paper electrophoresis in 7 M urea. J. biol. Chem. **237**, 3406 (1962)

SWOBODA, W.: Früh- und Spätergebnisse bei der Behandlung diabetischer Kinder mit Zinkinsulinen. Mod. Prob. Pädiat. **4**, 592 (1959)

SWOBODA, W., ZWEYMÜLLER, E.: Erfahrungen mit neuen Verzögerungsinsulinen beim Diabetes mellitus im Kindesalter. Schweiz. med. Wschr. **85**, 231 (1955a)

SWOBODA, W., ZWEYMÜLLER, E.: Neue Verzögerungsinsuline beim Diabetes mellitus im Kindesalter. Wien. klin. Wschr. **67**, 192 (1955b)

TANTILLO, J.J., KARAM, J.H., BURRILL, K.C., JONES, M.A., GRODSKY, G.M., FORSHAM, P.H.: Immunogenicity of "single peak" beef-pork insulin in diabetic subjects. Diabetes **23**, 276 (1974)

TEUSCHER, A.: Treatment of insulin lipoatrophy with monocomponent insulin. Diabetologia **10**, 211 (1974)

THOMSEN, O.F.: Studies of diabetic glomerulosclerosis using an immunofluorescent technique. Acta path. microbiol. scand. Section A **80**, 193 (1972)

TRAISMAN, H.S., NEWCOMB, A.L.: Management of juvenile diabetes mellitus. Saint Louis: C.V. Mosby Company 1965

TRAUMAN, K.J., WETZEL, U.: Klinische Erfahrungen mit Insulin Novo Rapitard in der Diabetes Therapie. Med. Klin. **59**, 27 (1964)

TRETENHAHN, W.: Die modernen Depot-Insuline. Wien. Z. inn. Med. **671**, 426 (1959)

TUTIN, M., COLLIN DE L'HORTET, G.: Étude clinique d'une nouvelle insuline retard: la durasuline. Gaz. méd. Fr. **76**, 4842 (1969)

ULRICH, H.: Clinical experiments with mixtures of standard and protamine zinc insulins. Ann. intern. Med. **14**, 1166 (1941)

UMBER, F.: Fortschritte in der Depotinsulinfrage. Verh. dtsch. Ges. Verdau.- u. Stoffwechselkr. **16**, XIV, 241 (1938)

UMBER, F., STÖRRING, F.K., FÖLLMER, W.: Erfolge mit einem neuartigen Depotinsulin ohne Protaminzusatz (Surfen-Insulin). Klin. Wschr. **17**, 443 (1938)

VENNING, G.R.: The insulin-zinc suspensions. Lancet **266**, 480 (1954)

VERMEULEN, A., BEKAERT, J.: Les insulines lentes dans le traitement des diabétiques. Brux.-méd. **38**, 291 (1958)

VOIT, K., KNICK, B.: Insulin-Zink-Suspensionen („Lente"-Insuline) in der klinischen Diabetesbehandlung. Dtsch. med. Wschr. **80**, 622 (1955)

WATSON, B.M., CALDER, J.S.: A treatment for insulin-induced fat atrophy. Diabetes **20**, 628 (1971)

WATSON, D., VINES, R.: Variations in the incidence of lipodystrophy using different insulins. Med. J. Aust. **5**, 248 (1973)

WAUCHOPE, G.M.: Zinc protamine insulin and soluble insulin interaction in combined doses. Lancet **1**, 962 (1940)

WEHNER, H., HUBER, H., KRONENBERG, K.H.: The glomerular basement membrane of the rabbit kidney on long-term treatment with heterologous insulin preparations of different purity. Diabetologia **9**, 255 (1973)

WEHNER, H., SCHADE, U., ASANTE, F.: Veränderungen an der Glomerulären Basalmembran des Meerschweinchens durch Fremdinsulin und ihre Beziehung zur Höhe der Insulin-Bindungsfähigkeit des Serums. Virchows Arch. Abt. A **348**, 164 (1969)

WEHNER, H., SCHADE, U., LIEBERMEISTER, E., VEIGEL, J.: Glomeruläre Veränderungen nach Immunisierung mit heterologem Insulin. Virchows Arch. Abt. A **349**, 345 (1970)

WEITZEDL, G.: Verzögerungs-Insuline. Ärztl. Forsch. **3**, 167 (1949)

WENIG, K.H., CALAP, J.: Auslösung allergischer Phänomene durch Insulin-Präparate. Münch. med. Wschr. **10**, 345 (1971)

WESTBERG, N.G., MICHAEL, A.F.: Immunohistopathology of diabetic glomerulosclerosis. Diabetes **21**, 163 (1972)

WHITEHOUSE, F.W., LOWRIE, W.L., REDFERN, E., BRYAN, J.B.: The lente insulin triad. With emphasis on the use of "lente combinations". Ann. intern. Med. **55**, 894 (1961)

WOLFF, H.O., MADDISON, T.G.: Insulin zinc suspension in childhood. Diabetes. Brit. med. J. **1955 II**, 413

ZACHAU-CHRISTIANSEN, B.: The relation between body weight and dosage of insulin in juvenile diabetes mellitus. Dan. med. Bull. **5**, 228 (1958)

ZWEYMÜLLER, E.: Erfahrungen mit neuen Verzögerungsinsulinen. Wien. med. Wschr. **105**, 1049 (1955)

Author Index

Page numbers in *italics* refer to the bibliography

Subject Index

Handbuch der experimentellen Pharmakologie / Handbook of Experimental Pharmacology

Heffter—Heubner, New Series

Vol. 4: **General Pharmacology**
ISBN 3-540-04845-6 DM 86,—; US $ 37.00

Vol. 10: **Die Pharmakologie anorganischer Anionen**
ISBN 3-540-01465-9 DM 280,—; US $ 120.40

Vol. 11: **Lobelin und Lobeliaalkaloide**
ISBN 3-540-01910-3 DM 24,—; US $ 10.40

Vol. 12: **Morphin und morphinähnlich wirkende Verbindungen**
ISBN 3-540-02158-2 DM 110,—; US $ 47.30

Vol. 13: **The Alkali Metal Ions in Biology.** Temp. out of print

Vol. 14:
Part 1 **The Adrenocortical Hormones I**
ISBN 3-540-02830-7 DM 290,—; US $ 124.70
Part 2 **The Adrenocortical Hormones II**
ISBN 3-540-03146-4 DM 90,—; US $ 38.70
Part 3 **The Adrenocortical Hormones III**
ISBN 3-540-04147-8 DM 180,—; US $ 77.40

Vol. 15: **Cholinesterases and Anticholinesterase Agents**
ISBN 3-540-02988-5 DM 360,—; US $ 154.80

Vol. 16: **Erzeugung von Krankheitszuständen durch das Experiment**
Part 2 **Atemwege**
ISBN 3-540-04517-1 DM 165,—; US $ 71.00
Part 4 **Niere, Nierenbecken, Blase**
ISBN 3-540-03305-X DM 195,—; US $ 83.90
Part 7 **Zentralnervensystem**
ISBN 3-540-02831-5 DM 165,—; US $ 71.00
Part 8 **Stütz- und Hartgewebe**
ISBN 3-540-04518-X DM 135,—; US $ 58.10
Part 9 **Infektionen I**
ISBN 3-540-03147-2 DM 195,—; US $ 83.90
Part 10 **Infektionen II**
ISBN 3-540-03531-1 DM 220,—; US $ 94.60
Part 11 A **Infektionen III**
ISBN 3-540-03840-X DM 195,—; US $ 83.90
Part 11 B **Infektionen IV**
ISBN 3-540-06290-4 DM 195,—; US $ 83.90
Part 12 **Tumoren I**
ISBN 3-540-03532-X DM 200,—; US $ 86.00
Part 13 **Tumoren II**
ISBN 3-540-03533-8 DM 120,—; US $ 51.60
Part 15 **Kohlenhydratstoffwechsel, Fieber/Carbohydrate Metabolism, Fever**
ISBN 3-540-03534-6 DM 195,—; US $ 83.90

Vol. 17:
Part 1 **Ions, alcalino-terreux I. Systèmes isolés**
ISBN 3-540-02989-3 DM 210,—; US $ 90.30
Part 2 **Ions, alcacino-terreux II. Organismes entiers**
ISBN 3-540-03148-0 DM 260,—; US $ 111.80

Vol. 18:
Part 1 **Histamine**
ISBN 3-540-03535-4 DM 230,—; US $ 98.90

Vol. 19: **5-Hydroxytryptamine and Related Indolealkylamines**
ISBN 3-540-03536-2 DM 230,—; US $ 98.90

Vol. 20:
Part 1 **Pharmacology of Fluorides I**
ISBN 3-540-03537-0 DM 175,—; US $ 75.30
Part 2 **Pharmacology of Fluorides II**
ISBN 3-540-04846-4 DM 165,—; US $ 71.00

Vol. 21: **Beryllium**
ISBN 3-540-03538-9 DM 60,—; US $ 25.80

Vol. 22:
Part 1 **Die Gestagene I**
ISBN 3-540-04148-6 DM 390,—; US $ 167.70
Part 2 **Die Gestagene II**
ISBN 3-540-04519-8 DM 390,—; US $ 167.70

Vol. 23: **Neurohypophysial Hormones and Similar Polypeptides**
ISBN 3-540-04149-4 DM 230,—; US $ 98.90

Vol. 24: **Diuretica**
ISBN 3-540-04520-1 DM 290,—; US $ 124.70

Vol. 25: **Bradykinin, Kallidin and Kallikrein**
ISBN 3-540-04847-2 DM 275,—; US $ 118.30

Vol. 26: **Vergleichende Pharmakologie von Überträgersubstanzen in tiersystematischer Darstellung**
ISBN 3-540-05132-5 DM 195,—; US $ 83.90

Vol. 27: **Anticoagulantien**
ISBN 3-540-05133-3 DM 240,—; US $ 103.20

Vol. 28:
Part 1 **Concepts in Biochemical Pharmacology I**
ISBN 3-540-05134-1 DM 190,—; US $ 81.70
Part 2 **Concepts in Biochemical Pharmacology II**
ISBN 3-540-05389-1 DM 275,—; US $ 118.30
Part 3 **Concepts in Biochemical Pharmacology III.**
ISBN 3-540-07001-X DM 248,—; US $ 106.70

Vol. 29: **Oral wirksame Antidiabetika**
ISBN 3-540-05554-1 DM 340,—; US $ 146.20

Vol. 30: **Modern Inhalation Anesthetics**
ISBN 3-540-05135-X DM 220,—; US $ 94.60

Vol. 31: **Antianginal Drugs**
Out of print

Vol. 32:
Part 1 **Insulin I**
ISBN 3-540-05470-7 DM 275,—; US $ 118.30

Vol. 33: **Catecholamines**
ISBN 3-540-05517-7 DM 396,—; US $ 170.30

Vol. 34: **Secretin, Cholecystokinin-Pancreozymin and Gastrin**
ISBN 3-540-05952-0 DM 180,—; US $ 77.40

Vol. 35:
Part 1 **Androgene I**
ISBN 3-540-05706-4 DM 320,—; US $ 137.60
Part 2 **Androgens II and Antiandrogens/Androgene II und Antiandrogene**
ISBN 3-540-06883-X DM 398,—; US $ 171.20

Vol. 36: **Uranium-Plutonium-Transplutonic Elements**
ISBN 3-540-06168-1 DM 374,—; US $ 160.90

Vol. 37: **Angiotensin**
ISBN 3-540-06276-9 DM 224,—; US $ 96.40

Vol. 38:
Part 1 **Antineoplastic and Immunosuppressive Agents I**
ISBN 3-540-06402-8 DM 258,—; US $ 111.00
Part 2 **Antineoplastic and Immunosuppressive Agents II**
ISBN 3-540-06633-0 DM 348,—; US $ 149.70

Vol. 40: **Organic Nitrates**
ISBN 3-540-07048-6 DM 97,—; US $ 41.80

Preisänderungen vorbehalten / Prices are subject to change without notice